AF342555

EMERGING TRENDS IN ORAL HEALTH SCIENCES AND DENTISTRY

Edited by **Mandeep Singh Virdi**

Emerging Trends in Oral Health Sciences and Dentistry

http://dx.doi.org/10.5772/58660
Edited by Mandeep Singh Virdi

Contributors

Maen Hussni Zreaqat, Preetika Chandna, Vivek Adlakha, Sukanya Tianviwat, Derek S J DSouza, Paulo Beltrão, Sukumaran Anil, Zühre Akarslan, Ilkay Peker, Belma Işık Aslan, Neslihan Üçüncü, Nao Suzuki, Masahiro Yoneda, Takao Hirofuji, Petra Surlin, Anne Marie Rauten, Constantin Daguci, Maria Bogdan, Mihai Raul Popescu, Marisa Diaz, Isabela Oliveira Carvalho, Kristina Goršeta, Dongliang Zhang, Rafael Da Silveira Moreira, Juan Antonio García-Nuñez, Ana Isabel García-Kass, Victoriano Serrano-Cuenca, Ticiana Sidorenko De Oliveira Capote, Marcela De Almeida Gonçalves, Andréa Gonçalves, Marcelo Gonçalves, Agim Begzati, Merita Berisha, Blerta Latifi-Xhemajli, Rina Prokshi, Valmira Maxhuni, Vala Hysenaj, Shefqet Mrasori, Feihm Haliti, Natalia Zamora Martinez, Monica Larrea, Vanessa Paredes, José-Luis Gandia, Rosa Cibrian, Mourad Sebbar, Ana Pejcic, Javier De La Fuente, Fatima Del Carmen Aguilar-Diaz, Ma. Carmen Villanueva-Vilchis, Andréa Cristina Barbosa Da Silva, Diego Romário Da Silva, Sabrina Ferreira, Andeliana Rodrigues, Allan Albuquerque, Sandra Marinho, Elena Preoteasa, Cristina Teodora Preoteasa, Marin Imre, Leandro Marques, Joana Ramos-Jorge, Maria Letícia Ramos-Jorge, Saul Martins Paiva, Hisashi Fujita, John Myers, Zorana Zoran Stamenkovic, Vanja Raickovic, Farid Bourzgui, Sanaa Alami, Sergio Sánchez-García, Fátima Del Carmen Aguilar-Díaz, Erika Heredia Ponce, Anna Maria Heikkinen, Catalina Pisoschi, Monica Banita, Anca Berbecaru-Iovan, Camelia Stanciulescu, Cristina Munteanu, Ana Marina Andrei, Fabio Sampaio, Jocianelle Fernandes, Valdenice Menezes, Marcos Oliveira, Karla Meira, Raimundo Junior, Mariana Braga, Isabela Floriano, Fernanda Rosche Ferreira, Alessandra Reyes, Daniela Procida Raggio, José Carlos Imparato, Fausto Medeiros Mendes, Juliana Mattos-Silveira, Tamara Kerber Tedesco, Koku Kahabuka

CBS, Edition **2017**

Published by InTech

Janeza Trdine 9, 51000 Rijeka, Croatia

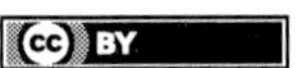

Notice

Statements and opinions expressed in the chapters are these of the individual contributors and not necessarily those of the editors or publisher. No responsibility is accepted for the accuracy of information contained in the published chapters. The publisher assumes no responsibility for any damage or injury to persons or property arising out of the use of any materials, instructions, methods or ideas contained in the book.

Publishing Process Manager Danijela Duric

Technical Editor InTech DTP team

Cover Designer InTech Design Team

Additional hard copies can be obtained from orders@intechopen.com

Emerging Trends in Oral Health Sciences and Dentistry, Edited by Mandeep Singh Virdi
p. cm.
ISBN 978-953-51-2024-7

Contents

Contents

Contents

Contents

Contents

Preface

This is the second book on Oral Health Science. The first book resulted in publication of Oral Health Care-Pediatric, Research, Epidemology and clinical Practices and Oral Health Care-Prosthodontics, Periodontology, Biology, Research and systemic Conditions in February 2012.

The present effort documents current developments in Oral Health Sciences in all major continents of the world and has contribution from authors and researchers from all over the world. This makes the present book reflection of the progress in Oral Health Science and Practices and indicates the direction in which this stream of education is likely to head forward.

The book covers areas of General Dentistry, Paediatric and Preventive Dentistry, Geriatric and Prosthodontics, Orthodontics, Periodontology, Conservative Dentistry and Radiology and Oral Medicine. The chapters of the book are grouped accordingly. The contributions to the book have been made from researchers and specialists from Europe, Americas and Asia.

It is hoped that chapters of this book will act as reference and initiators of further research in Oral Health Science and Dentistry.

This effort has been possible by the interest and untiring effort by InTech and its very energetic Head of Book Publishing Ms Danijela Duric. I sincerely thank for their imitative and efforts in making this publication possible. I will be failing in my duty if I do not acknowledge the contribution of my family specially my wife Dr. Harnit K. Virdi and my son Dharam Pratap for bearing with me during the development of this book.

Prof. (Dr.) Mandeep Singh Virdi
Department of Pediatric Dentistry
PDM Dental College and Research Institute
India

Pediatric and Preventive Dentistry

Chapter 1

Fissure Sealing in Occlusal Caries Prevention

Kristina Goršeta

Additional information is available at the end of the chapter

http://dx.doi.org/10.5772/59325

1. Introduction

In the modern world there is still a problem of dental caries. Dental caries is still the most common chronic childhood disease and the primary cause of tooth loss. Over the past 30 years, significant progress has been made in the prevention of dental caries in children and adolescents. While caries has decreased on interproximal surfaces, occlusal pit and fissure caries have increased [1, 2]. In general, research has demonstrated that caries on occlusal and buccal/lingual surfaces account for almost 90% of caries experienced in children and adolescents [3]. The caries process in the first and second molars usually starts soon after eruption. The occlusal surfaces of lateral teeth, especially molars have complicated morphology with many grooves (fissures) and pits on the occlusal surface and on the buccal and palatal surfaces (Figure 1). These molar teeth are considered the most susceptible teeth to dental caries due to the anatomy of the chewing surfaces of these teeth, which unfortunately inhibits protection from saliva and fluoride and instead favours plaque accumulation [4]. Pits and fissures don't cause caries process. They permit the entrance of microorganisms and food into this sheltered warm moist richly provided incubator and the dental plaque can be expected to form here. They instead provide a sanctuary to those agents, which cause caries. When carbohydrates in food come in contact with the plaque, acidogenic bacteria in the plaque create acid. This acid damages the enamel walls of the pits and fissures and caries results. Therefore, the most decay is concentrated on the occlusal surfaces of posterior molars.

Pits and fissures have variations in their appearance in cross section. They were described based on the alphabetical description of shape. According to Nango (1960) there were 4 types of pits and fissures: V&U type: self cleansing and somewhat caries resistant; U type: narrow slit like opening with a larger base-susceptible to caries and a number of different ranches K type: also very susceptible to caries [5]. These are the sites most susceptible to developing decay [6].

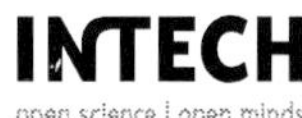

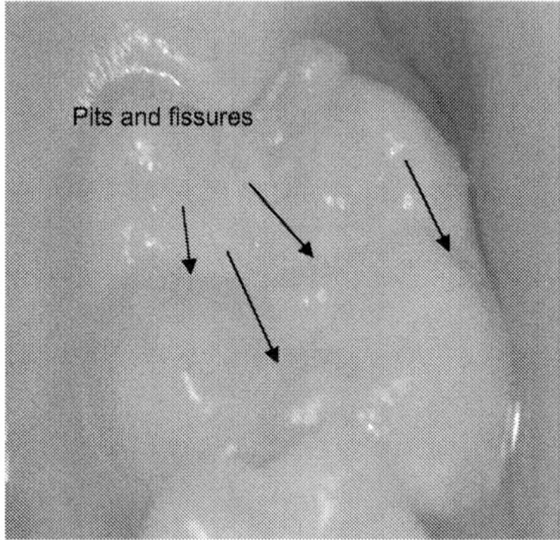

Figure 1. Occlusal morphology of molar teeth

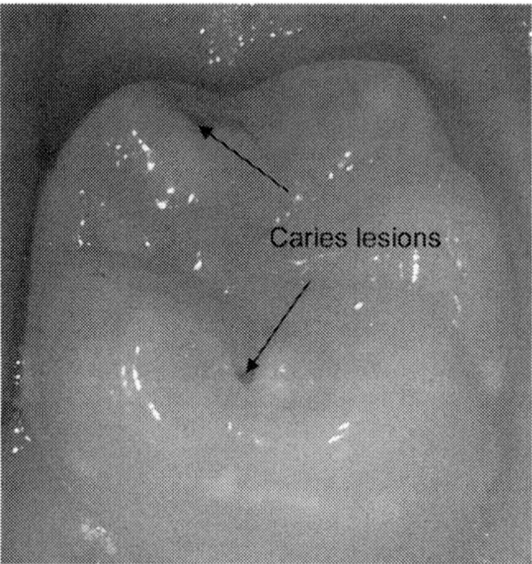

Figure 2. Caries lesions on the occlusal surface of molar tooth

In most cases the shape of the pit or fissure is such that it is impossible to clean, explaining the high susceptibility of pits and fissures to dental caries (Figure 2 and 3). Caries in the pits and fissures follows the direction of enamel rods and characteristically forms a triangular or cone shaped lesion with its apex at the outer surface and its base towards DEJ. Pits and fissures provide greater cavitations than smooth surface caries. Preventive measures for tooth decay include daily tooth brushing, topical fluoride application, chewing gums with xylitol and sealing of fissures which are applied by dental clinicians [7-10].

There have been many efforts made within past decades to prevent the development of caries, in particular occlusal caries as it was once generally accepted that pits and fissures of teeth

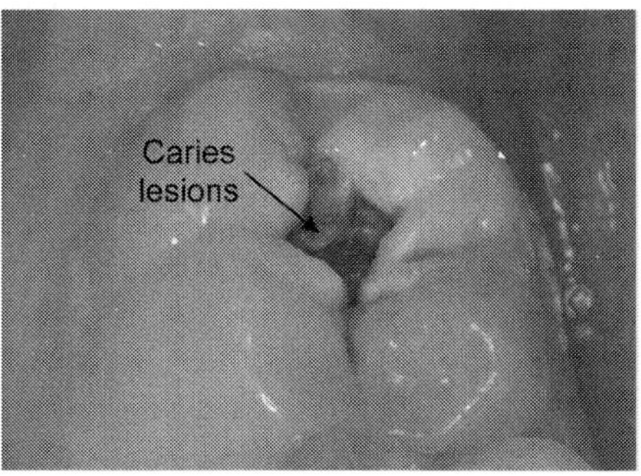

Figure 3. Caries lesion in the fissure of molar tooth

would become infected with bacteria within 10 years of erupting into the mouth [7-10]. G.V. Black, the creator of modern dentistry, informed that more than 40% of caries incidences in permanent teeth occurred in pits and fissures due to being able to retain food and plaque [9].There were many attempts to prevent occlusal caries. Willoughby D. Miller, a pioneer of dentistry, was applying silver nitrate with its antibacterial functions to surfaces of teeth to prevent occlusal caries in early 1905. It was chemically treating the biofilm against both Streptococcus mutans and Actinomyces naeslundii, which are both carious pathogens [7-9, 11]. Silver nitrate, which was also being practiced by H. Klein and J.W. Knutson in the 1940s, was being used in attempt to prevent and arrest occlusal caries [9,12].

In 1955, M.G. Buonocore gave insight to the benefits of etching enamel with phosphoric acid. [7-9] His studies demonstrated that resin could be bonded to enamel through acid etching, increasing adhesion whilst also creating an improved marginal integrity of resin restorative material [7,9]. Later, this bonding system leads to the future successful creation of fissure sealants [8-13].

By the late 1970s and early 1980s the clinical data on sealants and caries prevention was very positive. Studies have continued to demonstrate sealant success. One 4-year study showed an overall 43% decrease in the prevalence of caries effectiveness with significantly better sealant retention on premolars (84%) than molars (30%) [5]. A 7-year study reported 66% complete sealant retention and 14% partial retention [9]. Sealant loss was 20% while there was a 55% reduction in caries rate for the sealed teeth versus the unsealed teeth. One 10-year study showed that for over 8,000 sealants placed on permanent first molars, there was 41% complete sealant retention at 10 years and a 58%–63% retention rate over 7 to 9 years [10].

2. Sealants materials

Pit and fissure sealants proved to be an effective clinical intervention to prevent occlusal caries [13-15]. The aim of fissure sealants is to prevent or arrest the development of dental caries [15].

Preventing tooth decay from the pits and fissures of the teeth is achieved by the fissure sealants blocking these surfaces and therefore stopping food and bacteria from getting stuck in these grooves and fissures [15]. Fissure sealants also provide a smooth surface that is easily accessible for both our natural protective factor, saliva and the toothbrush bristles when cleaning our teeth. Fissure sealing prevents the growth of bacteria in fissures that cause tooth decay. There are several types of materials for fissure sealing.

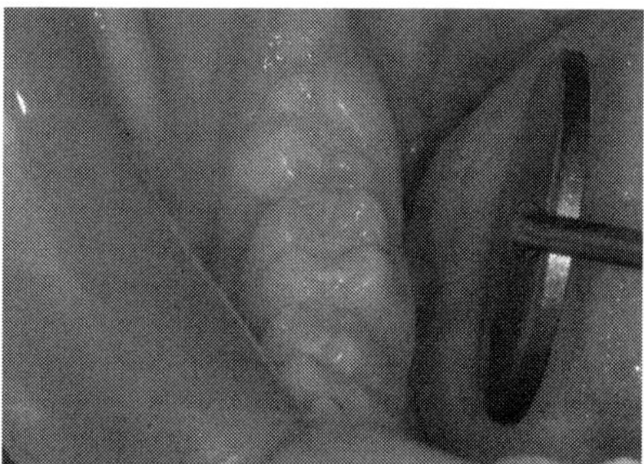

Figure 4. Fissure sealed with resin based sealant material

Caries in pits and fissures has responded less to routine preventive methods than caries on smooth surfaces. Pit and fissure sealant use is an effective clinical regime available for preventing occlusal caries. The most widely used pit and fissure sealants are based on bis-glycidyl methacrylate (Bis-GMA) resins. These resins were introduced in 1963 as restorative materials. The main types in use are resin-based sealants and glass ionomer cements [16, 17]. Cueto and Buonocore suggested the sealing of pits and fissures with an adhesive resin in 1967 [18,19]. E.I. Cueto created the first sealant material, which was methyl cyanoacrylate [7, 11,19]. However, this material was susceptible to bacterial breakdown over time, therefore was not an acceptable sealing material [18]. Bunonocore made further advances in 1970 by developing bisphenol-a glycidyl dimethacrylate, which is a viscous resin commonly known as BIS-GMA [13]. This material was used as the basis for many resin-based sealant/composite material developments in dentistry, as it is resistant to bacterial breakdown and forms a steady bond with etched enamel [13,19, 30].

A second group of materials used as fissure sealants are the glass ionomer cements (Figure 5). Glass ionomer cement is also the material of choice for fissure sealing. In 1974, glass ionomer cement fissure sealants (GIC) were introduced by J.W. McLean and A.D. Wilson [15,38]. GIC materials bond both to enamel and dentine after being cleaned with polyacrylic acid conditioner [15]. Some other advantages GIC's have is that they contain fluoride and are less moisture sensitive, with suggestions being made that despite having poor retention, they may prevent occlusal caries even after the sealant has fallen out due to their ability to release fluoride[7,13,14-16].

It has certain advantages over composite resins: less susceptible to moisture, easy handling and long-term release of fluoride ions [20,21]. These are all essential characteristics for materials handled in paediatric dentistry. However, various studies have shown a significantly lower level of retention compared with composite resins [22-25]. Mechanical properties of glass ionomer are significantly weaker than composite resin. Question about preventive effect of glass ionomer still gets controversial answers: Different studies have shown different preventive effects [22, 24, 21,26, 27].

Glass ionomer materials release fluoride over time and have the advantage of being less sensitive to moisture contamination than resin-based materials, making them a potential alternative to resin-based sealants when moisture control is an issue [28,29]. Hybrid materials which incorporate features of both resin and glass ionomer, e.g. polyacid-modified resins (compomers) and resin-modified glass ionomers, have also been developed and used as pit and fissure sealants [30].

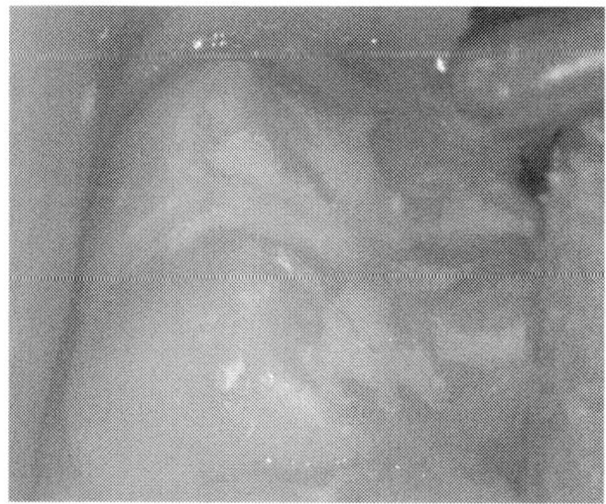

Figure 5. Fissure sealed with glass ionomer sealant material

3. Properties of fissure sealing materials

Resin-based fissure sealants are effective at preventing caries on pit and fissure surfaces in children and adolescents. A Cochrane systematic review of 16 trials found that first permanent molar teeth sealed with resin-based sealant had 78% less caries on occlusal surfaces after 2 years and 60% less after 4–4.5 years compared to unsealed molars [31]. Sealant retention is critical to the effectiveness of resin-based sealants and retention has become an important measure of sealant effectiveness. The Cochrane systematic review reported complete sealant retention rates and it ranged from 79% to 92% at 12 months, 71% to 85% at 24 months, 61% to 80% at 36 months, 52% at 48 months, 72% at 54 months and 39% at 9 years [31]. There was evidence of a clear trend for decreasing sealant retention with time. Some other systematic review on sealant effectiveness reported that the caries-preventive effect of sealants was influenced by sealant replacement, with relatively high reductions in caries risk found in those studies in which a sealant replacement strategy had been used [32].

To achieve effective caries prevention on occlusal surfaces, dental sealants should have several properties. Adhesion of material should be perfect during all kind of function and thermal challenges. Dimensional changes of material during setting should be minimal. Complete retention of sealant material in the occlusal fissures depends on the dimensional changes and resistance to wear and fracture. Good preventive effect today means substantial release of fluoride ions.

Glass ionomer cements (GICs) are also proposed for pit and fissure sealant materials. They have several advantages compared to classic resin sealant materials: easy handling, fluoride releasing at a continuous rate and they are not moisture sensitive.

For the best caries preventive effect in the fissures of lateral teeth, material for sealing should have the following properties:

1. Ideal adhesion of material should be maintained during setting and function, including the challenges of both thermal and mechanical cycling.

2. Complete retention of the sealant material in the occlusal fissures

3. Resistance to wear and fracture

4. Ease to handling and placement

5. Caries preventive effects

6. Biocompatibility.

Inclusion of fluoride ions in the material may be beneficial on the prevention of developing carious lesions, and the remineralization of any demineralized enamel adjacent to the sealant [33-37].

Some studies introduced additional treatment to improve mechanical properties of glass ionomer materials. So a few years ago a method of heating the glass ionomer was introduced. Material was heated with 60-70oC metal plates in order to improve the mechanical properties of materials [39]. Sidhu and colleagues have linked the contraction of the material and the loss of water from glass ionomer cement as a reason to improve the properties of materials[40]. Some studies have shown enhanced adhesion of glass ionomer for hard tissues [95].

Another study tried to increase the level of retention of glass ionomer sealants with heating during setting time of materials [41]. The results obtained for the resin sealing group as a control group in this study are consistent with previously published studies and their results [41-44]. Glass ionomer (Fuji VII) on the basis of the results obtained by monitoring of patient showed a relatively low percentage of retention after 12 months. The results did not differ when compared with the results obtained for the retention of classical (chemical) treated glass ionomer cement [45-50].

4. Caries preventive effect

There is good evidence that teeth sealed very early after eruption require more frequent reapplication of the FS than teeth sealed later [51,52]. Therefore, FS placement may be delayed until the teeth are fully erupted, unless high caries activity is present. Placement of FS even in the absence of regular follow-up is beneficial [53, 54].

Caries prevalence is relatively low in high-income and relatively high in low-and middle-income countries. Children from high-income countries have benefited from the available established caries preventive measures; such as the use of fluoride-containing products and awareness among their parents and caretakers of the importance of keeping tooth surfaces free from plaque [55].

The studies show that sealants work if applied correctly. Sealant success is multifactorial [56, 57]. Technique, fissure morphology, and the characteristics of the sealant contribute to clinical success [58]. When one reviews published sealant data, a basic concept of 5%–10% of sealant loss per year has been seen demonstrated [31, 32]. This data reveal the importance of re-evaluating teeth with sealants on a periodic basis and to reapply if necessary.

Discussion about caries preventive effect of glass ionomer sealants is still controversial: different studies have shown different preventive effects. It was reported that some material remnants in the fissures can maintain caries prevention. The treatment of glass ionomer material with thermo-curing was recently introduced and showed increase of the mechanical properties. Gorseta et al. showed increased bond strength of glass ionomers to hard dental tissues after thermo-curing during material setting [58]. Skrinjaric et al. investigated the retention rate of glass ionomer sealant material thermo-cured during setting time after 1-year clinical trial [41]. Some authors have pointed to the fact that the remains of SIC in the fissures may have some preventive effect in the development of caries [59, 60]. Skrinjaric et al. did not determine SIC remains in fissures. Increased cariostatic effect can be achieved by regular reapplication, but it increases the cost of such preventing procedure [61-64]. The Database Cochane Review could not find a conclusion on a comparison of glass ionomer sealants and resin sealants [63]. Therefore, it is an area that needs further investigation in order to obtain relevant conclusions.

Primary objective of the most studies is to evaluate the effectiveness of pit and fissure sealants in children and adolescents. It is very important that a different background level of caries in the population is related to obtained results. The diagnosis of the surface to be sealed was based on clinical examination in nine studies, one further study used also a DIAGNOdent device [65-68].

Studies which compare the retention of two or more nearly similar type of sealant materials and report the caries rates only on the sealed occlusal surfaces are not relevant. It is important to report on individual level. Information on the caries risk in the study population, the use of fluoridated water, toothpaste and general preventive methods as well as other preventive interventions should be reported in order to facilitate multivariate analysis of risk factors [69].

Comparing glass ionomers to resin sealants, where less than 10% of tooth surfaces had a small dentine caries lesion and most tooth surfaces were reported to be sound. Caries diagnosis of occlusal surfaces can be challenging. In general, using conventional visual, tactile and radiographic methods in occlusal caries lesion diagnosis, it is not accurate enough to identify whether a lesion extends into the dentine or not [70].

New technologies such as DIAGNOdent laser fluorescence devices may be more sensitive in detecting occlusal dentinal caries [71, 72]. However, the likelihood of false-positive diagnoses may increase when using laser-fluorescence compared with visual methods [71]. Regardless of the caries diagnostic method used, the condition of an occlusal surface to be sealed remains, however, in any case somewhat unclear.

5. Indications and contraindications

Post eruption period of the tooth is most caries susceptible. According to EAPD guidelines, fissure sealant should be placed as soon as possible if there is an indication for placement. However, teeth can be sealed at any age depending on assessment of caries risk factors. [15].

Indications for the use of dental sealants are individual and it depends on patients or teeth that are at high risk of dental caries.

This includes patients with:

- Patients with high risk of dental caries

- Poor oral hygiene

- Deep pits and fissures

- Enamel defects or hypomineralisation or hypoplasia

- Initial lesion of dental caries

- Orthodontics appliances.[73]

Contraindications for the use of dental sealants are individual patients or teeth that are at a low risk of dental caries:

This includes patients with:

- Teeth with shallow, self-cleansing fissures

- Adequate oral hygiene

- A balanced diet with low carbohydrates intake

- Partially erupted teeth without adequate moisture control (operators may choose to use GIC in these cases)

- Teeth with previously restored pits and fissures.[73]

6. Clinical procedure for fissure sealing

It includes:

1.   **Tooth selection** (Figure 6) and cleaning the occlusal surface (Figure 7).

Visual dental examination is the starting point for dental assessment and treatment planning. The assessment of occlusal surfaces is particularly challenging, due to their complex morphology. The basic prerequisites for visual caries detection are clean, dry teeth and good illumination [72, 74, 75].

The difficulty in detecting and correctly assessing occlusal caries by visual examination alone has led to the development of various caries detection methods to refine the diagnostic process, and to enhance the identification of early caries lesions [68, 71, 73]. These methods include dental radiography, light-based technologies e.g. fibre-optic transillumination, quantitative laser fluorescence (DIAGNOdent) or light induced fluorescence (QLF). Given the importance of the visual examination, a system for detailed visual examination of teeth – the International Caries Detection and Assessment System (ICDAS) – has been developed, which promotes the recording of the earliest changes in enamel as well as dentinal caries [76].

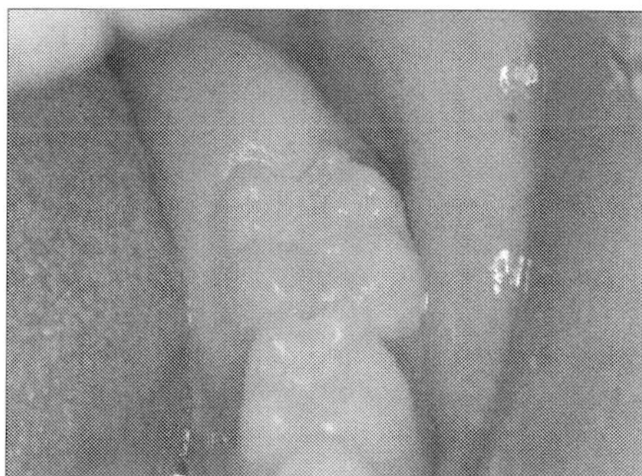

Figure 6. Tooth selected for sealing

There are different approaches for surface cleaning and the way of cleaning pits and fissures before sealing. It may seem to be controversial. Raadal et al. suggested careful removal of pellicle and plaque with pumice in order to achieve optimal acid-etch pattern of the enamel [77]. On the other hand, Harris and Garcia-Godoy keep that the enamel acid etching alone is sufficient for surface cleaning and provided soft plaque removal [78]. The literature is extensive on the effectiveness of different methods for cleaning prior to bonding [15]. Air abrasion also has been suggested for preparation of the occlusal surface before sealant application [79]. In this case a high-speed stream of purified aluminium oxide particles propelled by air pressure is used to clean the tooth surface. They can remove debris and excavate incipient decay in the fissures. A widening of the fissures with rotary instrumentation in order to remove superficial enamel and open the fissure to have the resin penetrate into it has been recommended before

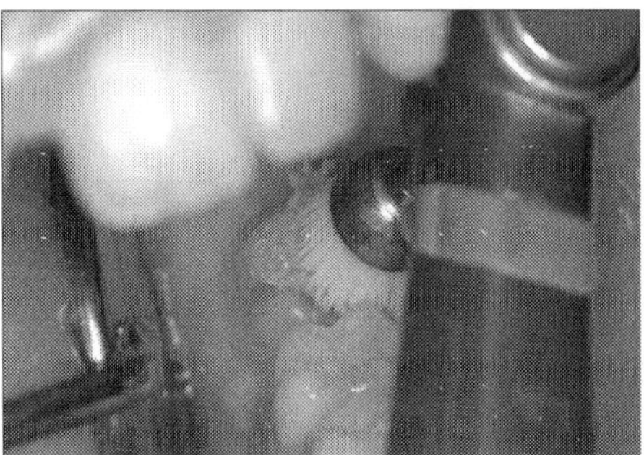

Figure 7. Cleaning the occlusal surface

etching and sealant application by Waggoner and Siegal. This is known as the invasive pit-and fissure technique [80, 81]. However, although cleaning the fissures with a bur has given superior retention in some studies [82, 83]. There is evidence in other studies that it provides no additional benefit [84]. Furthermore, purpose full removal of enamel or enameloplasty just to widen the base of a fissure in a sound occlusal surface is an invasive technique, which disturbs the equilibrium of the fissure system and exposes a child unnecessarily to the use of a handpiece or air abrasion. It is concluded, therefore, that there is a need for removal of most organic substance in order to obtain sufficient bonding, but that the removal of sound tooth tissue by the use of instruments, such as a bur, is unnecessary and undesirable. There is a significant volume of evidence of high fissure sealants retention without the use of a bur. Hydrogen peroxide (3%) also has been suggested for cleaning the occlusal fissures before etching, but there is no evidence that this improves clinical retention [85].

2.   Moisture control

Adequate isolation is the most critical aspect of the sealant application process [78]. Achieving good moisture control is one of the greatest challenges to successful sealant application. Salivary contamination of a tooth surface during or after acid etching will have a key effect on the bond quality between enamel and resin. Salivary contamination, also allows the precipitation of glycoprotein onto the enamel surface greatly decreasing bond strength. If the enamel porosity created by the etching procedure is filled by any kind of liquid, the formation of resin tags in the enamel is blocked or reduced [86, 87]. The circumstances that affect the control of moisture will vary from patient to patient, and may relate to the state of eruption of the tooth, the patient's ability to co-operate, the materials and equipment available for isolation, or a combination of these factors. The options considered by the Guideline Group for 'interim' treatment of teeth for which a sealant was indicated but for which adequate isolation could not be achieved were: resin-based sealant, fluoride varnish and glass ionomer sealant [15].

The rubber dam, when properly placed, provides the best, the safest way of moisture control, and for an operator working alone, it ensures properly isolation from start to finish. In young and partially erupted teeth this is usually not practical. There is evidence of difficulty in securely placing a clamp onto a partially erupted tooth, discomfort during clamp placement and it demands the use of local analgesia in some instances [7, 15]. On the other hand, there is sufficient evidence that careful isolation with cotton rolls gives similar retention results [83]. Cotton roll isolation offers some advantages over rubber dam isolation. No anaesthetic is necessary because no clamps are placed. Cotton rolls can be held in place with either cotton roll holders or fingers. The primary disadvantage to cotton roll isolation is that it is almost a practical necessity that an assistant be used to provide four-handed dentistry [88-90]. The maintenance of a dry field must therefore usually be achieved by the use of cotton rolls and isolation shields, in combination with a thoughtful use of the water spray and evacuation tip. The isolation procedure may frequently be extremely challenging, particularly in the partially erupted teeth or in those children with poor cooperation.

3.   Enamel cleaning(Figure 8)

The goal of etching is to produce a dry, uncontaminated and frosted surface [91]. There are various etching materials available, but the most frequently used is orthophosphoric acid, provided that its concentration lies between 30% and 50% by weight. This is available as both a liquid solution and a gel. Small variations in the concentration do not appear to affect the quality of the etched surface [81]. Duggal et al. showed no significant difference in retention of fissure sealant after one year follow-up on second primary and first permanent molars when 15, 30, 45 or 60 seconds etching times were used [92]. Liquid etching, likewise, is often applied by brush or a small cotton pledget. The application of the gel is often done either directly from the gel dispenser with special applicator tips or with a small disposable brush [7].

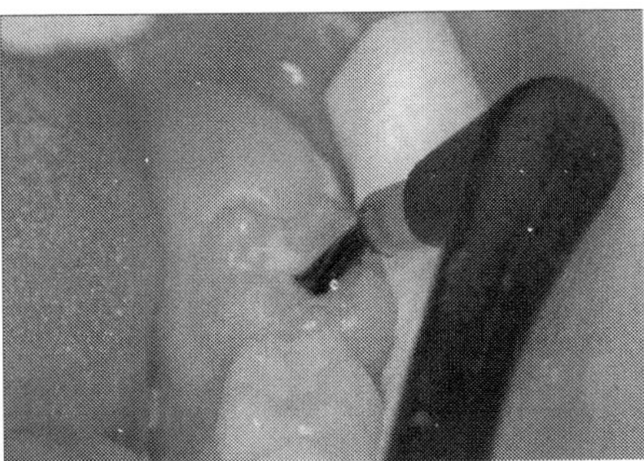

Figure 8. Etching the occlusal surface

4.   Rinsing and drying

Many of the sealant manufacturers recommend rinsing the tooth for 20 to 30 seconds to remove the etchant. The most important is ensuring that the rinse is long enough to remove all of the etchant from the surface. After drying the tooth with compressed air, the tooth exhibits a chalky, frosted appearance but if still no milky white appearance is seen, the tooth should be re-etched for 15 to 20 seconds [7, 81, 91].

5.   Sealant application (Figure 9)

During sealant application, all the susceptible pits and fissures should be sealed for maximum caries protection. The long-term clinical success of fissure sealants is closely related to their poor handling [93]. The sealant material can be applied to the tooth in a variety of methods. It may be applied with a small brush or on the tip of an explorer. Some common problems occur during sealant application. Small bubbles may form in the sealant material. If these are present, they should be teased out with a brush before polymerization. Many sealant kits have their own dispensers, which directly apply the sealant to the tooth surface. When using a dispenser, the dentist should allow the sealant to flow ahead into the pits and fissures. It reduces air entrapment [7].

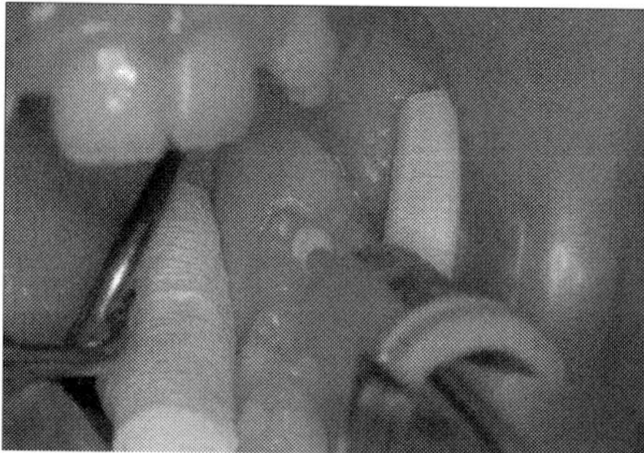

Figure 9. Application of glass ionomer fissure sealing material

6.   Application of surface gloss for glass ionomer sealants (Figure 10)

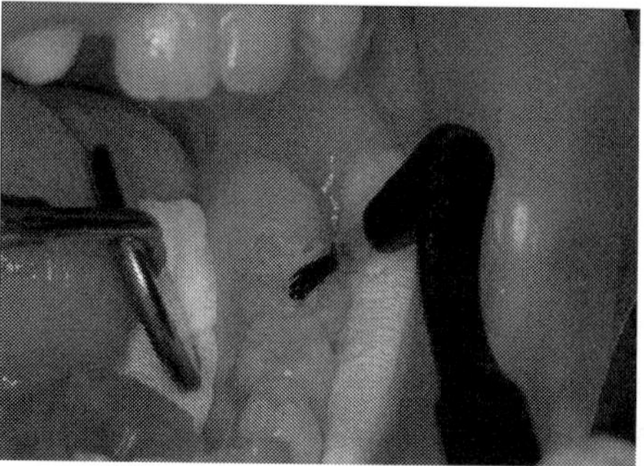

Figure 10. Application of surface gloss

7.   Polymerization of resin sealants or Thermo-curing of glass ionomer sealants (Figure 11)

For light cured sealants, polymerization should be initiated quickly after the sealant is placed on the etched surface to help minimize potential contamination. Some study found that the longer sealants were allowed to sit on the etched surface before being polymerized; the more the sealant penetrated the microporosities, creating longer resin tags, which are critical for micromechanical retention [94]. One of the key factors affecting polymerisation is the light intensity of the dental light curing unit. A Canadian study reported that 12.1% of light curing units tested in a sample of dental practices had intensities that would be considered inadequate (<300 mW/cm^2) [70]. Other factors that may influence polymerisation include curing time, distance of the light guide from the material being cured, and thickness, shade and composition of the material being cured.

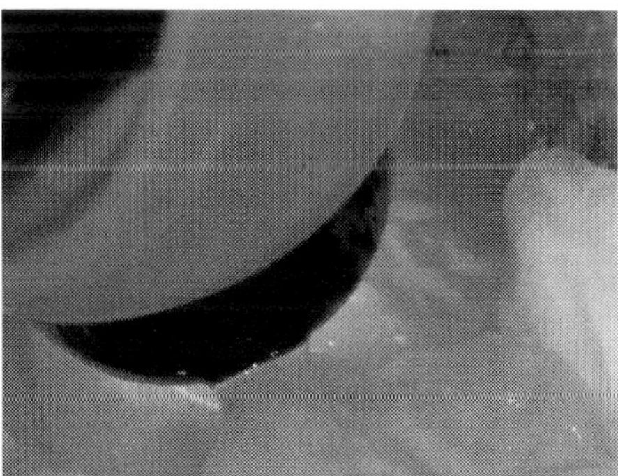

Figure 11. Thermo-curing with dental light

There are some tips for better fissure sealants:

a.   Cure each surface on the same tooth separately if more than one surface is being sealed

b.   Put the light-curing tip as close as possible to the surface and cure for at least the recommended curing time.

c.   Manufacturer's instructions for sealant materials and for curing lights should be available for every operator

d.   Check the light output and curing performance of dental curing units in accordance with the manufacturer's instructions

8.   Evaluation of the sealed tooth (Figure 12)

Sealant retention should be checked with a probe after application, and the sealant re-applied, if necessary, repeating each step of the sealant application procedure.

Regular evaluation of sealants for retention is critical to their success. During routine recall examinations, it is necessary to re-evaluate the sealed tooth surface both visually and tactually for loss of material, exposure of voids in the material and caries development. The need for reapplication of sealants is usually highest during the first six months after placement [95]. When sealants are partially lost and require repair, the clinician should vigorously attempt to dislodge the remaining sealant material with an explorer. If it remains intact to probing, there is no need to completely remove the old material before placing the new.

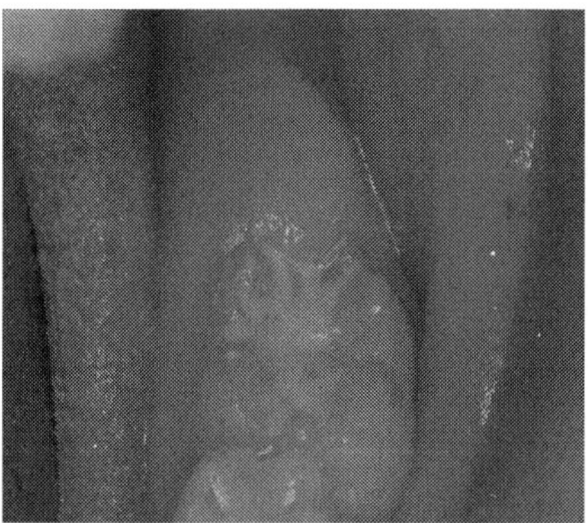

Figure 12. Occlusal view of fissure sealed with nano ionomer cement

7. Retention rates for the fissure sealing

One of the major problems when considering the success rates of sealant restorations is the variation in techniques and materials used. Short term studies indicate a high degree of success for sealant restorations [96-105]. However, longer term studies appear to indicate that success is less predictable [106-110].

Recent study by Gorseta et al. investigated retention of Glass Carbomer fissure sealant after six and twelve months of clinical trial [111]. Glass Carbomer is relatively new material developed from glass ionomer (GIC) and contains nano-sized powder particles and fluorapatite. Advantages of Glass Carbomer comparing to GIC are better mechanical properties and command setting through application of heat. Materials included forty eight teeth with well-delineated fissure morphology divided in two groups which were sealed with Glass Carbomer Sealant (Glass Carbomer Products, Netherlands) and Helioseal F (Vivadent, Liechtenstein) using split mouth design. Investigated materials were placed and set according to manufacturer's instruction using dental light Bluephase 16i (Vivadent, Liechtenstein) (Figure 10). Teeth in group A were sealed with Glass Carbomer material and in group B with Helioseal F. Evaluation criteria (Kilpatrick et al.) for retention of sealant was classified as: type 1: intact sealant; type 2: 1/3 of sealant missing; type 3: 2/3 of sealant missing; and type 4: whole sealant missing. Presence of new caries lesions was evaluated in two categories: 1-absent; 2-present.

Gorseta et al. used replicas for evaluation of fissure sealant retention rate. The impressions with polyvinylxyloxane impression material of Glass Carbomer-sealed teeth were taken in order to obtain replicas of occlusal surfaces (Figure 14). For that purpose, impression was taken and poured in acrylic resin (Citofix Kit, Struers) (Figure 13). The obtained replicas were analysed with SEM (Figure 15, 16).

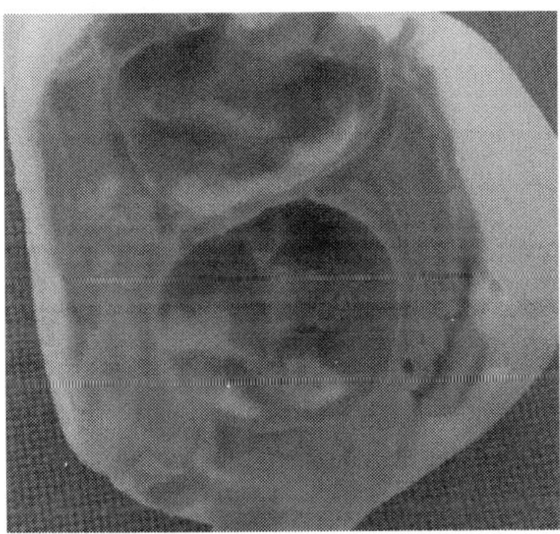

Figure 13. Impression of occlusal surface of molar

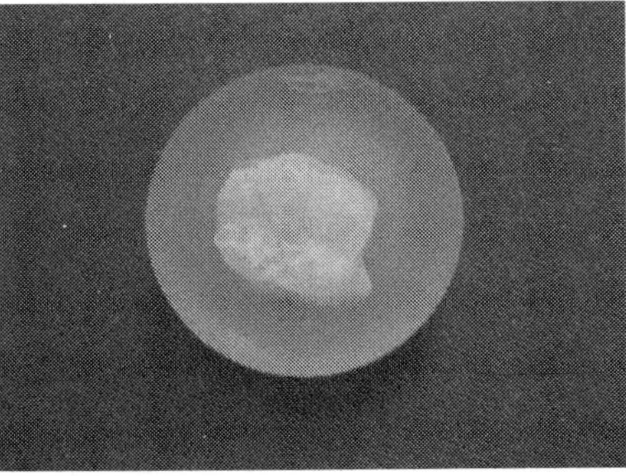

Figure 14. Replicas of occlusal surface of molar

Obtained data were statistically analyzed using non-parametric Mann-Whitney test.

Results showed that retention rate in-group A and B were 100% after six months of clinical service. There were no secondary caries lesions in either group. Results showed that complete retention in group A and B were 75% after 12 months of clinical service. There were two new caries lesions in each group. Mann-Whitney U test doesn't reveal significant statistical difference between groups. Glass Carbomer sealant material showed comparable retention rate to resin based sealant material and can also be recommended for every day practice [111].

In some studies which found statistically significantly more caries in group with glass ionomer sealed teeth at 36-48 months than in group with resin sealed teeth, the complete retention for resin sealants was about 80%, and for glass ionomers was very low (3%) [112, 113, 114].

Studies published by Karlzén-Reuterving and Williams reported similar retention rate did not show a difference between the materials in caries incidence [115, 116]. In next two studies, glass ionomers sealing were reported to be more effective regarding caries prevention [117, 118]. They reported retention of both sealant materials as low (resin-based sealants 28% to 40% and glass ionomers in 21% to 40% after 36 months). Conditioning with 10% polyacrylic acid as well as heating lamp polymerization during curing of cement had no effect on the level of retention of the tested glass ionomer cement (Fuji VII). Similar studies have been done in other parts of Europe, and all with the record of low retention rate of glass ionomer sealants, or the value does not significantly deviate from those of the observed in our study. The two-year Finnish study published the complete retention of polyalcenoic cement at 26% of the sealed teeth compared with 82% fully retained fissure sealants of bis-GMA materials [50].

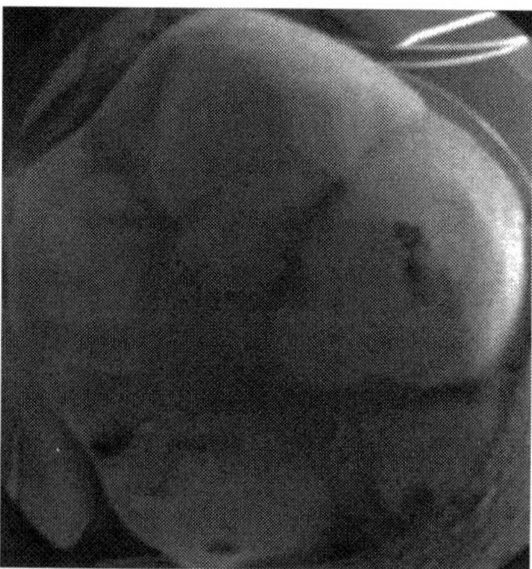

Figure 15. SEM analysis of glass ionomer sealant

After 28 months, Poulsen et al [45] have noted retention of Fuji III of less than 10%, and Pardi et al [46] only 3.5%. After nine months Weerheijm et al. [60] showed an overall retention of Fuji IX in the amount of 51% and only 15% for Fuji III. The incidence of new carious lesions in the group of sealing with glass ionomer cements was not statistically significant. The duration of study is only one year because of the small percentage of retention rate of glass ionomer sealants. Regardless of what is known that the most people prefer chewing on the right side, a control group of sealants (Helioseal F) placed on the right side of the jaw showed a high percentage of retention of 80%.

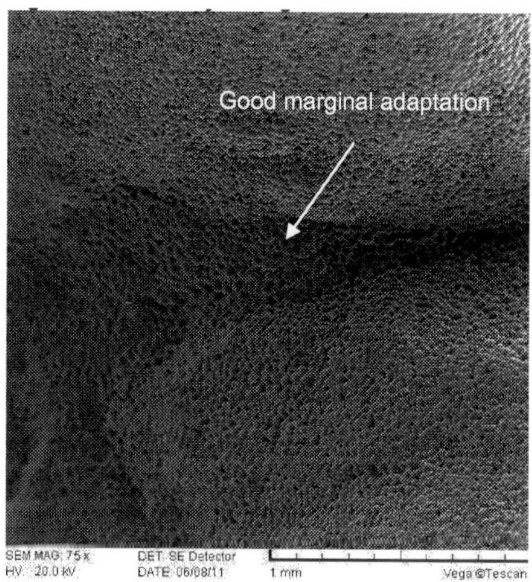

Figure 16. SEM analysis of glass ionomer sealant-higher magnification

Sidhu et al. studied contraction SIC after heating [40]. They concluded that the degree of contraction of the material depends on the porosity within the SIC. These dimensional changes can affect not only the marginal integrity between the enamel and the material, but also compromise the quality of adhesion between the glass ionomer and enamel. As the viscosity of glass ionomers used for sealing fissures greater than the viscosity of the resin sealants, Simonsen, McLean recommend use SIC only fissure having a diameter greater than 100 microns [119]. Also, solutions and gels for fluoridation may affect the surface SIC causing greater roughness [120]. This may induce microfractures on the surface of the material, then the fractures in the material and chained lead to loss of retention of material in the fissure.

The study of Pardi analyzed following sealant materials: flowable resin composite (Revolution), resin-modified glass ionomer (Vitremer) and compomer (DyractFlow) [121]. All occlusal surfaces were conditioned with 37% phosphoric acid. After 2 years, sealants were totally retained on 76% of the teeth sealed with Revolution, on 58% of teeth sealed with Dyract Flow and on 47% of the occlusal surfaces sealed with Vitremer. Recent studies comparing resins to resin-modified glass ionomers at 36 months, reported clearly better complete retention rates for resins (94%) than for resin-modified glass ionomers (5%) [122,123].

There might be many different causes behind the inconsistent results between the studies comparing resin-based materials to glass ionomers as sealants. Therefore, conclusion cannot be drawn based only on retention rate of material as sealants. However, information about caries prevalence in population is very important as diet and oral hygiene [122, 123].

Recent studies showed that the level of retention of glass ionomer sealants treated by heating during setting time is considerably lower than retention of conventional composite resin for sealing. Reduced time manipulation and adhesion of glass ionomer material for the wet surface of the tooth, unequivocally favours glass ionomer material as the material of choice for sealing partially erupted molars [124-130]. This procedure is especially warranted in high caries risk patients, uncooperative patients and those with special needs [121].

Griffin et al. evaluated the effectiveness of sealants in managing caries lesions in a meta-analysis, and found their effectiveness in preventing dentin caries to be in the range of 62% to 100% (median 74% for all; 83% for non-cavitated and 65% for cavitated lesions). They recommended the placement of sealants to arrest lesions in the early carious stages and also to surfaces where caries status is uncertain. The progression of non-cavitated occlusal lesions was slow also for surfaces that were not sealed indicating that such surfaces could either be monitored or sealed. Invasive treatment methods were not recommended [124, 126-131].

Sealant maintenance is an integrated part of the sealant approach – all sealed surfaces should be regularly monitored clinically and radiographically [132-133]. Bitewing radiographs are suggested to be taken at a frequency consistent with the patient's risk status especially in cases where there has been doubt about the surface caries status prior to sealant application [124]. Defective or lost sealants should be reapplied in order to maintain the marginal integrity of sealants.

8. Conclusion

A fissure sealant is a material that is placed in the pits and fissures of teeth in order to prevent or arrest the development of dental caries. As the integrity and retention of a sealant is considered crucial to the success of sealants in the long-term, resin based is the material of choice. Sealing over incipient caries lesions is both effective and practical – the dental profession should be encouraged to use sealants more in an interceptive manner rather than in a preventive or operative manner.) They recommended the placement of sealants to arrest lesions in the early carious stages and also to surfaces where caries status is uncertain. The progression of non-cavitated occlusal lesions was slow also for surfaces that were not sealed indicating that such surfaces could either be monitored or sealed.

Author details

Kristina Goršeta*

Address all correspondence to: kgorseta@sfzg.hr

Department of Pediatric and Preventive Dentistry, School of Dental Medicine, University of Zagreb, Croatia

References

[1] Eccles MFW. The problem of occlusal caries and its current management. N Z Dent J. 1989;85(380):50-55.

[2] Bohannan HM. Caries distribution and the case for sealants. J Public Health Dent. 1983; 43(3):200-204.

[3] Ripa LW, Leske GS, Sposato A. The surface-specific caries pattern of participants in a school-based fluoride mouthrinsing program with implications for the use of sealants. J Public Health Dent. 1985;45(2):90-94.

[4] Welbury R., Raadal M., & Lygidakis N.A. EAPD guidelines of the use of pit and fissure sealants. Paediatric Dentistry, 2004.

[5] Nagano T. The form of pits and fissure and the primary lesion of caries. Dent Abstr. 1961;Abstract 6:426.

[6] Slade GD, Spencer AJ, Davies MJ, Burrow D. Intra-oral distribution and impact of caries experience among South Australian School Children. Aust. Dent. J. 1996;41(5): 343–50.

[7] Avinash, J., Marya, C.M., Dhingra, S., Gupta, P., Kataria, S., Meenu, & Bhatia, H. P. Pit and Fissure Sealants: An Unused Caries Prevention Tool. Journal of Oral Health and Community Dentistry, 2010. 4(1), 1-6.

[8] Feigal, R. J., & Donly, K. J. The Use of Pit and Fissure Sealants. Pediatric Dentistry 2006, 28(2), 143-150.5. RE, Haugh LD, Grainger DA Conti AJ. Four-year clinical evaluation of pit and fissure sealant. J Am Dent Assoc. (2006). 1977;95(5):972-981.

[9] Mertz-Fairhurst EJ, Fairhurst CW, Williams JE, Della Giustina VE, Brooks JD. A comparative clinical study of two pit and fissure sealants: 7-year results in Augusta, Georgia. J Am Dent Assoc. 1984;109(2):252-255.

[10] Romcke RG, Lewis DW, Maze BD, Vickerson RA. Retention and maintenance of fissure sealants over 10 years. J Can Dent Assoc. 1990;56(3):235-237.

[11] Donovan, T. E., Anderson, M., Becker, W., Cagna, D. R., Carr, G. B., Albouy, J., Metz, J., Eichmiller, F., & McKee, J. R. Annual Review of selected dental literature: Report of the Committee on Scientific Investigation of the American Academy of Restorative Dentistry. The Journal of Prosthetic Dentistry, (2013). 110(3), 161-210.

[12] Knight, G. M., McIntyre, J. M., Craig, G. G., Zilm, P. S., & Gully, N. J. An in vitro model to measure the effect of a silver fluoride and potassium iodine treatment on the permeability of demineralized dentine to streptococcus mutans Australian Dental Journal, (2005). 50(4), 242-5.

[13] Zero, D. T. How the introduction of the acid-etch technique revolutionized dental practice. The Journal of the American Dental Association, (2013). 144(9), 990-994.

[14] Weintraub JA. The effectivness of pit and fissure sealants. J of Public Health Dent. 1989;49(5 Spec No):317-30.

[15] Welbury R, Raadal M, Lygidakis N. Guidelines on the use of Pit and Fissures Sealants in Paediatric Dentistry. An EAPD policy document. Eur J Paediatr Dent. 2004;3:179-84.

[16] Simonsen RJ. Pit and fissure sealant: review of the literature. Pediatr Dent 2002;24: 393-414.

[17] Adair SM. The role of sealants in caries prevention programs. J Calif Dent Assoc 2003;31:221-7.

[18] Cueto EI, Buonocore MG. Sealing pits and fissures with an adhesive resin. Its use in caries prevention. J Am Dent Assoc. 1967;75(1):121-128.

[19] Gwinnett AJ, Buonocore MG. Adhesives and caries prevention. A preliminary report. Br Dent J. 1965;119:77-80.

[20] Taifour D, Frencken JE, van't Hof MA, Beiruti N, Truin GJ. Effects of glass ionomer sealants in newly erupted first molars after 5 years: a pilot study. Community Dent Oral Epidemiol. 2003;31:314-9.

[21] Poulsen S, Laurberg L, Vaeth M, Jensen U, Haubek D. A field trial of resin-based and glass-ionomer fissure sealants: clinical and radiographic assessment of caries. Community Dent Oral Epidemiol. 2006;34:36-40.

[22] Pardi V, Pereira AC, Mialhe FL, Meneghim MC, Ambrosano GMB. A 5-year evaluation of two glass-ionomer cements used as fissure sealants. Community Dent Oral Epidemiol. 2003;31:386-91.

[23] Forss H, Halme E. Retention of a glass ionomer cement and a resin-based fissure sealant and effect on carious outcome after 7 years. Community Dent Oral Epidemiol. 1998;26:21-5.

[24] Poulsen S, Beiruti N, Sadat N. A comparison of retention and the effect on caries of fissure sealing with a glass-ionomer and a resin-based sealant. Community Dent Oral Epidemiol. 2001;29:298-301.

[25] Williams B, Laxton L, Holt RD, Winter GB. Fissure sealants: a 4-year clinical trial comparing an experimental glass polyalkenoate cement with a bis glycidyl metacrylate resin used as fissure sealants. Br Dent J. 1996;180:104-8.

[26] Mejare I, Major IA. Glass ionomer and resin based fissure sealants: a clinical study. Scand J Dent Res. 1990;98:345-50.

[27] Uribe S. The effectiveness of fissure sealants. Evid Based Dent. 2004;5:92.

[28] Yengopal V, Mickenautsch S, Bezerra A, Leal S. Caries-preventive effect of glass ion-omer and resin-based fissure sealants on permanent teeth: a meta analysis. J Oral Sci 2009;51(3):373–82.

[29] Seth, S. (2011). Glass ionomer cement and resin-based fissure sealants are equally ef-fective in caries prevention. JADA, 142(5), 551-552.

[30] Ahovuo-Saloranta, A., Forss, H., Walsh, T., Hiiri, A., Nordblad, A., Mäkelä, M., & Worthington, H. V. (2012). Sealants for preventing dental decay in the permanent teeth. The Cochrane database of systematic reviews, 3, 1-139.

[31] Ahovuo-Saloranta A, Hiiri A, Nordblad A, Mäkelä M, Worthington HV. Pit and fis-sure sealants for preventing dental decay in the permanent teeth of children and ado-lescents. Cochrane Database of Systematic Reviews 2008, Issue 4. [DOI: 10.1002/14651858.CD001830.pub3]

[32] Mejare I, Lingstrom P, Petersson L, Holm AK, Twetman S, Kallestal C, et al. Caries preventive effect of fissure sealants: a systematic review. Acta Odontol Scand 2003;61(6):321–30.

[33] Feigal RJ. The use of pit and fissure sealants. Pediatr Dent 2002; 24: 415-22.

[34] Feigal RJ. Sealants and preventive restorations: review of effectiveness and clinical changes for improvement. Pediatric Dent.1998;20(2):85-92.

[35] Seleeman JB, Owens BM, Johnson WW. Effect of preparation technique, fissure mor-phology, and material characteristics on the in vitro margin permeability and pene-trability of pit and fissure sealants. Pediatr Dent. 2007; 29(4):308-314.

[36] Llodra JC, Bravo M, Delgado-Rodriguez M, Baca P, Galvez R. Factors influencing the effectiveness of sealants-a metaanalysis. Community Dentistry and Oral Epidemiolo-gy 1993; 21(5):261–8.

[37] Splieth CH, Ekstrand KR, Alkilzy M, Clarkson J, MeyerLueckel H, Martignon S, et. al. Sealants in dentistry: outcomes of the ORCA Saturday Afternoon Symposium 2007. Caries Research 2010;44(1):3–13.

[38] McLean JW, Wilson AD. Fissure sealing and filling with an adhesive glass-ionomer cement. British Dental Journal 1974;136(7):269–76.

[39] Algera TJ, Kleverlaan CJ, de Gee AJ, Prahl-Andersen B, Feilzer AJ. The influence of accelerating the setting rate by ultrasound or heat on the bond strength of glass ion-omers used as ortodontic bracket cements. Eur J Orthod. 2005;27:472-6.

[40] Sidhu SK, Carrick TE, McCabe JF. Temperature mediated coefficient of dimensional change of dental tooth-colored restorative materials. Dent Mater 2004;20: 435–440.

[41] Skrinjaric K, Vranic DN, Glavina D, Skrinjaric I. Heat treated glass ionomer cement fissure sealants: retention after 1 year follow-up. International Journal of Paediatric-Dentistry 2008;18(5):368–73.

[42] Morphis TL, Toumba KJ. Retention of two fluoride pit-and-fissure sealants in comparison to a conventional sealant. Int J Paediatr Dent. 1998;8:203-8.

[43] Walker J, Floyd K, Jakobsen J. The effectiveness of sealants in pediatric patients. J Dent Child. 1996;63:268-70.

[44] Lygidakis NA, Oulis KI, Christodoulidis A. Evaluation of fissure sealants retention following four different isolation and surface preparation techniques: four years clinical trial. J Clin Pediatr Dent. 1994;19:23-5.

[45] Poulsen S, Laurberg L, Vaeth M, Jensen U, Haubek D. A field trial of resin-based and glass-ionomer fissure sealants: clinical and radiographic assessment of caries. Community Dent Oral Epidemiol. 2006;34:36-40.

[46] Pardi V, Pereira AC, Mialhe FL, Meneghim MC, Ambrosano GMB. A 5-year evaluation of two glass-ionomer cements used as fissure sealants. Community Dent Oral Epidemiol. 2003;31:386-91.

[47] Forss H, Halme E. Retention of a glass ionomer cement and a resin-based fissure sealant and effect on carious outcome after 7 years. Community Dent Oral Epidemiol. 1998;26:21-5.

[48] Poulsen S, Beiruti N, Sadat N. A comparison of retention and the effect on caries of fissure sealing with a glass-ionomer and a resin-based sealant. Community Dent Oral Epidemiol. 2001;29:298-301.

[49] Williams B, Laxton L, Holt RD, Winter GB. Fissure sealants: a 4-year clinical trial comparing an experimental glass polyalkenoate cement with a bis glycidyl metacrylate resin used as fissure sealants. Br Dent J. 1996;180:104-8.

[50] Forss H, Saarni M, Seppa L. Comparison of glass ionomer and resin based sealants. Community Dent Oral Epidemiol. 1994;22:21-4.

[51] Dennison JB, Straffon LH, More FG. Evaluating tooth eruption on sealant efficacy. J Am Dent Assoc 1990 Nov;121(5):610-4.

[52] Walker J, Floyd K, Jakobsen J, Pinkham JR. The effectiveness of preventive resin restorations in pediatric patients. ASDC J Dent Child 1996 Sep-Oct;63(5):338-40.

[53] Cueto EI, Buonocore MG. Sealing of pits and fissures with an adhesive resin: its use in caries prevention. J Am Dent Assoc 1967Jul;75(1):121-8.

[54] Chestnutt IG, Schafer F, Jacobson AP, Stephen KW. The prevalence and effectiveness of fissure sealants in Scottish adolescents. Br Dent J 1994 Aug 20;177(4):125-9.

[55] Jo E. Frencken. The ART approach using glass-ionomers in relation to global oral health care. Dental materials 2010;26:1–6.)

[56] Simonsen RJ. Retention and effectiveness of a single application of white sealant after 10 years. J Am Dent Assoc. 1987115(1):31-36.

[57] Simonsen RJ. Retention and effectiveness of dental sealant after 15 years. J Am Dent Assoc. 1991;122(10):34-42.

[58] Goršeta, Kristina; Škrinjarić, Tomislav; Glavina, Domagoj. The effect of heating and ultrasound on the shear bond strength of glass ionomer cement. // Collegium antropologicum. 36 (2012), 4; 1307-1312

[59] Uribe S. The effectiveness of fissure sealants. Evid Based Dent. 2004;5:92.

[60] Weerheijm KL, Kreulen CM, Gruythuysen RJM. Comparison of retentive qualities of two glass-ionomer cements used as fissure sealants. J Dent Child. 1996;63:265-7.

[61] Taifour D, Frencken JE, van't Hof MA, Beiruti N, Truin GJ. Effects of glass ionomer sealants in newly erupted first molars after 5 years: a pilot study. Community Dent Oral Epidemiol. 2003;31:314-9.

[62] Mejare I, Major IA. Glass ionomer and resin based fissure sealants: a clinical study. Scand J Dent Res. 1990;98:345-50.

[63] Ahovuo-Saloranta A, Hiri A, Nordblad A, Worthington H, Mäkelä M. Pit and fissure sealants for preventing dental decay in the permanent teeth of children and adolescents. Cohrane Database Syst Rev [serial on the internet]. 2004 [cited 2007 Apr 16]; Issue 3: CD001830.pub.2. DOI: 10.1002/14651858.CD00183.pub2. Available from: www.ncbi.nlm.mih.gov

[64] Hill RG, Wilson AD. Some structural aspects of glasses used in glass ionomer cements. Glass Technol. 1988;29:150-88.

[65] Pereira AC, Eggertsson H, Martinez-Mier EA, Mialhe FL, Eckert GJ, Zero DT. Validity of caries detection on occlusal surfaces and treatment decisions based on results from multiple caries-detection methods. Eur J Oral Sci 2009;117(1):51–7.

[66] Tranaeus S, Shi XQ, Angmar-Mansson B. Caries risk assessment: methods available to clinicians for caries detection. Community Dent Oral Epidemiol 2005;33(4):265–73.

[67] Zandona AF and Zero DT. Diagnostic tools for early caries detection. J Am Dent Assoc 2006;137(12):1675–84.

[68] Baelum V, Heidmann J, Nyvad B. Dental caries paradigms in diagnosis and diagnostic research. Eur J Oral Sci 2006;114(4):263–77.

[69] Beiruti N, Frencken JE, van't Hof MA, Taifour D, van Palenstein Helderman WH. Caries-preventive effect of a one-time application of composite resin and glass ionome-sealants after 5 years Caries Research 2006;40(1):52–9.

[70] McComb D, Tam LE. Diagnosis of occlusal caries: Part I. Conventional methods. Journal of Canadian Dental Association 2001;67(8):454–7.

[71] Bader JD, Shugars DA. A systematic review of the performance of a laser fluorescence device for detecting caries. Journal of the American Dental Association 2004;135 (10):1413–26.

[72] Lussi A, Hibst R, Paulus R. DIAGNOdent: an optical method for caries detection. Journal of Dental Research 2004;83(Spec Iss C):C80–3.

[73] Beauchamp J. CPW, Crall J.J., Donly K., Feigal R., Gooch B., Ismail A., Kohn W., Siegal M., Simonsen R. Evidence-based clinical recommendations for the use of pit-and-fissure sealants: A report of the American Dental Association Council on Scientific Affairs. JADA. 2008; 139

[74] Ekstrand KR, Martignon S, Ricketts DJN, Qvist V. Detection and activity assessment of primary coronal caries lesions: a methodologic study. Oper Dent 2007;32(3):225–35.

[75] Bader JD, Shugars DA, Bonito AJ. A systematic review of the performance of methods for identifying carious lesions. J Public Health Dent 2002;62(4):201–13.

[76] Ismail AI, Sohn W, Tellez M, Amaya A, Sen A, Hasson H, et al. The International Caries Detection and Assessment System (ICDAS): an integrated system for measuring dental caries. Community Dent Oral Epidemiol 2007;35(3):170–8.

[77] Raadal M, Espelid I, Mejare I. The caries lesion and its management in children and adolescents. In: Pediatric Dentistry: a clinical approach. Koch G, Poulsen S (eds). Copenhagen: Munksgaard; 2001. pp. 173-212.

[78] Harris NO, Garcia-Godoy F. Primary preventive dentistry. 5th edition. London: Asimon and Schuster Company; 1999.

[79] Goldstein RE, Parkins FM. Air-abrasive technology: its new role in restorative dentistry. JADA 1994;125:551-7.

[80] De Craene GP, Martens C, Dermaut R. The invasive pit and fissure sealing technique in pediatric dentistry: an SEM study of a preventive restoration. ASDC J Dent Child 1988;55(1):34-42.

[81] Waggoner WF, Siegal M. Pit and fissure sealant application: updating the technique. J Am Dent Assoc 1996 Mar;127(3):351-61, quiz 391-2.

[82] Shapira J, Eidelman E. Six-year clinical evaluation of fissure sealants placed after mechanical preparation: a matched pair study. Pediatr Dent 1986 Sep;8(3):204-5.

[83] Lygidakis NA, Oulis KI, Christodoulidis A. Evaluation of fissure sealants retention following four different isolation and surface preparation techniques: four years clinical trial. J Clin Pediatr Dent 1994 Fall;19(1):23-5.

[84] Blackwood JA, Dilley DC, Roberts MW, Swift EJ Jr. Evaluation of pumice, fissure enameloplasty and air abrasion on sealant microleakage. Pediatr Dent 2002 May-Jun; 24(3):199-203.

[85] Christensen GJ. Fluoride made it: why haven't sealants? JADA 1992;123(2):89-90.

[86] Donnan MF, Ball IA. A double-blind clinical trial to determine the importance of pumice prophylaxis on fissure sealant retention. Br Dent J 1988 Oct 22;165(8):283-6.

[87] Silverstone LM. State of the art on sealant research and priorities for further research. J Dent Educ 1984 Feb;48 (2 Suppl):10718.

[88] Cooper TM. Four-handed dentistry in the team practice of dentistry. Dent Clin North Am 1974;18(4):739-753.

[89] Robinson GE, Wuehrmann AH, Sinnett GM, McDevitt EJ. Fourhanded dentistry: the whys and wherefores. JADA 1968; 77(3):573-579.

[90] Wood AJ, Saravia ME, Farrington FH. Cotton roll isolation versus Vac-Ejector isolation. ASDC J Dent Child 1989;56:438-41.

[91] Manton DJ, Messer LB. Pit and fissure sealants: another major cornerstone in preventive dentistry. Aust Dent J 1995 Feb;40(1):22-9.

[92] Duggal MS, Tahmassebi JF, Toumba KJ, Mavromati C. The effect of different etching times on the retention of fissure sealants in second primary and first permanent molars. Int J Paediatr Dent 1997 Jun;7(2):81-6.

[93] Barroso JM, Lessa FC, Palma Dibb RG, Torres CP, Pecora J, Borsatto MC. Shear bond strength of pit and fissure sealants to saliva contaminated and non-contaminated enamel. J Dent Child 2005;72:95-9.

[94] Chosak A, Eidelman E. Effect of time from application until exposure to light on the tag lengths of a visible light-polymerized sealant. Dent Mater 1988;4:302-6.

[95] Dennison JB, Straffon LH, More FG.Evaluating tooth eruption on sealant efficacy. JADA 1990;121:610-4.

[96] Simonsen RJ, Stallard RE. Sealantrestorations utilizing a dilute filled composite resin: one year results. Quintessence Int 1977;23:307-315.

[97] Azhdari S, Sveen OB, Buonocore MG. Evaluation of a restorative preventive technique for localized occlusal caries. J Dent Res 1979;58(special issue A):330 Abstract 952.

[98] Walker JD, Jensen ME, Pickham JR. A clinical review of preventive resin restorations. ASDC J Dent Child 1990;57:257-259.

[99] Houpt M, Eidelman E, Shey Z, et al. Occlusal restoration using fissure sealant instead of 'extension for prevention', eighteen month results. J Dent Res 1982;61:214. Abstract 324.

[100] Gray G B. An evaluation of sealant restorations after 2 years. Br Dent J 1999;186:569-575.

[101] Walls AWG, Murray JJ, McCabe JF. The management of occlusal caries in permanent molars. A clinical trial comparing a minimal composite restoration with an occlusal amalgam restoration. Br Dent J 1988;164:288-292.

[102] Simonsen RJ, Jensen ME. Preventive resin restorations utilizing a diluted filled composite resins: 30 months results. J Dent Res 1979;58(special issue A):330(abstract No. 952).

[103] Raadal M. Follow-up study of sealing and filling with composite resins in the prevention of occlusal caries. Community Dent Oral Epidemiol 1978;6:176-180.

[104] Simonsen RJ. Preventive resin restorations. J Am Dent Assoc 1980;100:535-539.

[105] Houpt M, Eidelman E, Shey EZ. Occlusal restoration using fissure sealant instead of 'extension for prevention'. ASCD J Dent Child 1984;51:270-273.

[106] Houpt M, Eidelman E, Shey EZ. Occlusal composite restorations:4 year results. J Am Dent Assoc 1985;110:351-353.

[107] Welbury RR, Walls AGW, Murray JJ, McCabe JF. The management of occlusal caries in permanent molars. A 5-year clinical trial comparing a minimal composite with an amalgam restoration. Br Dent J 1990;169:361-366.

[108] Houpt M, Fuks A, Eidelman E. Composite/sealant restoration: 6.5 year results. Paed Dent 1988; 10: 304-306.

[109] Simonsen RJ, Landy NA. Preventive Resin Restorations: fracture resistance and 7-year clinical results. J Dent Res 1984; 63(special issue): 261(abstract No.175).

[110] Houpt M, Fuks A, Eidelman E. The preventive resin (composite resin/sealant) restoration:Nine-year results. Quintessence Int 1994;25:155-159.

[111] K. Gorseta, D. Glavina, A. Borzabadi-Farahani, R.N. Van Duinen, I. Skrinjaric, R.G. Hill and E. Lynch. One-Year Clinical Evaluation of a Glass Carbomer Fissure Sealant, a Preliminary Study European Journal of Prosthodontics and Restorative Dentistry. 22 (2014), 2; 67-71.

[112] Kervanto-Seppälä S, Lavonius E, Pietilä I, Pitkäniemi J, Meurman J, Kerosuo E. Comparing the caries-preventive effect of two fissure sealing modalities in public health care: a single application of glass ionomer and a routine resin-based sealant programme. A randomized split-mouth clinical trial. International Journal of Paediatric Dentistry 2008;18(1):56–61.

[113] Poulsen S, Beiruti N, Sadat N. A comparison of retention and the effect on caries of fissure sealing with a glassionomer and a resin-based sealant. Community Dentistry and Oral Epidemiology 2001;29(4):298–301.

[114] Rock WP, Foulkes EE, Perry H, Smith AJ. A comparative study of fluoride-releasing composite resin and glass ionomer materials used as fissure sealants. Journal of Dentistry 1996;24(4):275–80.

[115] Karlzén-Reuterving G, van Dijken JW. A three-year followup of glass ionomer cement and resin fissure sealants. Journal of Dentistry for Children 1995;62(2):108–10.

[116] Williams B, Laxton L, Holt RD, Winter GB. Fissure sealants: a 4-year clinical trial comparing an experimental glass polyalkenoate cement with a bis glycidyl methacrylate resin used as fissure sealants. British Dental Journal 1996; 180(3):104–8.

[117] Arrow P, Riordan PJ. Retention and caries preventive effects of a GIC and a resin-based fissure sealant. Community Dentistry and Oral Epidemiology 1995;23(5):282–5.

[118] Beiruti N, Frencken JE, van't Hof MA, Taifour D, van Palenstein Helderman WH. Caries-preventive effect of a one-time application of composite resin and glass ionome-sealants after 5 years. Caries Research 2006;40(1):52–9.

[119] McLean JW, Wilson AD. Fissure sealing and filling with an adhesive glass-ionomer cement. Br Dent J. 1974;136:269-76.

[120] De Witte AM, De Maeyer EA, Verbeeck RM. Surface roughening of glass ionomer cements by neutral NaF solutions. Biomater. 2003;24:1995-2000.

[121] Pardi V, Pereira AC, Ambrosano GMB, Meneghim MdeC. Clinical evaluation of three different materials used as pit and fissure sealant: 24-months results. Journal of Clinical Pediatric Dentistry 2005;29(2):133–8.

[122] Baseggio W, Naufel FS, Davidoff DC, Nahsan FP, Flury S, Rodrigues JA. Caries-preventive efficacy and retention of a resin-modified glass ionomer cement and a resin-based fissure sealant: a 3-year split-mouth randomised clinical trial. Oral Health & Preventive Dentistry 2010;8(3):261–8.

[123] Raadal M, Utkilen AB, Nilsen OL. Fissure sealing with light-cured resin-reinforced glass-ionomer cement (Vitrebond) compared with a resin sealant. International Journal of Paediatric Dentistry 1996;6(4):235–9.

[124] Griffin SO, Oong E, Kohn W, Vidakovic B, Gooch BF, CDC Dental Sealant Systematic Review Work Group, et al. The effectiveness of sealants in managing caries lesions. J Dent Res (2008). 87(2):169-74.

[125] Chen X, Du M, Fan M, Mulder J, Huysmans MC, Frencken JE. Effectiveness of two new types of sealants: retention after 2 years. Clinical Oral Investigations 2012;16(5): 1443–50.

[126] Barja-Fidalgo F, Maroun S, de Oliveira BH. Effectiveness of a glass ionomer cement used as a pit and fissure sealant in recently erupted permanent first molars. Journal of Dentistry for Children 2009;76(1):34–40.

[127] Liu BY, Lo ECM, Chu CH, Lin HC. Randomized trial on fluorides and sealants for fissure caries prevention. Journal of Dental Research 2012;91(8):753–8.

[128] Beiruti N, Frencken JE, van't Hof MA, Taifour D, van Palenstein Helderman WH. Caries-preventive effect of one-time application of composite resin and glass ionome-sealants after 5 years. Caries Research 2006;40(1):52–9.

[129] Antonson SA, Antonson DE, Brener S, Crutchfield J, Larumbe J, Michaud C, et al.Twenty-four month clinical evaluation of fissure sealants on partially erupted permanent first molars: glass ionomer versus resin-based sealant. Journal of the American Dental Association 2012;143(2): 115–22.

[130] Yilmaz Y, Beldüz N, Eyübo lu O. A two-year evaluation of four different fissure sealants. European Archives of Paediatric Dentistry: Official Journal of the European Academy of Paediatric Dentistry 2010;11(2):88–92.

[131] Yildiz E, Dörter C, Efes B, Koray F. A comparative study of two fissure sealants: a 2-year clinical follow-up. Journal of Oral Rehabilitation 2004;31(10):979–84.

[132] Yakut N, Sönmez H. Resin composite sealant vs. polyacidmodified resin composite applied to post eruptive mature and immature molars: two year clinical study. The Journal of Clinical Pediatric Dentistry 2006;30(3):215–8.

[133] Taifour D, Frencken JE, van't Hof MA, Beiruti N, Truin GJ. Effects of a glass ionomer sealant in newly erupted first molars after 5 years: a pilot study. Community Dentistry and Oral Epidemiology 2003;31(4):314–9.

Chapter 2

Early Childhood Caries (ECC) — Etiology, Clinical Consequences and Prevention

Agim Begzati, Merita Berisha, Shefqet Mrasori, Blerta Xhemajli-Latifi, Rina Prokshi, Fehim Haliti, Valmira Maxhuni, Vala Hysenaj-Hoxha and Vlera Halimi

Additional information is available at the end of the chapter

http://dx.doi.org/10.5772/59416

1. Introduction

Primary teeth are also known as milk or deciduous teeth. The 20 primary teeth start to appear in a baby's mouth around the sixth month and they stay in the mouth until they are gradually replaced by the permanent teeth between the ages of six to twelve years.

Primary teeth start to develop from the 6th to 7th week of fetal life from epithelial cells of the mouth that form the tooth buds. The cells of these initial tooth germs continue to differentiate during pregnancy, and, when the baby is born most teeth are already partially formed in the jaws.

The primary teeth play an important role in giving facial fullness and aesthetically pleasant facial shapes. Absence of teeth, due to any reason, not only hampers the masticatory activity of the individual, but also affect the facial features to great extent, affecting the concerned person physiologically, emotionally and socially.

Unfortunately, the primary teeth's function is disrupted when the demineralization process of hard tooth structures is involved – dental caries.

The oral health of children is especially aggravated with the occurrence of the so-called early childhood caries(ECC). ECC is an acute, rapidly developing dental disease occurring initially in the cervical third of the maxillary incisors, destroying the crown completely.

The presence of dental caries, especially of ECC, may reflect on the oral health status of children in countries with insufficient health system and inefficient primary dentistry. Early Childhood Caries (ECC) is a public health problem with biological, social and behavioral determinants.

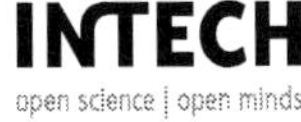

The preventive activities must start at an early age. Home-care methods are more than necessary.

1.1. Primary Teeth

The eruption of the primary teeth starts around the sixth month with the central incisors of the lower jaw and it is fully completed by the 3rd year of age with the appearance of the upper second molar. Normally, the first teeth that erupt are the two front teeth of the lower jaw (mandibular central incisors). After a few of months they are followed by the four front teeth of the upper jaw (maxillary central and lateral incisors). The last primary teeth that erupt are the upper second molars which are expected to appear around the age of 2½ years and not later than the completion of the 3rd year.

Teeth eruption is the process during which they move towards the surface of the jawbone and break through the gums, until they take their final position in the mouth with their crown fully visible. At this point the crown is completely formed, but the root of the tooth will continue to form for one more year.

The process of tooth eruption is usually accompanied with pain and discomfort for the baby. The associated symptoms such as drooling, disruptions in eating or sleeping patterns, irritability, swollen gums are referred as 'teething'.

When the primary dentition is completed, children have a set of 20 primary teeth, ten at every jaw. They belong to 3 different teeth types: 8 incisors, 4 canines, and 8 molars.

Eruption of the first permanent molar (age of 6 years), marks the end of the primary dentition period and the start of mixed dentition.

The anatomy and morphology of the primary teeth is also generally similar with that of permanent teeth. Externally the tooth is covered by a layer of enamel at the crown area and by cementum at the root area. Under the enamel there is a layer of dentine which surrounds the soft and alive dental pulp at the center of the tooth.

However some distinctive features of primary teeth are: smaller size, thinner and more translucent enamel, less mineralized enamel (which makes primary teeth more vulnerable to cavities, especially for early childhood caries), larger pulp chambers, narrower and smaller roots, etc.

1.2. Role/importance of the primary teeth

Parents commonly ask why they should worry about cavities in baby, since they will be replaced by the permanent teeth? The role of the primary teeth is just as important as the role of the permanent ones.

Humans use teeth to tear, grind, and chew food in the first step of digestion. Teeth also play a role in human speech. Additionally, teeth also provide structural support to muscles in the face and form the human smile and other facial expressions. So, broadly the main functions of the teeth can be summarized as follows: role in mastication (helps eating), aids in articulation and speech, role in aesthetics (gives shape and beauty to the face).

One of the main functions of teeth is the mastication of the food. The first step of digestion involves the mouth and teeth. Each type of tooth serves a different function in the chewing process. Depending on the shape, teeth enable cutting, grinding, chewing and preparing food for swallow and further digestion in the digestive tract. The Incisors cut foods when you bite into them. The sharper and longer canines tear food, while the wider molars grind the food.

Masticatory function, besides stimulating the development of the jaws, allows the child to learn the right way of eating. Toothache during mastication can affect the child's nutrition. According to some studies it has been found that children with more decayed teeth have less than 80% of average weight, which they are expected to have for their age (Acs et al 1999, Acs et al 1992). Children with toothache often after their recovery reach their normal weight and have tranquility during their sleep (Elice & Fields 1990).

The role of healthy primary teeth consists in clearly speaking and emphasizing the correct letters and sounds. The mouth, especially the teeth, lips, and tongue are essential for speech, one of the very important functions of teeth. The teeth, lips, and tongue are used to form words by controlling airflow through the mouth. Especially, the front teeth enable correct pronunciation of consonants: t, th, d, f, etc.

Primary teeth, among other roles, have one more extremely important role. As long as they are in the oral cavity, until their physiological loss, they will serve as space retention for permanent teeth. Their premature loss can be a cause of malocclusions in children. If we achieve to prevent their premature loss, malocclusion frequency will be reduced for 30%. Although early loss of primary incisors would not have a major consequence, a premature loss of primary molar and canine will be marked by a significant disorder in the development of occlusion during the eruption of the permanent teeth (Marković 1976).

Healthy teeth and full realization of their function, in fact, will allow a normal psycho-physical development of children, which for their age, is very important.

2. Dental caries — Definition, etiology and epidemiology

Dental caries is one of the most prevalent diseases in children worldwide. The Center for Disease Control and Prevention reports that dental caries is perhaps the most prevalent infectious diseases in children. Dental caries is five times more common than asthma and seven times more common than hay fever in children (US Department of Health and Human Services 2000).

Tooth decay is localized progressive disease, whose character consists in the destruction of tooth structures mainly under the influence of metabolic products of the oral microflora.

Dental caries is pathological destruction of tooth hard tissue with progressive effluence. Initially it appears in enamel, the dentin is involved after that, and later the pulp and the periodontium, with the possibility of complications that will affect the general health. The consequences of caries may be numerous, ranging from the morphological changes to functional ones, e.g. complete crown destruction (early childhood caries), chewing difficulties, speech impediments, digestive tract disorders, odentogenic focal points (Raiç 1985, Stosic 1991).

Dental caries usually begins as small, shallow holes; if left untreated, these holes can become larger and deeper and potentially lead to tooth destruction or loss. Complications of dental caries include: pain, dental abscess, difficulties during chewing, tooth damage or loss, tooth sensitivity.

There are numerous definitions on caries, depending on what is taken in consideration: etiology, pathogenesis, clinical features.

Dental caries may be defined as a bacterial disease of the hard tissues of the teeth characterized by demineralization of the inorganic and destruction of the organic substance of tooth (Soames & Southam 1999).

According to Douglas, dental caries is the most common chronic infectious disease of childhood, caused by the interaction of bacteria, mainly *Streptococcus mutans*, and sugary foods on tooth enamel. *S. mutans* breaks down sugars for energy, causing an acidic environment in the mouth and result in demineralization of the enamel of the teeth and dental caries (Douglass et al. 2004).

Since *S. mutans* is transmitted to the child, another definition is based in the transmissibility. Dental caries is defined as a transmissible localized infection caused by a multi-factorial etiology. In order for dental caries to develop, four interrelated factors must occur: the patient (host), substrate (carbohydrates), dental plaque (*S. mutans*), and the time factor.

2.1. Etiology

Dental caries is a disease that is not caused by one factor. If only one factor would cause this disease, its prevention would have been much easier and more controllable. Many studies like clinical studies, but mostly longitudinal epidemiological studies, show convincing evidence for a multi-factorial nature of this disease. Numerous factors affecting the appearance of caries act team-wise and not separately, make caries pathogenesis very complex but also hinder the possibility to undertake effective preventive measures.

There are several important factors that make up the dental caries etiological circle. Host respectively tooth, dental plaque respectively bacteria, and substrate respectively saliva carbohydrates, all in co-operation with the time factor, are vicious chain of dental caries development.

The hard tooth structure, the enamel, is the forefront part that undergoes the demineralization process, respectively caries. The development of caries in enamel surface as much as it is affected by the internal structure of the hard tissue build of the tooth, equally, perhaps even more it depends on the strength of external factors affect.

Sometimes for various reasons: local, general or even hereditary, tooth structure can be so poorly mineralized, that it would need a very small amount of external factors to cause dental caries.

The general opinion regarding the etiology of dental caries nowadays is that it is a very complex multifactorial disease, presented with high prevalence in all age groups. It has already been established that dental caries is a chronic infectious process with a multifactorial etiology. Dietary factors, oral microorganisms that can produce acids from sugars, and host susceptibility all need to coexist for caries to develop (Konig & Navia 1995).

There are some important factors that comprise the etiological circles of the dental caries: host or the tooth, dental or bacterial plaque, substrate – carbohydrates and saliva, and altogether co-react with the time factor. The hard dental structures, initially the enamel, undergo the demineralization process, respectively the caries. The caries development in the enamel surface is equally dependent from the inner hard dental structure and from the intensity of the extrinsic factors' action.

The newest concept in dentistry explains the cause of dental caries as a consequence of disruption of "Caries Balance" (Featherstone 2004) Dr. John Featherstone introduced the concept of the Caries Balance in 2002. The theory of "Caries Balance" defines dental caries as a disease of hard dental tissues, and the destruction of the enamel surface as a result of the disruption of the balance of demineralization and remineralization.

This misbalance may be manifested in the beginning of demineralization or during the process of remineralization. The defect in the enamel surface is a result of the domination of the demineralization process and such process has progressive course directed towards pulpar space. Which process will dominate depends on the proportions of the factors that constitute "Caries Balance", i.e. protective and pathological factors.

The balance disorder will be manifested with early demineralization process or eventually with remineralization process. This concept is that dental caries can be viewed as a balance of healthy or protective factors (factor of remineralization), and disease or pathogenic factors (factor of demineralization). Cavities are caused by an imbalance between risk factors for the disease and protective factors.

Pathological factors (risk factors) are: acid-producing bacteria, frequent eating/drinking of fermentable carbohydrates, sub-normal saliva flow and "function".

Protective factors are: saliva flow and its components; fluoride, calcium, phosphate remineralization; antibacterials (chlorhexidine, xylitol), etc.

The level of risk for dental caries depends on the domination of the certain group of factors that participate in the "Caries Balance". If there is domination of the pathological factors, the risk for dental caries will be higher and the treatment needs will require larger restorative interventions, as well as other consequences. If there is a domination of protective factors, then the invasive restorative dentistry will have fewer burdens, and concentrate in minimal restorations of superficial caries. Biological factors tend to be similar within all cultures and populations, although habit/environmental factors tend to be influenced specifically by the culture in place.

2.2. The prevalence of dental caries

It has already been mentioned that dental caries is the mostly spread disease in the world. Dental caries is a disease that affects all age groups, most commonly children.

Epidemiological data derived from the Oral Health Promotion Group of Kosovo showed a high prevalence of caries among children in Kosovo (89.2% among preschool children and 94.4% among school children). The mean dmft/DMFT index was 5.6 for preschool children and 4.9 for all school children (Begzati et al. 2011).

The results from the same previous study show that dental health of these children in Kosovo is worse than that of children in other European countries. Specifically, the mean dmft of five-year-olds at preschools in Kosovo (8.1) was found to be higher than the same value of preschool children in USA (1.7) and in many other European countries (1991-1995), including Ireland (0.9), Spain (1.0), Denmark (1.3), Norway (1.4), Finland (1.4), Netherlands (1.7), United Kingdom (2.0), France (2.5), and Germany (2.5). Our results are only comparable to the rates in Belarus (7.4), Sarajevo, Bosnia (7.53) (ages 5-7) and Albania (8.5), (Marthaler 1996, Kobaslia 2000). The low treatment rate of children in Kosovo (<2%) indicates a high treatment need. Also, the mean DMFT (5.8) of school children in Kosovo (age 12) was higher in comparison with school children (age 12) of the following developed countries: Netherlands (1.1), Finland (1.2), Denmark (1.3), USA (1.4), United Kingdom (1.4), Sweden (1.5), Norway (2.1), Ireland (2.1), Germany (2.6) and Croatia (2.6) (16). The mean DMFT of Kosovo's children (age 12) was similar to the mean values in Latvia (7.7), Poland (5.1) and a group of 12- to 14-year-olds in Sarajevo, Bosnia (7.18), (Marthaler 1996, Kobaslia 2000).

3. Early Childhood Caries (ECC)-definition

ECC is an acute, rapidly developing dental disease occurring initially in the cervical third of the maxillary incisors, destroying the crown completely. Early onset and rampant clinical progression makes ECC a serious public health problem. Due to varying clinical, etiological,

localization, and course features, this pathology is found under different names such as labial caries (LC), caries of incisors, nursing bottle mouth, rampant caries (RC), nursing bottle caries (NBC), nursing caries, baby bottle tooth decay (BBTD), early childhood caries (ECC), rampant early childhood dental decay, and severe early childhood caries (SECC) (James 1957, Goose 1967, Fass 1962, Winter et al.1966, Derkson & Ponti 1982, Ripa 1988, Arkin 1986, Bruered et al. 1989, Kaste & Gift 1995, Tinanoff et al. 1998, Horowitz 1998, Drury et al. 1999).

According to Davis, the definition of this pathology has always been complex and "difficult to be described, but when it is seen, you know what it's about" (Davis 1998).

In 1862, an American physician, Abraham Jacobi (Jacobi 1862) was the first to describe the clinical appearance of early childhood caries, which he observed in one of his own patients. Whereas, in 1932 Beltrami described this form of caries, as "Les dentes noires des tout petits" (black teeth in small children), (Beltrami 1952). Author Fass, created the term *nursing bottle mouth* (Fass 1962).

The literature contains a variety of other terms used to describe early childhood caries and its diagnostic criteria. Most of them relate to the use of a feeding bottle or prolonged breastfeeding (feeding bottle tooth decay, feeding bottle syndrome, nursing caries, nursing bottle mouth, and so on). The authors wish to highlight the danger of excessive drinking from a baby bottle, if it contains sweetened liquids, or prolonged on-demand breastfeeding (Schroth et al. 2007).

To inform the scientific community with internationally comparable data on the incidence of early childhood caries, delegates to a conference at the Centers for Disease Control and Prevention, invented the term *early childhood caries* in order to better the multi-factorial pathogenesis of the disease" (Kaste & Gift 1995).

Unfortunately, this term was seen to have its limitations. Three years later, a further conference on early childhood caries, organized by the National Health Institute (USA), added two further definitions/descriptions, which were *rampant infant caries* and *early childhood dental decay* (RIE, CDD), (Quartey & Williamson 1998). These differences in definition were due above all to diversity in diagnostic criteria.

3.1. Clinical diagnostic criteria of Early Childhood Caries (ECC)

Due to the early appearance, typical localization, rapid destruction of the hard tissue of tooth, early childhood caries is a specific form of primary tooth decay. Childhood caries appears in caries resistant regions, such as: labial surfaces of the upper incisors, in the upper and lower molars, more rarely in the upper canine, and even less or not at all in the lower canine and incisors. In addition, during bottle-feeding with sugar-containing drinks, the upper incisors bathe in these sugar-containing drinks but the saliva from minor salivary glands in the area of these teeth has only limited remineralising properties, whereas the lower incisors remain largely protected by the tongue during bottle-feeding.

Different authors propose different criteria to define or describe the early childhood caries. Author Amidi, studying the publications about ECC, has concluded that: in 27 publications, the criteria for defining ECC was the presence of labial surface caries in at least one frontal maxillary tooth, in 23 studies at least two frontal maxillary teeth while in 9 studies three frontal maxillary teeth (Soames & Southam 1999).

Below are some criteria's for defining early childhood caries from various researchers cited by authors Amid & Woosung 1999:

- involvement of one or more maxillary incisors, without the involvement of mandibular incisors- author Sewint;

- a white or black spot in the labial surface of the maxillary frontal teeth- author Bennitz;

- one or more carious lesions in maxillary incisors, along gingival margin- author Ayhan;

- carious lesions in labial-buccal surfaces at one or more maxillar incisors- author Ramos;

- two or more maxillar incisors- author Harrison.

In the literature we still can find some criteria's, for example:

- one or more frontal maxillary teeth that has evidence that the child was fed with a bottle (Al-Dashti 1995);

- maxillar incisors and the mesial surface of canine (O'Sallivan 1993);

- at least one carious maxillary incisor with the involvement of labial and proximal surface or only proximale surface (Kaste et al. 1996);

- one or more maxillary incisor with cervical crown caries (Lopez 1998).

Author Wynne 1999, classifies early childhood caries into three types:

Type I (moderately easy) - usually involves two upper central incisors.

Type II (moderate, severe) - includes incisors, first molar, canine, and does not include the lower incisors.

Type III (widespread, severe) - including the mandibular incisors.

3.2. ECC — Prevalence

Prevalence of ECC is different and it largely depends on the criteria set by the researcher and the place where the examination takes place. There are differences between the data for urban or rural places, rich or poor places, "flourished" or "non-flourished" places. Furthermore, the prevalence of ECC varies in different countries, which may depend on the diagnostic criteria. While in some developed countries having advanced programs for oral health protection, the prevalence of ECC is around 5% (Derkson & Ponti 1982, Ripa 1988, Kaste et al. 1996, Davenport 1990, Hinds & Gregory 1995). In some countries of Southeastern Europe (neighboring countries of Kosovo) this prevalence reaches 20% (Bosnia) and 14% (Macedonia) (Huseinbegović 2001, Apostolova et al. 2003). Much higher ECC prevalence has been reported for such places as Quchan, Iran (59%) (Mazhari et al. 2007) and Alaska (66.8%) (Kelly & Bruerd 1987). At American Indian children the preva-lence is 41.8% (Kelly & Bruerd 1987). Similarly, in North American populations, the prevalence at high-risk children ranges from 11% to 72% (Berkowitz 2003).

Data from relevant literature show different prevalence in different countries, cited by various authors (Berkowitz et al. 1993, McDonald 2000, Wendet 1995, Begzati et al. 2011, Barbakov et al. 1985, Harris & Garsia 1999, Huseinbegović 2001, Holt et al. 1996, Kaste 1991, Pettit et al. 2001, Bruered et al.1989, Reisine 1998, Wyne 1999, Apostolova 2003).

3.3. Etiology

Dental caries is an infectious and transmissible disease. Therefore, early childhood caries is an extremely aggressive form of the disease.

It was suggested that from the biological determinants, the three key causal factors for dental caries were: microorganisms, substrate, and host (Keyes 1962).

However, in the etiology of early childhood caries very special role given to dental plaque, respectively cariogenic bacteria. Of the great interest in the cariogenesis process are only two

Place (year)	Author	Age	Prevalence
England(1989)	Silver	3 years	4%
Sweden1991)	Wendet	12-14 months	4.7%
Finland (1993)	Paunio	3 years	6%
Irak (1990)	Yagoot	1-5 years	15.6%
Kosova (2011)	Begzati	2-6 y.	17.5%
Indonesia (1979)	Aldy, Siregar	Up to 5 years	48%
Bosnia (2001)	Huseinbegović	5 y.	29%
Nigeria (1985)	Salako	3-7 y.	38.4%
Canada (1987)	Budowski	1-5 y.	7.4%
USA (1976)	Kaste	One years	0.8-2%
USA(1991)	Kaste	5 y.	5%
USA (1991)	Kamp	4 y.	5.3%
USA (1987)	Brured	3-5y.,native Indians Amer., and Alaska's population,	41.8-66.8%
USA (1992)	Weinstetin,	Mexican American, 8-47 m.	29.6%
Italia (2002)	Petti, Iannazzo	3-5 y.	7.6%
Macedonia (2003)	Apostolova	3 y.	13.3%
Australia (1998)	Reisine	Aborigin children	50%
Saudi Arabia	Wynne	Preschool children	15%
Kuwait (1986)	Soparkar	4-5 y.	11.5%

bacterial genera: mutant streptococci and lactobacills (Norman & Franklin 1999). A very important role is attributed to the bacterium Streptococcus mutans-called "the window of infection" (Caufield et al. 1993), in that it is responsible for the primary oral infection in the first phase of ECC (Berkowitz 1980; Berkowitz et al. 1996).

The most important requirement is an early infection, usually with the mother's cariogenic bacteria, for example, between the age of 19-31 months. However, earlier and later infection is a possibility (Caufield et al. 1993, Wan 2001).

After transmission of cariogenic bacteria and a frequent supply of substrate (sucrose) to the plaque, usually given as a sugary drink (juices and so on from a feeding bottle) or in older children, in snacks in the form of solid-cariogenic foods such as sweets, chocolates, cakes, biscuits, the development of early childhood caries occurs. If this loading of the plaque with sugars occurs at bedtime (night) and there is no tooth brushing, caries can progress rapidly.

In addition to the other severe types of early childhood caries, feeding on demand with cariogenic food and liquids is regarded as a co-factor for early childhood caries (Wendt & Birkhed 1995). As mentioned earlier, many social and behavioral determinants are risk factors for early childhood caries.

Favoring risk factors are as follows: low socio-economic status, low educational attainment in parents, chronic non-communicable diseases, inadequate health literacy, are all risk factors for a early childhood caries. Social and behavioral factors have been described in association with early childhood caries in numerous publications (FDI 1988, Horowitz 1998, Reisine & Douglass 1998, Seow 1998).

3.3.1. Cariogenic bacteria

In one of our studies conducted in the clinic of Paediatric Dentistry, it was found that S.mutans had a crucial role in ECC. The prevalence of S.mutans at our children was around 90% (Begzati et al. 2014). These facultative anaerobes are commonly found in the human oral cavity, and are a major contributor of tooth decay. The result of decay can greatly affect the overall health of the individual (Whiley & Beighton 2013).

The mutans streptococci and some Lactobacillus species are the two groups of infectious agents most strongly associated with dental caries. Earlier clinical studies reported that MS could not be detected in the mouths of normal predentate infants (Berkowitz et al. 1975, Berkowitz et al. 1980, Stiles et al. 1976, Catalanotto et al. 1975, Caufield et al. 1993, Karn et al 1998).

More recent clinical investigations have demonstrated that MS can colonize in the mouths of predentate infants (Tanner et al. 2002; Wan et al. 2001).

According to Berkowitz transmission of S.mutans happens in two ways: vertical and horizontal transmission. Vertical transmission is the transmission of microbes from caregiver to child. The major reservoir from which infants acquire S.mutans is their mothers. A study conducted by Berkowitz and co-authors reported that, when mothers harbored greater than 10^5 colony forming units (cfu) of MS per mL of saliva, the frequency of infant infection was 58%. When mothers harbored 10^3 cfu of MS per mL of saliva or more, however, the frequency of infant infection was 9 times less (6%) (Berkowitz et al 1981). These data clearly demonstrate that mothers with dense salivary reservoirs of MS are at high risk for infecting their infants early in life.

Vertical transmission is not the only vector by which MS are perpetuated in human populations.

Horizontal transmission also occurs. Horizontal transmission is the transmission of microbes between members of a group (eg, family members of a similar age or students in a classroom). Based on appearance, ways of transmission and prevention, Berkowitz concludes that: primary oral infection by mutans streptococci (MS) may occur in predentate infants. Infants may acquire MS via vertical and horizontal transmission. Improvements in the prevention of dental caries may likely be realized through intervention strategies that focus on the natural history of this infectious disease.

Streptococcus mutans (SM)

Streptococcus mutans are gram-positive cocci shaped bacteria. SM is isolated from all tissues of the oral cavity and constitutes the largest number of inhabitants of the oral microflora. This bacteria belongs to the Viridans group of streptococci (Galdvin 2004). Traditionally oral streptococci are differentiated on the basis of simple biochemical and physiological tests. Many recent studies comparing homologous DNA, gave description of the whole protein content and detection of glicosidasis activity clarifying the relationship between many species.

Mutant streptococci represent a group of bacterial species that had previously been classified as serotypes of the same species. These bacteria are characterized by their ability to ferment manitol and sorbitol, producing extracellular glicanes from sucrose with cariogenic activity in animal models. Important for the human population are two species: S. mutans and S. sobrinus. Streptococcus mutans has got this name in 1924 when Clarke in England isolated the micro-organisms from human carious lesions. He noted that they are more oval shaped, not round and assumed that they are mutants of streptococcus.

Mutant streptococci, are now considered as the main pathogenic species involved in the caries process. It is noted that if they are seeded in the mouth of animals, including rats, rodents and monkeys, are able to cause caries. Some detailed studies have shown a correlation between the presence of S.mutans and caries. These findings are repeated in longitudinal studies of microbiology and caries incidence. Mutant streptococci are usually found in relatively large numbers in plaque formed immediately after the development of lesions at the superficial soft surfaces. During a longitudinal study samples are taken periodically for analysis of separate parts for S.mutans and teeth were examined simultaneously. Teeth destined to become decayed, showed a significant increase of the ratio of S.mutans 6 to 24 months before the eventual diagnosis of caries. In similar conditions SM isolated from dental plaque terrains on stained white lesions are characterized by a ratio greater than plaque by SM while probing enamel grounds. The increased number of SM in saliva has also gone hand in hand with the development of lesions in smooth surface. In another study of saliva analysis of 200 children showed that 93 percent of them were positive for caries evident S. mutant, while uninfected children were almost always unaffected by decay (Russell 2003).

S. mutans position as the primary agent of caries formation in favor of their certain physiological characteristics. These features include the ability to adhere in tooth surface, producing insoluble polysaccharides from sucrose, rapidly producing lactic acid substrates by a number of sugars, acid tolerance and formation of intracellular stores of polysaccharides. These features help cariogenic SM survival in an environment not suitable in terms of so-called "feast or famine" cycles or due to the low concentration of substrate (i.e between meals) or excess substrate concentrations (e.g during consumption of food rich in sugar). As a general rule, cariogenic bacteria metabolize sugars to produce energy they need for growth and multiplication. The products of this metabolism are acids, which are derived from bacteria in plaque fluid. Damage caused by S.mutans is mainly due to lactic acid, although other acids such as butyric and propionic was found within the plaque. Generally, S.mutans is the most common streptococcal mutant infectious agent in humans and strong evidences are presented as the most virulent cause of odontogenic infections. Another mutans bacteria from the group of so-called S.sobrinus, differs from S.mutans because they require sucrose for adherence and growth in the dental plaque.

Correlation between caries and S. mutans, based on the data described in the literature and based on experimental models that are performed, and based on certain conclusions (Russell 2003):

- Animal experiments: S. mutans causes caries among gnatobiotik animals in the presence of sugar;

- Virulence: S. mutans has properties that contribute to caries development. These properties are acidogenety, uric acid production, extarcelular production of glicanes and intracellular storage of polysaccharides;

- Cross-sectional studies in humans: an increase in the number of S. mutans found in the initial carious lesions;

- Longitudinal studies in humans: a large number of S. mutans in a number of tooth decays correlates with subsequent caries;

- Streptococci other "non mutans" with similar properties can also be cariogenic.

S.mutans, sugar and caries

Taking large amounts of sugar combined with low values of pH frequently leads to an increased number of S. mutans.These bacteria are characterized by these features:

- Capacity to adhere to tooth structure

- Sugar Transportation system

- Production of lactic acid from sugars

- Production of intra and extracellular polysaccharide

- Tolerance in acidic environment

S. mutans sugar transportation

S. mutans is equipped with a conveyor system more efficient to carry sugars within their cells. During the metabolic process in the cell, they produce different substances, which contribute sufficiently to their pathogenicity. When it received the greatest amount of sugars S. mutans produce mainly Lactic Acid (Hamada and Slade, 1980). Streptococcus mutans produces extracellular and intracellular polysaccharides. Extracellular polysaccharides are also produced during the enzymatic reactions. Their sticky properties are favorable for bacterial adherence capabilities on the surface of the teeth, helping their placement on smooth surfaces (Koga 1986, Loesch 1986).

Polysaccharides also help connectivity and multiplication of dental plaque. Moreover, their insolubility prevents natural protective effect of saliva. Polysaccharides ensure the survival of intracellular bacteria in nutritionally poor intervals, and are used by bacteria to produce acids (Hamada and Slade 1980).

S. mutans, tolerance to acidic environment

Bacteria multiply under certain environmental conditions and they have obvious advantages compared with other micro-organisms. Diet and lack of suppressive factors determine the composition of the oral flora.

The decrease in pH prevents many bacteria from growth, while streptococci are multiplying in this particular environment (Harper & Loesch 1984). Changes in bacterial flora are in favor of bacteria which can survive in acidic conditions on account of acid no-tolerant microorganisms and acidic production. Pathogenic micro-organisms produce acid, the pH of which is lower enough than the value below which the tooth enamel begins to melt. S. mutans is recognized as the initiator of caries. They affect the initiation of the process leading to loss of minerals, and this facilitates the bacteria to penetrate the tooth structure (Burne 1998).

3.3.2. Substrate (Carbohydrates)

The human body uses glucose as substrate food, while other carbohydrates under the action of relevant enzymes converted into glucose. Cariotic action of sugars depends on their fermenting potential, respectively as far as the highest level of acids produced by the their fermentation. It was found that carbohydrates are the major class fermentabile affecting ecological changes in the mouth. While carbohydrates are transformed into acids, sucrose under the action of bacterial enzymes (glykosiltransferasa-GTF, and fruktosyltransferasa-FTF) turns into two classes polymers (glukan and fruktan).

Glukan plays the role of infectious matter to the surface of the tooth, not dissolved in water. This attribute enables attachment of dental plaque and S.mutans for tooth surface. Levan under the influence of enzymes derived from S. mutans fermented in the acidic product (Pincaham 1994).

Dairy products (milk, cheese) has an influence in the ecology of the area of the mouth. Dairy products can protect teeth from decay. This can happen as a result of buffer capacity of milk proteins or because of decarboxylation of amino acids after proteolysis some bacteria can metabolise kazein. Milk protein (casein) and its derivatives can be absorbed on the surface of the tooth, modify the structure of pelicula which make it unsuitable for adhesion of S. mutans, but also enable establishing of calcium phosphate and initiate the process of remineralisation.

Some sugar substitutes that do not turn into acid, as xilitoli for example you add sweets, have a role in inhibiting the development of S. Mutans (Pincaham 1994, Marsh 2000).

Correlation between SM and consumption of sugars

Studies on the correlation between presence of SM in saliva and sweet diet is not entirely clear, even data from the literature are sometimes contradictory. While some studies such as those of Polish authors has shown that children with a SM presence is 94% while 56% LB and daily frequency of sweets consumption exceeds 5 times a day (Wierzbicka, 1987). But, so it does not happen with children in Mozambique where annual consumption of sugar for school children is very low (11 kg), while the presence of SM is 98%, 40% of their high value. Sudan is also similar in that although annual consumption is about 18 kg, SM was identified in 90%, moderate values and higher than 50% (Carlsson 1989).

4. Study report

In our previous study (Begzati et al. 2010), the prevalence of ECC and various caries risk factors such as quantity of cariogenic S mutans colonies, was evaluated.

Methods

In the study there were included 1,008 children of both sexes, from 1 to 6 years of age, from 9 kindergartens of Prishtina, capital city of Kosovo. The sample was random, representing 80% of all kindergarten children. The sample size was calculated with a confidence level of 95% and a confidence interval of 2.

Bacterial sampling — Determination of S.mutans

In our study the presence of S mutans was determined using the CRT bacteria test (Ivoclar Vivadent, Liechtenstein) on the saliva previously stimulated by chewing paraffin. Bacterial counts were recorded as colony-forming units per milliliter (CFU/mL) of saliva. The number of bacterial colonies was graded as follows: Class 0 and Class 1 (CFU < 105/mL saliva), and Class 2 and Class 3 (CFU ≥ 105/mL saliva), according to the manufacturers' scoring-card (Ivoclar-Vivadent, Lichtenstein). In younger subjects, with less saliva collected, the modified spatula method was used.

Dental examination and diagnostic criteria

The children were examined in well-lit premises, using a flashlight as the light source, and a dental mirror and dental probe. Diagnostic criteria were calibrated (Hunt 1986), with inter-examiner reliability resulting in kappa = 0.91, based on the examination of 35 children of different ages. Dental caries was scored as the number of decayed, missing, or filled primary teeth (dmft).

ECC was defined as "initial occurrence of caries in cervical region of at least two maxillary incisors." Using a careful lift-the-lip examination, the presence or absence of ECC was recorded depending on the presence of "noncavity caries/white spot lesions" or "cavity caries."

In order to study the clinical and etiological aspects of ECC, a sub-sample of children with ECC was included for further analysis. The latter part of the examination, which included the clinical study of ECC development (according to ECC stages), determination of bacterial colony sampling, oral hygiene index (OHI), and filling out of the questionnaire, was conducted in the Pediatric Dentistry Clinic of the School of Dentistry.Children with ECC were examined using the light of the dental unit, with dental mirror and probe.

Clinical course of ECC

In order to explain the clinical course of ECC, we propose the following stages in the occurrence and progression of carious lesions in ECC: ECCi (initial stage), ECCc (circular stage), ECC_d (destructive stage) and ECC_r (*radix relicta* stage).

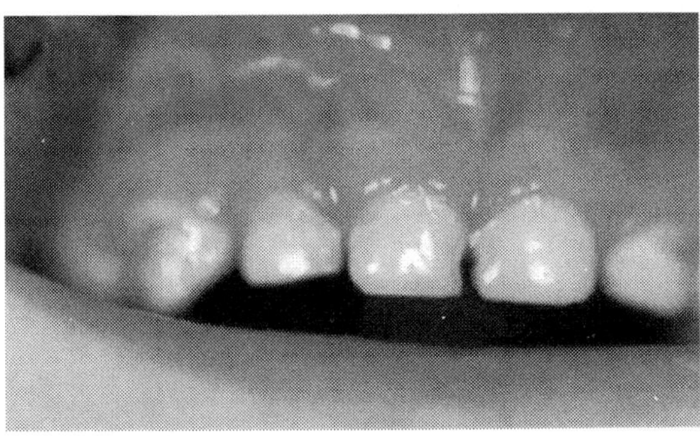

Figure 1. ECCi (initial stage) — white spot lesion or initial defect in enamel of cervix.

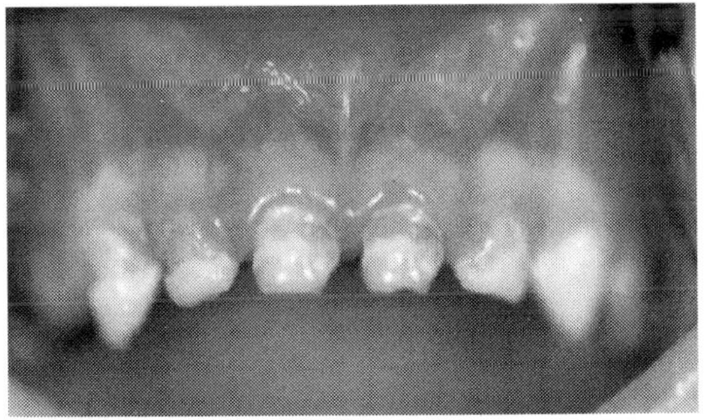

Figure 2. ECCc (circular stage) — lesion in the dentin and circular distribution of this lesion proximally.

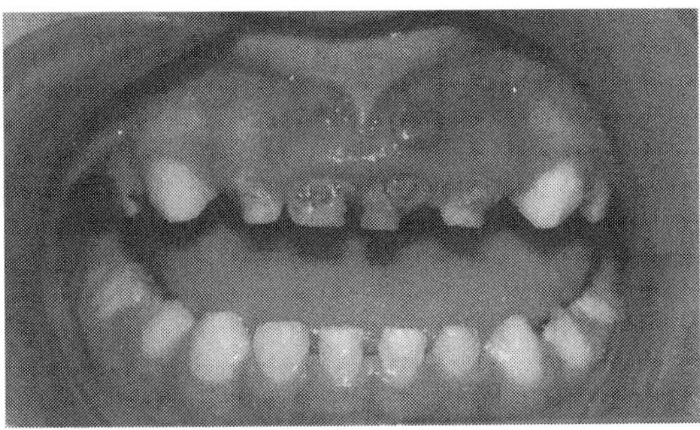

Figure 3. ECC$_d$ (destructive stage) — destruction of more than half the crown without affecting the incisal edge.

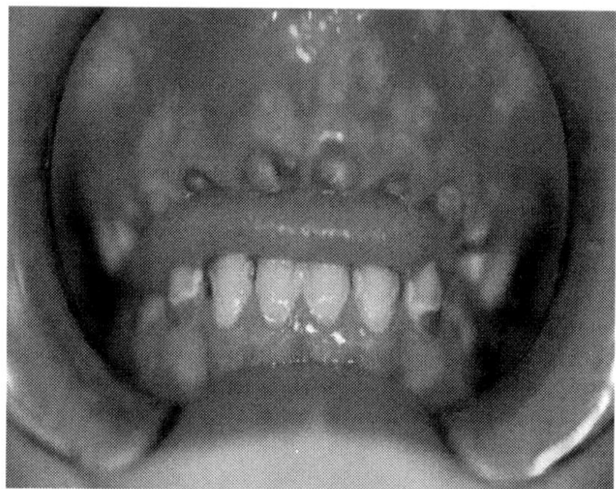

Figure 4. ECC$_r$ (*radix relicta* stage)—total destruction of the crown.

Results of study

From the total 1,008 examined children aged 1-6 years, the caries prevalence expressed in terms of the caries index per person, or dmft > 0, was 86.31%, with a mean dmft of 5.8. The prevalence of ECC was 17.36%, or 175 out of 1,008 examined children (Figure 1). The sub-sample of children with diagnosed ECC consisted of 150 children out of 175 invited for further analysis. Twentyfive children of this group from different kindergartens didn't show up in the Department. The mean age of children with ECC was 3.8 ± 1.2 years. The mean dmft in children with ECC was 11 ± 3.6. There was no statistical difference of ECC prevalence between genders (t test = 1.81, P = 0.07).

As expected, the lowest mean dmft score was found at age 2 (6.47 ± 2.13), with an age-related increase in dmft of 12.8 at age 6 (Table 1). In comparing the mean dmft in ECC children with respect to age, there was a significant statistical difference between age 2 and ages 4, 5, and 6. (One-Way ANOVA test F = 16, P < 0.001).

ECC stages

The ECC stages were not equally distributed. The most common stage present was that of radix relicta (41.7%), while the stage appearing least frequently was the initial stage (15.4%), or 27 out of 150 children with ECC.

There was a significant difference between the stages of ECC (c2 = 211.1, P < 0.0001). Twenty-five of the 27 children with ECC in the initial stage were reexamined 1 year after the baseline examination (2 children did not appear for reexamination dueto address change). The 1-year reexamination showed that the initial stage had advanced to the circular stage in 28% of cases, destructive stage in 20%, radix relicta stage in 36%, and having been extracted due to ECC in 16% of cases (Table 2). Mean age of subjects with initial stage of ECC was 2 ± 0.7. Mean dmft on reexamination showed an increase from 5.1 to 8.8 (P < 0.001).

4.1. Clinical specificities and progress

Even before the child is 2 years, in the gingival third of the labial surface of the upper front teeth, as a result of the enamel decalcification process a chalk colored stain ("white spot lesions") appears, which expands in the enamel of the cervical region of the tooth and for a short time it covers the entire tooth, destroying the whole hard tooth tissue. During this process, initially the enamel on the incisal region of the frontal tooth is resistant, especially canine, that shows that those parts of tooth enamel which are mineralized before birth, are more resistant to caries than the parts that are mineralized after birth (Thomas et al. 1999).

In the initial stage(Fig.1) there is a small loss of minerals from the hydroxylapatite crystals of enamel. As a result of tooth's hard tissue demineralization micropores start forming, which refract the light, and as a result it comes to the formation of so-called *white spots lesions*. Such spots are localized where the concentration of dental plaque is higher. If the destruction continues as a result of the demineralization effect of acids on enamel and apatite removal, the cavity starts to form. (Reisine & Douglass 1998).

This quick progress, helps the caries to quickly affect even the dentin layer, so for a short time the entire tooth crown is destroyed and all that remain are the roots (radix relicta)(Fig.4). Often it happens in 3 year old children, in the upper frontal region, where they have only roots remaining that resemble stumps.

Iritative formation of dentin, which makes the carious lesion get a brown color is a result of permanent irritation in the revealed dentin, while sclerotic tissue can make a full obliteration of tooth canal. The formation of iritative – sclerotic dentin can have an effect in this disease without symptoms, but with difficulties in feeding, speech and aesthetics. Also as a result of reflexive reaction (gums, tongue, lips injury etc.), a number of general symptoms is provoked such as digestive disorders, raised body temperature, increased saliva production, etc. The dental pain starts when the tooth pulp is revealed, in gangrenous teeth or when the infectious pathological process appears in periodoncium.

4.2. Complications and consequences

Early crown destruction – root remaining (radix relicta)

Sometimes, in the upper fornix we can see several changes that, in a quick glance, can lead us to the wrong diagnosis. Since the permanent teeth have palatine position, during their eruption process they put internal pressure in the apical part of the deciduous teeth, so that the deciduous tooth root tip can penetrate the bone and mucosa and erupt in the upper level of vestibular fornix (Fig.5). The erupted roots can make deep and painful decubitus at the upper lip (Fig. 8)

If in the root canal a purulent or gangrenous inflammatory process is present, then in the upper fornix we may encounter isolated purulent process (encapsulated) - abscess. (Fig. 6)

Extension of the inflammatory process - sometimes purulent inflammatory process involves gingiva, on all remaining roots, where the clinical symptoms become much more difficult.

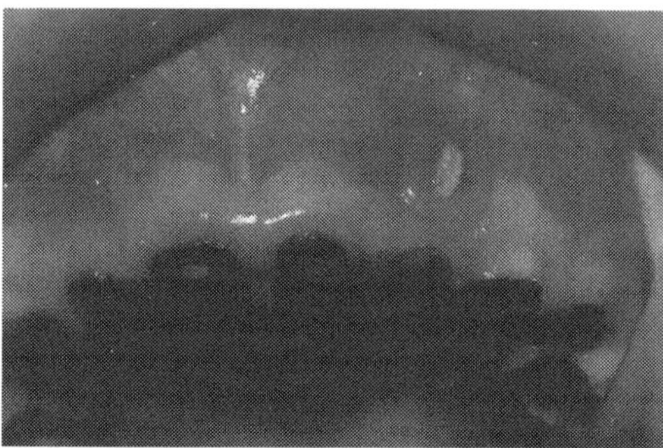

Figure 5. Radix relicta and bone penetration

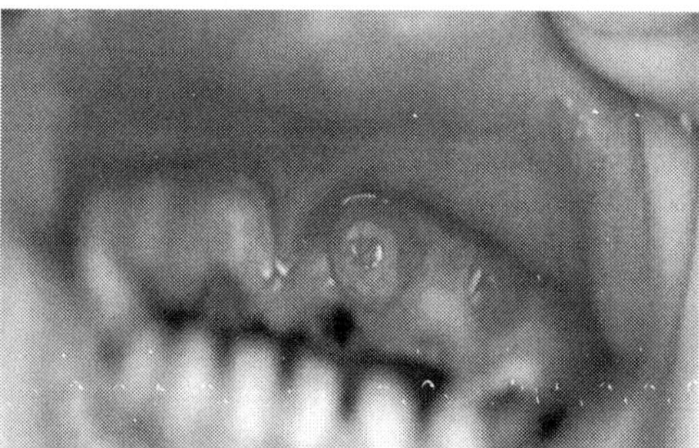

Figure 6. Abscess and fistula

Local situation – the gingiva is edematic, hyperemic and under pressure it is painful. Also while applying a slightly harder pressure from the gingival pocket purulent secret will come out. The tooth is extremely sensitive to palpation and percussion. (Fig.7)

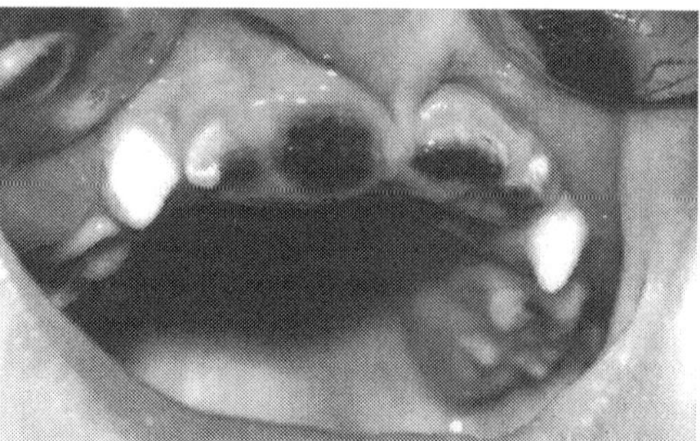

Figure 7. Edematic and hyperemic gingiva

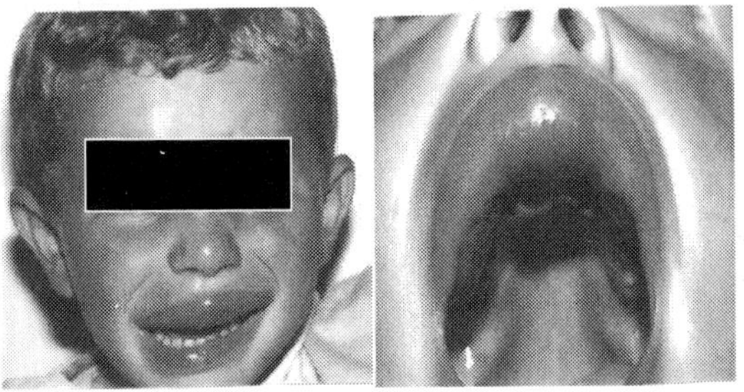

Figure 8. Spread of infection- result of ECC complications

General condition - pain, elevated temperature, fever, loss of appetite, the patient is pale and frightened. The patient cannot be fed as a result of edema of the lip and the gum inflammation. The food intake is affected due to the great sensitivity of the gangrenous roots in the upper front. (Fig.8)

Dental eruption disorders as a result of the remaining roots

As a result of root persistence, among others, it may have an effect in the eruption disorders of permanent teeth causing orthodontic abnormality (Fig. 9, 10.)

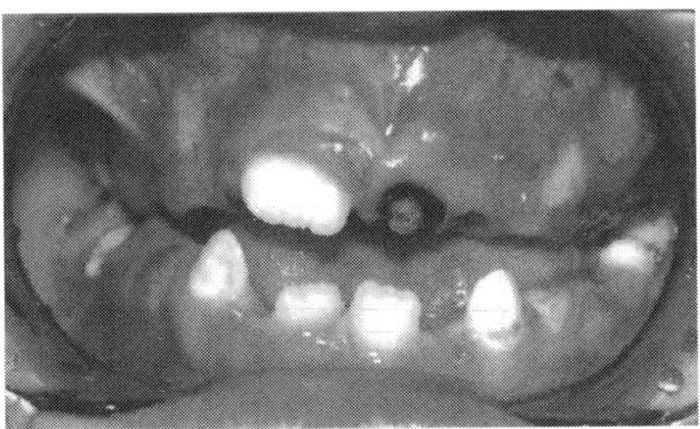

Figure 9. Persistence of radix relicta and disorders of permanent tooth eruption

Early Extraction

Consequence of an early childhood caries is the "loss" or extraction of teeth (Figure 11 & 12). Extraction of the teeth is approved when the clinical conditions become more serious, as a result of complications. But also: extraction may be due to unprofessional interference from the insisting parent, and the acceptance by the physician to do the extraction. The extraction, for example may be serial if it is decided by the therapist.

Consequences of Early extraction can be:

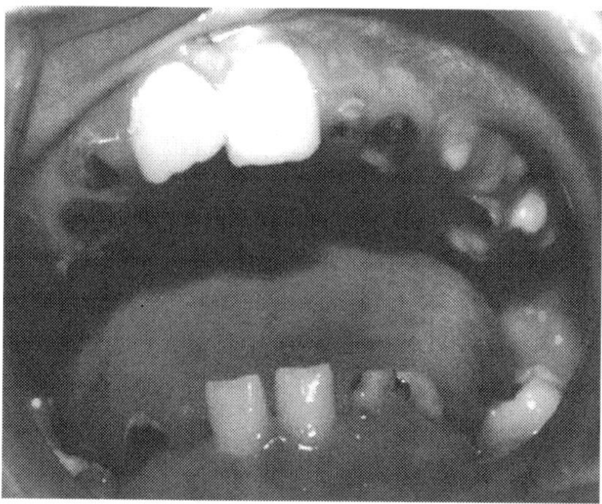

Figure 10. Orthodontic abnormality-result of radix relicta persistence

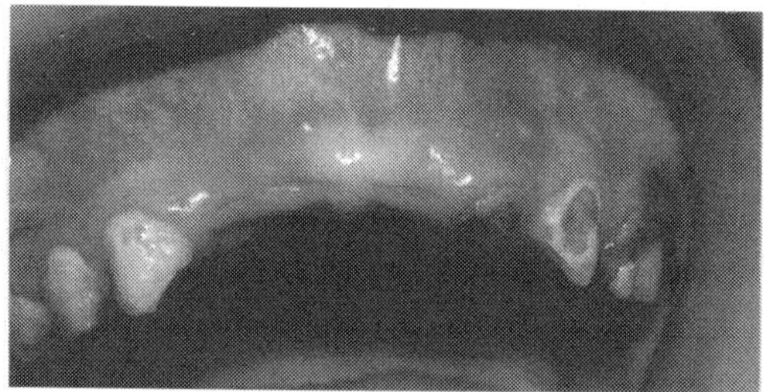

Figure 11. Early extraction of teeth

- abnormalities in the tooth eruption,

- speech impediment (incorrect pronunciation of letters),

- barriers in eating, poor aesthetics, etc.

Avoidance of these effects is done by prosthetic work, whose role would be: space mainte-nance, the normal pronunciation of letters, aesthetic improvement, etc.

5. Discussion

- *Risk factors of ECC*

Considering the data from the literature, the role of S mutans in the etiology of ECC, especially in the initial phase, is very crucial. These data also demonstrate the high prevalence of this

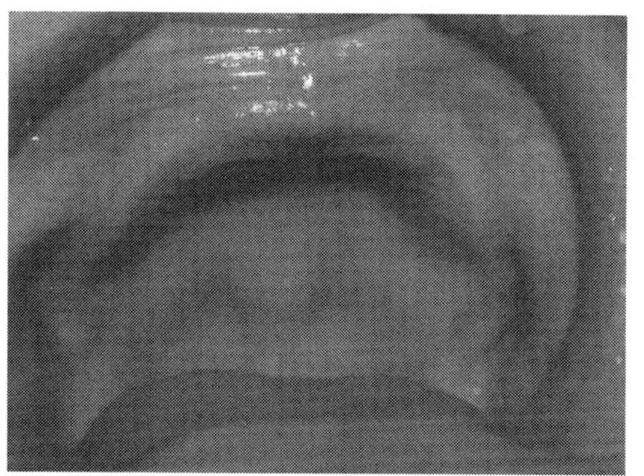

Figure 12. Total extraction of teeth-result of ECC complications

bacterium in preschool children. S mutans is found at the earliest ages, with the prevalence of 53% in 6- to 12-month-old children (Milgrom 2000), 60% in 15-month-olds (Karn 1998), 67% in 18-month-old Swedes (Hallonsten et al. 1995), and 94.7% in 3- to 4-year-old Chinese (Li et al. 1994). Almost all preschool urban Icelandic children were found to carry S mutans (Holbrook 1993). According to the studies of Ge and Caufield, all S-ECC children were S mutans–positive (Ge 2008). Borutta 2002, found that in 80% of children (3 years old) diagnosed with caries, the presence of S mutans was demonstrated, while higher counts of this bacterium were found in children with ECC.

The high prevalence of S mutans was also demonstrated in our study: 98% of preschool children. Expressed in colony-forming units (CFU/mL saliva), 93% of the ECC children in our study had a high S. mutans counts (CFU > 10^5). Higher salivary counts of *S. mutans* have been correlated with high dmft values (11.5) in our study. This significant correlation between high dmft or caries experience and high S mutans counts has been demonstrated in other studies (Köhler et al. 1995, Twetman & Frostner 1991, Maciel 2001).

In our study, the sweets consumption of children with ECC was very high. Almost 4/5 of ECC children have sweet snacks more than twice a day. It is of great concern that kindergartens as educational institutions do not have a more serious approach to a healthy diet and reduction of sugary food. On the contrary, at least once a day, sweet food (jam, chocolate, cream, biscuits, or cake) is served to children. Also, serving of this food is very common between meals. The literature also shows a high consumption of sweets between meals (Ölmez 2003) and high caries values in children who have frequent sweets (Holbrook 1989).

Another important factor in the etiology of ECC is bottle feeding, which is accompanied by high salivary counts of *S mutans*. The relationship between bottle usage and salivary counts of S mutans (Mohan 1998) has been reported. In the children that were in the study, the duration of bottle feeding with sweetened milk or juice was very long, wherein nearly 4/5 of children were bottle fed from 1 to 3 and more years.

Another harmful practice is putting children to sleep with a juice-filled bottle, which is practiced in 2/3 of children with ECC, although Johnsen has reported that 78% of parents of children with ECC had attempted to substitute water for a cariogenic liquid (e.g., apple juice, formula) in the bedtime nursing bottle [Johnsen]. A review of the literature from the etiological point of view of ECC shows that "the use of a bottle at night" is not the only cause of ECC (Plat 2000).

Oral hygiene habits established at the age of 1 can be maintained throughout early childhood (Wendt 1995). There is a high level of negligence in the oral hygiene of our children. More than half do not brush their teeth at all, exhibiting a very high oral hygiene index-OHI (1.52). The importance of the primary dentition of oral health promotion must be focused on the education of mothers to motivate their children for oral hygiene. Unfortunately, we found "bad conviction" of mothers regarding primary teeth that they will be replaced, thus neglecting the care for children's teeth. Data from the literature show that cooperation of mothers is very important in overcoming the belief that the deciduous dentition can be neglected (Rosamund 2003).

Mothers' knowledge and behaviours of oral hygiene are the key components for children's oral health care. The child imitates parental behaviours, including oral hygiene habits; thus, tooth brushing at an early age depends on maternal knowledge and behaviours. In our study, 38% of the mothers stated that their children did not brush their teeth at all. Only 11% of the interviewed mothers demonstrated proper techniques of tooth brushing. Unfortunately, a relatively low percentage of mothers (24%) stated that tooth brushing should last at least 2 to 3 minutes. The interviewed mothers rarely assisted their children during tooth brushing (5%).Even though fluoride and antimicrobial agents have a beneficial role in preventing caries, an insignificant number of interviewed mothers stated that they had knowledge regarding fluoride and they did not practice these preventive methods with their children (Begzati et al. 2014).

Besides fluoride treatments, an antimicrobial treatment option has become a serious consideration for many dental professionals. The data from the literature have confirmed the positive antibacterial role of chlorhexidine in the destruction of S. mutans colonies and inhibiting caries (Featherstone 2004, Zhang et al. 2006).

From the answers of mothers concerning fluoride use, we ascertained a marked lack of knowledge about the benefits of this agent in maintaining healthy tooth structure. This information gap can be inferred from their answers. When asked, "Do you give fluoride tablets to your child?" their answers were stated as if they have been asked about some medication: "I give those tablets to my child as needed." The absence of fluoride in Kosovo's municipal drinking water may highly influence caries prevalence rates in children.

Nutritional counseling, fluoride therapy, and oral hygiene may be required to prevent development of carious lesions in children. In the case of high-risk patients such as ECC children with a predominance of high salivary counts of S mutans, the use of either the antibacterial rinse chlorhexidine gluconate or the oral health care gel chlorhexidine has been suggested (Featherstone 2004).

The oral health promotion and preventive measures are also influenced by social and economic factors. Statistical data from Kosovo are as follows: large families (with average size of 6.5 members), high unemployment rate (in 2008 it marked 45.4%, for female 56.4%), high birth rate (16%) and the lowest economic growth in the region [56], represent some of the aggravating factors when dealing with the health issues of the population, including oral health issues (Ministry of Public Administration. Statistical Office of Kosovo 2010).

Given the complexity of factors associated with ECC, it is unfortunate that most of the interest has only been from dental organizations. The critical change needed to accomplish the necessary research related to prevention of ECC is to expand our network through inclusion other health professionals, community leaders, national organizations serving children, and political leaders (Ismaili 1998).

- *Consequences of ECC*

Scientific research suggests that the development of ECC occurs in 3 stages. The first stage is characterized by a primary infection of the oral cavity with ECC. The second stage is the proliferation of these organisms to pathogenic levels as a consequence of frequent and prolonged exposure to cariogenic substrates. Finally, a rapid demineralization and cavitation of the enamel occurs, resulting in rampant dental caries (Wyne 1998). A 1-year follow-up of ECC development from the initial stage, representing decay at the enamel level and its progression to more destructive stages, shows even development in all affected teeth. It is quite an acute development, because in 2/3 of the children, the ECC has progressed to more complicated stages (destructive and radix relicta stages). Within 1 year, the dmft values have increased to 3.7. Consecutively, these children commonly experience pain from pulpitis, gangrene, and apical periodontitis. Also, these conditions are often followed by abscesses and cellulitis, sometimes with phlegmona, seriously endangering the child's general health. De Grauwe, in describing the progression of ECC, has noticed that the development of caries from the enamel to the dentin level can occur within 6 months (De Grauwe et al. 2004). The rapid development of ECC and its clinical appearance, especially in primary incisors, identifies it in its initial stages as a risk factor for future caries in the primary and permanent dentitions (Al-Shalan et al. 1997).

Children with congenital heart anomalies are frequent patients in our departments, some of them exhibiting severe ECC. There is strong evidence that untreated dental disease is an important etiological factor in the pathogenesis of infective endocarditis, a condition that still carries a high risk of mortality (Child 1996).

Preventive measures for ECC (Begzati et al. 2012)

Early childhood caries (ECC) is a health problem with biological, social and behavioral determinants. Intervention treatment does not resolve this problem. It is difficult, sometimes impossible and expensive.

The only safest way is prevention of this complex pathology. European Academy of Pediatric Dentistry (2008) has recommended general strategies for ECC prevention:

- Oral health assessments with counseling at regularly scheduled visits during the first year of life are an important strategy to prevent ECC

- Children's teeth should be brushed daily with a smear of fluoride toothpaste as soon as they erupt

- Professional applications of fluoride varnish are recommended at least twice yearly in groups or individuals at risk.

- Parents of infants and toddlers should be encouraged to reduce behaviours that promote the early transmission of mutans streptococci.

Based on these recommendations, we will describe detailed preventive measures: primary prevention – prenatal and postnatal care; and secondary prevention – parents' and dental professionals' role.

- **Primary prevention**

It should begin during prenatal period and it consists of pregnant woman's needs' fulfillment with necessary and healthy products;

Proper quality of food for the newborn during the enamel maturation phase;

Fluoridation of newly-erupted teeth;

Antimicrobial therapy with chlorhexidine.

- **Secondary prevention**

Mothers' education on recognizing the first signs of ECC using "lift-the-lip" technique. The aim of this measure is early detection of the so-called "white spot".

Parents should be encouraged to avoid bad feeding habits of their children and give effort for proper feeding:

- breast-feeding of the baby;

- the use of cup instead of the bottle as early as possible;

- not sleeping with bottle in mouth;

- avoid the use of fabricated juices or soda;

- the use of natural, a little sweetened, juice or tea, or just water;

- avoid the discontinuation of bottle use by the method "bottle is gone";

- reduce the liquid in the bottle, gradually by night,

- reduce sweets as much as possible;

- no sweets between meals;

- daily tooth brushing, at least twice a day, obligatory before going to bed.

Necessary consultations with the dentist -

Professional education activity targeting primary care health providers (pediatricians, internists, family physicians, obstetricians, mid-level medical practitioners):

- early identification of disease,

- fluoride supplements as appropriate,

- healthful feeding practices,

- snacking behaviors that promote good oral health, and

- referral to the dentist by 12 months of age.

6. Conclusions

Oral health is integral to general health and should not be considered in isolation. Oral diseases have detrimental effects on an individual's physical and psychological well-being and reduce quality of life. The commonest disease is dental caries. Caries progression or reversal is determined by the balance between protective and pathological factors in the mouth. The most important component in the treatment of the caries disease is prevention. Understanding the balance between pathological factors and protective factors is the key to successful prevention of caries. Analyzing the etiology, prevalence, clinical specifics, consequences and complications, caries in general and ECC in particular are estimated as serious diseases, which represent not only health problem, but also a great serious social and economic problem.

Consequence of an early childhood caries, especially in underdeveloped countries, can be very severe, spanning from tooth loss to general health disorders. One of the complications of untreated ECC is the "loss" or extraction of teeth. Consequences of early extraction can be: abnormalities in the tooth eruption, speech impediment (incorrect pronunciation of letters), barriers in eating, poor aesthetics, etc.

The rapid development of ECC, especially in primary incisors, identifies it in its initial stages as a risk factor for future caries in the primary and permanent dentitions. There is strong evidence that untreated dental disease is an important etiological factor in the pathogenesis of infective endocarditis, a condition that still carries a high risk of mortality.

The risk factors for early childhood caries include a number of social and behavioural determinants.

Primary prevention must start in the prenatal stage to fulfill the needs of pregnancy. Parents should be encouraged to avoid bad feeding habits and to instruct and supervise their children in tooth brushing. Mothers should be instructed to use the lift-the-lip technique to spot the white-spot lesions as first signs of dental caries. Newly erupted teeth must be treated with fluoride agents, and, as needed, antimicrobial agents containing chlorhexidine and thymol. Further investigation is needed to assess the effectiveness of new intervention strategies beyond traditional measures that are not strictly dependent on access to dental professional providers.

Permanent and sustained oral health promotion organized with the participation of the entire civil society, with the mandatory presence of key stakeholders in the areas of education and healthcare, represent one of the highest priorities. The WHO strategies and objectives implementation regarding oral health promotion should be understood in the right manner and should be implemented continuously.

Author details

Agim Begzati[1*], Merita Berisha[3], Shefqet Mrasori[2], Blerta Xhemajli-Latifi[1], Prokshi[1], Haliti[1], Valmira Maxhuni[1], Vala Hysenaj-Hoxha[1] and Vlera Halimi[1]

*Address all correspondence to: agimbegzati@yahoo.com

1 Department of Pedodontics and Preventive Dentistry, School of Dentistry, Medical Faculty, University of Prishtina, Prishtina, Republic of Kosovo

2 Department of Endodnintic, Medical Faculty, University of Prishtina, Prishtina, Republic of Kosovo

3 National Institute of Public Health of Kosovo, Department of Social Medicine, Medical Faculty, University of Prishtina, Prishtina, Republic of Kosovo

References

[1] Arkin, E.B. (1986). The Healthy Mothers, Healthy Babies Coalition: four years of progress. *Public Health Repository,* Vol. 101, pp. 147-156.

[2] Acs, G., Shulman, R., Wai, M. & Chussid' S. (1999). The effect of dental rehabilitation on the body weight of children with early childhood caries. *Pediatric Dentistry,* Vol. 21, pp.109-113.

[3] Acs, G., Lodolini, G., Kaminsky, S. & Cisneros, G.J.(1992). Effect of nursing caries on body weight in a pediatric population. *Pediatric Dentistry,* Vol. 14, pp:302-305.

[4] Al-Dashti, A.A., Williams, S.A. & Curzon, M.E.(1995). Breast feeding, bottle feeding and dental caries in Kuwait, a country with low-fluoride levels in the water supply. *Community Dental Health.* Vol.12, pp.42–47.

[5] Apostolova, D., Asprovsa, V. & Simovska N (2003). Circular caries-ECC-a problem at the earliest age. *8th Congress of the Balkan Stomatological Society,* (Abstract Book) Tirana, 2003.

[6] Al-Shalan, T.A., Erickson, P.R. & Hardie, N.A.(1997). Primary incisor decay before age 4 as a risk factor for future dental caries. *Paediatric Dentistry*,Vol.19, No.1, pp. 37-41.

[7] Begzati, A., Meqa, K., Siegenthaler, D., Berisha, M. & Mautsch, W. (2011). Dental health evaluation of children in Kosovo. *European Journal of Dentistry*, Vol. 5, pp. 32-39

[8] Begzati, A., Bytyci, A., Meqa, K., Latifi-Xhemajli, B. & Berisha, M. (2014). Mothers' Behaviours and Knowledge Related to Caries Experience of Their Children, *Oral Health & Preventive Dentistry*, Vol.2, pp.133-140

[9] Begzati, A., Meqa, K. & Berisha, M. Early childhood caries in preschool children of Kosovo - a serious public health problem . *BMC Public Health* 2010, 10:788

[10] Begzati, A., K. Meqa, K., Azemi, M., Begzati, Aj., Kutllovci, T., Xhemajli, B. & Berisha, M.(2012) Oral health care in children - a preventive perspective, In: *Oral health Care-Pediatric, Research, Epidemiology and Clinical Practices*, Published by InTech, 2012; 19-59.

[11] Bruered, B., Kinney, M.B. & Bothwell, E. (1989). Preventing baby bottle tooth decay in American Indian and Alaska native communities: a model for planning. *Public Health Repository*, Vol. 104, No. 6, pp. 631-640.

[12] Beltrami, G.(1952) .Black teeth in toddlers. Siècle Medical 1932 Apr 4. Cited in Beltrami, G. *La mélanodontie infantile* . Marseilles, By Leconte Editeur.

[13] Berkowitz. R.J., Turner, J. & Green, P. (1980). Primary oral infection of infants with Streptococcus mutans. *Archives of Oral Biology*, Vol. 25, pp. 221-224.

[14] Barbakov. F., Scheil. W. & Imfel, T.(1985). Observations of SnF2-treated Human Enamel Using the Scanning Electron microscope, *Journal of Dentistry for Children*, Vol.52, pp.279-287.

[15] Berkowitz, R.J. (1996). Etiology of nursing caries; a microbiologic perspective. *Journal of Public Health Dentistry*, Vol. 56, No. 1, pp. 51-54.

[16] Berkowitz, R.J., Jordan, H.V. & White, G. (1975). The early establishment of Streptococcus mutans in the mouths of infants. *Archives of Oral Biology*, Vol.20, pp.171-174.

[17] Burne, R.A.(1998). Oral streptococci products of their environment, *Journal of Dental Research*, Vol.77, pp.445-452.

[18] Borutta, A., Kneist, S. & Eherler, D.P. (2002). Oral health and Occurrence of Salivary S. mutans in Small Children, *Journal of Dental and Oral Medicine*, Vol. 4, No. 3, Poster 128.

[19] Berkowitz, R.J., Turner, J. & Green P.(1981). Maternal salivary levels of Streptococcus mutans: The primary oral infection in infants. *Archives of Oral Biology*, Vol.26, pp. 147-149.

[20] Carlsson, P.(1989). Distribution of mutans streptococci in populations with different levels of sugar consumption. *Scandinavian journal of dental research*, Vol.97 No.2, pp. 120-125.

[21] Centers for Disease Control and Prevention (CDCP), conference. Atlanta, GA, September 1994.

[22] Caufield, P.W., Cutter, G.R. & Dasanayake A.P.(1993). Initial acquisition of mutans streptococci by infants: evidence for a discrete window of infectivity. *Journal of Dental Research* , Vol.72, pp. 37-45.

[23] Catalanotto, F.A., Shklair, I.I. & Keene, H.J.(1975). Prevalence and localization of Streptococcus mutans in infants and children. *Journal of the American Dental Association*, Vol.91, pp:606-609.

[24] Child, J.S. (1996). Risks for and prevention of infective endocarditis. In: Child JS, ed. *Cardiology Clinics—Diagnosis and Management of Infective Endocarditis*. Philadelphia, Pa: WB Saunders Co, Vol. 14, pp. 327-343.

[25] Drury, Th.F., Horowitz, A.M., Ismail, A.I., Maertens, M.P., Rozier, R.G. & Selwitz, R.H. (1999). Diagnosing and reporting Early Childhood Caries for Research Purposes. *Journal of Public Health Dentistry*, Vol. 59, pp. 192-197.

[26] Davis, G.N. (1998). Early childhood caries-a synopsis. *Community Dentistry and Oral Epidemiology*,Munksgaard , Vol. 26, pp.106-116.

[27] Derkson, G.D. & Ponti, P. (1982). Nursing bottle syndrome: prevalence end etiology in a non fluoridated city. *Journal of the Canadian Dental Association*, Vol. 6, pp. 389-393.

[28] Douglass, J.M., Douglass, A.B. & Silk HJ.(2004). A practical guide to infant oral health. *Am Fam Physician.* Vol.70, pp.2113–2120.

[29] Elice, C.E. & Fields, C.W.(1990). Failure to thrive: Rewire of literature, case reports and implications for dental treatment. *Pediatric Dentistry*, Vol.12, pp.185-189.

[30] European Academy of Paediatric Dentistry (EAPD 2008). *Guidelines on Prevention of Early Childhood Caries: An EAPD Policy Document.* Dublin, Ireland.

[31] Featherstone, J.D.B. (2004). The Caries Balance: The Basis for Caries Management by Risk Assessment. *Oral Health and Preventive Dentistry*, Vol. 2, No 1, pp. 259-264

[32] Fass, E.(1962). Is bottle feeding of milk a factor in dental caries? *Journal of Dentistry for Children* Vol.29, pp. 245-251.

[33] Fédération Dentaire Internationale –FDI(1988). Technical report No. 31. Review of methods of identification of high caries groups and individuals. *International Dental Journal, Vol.38*, pp. 177-189.

[34] Ge. Y., Caufield, P.W., Fisch, G.S. & Li. Y.(2008). Streptococcus mutans and Streptococcus sanguinis Colonization Correlated with Caries Experience in Children. *Caries Res*, Vol.42, pp.444-448.

[35] De Grauwe, A., Aps, J.K. & Martens, L.C. (2004). Early Childhood Caries (ECC): What's in a name? *European Journal of Pediatric Dentistry*, Vol. 5, No. 2, pp. 62-70.

[36] Goose, D.H.(1967). Infant Feeding and Caries of the Incisors: an epidemiological Approach. *Caries Research*, Vol.1 , pp.167-173.

[37] Galdvin, M. & Trattler, B.(2004) Clinical Microbiology, MedMaster, Inc., Miami, Florida-USA.

[38] Horowitz, H.S.(1998). Research issues in early childhood caries. *Community Dentistry and Oral Epidemiology, Vol.17*, pp. 292-295.

[39] Hamada, S. & Slade, H.D.(1980). Biology, immunology and Cariogencity of Streptococcus mutans; *Microbiology Reviews*, Vol.44, pp. 331-384.

[40] Harris, O.N. & Garsia, F. (1999). Primary Preventive Dentistry, by Applenton & Lange, Stamford.

[41] Holt, R.D., Winter, G.B., Downer, M.C. & Bellis, W.J. (1996). Caries in pre-school children in Camden 1993/94. *British Dental Journal*, Vol. 181, pp. 405-410.

[42] Hunt, R.J. (1986). Percent agreement, Pearson's correlation, and kappa as measures of inter-examiner reliability. *Journal of Dental Research*, Vol. 65, pp.128-130

[43] Hallonsten, A.L., Wendt, L.K., Mejar, I., Birkhed, D., Hakansson, C., Lindwall, A.M., Edwardsson, S., Koch, G. (1995). Dental Caries and prolonged breast-feeding in 18-month- old. Swedish children. *International Journal of Paediatric Dentistry*, Vol.5, No.3, pp.149-155.

[44] Holbrook, W.P.(1993). Dental caries and cariogenic factors in pre-school urban Icelandic children. *Caries Res*,Vol. 27, No.5, pp.431-437.

[45] Holbrook, W.P., Kristinsson, M.J., Gunnarsdóttir, S. & Briem, B. (1989). Caries prevalence, Streptococcus mutans and sugar intake among 4-year-old urban children in Iceland. *Community Dentistry and Oral Epidemiology*, Vol. 17, No. 6, pp. 292-295.

[46] Harper, D.S. & Loesche, W.J.(1984). Growth and acid tolerance of human dental plaque bacteria. *Archives of Oral Biology*, Vol. 29, pp.843-848.

[47] Huseinbegović, A. (2001). Social and medical aspects of primary dentition caries in urban conditions. Master degree- Sarajevo.

[48] Horowitz, H.S. (1998). Research issues in early childhood caries. *Community Dentistry and Oral Epidemiology*, Vol. 26, No. 1, pp. 67-81.

[49] Ismail, A.I. & Sohn, W. (1999). A Systematic Review of Clinical Diagnostic Criteria of Early Childhood Caries. *Journal of Public Health Dentistry*, Vol. 59, No. 3, pp. 171-191.

[50] Ismail, A.I. (1998). Prevention of early childhood caries. *Community Dentistry and Oral Epidemiology*, Vol. 26, No.1, pp. 49-61.

[51] Johnsen, D.C. (1982). Characteristics and backgrounds of children with "nursing caries." *Pediatric Dentistry*, Vol. 4, No. 3, pp. 218–224.

[52] Jacobi, A. (1862). Dentition. *Its Derangements. A Course of Lectures Delivered in the New York Medical College.* New York: Ballière Brothers

[53] James, P.M.C., Parfitt, G.J. & Falkner, F. (1957). A study of the aetiology of labial caries of the deciduous incisor teeth in small children. *British Dental Journal*, Vol. 103, No. 2, pp.37–40.

[54] Kobaslia, S., Maglaic, N. & Begovic, A. (2000). Caries prevalence of Sarajevo children. *Acta Stomatologica Croatica*, Vol. 34, pp. 83-85

[55] Konig, K.G. & Navia, E.M. (1995). Nutritional role of sugars in oral health. *American Journal of Clinical Nutrition*, Vol. 62, Suppl. pp. 275S-83S.

[56] Keyes, P.H.(1962). Recent advances in dental caries research. *International Dental Journal, Vol.* 12, pp. 443-464.

[57] Kaste, L.M. & Gift, H.C. (1995). Inappropriate infant bottle feeding: Status of the Healthy People 2000 Objective. *Archives of Pediatrics & Adolescent Medicine.* Vol. 149, pp.786-791.

[58] Kaste, L.M., Selwitz, R.H., Oldakowski, R.J., Brunelle, J.A., Win, D.M. & Brown, L.J. (1996). Coronal Caries in the Primary and Permanent Dentition of Children and Adolescents 1-17 Years of Age: United States, 1988-1991, *Journal of Dental Research,*Vol. 75, pp. 631-641.

[59] Karn, T.A., O'Sullivan, D.M. & Tinannoff N. (1988). Colonization of mutans streptococci in 8- to 15- month-old children. *Journal of Public Health Dentistry,*, Vol. 58, No.3. pp. 248-249.

[60] Köhler, B., Andreen, I. & Jonsson, B. (1988). The earlier the colonization by mutans streptococci, the higher the caries prevalence at 4 years of age. *Oral Microbiology and Immunology*, Vol. 3, pp. 14-17.

[61] Köhler, B., Bjarnason, S., Care, R., Mackevica, I. & Rence, I. (1995). Mutans streptococci and dental caries prevalence in a group of Latvian preschool children. *European Journal of Oral Sciences*, Vol. 103, No. 4, pp. 264-266.

[62] Koga, T., Asakawa, H., Okahashi, N. & Hamada, S.(1986). Sucrose –dependent cell adherence and cariogenicity of serotype-c streptococcus mutans *Journal of general microbiology,* . Vol.132, pp.2873-2883.

[63] Lopez, L., Berkowitz, R.J., Moss, M.E. & Weinstein, P. (2000). Mutans streptotocci prevalence in Puerto Rican babies with cariogenic feeding behaviors. *Pediatric Dentistry*, Vol. 22, No. 4, pp. 299–301.

[64] Li, Y., Navia, J.M. & Caufield, P.W.(1994). Colonization by mutans streptococci in mouths of 3- and 4- year -old Chinese children with or without enamel hypoplasia. *Archives of Oral Biology, ,* Vol.39, N.12, pp.1057-1062.

[65] Loesche, W.J.(1986). Role of Streptococcus mutans in human dental decay; *Microbiological reviews,* Vol.50, pp. 353-380.

[66] Maciel, S.M., Marcenes, W. & Sheiham, A. (2001). The relationship between sweetness preference, levels of salivary mutans streptococci and caries experience in Brazilian pre-school children. *International Journal of Paediatric Dentistry,* Vol. 11, pp. 123-130.

[67] Mohan, A.M., O'Sallivan, D.M. & Tinanoff, N. (1998). The relationship between bottle usage/content, age and number of teeth with mutans streptococci colonization in 6-24 – month-old children. *Community Dentistry and Oral Epidemiology* Vol. 26, Suppl. 1, pp. 12-20.

[68] Ministry of Public Administration. Statistical Office of Kosovo. (http://esk.rksov.net/eng/index.php? option=com_docman&task=doc_download&gid=870&Itemid=8). Accessed on October 20th, 2010.

[69] Marthaler, M., O'Mullane, M. & Vrbic, V. (1996). The prevalence of dental caries in Europe 1990-1995. *Caries Research,* Vol. 30, pp. 237-255

[70] Marković, M.(1976). Etiologija malokluzija-book. Beograd, pp. 141-171

[71] Milgrom, P., Riedy, C.A., Weinstein, P., Tanner, A.C., Manibusan, L.& Bruss J(2000). Dental caries and its relationship to bacterial infection, hypoplasia, diet, and oral hygiene in 6- to 36-month-old children. *Community Dent Oral Epidemiol,* Vol. 28, pp: 295-306.

[72] Mcdonald, R. & Avery, D.A.(2000). Dentistry for the Child and Adolescent, Mosby.

[73] Norman, O.H. & Franklin, G. (1999). *Primary Preventive Dentistry.* Appleton & Lange, Stamford, Connecticut.

[74] O'Sullivan, D.M. & Tinanoff, N. (1993). Social and biological factors contributing to caries of the maxillary anterior teeth. *Pediatric Dentistry,* Vol. 15, pp. 41-44.

[75] Ölmez, S., Uzamis, M. & Erdem, G. (2003). Association between early childhood caries and clinical, microbiological, oral hygiene and dietary variables in rural Turkish children. *The Turkish Journal of Pediatrics,* Vol. 45, pp. 231-236.

[76] Plat, L. & Cebazas, M.C. (2000). Early childhood dental caries. Building community system for young children. Los Angeles, CA: University of California-Los Angeles Center for Healthier Children, Families and Communities, Vol. 32, exec. summ. (4 pp.).

[77] Petti, S., Iannazzo, S., Gemelli, G., Rocchi, R., Novello, M.R., Ortensi, V., Nicolussi, A., Simonetti D'Arca, A. & Tarsitani, G. (2001). Incidence of caries in a sample of 3-7-

year old children in Rome who were not included in population prevention programs. Ann Ig. Vol.13, No.4, pp.329-38.

[78] Quartey, J.B. & Williamson, D.D.(1998). Prevalence of early childhood caries at Harris County clinics. *Journal of Dentistry for Children. Vol.* 7, pp.127-131.

[79] Raiç, Z.(1985). Deçija i preventivna stomatologija-book, Zagreb.

[80] Reisine, S., Douglass, J.M. (1998). Psychosocial and behavioral issues in early childhood caries. *Community Dentistry and Oral Epidemiology*; Vol. 26, No.1, pp. 32-44.

[81] Rosamund, L.H. & Tracy, W. (2003). An oral health promotion program for an urban minority population of preschool children. *Community Dentistry and Oral Epidemiolology*, Vol. 31, No. 5, pp. 392-399.

[82] Russell, R.(2003). Microbiological aspects of caries prevention, Prevention of oral disease, Oxford.

[83] Ripa, L.W. (1988). Nursing caries: a comprehensive review. *Pediatric Dentistry*, Vol. 10, pp. 268-282.

[84] Soames, J.V. & Southam, J.C. (1999). Oral Pathology-book, by Oxford University press.

[85] Stile, H.M., Loesche, W.J. & O'Brien T.C. (1976). Microbial Aspects of Dental Caries. London, England: Information Retrieval; Vol. 1. pp:187-199.

[86] Schroth, R.J., Brothwell, D.J. & Moffatt, M.E.K.(2007). Caregiver knowledge and attitudes of preschool oral health and early childhood caries (ECC). *International Journal of Circumpolar Health* Vol. 66, pp. 153-167.

[87] Stosiç, P.(1991). Deçja i preventivna stomatologija-book. Beograd.

[88] Soames, J.V. & Southam, J.C. (1999). Oral Pathology. 3rd ed. Oxford

[89] Seow, W.K.(1998). Biological mechanisms of early childhood caries. *Community Dentistry and Oral Epidemiology, Vol.* 26, pp. 8-27.

[90] Tinanoff, N., Kaste, L.M. & Corbin, S.B. (1998). Early childhood caries: a positive beginning. *Community Dentistry and Oral Epidemiolology*, Vol. 26, No. 1, pp. 117-119.

[91] Twetman, S. & Frostner, N. (1991). Salivary mutans streptococci and caries prevalence in 8-year-old Swedish schoolchildren. *Swedish Dental Journal*, Vol. 15, No. 3, pp. 145-151.

[92] Tanner, ACR.(2002). The microbiota of young children from tooth and tongue samples. *Journal of Dental Research*, Vol.81, pp:53-57.

[93] Thomas, F.D., Alice, M.H., Amidi, I.I., Marco, P.M., Rozier, G.R. & Robert, H.(1999). Diagnosing and Reporting Early Childhood Caries for Research Purposes, *Journal of Public Health Dentistry*, Vol.59, pp.192-197.

[94] Thomas, A.K., David, M.O. & Norman, T.(1998). Colonization of Mutans Streptococci in 8 to 15 month-old Children. *Journal of Public Health Dentistry*, Vol.58, pp:248-249.

[95] Tsai, I.A., Johnsen, C.D., Lin, Y. & Kuang-Hung, H.(2001). A study of risk factors associated with nursing caries in Taiwanes children aged 24-48 months. *International Journal of Pediatric Dentistry*, Vol.11, pp.147-149.

[96] US Department of Health and Human Services. (2000). *Oral Health in America*: A Report of the Surgeon General. Rockville, MD: US Department of Health and Human Services, National Institute of Dental and Craniofacial Research, National Institutes of Health.

[97] Wan, A.K.L.(2001). Oral colonization of *Streptococcus mutans* in six-month-old predentate Infants. *Journal of Dental Research,* Vol.12, pp.2060-2065.

[98] Wyne, A.H. (1999). Early chlidhood caries: nomenclatur and case definition. *Community Dentistry and Oral Epidemiology*, Vol. 7, pp. 313-315.

[99] Wendt, L.K. & Birkhed, D.(1995). Dietary habits related to caries development and immigrant status in infants and toddlers living in Sweden. *Acta Odontologica Scandinavica, Vol.*53, pp. 339-344.

[100] Wendt, L.K. (1995). On oral health in infants and toddlers. *Swedish Dental Journal,* Vol. 19, Suppl., pp. 106:1-62.

[101] Winter, G.B., Hamilton, M.C. & James, P.M.C. (1966). Role of comforter as en etiological factor in rampant caries of deciduous dentition. *Archives of Diseases in Children,* Vol. 417, pp. 207-212.

[102] Whiley, R.A., & Beighton, D.(2013) "Streptococci and Oral Streptococci." Bite-Sized Tutorials. N.p. Web. 2013 *https://microbewiki.kenyon.edu/index.php/Streptococcus_mutans-_Tooth_Decay_References*

[103] Wierzbicka, M., Carlsson, P., Struzycka, I., Iwanicka-Frankowska, E. & Bratthall, D. (1987). Oral health and factors related to oral health in Polish schoolchildren. *Community Dentistry and Oral Epidemiology*, Vol. 15, No. 4, pp.177-239.

[104] Wan, A.K.L., Seow, K.(2001). Association of Streptococcus mutans infection and oral developmental nodules in predentate infants. *Journal of Dental Research*, Vol.80, pp. 1945-1948.

Chapter 3

Improving Antimicrobial Activity of Dental Restorative Materials

J.M.F.A. Fernandes, V.A. Menezes,
A.J.R. Albuquerque, M.A.C. Oliveira, K.M.S. Meira,
R.A. Menezes Júnior and F.C. Sampaio

Additional information is available at the end of the chapter

http://dx.doi.org/10.5772/59252

1. Introduction

The oral cavity harbors a great diversity of microbial species that have a strong tendency to colonize dental surfaces, tongue and oral mucosa [1,2]. These accumulations of oral bacteria on dental surfaces are natural forms of biofilm growth in humans. They are also known as dental plaque and in spite of several favorable conditions (e.g. temperature, humidity) these biofilms are constantly challenged by host factors. It is recognized that structural organization of a dental biofilm are influenced by the interplay of many unfavorable and also several favorable ones such as the chemical nature of the substrate and the type of the surface where the biofilm develops [3].

In dentistry, restoration failure is generally attributed to a combination of oral bacteria and inappropriate features of dental materials. Efficient dental restorative materials are important for an adequate recovery of masticatory and esthetic functions. However, these materials are prone to biofilm formation, affecting oral health. It is well accepted that under *in vivo* conditions, rough surfaces attract more biofilm than smooth ones, but the variables that influence bacterial adhesion to dental materials are still a matter of debate.

Dental caries is the most prevalent disease found in the oral cavity of humans. It is regarded as multifactorial chronic and complex disease which is dependent of a cariogenic biofilm [4,5]. Thus, a carious lesion takes some time to develop. However, initial carious lesions are easily and rapidly formed during a three-day of high sucrose regime and poor oral hygiene conditions. So, as long as there is a cariogenic microbial biofilm attached to a dental surface there is a great chance to find a carious lesion on this tooth spot [6]. Growth of oral

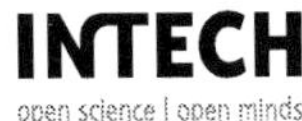

bacteria on dental surfaces requires adhesion strategies because there is a constant flow of host secretions (e.g. saliva) that can interfere on the ability of planktonic cells (non-attached bacteria). As a result, the formation of the oral biofilm is not homogenous and it contains multiple bacterial species [4,7,8].

Oral bacteria can adhere to hydrophobic as well as to hydrophilic surfaces and many explanatory theories are suggested including the influence of complex electrostatic mechanisms such as van der Waals energy. After biofilm establishment on restorations, surface deterioration of materials (e.g.: resin composites and glass-ionomer cements) will take place facilitating the development of a mature biofilm resulting in dental carious lesions. The microflora from these diseased teeth sites is significantly different from healthy sites on a tooth [10]. The frequent changes in environmental conditions can lead to shifts in biofilm microflora and as a result the microbial homeostasis breaks down in dental plaque (e.g. low pH), and disease occurs.

It must be pointed out that the presence of these oral microbes in the mouth is natural, and is also essential for the normal development of the physiology of the oral cavity [9]. Hence, any antimicrobial strategy has to consider the perspective of restoring some microbial equilibrium and not a complete depletion of oral bacterial from the mouth. Many antimicrobial substances, compounds or mixture of antibacterial agents (e.g. bisbiguanides, metal ions, quaternary ammonium compounds, essential oils) have been successfully formulated into home care products to control oral biofilms. Several investigations have proved their efficacy in controlling the development of oral biofilms despite important drawbacks as tooth staining, bad taste, etc. [3,4]. Moreover, at moderate or high concentrations, these antimicrobial mouthwashes and toothpastes can inhibit bacterial growth in many different modes and truly affect biofilm-forming capacity of some pathogenic traits. Hence, to be considered a successful antimicrobial agent a substance, compound or the mixture of both must be able of maintaining the oral biofilm at "normal" cariogenic bacterial levels which are compatible with the individual oral health. Simultaneously, the material must be effective without any interference on the beneficial properties of the resident oral microflora.

Mouthwashes and toothpastes are accepted methods to deliver antimicrobials into the oral mouth. However, they are completely dependent on the discipline and compliance of the patient to the oral treatment. In addition, many of these antimicrobials are prescribed for short periods to avoid any risk of disturbing the resident oral microflora [3,10]. Hence, one strategy is to incorporate antimicrobials into dental materials. The possibility that dental restorative material may release antimicrobial compounds are regarded as an interesting strategy for overcoming the development of cariogenic dental biofilms and the risk for secondary dental caries. In addition, there is a chance that under less biofilm stress dental materials could increase longevity. This strategy is of great importance since dental restorations properties may be improved if an antibiotic-dental material is used.

The aim of the present review is to shed light on the techniques and effectiveness on improving antibacterial activities of dental restorative materials. The main focus is on incorporation and subsequent slow-release of antimicrobial chemical species, molecules, compounds and low molecular weight antibacterial agents such as metal ions, iodine, antibiotics, chlorhexidine and natural products such as essential oils. The *in vitro* and *in vivo* techniques used in microbiology are also explored taking into account that main bacteria involved are Gram-positive cocci shaped bacteria such as *Streptococcus sobrinus, Streptococcus mutans* and Lactobacillus sp.

2. *In vitro* and *in vivo* techniques for studying biofilms

In 1940´s microbiologists described an interesting phenomenon that occurs when fresh sea water is kept in a glass bottle, the so-called "bottle effect". It was observed that the number of microorganisms attached a glass surface increase while at the same time there is a reduction in free-living microorganisms [11]. This is a relevant historical landmark because it represents the starting point of a paradigm shift that is still valid these days. In fact, only 30 years later, scientific community understood that the biofilm mode of life is the rule rather the exception when bacteria and fungi species are collected, studied and investigated in nature under real life conditions. Biofilms are defined as complex consortia of microorganisms that are attached to a surface that can be of biotic or abiotic nature [12].

The microbial biofilm formation involves a multi-stage process in which bacterial and fungi adhere to the surface. For more details see figure 1 which is based in several reports [13-16].

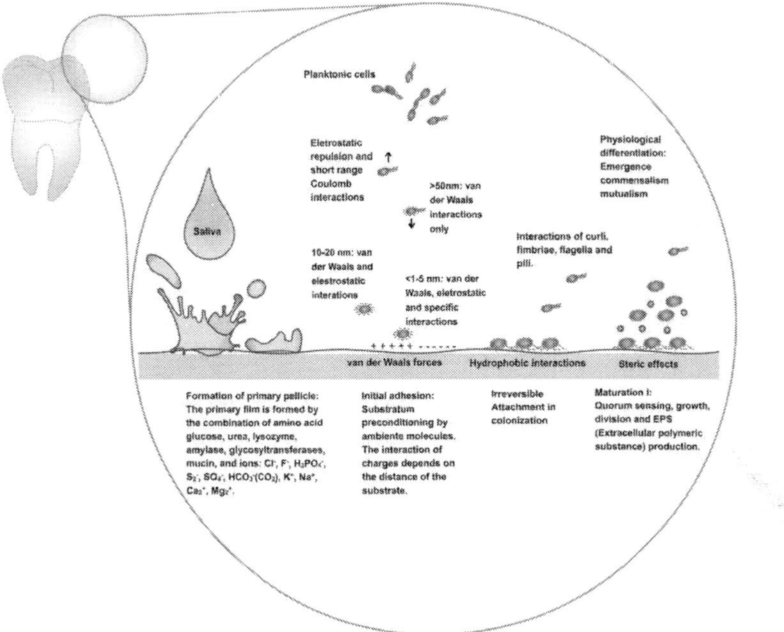

Figure 1. The multi-stage process of biofilm formation by oral microorganisms.

At this stage only weak forces are operating. Therefore it is also known as the initial reversible attachment stage. Subsequently, there is a production of an extracellular matrix (containing polysaccharides, proteins and DNA) that results in a stronger attachment which is also known as the irreversible attachment stage [16]. In general, after attachment, biofilm growth follows two other distinct phases or behavior: spreading and dispersal of microorganisms.

Basically, the attachment process involves equilibrium of electrostatic forces. Microbes and tooth surfaces are negatively charged. As they are immersed in a fluid (saliva) system which is rich in calcium and other counterions, these negative charged surfaces attract and mobilize cations. As a result, a double charged layer is formed (electrical double layer) and this overlap causes a repulsive electrostatic force. Simultaneously, as the bacterium approaches the tooth surface, they also experience a repulsive force (van der Waals force). Finally, the combinations of repulsive and attraction forces known as DLVO theory modulate the microorganism adherence to dental surfaces. This is valid for dental restorative materials as well, and one must consider the fact that it can be more favorable if a porous or irregular surface is facilitating bacterial adherence [3,13-16].

The first bacteria to attach to the acquired pellicle (layer of glycoproteins) on the tooth surface are called the pioneer species (*Streptococcus oralis, Streptococcus mitis, Streptococcus sanguis*). Surprisingly, *S. mutans* is not a first colonizer despite its high cariogenic nature. In fact, *S. mutans* is the most studied bacteria in oral microbiology but under clinical environment one must consider that a multispecies biofilm is operating [3,9].

Historically, in Dentistry, the examination of mature oral biofilms started when electron microscope became available for microbiologists [19]. Later, molecular biological tools became popular and new insights about how microbes attach and develop on tooth surfaces were finally confirmed. One "striking" observation was actually a confirmation of an obvious theory that microbes stick to a surface many benefits are obtained: a) selection of sites where they stay in favorable environments, b) these surfaces may have enough substrate or can contribute to diffuse some nutrient and c) the different species often work together and this consortium provides physical support and protection [20-29].

More recently, zeta potential, confocal laser scanning microscopy (CLSM) together with fluorescence techniques received attention and became useful techniques to study bacteria adhesion to surfaces [29]. In spite of the great evolution in techniques, many limitations have to be considered when comes to the evaluation of an antimicrobial substances against biofilms development. First, there is still the gap of *in vitro* and *in vivo* environments. *In situ* studies can overcome some of these limitations but other drawbacks cannot be ruled out. Most studies on bacteria adhesion to surfaces were carried out under *in vitro* conditions which do not reflect the real life. Secondly, there is the paradox of testing planktonic cells but interpretations are generalized to conditions of biofilm formation. It is well established that biofilms express genes different from those of planktonic cells. Moreover, it has been observed that biofilm cells are generally believed to closely resemble planktonic cells in stationary phase. However, biofilms were found to more closely resemble to planktonic cells at exponentially growing than those of planktonic cells in the stationary phase [19,20]. In addition, it cannot be ruled out the differences between single species biofilm versus multispecies biofilms since under laboratory

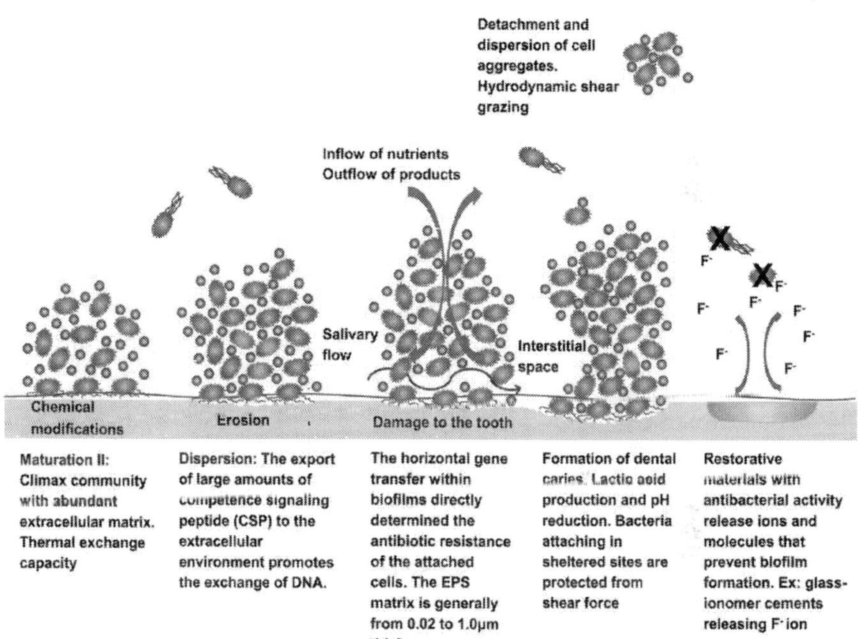

Figure 2. Schematic representation of the development of an oral biofilm and the potential of antimicrobials to interfere on this process when releasing some antimicrobial element or substance [13-18]

conditions monospecies biofilm can survive for only 72 hours in absence of sugar. The duration of survival can be extended with addition of mucin, but how close is this to the real oral mouth of a patient? [21] Another flow systems versus static models, pre-treatment of acquired pellicle or no pre-treatment at all. [22]. Finally, a crucial point is: how to validate microbial growth? BacLight staining techniques only measure the presence of intact membranes and may not correlate with the culturability or viability of bacteria from oral biofilms [23].

After all these relevant methodological points, more questions marks can be attributed on how to evaluate antimicrobial agents against biofilms. In addition to evaluate the effects in biofilms itself, one must consider the understanding of suitable methods related to the incorporation of antimicrobials into these dental restorative materials. For instance, the concentration of the antimicrobial agent, the volume or amount of material to be included and how far these substances can interfere on mechanical and esthetic features of a restoration [21-26].

Considering the presence of a mature biofilm covering a dental restoration, it must be pointed out that a major requirement of the final formulation is to deliver sufficient concentration of the inhibitor in the surroundings. Moreover, the antimicrobial effect must be kept on a prolonged time or at least for a enough period of time that will maintain an effective dose operating. This point is quite important since oral bacteria do not live as independent entities. So, as highlighted previously, a high resistance to antibiotics is likely to occur [27-30].

Along the last decades biofilms have been studied extensively because they are present in several surfaces, such as all solid surfaces in the oral cavity, in biomateriais implanted in the human body, in catheter surfaces, in water pipes [24]. After the establishment of a biofilm on dental restorations, deterioration of the outer layer surface of these materials will take place and facilitate bacteria adhesion [25]. On the other hand, the possibility that dental restoring materials can deliver antimicrobials may reduce considerably the risk of secondary caries in spite of the limitations of some dental materials.

3. Antimicrobials in dental materials: How much is enough versus how much is safe?

Oral bacteria can attach to many restorative materials like amalgam, gold, ceramics, resin composite, glass ionomer cements. In order to achieve long-term success of dental fillings there are many requirements. Some are related to the professional ability in manipulating and polishing these materials. However, some considerations rely on physical, chemical and biological characteristics of the dental material used. Surface roughness is not the focus of this review, but it may be influenced by the interplay of professionals' ability as well as dental materials features.

The incorporation of 5, 10, 15 up to 30% of antimicrobial compounds or substances into dental materials have been proposed [24-30]. However, the higher amount of antimicrobial agents, the higher is the risk to loose important features in dental restoration as biocompatibility and resistance. Hence, how much is enough and how much is safe? In the literature, addition of 1.5% can be effective if the antimicrobial is potent enough [27].

Figure 3 presents this dilemma related to the interference of "extra" substances to be incorporated into dental materials and limitations regarding the loss of important features of the material.

An interesting report showed that incorporation of 1% chlorhexidine (CHX) diacetate in GIC (glass ionomer cements) is optimal for clinical use. This is valid in terms of antimicrobial activities, CHX-release pattern, physical properties and bonding ability to tooth surfaces [28]. An additional valuable information was the conclusion that incorporation of CHX diacetate at 2% or greater values of percentage participation significantly decreased compressive strength and adversely affected bond strength to dentin.

It has been observed that some dental materials (e.g. gold and its alloys) are naturally able to kill bacteria in the adhering biofilms [29]. Glass ionomer cements (GIC) are recognized for releasing fluoride ions that can modulate biofilm formation [27,30]. The point is that this is not enough since GIC reduces its ability to release fluoride in short periods. So, it is expected that dental restoration with antimicrobial properties may have extended potential for inhibiting biofilm formation in a long-term basis.

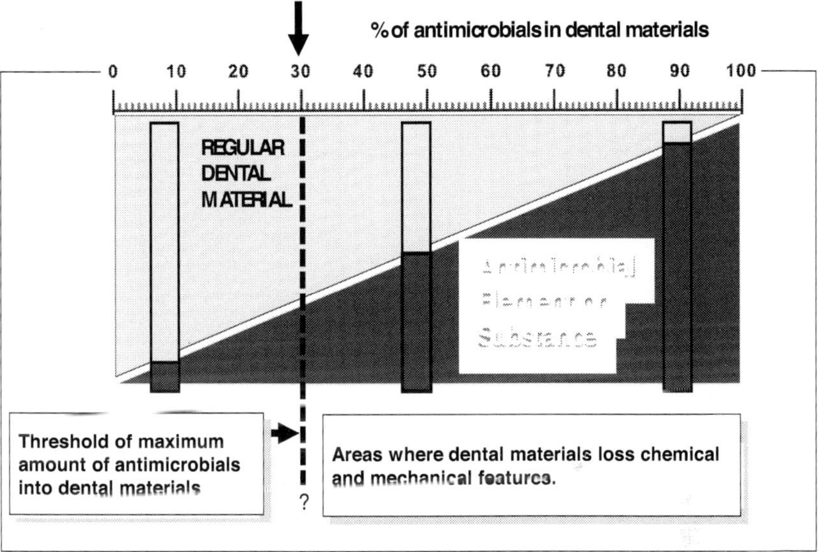

Figure 3. Schematic representation for understanding the effects of external substances and compounds when incorporated into regular dental materials.

In addition to chemical changes due to incorporation of antimicrobials into dental restorative materials, there is also the problem of chemical changes also interfere in the distribution of masticatory forces applied on a tooth. For instance, the presence of a carious lesion in molar tooth can demand fast treatment protocol for the affected area and depending on the lesion extension, it must receive a temporary filling [31-34]. In general, temporary filling materials are typically made from a combination of zinc oxide and eugenol which has good antimicrobial activity. Eugenol is also important due to its sedative properties. The zinc oxide powder is a very versatile compound that can present different properties when combined with various agents. When mixed together, the material starts off soft and in few minutes it becomes more hard and brittle. However, this mixture is not harder enough to be compared to regular dental fillings and its far from restoring tooth hardness. This material is classified as intermediate restorative material (IRM) and it is a good example that the beneficial aspects of antimicrobial and anti-inflammatory properties are achieved while mechanical properties of resistance become very low. Therefore, this material must be accepted as a temporary and not a definite filling material. Under the influence of masticatory forces, as previously mentioned, there will be a stress in the remaining parts of the dental element that will certainly compromise the longevity of the restoration as well as the whole tooth structure [31-34].

A comparative study analysing deformations done through Finite Element Method (FEM) and applying the software ANSYS shows the differences in compressive loads between sound and restored teeth with intermediate restorative materials (IRM), see figure 4A and 4B. It is shown that the restored tooth IRM (figure 4B) is deformed in a different way when compared to the sound tooth (4A). Figure 5 shows this simulation evaluating a map of tension for both conditions: A (sound tooth) and B (restored).

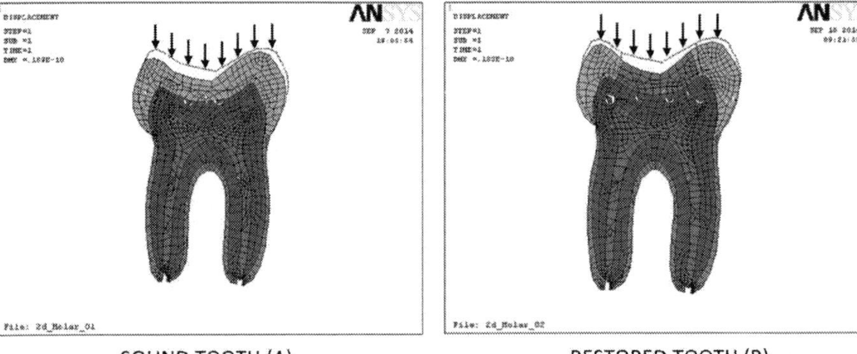

Figure 4. Sites of deformations in sound and IRM restored teeth.

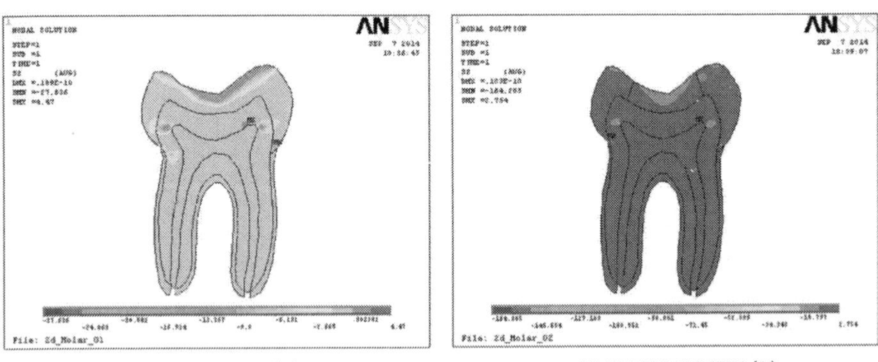

Figure 5. Sites of tensions in sound and IRM restored teeth.

As expected, the analysis shows that the distribution of forces in the interior of the teeth flows in different patterns. As a result, the restored tooth experiences a higher stress in some parts. Basically, these maps show compressive forces throughout the whole sound tooth (A) whereas for restored teeth tensile stress forces are observed.

It well is established that development of a numerical model as FEM makes it possible to quantify and evaluate masticatory loads [34]. However, few studies have considered the influence of antimicrobials in dental restorations. One must bear in mind that a good balance has to be achieved between the beneficial aspects of having an "antibacterial restoration" compared do a regular one. Certainly the size and shape of the restoration are important variables but interesting results can be obtained by these simulations.

It is important to realize that the changes in the map of tensions are directly related to the changes in the physical constitution of the tooth because in this case, the dental enamel was substituted by a restorative material. This change cannot necessarily be attributed to a change of forces because the molar frequently will be constantly submitted to the same masticatory forces it was receiving before the carious lesion. As shown in figure 5, the red colour of the figure 5B indicates a significant higher tension the 5A. The structural fatigue is the main mechanism of collapse of the reminiscent dental tissue and this process can be aggravated when it is submitted to long treatment periods, particularly if IRM is used. In other words, the IRM used as temporary fillings must have a short life because they reduce the mechanical efficiency of the teeth in spite of its beneficial support to control biofilm formation.

According to Noort (2013) [35], there is a subtle distinction between safety and biocompatibility two important features of dental materials. Safety is concerned with the fact that materials when in contact with the human body should not cause any adverse effect, whereas biocompatibility is the quality of being non-destructive in the biological environment maintaining the beneficial effect to the patient. So far, few materials can be regarded as completely safe and fully biocompatible in the oral environment. Most dental materials interact with the oral environment and this interaction might be a release of components with undesirable side effects for oral tissues.

4. Dental restorative materials with antimicrobials

Dental materials must simulate dental structure and have to restore the anatomy and the function of affected dental surfaces due to dental caries or trauma. However, the desirable aesthetics and the concerns with biocompatibility have not been forgotten and this is valid for resin composite, glass ionomer cements and IRM (MJÖR et al., 1990). It must be highlighted that bone and dentin can be considered as natural composites, whose main constituents are collagen (polymer) and apatite (a ceramic) [35].

Metals have been used for centuries as antimicrobial agents and they continue to be useful at the present time. Silver, copper, gold, titanium and zinc are the most common examples in Dentistry [36]. Dioxide of titanium has been used as whitening agent. However, silver and copper has been receiving larger attention due to their antimicrobial properties. As a result, these metals are incorporate to several dental products to control halitosis and dental biofilms [5].

As for dental resins, GIC and IRM, these materials are probably the best examples of improvement of restorative materials that has contributed to the recovery of ideal anatomical form and function with less removal of tooth structure. The use of "fluoride-release" materials, "smart-materials" and "bio-active" materials are some desirable features that are becoming necessary in many clinical situations because minimally invasive treatment of carious lesions is much more acceptable nowadays. Probably, the first experiences to produce a useful "smart-material" were related to the concept that fluoride-releasing materials. Glass ionomer cements do not undergo great dimensional changes in a moist environment and exhibit noticeable shrinkage in a dry environment at temperatures higher than 50°C, which is similar to the behavior of dentin [37]. This is a good example of biocompatibility.

Attempts to improve GIC have been quite successful. There is one report indicating that zinc addition to GIC can decrease microorganisms growth and improve fluoride release, without significantly affecting the materials' flexural strength and solubility [38]. In another report, conventional glass ionomer cement (GIC) liner was mixed with different antibiotics such as metronidazole, ciprofloxacin and cefaclor to produce an antibacterial GIC. After an *in vitro* evaluation of infected dentin sealed with this product, there was a 98.6% decrease in micro-organisms, bacterial aggregates, and intertubular dentin with exposed collagen fibers and dentinal tubules [41]. When conventional GIC was added with 1.5, 3.0 and 4.5% of ciprofloxacin, metronidazole and minocycline this material was effective for inhibiting *S. mutans* and *L. casei*, and the addition of a 1.5% antibiotic mixture was optimal to provide appropriate physical and bonding properties [39]. For more than a decade, several reports in the literature has been demonstrating antibacterial activity against *S. mutans*, *S. oralis*, *S. salivarius* and Streptococcus sp when GIC are reinforced with antimicrobials or due to fluoride or pH equilibrium [7, 40-44]. It has been claimed that GIC has the ability to increase pH and this is likely to be an important mechanism of caries protection under clinical conditions since oral bacteria can produce lactic acid [43].

The resin composites have been used, frequently, as restoring material due to its great aesthetics and physiologic properties [44]. More recently, incorporation of 12-methacryloyloxydodecylpyridinium bromide, a monomer also known as MDPB showed good results for its antibacterial activity when incorporated in bonding agents [28].

However, instead of releasing an antimicrobial substance, the strategy to incorporate them to act as part of its structure is also possible. In this perspective, nanoparticles can provide good optical properties for conventional and hybrid composites [45]. However, there is still a lack of studies in the literature showing the beneficial aspects for placing such material in a dental cavity. For instance, it is still unknown how effective these materials can inhibit caries activity close to restorations when active bioparticles are incorporated into these resins [46-48]. As a general observation, it must be highlighted that there are many in vitro studies but very few clinical trials to support their use under regular clinical activity [46].

Finally, it can be stated that two main approaches can be presented when antimicrobial bioactive materials are prepared. One approach is to prepare a substance-release material (e.g. GIC). Another perspective is to incorporate the antimicrobial to be active being part of its structure without any release of active component. Basically, this latter option is of outmost importance since the release of a substance implies in loss of matter and in theoretical basis this means some loss in mechanical properties. Taking into account that GIC acts as battery charges for fluoride, it must be pointed out that "recovery" of fluoride ions does not reach original levels [47-49]. Hence, other advantages have to be operating to consider this material as a good option for dental restorations.

Another point to be considered is the fact concentrations of substances released from some dental materials such as GIC materials were not different, regardless of the amount of antimicrobial substance incorporated. Thus, as long as the antimicrobial is not interfering in the mechanical properties, an increase in the amount of antimicrobial drug will not provide additional benefits.

5. Dental restorative materials with nanoparticles

Nanoparticles are generally defined as particles that are smaller than 100 nanometers in diameter. So, in order to provide a good perspective, it can be emphasized that nanotechnology deals with structures as small as 10^{-9} m while oral bacteria reach a size of 10^{-6} m. Although there is a large difference in size, the improvements of many technologies in the 1980s made possible the combination of these two worlds. Many researchers' points out that nanotechnology has been applied for dental materials as an innovative concept for the development of materials with better properties including the anti-caries effect [5,45,49].

It is recognized that many nanoparticles do have a great antimicrobial activity, particularly if it is a metallic nanoparticles. The antimicrobial activity of many types of nanoparticle is certainly a function of their size but other features are important such as high surface area, unusual crystal morphologies (edges and corners) and reactive sites.There is a great difference of a regular metal and a 10^{-9} m particles when incorporated into dental materials. Consequently, their properties can radically change, as hardness, area of active surface, chemical reactivity and biological activity [26].

The inverse relationship between the size of some particles and its antimicrobial activity has been demonstrated for particles of up to 10 nm were tested against *Escherichia coli* [50]. Thus, this might be valid for nanoparticles as well. The main mechanism or mechanisms behind the antimicrobial activity of nanoparticles are not fully elucidated. Hence, several studies focusing on the antimicrobial activity of different metals and metallic nanoparticles against oral microorganisms have to be performed for a clear picture on this matter. Another point to be considered is the effectiveness of these nanoparticles to control the development of a biofilm. Considering that biofilms are rather organized and can avoid the penetration of big molecules (e.g. chlorhexidine) the small size of these particles can be advantageous. However, so far these particles have been introduced into prosthetic devices coatings and oral care products. The strategy for placing them within dental materials is currently being explored in vitro and more research is needed to consider their regular use in the dental clinic.

Basically, the most promising nanoparticles are: silver, zinc oxide, calcium-phosphates [5]. Nevertheless, is must be also known that an interesting systematic map demonstrated that there is currently a limited amount of information concerning the release of nanoparticles from polymer-based dental materials. After reviewing 140 full-text articles on this matter, only 3 were regarded as methodological sound. Actually, a passive release of nanoparticles from a polymer-based dental material was not observed by the investigated reports. [51]. Table 1 summarizes some important features of these materials when present within dental materials.

Nanoparticles	Observations	References
Silver	• It may provoke structural changes and damage bacterial membranes, resulting in cell death. • Incorporated into dental adhesives could reduce *S. mutans* close to orthodontic brackets. • Concentrations of 0.5-1% provided antimicrobial activity with preservation of aesthetic and mechanical properties of dental materials (resin composites). • Future research must focus on silver-biofilm interaction and silver-polimerization processes of dental materials.	[5,26,49, 52-59]
Zinc oxide	• The mechanism of action may be attributed to oxidative stress by H_2O_2 and structural changes in cell wall. • Incorporated into dental materials ZnO may release Zn^{2+} which interferes in sucrose metabolism and magnesium depletion that is important for biofilm equilibrium. • Future research must focus on the determination of ideal concentrations of nanoparticles in order to have antimicrobial activity without compromising mechanical properties of the materials.	[5,26,49, 58, 60, 61]
Quaternary Ammonium	• This compound was selected due to its good antimicrobial activity and because it can be copolymerized with other monomers providing a strong bonding system with the material. However, difficulties in controlling the release of such agents may be a potential drawback. • The hydrophobic nature and positive charge of these nanoparticles may enhance the antimicrobial activity. • Future research must focus on kinetics to optimize the release characteristics.	[5,26,63-65]
Calcium-phosphates	• These compounds can interfere on adherence and growth of *Streptococcus mutans*. • The resin composites with these nanoparticles can increase up to four times the capacity of remineralization of the enamel in comparison with the composites with fluoride. • Hydroxyapatite nanocrystals may interact with bacterial adhesins and can reduce bacterial adherence to dental surfaces. • Future research must focus on efficacy of products that are already available in the market such as casein phosphopeptide (CPP)-amorphous and calcium phosphate (ACP) nanocomplex.	[5,26,66-71]

Table 1. Observations and conclusions related to nanoparticles incorporated into dental materials.

6. Final considerations

The oral environment imposes difficulties when it is designed a study for evaluating dental materials [3,9,10,25]. Since 1950's it is know that microbial microleakage at the cavity wall/

material interface is a problem to restoration survival. The persistence of microorganisms underneath fillings is also recognized as a serious problem in restorative dentistry. The antibacterial properties of restorative materials can substantially influence the success of a dental filling in the oral cavity. The frequent problem is that dental materials "natural" antibacterial properties are not enough to cope with the facility of biofilm formation. Thus, the incorporation of antimicrobials in restorative materials has to take into account the properties of each dental material. For instance, restorations of glass-ionomer cements are based on an acid-base reaction between a polyacrylic acid solution and fluoroaminosilicate glass particles. This reaction yields a structure that is more stable than composites. As a result, by adhering to tooth structure the glass-ionomer cements potentially reduces microleakage. This is an important property since it can enhance fluoride release. So, why not incorporating antibiotics as well? Hence, glass ionomer cements are strong candidates to have antimicrobials incorporated as long as it does not disturb the acid-base reaction. On the other hand, resin composites are much better materials considering aesthetic properties. Finally, coatings killing bacteria upon contact seems to be more promising than antimicrobial-releasing coatings. However, many in vitro studies cannot support the findings that are observed *in vivo*. This observation suggests that more clinical research is needed to clarify this issue. Hence, clinical research on this topic is of outmost relevance for minimum intervention restorative techniques in dentistry and for promoting oral health. Another point to consider is the challenge for the future dental materials with antimicrobials properties: to develop even more effective materials that are able to improve clinical antimicrobial efficacy while still preserving the benefits of the normal, resident oral microflora.

Author details

J.M.F.A. Fernandes[1], V.A. Menezes[1], A.J.R. Albuquerque[2], M.A.C. Oliveira[3], K.M.S. Meira[3], R.A. Menezes Júnior[4] and F.C. Sampaio[2,3*]

*Address all correspondence to: fcsampa@gmail.com

1 Post-graduation in Pediatric Dentistry, Faculty of Dentistry, University of Pernambuco, Camaragibe, Pernambuco, Brazil

2 RENORBIO, Northeast Network of Biotechnology, Federal University of Paraiba, Biotechnology Centre, Campus I, Joao Pessoa, Paraiba, Brazil

3 Post-graduation in Dentistry, Health Science Center, University of Paraíba, João Pessoa, Paraíba, Brazil

4 Alternative and Renewable Energy Center, Department of Renewable Energy Engineering, Federal University of Paraíba, João Pessoa, Paraíba, Brazil

References

[1] Gharechahi M, Moosavi H, Forghani M. Effect of surface roughness and materials composition on biofilm formation. JBNB 2012; 3:541-6.

[2] Marsh PD. Contemporary perspective on plaque control. Br Dent J 2012; 22:601-6

[3] Marsh PD, Martin M. Oral microbiology, 5th ed. Oxford, UK: Churchill; Livingstone; 2009.

[4] Fejerskov O, Kidd E. Dental caries: the disease and its clinical management. 2nd ed. Oxford, UK: Blackwell Munksgaard; 2011.

[5] Allaker RP. The use of nanoparticles to control oral biofilm formation. J Dent Res 2010; 89:1175–86.

[6] von der Fehr FR, Löe H, Theilade E. Experimental caries in man. Caries Res 1970; 4:131-48.

[7] Naik S, Sureshchandra B. Antimicrobial efficacy of glass ionomers, composite resin, liners & polycarboxylates against selected stock culture microorganisms: an in vitro study. Endodontology 2012; 24(2):21-8.

[8] Selwitz RH, Ismail AI, Pitts NB. Dental caries. Lancet 2007; 369:51-9.

[9] Marsh PD. Dental plaque: biological significance of a biofilm and community lifestyle. J Clin Periodontol 2005; 32:7–15.

[10] Fine DH, Markowitz K, Furgang D, Goldsmith D, Ricci-Nittel D, Charles CH, et al. Effect of rinsing with an essential oil-containing mouthrinse on subgingival periodontopathogens. J Periodontol 2007; 78:1935–42.

[11] Zobell CE. The effect of solid surfaces upon bacterial activity. J Bacteriol 1943; 46:39-56.

[12] Costerton JW, Stewart PS, Greenberg EP. Bacterial biofilms: a common cause of persistent infections. Science 1999; 284:1318-22.

[13] Tuson HH, Weibel DB. Bacteria–surface interactions. Soft Matter 2013; 9:4368-80.

[14] Renner LD, Weibel DB. Physicochemical regulation of biofilm formation. MRS Bull 2011 May; 36(5):347-55.

[15] Petersen FC, Tao L, Scheie AA. DNA binding-uptake system: a link between cell-to-cell communication and biofilm formation. J. Bacteriol 2005; 187:4392.

[16] Witchurch CB, Tolker-Nielsen T, Ragas PC, Mattick JS. Extracellular DNA required for bacterial biofilm formation. Science 2002; 295:1487.

[17] Bowen WH, Koo H. Biology of Streptococcus mutans-Derived Glucosyltransferases: Role in Extracellular Matrix Formation of Cariogenic Biofilms. Caries Research 2011; 45:69-86.

[18] Lembre P, Lorentz C, Di Martino P. Exopolysaccharides of the Biofilm Matrix: A Complex Biophysical World. In: Karunaratne DN. (ed). The Complex World of Polysaccharides. Rijeka: InTech; 2012. p371-392. Available from http://www.intechopen.com/books/the-complex-world-of-polysaccharides/exopolysaccharides-of-the-biofilm-matrix-a-complex-biophysical-world (accessed 27 August 2014).

[19] Palmer RJ. Oral bacterial biofilms–history in progress. Microbiology 2009; 155:2113-4.

[20] Mikkelsen H, Duck Z, Lilley KS, Welch M. Interrelationships between colonies, biofilms, and planktonic cells of *Pseudomonas aeruginosa*. J Bacteriol. 2007; 189(6): 2411-6.

[21] Renye JA, Piggot PJ, Daneo-Moore L, Buttaro BA. Persistence of Streptococcus mutans in Stationary-Phase Batch Cultures and Biofilms, Applied Environm Microbiol 2004; 70(10):6181-7.

[22] Guggenheim B, Giertsen E, Schüpbach P, Shapiro S. Validation of an *in vitro* biofilm model of supragingival plaque. J Dent Res. 2001; 80(1):363-70.

[23] Netuschil L, Auschill TM, Sculean A, Arweiler NB. Confusion over live/dead stainings for the detection of vital microorganisms in oral biofilms-which stain is suitable? BMC Oral Health 2014; 14:2.

[24] Teughels W, Van Assche N, Sliepen I, Quirynen M. Effect of material characteristics and/or surface topography on biofilm development. Clin Oral Implants Res 2006; 17(2):68-81.

[25] Busscher HJ, Rinastiti M, Siswomihardjo W, van der Mei HC. Biofilm formation on dental restorative and implant materials. J Dent Res 2010; 89(7):657-65.

[26] Allaker RP, Ren G. Potential impact of nanotechnology in the control of infectious diseases. Trans R Soc Trop Med Hyg 2008; 102:1-2.

[27] Pinheiro SL, Simionato MR, Imparato JC, Oda M. Antibacterial activity of glass-ionomer cement containing antibiotics on caries lesion. Am J Dent 2005; 18(4):261-6.

[28] Imazato S. Bio-active restorative materials with antibacterial effects: new dimension of innovation in restorative dentistry. Dental Materials J. 2009; 28(1):11-19.

[29] Auschill TM, Arweiler NB, Brecx M, Reich E, Sculean A, Netuschil L: The effect of dental restorative materials on dental biofilm. Eur J Oral Sci. 2002; 110:48-53.

[30] Chen M. Novel strategies for the prevention and treatment of biofilm related infections. Int J Mol Sci 2013; 14(9):18488-501.

[31] Lin CL, Chang CH, Wang CH, Ko CC, Lee HE. Numerical investigation of the factors affecting interfacial stresses in an MOD restored tooth by auto-meshed finite element method. J Oral Rehabil 2001; 28:517-25.

[32] Toparli M, Gokay N, Aksoy T. Analysis of a restored maxillary second premolar tooth by using three-dimensional finite element method. J Oral Rehabil 1999; 26:157-64.

[33] Farah JW, Craig RG. Finite element stress analysis of restored axisymmetric first molar. J Dent Res 1974; 53:859-66.

[34] Williams KR, Edmundson JT, Rees JS. Finite element stress analysis of restored teeth. Dent Mater 1987; 3:200-6.

[35] Noort R. Introduction to dental materials. 4th ed. Edinburgh; New York: Mosby Elsevier, 2013.

[36] Giertsen E. Effects of mouthrinses with triclosan, zinc ions, copolymer, and sodium lauryl sulphate combined with fluoride on acid formation by dental plaque in vivo. Caries Res 2004; 38(5):430-5.

[37] Khoroushi M, Keshani F. A review of glass-ionomers: From conventional glass-ionomer to bioactive glass-ionomer. Dent Res J. 2013; 10(4): 411-20.

[38] Osinaga PW, Grande RH, Ballester RY, Simionato MR, Delgado Rodrigues CR, Muench A. Zinc sulfate addition to glass-ionomer-based cements: Influence on physical and antibacterial properties, zinc and fluoride release. Dent Mater. 2003; 19:212–7

[39] Yesilyurt C, Er K, Tasdemir T, Buruk K, Celik D. Antibacterial activity and physical properties of glass-ionomer cements containing antibiotics. Oper Dent 2009; 1:18-23.

[40] Nakajo K, Imazato S, Takahashi Y, Kiba W, Ebisu S, Takahashi N. Fluoride Released from Glass-Ionomer Cement Is Responsible to Inhibit the Acid Production of Caries-Related Oral Streptococci. Dental Materials 2009; 25(6):703-8.

[41] Ferreira JMS, Pinheiro SL, Sampaio FC, Menezes VA. Use of glassionomer cement containing antibiotics to seal off infected dentin: a randomized clinical trial. Brazilian Dental Journal. 2013; 24(1):68-73.

[42] Jedrychowski JR, Caputo AA, Kerper S. Antibacterial and mechanical properties of restorative materials combined with chlorhexidines. J Oral Rehabil 1983; 10:373-381.

[43] Nicholson JW, Aggarwal A, Czarnecka B, Li-manowska-Shaw H. The rate of change of pH of lactic acid exposed to glass-ionomer dental cements. Biomaterials 2000; 21(19):1989-93.

[44] Konradsson K. Influence of a dental ceramic and a calcium aluminate cement on dental biofilm formation and gingival inflammatory response. Dissertation (Master Degree in Odontology). Umeå University, Sweden; 2007.

[45] Hamouda IM. Current perspectives of nanoparticles in medical and dental biomaterials. J Biomed Res 2012;26:143–151. http://www.readcube.com/articles/10.7555/JBR.26.20120027 (accessed 02 September 2014).

[46] Luna DMN, Andrade CAS. Nanotecnologia aplicada à odontologia. Int J Dent 2011; 10(3):161-8.

[47] Weng Y, Guo X, Gregory R, Xie D. A novel antibacterial dental glassionomer cement. Eur J Oral Sci 2010; 118:531-4.

[48] Frencken J, Pilot T, Songpaisan Y, Phantumvanit P. Atraumatic restorative treatment (ART): rationale, technique, and development. J Public Health Dent 1996; 56:135-40.

[49] Melo MAS, Guedes SFF, Xu HHK, Rodrigues LKA. Nanotechnology-based restorative materials for dental caries management. Trends Biotechnol 2013; 31(8):2-18.

[50] Verran J, Sandoval G, Allen NS, Edge M, Stratton J Variables affecting the antibacterial properties of nano and pigmentary titania particles in suspension. Dyes and Pigments. 2007; 73:298-304.

[51] Rehnman J. Release of nanoparticles from dental materials. A systematic map. Socialstyrelsen: Nordic Institute of Dental Materials. 2013.

[52] Sotiriou GA, Pratsinis SE. Antibacterial activity of nanosilver ions and particles. Environ Sci Technol 2010; 44:5649-54.

[53] Peng JJ, et al. Silver compounds used in dentistry for caries management: a review. J Dent 2012; 40:531-41.

[54] Chaloupka K, Malam Y, Seifalian AM. Nanosilver as a new generation of nanoproduct in biomedical applications. Trends Biotechnol Nov 2010; 28(11):580-8.

[55] Ahn SJ. Experimental antimicrobial orthodontic adhesives using nanofillers and silver nanoparticles. Dent Mater 2009; 25:206–13.

[56] Radzig MA, et al. Antibacterial effects of silver nanoparticles on gram-negative bacteria: Influence on the growth and biofilms formation, mechanisms of action. Colloids Surf B: Biointerfaces 2013; 102:300–6.

[57] Silver S. Bacterial silver resistance: molecular biology and uses and misuses of silver compounds. FEMS Microbiol Rev 2003; 27:341-53.

[58] Cheng L, Weir MD, Xu HH, Antonucci JM, Lin NJ, Lin-Gibson S, Xu SM, Zhou X. Effect of amorphous calcium phosphate and silver nanocomposites on dental plaque microcosm biofilms. J Biomed Mater Res B: Appl Biomater 2012; 100:1378-86.

[59] Espinosa-Cristóbal LF. Antimicrobial sensibility of Streptococcus mutans serotypes to silver nanoparticles. Mater Sci Eng C 2012; 32:896–901.

[60] Jones N, et al. Antibacterial activity of ZnO nanoparticle suspensions on a broad spectrum of microorganisms. FEMS Microbiol Lett 2008; 279:71-6.

[61] Gu H, et al. Effect of ZnCl₂ on plaque growth and biofilm vitality. Arch Oral Biol 2012; 57:369-75.

[62] Vaidyanathan M, et al. Antimicrobial properties of dentine bonding agents deter-mined using *in vitro* and *ex vivo* methods. J Dent 2009; 37:514-21.

[63] Imazato S, et al. Antibacterial resin monomers based on quaternary ammonium and their benefits in restorative dentistry. Jpn Dent Sci Rev 2012; 48:115–25.

[64] Zhang K, et al. Effect of water-ageing on dentine bond strength and anti-biofilm ac-tivity of bonding agent containing new monomer dimethylaminododecyl methacry-late. J Dent 2013; 41:504-13.

[65] Cheng L, Weir MD, Xu HHK, Antonucci JM, Kraigsley AM, Lin NJ, Lin-Gibson S, Zhou X. Antibacterial amorphous calcium phosphate nanocomposites with a quater-nary ammonium dimethacrylate and silver nanoparticles. Dent Mater 2012; 28:561-72.

[66] Xu HHK, Moreau JL, Sun L, Chow LC. Strength and fluoride release characteristics of a calcium fluoride based dental nanocomposite. Biomaterials Nov 2008; 9(32): 4261-7.

[67] Moreau JL, Sun L, Chow LC, Xu HHK. Mechanical and acid neutralizing properties and bacteria inhibition of amorphous calcium phosphate dental nanocomposite. J Bi-omed Mater Res B Appl Biomater Jul 2011; 98(1):80-8.

[68] Hannig C, Hannig M. Natural enamel wear: a physiological source of hydroxylapa-tite nanoparticles for biofilm management and tooth repair? Medical Hypothese. 2010; 74:670-2.

[69] Venegas SC, Palacios JM, Apella MC, Morando PJ, Blesa MA. Calcium modulates in-teractions between bacteria and hydroxyapatite. J Dent Res 2006; 85:1124-8.

[70] Arcís RW, López-Macipe A, Toledano M, Osorio E, Rodríguez-Clemente R, Murtra J, Fanovich MA, Pascual CD. Mechanical properties of visible light-cured resins rein-forced with hydroxyapatite for dental restoration. Dent Mater Jan 2002; 18(1):49-57.

[71] Chen M. Novel strategies for the prevention and treatment of biofilm related infec-tions. Int J Mol Sci 2013; 14(9):18488-501.

Chapter 4

Are the Approximal Caries Lesions in Primary Teeth a Challenge to Deal With? — A Critical Appraisal of Recent Evidences in This Field

Mariana Minatel Braga, Isabela Floriano, Fernanda Rosche Ferreira,
Juliana Mattos Silveira, Alessandra Reyes, Tamara Kerber Tedesco,
Daniela Prócida Raggio, José Carlos Pettorossi Imparato and
Fausto Medeiros Mendes

Additional information is available at the end of the chapter

http://dx.doi.org/10.5772/59600

1. Introduction

Approximal surfaces have been pointed as a challenge regarding the control of caries lesions in primary teeth, specially due to the larger area of contact between adjacent teeth and limited salivary access [1, 2]. In addition, children can present less dexterity to using dental floss and depend on parent's collaboration to remove interproximal dental plaque [3]. Therefore, poor compliance to flossing by children [4] seems to contribute to make the arrestment of approximal caries lesions more difficult. Consequently, identifying and understanding attitudes towards flossing are very important tasks to aid health professionals for flossing orientation and its incentive [4].

Several evidences have been published recently as promising alternatives in order to deal with approximal caries lesion in primary teeth and minimize the effects of poor compliance with flossing and/or repair eventual irreversible dental decay caused by caries progression.

Minimally invasive interventions have been proposed to caries lesion management, comprising early detection, preventive procedures and minimal invasion [5]. This approach also proposes to minimize the discomfort of patient [6], specially to deal with pediatric patients' dental anxiety and fear [7]. However, even considering minimal invasive treatments, there are operational differences among them that could interfere on children's discomfort and acceptability. Indeed, when exploring options for dental treatment, not only the efficacy/effectiveness

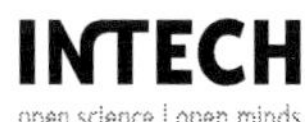

but also the cost-efficacy/effectiveness and the patient's discomfort/satisfaction should also be comparatively investigated for available approaches.

Based on the exposed above, this chapter aims to present the particularities of dealing with approximal caries lesions and make a critical appraisal concerning effectiveness/efficacy, applicability, utility and clinical relevance of recent published studies and their findings. In this way, we expect to permit the clinicians to choose the best option for treating initial and advanced approximal caries lesions in primary teeth basing your decision-making process on relevant scientific evidences.

2. Approximal caries

Caries lesions (clinical signs of the disease) are developed on the biofilm-tooth interface [8-10] and the key factor of their formation is the presence acid-producing biofilm of the tooth surface [11]. Usually, minerals from oral fluids and tooth are in balance. However, when a tooth surface has biofilm accumulated for some period, changes in pH occur, caused by biofilm bacterial metabolism [8]. These pH fluctuations at biofilm-tooth interface may cause tooth mineral loss when the pH is decreasing (demineralization) or mineral gain when the pH is increasing (remineralization) [12]. When there is a prevalence of demineralization over remineralization, mineral loss is observed and this leads to a caries lesion [8, 13]. Thus, caries lesions start with mineral loss from the tooth surface and, if the biofilm is not removed, they progress until cavitation and tooth destruction.

Considering that the demineralization/remineralization processes occur on the biofilm-tooth interface, special attention should be given to the main biofilm stagnation areas, as occlusal surfaces, approximal surfaces and smooth surfaces along the gingival margin. These areas are relatively protected from mechanical wear by tongue, cheeks, abrasive food, and toothbrushing [13].

Since mechanical removal of the stagnated biofilm does not occur, the lactic acid produced by this biofilm acts on enamel and may cause demineralization. As the enamel is constituted by hydroxyapatite crystals, separated from each other by small intercrystalline spaces filled with water and organic material [14], the mineral loss due to caries results on an increase of these intercrystalline spaces, increasing the enamel porosity [15]. The mineral loss is higher in the subsurface of caries lesions and the surface layer thickness of the lesions ranged from 35 to 130 μm. The maximum mineral content in this layer corresponds to 74% to 100% of that of sound enamel [16]. This histopathological process is observed clinically as the formation of white spot lesions. The mentioned mineral loss results in the loss of translucence of the enamel and the opaque appearance of the white-spot lesion [17]. On the approximal surfaces, these lesions developed between the contact point and the gingival margin, resulting in a kidney-shaped white spot lesion (Figure 1). This area is the one most prone to biofilm accumulation on approximal surfaces (Figure 2).

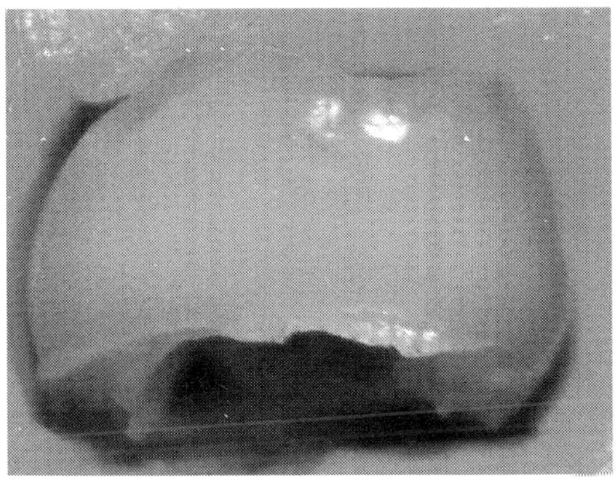

Figure 1. Approximal caries lesions. Note the shape of this lesion, located contouring the contact point, which is the area where the biofilm usually stagnates

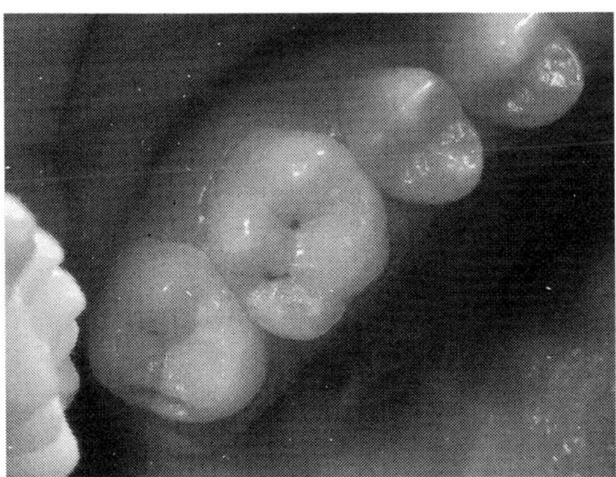

Figure 2. Biofilm accumulation on approximal surfaces. Note other dental surfaces are clean, but the biofilm remains stagnated in approximal areas.

The progression of enamel caries takes place along the enamel prisms, and in the approximal surfaces results on a conical shape [18] (Figure 3 and 4). If the plaque stagnation on caries lesions does not succeed, the lesion may reach the dentinoenamel junction and progress into the dentin [11] (Figure 3). The progression of an enamel lesion into dentine in primary teeth is faster than the observed in permanent ones [19].

There is no consensus in the literature about how does the progression of caries lesions when it reaches the dentinoenamel junction [11, 20]. Nevertheless, it is known that in lesions that reach the dentinoenamel junction, demineralized dentine is present, as part of the progression of enamel lesions [21]. On the other hand, the level of bacterial invasion is very low [22], especially because there is no cavitation. Therefore, it is expected a lower progression compared to cavitated lesions [23]. As dentine is composed of about 50% of mineral [24], caries progression into dentine tends to be faster than in enamel. As the less demineralized areas are the intertubular dentin composed of a matrix of collagen reinforced by apatite, the demineralization process tends to follow the direction of dentine tubules, resulting in the typical histology of dentine caries lesions, as you can see in Figure 3.

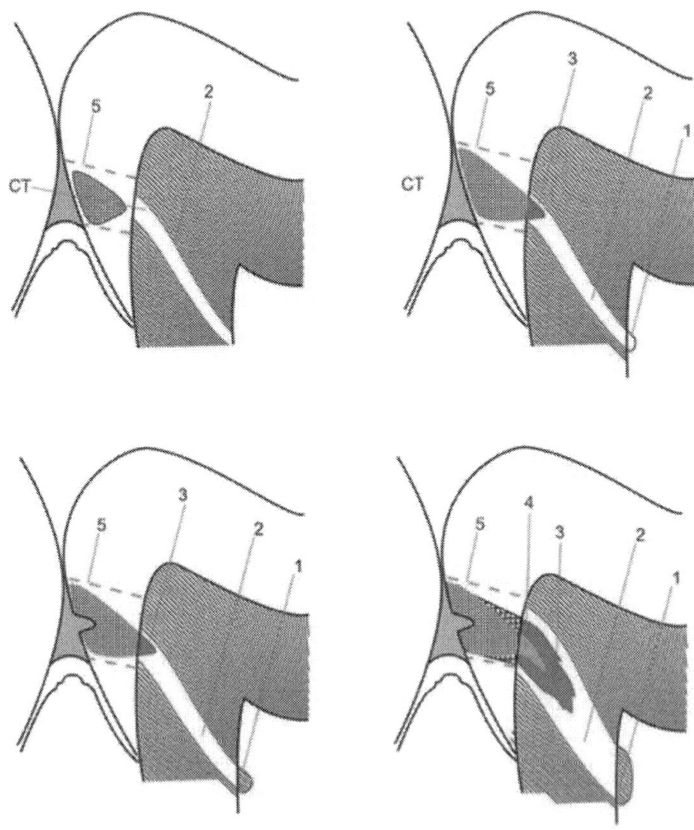

Figure 3. Schematic diagram of approximal caries progression. Different numbers symbolize different areas observed during caries lesion progression. (1- tertiary or reparative dentine, 2 - dentine tubules, 3- affected layer of carious dentine, 4-infected layer of carious dentine 5- enamel lesion) - adapated from Fejerskov et al., 2008 [14].

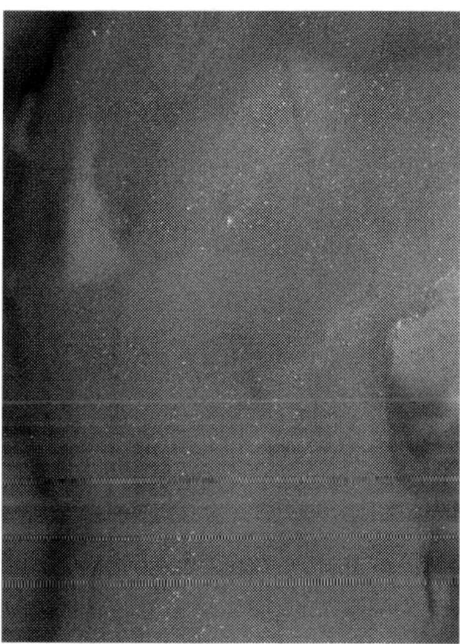

Figure 4. Histological exam of an enamel caries lesion. Note its conical shape, since progression follows the interprismatic spaces.

Substantial demineralization into dentin may be observed despite the absence of cavitation [25]. Nevertheless, if caries lesion progresses continuously into dentine, demineralized enamel may collapse and the intact surface may become cavitated. Thus, bacterial invasion into enamel and proteolytic action of bacterial enzymes mainly on the collagen may occur. If the biofilm stagnation is not controlled, an increase of the cavity size and further biofilm invasion could be expected [26]. When the cavity is present, a most infected dentine could be expected [23], which contribute to faster caries progression.

Two altered zones of dentine could be found in a dentine caries lesion: a superficial infected and a deeper affected layer [27] (Figure 3). The infected dentine consists of irreversibly acid-demineralized dentine, with its collagen degraded and highly contaminated with bacteria [28]. The affected dentine is only minimally infected and has potential to repair under suitable conditions, since their collage structure is maintained [29, 30]. Clinically, the main difference between these zones is the consistency due to the amount of collagen degradation observed in each one. The infected dentine tends to be soft and easily removed with excavators, while the affected dentine is usually harder [29] (Figure 5).

Since the progression of caries lesions is slow, the dentine may react in order to minimize the chance of occurrence of pulp exposition/inflammation. Therefore, highly mineralized peri-tubular dentin is secreted and reduces the tubules diameter, decreasing the dentine permeability and the chance for bacterial contamination [11]. This reaction is usually started since the caries lesion reaches the dentinoenamel junction. However, even considering the slow progression of caries lesions and pulp mechanisms for preventing pulp damage, it is not always possible to avoid the pulp exposure. When the reaction takes time to succeed, this

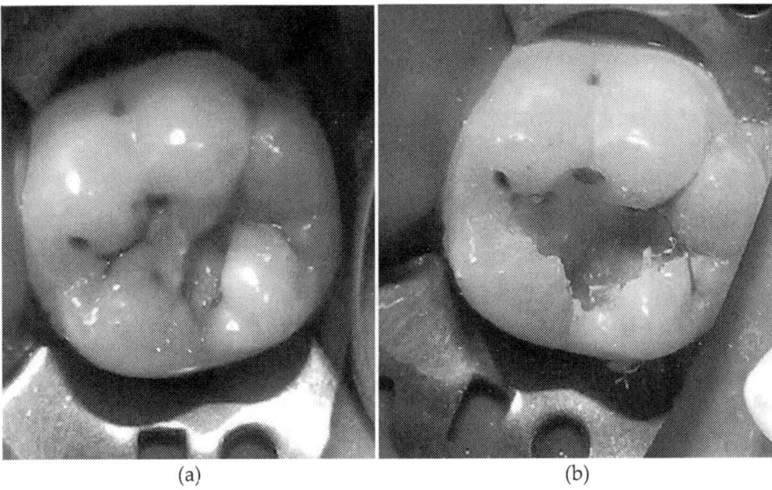

(a)   (b)

Figure 5. Clinical aspect of infected (a) and affected dentine (b) in dentine caries lesion.

highly mineralized dentine (Figure 6), also called as sclerotic dentine [31], is found in the bottom of the cavities, showing a hard consistency and usually a darker coloration.

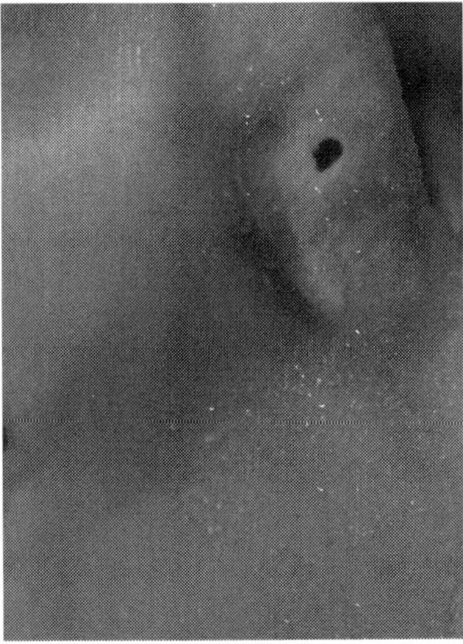

Figure 6. Histological appearance of sclerotic dentine. Note the different appearance of dentine, evidencing the hyper-mineralization of peritubular dentine.

Despite the stage of caries lesion, the presence of biofilm at the tooth surface determines caries progression [32]. Since this biofilm may be controlled, the lesion may be arrested. Therefore, both for non-cavitated and cavitated lesions, the inactivation of caries lesions would be possible, when the control of the biofilm is possible [33]. Since the biofilm control is achieved, the redeposition of mineral is facilitated. This mineral gain tend to reduce enamel porosities [34, 35]. Therefore, active lesions generally exhibits a more porous surface layer than the inactive lesions [16]. In addition, the surface wear/polishing may occur and differences in enamel surface roughness may occur [34, 35]. Due to that, active and inactive lesions tend to be different due to enamel porosity and surfaces wear/polishing (Figure 7). Besides, dentine caries may also be arrested. In these cases, there is an increase in the mineral content in the surface layer of the dentine lesions. The arrested dentine caries lesion presents more mineralized dentine, the surface is not always infected surface layer and may present sclerotic, harder

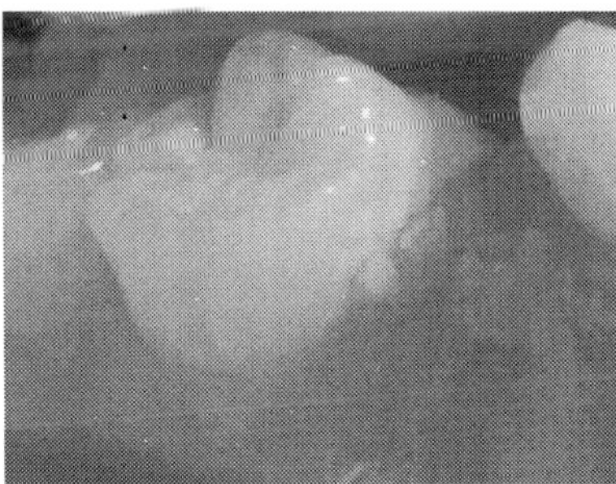

Figure 7. Active enamel caries on mesial surface of a second primary molar. Note characteristics usually associated with active lesions caused by biofilm stagnation in this area. Despite the absence of the adjacent primary molar, note the remained fragments that make the plaque removal and lesion arrestment more difficult.

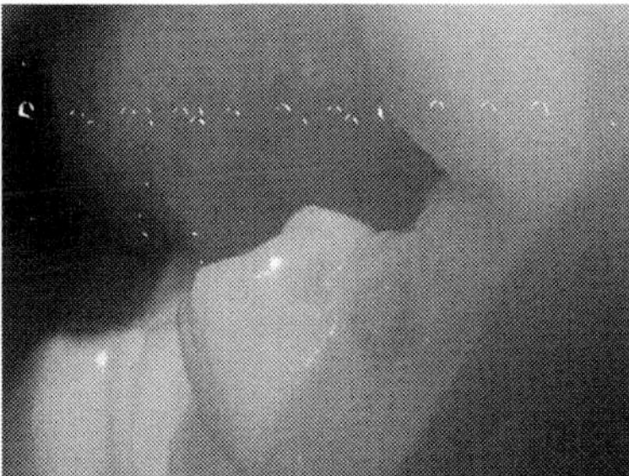

Figure 8. Active dentine caries on mesial surface of a second primary molar. Note characteristics usually associated with active lesions caused by biofilm stagnation in this area. Despite the absence of the adjacent primary molar, which will permit the mechanical control of local biofilm, this lesion did not have time enough to arrest. In this situation (absence of the adjacent tooth), this lesion tend to be arrested. That is why the picture still evidences characteristics of a dentine active lesion.

consistency and, usually, dark colour [36] (Figure 8). Changes observed in inactive dentine lesions may be detected after 6 months. However, hard consistency is usually observed after total arrestment of the lesion, which generally takes years [36].On the other hand, it is worth to state that due to difficulties in controlling the biofilm on approximal lesions, few assessed lesions present the characteristic above, as we are going to discuss in further sections of this chapter (Figures 7 and 8).

3. The challenge: Controlling approximal caries lesions

Approximal surfaces of primary molars present some particularities that expose them to a greater risk of developing caries [1, 37], and, consequently, it is a challenge when controlling caries lesion is needed.

Firstly, approximal surfaces in primary teeth present a large area of contact between them, favoring stagnation of carbohydrates and hindering biofilm removing [1, 2]. Moreover, the salivary access is limited, which contributes to further reduction of the biofilm pH compared to more accessible surfaces, promoting a more acidogenic environment and propitious to the development of caries lesions [1]. In addition, the limited salivary access reduces the exposition of these surfaces to fluorides.

Despite young children usually present wider approximal spaces [38], in most children, the anatomical conditions do not allow that approximal surfaces are cleaned only with brushing, requiring the use of dental floss to remove the biofilm. Besides, the patients' adherence to using dental floss seems to be low [39], mainly regarding children, since they could present less dexterity to flossing and depend on parent's collaboration to remove interproximal biofilm [3, 40]. In fact, a systematic review showed that interproximal caries risk decrease when children's flossing is performed by professional. However, authors suggest these findings cannot be extrapolated, since flossing has only failed when used by the children by themselves [41]. A recent study of our group showed motivational issues are more associated with non compliance with flossing by children (Figure 9).

The challenge becomes even greater when the initial lesion progresses to cavitated lesion (Figure 10). In addition, the biofilm accumulates inside the lesion and it is not possible to be removed by flossing. Consequently, the dentine inside this cavity tend to become more infected [23] and caries progression is faster. Indeed, the inactivation of cavitated lesions (only by self-removal of biofilm) is usually more observed in smooth or occlusal surfaces. We usually observe that in very small cavities or very large decays, for example. On approximal surfaces, most cavitated caries lesions hardly ever present favorable conditions to be arrested (Figure 10).

For all these reasons the approximal surfaces of primary molars are the most affected by caries lesions in some populations [1, 42]. Even in regions where this is not occurring, controlling interproximal caries lesions is still a challenge, especially due to the difficulty of the mechanical control of biofilm on such surfaces. That is why many approximal lesions are active lesions,

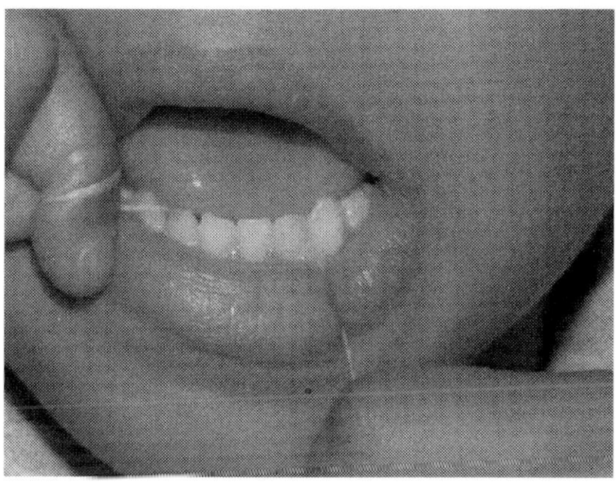

Figure 9. Child using dental floss. Sometimes, children present difficulties in dexterity for flossing. However, motivation is often the biggest problem.

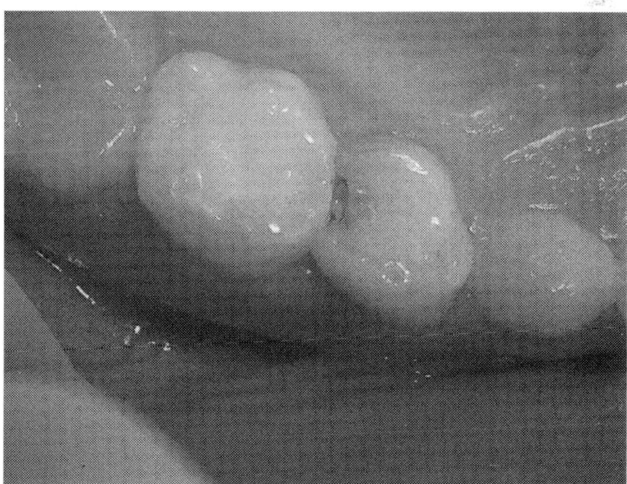

Figure 10. Cavitated lesion on distal surface of the first primary molar. Note the plaque stagnation inside the cavity, which makes difficult the control of such lesions.

although other surfaces have presented higher rates of caries progression [43]. In fact, smooth surfaces are cleaned easily [43] and lesions are easier to be controlled [44]. Besides, the occlusal surfaces, despite their morphology, are favored by the attrition [43]. In the Figure 2, it is possible to notice the remained biofilm on approximal surface, despite presenting smooth and occlusal surfaces with absence of visible plaque, complicating the control of approximal caries, even in initial stages.

Rates ranging from 70% to 90% of approximal caries progression have been shown for primary teeth after 1 or 2-year-follow-up [45, 46]. These figures have been superior to rates found for permanent teeth [47], that is comprehensible since a faster progression is expected in these teeth [48].

Based on the rationale detailed above, it is evident that controlling approximal caries lesions is really an actual challenge in pediatric clinic. Further, we will discuss about important aspects concerning detection and management of approximal caries lesions in primary teeth.

4. How may approximal caries be accurately detected? — Difficulties and important aspects

Detection of approximal caries lesions has not been a simple task. The simplest and most accepted method for caries detection among children is the visual inspection [49]. On the other hand, it is obvious that the contact between adjacent teeth makes caries detection by visual inspection more difficult. Ideally, approximal surfaces should be examined after cleaning by dental floss (Figure 11). When assessing approximal surfaces looking for caries lesions, it is important to examine, firstly, by an occlusal view. In this view, the dentist will observe the integrity and appearance of the marginal ridge. If a caries lesion is present (usually more advanced ones), cavities (Figure 10) or shadows (Figure 12) may be seen in this area. Further, the surface should be examined by buccal and lingual/palatal view. If caries lesion reaches these areas, it may be also detected by visual inspection (Figure 13). The direct examination of this surface is rare and may only occur when the adjacent tooth is not present (Figure 14).

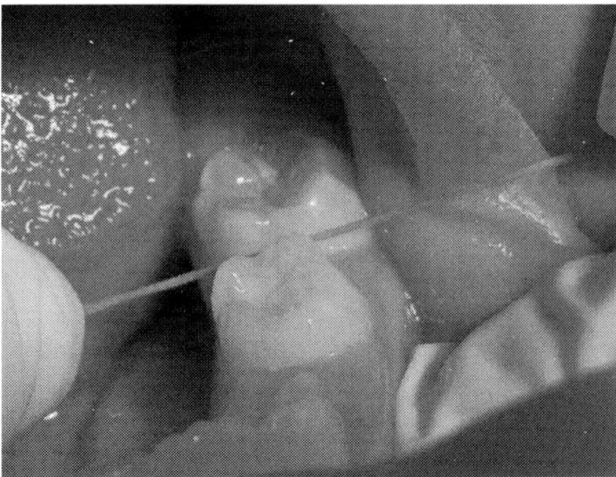

Figure 11. Cleaning the approximal surface before visual examination – note the use of dental floss.

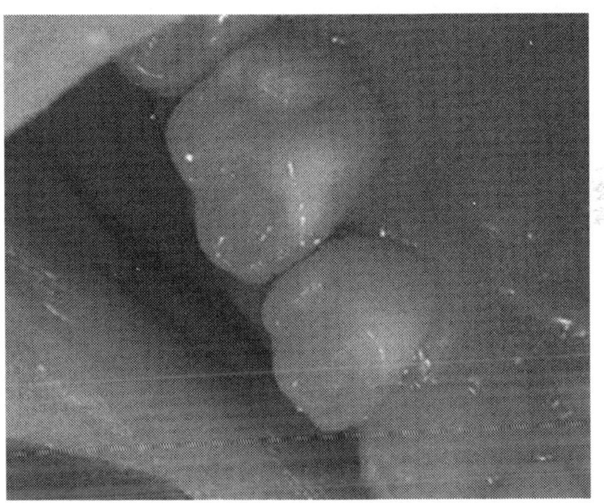

Figure 12. Approximal caries lesion evidenced by the shadow we can see above the marginal bridge.

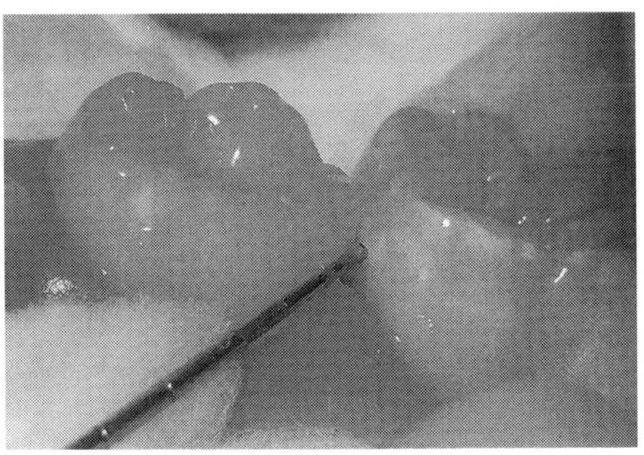

Figure 13. Buccal view – lesion may be detected since is extended from mesial into buccal surface.

The visual inspection using a scoring visual system has shown high specificity in caries detection on approximal surfaces [50]. However, lower values of sensitivity should be expected [50]. In other words, most part of non-cavitated approximal caries, as well other several cavitated lesions, cannot be detected when visual inspection is used. Radiographs have shown to increase the sensitivity of caries detection [50, 51]. On the other hand, although some clinical guidelines have recommend taking bitewing radiographs in all children to detect caries lesions in primary molars[52], its utility has been recently questioned, since no additional benefit was observed in comparison to only the visual inspection being performed [53].

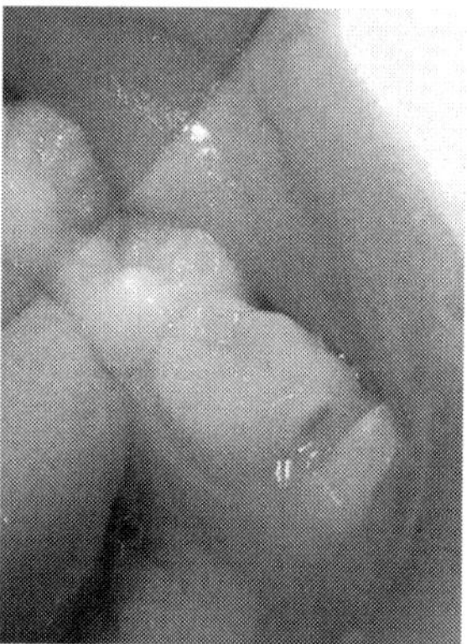

Figure 14. Direct examination of an approximal caries lesion due to the absence of the adjacent tooth.

Actually, using only visual inspection may lead to higher number of false negatives (some non-evident lesions may be missed). However, these lesions may be arrested by preventive measurements. On the other hand, the radiographs may result in higher number of false positive results, what may be worse, since it might lead to unnecessary operative treatment [53]. In addition, several non-cavitated lesions may have the radiographic appearance of a cavitated lesion (Figure 15). As a consequence of radiographic examination, they might receive unnecessary operative treatment. Weighing the pros and cons of bitewing radiographs for caries detection, it seems more useful to take bitewing radiographs in order to confirm the presence of approximal caries, in cases in which visual signs have been identified (instead of detecting non-evident caries) or to help the choice for the best option for treating an approximal caries [54]. In the last situation, radiographs may help in caries depth assessment and also, in evaluation of the periapical tissue [54].

The presence of cavities has been another concern regarding approximal caries detection, since the cavitation has been considered an important point in the prognosis of these caries lesions. As mentioned, some cavities are not detected by visual examination. Besides, radiographs do not aid in this issue, as exposed before. The temporary separation using orthodontic rubbers is an available alternative [55, 56], which permit the direct visual inspection and tactile examination of the approximal surfaces (Figures 15 to 17). This technique is well-accepted by children [49]. However, it is necessary two appointments to permit the conclusion of diagnostic using this method. Even visuo-tactile assessment of approximal surface is possible; doubts in diagnosis may remain. The inderdental space created after temporary separation is around 0.8 mm [38] and may not always be large enough to guarantee there is no cavity on the surface, nor to affirm the cavity is clinically within enamel. In fact, several dentine lesions are not cavitated. Other dentine lesions may may be associated with microcavities; however, without exposing the dentine. On the other hand, we believe that some cavitations which present radiographic image into dentine may be wrongly scored as cavity clinically restricted to enamel. This is why the limited space reached after teeth separation may be not enough to the

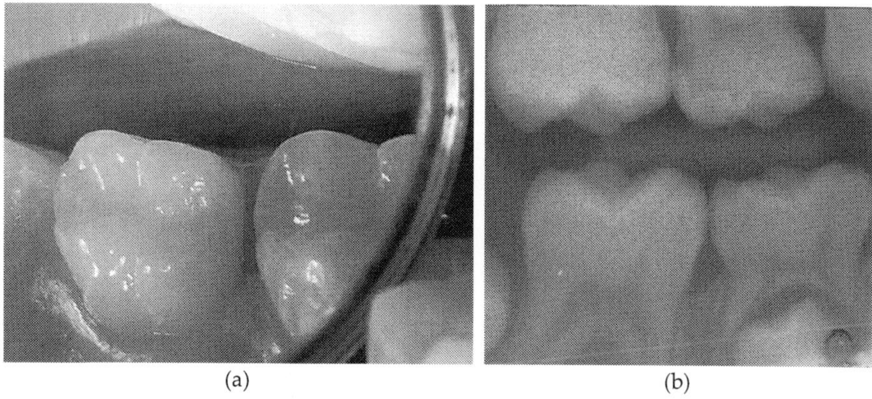

(a)   (b)

Figure 15. Direct visual inspection (a) and radiograph (b) of the same surface (distal surface of the second primary molar). Clinically, we can see a white spot on the approximal surface (absence of shadows in the marginal bridge) – (a). Radiographically, we evidence a radiolucid image suggestive of caries lesion in dentine. The image might also suggest the presence of cavity (b), that is definitely not evidenced in clinical examination (a). This case represents a false-positive result for caries in dentine that could occur in some radiographic examinations.

dentist being able to actually felt the bottom of these cavities, in order to confirm if he/she is felling enamel or dentine surface. These are limitations of this method. However, since there is no other available possibility to detect the presence of cavities, we have used the temporary separation when we suspect that a cavity is present, especially if dentine involvement is confirmed by visual signs or radiographs.

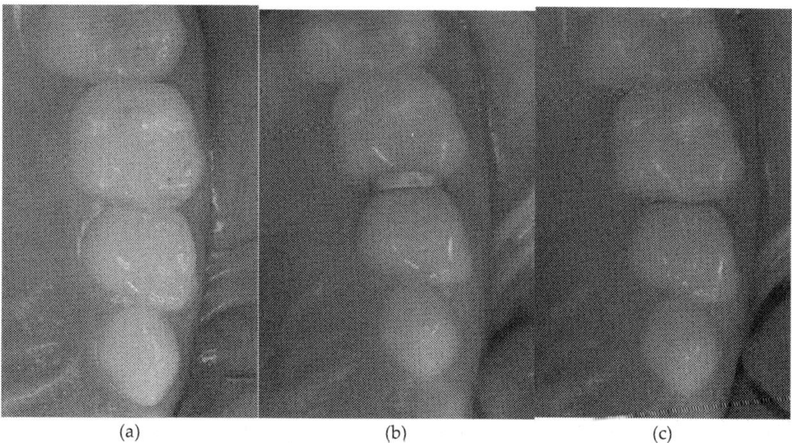

(a)   (b)   (c)

Figure 16. Temporary tooth separation using orthodontic rubbers. (a) before placing the rubber between adjacent teeth; (b) after placing the rubber; (c) after removing the rubber – note the wide space for direct examination.

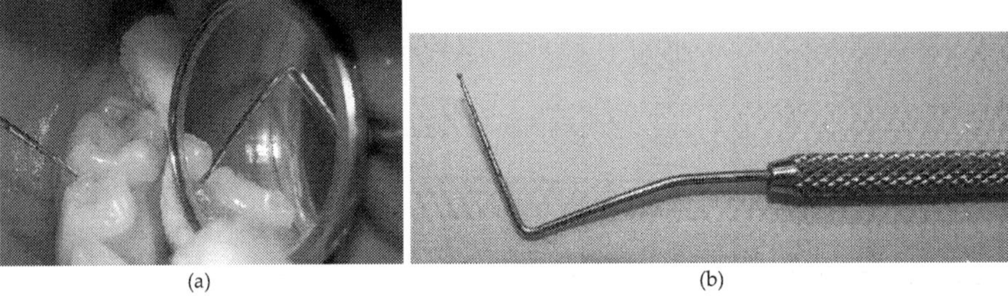

(a)   (b)

Figure 17. Temporary tooth separation using orthodontic rubbers – visual and tactile assessment of separated surfaces (a); WHO probe (ballpoint probe) used to tactile assessment of surfaces.

The activity status is not usually a differential in caries lesions assessment, especially in children. In fact, as exposed before, most part of detected approximal lesions tend to be active [43]. It is not impossible to find inactive approximal caries. However, especially among children, the interproximal plaque control is still very deficient and make the lesions arrestment more difficult. Thus, activity assessment is not a real concern in primary teeth. In some situations, when the adjacent tooth have exfoliated, we may observe a natural process of lesion inactivation of an approximal caries due to the possibility of controlling biofilm only by toothbrushing such area (see Figures 8 and 14).

5. Is it possible to control approximal caries lesions?

In theory, controlling dental caries in any surface is related to controlling of dental plaque over the lesion [32]. As the activity status of approximal caries is not usually a differential factor, we will not discuss it here. However, it is obvious that, if an approximal caries lesion is arrested, it would not demand any measure to be controlled. Considering this situation, we may guide the management of approximal caries lesions basically according to depth and severity, assessed during examination of caries lesions. The conceptual tree for managing caries lesions on approximal surfaces is presented below (Figure 18).

Non-cavitated approximal caries lesions tend to be easier to be controlled since there is no cavity to complicate biofilm removal. Besides, if these lesions are restricted to the enamel, they have a slower progression compared to dentine [45]. Therefore, several possibilities are available in order to controlling them, from the dental flossing to the use of resin infiltration.

Cavitated enamel lesions (Figure 19) are expected to progress faster than those which present intact surface. However, most part of these lesions cannot be detected clinically, neither by visual, nor by tactile assessment. If detected by tooth separation, both non-invasive and invasive treatments would be available for such cases, but there is no strong evidence of the best option in this case. Choosing the non-invasive treatment may permit to postpone invasive interventions. Otherwise, since the presence of cavity is detected, the use of restoration as a

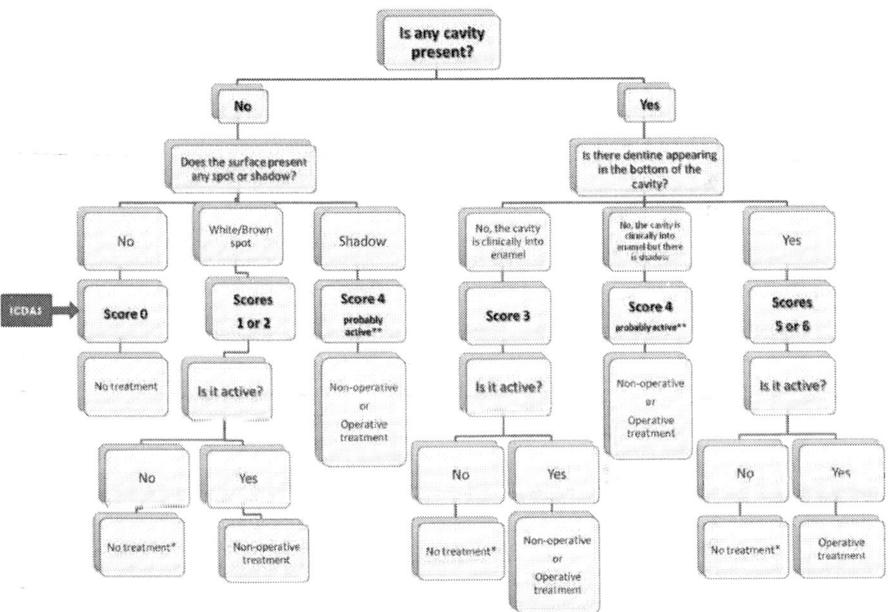

Figure 18. Conceptual tree for managing approximal caries, correlating the caries detection and activity assessment based on ICDAS and clinical decision-making. (* situations in which is usually difficult to affirm caries lesions are really inactive; ** the ICDAS activity assessment always considers lesions score 4 as probably active)

manner to control biofilm at the lesion would be necessary [57]. On the other hand, high amount of sound tissue would be acceptable in order to restore this surface adequately. Therefore, depending on patients' and professional's preferences and particularities of the clinical case, both options are possible. Considering the minimal invasive philosophy, maybe, opting for the non-restorative approach would be interesting since the children's comfort and preservation of dental structures would be maximized.

For approximal dentine caries lesions, the detection of cavities may be more relevant. If the cavitation is not easily visible or not felt by probing, the temporary separation could aid in seeking for cavities (see Figure 15). A dentine lesion progress faster than an enamel lesion. However, if the lesion is not cavitated, this progression is slower than for cavitated lesions [23], since the level of bacterial invasion is very low [22]. Based on that, we may argue the control of several outer non-cavitated dentine lesions would be possible. However, this is not so frequent. Actually, most dentine caries lesions in primary teeth are cavitated [58]. On the other hand, when the cavity is present, some approach that avoids the stagnation of the biofilm over the lesion seems to be indispensable. In this sense, any intervention which prevents biofilm accumulation on these lesions or facilitates is removal could be useful. Otherwise, it is important to clarify that mechanical removal of biofilm by flossing might not be a good choice in these cases, since the cavity may hide the plaque and interfere with caries lesion control.

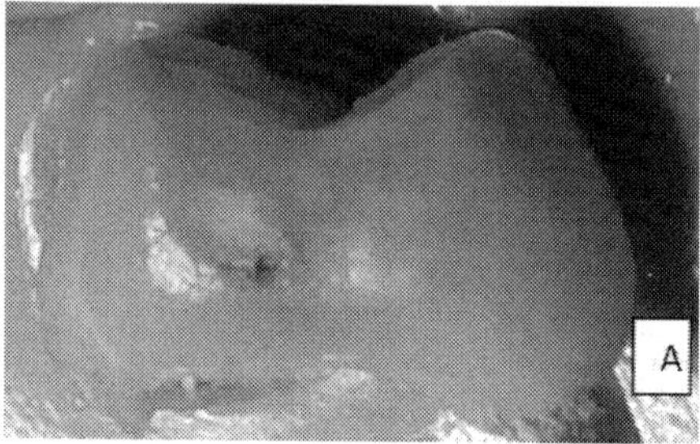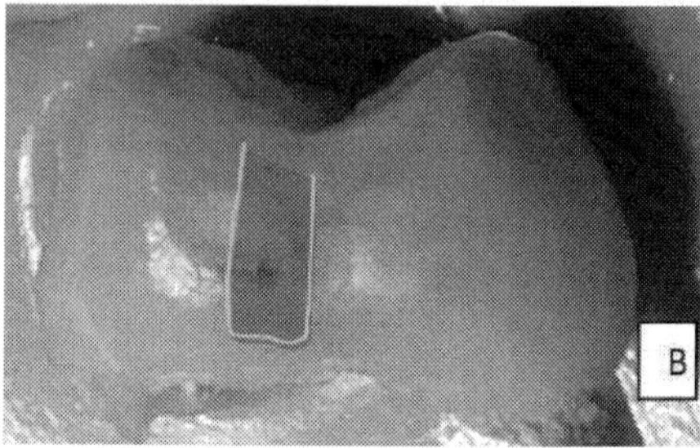

Figure 19. a) Cavitated caries lesion into enamel (direct examination). This cavity probably would not be seen when surface was assessed in the oral cavity due to the presence of the adjacent tooth. Using the temporary separation might help in detecting this cavity. Regarding treatment, we have to ponder if this lesion was detected and the option was operative treatment, a high amount of sound tissue would have to be removed. (b) Schematic representation of how accessing the mentioned cavity if the tooth was actually in the arch.

6. Options (interventions) to control initial approximal caries

Despite flossing is the most suitable method for mechanical removal of biofilm from the interproximal area [59, 60], controlling approximal caries just by flossing has not been shown to be effective [41], probably because its flossing by children and adolescents is not constant and adequate [4]. Controlling approximal caries by just flossing is a simple intervention, however, patient might be instructed and constantly motivated by professional [61]. Although dentist should never give up instructing and motivating to floss, choosing only this approach could be not enough for some approximal caries lesions. In fact, depending on children's compliance with flossing this option may not succeed, especially considering problems with motivation to flossing discussed earlier in this chapter. Thus, early interventions to initial caries lesions become even more important to arrest these lesions and prevent cavitations or lesions progression into dentine.

Initial caries lesion may be managed by remineralizing agents. A recent systematic review has shown the fluorides, in its different vehicles, present the most consistent benefit in controlling progression of initial caries lesions [62]. However, this review did not include any study which had used fluorides for approximal caries lesions in primary teeth. Actually, few studies have been performed aiming to investigate the management of initial caries in primary teeth and the evidence is inconclusive when we consider the most effective vehicle to be used, the frequence of use and the cost-effectiveness of using fluorides in primary teeth[63]. The fluoride varnish reduced in 25% the caries progression on approximal caries of primary molars [45] (Figure 20). Other fluorides vehicles, as gels and foams, have been associated with caries reduction on approximal surfaces [64]. However, they were tested in permanent teeth. The use of interdental brush or dental floss dipped in fluoride gel has been also advocated to using fluorides for approximal areas [65, 66] (Figure 21).

Another option tested for the same purpose was an association AgF followed by SnF2, resulting in a arrestment of 74% of approximal caries lesions [46]. At the moment, our group is testing

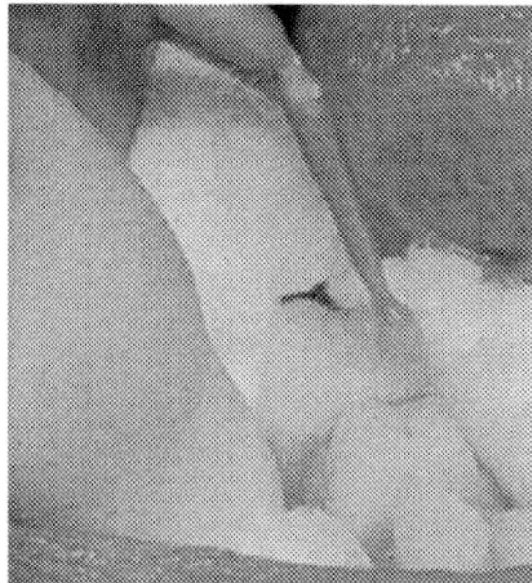

Figure 20. Application of fluoride varnish on approximal surfaces which present initial caries lesions.

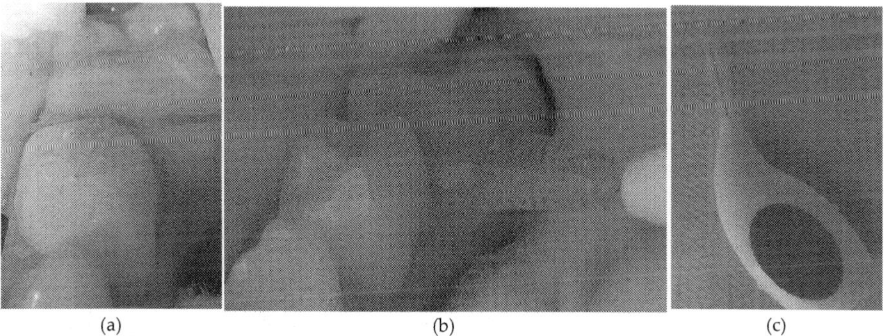

(a)   (b)   (c)

Figure 21. Use of fluoride gel on approximal initial caries lesions. (a) dental floss dipped in fluoride gel. (b) interdental toothbrush dipped in fluoride gel. (c) interdental toothbrush (note some natural space/separation is need for its introduction into approximal areas.

the use of the silver diamine fluoride (SDF) to control approximal caries in primary teeth [67] (Figure 22 and 23). A previous study of our group pointed to the possibility of using the silver diamine fluoride (SDF) in children for arrestment of enamel caries lesions on occlusal surfaces of permanent erupting molar [68]. As erupting occlusal surfaces, approximal surfaces challenge by making the mechanical control biofilm more difficult. In addition, some studies have shown that the SDF is more effective than fluoride varnish to prevent and arrest caries [69-71]. Even showing success since 1960 [69], its effectiveness had not been tested in approximal lesions of primary teeth. It is expected after SDF application, some staining may be seen on treated surfaces. The staining is probably caused by the precipitation of insoluble silver phosphates [72] (Figure 23).

Besides the remineralizing agents, another possibility in order to treat initial caries is sealing or infiltrating caries lesions [74]. Sealants have been used for several years in prevention of dental caries [75]. However, its therapeutic effect may be more expressive than the preventive one [76]. Sealing a caries lesion avoid its contact with biofilm, permitting its arrestment.

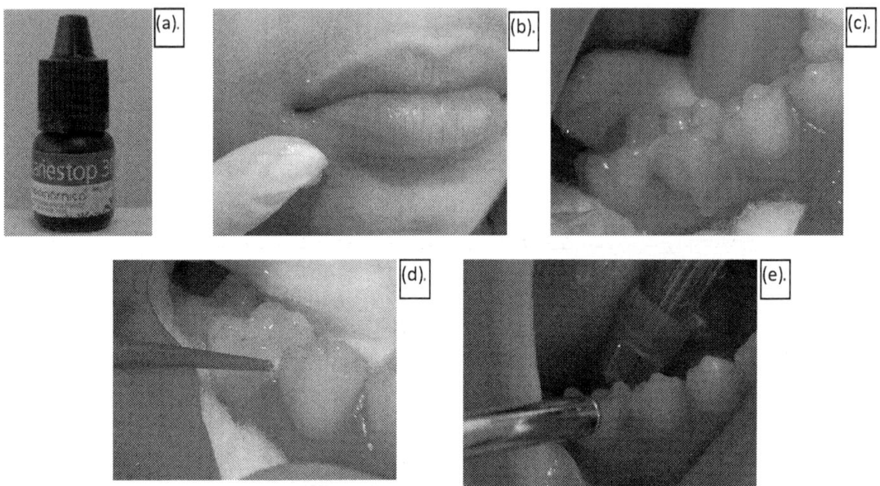

Figure 22. Application of silver diamine fluoride (SDF) in approximal caries lesions of primary teeth. (a) 30% SDF (Cariestop 30%,Biodinâmica Química e Farmacêutica LTDA, Ibiporã, Paraná, Brazil); (b) and (c) Extra-oral and intra-oral protection of soft tissues with petroleum jelly to avoid staining and mucosal irritation [73]; (d) application of SDF using a small disposable brush for 3 min – moisture was controlled by using cotton rolls and saliva ejectors. (e) washing for 30s to remove soluble final products of reaction between SDF and hydroxapatite.

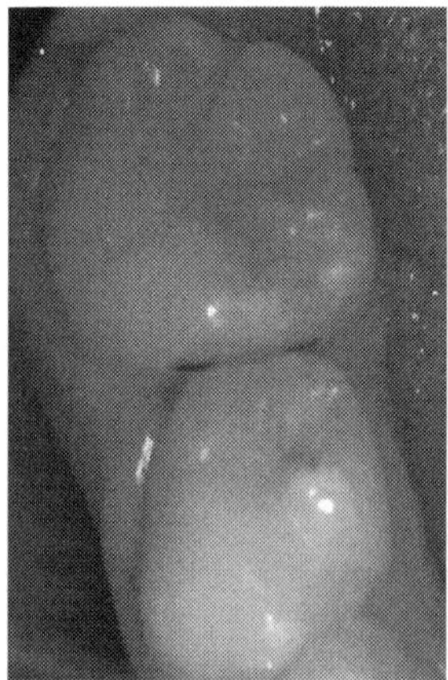

Figure 23. Staining caused by the SDF application after follow-up. The staining is probably due to deposition of silver phosphate that is a insoluble salt, responsible to the dark colour when exposed to the light [72]. Note the staining is hardly visible on treated approximal surfaces.

Sealants were initially devised for occlusal surfaces, which present a complex morphology and difficult mechanical plaque removal, especially in non-motivated or collaborative patients.

However, the principle of sealing has been extended to other surfaces in which controlling the biofilm is a challenge, as approximal surfaces [77]. The idea is the same: preventing caries lesion progression by eliminating the direct contact between the lesion and the biofilm. A previous study showed a 25% reduction in caries progression on approximal surfaces of primary teeth when sealed (comparatively to surfaces in which patients only flossed) [42]. These findings were comprehensible since when sealants are used, the poor children's compliance with flossing tends to be minimized.

Resin infiltration is other available option to "seal" caries lesions [78]. The infiltrant is a low-viscosity resin that promotes sealing into the lesion [78]. Differently from sealing, for infiltrating caries lesions, the superficial layer of caries lesion is removed by acid conditioning. Further, the lesion is infiltrated with a low-viscosity resin. Therefore, the barrier against biofilm would be created inside the lesions, instead of in the surface of caries lesions [79]. In addition, the tooth separation is not required for infiltrating caries lesions. On the other hand, if tooth separation is not performed, some doubts concerning diagnosis may remain. Besides, a kit for resin infiltration is sold containing all products used in the process and specifically designed applicators for approximal surfaces. (Figure 24). Despite these differences compared to the traditional sealants, we believe they exert similar roles in controlling caries lesions progression, since the contact between lesion and biofilm is avoided. Infiltration has been showed as an efficacious treatment for permanent teeth [79-81], but only one study was conducted in primary teeth [82]. In this study, resin infiltration was more efficacious than fluoride varnish in the arrestment of proximal lesions [82]. Although no study has compared sealing and infiltrating caries lesions on approximal surfaces of primary teeth, results in permanent teeth permit to guess that sealants and infiltrants tend to have similar efficacy when the deal is treating initial caries lesions [81].

Besides effectiveness/efficacy in controlling caries lesions, the patients' acceptance regarding the available treatments should be considered in clinical decision-making, especially treating children. Few studies have assessed patient-centered outcomes related to enamel caries lesions treatments. Sealing using relative isolation was well-accepted by most children [42]. In this study, the non-use of rubber dam was pointed as a possible concern [42]. On the other hand, when local anesthesia and rubber dam were used for infiltrating lesions in primary teeth, children reported higher levels of discomfort than when other non-invasive approaches were used [83]. Therefore, we consider that those techniques that cause less discomfort should be preferred and considered by clinicians. In addition, patient's and parents' satisfaction with treatments for initial caries lesions have not been evaluated. Staining caused by inactivation of caries lesions and/or using of SDF has not been systematically assessed. That is one of our concerns when testing the SDF as a possibility to treat initial caries [67]. Based on some preliminary findings, we believe this consequence of the mentioned treatment will not impact on patient's and parent's perceptions, especially due to the position of the surface, which hides the effect of SDF application (see Figure 23).

Finally, cost-efficacy of the mentioned treatment should be considered. More complex treatments as sealing or infiltrating caries lesions are more time-consuming [83], which will certainly lead to higher costs. Thus, even being equally effective, simpler procedures tend to

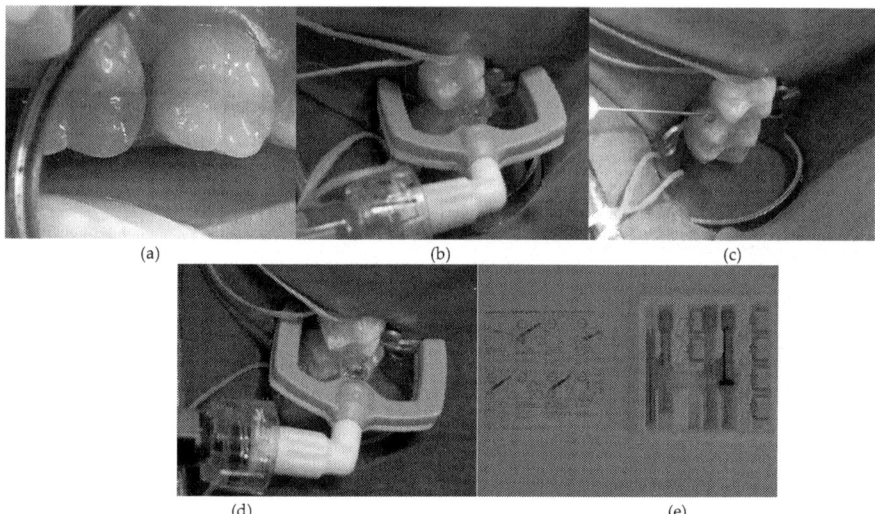

(a)   (b)   (c)

(d)   (e)

Figure 24. Resin infiltration of an initial caries lesion – (a) direct visual inspection after tooth separation - distal surface of element 54 presented a white spot lesion without any cavity. (b) After local anesthesia and adaptation of the rubber dam, 15%hydrochloric acid was applied on the lesion for 120s, followed by washing and air-drying. (c) Dehydration using 95% ethanol, followed by air-drying. (d) Resin infiltrant application on the lesion for 120s, followed by excess removal and light-curing for 40s. Further, resin is applied for more 30s and light-cured again. (e) All products used in resin infiltration are included in a specific kit commercialized for this purpose by the manufacturers (Icon® - Dental Milestones Guaranteed – DMG, Germany). *Note: For caries sealing, the steps A, B and D will be the same, but without the use of special applicators and using other materials (dental adhesives and resin sealants).*

be more cost-efficacious than complex ones. This is another point to be weighed in the decision-making process. Although our investigation is ongoing, we believe the SDF may be a more cost-efficacious/effective approach to be used in treating initial caries compared to other available treatments.

In summary, the scientific evidence regarding the effectiveness for treating initial caries on approximal surfaces in primary teeth is still scarce. However, some possible alternatives may be used until stronger evidences may be available. Additionally, it is important to consider the simplest techniques are cheaper and seem to be more accepted by children. Therefore, all these properties of the technique chosen for treating enamel caries on approximal surfaces in primary teeth should be considered conjointly.

7. Options to be used when cavitated

As discussed earlier, the greater susceptibility to caries experience of the approximal surface [1] linked to the faster progression rate for enamel to reach the dentin in primary teeth [19] results in a high prevalence of cavitated dentin caries lesions. These lesions need procedures that allow to arrest them and, especially, to reestablish the previous anatomy.

The treatments recommended to cavitated dentin lesion in approximal surfaces can be assigned according to depth and extent of the lesions.

Initially, when observed one cavitated lesion reaching outer dentin of approximal surface in primary teeth, without breaking the marginal ridge (see Figure 15), the utilization of infiltrating technique [82] or the sealing with adhesive system [42] or fissure sealants [77] has been proposed. These materials, as discussed for initial lesions, mechanically block the biofilm accumulation over the lesion. Previous studies have shown that both treatments seem to be good option to control caries progression in outer third of dentin [42, 82]. These previous studies included cavitated caries lesions clinically into enamel (despite their radiographic extension into dentin) [42, 82]. However, as few lesions with this severity were included in the samples, we could not draw definitive conclusions on the efficacy of these techniques or dental materials for cavitated lesions.

Sealing has been proved to be an option for small occlusal cavities exposing dentine [84]. Once more, the purpose of preventing the contact with cariogenic biofilm and enabling plaque removal from the surface instead is performing operative procedure care [84]. The same approach, if used on approximal surfaces, would avoid removal of sound enamel to access small lesions into dentine with preserved marginal bridge (Figure 25). A pilot study that compared the sealing to restoration for approximal cavitated dentin lesions showed almost 70% of sealed lesions have failed after 18 months compared to 11% of the restorations [85]. Besides, 54% of sealed lesions showed progression [85]. This finding seems to be linked with the technical difficulties in performing approximal caries sealing. Since the resin-based sealant is hydrophobic, there is a need to use rubber dam; however, sometimes there is a difficulty to maintain the work area without water (saliva, fluid) contamination [85]. Moreover, inserting both acid phosphoric and resin-based sealant into approximal cavities may have been a challenge which may justify the high proportion of observed failures [85]. Thus, although resin-based sealing represents the most conservative option to control cavitated dentin lesions, until the present moment, it is still not a satisfactory option to treat approximal cavitated caries lesions.

Depending on the size of the cavity and its location, it is also possible to improve the plaque removal from the cavity in order to promote caries lesions arrestment. This choice is especially interesting in areas in which restoration may be a greater challenge to deal than the mechanical control of the biofilm. Small approximal cavities in anterior primary teeth may be one indication for that, since restorations in these teeth may require sound tissue removal in order to access the cavity (Figure 26). Slicing has been also tested to approximal caries in posterior primary teeth [86]. Although, this technique seems to be a most conservative option for such cases, strongest evidences are necessary concerning it.

A recent systematic review showed that there is no difference concerning the choice of restorative material to treat occlusoproximal dentin cavities [87]. In this study, both conventional approaches as amalgam and composite resin were compared to Atraumatic Restorative

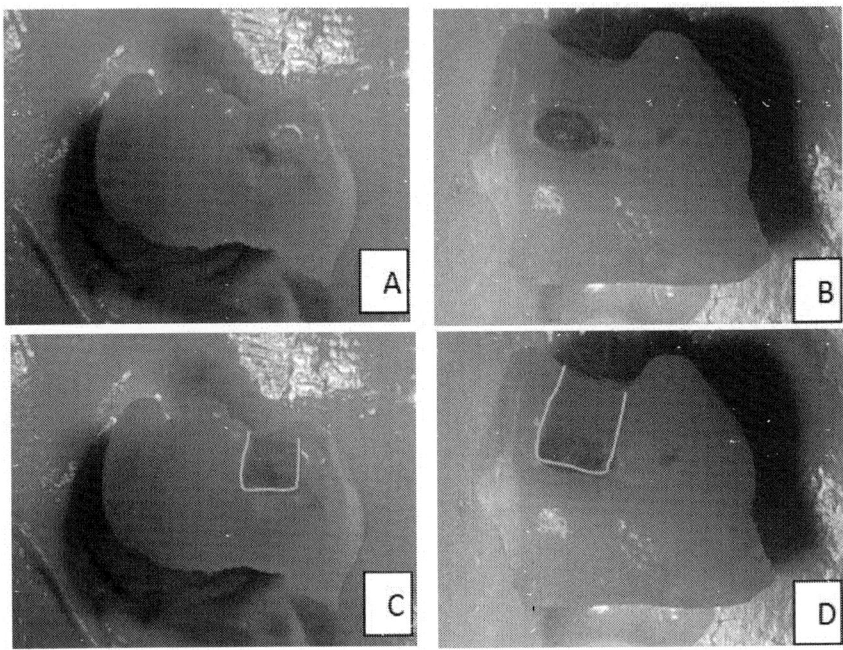

Figure 25. Cavitated dentine caries lesions (a-b). To restore these lesions, sound tissues should have to be removed, as schematically drawn (c-d).

Treatment (ART) performed with high-viscous glass ionomer cement (GIC), demonstrating similar results and satisfactory options to treating these lesions in primary teeth, until 3 years of follow up. However, when we think about the minimal intervention, which has the partial caries removal as one of its concepts, there is no reason to perform the amalgam restoration. Due to that, this procedure will not be discussed in this chapter.

Worldwide, the composite resin associated to adhesive system is, in approximately 25% of cases, the material of choice for restoring primary teeth [88-90]. This material shows satisfactory efficacy when used under local anesthesia and rubber dam, regardless of the brand of composite resin [91], demonstrating a success rate around 90% on occlusal and occlusal-proximal surface of primary teeth [92]. On the other hand, when it is considered the adhesive system, a systematic review reported that both three-step etch-and-rinse and two-step self-etching adhesive system present the best clinical performances [93]. However, this systematic review only considered the clinical trials performed in permanent teeth and these results should be interpreted with caution to primary teeth.

Some specific protocols to be applied in primary teeth in order to obtain similar results that observed to permanent teeth have been suggested. One of the proposals is shortening the etching time in dentin, for etch-and-rinse adhesive systems in order to increase the bond

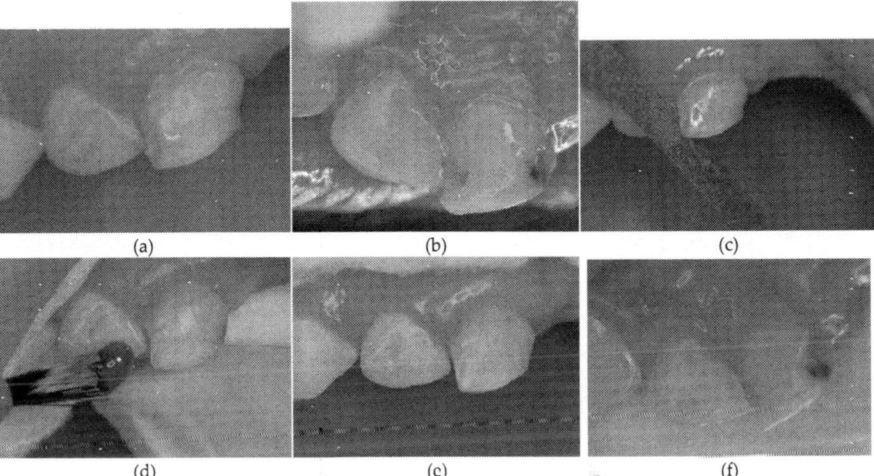

Figure 26. Small cavity on distal surface of upper primary central incisor – buccal (a) and palatal (b) view. Treatment: (c) access to the cavity to facilitate the mechanical removal of the biofilm; (d) application of fluoride varnish to enhance the remineralization. (e/f) follow-up after two weeks evidences the best control of the biofilm in the region.

stability of the restorations in primary teeth [94]. This protocol is based on previous studies that demonstrated the primary dentin is more reactive to acid etching [95, 96] and showed good results *in vitro* studies [94, 97]. Thus, the authors suggest the dentin etching of 35-37% acid phosphoric for 7 seconds before the adhesive system application [94]. Etching enamel remains in 15 seconds.

One important point to be pondered is that the main reason to failure of resin composite restorations is caries around restorations [92]. Due to that, other options of restorative materials may be considered. A previous study evidenced the effect of the resin-modified GIC restoration in prevention of secondary caries when compared to resin composite [98], probably due to fluoride release and uptake of the glass ionomer cements. The resin-modified GIC may be a good alternative, since presents a similar behavior of resin composite in clinical situation [91]. Its longevity is on average 5 years in occlusoproximal cavities [99]. However, this material contains resin monomers in its composition and may increase susceptibility to the presence of humidity compared to other ionomers. This characteristic associated to the need of a light source to polymerization of the material can be pointed as disadvantages of using resin-modified GIC.

On the other hand, similar trend regarding the protection of the margin of restorations can be observed with ART (Figure 26), since this treatment has high-viscous GIC as the material of choice. The GIC shows results such like the RMGIC in prevention of new caries lesion [100]. Moreover, studies have considered GIC as a viable alternative due to the similar survival rates compared to others restorative materials/techniques [87]. Other proprieties of GIC may also contribute to this choice, i.e., ability to chemically bond to enamel and dentine with insignificant heat formation or shrinkage, biocompatibility with the pulp and periodontal tissues and a similar coefficient of thermal expansion to tooth structure [101].

More recently, a new advantage related to GIC in occlusoproximal restoration has been addressed. Studies have claimed the contact with an approximal cavity offers a higher risk to the adjacent surfaces developing caries lesion [1]. In these cases, GIC restoration could prevent the new lesions and even to arrest the initial ones [102]. This hypothesis has been confirmed by a practice-based research, which showed that the progression rate of caries lesion on tooth surfaces adjacent to amalgam restorations was 30%, whilst to GIC restorations was only 16% [103]. These premises associated with no need of local anesthesia and rubber dam application have contributed for indicating GIC restoration associated to partial caries removal as the best option to treat cavitated lesions in children (Figure 27).

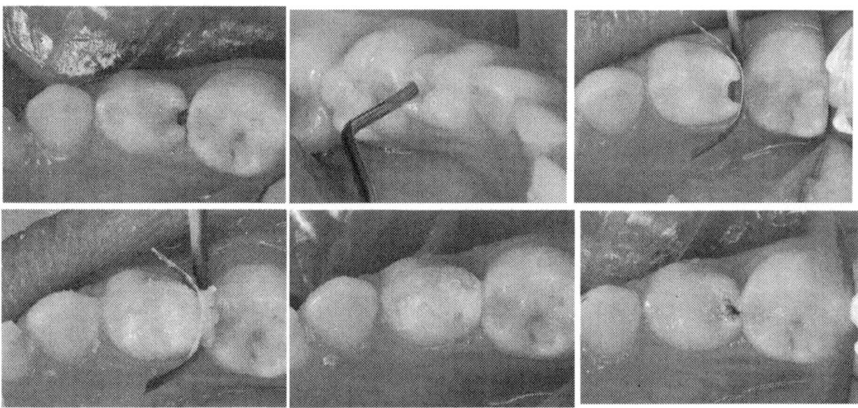

Figure 27. Step-by-step of an occlusoproximal restoration based on atraumatic restorative treatment, using partial caries removal and high-visous glass ionomer cement (GIC). (a) cavity into dentine; (b) accessing the cavity using a manual instrument; (c) preparing for restoration – to restore the contact point and avoid marginal excess; (d) after inserting the GIC and using finger pressure over the material; (e) final restoration; (f) checking the occlusal contacts. *(images gently donated by Dr. Isabel Olegario)*

8. Final considerations

It is evident, based on topics discussed in this paper, that approximal caries lesions are an actual challenge to dentists deal with. Indeed, the detection of caries lesion on these surfaces presents a duality. On one hand, the surfaces position in oral cavity makes the direct visual inspection almost impossible. On the other hand, if additional caries detection methods are used sequentially, they may lead to overtreatment in some situations (e.g. indiscriminate use of bitewings) or result in a greater doubt regarding options for treating those lesions (e.g. temporary tooth separation), since weak scientific evidences have been found for corroborating some available for clinical decision-making for approximal cavities clinically restricted to enamel.

Even if caries detection has been an overcome stage, treating approximal caries is not a simple task. Unfortunately, few strong evidences are available to support these treatments. Therefore, clinicians should try to use the best available evidences at the occasion. Based on that, we tried to contribute to clinical decision-making process joining the description of present evidences to a critical appraisal of them. We believe the critical judgment of the published evidences is crucial to guide the better clinicians' conduct to their patients.

Nowadays, the adoption of the minimal intervention philosophy has been a reality. Based on that, we have looked into evidences that may support our clinical decision-making not only based on effectiveness or efficacy of therapies used. We have also looked for manners of treating our children minimizing destruction/loss of healthy or reparable structures and guaranteeing higher levels of comfort and satisfaction to them. Due to that, we have insisted on situations in which treatments present similar effectiveness/efficacy, the simplest, the most cost effective/efficacious or the most acceptable approaches should be preferable by dentists for treating their patients. We believe the conjoint critical appraisal of these requisites may be helpful when dealing with the challenge that approximal caries lesions in primary teeth represents.

Acknowledgements

Authors would like to thank the CNPq, Capes and Fapesp (Protocol 2012/50716-0 and 2014/00271-7), which have given financial support for investigations performed in this field. They were also very thankful to Dr. O'Such for English revision and to Dr. Olegario to donation of some images for illustrating this chapter.

Author details

Mariana Minatel Braga[1*], Isabela Floriano[1], Fernanda Rosche Ferreira[1], Juliana Mattos Silveira[1], Alessandra Reyes[1], Tamara Kerber Tedesco[1], Daniela Prócida Raggio[1], José Carlos Pettorossi Imparato[2] and Fausto Medeiros Mendes[1,2]

*Address all correspondence to: mmbraga@usp.br

1 Dental School, Department of Pediatric Dentistry, University of São Paulo, São Paulo, Brazil

2 University Camilo Castelo Branco, São Paulo, Brazil and CPO São Leopoldo Mandic, Campinas, Brazil

References

[1] Cagetti MG, Campus G, Sale S, Cocco F, Strohmenger L, Lingström P. Association between interdental plaque acidogenicity and caries risk at surface level: a cross sectional study in primary dentition. Int J Paediatr Dent. 2011 Mar;21(2):119-25. PubMed PMID: 20731733. eng.

[2] Seki M, Karakama F, Terajima T, Ichikawa Y, Ozaki T, Yoshida S, et al. Evaluation of mutans streptococci in plaque and saliva: correlation with caries development in preschool children. J Dent. 2003 May;31(4):283-90. PubMed PMID: 12735923. Epub 2003/05/09. eng.

[3] Choo A, Delac DM, Messer LB. Oral hygiene measures and promotion: review and considerations. Aust Dent J. 2001 Sep;46(3):166-73. PubMed PMID: 11695154. eng.

[4] Ashkenazi M, Bidoosi M, Levin L. Factors associated with reduced compliance of children to dental preventive measures. Odontology. 2011 Jun. PubMed PMID: 21698350. ENG.

[5] Longbottom CL, Huysmans MC, Pitts NB, Fontana M. Glossary of key terms. Monogr Oral Sci. 2009;21:209-16. PubMed PMID: 19494688. eng.

[6] Rao A, Malhotra N. The role of remineralizing agents in dentistry: a review. Compend Contin Educ Dent. 2011 2011 Jul-Aug;32(6):26-33; quiz 4, 6. PubMed PMID: 21894873. eng.

[7] Milsom KM, Tickle M, Humphris GM, Blinkhorn AS. The relationship between anxiety and dental treatment experience in 5-year-old children. Br Dent J. 2003 May; 194(9):503-6; discussion 495. PubMed PMID: 12835786. eng.

[8] Fejerskov O. Concepts of dental caries and their consequences for understanding the disease. Community Dent Oral Epidemiol. 1997 Feb;25(1):5-12. PubMed PMID: 9088687.

[9] Fejerskov O. Changing paradigms in concepts on dental caries: Consequences for oral health care. Caries research. 2004;38(3):182-91.

[10] Featherstone JD. The continuum of dental caries--evidence for a dynamic disease process. J Dent Res. 2004;83 Spec No C:C39-42. PubMed PMID: 15286120. eng.

[11] Bjørndal L, Mjör IA. Pulp-dentin biology in restorative dentistry. Part 4: Dental caries--characteristics of lesions and pulpal reactions. Quintessence Int. 2001 Oct;32(9): 717-36. PubMed PMID: 11695140. eng.

[12] Manji F, Fejerskov O, Nagelkerke NJ, Baelum V. A random effects model for some epidemiological features of dental caries. Community Dent Oral Epidemiol. 1991 Dec;19(6):324-8. PubMed PMID: 1764899. eng.

[13] Kidd EA, Fejerskov O. What constitutes dental caries? Histopathology of carious enamel and dentin related to the action of cariogenic biofilms. Journal of dental research. 2004;83 Spec No C:C35-8. PubMed PMID: 15286119.

[14] Fejerskov O, Nyvad B, Kidd E. Pathology of Dental Caries. In: Fejerskov O, Kidd E, editors. Dental Caries: The Disease and Its Clinical Management. 2nd ed. Oxford: Wiley; 2008.

[15] Holmen L, Thylstrup A, Ogaard B, Kragh F. A scanning electron microscopic study of progressive stages of enamel caries in vivo. Caries Res. 1985;19(4):355-67. PubMed PMID: 3861258. eng.

[16] Cochrane NJ, Anderson P, Davis GR, Adams GG, Stacey MA, Reynolds EC. An X-ray microtomographic study of natural white-spot enamel lesions. Journal of dental research. 2012 Feb;91(2):185-91. PubMed PMID: 22095069.

[17] Holmen L, Thylstrup A, Artun J. Clinical and histological features observed during arrestment of active enamel carious lesions in vivo. Caries research. 1987;21(6): 546-54 PubMed PMID: 3479261.

[18] Bjørndal L, Thylstrup A. A structural analysis of approximal enamel caries lesions and subjacent dentin reactions. Eur J Oral Sci. 1995 Feb;103(1):25-31. PubMed PMID: 7600246. eng.

[19] Vanderas AP, Manetas C, Koulatzidou M, Papagiannoulis L. Progression of proximal caries in the mixed dentition: a 4-year prospective study. Pediatric dentistry. 2003 May-Jun;25(3):229-34. PubMed PMID: 12889698.

[20] Ekstrand KR, Ricketts DN, Kidd EA. Do occlusal carious lesions spread laterally at the enamel-dentin junction? A histolopathological study. Clin Oral Investig. 1998 Mar;2(1):15-20. PubMed PMID: 9667149. eng.

[21] Bjørndal L, Kidd EA. The treatment of deep dentine caries lesions. Dent Update. 2005 Sep;32(7):402-4, 7-10, 13. PubMed PMID: 16178284. eng.

[22] Bjørndal L. Buonocore Memorial Lecture. Dentin caries: progression and clinical management. Oper Dent. 2002 2002 May-Jun;27(3):211-7. PubMed PMID: 12022450. eng.

[23] Ratledge DK, Kidd EA, Beighton D. A clinical and microbiological study of approximal carious lesions. Part 1: the relationship between cavitation, radiographic lesion depth, the site-specific gingival index and the level of infection of the dentine. Caries research. 2001 Jan-Feb;35(1):3-7. PubMed PMID: 11125189.

[24] Marshall GW, Marshall SJ, Kinney JH, Balooch M. The dentin substrate: structure and properties related to bonding. J Dent. 1997 Nov;25(6):441-58. PubMed PMID: 9604576. eng.

[25] Pitts NB, Rimmer PA. An in vivo comparison of radiographic and directly assessed clinical caries status of posterior approximal surfaces in primary and permanent teeth. Caries Res. 1992;26(2):146-52. PubMed PMID: 1521308. eng.

[26] González-Cabezas C. The chemistry of caries: remineralization and demineralization events with direct clinical relevance. Dent Clin North Am. 2010 Jul;54(3):469-78. PubMed PMID: 20630190. eng.

[27] Almahdy A, Downey FC, Sauro S, Cook RJ, Sherriff M, Richards D, et al. Microbiochemical analysis of carious dentine using Raman and fluorescence spectroscopy. Caries Res. 2012;46(5):432-40. PubMed PMID: 22739587. eng.

[28] Banerjee A, Watson TF, Kidd EA. Dentine caries: take it or leave it? Dent Update. 2000 2000 Jul-Aug;27(6):272-6. PubMed PMID: 11218463. eng.

[29] Fusayama T. Two layers of carious dentin; diagnosis and treatment. Operative dentistry. 1979 Spring;4(2):63-70. PubMed PMID: 296808.

[30] Bjørndal L, Larsen T, Thylstrup A. A clinical and microbiological study of deep carious lesions during stepwise excavation using long treatment intervals. Caries Res. 1997;31(6):411-7. PubMed PMID: 9353579. eng.

[31] Schupbach P, Lutz F, Guggenheim B. Human root caries: histopathology of arrested lesions. Caries research. 1992;26(3):153-64. PubMed PMID: 1628289.

[32] Kidd EA. How 'clean' must a cavity be before restoration? Caries research. 2004 May-Jun;38(3):305-13. PubMed PMID: 15153704.

[33] Mejare I, Stenlund H, Zelezny-Holmlund C. Caries incidence and lesion progression from adolescence to young adulthood: a prospective 15-year cohort study in Sweden. Caries research. 2004 Mar-Apr;38(2):130-41. PubMed PMID: 14767170.

[34] Holmen L, Thylstrup A, Artun J. Surface changes during the arrest of active enamel carious lesions in vivo. A scanning electron microscope study. Acta odontologica Scandinavica. 1987 Dec;45(6):383-90. PubMed PMID: 3481156.

[35] Artun J, Thylstrup A. A 3-year clinical and SEM study of surface changes of carious enamel lesions after inactivation. American journal of orthodontics and dentofacial orthopedics : official publication of the American Association of Orthodontists, its constituent societies, and the American Board of Orthodontics. 1989 Apr;95(4):327-33. PubMed PMID: 2705413.

[36] Nyvad B, Fejerskov O. Assessing the stage of caries lesion activity on the basis of clinical and microbiological examination. Community Dent Oral Epidemiol. 1997 Feb;25(1):69-75. PubMed PMID: 9088694.

[37] Igarashi K, Lee IK, Schachtele CF. Comparison of in vivo human dental plaque pH changes within artificial fissures and at interproximal sites. Caries Res. 1989;23(6): 417-22. PubMed PMID: 2598230. Epub 1989/01/01. eng.

[38] Novaes TF, Matos R, Celiberti P, Braga MM, Mendes FM. The influence of interdental spacing on the detection of proximal caries lesions in primary teeth. Brazilian oral research. 2012 Jul-Aug;26(4):293-9. PubMed PMID: 22790495.

[39] Martignon S, Ekstrand KR, Ellwood R. Efficacy of sealing proximal early active lesions: an 18-month clinical study evaluated by conventional and subtraction radiography. Caries Res. 2006;40(5):382-8. PubMed PMID: 16946605. Epub 2006/09/02. eng.

[40] Schüz B, Sniehotta FF, Wiedemann A, Seemann R. Adherence to a daily flossing regimen in university students: effects of planning when, where, how and what to do in the face of barriers. J Clin Periodontol. 2006 Sep;33(9):612-9. PubMed PMID: 16856896. eng.

[41] Hujoel PP, Cunha-Cruz J, Banting DW, Loesche WJ. Dental flossing and interproximal caries: a systematic review. Journal of dental research. 2006 Apr;85(4):298-305. PubMed PMID: 16567548. Epub 2006/03/29. eng

[42] Martignon S, Tellez M, Santamaria RM, Gomez J, Ekstrand KR. Sealing distal proximal caries lesions in first primary molars: efficacy after 2.5 years. Caries research. 2010;44(6):562-70. PubMed PMID: 21088401.

[43] Guedes RS, Piovesan C, Ardenghi TM, Emmanuelli B, Braga MM, Ekstrand KR, et al. Validation of Visual Caries Activity Assessment: A 2-yr Cohort Study. J Dent Res. 2014 Apr;93(7 suppl):101S-7S. PubMed PMID: 24713370. ENG.

[44] Nyvad B, Machiulskiene V, Baelum V. Construct and predictive validity of clinical caries diagnostic criteria assessing lesion activity. Journal of dental research. 2003 Feb;82(2):117-22. PubMed PMID: 12562884.

[45] Peyron M, Matsson L, Birkhed D. Progression of approximal caries in primary molars and the effect of Duraphat treatment. Scandinavian journal of dental research. 1992 Dec;100(6):314-8. PubMed PMID: 1465563.

[46] Craig GG, Powell KR, Cooper MH. Caries progression in primary molars: 24-month results from a minimal treatment programme. Community dentistry and oral epidemiology. 1981 Dec;9(6):260-5. PubMed PMID: 6955124.

[47] Foster LV. Three year in vivo investigation to determine the progression of approximal primary carious lesions extending into dentine. British dental journal. 1998 Oct 10;185(7):353-7. PubMed PMID: 9807919.

[48] Sonju Clasen AB, Ogaard B, Duschner H, Ruben J, Arends J, Sonju T. Caries development in fluoridated and non-fluoridated deciduous and permanent enamel in situ examined by microradiography and confocal laser scanning microscopy. Adv Dent Res. 1997 Nov;11(4):442-7. PubMed PMID: 9470502.

[49] Novaes TF, Matos R, Raggio DP, Braga MM, Mendes FM. Children's discomfort in assessments using different methods for approximal caries detection. Brazilian oral research. 2012 Mar-Apr;26(2):93-9. PubMed PMID: 22473342.

[50] Abazov VM, Abbott B, Abolins M, Acharya BS, Adams M, Adams T, et al. Search for resonant pair production of neutral long-lived particles decaying to bb in pp collisions at square root(S)=1.96 TeV. Phys Rev Lett. 2009 Aug 14;103(7):071801. PubMed PMID: 19792632. Epub 2009/10/02. eng.

[51] Bader JD, Shugars DA, Bonito AJ. A systematic review of the performance of methods for identifying carious lesions. J Public Health Dent. 2002 Fall;62(4):201-13. PubMed PMID: 12474624.

[52] Espelid I, Mejare I, Weerheijm K, Eapd. EAPD guidelines for use of radiographs in children. European journal of paediatric dentistry : official journal of European Academy of Paediatric Dentistry. 2003 Mar;4(1):40-8. PubMed PMID: 12870988.

[53] Mendes FM, Novaes TF, Matos R, Bittar DG, Piovesan C, Gimenez T, et al. Radiographic and laser fluorescence methods have no benefits for detecting caries in primary teeth. Caries research. 2012;46(6):536-43. PubMed PMID: 22907166.

[54] Braga MM, Mendes FM, Ekstrand KR. Detection activity assessment and diagnosis of dental caries lesions. Dental clinics of North America. 2010 Jul;54(3):479-93. PubMed PMID: 20630191.

[55] Rimmer PA, Pitts NB. Temporary elective tooth separation as a diagnostic aid in general dental practice. British dental journal. 1990 Aug 11-25;169(3-4):87-92. PubMed PMID: 2206652.

[56] Mialhe FL, Pereira AC, Pardi V, de Castro Meneghim M. Comparison of three methods for detection of carious lesions in proximal surfaces versus direct visual examination after tooth separation. The Journal of clinical pediatric dentistry. 2003 Fall;28(1): 59-62. PubMed PMID: 14604144.

[57] Ridell K, Olsson H, Mejàre I. Unrestored dentin caries and deep dentin restorations in Swedish adolescents. Caries Res. 2008;42(3):164-70. PubMed PMID: 18446024. eng.

[58] Mendes FM, Braga MM. Caries detection in primary teeth is less challenging than in permanent teeth. Dental Hypotheses. 2013;4:17-20.

[59] Corby PM, Biesbrock A, Bartizek R, Corby AL, Monteverde R, Ceschin R, et al. Treatment outcomes of dental flossing in twins: molecular analysis of the interproximal microflora. J Periodontol. 2008 Aug;79(8):1426-33. PubMed PMID: 18672992. Epub 2008/08/05. eng.

[60] Merchant AT. Flossing for 2 weeks reduces microbes associated with oral disease. J Evid Based Dent Pract. 2009 Dec;9(4):223-4. PubMed PMID: 19913742. Epub 2009/11/17. eng.

[61] Schüz B, Wiedemann AU, Mallach N, Scholz U. Effects of a short behavioural intervention for dental flossing: randomized-controlled trial on planning when, where and how. J Clin Periodontol. 2009 Jun;36(6):498-505. PubMed PMID: 19453572. eng.

[62] Tellez M, Gomez J, Kaur S, Pretty IA, Ellwood R, Ismail AI. Non-surgical management methods of noncavitated carious lesions. Community dentistry and oral epidemiology. 2013 Feb;41(1):79-96. PubMed PMID: 23253076.

[63] Vanderas AP, Skamnakis J. Effectiveness of preventive treatment on approximal caries progression in posterior primary and permanent teeth: a review. European journal of paediatric dentistry : official journal of European Academy of Paediatric Dentistry. 2003 Mar;4(1):9-15. PubMed PMID: 12870982.

[64] Jiang H, Bian Z, Tai BJ, Du MQ, Peng B. The effect of a bi-annual professional application of APF foam on dental caries increment in primary teeth: 24-month clinical trial. Journal of dental research. 2005 Mar;84(3):265-8. PubMed PMID: 15723868.

[65] Sarner B, Lingstrom P, Birkhed D. Fluoride release from NaF- and AmF-impregnated toothpicks and dental flosses in vitro and in vivo. Acta odontologica Scandinavica. 2003 Oct,61(5):289-96. PubMed PMID: 14763781.

[66] Sarner B, Birkhed D, Huysmans MC, Ruben JL, Fidler V, Lingstrom P. Effect of fluoridated toothpicks and dental flosses on enamel and dentine and on plaque composition in situ. Caries research. 2005 Jan-Feb;39(1):52-9. PubMed PMID: 15591735.

[67] Mattos-Silveira J, Floriano I, Ferreira FR, Viganó ME, Frizzo MA, Reyes A, et al. New proposal of silver diamine fluoride use in arresting approximal caries: study protocol for a randomized controlled trial. Trials 2014 15:448.

[68] Braga MM, Mendes FM, De Benedetto MS, Imparato JC. Effect of silver diammine fluoride on incipient caries lesions in erupting permanent first molars: a pilot study. J Dent Child (Chic). 2009 Jan-Apr;76(1):28-33. PubMed PMID: 19341576. Epub 2009/04/04. eng.

[69] Chu CH, Lo EC, Lin HC. Effectiveness of silver diamine fluoride and sodium fluoride varnish in arresting dentin caries in Chinese pre-school children. Journal of dental research. 2002 Nov;81(11):767-70. PubMed PMID: 12407092. Epub 2002/10/31. eng.

[70] Rosenblatt A, Stamford TC, Niederman R. Silver diamine fluoride: a caries "silver-fluoride bullet". J Dent Res. 2009 Feb;88(2):116-25. PubMed PMID: 19278981. eng.

[71] Beltrán-Aguilar ED. Silver diamine fluoride (SDF) may be better than fluoride varnish and no treatment in arresting and preventing cavitated carious lesions. J Evid Based Dent Pract. 2010 Jun;10(2):122-4. PubMed PMID: 20466328. eng.

[72] Yamaga R, Nishino M, Yoshida S, Yokomizo I. Diammine silver fluoride and its clinical application. The Journal of Osaka University Dental School. 1972 Sep;12:1-20. PubMed PMID: 4514730.

[73] Llodra JC, Rodriguez A, Ferrer B, Menardia V, Ramos T, Morato M. Efficacy of silver diamine fluoride for caries reduction in primary teeth and first permanent molars of schoolchildren: 36-month clinical trial. J Dent Res. 2005 Aug;84(8):721-4. PubMed PMID: 16040729. Epub 2005/07/26. eng.

[74] Ammari MM, Soviero VM, da Silva Fidalgo TK, Lenzi M, Ferreira DM, Mattos CT, et al. Is non-cavitated proximal lesion sealing an effective method for caries control in primary and permanent teeth? A systematic review and meta-analysis. Journal of dentistry. 2014 Oct;42(10):1217-27. PubMed PMID: 25066832.

[75] Ahovuo-Saloranta A, Forss H, Walsh T, Hiiri A, Nordblad A, Makela M, et al. Sealants for preventing dental decay in the permanent teeth. The Cochrane database of systematic reviews. 2013;3:CD001830. PubMed PMID: 23543512.

[76] Heller KE, Reed SG, Bruner FW, Eklund SA, Burt BA. Longitudinal evaluation of sealing molars with and without incipient dental caries in a public health program. J Public Health Dent. 1995 Summer;55(3):148-53. PubMed PMID: 7562727. Epub 1995/01/01. eng.

[77] Gomez SS, Basili CP, Emilson CG. A 2-year clinical evaluation of sealed noncavitated approximal posterior carious lesions in adolescents. Clinical oral investigations. 2005 Dec;9(4):239-43. PubMed PMID: 16167153.

[78] Phark JH, Duarte S, Jr., Meyer-Lueckel H, Paris S. Caries infiltration with resins: a novel treatment option for interproximal caries. Compend Contin Educ Dent. 2009 Oct;30 Spec No 3:13-7. PubMed PMID: 19891346. Epub 2009/11/07. eng.

[79] Paris S, Hopfenmuller W, Meyer-Lueckel H. Resin infiltration of caries lesions: an efficacy randomized trial. Journal of dental research. 2010 Aug;89(8):823-6. PubMed PMID: 20505049. Epub 2010/05/28. eng.

[80] Meyer-Lueckel H, Bitter K, Paris S. Randomized controlled clinical trial on proximal caries infiltration: three-year follow-up. Caries Res. 2012;46(6):544-8. PubMed PMID: 22922306. eng.

[81] Martignon S, Ekstrand KR, Gomez J, Lara JS, Cortes A. Infiltrating/sealing proximal caries lesions: a 3-year randomized clinical trial. Journal of dental research. 2012 Mar; 91(3):288-92. PubMed PMID: 22257664. Epub 2012/01/20. eng.

[82] Ekstrand KR, Bakhshandeh A, Martignon S. Treatment of proximal superficial caries lesions on primary molar teeth with resin infiltration and fluoride varnish versus fluoride varnish only: efficacy after 1 year. Caries research. 2010;44(1):41-6. PubMed PMID: 20090327. Epub 2010/01/22. eng.

[83] Mattos-Silveira J, Floriano I, Ferreira FR, Vigano ME, Mendes FM, Braga MM. Children's discomfort may vary among different treatments for initial approximal caries lesions: preliminary findings of a randomized controlled clinical trial. Int J Paediatr Dent. 2014 Sep 17. PubMed PMID: 25229641.

[84] Hesse D, Bonifacio CC, Mendes FM, Braga MM, Imparato JC, Raggio DP. Sealing versus partial caries removal in primary molars: a randomized clinical trial. BMC Oral Health. 2014;14:58. PubMed PMID: 24884684. Pubmed Central PMCID: 4045925.

[85] Celiberti P. Novas possibilidades de manejo e monitoramento de lesões de cárie em superfícies proximais.. São Paulo: Dental School, University of São Paulo; 2011.

[86] Hansen HV, Heidmann J, Nyvad B. Non-Operative Control of Cavitated Approximal Caries Lesions in Primary Molars Over 6–24 Months: A Practice-Based Approach. Caries Res 2014. p. 414.

[87] Raggio DP, Hesse D, Lenzi TL, C ABG, Braga MM. Is Atraumatic restorative treatment an option for restoring occlusoproximal caries lesions in primary teeth? A systematic review and meta-analysis. Int J Paediatr Dent. 2013 Nov;23(6):435-43. PubMed PMID: 23190278.

[88] Guelmann M, Mjor IA. Materials and techniques for restoration of primary molars by pediatric dentists in Florida. Pediatr Dent. 2002 Jul-Aug;24(4):326-31. PubMed PMID: 12212875.

[89] Pair RL, Udin RD, Tanbonliong T. Materials used to restore class II lesions in primary molars: a survey of California pediatric dentists. Pediatr Dent. 2004 Nov-Dec; 26(6):501-7. PubMed PMID: 15646912.

[90] Buerkle V, Kuehnisch J, Guelmann M, Hickel R. Restoration materials for primary molars-results from a European survey. Journal of dentistry. 2005 Apr;33(4):275-81. PubMed PMID: 15781135.

[91] Casagrande L, Dalpian DM, Ardenghi TM, Zanatta FB, Balbinot CE, Garcia-Godoy F, et al. Randomized clinical trial of adhesive restorations in primary molars. 18-month results. Am J Dent. 2013 Dec;26(6):351-5. PubMed PMID: 24640441.

[92] dos Santos MP, Passos M, Luiz RR, Maia LC. A randomized trial of resin-based restorations in class I and class II beveled preparations in primary molars: 24-month results. J Am Dent Assoc. 2009 Feb;140(2):156-66; quiz 247-8. PubMed PMID: 19188412.

[93] Peumans M, Kanumilli P, De Munck J, Van Landuyt K, Lambrechts P, Van Meerbeek B. Clinical effectiveness of contemporary adhesives: a systematic review of current clinical trials. Dent Mater. 2005 Sep;21(9):864-81. PubMed PMID: 16009415.

[94] Lenzi TL, Braga MM, Raggio DP. Shortening the etching time for etch-and-rinse adhesives increases the bond stability to simulated caries-affected primary dentin. J Adhes Dent. 2014 Jun;16(3):235-41. PubMed PMID: 24669366.

[95] Senawongse P, Harnirattisai C, Shimada Y, Tagami J. Effective bond strength of current adhesive systems on deciduous and permanent dentin. Oper Dent. 2004 Mar-Apr;29(2):196-202. PubMed PMID: 15088732.

[96] Nor JE, Feigal RJ, Dennison JB, Edwards CA. Dentin bonding: SEM comparison of the dentin surface in primary and permanent teeth. Pediatr Dent. 1997 May-Jun; 19(4):246-52. PubMed PMID: 9200195.

[97] Lenzi TL, Mendes FM, Rocha Rde O, Raggio DP. Effect of shortening the etching time on bonding to sound and caries-affected dentin of primary teeth. Pediatr Dent. 2013 Sep-Oct;35(5):E129-33. PubMed PMID: 24290541.

[98] Yengopal V, Mickenautsch S. Caries-preventive effect of resin-modified glass-ionomer cement (RM-GIC) versus composite resin: a quantitative systematic review. Eur Arch Paediatr Dent. 2011 Feb;12(1):5-14. PubMed PMID: 21299939.

[99] Qvist V, Laurberg L, Pouisen A, Teglers PT. Class II restorations in primary teeth: 7-year study on three resin-modified glass ionomer cements and a compomer. Eur J Oral Sci. 2004 Apr;112(2):188-96. PubMed PMID: 15056118.

[100] Mickenautsch S, Tyas MJ, Yengopal V, Oliveira LB, Bonecker M. Absence of carious lesions at margins of glass-ionomer cement (GIC) and resin-modified GIC restorations: a systematic review. Eur J Prosthodont Restor Dent. 2010 Sep;18(3):139-45. PubMed PMID: 21077424.

[101] Anusavice KJ. Phillips' Science of Dental Materials. 12.ed. ed. Philadelphia: Saunders; 2012.

[102] Guglielmi CA. Efeito de materiais restauradores em contato proximal com lesões de cárie em dentes decíduos São Paulo: Dental School, University of São Paulo, 2013.

[103] Qvist V, Laurberg L, Poulsen A, Teglers PT. Eight-year study on conventional glass ionomer and amalgam restorations in primary teeth. Acta odontologica Scandinavica. 2004 Feb;62(1):37-45. PubMed PMID: 15124781.

Chapter 5

Dental Caries and Quality of Life Among Preschool Children

Joana Ramos-Jorge, Maria Letícia Ramos-Jorge,
Saul Martins de Paiva, Leandro Silva Marques and
Isabela Almeida Pordeus

Additional information is available at the end of the chapter

http://dx.doi.org/10.5772/59515

1. Introduction

Dental caries (tooth decay) is an adverse oral condition with a multifactor etiology involving genetic, behavioral and environmental aspects (Reisine and Psoter, 2001; Petersen *et al.*, 2005). Socioeconomic factors have been associated with caries experience and the distribution of this condition among individuals (Pereira *et al.*, 2007; Traebert *et al.*, 2009). Understanding the influence of lifestyle and social aspect on the occurrence and progression of dental caries can contribute to improvements in preventive and restorative treatment (Petersen *et al.*, 2005).

Although not a fatal condition, dental caries can lead to pain as well as problems with sleeping, eating, socializing and self-esteem. Thus, tooth decay can exert a negative impact on activities of daily living and, consequently, quality of life (Patel *et al.*, 2007). Quality of life is often evaluated by means of the investigation into the consequences of an adverse health condition and its treatment from the standpoint of the affected individual (Tamanini *et al.*, 2004). The association between oral health and quality of life is considered by many researchers to be a complement to clinical indicators (Martins-Júnior *et al.*, 2012a).

There are few assessment tools for measuring the impact of oral problems on the quality of life of children. As adults are responsible for decisions involving the health of their children (Pahel *et al.*, 2007), evaluating the perceptions of parents/caregivers regarding oral health problems that affect the quality of life of children is fundamental to planning health promotion strategies.

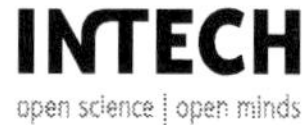

2. Problem statement

The concept of oral health-related quality of life (OHRQoL) regards the impact that oral problems have on the performance of activities of daily living, wellbeing and quality of life (Slade, 1997). It is therefore important to assess OHRQoL in different populations to understand the oral health problems that affect individuals and design public health programs and strategies directed at prevention and treatment.

Despite the growing interest and consequent increase in the number of publications on this issue, the evaluation of the impact of dental caries in preschool children has only recently been the focus of investigation. As young children may not be capable of remembering events that occurred more than 24 hours earlier (Rebok *et al.*, 2001) and have limitations regarding the expression of emotions and anguish (Talekar *et al.*, 2005), this investigation is often performed with the aid of parents/caregivers. It is therefore important to explore the perceptions of parents/caregivers that affect the preventive care children receive at home as well as the use of dental services (Filstrup *et al.*, 2003). Moreover, the perceptions of parents/caregivers may offer insight into some of the reasons why preschool children often do not receive the dental treatment they need.

The Early Childhood Oral Health Impact Scale (ECOHIS) was developed for parents/caregivers of young children (Pahel *et al.*, 2007). The use of this questionnaire in epidemiological studies has allowed broadening knowledge on adverse oral conditions that affect the quality of life of children as well as strengthening scientific evidence on this issue and demonstrating the need for oral health programs directed at preschool children.

Based on evidence that children aged four to six years can reliably report on their own quality of life (Filstrup *et al.*, 2003), the Scale of Oral Health Outcomes for Five-Year-Old Children (SOHO-5) has recently been developed in the United Kingdom (Tsakos *et al.*, 2012). However, studies employing this instrument have been limited to evaluating its reliability and validity.

Dental caries is the oral condition most often associated with a negative impact on the quality of life of preschool children (Abanto *et al.*, 2011; Scarpelli *et al.*, 2012; Ramos-Jorge *et al.*, 2014), the consequences of which include pain, decreased appetite, difficulty chewing, difficulty eating some foods and drinking hot or cold beverages, weight loss, difficulty sleeping, changes in behavior and a poor academic performance (Abanto *et al.*, 2011; Acs *et al.*, 1992; Ayhan *et al.*, 1996; Filstrup *et al.*, 2003; Feitosa *et al.*, 2005; Oliveira *et al.*, 2008; Martins-Júnior *et al.*, 2012b). Studies carried out in China (Wong *et al.*, 2011) and Brazil (Abanto *et al.*, 2011; Scarpelli *et al.*, 2012; Martins-Júnior *et al.*, 2012b) using the ECOHIS report that dental caries has a negative impact on the quality of life of preschool children and their parents/caregivers and this impact is greater in the presence of six or more carious lesions.

A study conducted in Canada found that dental surgery is the most common surgical procedure at most pediatric hospitals (Canadian Paediatric Decision Support Network, 2004), which indicates that the treatment of dental caries in children is costly. Moreover, the need for restorative treatment can lead to the establishment of a repetitive restorative cycle (Elderton *et al.*, 1990), which further raises treatment costs (Zero *et al.*, 2011). However, caries can be detected in the early stages, when restorative treatment is not necessary. The International Caries Detection and Assessment System (ICDAS) allows the standardization and diagnosis of dental caries in different settings and situations (Pitts, 2004). The integration of criteria from other caries detection and diagnostic systems involving non-cavitated enamel lesions and the staging of the disease process (Ekstrand *et al.*, 1997; Fyffe *et al.*, 2000; Chesters *et al.*, 2002; Rickets *et al.*, 2002) led to the current system, denominated ICDAS II (Shoaib *et al.*, 2009), which contributes to the preventive management of tooth decay.

Despite the decline in the prevalence of dental caries beginning in the 1970s, the control of this condition continues to pose a challenge to public health authorities (Petersen *et al.*, 2005; Dye *et al.*, 2007). Moreover, increasing polarization is seen due to social inequalities in oral health (Sabbah *et al.*, 2007), which has led to a greater prevalence rate of dental caries in some minorities (Antunes *et al.*, 2004).

The difficulty in controlling dental caries affects both developed and developing nations. Successive national child dental health surveys in the United Kingdom have shown little change in the prevalence of caries among five-year-old children over the last 20 years (Lader *et al.*, 2004). Data from the United States of America tells a similar story, as no significant changes in the prevalence of dental caries among children aged two to 11 years was found from 1988-1994 to 1999-2002 (Beltran-Aguilar *et al.*, 2005).

The monitoring of the early stages of caries progression requires the assessment of a dentist. However, this is not a common occurrence among preschool children. Indeed, a Brazilian study found that only 13.3% of a sample of 1092 children aged zero to five years had visited a dentist at least once (Kramer *et al.*, 2008). This low rate of access to dental treatment can contribute to the greater prevalence of severe tooth decay in comparison to less advanced stages of pro‐ gression (Ramos-Jorge *et al.*, 2014). Furthermore, among older preschoolers, the negative impact on OHRQoL (Ramos-Jorge *et al.*, 2014) seems to stem from the fact that these individuals have caries in more advanced stages of decay and also have a greater capacity to communicate the effect of oral health conditions on their quality of life to parents/caregivers (Ramos-Jorge *et al.*, 2014). Consequently, the prevention and management of dental caries should begin at an early age, as this is an evident public health problem among preschool children.

The diminished appetite, difficulty chewing, weight loss and difficulty sleeping stemming from dental caries can compromise growth and development. Moreover, children with severe caries appear to be at significantly greater odds of having low vitamin D status compared to their caries-free counterparts and are likely malnourished, as they display significantly lower levels of calcium and serum albumin as well as higher levels of PTH compared to a control group (reference).

OHRQoL assessment tools designed for preschool children are useful for the evaluation of public oral health strategies and interventions. Such tools should have properties that enable the detection of clinical changes following treatment. Responsiveness is a key technical property that allows researchers to choose the most appropriate measures for clinical trials, provides a basis for estimating sample sizes and facilitates the interpretation of changes occurring after treatment (Guyatt *et al.*, 2002; Malden *et al.*, 2008).

The aim of health interventions should be to improve quality of life. Despite the tendency to consider oral health as a separate concept, it is an integral part of general health (Cunningham and Hunt, 2001). Thus, the complex multidimensional interrelationship between general and oral health is essential to quality of life (Kieffe and, Hoogstraten, 2008). In this context, the use of subjective measures considering individual viewpoints has become increasingly important to the evaluation of general and oral health (Kieffer and Hoogstraten, 2008).

3. Application area

The findings of studies on OHRQoL and dental caries in preschool children are useful to the fields of pediatrics and pediatric dentistry and can be employed by public health administrators for the definition of strategies directed at improving the oral health status of this population.

4. Research course

According to a large number of the aforementioned studies, scientific evidence indicates that dental caries has a negative impact on quality of life among preschool children, especially those with six or more carious lesions or lesions in a more advanced stage of progression. The aim of the study reported herein was to evaluate the association between different stages of dental caries and the impact on the quality of life of preschool children.

5. Method used

A population-based, cross-sectional study was conducted involving preschool children. The inclusion criteria age between three and five years, enrolment in a preschool/daycare center in the city of Diamantina, Brazil, and parents/guardians fluent in Brazilian Portuguese who live with the child at least 12 hours per day. The exclusion criteria were current orthodontic treatment, systemic disease, having all carious lesions treated satisfactorily and the presence of tartar. The sample size was calculated using a 37.8% prevalence rate of impact from dental caries on the quality of life of preschool children (Martins-Júnior *et al.*, 2013), a 95% confidence interval and 5% standard error. The minimum sample was defined as 346 preschool children. A 1.2 correction factor was applied to enhance the precision and an additional 84 children were added to compensate for possible losses, resulting in a sample of 499 preschool children. To ensure representativeness, the sample was stratified based on the type of preschool (public or private) and the distribution of the sample was proportional to the total population enrolled in private and public preschools in the city.

Parents/caregivers were asked to answer the Brazilian version of the ECOHIS (B-ECOHIS) (Martins-Júnior *et al.*, 2012) and fill out a form addressing socio-demographic information, such as mother's schooling (years of study), whether the mother worked outside the home, monthly household income (categorized based on the Brazilian minimum wage = US$304.38), duration of salary (in weeks), family provider and number of individuals who depend on the income.

The B-ECOHIS was used to assess the negative impact of the progression stage and activity of dental caries on the quality of life of the preschool children. This questionnaire is composed of 13 items distributed in a Child Impact Section (CIS) and Family Impact Section (FIS). The former section has four domains (symptoms, function, psychology and self-image/social interaction) and the latter has two domains (parental distress and family function). The scale has five response options for recording how often an event has occurred in a child's life. The CIS and FIS scores are calculated through a simple sum of the scores on all items in each section, ranging from 0 to 36 and 0 to 16, respectively. The total score ranges from 0 to 52, with higher scores denoting greater oral health impact and poorer OHRQoL.

The clinical oral examination of the children was performed by a single dentist who had undergone a calibration exercise at a public preschool, during which inter-examiner and intra-examiner Kappa values were greater than 0.8 for all oral conditions evaluated. The examination was carried out after brushing performed by the dentist, with the aid of a head lamp (PETZL®, Tikka XP, Crolles, France), mouth mirrors (PRISMA, São Paulo, SP, Brazil), WHO probes (Golgran Ind. e Com. Ltda., São Paulo, SP, Brazil) and dental gauze for drying the teeth. During the examination, the children remained lying on a portable stretcher.

The ICDAS II criteria and Activity Lesion Assessment, which measures visual appearance, local susceptibility to plaque buildup and surface texture, were used for the determination of dental caries. Dental caries was recorded as follows: distinct visual change in enamel – ICDAS code 2 (active and inactive); localized enamel breakdown – ICDAS code 3 (active and inactive); underlying dentin shadow – ICDAS code 4 (active and inactive); distinct cavity within visible dentin – ICDAS code 5 (active and inactive); and extensive cavity within visible dentin – ICDAS code 6, without pulp exposure (active and inactive), with pulp exposure (with absence or presence of fistula and root remnants). The first visual change in enamel (ICDAS code 1, when there is no pigmentation) is detected only after drying with compressed air. As drying was performed with dental gauze in the present study, the decision was made to exclude the evaluation of this condition. When the characteristic pigmentation of this stage of carious lesion was detected on any face with the tooth either wet or dried with gauze, the tooth was recorded as "sound".

Malocclusion, traumatic dental injury (TDI) and physiological tooth mobility were evaluated as possible confounding variables. Malocclusion was recorded in the presence of anterior open bite, posterior open bite, increased overjet, deep bite, anterior crossbite or posterior crossbite. The clinical diagnosis of TDI was performed using the criteria proposed by Andreasen (Andreasen et al., 2007) and the assessment of tooth discoloration. Physiological tooth mobility was considered only when the tooth was nearing exfoliation. All confounding variables were categorized as absent or present.

Statistical analysis was performed using the SPSS 20.0 program for Windows (SPSS Inc, Chicago, IL, USA). Descriptive analysis (including frequency distribution) was performed for mean total B-ECOHIS scores. Scores for the individual domains were analyzed for differences between oral conditions and socioeconomic/demographic factors. In cases of children with a tooth exhibiting different stages of dental caries, the worst condition was considered. Poisson regression analysis with robust variance was performed to associate the mean total B-ECOHIS score with each clinical oral condition, socioeconomic factor and characteristic of the child. Prevalence rates (PR) and 95% confidence intervals (95% CI) were calculated.

6. Status

This study was completed and published in Community Dentistry and Oral Epidemiology.

7. Results

A total of 499 preschool children were initially enrolled in the study, 451 (90.4%) of whom participated through to the end of the study. The main reason for losses was the absence of a questionnaire filled out by the parents. Mean age (standard deviation) of the preschool children was 4.25 (0.83) years. The female sex accounted for 53.9% of the sample. The prevalence of untreated caries was 51.2%. A total of 60.6% of the teeth with caries exhibited severe decay. Malocclusion, TDI and physiological tooth mobility were present in 28.4%, 17.5% and 2.0% of the preschool children, respectively.

The majority of parents/caregivers reported no impact on quality of life (52.8%) (i.e., B-ECOHIS score: 0). The most frequently reported items were pain, difficulty eating and drinking, irritability, trouble sleeping and smiling.

In the final multivariate model, negative impact on quality of life was associated with the age of the child and a lower level of mother's schooling. More advanced stages of caries were associated with an increased negative impact on the quality of life of the children. Among inactive lesions, only extensive cavity without pulp exposure had an increased negative impact on quality of life (PR = 3.68; 95% CI: 1.74 to 7.81; p = 0.001).

8. Further research

Future investigations should be conducted to evaluate the results of intervention strategies on both the individual and population levels.

9. Conclusion

Dental caries exerts a negative impact on the quality of life of preschool children, especially those with a greater number of carious lesions or lesions in a more advanced stage of progression.

Author details

Joana Ramos-Jorge[1*], Maria Letícia Ramos-Jorge[1], Saul Martins de Paiva[2], Leandro Silva Marques[1] and Isabela Almeida Pordeus[2]

*Address all correspondence to: joanaramosjorge@gmail.com

1 Universidade Federal dos Vales do Jequitinhonha e Mucuri, Diamantina, Minas Gerais, Brazil

2 Universidade Federal de Minas Gerais, Belo Horizonte, Minas Gerais, Brazil

References

[1] Abanto J, Carvalho TS, Mendes FM, Wanderley MT, Bönecker M, Raggio DP. Impact of oral diseases and disorders on oral health-related quality of life of preschool children. Community Dent Oral Epidemiol 2011;39:105-14.

[2] Acs G, Lodolini G, Kaminsky S, Cisneros GJ. Effect of nursing caries on body weight in a pediatric population. Pediatr Dent 1992;14:302-5.

[3] Andreasen JO, Andreasen FM, Andersson LC. Textbook and color atlas of traumatic injuries to the teeth. Copenhagen: Munskgaard, 4 2007.

[4] Antunes JL, Narvai PC, Nugent ZJ. Measuring inequalities in the distribution of dental caries. Community Dent Oral Epidemiol 2004; 32: 41-48.

[5] Assaf AV, de Castro Meneghim M, Zanin L, Tengan C, Pereira AC. Effect of different diagnostic thresholds on dental caries calibration - a 12 month evaluation. Community Dent Oral Epidemiol 2006; 34: 213-9.

[6] Ayhan H, Suskan E, Yildrim S: The effect of nursing or rampant caries on height, body weight and head circumference. J Clin Pediatr Dent 1996;20:209-12.

[7] Beltrán-Aguilar ED, Barker LK, Canto MT, Dye BA, Gooch BF, Griffin SO, Hyman J, Jaramillo F, Kingman A, Nowjack-Raymer R, Selwitz RH, Wu T; Centers for Disease Control and Prevention (CDC). Surveillance for dental caries, dental sealants, tooth

retention, edentulism, and enamel fluorosis--United States, 1988-1994 and 1999-2002. MMWR Surveill Summ. 2005;54:1-43.

[8]   Chesters RK, Pitts NB, Matuliene G, Kvedariene A, Huntington E, Bendinskaite R, Balciuniene I, Matheson JR, Nicholson JA, Gendvilyte A, Sabalaite R,Ramanauskiene J, Savage D, Mileriene J. An abbreviated caries clinical trial design validated over 24 months. J Dent Res 2002; 81:637-40.

[9]   Cunningham SJ, Hunt NP. Quality of life and its importance in orthodontics. J Orthod 2001; 28:152-8.

[10]   Dye BA, Tan S, Smith V, Lewis BG, Barker LK, Thornton-Evans G, Eke PI, Beltrán-Aguilar ED, Horowitz AM, Li CH. Trends in oral health status: United States, 1988-1994 and 1999-2004. Vital Health Stat 2007; 11:1-92.

[11]   Elderton RJ. Clinical studies concerning re-restoration of teeth. Adv Dent Res 1990; 4:4-9.

[12]   Ekstrand KR, Ricketts DN, Kidd EA. Reproducibility and accuracy of three methods for assessment of demineralization depth of the occlusal surface: an in vitro examination. Caries Res 1997; 31:224-31.

[13]   Feitosa S, Colares V, Pinkham J: The psychosocial effects of severe caries in 4-year-old children in Recife, Pernambuco, Brazil. Cad Saude Publica 2005;21:1550-6.

[14]   Filstrup SL, Briskie D, da Fonseca M, Lawrence L, Wandera A, Inglehart MR: Early childhood caries and quality of life: child and parent perspectives. Pediatr Dent 2003; 25:431-40.

[15]   Fyffe HE, Deery C, Nugent ZJ, Nuttall NM, Pitts NB. Effect of diagnostic threshold on the validity and reliability of epidemiological caries diagnosis using the Dundee Selectable Threshold Method for caries diagnosis (DSTM). Community Dent Oral Epidemiol 2000; 28: 42-51.

[16]   Guyatt G, Osoba D, Wu A, Wyrwich K, Norman G: Methods to explain the significance of health status measures. Hamilton, Ontario: Clinical Significance Consensus Meeting Group, Unpublished paper; 2002.

[17]   Kramer PF, Ardenghi TM, Ferreira S, Fischer LA, Cardoso L, Feldens CA. Use of dental services by preschool children in Canela, Rio Grande do Sul State, Brazil. Cad. Saúde Pública 2008;24:150-6.

[18]   Kieffer JM, Hoogstraten J. Linking oral health, general health, and quality of life. Eur J Oral Sci. 2008;116:445-50

[19]   Lader D, Chadwick B, Chestnutt, Harker R, Morris J, Nuttal N, Pitts N, Steele J, White D: Children's Dental Health in the United Kingdom, 2003 London: Office for National statistics; 2004.

[20] Malden PE, Thomson WM, Jokovic A, Locker D: Changes in parente assessed oral health-related quality of life among young children following dental treatment under general anaesthetic. Community Dent Oral Epidemiol 2008, 36:108–117.

[21] Martins-Júnior PA, Ramos-Jorge J, Paiva SM, Marques LS, Ramos-Jorge ML: Validations of the Brazilian version of the Early Childhood Oral Health Impact Scale (ECOHIS). Cad Saude Publica 2012a;28:367-74.

[22] Martins-Júnior PA, Vieira-Andrade RG, Corrêa-Faria P, Oliveira-Ferreira F, Marques LS, Ramos-Jorge ML. Impact of early Childhood caries on the oral health-related quality of ife of preschool children and their parents. Caries Res 2012b;47:211-8.

[23] Oliveira LB, Sheiham A, Bönecker M: Exploring the association of dental caries with social factors and nutritional status in Brazilian preschool children. Eur J Oral Sci 2008;116:37-43.

[24] Pahel BT, Rozier RG, Slade GD. Parental perceptions of children's oral health: The Early Childhood Oral Health Impact Scale (ECOHIS). Health Qual Life Outcomes 2007; 5:6.

[25] Patel RR, Tootla R, Inglehart MR. Does oral health affect self perceptions, parental ratings and video-based assessments of children's smiles? Community Dent Oral Epidemiol 2007; 35: 44-52.

[26] Pereira SM, Tagliaferro EP, Ambrosano GM, Cortelazzi KL, Meneghim MC, Pereira AC. Dental caries in 12-year-old schoolchildren and its relationship with socioeconomic and behavioural variables. Oral Health Prev Dent 2007; 5: 299-306.

[27] Petersen PE, Bourgeois D, Ogawa H, Estupinan-Day S, Ndiaye C. The global burden of oral diseases and risks to oral health. Bull World Health Organ 2005; 83: 661-69.

[28] Pitts NB. Are we ready to move from operative to non-operative/preventive treatment of dental caries in clinical practice? Caries Res 2004; 38: 294-304. Review.

[29] Ramos-Jorge J, Pordeus IA, Ramos-Jorge ML, Marques LS, Paiva SM: Impact of untreated dental caries on quality of life of preschool children: diferent stages and activity. Community Dent Oral Epidemiol 2014; 42:311-22.

[30] Rebok G, Riley A, Forrest C, Starfield B, Green B, Robertson J, Tambor E. Elementary school-aged children's reports of their health: a cognitive interviewing study. Qual Life Res 2001;10:59-70.

[31] Reisine ST, Psoter W. Socioeconomic status and selected behavioral determinants as risk factors for dental caries. J Dent Educ 2001; 65: 1009-16.

[32] Ricketts DN, Ekstrand KR, Kidd EA, Larsen T. Relating visual and radiographic ranked scoring systems for occlusal caries detection to histological and microbiological evidence. Oper Dent 2002; 27:231-7.

[33] Sabbah W, Tsakos G, Chandola T, Sheiham A, Watt RG. Social gradients in oral and general health. J Dent Res 2007;86:992-6.

[34] Scarpelli AC, Paiva SM, Viegas CM, Carvalho AC, Ferreira FM, Pordeus IA: Oral health-related quality of life among Brazilian preschool children. Community Dent Oral Epidemiol 2012;41:336-44.

[35] Schroth RJ, Levi JA, Sellers EA, Friel J, Kliewer E, Moffatt ME. Vitamin D status of children with severe early childhood caries: a case-control study. BMC Pediatr 2013;13:174.

[36] Shoaib L, Deery C, Ricketts DN, Nugent ZJ. Validity and reproducibility of ICDAS II in primary teeth. Caries Res 2009;43:442-8.

[37] Slade GD. Derivation and validation of a short-form oral health impact profile. Community Dent Oral Epidemiol 1997; 25:284-90.

[38] Tamanini JTN, Dambros M, D'ancona CAL, Palma PCR, Netto Jr NR. Validation of the International Consultation on Incontinence Questionnaire – Short Form" (ICIQSF) for Portuguese. Rev Saude Publica 2004; 38:438-444.

[39] Talekar BS, Rozier RG, Slade GD, Ennett ST. Parental perceptions of their preschool-aged children's oral health. J Am Dent Assoc 2005;136:364-72.

[40] Traebert J, Guimarães LA, Durante EZ, Serratine AC. Low maternal schooling and severity of dental caries in Brazilian preschool children. Oral Health Prev Dent 2009; 7:39-45.

[41] Tsakos G, Blair YI, Yusuf H, Wright W, Watt RG, Macpherson LMD. Developing a new self-reported scale of oral health outcomes for 5-year-old children (SOHO-5). Health Qual Life Outcomes 2012;10:62.

[42] Wong HM, McGrath CP, King NM, Lo EC: Oral health-related quality of life in Hong Kong preschool children. Caries Res 2011;45:370-6.

[43] Zero DT, Zandona AF, Vail MM, Spolnik KJ: Dental caries and pulpal disease. Dent Clin North Am 2011;55:29-46.

Chapter 6

Herbal Dentifrices for Children

Marisa Alves Nogueira Diaz,
Isabela de Oliveira Carvalho and Gaspar Diaz

Additional information is available at the end of the chapter

http://dx.doi.org/10.5772/59812

1. Introduction

The use of plant extracts as antimicrobial agents has been increasing every daily. Currently, these applications are mainly found in dentistry with the increased use of plant extracts in toothpastes for both adults and children. This finding results from the fact that the oral cavity is considered a favorable environment for the colonization and growth of a wide range of microorganisms, bacteria being the most common [1, 2]. One of the core arguments for the pharmaceutical industry to use toothpastes made from plant extracts is that they can act as antibiotics, analgesics, sedatives, and anti-inflammatories, in addition to being less likely to cause side effects. In the case of toothpastes for children's use where the presence of fluoride can lead to fluorosis, the presence of extracts with antimicrobial activity is quite interesting, given that these combat microorganisms by preventing the formation of biofilms [3].

The presence of microorganisms in the physiology of the oral cavity is essential for normal development, since most species are commensal microorganisms. In some cases, these microorganisms contribute to preventing the establishment of pathogenic microorganisms [4]. However, some of these microorganisms are considered to be opportunistic pathogens that play an important role in the etiology of periodontitis and dental caries, which are believed to be the most prevalent diseases in the world [5]. These microorganisms have also regularly been involved in the etiology of a number of systemic diseases, such as respiratory infections, infective endocarditis, and cardiovascular diseases [6, 7].

Dental caries is a complex oral disease, caused mainly by dental plaque. Dental plaque has been described as an ordered structure in which the primary colonizers are *Actinomyces* and *Streptococci*. These microorganisms bind tightly to one another, in addition to the solid tooth surface, by means of an extracellular matrix consisting of polymers of both host and microbial origin [8-10]. The formation of dental plaque includes a series of steps that begins with the

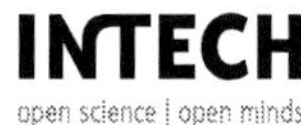

initial colonization of the pellicle and ends with the complex formation of a mature biofilm. Additionally, through the growth process of the biofilm, the microbial composition changes from one that is primarily Gram-positive and *Streptococcus*-rich to a structure filled with Gram-negative anaerobes in its more mature state [11]. It is widely accepted that the accumulation of microorganisms plays a key role in the initiation and progression of gingivitis and other oral diseases [12].

Gram-positive bacteria, such as *Lactobacilli* and the *Streptococci* species are associated with the formation of dental caries. As a result, strategies for treating this disease must concentrate on controlling the growth of these bacteria [13-15].

According to data from the World Health Organization (WHO), the prevalence of caries in schoolchildren is 60-90%, while among adults it is universal in most countries [16]. Biofilm formation is a natural process in the oral environment, and its control should be done through chemical and mechanical means. Brushing is a preventive measure considered essential for the prevention of caries and periodontal diseases, and can be effectively increased by using the toothpaste formulations containing antimicrobial agents [17-19].

1.1. Dental fluorosis

Dental fluorosis is the exposure of the tooth germ during its formation process at high concentrations of fluoride, resulting in defects of enamel mineralization with severity directly linked to the amount ingested. Clinically, the formation of opaque spots on the enamel of homologous teeth turning to a yellow or brown color, can be observed in more severe cases. In addition to the high dosage of fluoride, other factors contribute to the onset of fluorosis: low body weight, nutritional status, rate of skeletal growth and bone remodeling periods. In this sense, dental fluorosis is a more common disease in teeth of late mineralization (permanent teeth) in children with a low weight or poor nutritional state, occurring mainly at the ages of the first to second stages of childhood where there is a high incidence of systemic fluoride intake and subsequent harmful effects [20].

The decrease in the prevalence of dental caries has been attributed in large part to the use of fluoride toothpastes when brushing, one of the most accepted measures for the control of dental caries [21, 22]. By contrast, the prevalence of dental fluorosis has increased worldwide. The use of fluoride toothpaste before 6 years of age has been identified as one of the main risk factors for dental fluorosis [23]. However, other factors have also been found to cause fluorosis, especially commercially sold drinks, such as mineral water and soft drinks, among others, a fact that has increased the incidence of fluorosis in both places with fluoridated water consumption as well as in areas with non-fluoridated water consumption. This finding indicates that there is an intake of fluoride from other sources as well, in addition to the public water supply. Several studies have been conducted in many countries to determine the amount of fluoride in mineral waters, especially in soft drinks. The values obtained range from 0.007 mg/L to more than 4.1 mg/L for mineral waters and from 0.02 to 1.28 ppm, an average level of 0.72 ppm, for soft drinks, with no significant difference when the tastes of diet sodas are compared [24].

Depending on its severity, dental fluorosis may not only have aesthetic consequences, but it may also cause pain and affect masticatory efficiency [25]. Due to these facts, it is necessary to develop alternative formulations of toothpaste based on plant extracts with proven antimicrobial activity for use in children's dentistry to minimize the risk of dental fluorosis in infants and children from 1 to 6 years of age. Thus, many plant extracts with antimicrobial activity have been incorporated into toothpastes to prevent oral diseases. The plant extracts of the *Chordata macleya* and *Prunella vulgaris* species are examples of plants with an anti-inflammatory activity used in the international toothpaste market [26].

2. Toothpastes and antimicrobial agents

Common antimicrobial compounds added to toothpastes include: triclosan, stannous fluoride, and chlorhexidine. Nevertheless, despite the effectiveness of many formulations of toothpaste with antibacterial properties, the search for natural products with these properties has been increasing. Thus, plant extracts are being investigated as potential sources of new antibacterial compounds [27-29]. Dental plaque is considered an essential factor linked to the onset of caries, thus justifying the measures taken to control it. It is well-known that many metabolites produced by plants, such as tannins, terpenoids, flavonoids, and alkaloids, may represent a new source of antimicrobial substances [30, 31].

Natural toothpastes are considered to be those that do not incorporate the antimicrobial triclosan and fluoride. These toothpastes contain natural ingredients, such as the salts of sodium fluoride and sodium chloride and plant extracts, such as lemon, eucalyptus, rosemary, chamomile, sage, and myrrh [32]. Chamomile extract, for example, exhibits anti-inflammatory properties. By contrast, salvia extract decreases the tissue bleeding, whereas the extract of myrrhis, a natural antiseptic and extract of mentha, presents antiseptic, anti-inflammatory, and antimicrobial activities [33, 34]. Terpenoid compounds derived from medicinal plants and natural products, such as ursolic acid (UA) and oleanolic acid (OA), inhibited the growth of cariogenic microorganisms in a study conducted by Zhou and co-workers [35], suggesting that both compounds have the potential for use as antibacterial agents in the prevention of dental caries. Oral care products that are incorporated together with plant extracts are widely used due to their low toxicity, as compared to oral care products that contain antimicrobials, such as triclosan, cetyl pyridinium chloride, chlorhexidine, and fluoride [36, 37].

Toothpastes for children's use have had their contents changed in the name of progress and development in dentistry. In the past, toothpastes consisted of creams with a high fluorine content, masked by packaging illustrated with children's themes and flavored goodies that attracted children to the product. Nowadays, the cosmetics industry has reduced the fluorine content in these toothpastes to minimize the risk of fluorosis in children of less than 5 years of age, where fluorosis primarily affects the aesthetic appearance of their teeth [38].

3. Medicinal plants with antibacterial activity used in dentistry

The use of medicinal plants for the treatment of dental problems has widely been discussed by many researchers. Many cultures still use medicinal plants for the treatment of oral diseases, including caries for the cleaning and brushing of teeth, especially in rural areas of underdeveloped countries where people still brush their teeth without toothpaste [39]. The scientific field that uses the knowledge of medicinal plants for use in oral health is called Ethno-dentistry, which combines the knowledge of plants used by rural populations, indigenous populations, and communities in general. A brief description of some of the most common plants used in oral health was compiled, as described below.

3.1. *Myristica fragrans*

Myristica fragrans (Myristicaceae) is grown to be used as a spice and for medicinal purposes [40]. Its main constituents include alkylbenzenes (myristicin, elemicin, safrole, etc.); terpenes (α-pinene, β-pinene, myristic acid, trimyristin); and neolignans (myrislignan and macelignan) [41-43]. Its seed (known as nutmeg) is widely used in traditional medicine as an antithrombotic and antifungal drug, for the treatment of nausea and dyspepsia, and as an anti-inflammatory drug [44-46].

Studies have shown that *M. fragrans* has a great potential benefit in the field of dentistry, as its ethanol extract has proven to provide antibacterial activity against cariogenic bacteria [47]. According to Chung [42], the macelignan, an active compound isolated from *M. fragrans*, also presents an antibacterial activity against *Streptococcus mutans* and other oral microorganisms, such as *Streptococcus sobrinus*, *Streptococcus salivarius*, *Streptococcus sanguinis*, *Lactobacillus acidophilus*, and *Lactobacillus casei*, which indicates that it can be used as a natural antibacterial agent in oral hygiene products.

3.2. Propolis

Propolis, a natural antibiotic, is a resinous yellowish-brown to dark-brown substance collected by bees (*Apis mellifera*) from tree buds and is mixed with secreted beeswax. Bees use propolis as a glue to seal the opening of the hives protecting it from outside contaminants, which features over 300 compounds in its composition [48]. Among these constituents, one can find: flavonoids, steroids, sugars, and amino acids. The composition depends on the vegetation of the place from which it was collected and the season [48-50]. Thus, its biological activity is related to the plant ecology of the region visited by bees [51, 52]. Propolis has been outstanding for its anesthetic anti-inflammatory, healing, anti-trypanosome, and anti-cariogenic activities [53-56]. Brazilian propolis is one of the most active resinous substance, whose major components include diterpenes, lignans, *p*-coumaric acid, and flavonoids. A flavonoid is a compound with a wide range of biological activities, mainly antioxidant, anti-inflammatory, and antimicrobial activities [57, 58, 49].

Ikeno *et al.* [59] and Park *et al.* [60], respectively, have shown that propolis has *in vitro* effects on bacterial growth as well as on the activity of the glucosyltransferase enzyme (GTF), responsible for the formation of *S. sobrinus*, *S. mutans*, and *S. cricetus* biofilms in caries developed in rats. These studies demonstrate that propolis may well become a promising alternative for the prevention of caries and other oral diseases [61-63].

3.3. Chitosan

Chitin and chitosan are copolymers consisting of *N*-acetyl-D-glucosamine and D-glucosamine units in varying proportions. Chitin is the second most abundant polysaccharide in nature and is the main component of the exoskeleton of crustaceans and insects, but can also be found in nematodes, fungal cell walls, and yeasts. Chitosan has interesting medicinal properties, especially the antimicrobial activity *in vitro* against oral biofilm formations. This finding was reported in studies conducted by Verkaik *et al.* [64-66], who found that chitosan-based toothpaste, when compared with chlorhexidine-based toothpaste, traditionally used as an antimicrobial agent in toothpastes, may be equally as effective.

Chitosan showed a significant action in reducing dental plaque and presented antimicrobial activity *in vitro* against several pathogens in the oral cavity associated with the formation of dental plaque and periodontal disease, such as *Actinobacillus*, *S. mutans*, and *P. gingivalis* [67, 68]. Tarsie *et al.* [69] demonstrated that chitosan could influence the adherence of *S. mutans* to tooth surfaces, thus confirming the possibility of using this polysaccharide as a preventive agent in the formation of biofilms. According to the literature [70, 71], chitosan mouthwash was quite effective in reducing plaque that adheres to the teeth and reducing the count of *S. mutans* in saliva.

According to Mohiree Yadav [72], the addition of chitosan to toothpastes reduced plaque levels by 70% and caries caused by bacteria by 85%, respectively. Thus, toothpastes containing plant extracts and chitosan present an antibacterial efficacy comparable to those containing chlorhexidine [65]. The proven antimicrobial, anti-inflammatory, and healing effects of chitosan, coupled with their ability to inhibit the formation of biofilms, may well represent a formidable advantage in the treatment of diseases associated with the oral cavity [73].

3.4. *Punica granatum* Linn.

Punica granatum Linn. (Punicaceae), known in Brazil as "romã", is a small shrub cultivated worldwide in tropical and subtropical climates, has been used in traditional medicine as an astringent, hemostatic agent, and in the control of diabetes [74]. It is also commonly used to treat throat infections, cough and fever due to its anti-inflammatory and antimicrobial potential [75]. The antibiotic activity of the *P. granatum* extract is associated with its chemical constituents, including tannins and alkaloids found in the leaves, roots, stems and fruits [76, 77]. The alcoholic extract obtained from the fruit of *P. granatum* has shown effective antimicrobial activity against cariogenic bacteria, such as *S. mitis*, *S. mutans*, *S. sanguinis*, *S. sobrinus*, and *L. casei* [78, 79]. Toothpaste obtained from the alcoholic extract of *P. granatum* showed activity against cariogenic *S. mutans*, *S. sanguinis*, and *S. mitis* bacteria, demonstrating its antibacterial effect, suggesting the effective use of this herbal agent in the control of the adherence of different microorganisms within the oral cavity [80].

3.5. *Lentinus edodes* and *Cichorium intybus*

Lentinula edodes is the second most cultivated species of edible mushroom in the world, behind only champignon (*Agaricus bisporus*) [81]. It can be grown on tree trunks or on prepared substrates, and has attracted the interest of researchers, as it presents scientifically proven nutritional and therapeutic qualities [82].

Cichorium intybus (Compositae) has been used by humans as food since the dawn of civilization. It is a native plant of Europe that can be grown virtually everywhere [83, 84]. Studies have shown that various plant foods contain components with antibacterial and anti-dental plaque activity [85], including the alcoholic extracts of edible mushrooms, namely *L. edodes* and *C. intybus*, which can be used in products formulated for daily oral hygiene, such as mouthwashes and toothpastes [86-88].

3.6. *Copaifera officinalis* L.

Copaifera officinalis L. (Fabaceae) is a tree found mainly in Latin America and West Africa, also known as "Copaiba", copaiba balsam, Jesuit's balsam, copal, and capivi [89-91]. The copaiba oil has been documented to contain antibacterial activity. It corresponds to an excretion product, whose purpose is most likely to protect the plant against animals, fungi, and bacteria [92]. It is a liquid of varying viscosity and color, which can vary from yellow to brown [93, 94]. The extracted oil can vary in relation to its concentration of diterpenes and sesquiterpenes [95]. It is popularly used as an anti-inflammatory and healing agent whose actions are related to the presence of diterpenes within its composition [96]. Pieri *et al.* [97] studied the antimicrobial activity of copaiba oil on plaque-forming bacteria in dogs. The results showed that the oil was active against cariogenic bacteria, presenting an inhibitory effect on the adhesion of plaque-forming bacteria.

3.7. *Rosmarinus officinalis* Linn.

Rosmarinus officinalis Linn. (Labiatae) is a small shrub whose leaves have small glands containing essential oils. Tests performed *in vitro* with the essential oil showed an inhibitory effect on the adherence of *S. mutans* and the inhibitory growth activity of Gram-negative bacteria [98-100]. This plant has great potential in inhibiting bacterial growth and in the synthesis of glucan, suggesting its potential use in the control of cariogenic bacteria, whose activities were observed when its hydro-alcoholic extract showed significant activity on the glucosyltransferase enzyme produced by *S. mutans* [101-103]. It could also be observed that the alcoholic extract proved to be efficient in inhibiting the adherence of *S. mitis*, *S. mutans* and *S. sobrinus*, which suggests that it contains compounds with antibacterial activity against oral bacteria [104].

3.8. *Lippia sidoides* Cham.

Lippia sidoides Cham. (Verbenaceae) is a shrub originating from northeastern Brazil, popularly known as "alecrim pimenta". It is used in the treatment of allergic rhinitis, sore throat, gum inflammation, and the treating of skin wounds and cuts [105, 106]. *L. sidoides* contains an essential oil rich in thymol, which contains bactericidal properties [107, 108]. Tests performed *in vivo* have proven the effectiveness of a mouthwash and toothpaste-based essential oil of *L. sidoides*. An inhibition of approximately 12% of the microorganisms could be observed, with a 6% of reduction in the biofilm formation rate, thus demonstrating the efficiency of this essential oil in oral-based hygiene products [109, 110].

3.9. *Calendula officinalis* L.

Calendula officinalis L. (Asteraceae) is an herbaceous plant that is widely cultivated in many parts of the world for ornamental, medicinal, and cosmetic purposes [111]. In the dental field, this plant has been tested as regards its capacity to control the growth of biofilm-forming bacteria. Tests performed *in vivo* have demonstrated the effect of a 10% tincture of *C. officinalis* against chronic gingivitis, presenting significant improvement in the gingival tissues, with no apparent side effects [112, 19]. From these results, a toothpaste and a mouthwash containing 10% tincture of *C. officinalis* was developed. Tests performed *in vivo* using the type of toothpaste have demonstrated the effectiveness of this dental cream on gingival inflammation and the reduction of biofilm formation caused by *S. mutans* [113, 103]. Tests performed *in vivo* using a mouthwash containing 10% tincture of *C. officinalis* verified its efficiency in improving periodontal health, concluding that the performance was similar to mouthwashes prepared with 0.12% chlorhexidine in most evaluated parameters [114]. Another test performed *in vivo* using a toothpaste containing hydroalcoholic extracts of *C. officinalis* and *C. sylvestris* also showed bacteriostatic and fungistatic actions against microorganisms, such as *S. aureus*, *S. mutans*, and *C. albicans*, showing the associated therapeutic properties of these extracts [115].

3.10. *Schinus terebinthifolius* Raddi and *Myracrodruon urundeuva* Fr. All.

Schinus terebinthifolius Raddi and *Myracrodruon urundeuva* Fr. All. (Anacardiaceae), known in Brazil as "aroeira da praia" and "aroeira do sertão", respectively, are plants that are commonly found in South America. These plants are still used in traditional medicine in the northeastern regions of Brazil [116-119]. A 10% tincture of *S. terebinthifolius* showed efficacy in controlling biofilms formed by *S. mutans*, with a significant reduction in colony-forming units, as well as in the treatment of chronic gingivitis, presenting similar results when compared to 0.12% chlorhexidine-based toothpastes. This tincture also showed anti-inflammatory and antifungal activities against *Candida albicans*, suggesting its potential as an antibacterial agent, especially in the prevention oral cavity disease [120-123]. By contrast, the alcoholic extract of *M. urundeuva* also showed significant antimicrobial and anti-adherent activities against microorganisms that form biofilms [124].

3.11. *Matricaria recutita* Linn.

Matricaria recutita Linn. (Compositae) is a native plant of Europe and western Asia and is known for its variety of active flavonoids as well as for its essential oil, which is rich in terpenoids and is responsible for its anti-inflammatory and antibacterial activities [125, 126]. This plant has been widely used in inflammatory and infectious processes of the oral cavity [127]. Costa *et al.* [128] found that the alcoholic extract of *M. recutita* has antibacterial and anti-adherent activities against cariogenic bacteria *S. mutans*, *S. sanguinis* and *L. casei* [129]. According to studies performed by Lins *et al.* [130], a simple application of a mouthwash based on the hydroalcoholic extract of *M. recutita* proved effective in controlling biofilm formations caused by microorganisms, such as *S. mutans* and *S. sanguinis*, found in the oral cavity. In addition, this plant has been used in commercial toothpastes formulations for adults and children.

3.12. *Eugenia uniflora* L.

Eugenia uniflora L. (Myrtaceae), popularly known as "pitangueira", is a fruitful plant that is native to Brazil but can also be found in northern Argentina and Uruguay. [131]. Its leaves have been related to the treatment of various ailments, including fever, stomach ailments, hypertension, and obesity [132]. Antimicrobial activity was observed in this plant's leaves and cherries against *S. mutans*, *S. sanguinis*, *S. salivarius*, *S. mitis*, and *S. oralis* bacteria. Toothpastes containing the alcoholic extract of the ripe fruit of *E. uniflora* showed a similar efficacy to the Colgate Total 12 toothpaste, used as controlling agents in tests performed *in vivo* by Jovito *et al.* [133]. Castro *et al.* [134] demonstrated that hydroalcoholic extracts of *E. uniflora* showed antibacterial activity against *L. casei*.

3.13. *Myrciaria cauliflora* (Mart.) O. Berg.

Myrciaria cauliflora (Mart.) O. Berg. (Myrtaceae) is a native plant from Brazil and can be found throughout the country [135]. Tests performed *in vitro* using the alcoholic extract of this plant's leaves against *S. mutans* demonstrated that this extract acts on biofilm formation and could be an alternative for use in toothpastes [136, 137].

3.14. *Syzygium aromaticum*

Syzygium aromaticum (Myrtaceae), an aromatic flower bud of a tree that is native to the Maluku Islands in Indonesia, is commonly used as a spice. Cloves are commercially harvested primarily in Indonesia, India, Madagascar, Zanzibar, Pakistan, and Sri Lanka. The essential oil of *S. aromaticum* is used for flavoring and as a natural food preservative, as it presents antifungal and antibacterial activities [138, 139]. Its essential oil is rich in the compound eugenol, which is the most abundant substance in the tree's bark and is widely used in dentistry as an anesthetic in dental hygiene and to relieve toothaches [140]. This tree's branches contain a predominance of α and β-pinene, α-phellandrene, *p*-cymene, limonene, linalool, α-sequiterpenes copaene, β-caryophyllene, caryophyllene oxide, alilbenzenos ε-cinnamaldehyde, and aceto of ε-cinnamyl monoterpenes [141]. Tests performed *in vitro* demonstrated that the essential oil of *S. aromaticum*, when pure and incorporated into a toothpaste, presented antibacterial activity against *S. mutans* [142].

3.15. *Cinnamomum zeylanicum*

Cinnamomum zeylanicum (Lauraceae), native to Sri Lanka in South Asia, is a small or medium sized tree, commonly reaching 20 to 40 ft. in height. *C. zeylanicum* was widely used in ancient times as a spice. It is currently used as a flavoring in cooking food as well as in medicine as an antimicrobial agent. The essential oil extracted from its leaves contain a greater quantity of an aldehyde called cinnamaldehyde. Oliveira *et al.* [142] evaluated the essential oil of this plant against *S. mutans* and *L. casei*. These authors observed that the essential oil of *C. zeylanicum* showed inhibition zones of close to or above those of standard chlorhexidine, which was the same result observed for toothpastes formulated with the oil. Other studies have demonstrated the action of this essential oil on yeasts, such as *C. albicans* and *C. tropicalis*, which produce oral candidiasis in denture users [143].

3.16. *Cymbopogon citratus*

Cymbopogon citratus (Poaceae) is a herbaceous plant that is, native to the tropical regions of Asia, especially India. Also known as *Cymbopogon (nardus)* or by synonyms, such as *Andropogon citratus ceriferus, Andropogon citratus, Andropogon citriodorum, Andropogon nardus ceriferus, Andropogon roxburghiie*, and *Andropogon schoenanthus*. The essential oil extracted from this plant's leaves contains the main components of citral, geraniol, methyleugenol, myrcene, and citronellal [144]. Oliveira *et al.* [142] evaluated this plant's essential oil against *S. mutans* and *L. casei* and noted that it presented inhibition zones of close to those of standard chlorhexidine against the microorganism *S. mutans*. However, when analyzing the formulation of toothpastes containing the essential oil, it was found that this oil proved ineffective in the concentration tested to inhibit the growth of microorganisms. Perazzo *et al.* [145] also evaluated the essential oil of *C. citratus* on bacterial biofilm formation, especially in strains of *S. mutans* (ATCC 25175), *S. salivarius* (ATCC7073), and *S. oralis* (ATCC1055) and observed that this essential oil was more effective against *S. mutans*.

3.17. *Malva sylvestris*

Malva sylvestris (Malvaceae) is a biennial or perennial erect herbaceous species that is native to Europe and is widely known for its anti-inflammatory and antimicrobial properties [146]. Its phytochemical composition includes tannins, glycolipids, and flavonoids, which were tested as regards their capacity to control the growth of bacteria and biofilm formation [147, 18]. *M. sylvestris* has proven to be so effective that it already exists on the commercial market, called Malvatricin®, which is widely used as an antimicrobial agent against cariogenic bacteria. This effect is most likely due to the action of quinosol, a substance present in its composition [148].

3.18. *Nasturtium officinale*

Nasturtium officinale (Cruciferaceae) is a native plant of Europe and Asia that has many uses in medicine and pharmacology [149]. It is rich in vitamins and active substances, and is most commonly used in the treatment of urinary tract infections in children [150]. Tests performed *in vitro* with a mouthwash containing 10% hydroalcoholic extract of *N. officinale* was effective in controlling the growth of the microorganisms present in the oral cavity and dental plaque [151].

3.19. *Aloe vera*

Aloe vera (L.) Burm and *Aloe barbadensis* Miller (Asphodelaceae), popularly known as "aloe", are native from Africa and are widely used in traditional medicine. The gel of this plant contains healing, antibacterial, and antifungal activities due to the presence of anthraquinones, such as aloenin, barbaloin, and isobarbaloin in its chemical composition [152-155]. Studies have demonstrated the antimicrobial activity of toothpastes containing *A. vera* on oral microorganisms, such as *S. mutans, S. sanguis, A. viscosus,* and *C. albicans* [27].

3.20. *Magnolia officinalis*

Magnolia officinalis (Magnoliaceae) is a native plant of the mountains and valleys of China at altitudes of 300-1500 meters. The highly aromatic bark is stripped from the stems, branches, and roots, and is used in traditional Chinese medicine, where it is known as "hou po" [156]. The traditional use indications are to eliminate the dampness and phlegm, and relieve the distension. Huang *et al.* [157] have shown that the magnolol isolated from this plant was able to inhibit the growth of cariogenic bacteria.

Plants	Pharmaceutical form	Use
Salvia officinalis	mouthwash	plaque and bleeding on probing
Plantago psyllium L	mouthwash	periodontitis
Punica granatum Linn. and *Centella asiatica*	mouthwash	periodontitis
Aloe ferox Mill	mouthwash	gingivitis
Calendula officinalis L	mouthwash	Gengivite and periodontitis
Lippia sidoides Cham	mouthwash	plaque and bleeding on probing
Punica granatum Linn.	toothpaste	gingivitis
M. recutita L./Enchinacea angustifólia/ Krameria triandria Ruíze Pavon	toothpaste	gingivitis
Calendula officinalis L	toothpaste	gingivitis
Punica granatum Linn.	Gel	candidiasis, plaque and gingivitis

Table 1. Medicinal plants use in the treatment of oral diseases clinical studies.

3.21. *Salvia officinallis*

Salvia officinallis (Labiatae) is plant that is native to the Mediterranean region, though it has been naturalized in many places throughout the world. It is a perennial, evergreen subshrub that has a long history of medicinal and culinary uses. Its essential oil contains cineole, borneol, and thujone. Sage leaf contains tannic acid, oleic acid, ursonic acid, ursolic acid, carnosol, carnosic acid, fumaric acid, chlorogenic acid, caffeic acid, niacin, nicotinamide, flavones, flavonoid glycosides, and estrogenic substances [158]. Tests performed *in vivo* by Celeste *et al.* [159] have shown that a mouthwash containing a 10% alcoholic extract of *S. officinalis* reduced the visible plaque index (VPI) of the volunteers in 15.3% and the gingival index (GI) in 9.3% when compared to the chlorhexidine control.

3.22. *Azadirachta indica*

Azadirachta indica (Meliaceae) is native plant of India and the Indian subcontinent including Nepal, Pakistan, Bangladesh, and Sri Lanka. The tree can reach a height of 15 to 20 m (49 to 66 ft.). It has been used in India for decades in the treatment of several diseases in medicine and dentistry. Chatterjee *et al.* [160] evaluated a 0.19% *A. indica* mouthwash in tests performed *in vivo* and observed that the *A. indica* mouthwash is as effective in reducing periodontal indices as is chlorhexidine, which was used as the control, showing a significant reduction in gingival bleeding, and plaque indices.

4. Conclusion

The decrease in the amount of fluoride associated with the presence of plant extracts with proven antimicrobial activity is a positive factor for the reduction of fluorosis. For babies, we recommend the use of toothpastes containing only plant extracts, with no fluoride, since there is no risk of caries at this age. In such cases, these toothpastes can be used to adapt the babies to a proper hygiene of their oral cavity as well as maintain their beneficial microbiota.

Acknowledgements

The authors are grateful to CNPq, CAPES and FAPEMIG for their financial support.

Author details

Marisa Alves Nogueira Diaz[1*], Isabela de Oliveira Carvalho[1] and Gaspar Diaz[2]

*Address all correspondence to: marisanogueira@ufv.br

1 Departament of Biochemistry and Molecular Biology, Federal University of Viçosa, Viçosa, Minas Gerais, Brazil

2 Departament of Chemistry, Federal University of Minas Gerais, Belo Horizonte, Minas Gerais, Brazil

References

[1] Aas JA, Paster BJ, Stokes LN, Olsen I, Dewhirst FE. Defining the normal bacterial flora of the oral cavity. Journal of Clinical Microbiology 2005;43(5) 721–732.

[2] Zaura E, Keijser BJ, Huse SM, Crielaard W. Defining the healthy "core microbiome" of oral microbial communities. BMC Microbiology 2009;9(1) 259-271.

[3] Groppo FC, Bergamaschi CC, Cogo K, Franz-Montan M, Motta RHL, Andrade ED. Use of Phytotherapy in Dentistry. Phytotherapy Research 2008; 22 993–998.

[4] Marsh PD, Moter A, Devine DA. Dental plaque biofilms: communities, conflict and control. Periodontology 2011;53(1) 16-35.

[5] Meyer DH, Fives-Taylor PM. Oral pathogens: from dental plaque to cardiac disease. Current Opinion in Microbiology 1998;1(1) 88-95.

[6] Barrau K, Boulamery A, Imbert G, Casalta JP, Habib G, Messana T, Bonnet JL, Rubinstein E, Raoult D. Causative organisms of infective endocarditis according to host status. Clinical Microbiology and Infection 2004;10(4) 302-308.

[7] Okuda K, Kato T, Ishihara K. Involvement of periodontopathic biofilm in vascular diseases. Oral Diseases 2004;10(1) 5-12.

[8] Kolenbrander PE. Intergeneric coaggregation among human oral bacteria and ecology of dental plaque. Annual Review of Microbiology 1988;42(1) 627-656.

[9] Bowenand WH, Koo H. Biology of *Streptococcus mutans* derived glucosyltransferases: role in extracellular matrix formation of cariogenic biofilms. Caries Research, 2011;45(1) 69-86.

[10] Bradshaw DJ, Marsh PD, Watson GK, Allison C. Role of *Fusobacterium nucleatumand* coaggregation in anaerobe survival in planktonic and biofilm oral communities during aeration. Infection and Immunity 1998;66(10) 4729-4732.

[11] Marsh PD. Dental plaque as a biofilm and a microbial community-implications for health and disease. BMC Oral Health 2006;6(suppl 1) S14.

[12] Socransky SS, Haffajee AD. Periodontal microbial ecology. Periodontol 2000. 2005;38(1) 135-187.

[13] Thibodeau EA, O'Sullivan DM. Salivary *mutans* streptococci and caries development in the primary and mixed dentitions of children. Community Dentistry and Oral Epidemiology 1999;27(6) 406-412.

[14] Loesche W. Dental caries and periodontitis: contrasting two infections that have medical implications. Infectious Disease Clinics of North America 2007;21(2) 471-502.

[15] Featherstone JDB. Dental caries: a dynamic disease process. Australian Dental Journal 2008;53(3) 286-291.

[16] Petersen PE, Bourgeois D, Ogawa H, Estupinan-Day S, Ndiaye C. The global burden of oral disease and risks to oral health. Bulletin of the World Health Organization 2005;83(9) 661-669.

[17] Long SR, Santos AS, Nascimento CMO. Avaliação da contaminação de escovas dentais por enterobactérias. Revista de Odontologia da Universidade de Santo Amaro 2000;5(1) 21-25.

[18] Buffon MCM, Lima MLC, Galarda L, Cogo L. Avaliação da eficácia dos extratos de *Malva sylvestris*, *Calendula officinalis*, *Plantago major* e *Curcuma zedoarea* no controle do crescimento das bactérias da placa dentária. Estudo *"in vitro"*. Revista Visão Acadêmica 2001;2(1) 31-38.

[19] Van Rijkom HM, Truin GJ, Van't Hof MA. A meta-analysis of clinical studies on the caries-inhibiting effect of chlorhexidine treatment. Journal of Dental Research 1996;75(2) 790 795.

[20] Cangussu MCT, Narvai PC, Castellanos Fernandez R, Djehizian V. A fluorose dentária no Brasil: uma revisão crítica. Cadernos de Saúde Pública 2002;18(1) 7-15.

[21] Cury JA, Tenuta LMA, Ribeiro CCC, Paes Leme AF. The importance of fluoride dentifrices to the current dental caries prevalence in Brazil. Brazilian Dental Journal 2004;5(3) 167-174.

[22] Ricomini Filho AP, Tenuta LMA, Fernandes, FSF, Calvo SCK, Cury JA. Fluoride concentration in the top-selling Brazilian toothpastes purchased at different regions. Brazilian Dental Journal 2012;23(1) 45-48.

[23] Mascarenhas AK. Risk factors for dental fluorosis: A review of the recent literature. Pediatric dentistry 2000;22(4) 269-277.

[24] Moysés SJ, Moysés ST, Allegretti AC, Argenta M, Werneck R. Dental fluorosis: epidemiological fiction?. Revista Panamericana de Salud Pública 2002;12(5) 339-346.

[25] National Research Council. Fluoride in drinking water: a scientific review of EPA's standards. The National Academies Press, 2006.

[26] Adamkova H, Vicar J, Palasova J, Ulrichova J, Simanek V. Macleya cordata and Prunella vulgaris in oral hygiene products – their efficacy in the control of gingivitis. Biomed Pap Med Fac Univ Palacky Olomouc Czech Repub. 2004;148(1) 103-105.

[27] Lee SS, Zhang W, Li Y. The antimicrobial potential of 14 natural herbal dentifrices: results of anin vitro diffusion method study. The Journal of the American Dental Association 2004;135(8) 1133-1141.

[28] Gunsolley JC. A meta-analysis of six-month studies of antiplaque and antigingivitis agents. The Journal of the American Dental Association 2006;137(12) 1649-1657.

[29] Allaker RP, Douglas CW. Novel anti-microbial therapies for dental plaque-related diseases. International Journal of Antimicrobial Agents 2009;33(1) 8-13.

[30] DenBesten P, Berkowitz RJ. Early childhood caries: an overvview with reference to our experience in California. Journal of California Dental Association 2003;31(1) 139-143.

[31] Agarwala M, Yadav RNS. Phytochemical analysis of some medicinal plants. Journal of Phytology 2011;3(12) 10-14.

[32] Okpalugo J, Ibrahim K, Inyang US. Toothpaste formulation efficacy in reducing oral flora. Tropical Journal of Pharmaceutical Research 2009;8(1) 71-77.

[33] Pistorius A, Willershausen B, Steinmeier EM, Kreislert M. Efficacy of subgingival irrigation using herbal extracts on gingival inflammation. Journal of Periodontology 2003;7 4616–622.

[34] Pannuti CM, Mattos JP, Ranoya PN, Jesus AM, Lotufo RF, Romito GA. Clinical effect of a herbal dentifrice on the control of plaque and gingivitis: a double-blind study. Pesquisa Odontológica Brasileira 2003;17(4) 314-318.

[35] Zhou L, Ding Y, Chen W, Zhang P, Chen Y, Lv X. Thein vitro study of ursolic acid and oleanolic acid inhibiting cariogenic microorganisms as well as biofilm. Oral Diseases 2013;19(5) 494-500.

[36] Knoll-Kohler E, Stiebel J. Amine fluoride gel affects the viability and the generation of superoxide anions in human polymorphonuclear leukocytes: an in vitro study. European Journal of Oral Sciences 2002;110(4) 296-301.

[37] Neumegen RA, Fernández-Alba AR, Chisti Y. Toxicities of triclosan, phenol, and copper sulfate in activated sludge. Environmental Toxicology 2005;20(2) 160-164.

[38] Vieira MD, Hirata Júnior R, Barbosa ARS. Avaliação antimicrobiana de três dentifrícios para uso infantil: estudo in vitro. Revista Brasileira de Odontologia 2008;65(1) 52-56.

[39] Jose M, Deepa KC, Prabhu V. Ethnomedicinal Practices for Oral health and hygiene of Tribal population of Wayanad Kerala. In International Journal of Research in Ayurveda & pharmacy (IJRAP) 2011;2(4) 1246-1250.

[40] Jaiswal P, Kumar P, Singh VK., Singh D.K. Biological effects of *Myristica fragrans*. Annual Review of Biomedical Sciences 2009;11(1) 21-29.

[41] Qiu Q, Zhang G, Sun X, Liu X. Study on chemical constituents of the essential oil from *Myristica fragrans* Houtt. by supercritical fluid extraction and steam distillation. Journal of Chinese Medicinal Materials 2004; 27(11) 823-826.

[42] Chung JY, Choo JH, Lee MH, Hwang JK. Anticariogenic activity of macelignan isolated from *Myristica fragrans* (nutmeg) against *Streptococcus mutans*. Phytomedicine 2006;13(4) 261-266.

[43] Yang XW, Huang X, Ahmat M. "New neolignan from seed of *Myristica fragrans*," Zhongguo Zhongyao Zazhi 2008;33(4) 397-402.

[44] Sonavane GS, Sarveiya VP, Kasture VS, Kasture SB. Anxiogenic activity of *Myristica fragrans* seeds. Pharmacology Biochemistry and Behavior 2002;71(1-2) 239-244.

[45] Zaidi SFH, Yamada K, Kadowaki M, Usmanghani K, Sugiyama T. Bactericidal activity of medicinal plants, employed for the treatment of gastrointestinal ailments, against *Helicobacter pylori*. Journal of Ethnopharmacology 2009;121(2) 286-291.

[46] Ozaki Y, Soedigdo S, Wattimena YR, Suganda AG. Anti-inflammatory effect of Mace, aril of *Myristica fragrans* Houtt. and its active principles. Japanese Journal of Pharmacology 1989;49(2) 155-163.

[47] Shafiei Z, Shuhairi NN, Yap NMFS, Sibungkil C-AH, Hindawi JL. Antibacterial activity of *Myristica fragrans* against oral pathogens.vol. 2012, Article ID 825362, 7 pages, 2012. doi:10.1155/2012/825362.

[48] Burdock GA. Review of the biological properties and toxicity of bee propolis (propolis). Food and Chemical Toxicology 1998;36(4) 347-363.

[49] Tosi EA, Ré E, Ortega ME, Cazzoli AF. Food preservative based on propolis: bacteriostatic activity of propolis polyphenols and flavonoids upon *Escherichia coli*. Food Chemistry 2007;104(3) 1025-1029.

[50] Valencia D, Alday E, Robles-Zepeda R, Garibay-Escobar A, Galvez-Ruiz JC, Salas-Reyes M, Jiménez-Estrada M, Velázquez-Contreras E, Hernández J, Velázquez C. Seasonal effect on chemical composition and biological activities of Sonoran propolis. Food Chemistry 2012;131(2) 645-651.

[51] Park YK, Ikegaki M, Alencar SM, Moura FF. Evaluation of brazilian propolis by both physicochemical methods and biological activity. Honeybee Science 2000;21(2) 85-90.

[52] Marcucci MC, Ferreres F, Custódio AR, Ferreira MMC, Bankova VS, García-Viguera C, Bretz WA. Evaluation of phenolic compounds in Brazilian propolis from different geographic regions. Zeistchrift fur Naturforschung, 2000;55(1/2) 76-81.

[53] Cunha IBDS, Salomao K, Shimizu M, Bankova VS, Custodio AR, De Castro SL, Marcucci MC. Anti-trypanosomal activity of Brazilian propolis from *Apis mellifera*. Chemical & pharmaceutical Bulletin 2004;52(5) 602-604.

[54] Koo H, Rosalen PL, Cury JA, Park YK, Ikegaki M, Sattler A. Effect of *Apis mellifera* propolis from two Brazilian regions on caries development in desalivated rats. Caries Research 1999;33(5) 393-400.

[55] Koo H, Rosalen PL, Cury JA, Ambrosano GMAB, Murata RM, Yatsuda R, Ikegaki M, Alencar SM, Park YK. Effect of a new variety of *Apis mellifera* propolis on mutans Streptococci. Current Microbiology 2000;41(3) 192-196.

[56] Duarte S, Rosalen PL, Hayacibara MF, Cury JA, Bowen WH, Marquis RE, Rehder VLG, Sartoratto A, Ikegaki M, Koo H. The influence of a novel propolis on mutans

streptococci biofilms and caries development in rats. Archives of Oral Biology 2006;51(1) 15-22.

[57] Bankova V. Chemical diversity of propolis and the problem of standardization. Journal of Ethnopharmacology 2005;100(1-2) 114-117.

[58] Piccinelli AL, Fernández MC, Cuesta-Rubio O, Hernández IM, De Simone F, Rastrelli L. Isoflavonoids isolated from Cuban propolis. Journal of Agricultural and Food Chemistry 2005;53(23) 9010-9016.

[59] Ikeno K, Ikeno T, Miyazawa C. Effects of propolis on dental caries in rats. Caries Research 1991;25(5) 347-351.

[60] Park YK, Koo MH, Abreu JA, Ikegaki M, Cury JA, Rosalen PL. Antimicrobial activity of propolis on oral microorganisms. Current Microbiology 1998;36(1) 24-28.

[61] Duailibe SA, Gonçalves AG, Ahid FJ. Effect of a propolis extract on *Streptococcus mutans* counts *in vivo*. Journal of Applied Oral Science 2000;15(5) 420-423.

[62] Arslan S, Silici S, Perçin D, Ko AN, Er Ö. Antimicrobial activity of poplar propolis on mutans streptococci and caries development in rats. Turkish Journal of Biology 2012;36(1) 65-73.

[63] Barrientos L, Herrera CL, Montenegro G, Ortega X, Veloz J, Alvear M, Cuevas A, Saavedra N, Salazar LA. Chemical and botanical characterization of Chilean propolis and biological activity on cariogenic bacteria *Streptococcus mutans* and *Streptococcus sobrinus*. Brazilian Journal of Microbiology 2013;44(2) 577-585.

[64] Kubota N, Tastumoto N, Sano T, Toya K. A simple preparation of half N-acetylated chitosan highly soluble in water and aqueous organic solvents. Carbohydrate Research 2000;324(4) 268-274.

[65] Kittur FS, Kumar ABV, Varadaraj MC, Tharanathan RN. Chitooligosaccharides-preparation with the aid of pectinase isozyme from *Aspergillus nigerand* their antibacterial activity. Carbohydrate Research 2005;340(6) 1239-1245.

[66] Verkaik MJ, Busscher HJ, Jager D, Slomp AM, Abbas F, van der Mei HC. Efficacy of natural antimicrobials in toothpaste formulations against oral biofilms *in vitro*. Journal of dentistry 2011;39(3) 218-224.

[67] Choi BK, Kim KY, Yoo YJ, Oh SJ, Choi JH, Kim CY.*in vitro* antimicrobial activity of a chitooligosaccharide mixture against *Actinobacillus actinomycete comitans* and *Streptococcus mutans*. International Journal of Antimicrobial Agents 2001;18(6) 553-557.

[68] İkinci G, Şenel S, Akıncıbay H, Kaş S, Erciş S, Wilson CG, Hıncal AA. Effect of chitosan on a periodontal pathogen *Porphyromonas gingivalis*. International Journal of Phamaceutics 2002; 235(1/2) 121-127.

[69] Tarsi R, Muzzarelli R, Guzmàn C, Pruzzo C. Inhibition of *Streptococcus mutans* adsorption to hydroxyapatite by low-molecular-weigth chitosans. Journal of Dental Research 1997;76(2) 665-672.

[70] Sano H, Shibasaki KI, Matsukubo T, Takaesu Y. Effect of chitosan rinsing on reduction of dental plaque formation. The Bulletin of Tokyo Dental College 2003;44(1) 9-16.

[71] Decker EM, von Ohle C, Weiger R, Wiech I, Brecx M. A synergistic chlorhexidine/chitosan combination for improved antiplaque strategies. Journal of Periodontal Research 2005;40(5) 373-377.

[72] Mohire NC, Yadav AV. Chitosan-based polyherbal toothpaste: As novel oral hygiene product. Indian Journal of Dental Research 2010;21(3) 380-384.

[73] Tavaria FK, Costa EM, Pina-Vaz L, Carvalho MF, Pintado MM. A quitosana como biomaterial odontológico: estado da arte. Brazilian Journal of Biomedical Engineering 2013;29(1) 110-120.

[74] Ross RG, Selvasubramanian S, Jayasundar S. Immunomodulatory activity of *Punica granatum* in rabbits-a preliminary study. Journal of Ethnopharmacology 2001;78(1) 85-87.

[75] Machado TB, Pinto MCFR, Leal LCR, Silva MG, Amaral ACF, Kuster RM, Netto-Dos-Santos KR. In vitro activity of Brazilian medicinal plants, naturally occurring naphthoquinones and their analogues, against methicillin-resistant *Staphylococcus aureus*. International Journal of Antimicrobial Agents 2003;21(3) 279-284.

[76] Nawwar MAM, Hussein SAM, Merfort L. Leaf phenolics of *Punica granatum*. Phytochemistry 1994;37(4) 1175-1177.

[77] Machado TB, Leal LCR, Amaral ACF, Santos KRN, Silva MG, Kuster RM. Antimicrobial ellagitannin of *Punica granatum* fruits. Journal of the Brazilian Chemical Society 2002;13(5) 606-610.

[78] Pereira JV, Pereira MSV, Higino JS, Sampaio FC, Alves PM, Araújo CRF. Estudos com o extrato da *Punica granatum* Linn. (romã): efeito antimicrobiano in vitro e avaliação clínica de um dentifrício sobre microrganismos do biofilme dental. Revista Odonto Ciência 2005;20(49) 262-269.

[79] Pereira JV, Pereira MSV, Sampaio FC, Correia MC, Alves PM, Araújo CRF, Higino JS. Efeito antibacteriano e antiaderente *in vitro* do extrato da *Punica granatum* Linn.sobre microrganismos do biofilme dental. Revista Brasileira de Farmacognosia 2006;16(1) 88-93.

[80] Vasconcelos LCS, Sampaio FC, Sampaio MCC, Pereira MSV, Higino JS, Peixoto MHP. Minimum inhibitory concentration of adherence of *Punica granatum* Linn (pomegranate) gel against *S. mutans*, *S. mitis* and *C. albicans*. Brazilian Dental Journal 2006;17(3) 223-227.

[81] Chang ST, Kwan HS, Kang YN. Collection, characterization and utilization of germ plasm of *Lentinula edodes*. Canadian Journal of Botany 1995;73(1) 955-961.

[82] Eira AF, Kaneno R, Rodrigues Filho E, Barbisan LF, Pascholati SF, Di Piero RM, Salvadori DMF, Lima PLA, Ribeiro LR. Farming technology, biochemistry characterization, and protective effects of culinary-medicinal mushrooms *Agaricus brasiliensis* and *Lentinus edodes*: five years of research in Brazil. International Journal of Medicinal Mushrooms 2005;7(1/2) 281-300.

[83] Galvão G. Almeirão. Natureza 1995;8(7) 53-55.

[84] Van Lo J, Coussement P, Leenheer L, Hoebregs H, Smits G. On the presence of inulin and oligofructose as natural ingredients in the western diet. Critical Reviews in Food Science and Nutrition 1995;35(6) 525-552.

[85] Signoretto C, Canepari P, Pruzzo C, Gazzani G. Anticaries and antiadhesive properties of food constituents and plant extracts and implications for oral health. In: Wilson M. (ed) Food constituents and oral health: current status and future prospects. Cambridge: Woodhead Publishing Limited; 2009.

[86] Daglia, M, Papetti A,Mascherpa D,Grisoli P, Giusto G, Lingström P, Pratten J, Signoretto C, Spratt DA, Wilson M, Zaura E, Gazzan G. Plant and fungal food components with potential activity on the development of microbial oral diseases. Journal of Biomedicine and Biotechnology 2011;1-9.

[87] Spratt DA, Daglia M, Papetti A, Stauder M, Donnell DO, Ciric L, Tymon A, Repetto B, Signoretto C, Houri-Haddad Y, Feldman M, Steinberg D, Lawton S, Lingström P, PrattenJ, Zaura E,Gazzani G,Pruzzo C,Wilson M. Evaluation of plant and fungal extracts for their potential antigingivitis and anticaries activity. Journal of Biomedicine and Biotechnology 2012;1-12.

[88] Signoretto AM, Bertoncelli A, Burlacchini G, Tessarolo F, Caola L, Pezzati E, Zaura E, Papetti A, Lingstrom P, Pratten J, Spratt DA, Wilson M, Canepari P. Effects of mushroom and chicory extracts on the physiology and shape of *Prevotella intermedia*, a periodonto pathogenic bacterium. Journal of Biomedicine and Biotechnology 2011;1-8.

[89] Veiga Junior VF, Pinto AC, Calixto JB, Zunino L, Patitucci ML. Phytochemical and antiedematogenic studies of commercial copaíba oils available in Brazil. Phytotherapy Research 2001;15(6) 476-480.

[90] Lima SRM, Veiga Junior VF, Christo HB, Pinto AC, Fernandes PD. *In vivo* and *in vitro* studies on the anticancer activity of *Copaifera multijuga* Hayne and its fractions. Phytotherapy Research 2003;17(9) 1048-1053.

[91] Francisco SG. Uso do óleo de copaíba (*Copaifera officinalis*) em inflamação ginecológica. Femina 2005;33(2) 89-93.

[92] Pontes AB, Correia DZ, Coutinho MS, Mothé CG. Emulsão dermatológica a base de copaíba. Revista Analytica 2003; 7(7) 36-42

[93] Cascon V, Gilbert B. Characterization of the chemical composition of oleoresins of *Copaifera guianensis* Desf.,*Copaifera duckei* Dwyer and *Copaifera multijuga* Hayne. Phytochemistry 2000;55(7) 773-778.

[94] Pinto AC, Braga WF, Rezende CM, Garrido FMS, Veiga Júnior VF, Bergyer L, Patitucci ML, Antunes AC. Separation of acid diterpenes of *Copaifera cearenses* Huber ex Duke by flash chromatography using potassium hydroxide impregnated silica gel. Journal of the Brazilian Chemical Society 2000;11(4) 355-360.

[95] Veiga Junior VF, Pinto AC, Maciel MAM. Plantas medicinais: cura segura?. Química nova 2005;28(3) 519-528.

[96] Brito MVH, Oliveira RVB, Reis JMC. Estudo macroscópico do estômago de ratos após administração do óleo de Copaíba. Revista Paraense de Medicina 2000;14:(3) 29-33.

[97] Pieri FA, Mussi MC, Fiorini JE, Schneedorf JM. Efeitos clínicos e microbiológicos do óleo de copaíba (*Copaifera officinalis*) sobre bactérias formadoras de placa dental em cães. Arquivo Brasileiro de Medicina Veterinária e Zootecnia 2010;62(3) 578-585.

[98] Al-Sereiti MR, Abu-Amer KM, Sen P. Pharmacology of rosemary (*Rosmarinus offi cinalis* Linn.) and its therapeutic potentials. Indian Journal of Experimental Biology 1999;37(2) 124-130.

[99] Newall CA, Anderson LA, Phillipson JD. Plantas Medicinais: guia para profissional de saúde. São Paulo: Premier 2002.

[100] Takarada K, Kimizuka R, Takahashi N, Honma K, Okuda K, Kato T. A comparison of the antibacterial efficacies of essential oils against oral pathogens. Oral Microbiology and Immunology 2004;19(1) 61-64.

[101] Alves MP, Pereira VJ, Higino JS, Pereira MSV, Queiroz, MG. Atividade antimicrobiana e antiaderente in vitro do extrato de *Rosmarinus officinalis* Linn. (alecrim) sobre microrganismos cariogênicos. Arquivos em Odontologia 2008;44(2) 5-10.

[102] Battagin J. Cinética enzimática e efeito de extratos naturais na atividade da enzima glicosiltransferase de *Streptococcus mutans*. Master thesis. Universidade São Francisco; 2010.

[103] Pinheiro, MA, Brito DBA, Almeida LFD, Cavalcanti YW, Padilha WWN. Efeito antimicrobiano de tinturas de produtos naturais sobre bactérias da cárie dentária. Revista Brasileira em Promoção da Saúde, 2012;25(2) 197-201.

[104] Silva MSA, Silva MAR, Higino JS, Pereira MSV, Carvalho AAT. Atividade antimicrobiana e antiaderente in vitro do extrato de *Rosmarinus officinalis* Linn. sobre bactérias orais planctônicas. Revista Brasileira de Farmacognosia 2008;18(2) 236-240.

[105] Lemos TL, Craveiro AA, Alencar JW, Matos FJ, Clarck AM, Macchesney JD. Antimicrobial activity of essential oil of Brazilian plants. Phytotherapy Research 1990;4(2) 82-84.

[106] Nunes RS. Desenvolvimento galênico de produtos de uso odontologico (creme dental e enxaguatorio bucal) a base de *Lippia sidoides* Cham (verbenaceae) Master thesis. Universidade Federal de Pernambuco; 1999.

[107] Girão VCC, Nunes-Pinheiro DCS, Morais SM, Sequeira JL, Gioso MA. A clinical trial of the effect of a mouthrinse prepared with *Lippia sidoides* Cham essential oil in dogs with mild gingival disease. Preventive Veterinary Medicine 2003;59(1/2) 95-102.

[108] Cavalcanti ESB, Morais SM, Lima MA, Santana EWP. Larvicidal activity of essential oils from Brazilian plants against *Aedes aegypti* L. Memórias do Instituto Oswaldo Cruz 2004;99(5) 541-544.

[109] Sobreira FFE, Morais SM, Fonseca SGC, Mota OML. Preparation and clinical evaluation of an antiseptic mouthrinse using *Lippia sidoides* Cham (Alecrim pimenta) essencial oil. Revista ABO Nacional 1998;6(5) 323-325.

[110] Nunes RS, Lira AAM, Lacerda CM, Silva, DOB, Silva JA, Santana DP. Obtenção e avaliação clínica de dentifrícios à base do extrato hidroalcoólico da *Lippia sidoides* Cham (Verbenaceae) sobre o biofilme dentário Revista de Odontologia 2006;35(4) 275-283.

[111] Ramos A, Edreira A, Vizoso A, Betancourt J, López M, Décalo M. Genotoxicity of extract of *Calendula officinalis* L. Journal of Ethnopharmacology 1998;61(1) 49-55.

[112] Lorenzo MRO, Madrigal RG, Pineda PJ. Efectos de la tintura de calendula al 10 por ciento en adolescentes afectados por gingivitis crónica. Mediciego 1997;3(2) 33-36.

[113] Amoian B, Moghadamnia AA, Mazandarani M. The effect of calendula extract toothpaste on the plaque index and bleeding in gingivitis. Research Journal of Medicinal Plant 2010;4(3) 132-140.

[114] Vinagre NPL, Farias CG, Araújo RJG, Vieira JMS, Silva Júnior JOC, Corrêa AM. Clinical efficacy of a phytotherapic mouthrinse with standardized tincture of *Calendula officinalis* in the maintenance of periodontal health. Revista de Odontologia da UNESP 2011;40(1) 30-35.

[115] Arantes AB, Luz MMS, Santos CAM, Sato MEO. Desenvolvimento de dentifrícios com extratos fluídos de *Calendula officinalis* L. (Asteraceae) e *Casearia sylvestris* Sw. (Flacourtiaceae) destinado ao combate à placa bacteriana. Revista Brasileira de Farmacognosia 2005;86(2) 61-64.

[116] Kato ETM, Akisue G. Estudo farmacognóstico de cascas *Myracrodruon urundeuva* Fr. All. Revista Lecta 2002;20(1) 69-76.

[117] Santin DA, Leitão HF. Restabelecimento e revisão taxonômica do gênero *Myracro-druon* Freire Allemão (Anacardiacea). Revista Brasileira de Botânica 1991;14(2) 133-145.

[118] Deharo E, Baelmans R, Gimenez A, Quenevo C, Bourdy G. *In vitro* immunomodulatory activity of plants used by the *Tacana* ethnic group in Bolívia. Phytomedicine 2004;11(6) 516-522.

[119] Biavatti M, Marensi V, Leite SN, Reis A. Ethnopharmacognostic survey on botanical compendia for potential cosmeceutic species from Atlantic Forest. Revista Brasileira de Farmacognosia 2007;17(4) 640-653.

[120] Brandão EHS, Oliveira LD, Landucci LF, Koga-Ito CY, Cardoso JAO. Antimicrobial activity of coffee based solutions and their effects on *Streptococcus mutans* adherence. Brazilian Journal of Oral Science 2006;6(20) 1274-1277.

[121] Soares DGS, Oliveira CB, Lcali C, Drumond MRS, Padilha WWN.Atividade antibacteriana *in vitro* da tintura de aroeira (*Schinus terebinthifolius*) na descontaminação de escovas dentais contaminadas pelo *S. mutans*. Odontologia Clínico-Científica 2007;7(3) 253-257.

[122] Freires IA, Alves LA, Jovito VC, Almeida LFD, Castro RD, Padilha WWN. Atividades antibacteriana e antiaderente *in vitro* de tinturas de *Schinus terebinthinfolius* (Aroeira) e *Solidago microglossa* (Arnica) frente a bactérias formadoras do biofilme dentário. Odontologia Clínico-Científica 2010;9(2) 139-143.

[123] Lins R, Vasconcelos FHP, Leite RB, Coelho-Soares RS, Barbosa DN. Avaliação clínica de bochechos com extratos de Aroeira (*Schinus terebinthifolius*) e Camomila (*Matricaria recutita* L.) sobre a placa bacteriana e a gengivite. Revista Brasileira de Plantas Medicinais 2013;15(1) 112-120.

[124] Alves PM, Queiroz LMG, Pereira JV, Pereira MSV. Atividade antimicrobiana, antiaderente e antifúngica *in vitro* de plantas medicinais brasileiras sobre microrganismos do biofilme dental e cepas do gênero *Candida*. Revista da Sociedade Brasileira de Medicina Tropical 2009;42(2) 222-224.

[125] Mulinacci N, Romani A, Pinelli P, Vincieri FF, Prucher D. Characterization of *Matricaria recutita* L. flower extracts by HPLC-MS and HPLC-DAD analysis. Chromatography 2000;51(5/6) 301-307.

[126] McKay DL, Blumberg JBA. Review of the bioactivity and potential health benefits of chamomile tea (*Matricaria recutita* L.). Phytotherapy Research 2006;20(7) 519-530.

[127] Paixão CCB, Santos AA, Oliveira CCC, Silva LG, Nunes MAR. Uso de plantas medicinais em pacientes portadores de afecções bucais. Odontologia Clinica Científica, 2002;1(1) 23-27.

[128] Costa MR, Albuquerque AC, Pereira L, Vieira A, Diniz DN, Pereira MSV, Pereira JV, Trevisan LFA. Efeito antimicrobiano do extrato da *Myrciaria cauliflora* Berg e *Matrica-*

ria recutita Linn. sobre microrganismos do biofilme dental. Revista de Biologia e Farmácia 2010;4(1) 19-25.

[129] Albuquerque ACL, Pereira MSV, Pereira JV, Pereira LF, Silva DF, Macedo-Costa MR, Higino JS. Efeito antiaderente do extrato da *Matricaria recutita* Linn. sobre microrganismos do biofilme dental. Revista de Odontologia da UNESP 2010; 39(1) 21-25.

[130] Lins R, Vasconcelos FHP, Leite RB, Coelho-Soares RS, Barbosa DN. Avaliação clínica de bochechos com extratos de Aroeira (*Schinus terebinthifolius*) e Camomila (*Matricaria recutita* L.) sobre a placa bacteriana e a gengivite. Revista Brasileira de Plantas Medicinais 2013;15(1) 112-120.

[131] Bezerra JEF, Lederman IE, Silva Júnior JF, Alves MA. Comportamento da pitangueira (*Eugenia uniflora*) sob Irrigação na Região do Vale do Rio Moxotó, Pernambuco. Revista Brasileira de Fruticultura 2004;26(1) 177-179.

[132] Schmeda-Hirschmann G, Theoduloz C, Franco L, Ferro E, Arias AR. Preliminary pharmacological studies on *Eugenia uniflora* leaves: xanthine oxidase inhibitory activity. Journal of Ethnopharmacology 1987;21(2) 183-186.

[133] Jovito VC, Almeida LFD, Ferreira DAH, Moura D, Paulo MQ, Padilha WWN. Avaliação *in vivo* de dentifrício contendo extrato da *Eugenia uniflora* L. (Pitanga) sobre Indicadores de saúde bucal. Pesquisa Brasileira em Odontopediatria e Clínica Integrada 2009;9(1) 81-86.

[134] Castro RD, Freires IA, Ferreira DAH, Jovito VC, Paulo, MQ. Atividade antibacteriana *in vitro* de produtos naturais sobre *Lactobacillus casei.* International Journal of Dentistry 2010;9(2) 74-77.

[135] Agra MF, França PF, Barbosa-Filho JM. Synopsis of the plants known as medicinal and poisonous in Northeast of Brazil. Revista Brasileira de Farmacognosia 2007;17(1) 114-140.

[136] Carvalho CM, Macedo-Costa MR, Pereira MSV, Higino JS, Carvalho LFPC, Costa, LJ. Efeito antimicrobiano in vitro do extrato de jabuticaba (*Myrciaria cauliflora* (Mart.) O. Berg.) sobre *Streptococcus* da cavidade oral. Revista Brasileira de Plantas Medicinais 2009;11(1) 79-83.

[137] Costa, MR, Diniz, DN, Carvalho, CM, Pereira MSV, Pereira JV, Higino JS. Eficácia do extrato de *Myrciaria cauliflora* (Mart.) O. Berg. (jabuticabeira) sobre bactérias orais. Revista Brasileira de Farmacognosia 2009;19(2B) 565-571.

[138] Lima IO, Oliveira RAG, Lima EO, Farias NMP, Souza EL. Antifungal activity from essential oils on Candida species. Revista Brasileira de Farmacognosia 2006;16(2) 197-201.

[139] Matan N, Rimkeeree H, Mawson AJ, Chompreeda P, Haruthaithanasan V, Parker M. Antimicrobial activity of cinnamon and clove oils under modified atmosphere conditions. International Journal of Food Microbiology 2006;107(2) 180-185.

[140] Chong BS, Ford TRP, Kariyawasam SP. Short-term tissue response to potential root-end filling materials in infected root canals. International Endodontic Journal 1997;30(4) 240-249.

[141] Lima MP, Zoghbi MGB, Andrade EHA, Silva TMD. Fernandes CS. Constituintes voláteis das folhas e dos galhos de *Cinnamonum zeylanicum* Blume (Lauraceae). Acta Amazônica 2005;35(3) 363-366.

[142] Oliveira SMM, Lorscheider JA, Nogueira MA. Avaliação da ação *in vitro* de gel dentifrício contendo óleos essenciais sobre bactérias cariogênicas. Latin American Journal of Pharmacy 2008;27(2) 266-269.

[143] Castro RD, Lima EO. Screening of essential oils antifungal activity on candida Strains. Pesquisa Brasileira em Odontopediatria e Clínica Integrada 2011;11(3) 341-345.

[144] Brito ES, Garruti DS, Alves PB, Blank AF.Caracterização odorífera dos componentes do óleo essencial de capim-Santo (*Cymbopogon citratus* (DC.) Stapf., Poaceae) por cromatografia gasosa (CG) – Olfatometria. Fortaleza: Empresa Brasileira de Pesquisa Agropecuária; 2011.

[145] Perazzo MF, Costa Neta MC, Cavalcanti YW, Xavier AFC, Cavalcanti AL. Antimicrobial effect of *Cymbopogon citratus* essential oil on dental biofilm-forming bacteria. Revista Brasileira de Ciências da Saúde 2012;16(4) 553-558.

[146] Alzugaray D, Alzugaray C. Plantas que curam. São Paulo: Três; 1996.

[147] Torres CRG, Cubo CH, Anido AA, Rodrigues JR. Agentes antimicrobianos e seu potencial de uso na odontologia. Revista da Faculdade de Odontologia de São José dos Campos 2000;3(2) 43-52.

[148] Moreira MJS, Ferreira MBC, Hashizume LN. Avaliação in vitro da atividade antimicrobiana dos componentes de um enxaguatório bucal contendo malva. Pesquisa Brasileira em Odontopediatria e Clínica Integrada 2012;12(4) 505-509.

[149] Carvalho JLS. Contribuição ao estudo fitoquímico e analítico no *Nasturtium officinale* R. Br., Brasicaceae. Master thesis. Universidade Federal do Paraná; 2001.

[150] Blumenthal M, Goldberg A, Brinckmaann J. Herbal medicine In: Hardcover (ed) Integrative Medicine Communications.2000. p 404-407.

[151] Cordeiro CHG, Sacramento LVS, Corrêa MA, Pizzolitto AC, Bauab TM. Análise farmacognóstica e atividade antibacteriana de extratos vegetais empregados em formulação para a higiene bucal. Revista Brasileira de Ciências Farmacêuticas 2006;42(3) 395-404.

[152] Schimid R. An old medicinal plant: *Aloe vera*. Parfümerie und kosmetik 1991;72(3) 146-150.

[153] Okamura N, Asai M, Hine N, Yagi A. High-performance liquid chromatographic determination of phenolic compounds in Aloe species. Journal of Chromatography 1996;746(2) 225-231.

[154] Kuzuya H, Tamai I, Beppu H, Shimpo K, Chihara T. Determination of aloenin, barbaloin and isobarbaloin in Aloe species by micellar electrokinetic chromatography. Journal of Chromatography 2001;752(1) 91-97.

[155] Steinert J, Khalaj S, Rimpler M. High-performance liquid chromatographic separation of some naturally occurring naphthoquinones and anthraquinones. Journal of Chromatograhy A 1996;723(1/2) 206-209.

[156] Ho KY, Tsai CC, Chen CP, Huang JS, Lin CC. Antimicrobial activity of honokiol and magnolol isolated from *Magnolia officinalis*. Phytotherapy Research 2001;15(2) 139-141.

[157] Huang BB, Fan MW, Wang SL, Huang YB, Zhou J, Wang Q. Inhibitory effect of *Magnolia officinalis* extract on growth of *Streptococcus mutans*. The Chinese Journal of Dental Research 2004;7(2) 15-9.

[158] Oliveira FQ, Gobira B, Guimarães C, Batista J, Barreto M, Souza M. Espécies vegetais indicadas na odontologia. Revista Brasileira de Farmacognosia 2007;17(3) 466-476.

[159] Celeste RK, Slavutzky SMB, Van PGL. Ação preventiva do bochecho de sálvia: efeitos sobre placa dental e gengivite. Revista Gaúcha de Odontologia 1998;46(2) 97-99.

[160] Chatterjee A, Saluja M, Singh N, Kandwal A. To evaluate the antigingivitis and antipalque effect of an Azadirachta indica (neem) mouthrinse on plaque induced gingivitis: A double-blind, randomized, controlled trial. Journal of Indian Society of Periodontology 2011;15(4) 398–401.

Chapter 7

Infant Oral Health

Preetika Chandna and Vivek K. Adlakha

Additional information is available at the end of the chapter

http://dx.doi.org/10.5772/59245

1. Introduction

Infancy is the first year of life after birth and a newborn child is called an infant from birth till the completion of the first year of life. In the initial half of infancy, the oral cavity has gum pads alone and towards the later half there is the eruption of primary teeth in the oral cavity. Preventive oral care in infancy is the basis of future oral health. The primary aim of a dentist or pediatric dentist at this stage is to educate and motivate the new parents to maintain good oral hygiene of the infant. An infant is completely dependent on the parents/caregivers to fulfil his basic needs. Thus, the entire responsibility of preventive care for optimal oral health lies in the hands of the infant's parents/ caregivers.

1.1. Importance of infant oral health care

Infant oral health is the foundation upon which education and motivation regarding dental hygiene and other preventive dental care must be built on, to augment the prospect of a lifetime free of preventable dental diseases. Infant oral health is an integral part of general well being of an infant, as he or she increases in age. It encompasses the care of the oral cavity and monitoring of the development of the teeth. Unfortunately, pregnant women, parents and caregivers of infants often do not receive timely and accurate education about preventive oral and dental health care [1].

1.2. Role of infant oral health care in preventive dentistry

Prevention is the primary focus of infant oral health care and prevention of dental diseases should be initiated in infancy itself. For diseases that occur early in life such as early childhood caries (ECC) prevention of diseases and the promotion of healthy behavior among parents/ caregivers must be given importance [2]. Preventive oral healthcare must be initiated in infancy because of the following reasons:

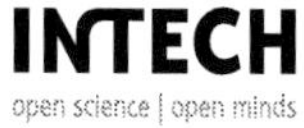

1. Poor oral hygiene and improper infant feeding practices create an environment that promotes the colonization of cariogenic bacteria such as *Streptococcus mutans* in the infant's mouth. Thus, when a tooth erupts in an infant's mouth, it is in an undesirable oral environment that promotes demineralization.

2. Risk factors such as improper feeding practices and poor oral hygiene that may lead to early childhood caries (ECC) may be identified at an early age and appropriate intervention may be planned.

3. Parents/caregivers may be educated regarding good oral health care practices to maintain the infant's mouth in a state of good dental health.

4. Undesirable consequences of poor dental health such as ECC may be avoided and the infant may escape its complications such as dental pain and poor nutrition.

5. Psychologic health of the child can be maintained as unesthetic appearance of teeth negatively impacts the psychology of a child.

1.3. Causes and risk factors leading to poor infant oral health

Evidence suggests that early-in-life risk factors play a significant role as predictors of future dental caries in children [3-6]. These risk factors include the extent of parental knowledge, attitude and practices (KAP) and an infant's oral hygiene status, medical history, oral medications and feeding habits. Thus it is important to understand the causes and risk factors of poor infant oral health to avoid the risk of early childhood caries later in life. A major factor contributing to poor infant oral health is insufficient or improper knowledge, attitudes and practices (KAP) related to infant feeding practices and oral care. Evidence gathered from both global and Indian studies shows that both pregnant mothers and parents/caregivers of infants have inadequate KAP regarding infant feeding, weaning, and bottle feeding practices and cleaning of the mouth [7-10]. Lower socio economic status has also been correlated to a low dental KAP [11, 12]. The age group of parents does not show a consistent correlation with lack of dental KAP, with different studies reporting varying results [7, 13]. In addition to the lack of KAP regarding infant oral health, pregnant women seldom attain regular dental care and have dental care needs that are not satisfactorily dealt with [14].

Infants with medically compromised health such as congenital heart disease (CHD) may also be prone to poor oral health. Despite good dental care and intensive prevention, poorer dental health has been seen in children with CHD than in healthy children [15]. Medically compromised children may also have poor oral hygiene since in the presence of life threatening conditions, oral hygiene takes on low priority.

Medical illness and long term medication for it, is another risk factor for poor infant oral health [16-7]. Medically compromised infants are often on long term medication that may have side effects of xerostomia or alteration of salivary properties such as flow, buffering capacity or rate. For example, diuretics are used in congenital heart disease since they increase the excretion of water from the circulatory system. Reduced saliva and altered salivary flow are known side effects of diuretics [18]. Disturbed mineralization in teeth has also been reported

[19]. Additionally, medications in syrup form for infants are often sweetened and this may result in a caries promoting oral environment. Sucrose is still used as a sweetener in some drugs, to enhance flavor [20-1].

Inappropriate infant feeding practices related to bottle feeding, breastfeeding and sweetened pacifiers/ liquids may be another cause of early childhood caries (ECC) as the teeth in the infant [22]. Nighttime bottle feeding with sweetened or sweet liquids is a risk factor for ECC due to salivary reduction and prolonged exposure of the teeth to fermentable carbohydrates [22]. The American Academy of Pediatrics (AAP) recommends breastfeeding as the ideal method of feeding and nurturing infants and recognizes the role of breastfeeding as primary in achieving optimal infant growth and development [23]. Further, the AAP recommends exclusive breastfeeding for the first 6 months followed by the addition of iron-enriched solid foods between 6 to 12 months of age [23]. Though breastfeeding serves several health and immuno-logic advantages to the infant, certain breastfeeding practices may result in ECC. The factors associated with breastfeeding that may result in ECC are ad libitum or at-will feeding, prolonged breastfeeding and frequent breastfeeding during the night, resulting in accumula-tion of milk in the teeth, which, combined with reduced salivary flow and lack of oral hygiene, may produce tooth decay [24-5].

1.4. Consequences of poor infant oral health

Dental caries remains the most widespread chronic disease of childhood and can have damaging effects on growth and development when it progresses to severe forms [26]. Early childhood caries is a public health problem with its etiologic factors playing a role from infancy itself. Low income and minority children experience disproportionately more dental caries than other groups because of their added barriers, such as limited access to dental services [27].

Poor infant oral health may lead to early childhood caries which is an infectious disease, and *S. mutans* is the most likely causative agent. Early acquisition, i.e., in infancy, of *S. mutans* is a crucial event in the natural history of ECC [28].

2. The infant's mouth

Oral microbial colonization of an infant's mouth begins shortly after birth [29]. The infants mouth consists only of gum pads in the pre-dentate stage, i.e., till about 6-7 months of age. As the teeth begin to erupt into the oral cavity (as the infant enters dentate stage), the colonization changes as the teeth present additional hard tissue surfaces for colonization. Influences from the mother/caregiver and siblings also play a role in the type of colonization of an infant's mouth.

2.1. Infant Oral Microbiology

The initial microbial microorganisms that colonize an infant's mouth are *Streptococcus salivar-ius, Streptococcus mitis* and *Streptococcus oralis* which belong to the group Mutans streptococcus

[30-3]. Of interest to the dentist is the acquisition of another species of the group Mutans streptococcus – *Streptococcus mutans* (*S. mutans*), which is strongly implicated in the etiology of dental caries [34]. Early-in-life or infant colonization by *S. mutans* is a chief risk factor for early childhood caries and future dental caries [28]. *Streptococcus mutans* was believed to show feeble adhesion to epithelial surfaces found in the pre-dentate infant's mouth [35-6]. The infants' mouth in the pre-dentate stage was thus considered unlikely to harbor *S. mutans* colonization. However, more recent evidence has shown that *S. mutans* colonization does occur in pre-dentate infants and the tongue may serve as an ecological niche in such cases [37-9]. Recently, a new microorganism *Scardovia wiggasiae* has been isolated from the plaque of ECC affected children using polymerase chain reaction (PCR) technology and research in this area is in progress [40].

2.2. Clinical aspects: Acquisition and transmission of *Streptococcus mutans*

Early-in-life acquisition of *Streptococcus mutans* has an impact on the future oral health of infants [28]. Infants may develop oral colonization with *S. mutans* colonization from their colonized parents [41]. The mother is the main source of transmission of S. mutans to a child as seen from clinical and microbiologic studies [42]. Mother-to-child or maternal transmission of *S. mutans* is one of the primary sources of transmission of *S. mutans* to an infant's mouth. This type of transmission of *S. mutans* is also known as *vertical transmission* [43]. In support of this route of transmission, several studies have reported identical bacteriocin profiles [44-5] and plasmid or chromosomal DNA patterns [46-7] of *S. mutans* strains in mother-child pairs. One study reported that when maternal salivary reservoirs exceed 10^5 colony forming units (CFU) the frequency of transmission of *S. mutans* to the infant was 9 times greater than when the maternal salivary levels of *S. mutans* were less than or equal to 10^3 CFU [48].

Horizontal transmission is the other major mode of transmission of *S. mutans* which occurs thorough sharing of spoons, glasses and interpersonal contact between the infant and other members of his/her environment such as siblings, daycare supervisors etc. Evidence for this mode of microbial transmission comes from several studies which have shown that infants and children in the same environment shared *S. mutans* isolates [49, 50]. Accordingly, vertical and horizontal transmission of *S. mutans* needs to be evaluated when taking into account risk factors for dental caries in an infant.

3. Dental home: Concept and advantages

The first step towards promotion of good infant oral health is the creation and maintenance of a dental home. This concept is derived from the concept of medical home that was proposed by the American Academy of Pediatrics in 1992 [51]. The premise behind the medical home was that the best care may be offered to a child when the child in focus and his/her family has a good relationship with the doctor.

The American Academy Pediatric Dentistry (AAPD) recommends that a dental home may be designed for the infant on the same lines as the medical home concept. The characteristics of an ideal dental home are the following [52]:

1. **Accessible:** This implies that dental care should be reachable to the infant and family

2. **Family Centered:** The importance of the family is recognized and behavior management techniques acceptable to the family are utilized.

3. **Continuous:** A dental home should be designed to look after the needs of a child from infancy through adolescence so that continuous care may be provided to the infant at all stages of childhood and adolescence.

4. **Comprehensive:** A dental home provides round-the-clock dental care for a child and includes primary, secondary and tertiary care for the infant.

5. **Coordinated:** An ideal dental home setup works in coordination with school and family of a child so that information may be shared for the benefit of the child in focus.

6. **Compassionate:** In a dental home, good relationships are established with a child's family a community with a concerned and compassionate approach for the child receiving dental care and his/her family.

7. **Culturally Competent:** Since children at a dental home come from varying backgrounds and cultures, an ideal dental home recognizes, values and respects the varied cultures and ethnic backgrounds of children.

There are several advantages of developing a dental home for an infant. Most importantly, the timing of the first dental visit of an infant may be planned within 1 year of age of an infant. This is in accordance with AAPD recommendations for the first dental visit of the child. Early-in-life risk factors can thus be identified at an early stage and appropriate intervention through increase in KAP related to infant feeding and oral hygiene suggested to the parents/caregivers [52]. Moreover, a dental home personalized or tailored preventive program may be designed to suit the specific oral health needs of a child at every stage.

4. Anticipatory guidance

The dental home provides scope for anticipatory guidance at every stage of a child's development. Anticipatory guidance is the process of providing practical, developmentally appropriate information about children's health to prepare parents for the significant physical, emotional and psychological milestones [43, 53]. Anticipatory guidance encompasses 3 types of responsibilities: (1) gathering information, (2) establishing a therapeutic alliance, and (3) providing education and guidance [43, 54].

5. Prenatal oral health counseling

Prenatal oral health counseling for parents is the first step to infant oral healthcare. The rationale of prenatal oral health counseling is to generate awareness among expectant mothers about dental disease, its prevention and the means to promote good oral health in the infant [54]. A mother's DMFS scores, education, and feeding habits are strong risk indicators for the colonization of caries-related micro-organisms and ECC [55].

5.1. Importance of prenatal oral health care (during pregnancy)

Ideally, optimization of infant oral health begins prenatally and continues with the monitoring and counseling of the mother and child, beginning when the infant is approximately 6 months of age, with the eruption of the first tooth [56]. Infants with low birth weight and malnourished infants are at risk for development of enamel hypoplasia [22, 57-8]. Enamel hypoplasia may result in a rough enamel surface which can result in areas more prone to plaque accumulation and resultant caries [57, 59]. Thus, expecting mothers should be advised to optimize nutrition during the third trimester and the infant's first year, when the enamel is undergoing maturation [54]. Recent literature also reports an association between periodontitis in the mother and preterm birth [60] and between *S. mutans* levels in mothers and caries experience in their children [42].

Evaluation of the oral status of expectant mothers followed by pre-and perinatal counseling regarding the expectant mothers' nutrition, oral hygiene, caries experience and KAP regarding infant feeding practices can have a significant impact on the child's caries rate in the future [54]. A dental home can address these needs, if developed at the prenatal stage itself. Pediatric dentists, pediatricians and nutritionists have a combined role in relation to prenatal counseling with a goal to providing the best oral and overall health for the newborn and infant. Future parents should be monitored on a regular basis to ensure effective oral hygiene and dietary habits have been established through regular pre-and perinatal parent counseling.

5.2. Anticipatory guidance for the pregnant mother

Anticipatory guidance has been recommended for the pregnant mother to avoid caries and gingival problems and promote later oral health for the child. These include the following [43, 61-2]:

a.   Education concerning development and prevention of dental disease and also demonstration of oral hygiene procedures.

b.   Counseling to instill preventive attitudes and motivation among mothers.

c.   Providing information to pregnant women about pregnancy gingivitis.

d.   Visiting a dentist for an examination and restoration of all active decay as soon as feasible and to decrease chances of developing pregnancy gingivitis.

e.   Eating healthy foods such as fruits, vegetables, grain products (especially whole grain), and dairy products (milk, cheese) during meals and snacks. Limit eating between meals.

f.   Eating foods containing only sugar at mealtimes, and limiting the amount.

g.   Brushing teeth thoroughly twice a day (after breakfast and before bed) with fluoridated toothpaste and flossing daily.

h.   Rinsing every night with an alcohol-free, over-the-counter fluoridated mouth rinse.

i.   Not smoking cigarettes or chewing tobacco.

6. Infant oral health care: Strategies and methods

An effective approach toward primary prevention of early childhood caries is to develop an approach that targets its infectious element, for example by preventing or delaying primary acquisition of *S. mutans* at an early age or infancy, through suppression of maternal reservoirs of *S. mutans* [63]. Mothers with dense salivary or plaque reservoirs of *S. mutans* are at high risk for transmitting the microorganism to their infants early-in-life [54].

6.1. Parent oral health counseling and education

Parent education and increase in knowledge, attitude and practices (KAP) regarding infant oral health care may provide long lasting benefits on an infant's oral health. Maternal/ Caregiver KAP [7-9] is an area where several lacunae exist regarding infant nutrition, feeding practices and first dental visit. Emphasis must be placed on behavioral approaches to conditions such as ECC that begin early in life the prevention of diseases and the promotion of healthy behavior among mothers and their children [2]. Low-cost health education combined with external motivation proved to be a valuable tool for promoting health behavior in mothers and their children [64].

6.2. Infant feeding related behavior

Infant feeding practices related to breastfeeding, bottle feeding and their timing of cessation must be given importance. Infant formulas are acidogenic and possess cariogenic potential [65-6]. Prenatal and postnatal counseling is essential to generate awareness about the unfavorable consequences of inappropriate infant feeding practices on infant oral health. Recommendations for appropriate infant feeding practices behaviors include [54, 67-8]:

- Infants should not be put to sleep with a bottle containing fermentable carbohydrates.

- At-will breast-feeding should be avoided after the first primary tooth begins to erupt and other dietary carbohydrates are introduced.

- Parents should be encouraged to have infants drink from a cup as they approach their first birthday.

- Infants should be weaned from the bottle at 12 to 14 months of age.

- Repetitive consumption of any liquid containing fermentable carbohydrates from a bottle or training cup should be avoided.

- Between-meal snacks and prolonged exposures to foods and juice or other beverages containing fermentable carbohydrates should be avoided.

6.3. Oral hygiene for the infant

Oral hygiene measures must be implemented no later than the time of eruption of the first primary tooth. These measures include the following [25, 68]:

- If an infant falls asleep while feeding, the teeth should be cleaned before placing the child in bed.

- Tooth brushing of all dentate children should be performed twice daily with a fluoridated toothpaste and a soft, age-appropriate sized toothbrush.

- Parents should use a 'smear' of toothpaste to brush the teeth of a child less than 2 years of age and perform or assist with their child's tooth brushing.

6.4. Fluoride supplementation

Fluoride is a well documented agent in caries control and it may be used for infants also. As per the AAPD, daily fluoride exposure for all children is recommended as a primary preventive procedure [69]. An infant's exposure to drinking water fluoride should be determined based on access to fluoridated water in community water supplies or through water analysis for those drinking well water [69]. A comprehensive knowledge of high fluoride belts and regions with endemic fluorosis is also important especially in countries like India with several geographic high fluoride belts. For infants older than 6 months of age who are exposed to water with less than 0.3 ppm fluoride, dietary fluoride supplements of 0.25 mg fluoride per day should be prescribed [69]. Irrespective of fluoride exposure in water, dietary supplements should not be prescribed for infants under the age of 6 months [69].

7. First dental visit: timing and its relevance

To promote early detection of dental caries and the establishment of a dental home, both the American Academy of Pediatrics (AAP) and American Academy of Pediatric Dentistry recommend the first dental visit by 1 year old. The AAPD recommends that the first oral evaluation visit should occur within 6 months of the eruption of the first primary tooth and no later than 12 months of age [70]. Since *S. mutans* begins to colonize an infant's mouth even prior to tooth eruption, a good dental care regime complemented by a dental home that is established at an initial stage of infancy may lead to long term oral health benefits for the infant.

8. Conclusion

Infant oral health forms the basis of a lifetime of good oral health. The primary focus of infant oral health is prevention and every effort must be made to prevent and promote oral health at this crucial stage of infancy. A dental home must be developed for each child, which provides anticipatory guidance from infancy through adolescence. Maternal education and emphasis on good maternal oral health should also be encouraged at pre-and perinatal stages to further prevent early colonization of cariogenic microorganisms.

Author details

Preetika Chandna* and Vivek K. Adlakha

*Address all correspondence to: drpreetikachandna@gmail.com

Department of Paedodontics and Preventive Dentistry, Subharti Dental College, Meerut, Uttar Pradesh, India

References

[1] Fitzsimons D, Dwyer JT, Palmer C, Boyd LD. Nutrition and oral health guidelines for pregnant women, infants, and children. J Am Diet Assoc. 1998 Feb;98(2):182-6, 189; quiz 187-8.

[2] Hobdell MH, Oliveira ER, Bautista R, Myburgh NG, Lalloo R, Narendran S, Johnson NW. Oral diseases and socioeconomic status (SES). British Dent J 2003:194;91–6.

[3] Alaluusua S, Malmivirta R. Early plaque accumulation: a sign for caries risk in young children. Community Dent Oral Epidemiol. 1994;22:273-6.

[4] Grindefjord M, Dahllof G, Nilsson B, Modeer T. Prediction of dental caries development in 1-year-old children. Caries Res. 1995;29:343-8.

[5] Wendt LK, Hallonsten AL, Koch G, Birkhed D. Analysis of cariesrelated factors in infants and toddlers living in Sweden. Acta Odontol Scand. 1996;54(2):131-7.

[6] Watson MR. Validity of various methods of scoring visible dental plaque as ECC risk measure (abstract 771). J Dent Res. 2001;80:132.

[7] Nagarajappa R, Kakatkar G, Sharda AJ, Asawa K, Ramesh G, Sandesh N. Infant oral health: Knowledge, attitude and practices of parents in Udaipur, India. Dent Res J. 2013;10:659-65.

[8] Nagaraj A, Pareek S. Infant Oral Health Knowledge and Awareness: Disparity among Pregnant Women and Mothers visiting a Government Health Care Organization. Int J Clin Pediatr Dent. 2012;5(3):167-172.

[9] Shivaprakash PK, Elango I, Baweja DK, Noorani HH. The state of infant oral health-care knowledge and awareness: Disparity among parents and healthcare professionals. J Indian Soc Pedod Prev Dent. 2009;27:39-43.

[10] Hoeft KS, Masterson EE, Barker JC. Mexican American mothers' initiation and understanding of home oral hygiene for young children. Pediatr Dent. 2009 Sep-Oct; 31(5):395-404.

[11] Suresh BS, Ravishankar TL, Chaitra TR, Mohapatra AK, Gupta V. Mother's knowledge about pre-school child's oral health. J Indian Soc Pedod Prev Dent. 2010;28:282-7.

[12] Williams NJ, Whittle JG, Gatrell AC. The relationship between socio-demographic characteristics and dental health knowledge and attitudes of parents with young children. Br Dent J 2002;193:651-4.

[13] Rwakatema DS, Ng'ang'a PM. Oral health knowledge, attitudes and practices of parents/guardians of pre-school children in Moshi, Tanzania. East Afr Med J 2009;86:520-5.

[14] Villa A, Abati S, Pileri P, Calabrese S, Capobianco G, Strohmenger L, Ottolenghi L, Cetin I, Campus GG. Oral health and oral diseases in pregnancy: a multicentre survey of Italian postpartum women. Aust Dent J. 2013 Jun;58(2):224-9.

[15] Stecksen-Blicks C, Rydberg A, Nyman L, Asplund S, Svanberg C. Dental car-ies experience in children with congenital heart disease: a case-control study. Int J Paediatr Dent 2004;14:94-100.

[16] Moore PA, Guggenheimer J. Medication-induced hyposalivation: etiology, diagnosis, and treatment. Compend Contin Educ Dent. 2008;29:50-5.

[17] Maupome G, Shulman JD, Medina-Solis CE, Ladeinde O. Is there a relation-ship between asthma and dental caries?: a critical review of the literature. J Am Dent Assoc. 2010;141:1061-74.

[18] Scully C, Felix DH. Oral medicine-update for the dental practitioner lumps and swellings. Br Dent J. 2005;199:763-70.

[19] Hakala PE, Haavikko K. Permanent tooth formation of children with congenital cyanotic heart disease. Proc Finn Dent Soc 1974;70:63-6.

[20] Bigeard L. The role of medication and sugars in Paediatric dental patients. Dent Clin North Am. 2000; 44:443-56.

[21] Moursi AM, Fernandez JB, Daronch M, Zee L, Jones CL. Nutrition and oral health considerations in children with special health care needs: implications for oral health care providers. Pediatr Dent. 2010; 32:333-42.

[22] Seow WK. Biological mechanisms of early childhood caries. Community Dent Oral Epidemiol. 1998; 26 (1 Suppl):8-27.

[23] Breastfeeding and the use of human milk. Pediatrics. 2012 Mar;129(3):e827-41.

[24] Schafer TE, Adair SM. Prevention of dental disease. Pediatr Clin North Am. 2000;47:1021-42

[25] McDonald R, Avery D, Dean J Mosby. Dentistry for the Child and the Adolescent. 8th Ed St. Louis, Missouri: Mosby; 2004.

[26] Dela Cruz GG, Rozier G, Slade G. Dental screening and referral of young children by pediatric primary care providers. Pediatrics. 2006;114:642-52.

[27] Lewis CW, Grossman DC, Domoto PK, Deyo RA. The role of the pediatrician in the oral health of children: A national survey. Pediatrics. 2002;106:84-90.

[28] Berkowitz RJ. Causes, treatment and prevention of early childhood caries: a micro-biologic perspective. J Can Dent Assoc. 2003 May;69(5):304-7.

[29] Law V, Seow WK, Townsend G. Factors influencing oral colonization of mutans streptococci in young children. Aust Dent J. 2007 Jun;52(2):93-100; quiz 159.

[30] Pearce C, Bowden GH, Evans M, et al. Identification of pioneer viridans streptococci in the oral cavity of human neonates. J Med Microbiol. 1995;42:67-72.

[31] Kononen E, Asikainen S, Saarela M, Karjalainen J, Jousimies-Somer H. The oral gram-negative anaerobic microflora in young children: longitudinal changes from edentulous to dentate mouth. Oral Microbiol Immunol. 1994;9:136-41.

[32] Rotimi VO, Duerden BI. The development of the bacterial flora in normal neonates. J Med Microbiol. 1981;14:51-62.

[33] Carlsson J, Grahnen H, Jonsson G. Lactobacilli and streptococci in the mouth of children. Caries Res. 1975;9:333-9.

[34] van Houte J. Role of micro-organisms in caries etiology. J Dent Res 1994;73:672-681.

[35] Gibbons RJ. Bacteriology of dental caries. J Dent Res. 1964;43:1021–8.

[36] Gibbons RJ, Houte JV. Bacterial adherence in oral microbial ecology. Annu Rev Microbiol. 1975;29:19–44.

[37] Wan AK, Seow WK, Purdie DM, Bird PS, Walsh LJ, Tudehope DI. Oral colonization of *Streptococcus mutans* in six-month-old predentate infants. *J Dent Res* 2001; 80(12): 2060–5.

[38] Ramos-Gomez FJ, Weintraub JA, Gansky SA, Hoover CI, Featherstone JD. Bacterial, behavioral and environmental factors associated with early childhood caries. J Clin Pediatr Dent 2002; 26(2):165–73.

[39] Tanner AC, Milgrom PM, Kent R Jr, Mokeem SA, Page RC, Riedy CA, Weinstein P, Bruss J. The microbiota of young children from tooth and tongue samples. J Dent Res. 2002 Jan;81(1):53-7.

[40] Tanner AC, Mathney JM, Kent RL, Chalmers NI, Hughes CV, Loo CY, Pradhan N, Kanasi E, Hwang J, Dahlan MA, Papadopolou E, Dewhirst FE Cultivable anaerobic microbiota of severe early childhood caries. J Clin Microbiol. 2011 Apr;49(4):1464-74.

[41] Douglass JM, Li Y, Tinanoff N. Association of mutans streptococci between caregivers and their children. Pediatr Dent 2008; 30:375-87.

[42] Berkowitz R. Mutans streptococci: Acquisition and transmission. Pediatr Dent. 2006;28:106-9.

[43] Pinkham J, Casamassimo P, Fields H, McTigue D, Nowak A. Pediatric Dentistry: Infancy through Adolescence. 4th Ed. Philadelphia: Saunders; 2005.

[44] Berkowitz RJ, Jordan H. Similarity of bacteriocins and Streptotoccus mutans from mother and infant. Arch Oral Biol. 1975; 20(11):725–30.

[45] Davey AL, Rogers AH. Multiple types of the bacterium *Streptococcus mutans* in the human mouth and their intra-family transmission. Arch Oral Biol. 1984; 29(6):453–60.

[46] Caufield PW, Wannemuehler Y, Hensen J. Familiar clustering of the *Streptococcus mutans* cryptic plasmid strain in a dental clinic population. Infect Immun. 1982; 38(2): 785–7.

[47] Kulkarni GV, Chan KH, Sandham HJ. An investigation into the use of restriction endonuclease analysis in the study of transmission of mutans streptococci. J Dent Res. 1989; 68(7):1155–61

[48] Berkowitz RJ, Turner J, Green P. Maternal salivary levels of *Streptococcus mutans* and primary oral infection in infants. Arch Oral Biol 1981; 26(2):147–9.

[49] Mattos-Graner RO, Smith DJ, King WF, Mayer MP. Water insoluble glucan synthesis by mutans streptococcal strains correlates with caries incidence in 12-to 30-month-old children. J Dent Res. 2000;79:1371-7.

[50] van Loveren C, Buijs JF, ten Cate JM. Similarity of bacteriocin activity profiles of mutans streptococci within the family when the children acquire the strains after the age of 5. Caries Res 2000; 34(6):481–5.

[51] The American Academy of Pediatrics Ad Hoc Task Force on Definition of the Medical Home. The medical home. Pediatr. 1992;90:774.

[52] Nowak AJ, Casamassimo PS. The dental home: a primary care oral health concept. J Am Dent Assoc. 2002 Jan;133(1):93-8.

[53] Lewis CW, Grossman DC, Domoto PK, Deyo RA. The role of the pediatrician in the oral health of children: A National survey. Pediatr. 2000;106:E84.

[54] Chandna P, Adlakha VK. Oral health in children guidelines for pediatricians. Indian Pediatr. 2010 Apr;47(4):323-7.

[55] Ersin NK, Eronat N, Cogulu D, Uzel A, Aksit S. Association of maternal-child characteristics as a factor in early childhood caries and salivary bacterial counts. J Dent
Child (Chic). 2006 May-Aug;73(2):105-11.

[56] Gomez SS, Weber AA. Effectiveness of a caries preventive program in pregnant
women and new mothers on their offspring. Int J Paediatr Dent. 2001;11:117-22.

[57] Seow WK, Humphrys C, Tudehope DI. Increased prevalence of developmental dental defects in low birth-weight, prematurely born children: a controlled study. Pediatr Dent. 1987;9:221-5.

[58] Davies GN. Early childhood caries–a synopsis. Community Dent Oral Epidemiol
1998;26(1 Suppl):106-16.

[59] Horowitz HS. Research issues in early childhood caries. Community Dent Oral Epidemiol 1998;26(1 Suppl):67-81.

[60] McGaw T. Periodontal disease and preterm delivery of low-birth-weight infants. J
Can Dent Assoc. 2002;68:165-9.

[61] Brambilla E, Felloni A, Gagliani M, Malerba A, García-Godoy F, Strohmenger L. Caries prevention during pregnancy: results of a 30-month study. J Am Dent Assoc.
1998;129:871-7.

[62] Nowak AJ, Casamassimo PS. Using anticipatory guidance to provide early dental intervention. J Am Dent Assoc. 1995;126.1156-63.

[63] Kohler B, Bratthall D, Krasse B. Preventive measures in mothers influence the establishment of the bacterium *Streptococcus mutans* in their infants. *Arch Oral Biol* 1983;
28(3):225–31.

[64] Mohebbia SZ, Virtanen JI, Vehkalahtic MM. Improvements in the Behaviour of
Mother-Child Pairs Following Low-cost Oral Health Education. Oral Health Prev
Dent 2014;1:13-1.

[65] Sheikh C, Erickson PR. Evaluation of plaque pH changes following oral rinse with
eight infant formulas. Pediatr Dent. 1996;18:200-4.

[66] Bowen WH, Pearson SK, Rosalen PL, Miguel JC, Shih AY. Assessing the cariogenic
potential of some infant formulas, milk and sugar solutions. J Am Dent Assoc.
1997;128:865-71.

[67] American Academy on Pediatric Dentistry Council on Clinical Affairs. Policy on early childhood caries (ECC): unique challenges and treatment option. Pediatr Dent.
2008-2009;30(7 Suppl):44-6.

[68] American Academy on Pediatric Dentistry Council on Clinical Affairs. Policy on early childhood caries (ECC): classifications, consequences, and preventive strategies.
Pediatr Dent. 2008-2009;30(7 Suppl):40-3.

[69] American Academy on Pediatric Dentistry Liaison with Other Groups Committee; American Academy on Pediatric Dentistry Council on Clinical Affairs. Guideline on fluoride therapy. Pediatr Dent. 2008-2009;30(7 Suppl):121-4.

[70] American Academy of Pediatric Dentistry. Clinical Affairs Committee-Infant Oral Health Subcommittee. Guideline on infant oral health care. Pediatr Dent. 2012 Sep-Oct;34(5):148-52

Comparative School Dental Sealant Program to Alleviate Dental Caries Problem — Thai versus International Perspective

Sukanya Tianviwat

Additional information is available at the end of the chapter

http://dx.doi.org/10.5772/59516

1. Introduction

The application of dental sealant has been recommended for caries prevention in pit and fissure surfaces. For school dental sealant programes, the Community Preventive Services Task Force recommends the implementation of school dental sealant delivery programs based on strong evidence of their effectiveness in preventing dental caries among children [1]. In the United States, school-based dental sealant programs have been implemented successfully around the country, and the American Association for Community Dental Programs and the National Maternal and Child Oral Health Resource Center have published the guideline of "Seal America" to promote the implementation of this program [2]. School dental sealant program offer several advantages over other approaches [2, 3]: increasing access to dental service among deprived children, strengthening the relationship between schools and health care institutions, and establishing the follow-up and maintenance system of the dental sealant program.

The implementation of school dental sealant programs differs from country to country. Most of the evidence of effectiveness of these programs are found in well-equipped studies conducted in developed countries. This chapter will present more than fifteen years of scientific experience of the program operating among rural primary school children in Thailand and make comparisons with scientific data published in international journals. The scope of this chapter will include several topics related to school dental sealant programs: their effectiveness, factors related to effectiveness, critical findings and most common failures, and the impact of the program on oral health status.

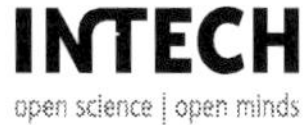

2. Background

In Thailand, the dental sealant program was initiated in 1996 and has been delivered to children on either a "school-based" or a "school-linked" pattern [3, 4]. In the school-based pattern, dental equipment is carried out by the dental health section of the community hospital, which visits all schools in the area under its responsibility at least once a year. Each school visit lasts 1-2 days. The mobile dental clinic, with portable field equipment, is transported from the hospital to schools by van. The equipment includes a patient chair, a portable artificial light, an operator stool, a master unit with slow-speed and high-speed handpieces with a triple syringe, a portable suction and a light polymerization unit. A temporary clinic is usually set up in an available area at each school (Figures 1 and 2). In the school-linked or hospital-based pattern, by contrast, the children receive dental sealant at the district or sub-district hospital (Figure 3). Children are screened by dentists or dental nurses at school and the parents requested to bring their children to the hospital to receive sealant. Some hospitals, however, request school teachers to bring the group of children whose parents have given permission for the child to receive dental sealant to the hospital. Some hospitals combine the two patterns of dental sealant delivery program – a school-based pattern for children in areas remote from a hospital and a school-linked pattern for children who live nearby.

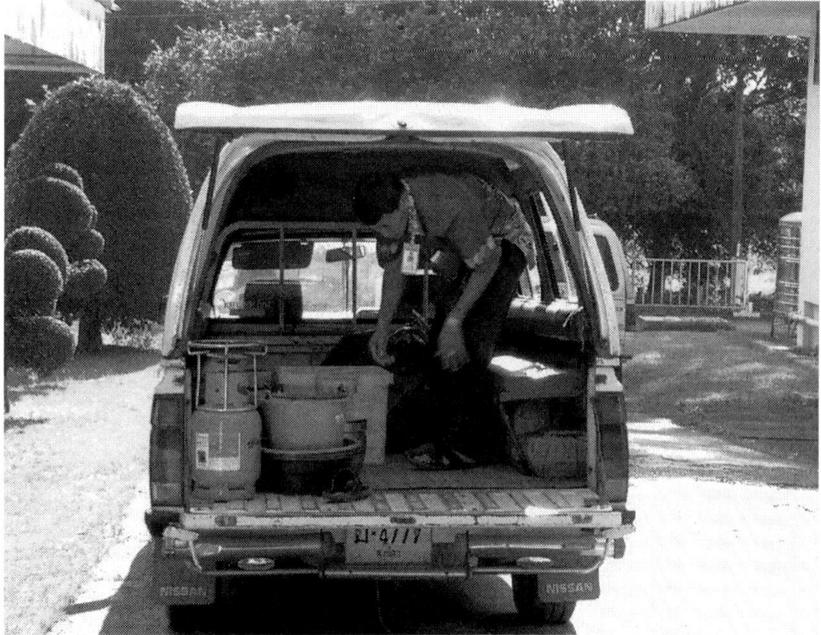

Figure 1. Mobile dental equipment delivered to school by van.

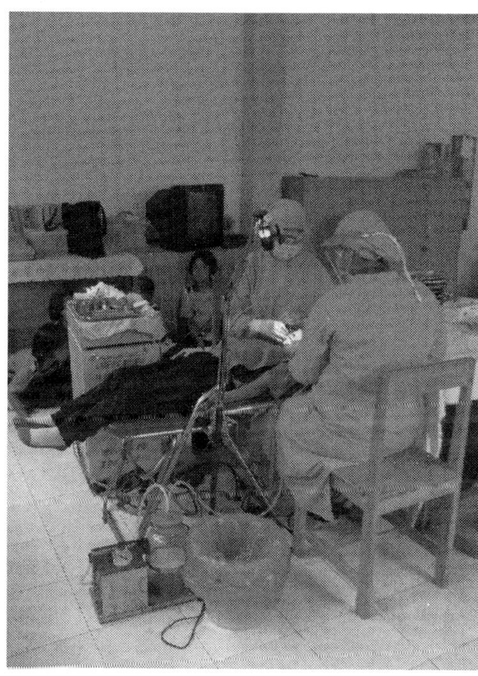

Figure 2. Mobile dental equipment set up in an available area at a school where dental services are delivered.

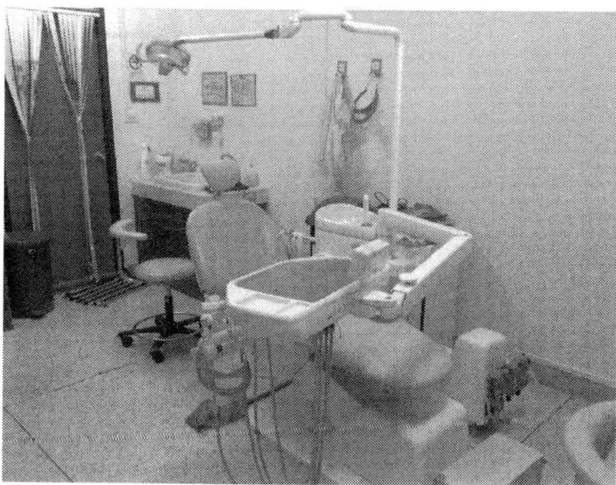

Figure 3. Dental equipment at a district or a sub-district hospital

In 2005, the Dental Health Division, Ministry of Public Health, Thailand, initiated the Oral Health Promotion and Prevention in School Children Project under the National Health Security with the slogan "Yim Sodsai Dek Thai Fun Dee" project, which can be translated as "Bright Smile and Healthy Teeth in Thai Children" [5]. One of the objectives of this project is to achieve 50% of the first grade children with an average 2.5 teeth that have received dental sealant, especially the first permanent molars. Due to this universal coverage project the number of 12-year-old children whose teeth were sealed increased from 12.7% in the year 2007 [6] to 35.2% in the year 2012 [7].

In the following text, the phrase "school dental sealant program" is used to refer to both "school-based and school-linked dental sealant programs". The content of this chapter is based mainly on reports of the sealant program implementation published since 1996, which was the year of that marked the beginning of the school dental sealant program. Experimental studies, such as those concerned with sealant materials or properties, are not included. The main content is based on resin sealant, which is in widespread use in the school programs.

3. Effectiveness of the school dental sealant program

Evaluation of the effectiveness of school dental sealant programs has been evaluated mostly on the basis of the percentage of full retention sealant and/or percentage of caries on sealed surfaces. Tables 1 and 2 compare such rates between Thailand [8-17, 25] and other countries [18-24]. Because of differences in the pattern of dental sealant delivery, in the summary of the setting, the terms "hospital" or "clinical setting" are used to represent the use of stationery dental equipment and "mobile clinic" to represent the use of mobile van or mobile dental equipment.

Major differences in sealant effectiveness between Thailand and other countries are evident. International publications report high percentages of full sealant retention within 1 to 5 years; 52.7-91.0 % [18-20, 22, 24], 74.7-85.0 % [20, 22, 24], 61.7-81.0 % [22, 24], 76 % [22] and 69% [22]. Very high long-term sealant retention at 15 and 20 years of 65% has also been reported [21]. In that study, the children had continuous access to comprehensive dental services. Moreover, the caries rate on sealed surfaces was generally low: 0.8-10.7% of the sealed teeth at one year [18-20]. Within 2 years, 0.9% of sealed surfaces had caries [20] and at 5 years 8% [22]. Very low long-term caries rate has also been reported 5.0 and 13.0% at 15 and 20 years respectively [21]. Results from Australia [23] are difficult to compare because of variation in follow-up time for evaluation of sealant retention in the study.

In Thailand, school dental sealant programs present a major difference from international results. Full sealant retention at one year in Thailand has varied between 19.6 and 67.7% [8, 9, 12, 13, 16] and that at 2 and 3 years from 8.9 to 41.8% [11, 14 - 17] and from 0 to 52.1% [9, 10, 12, 17], respectively. Moreover, higher rates of caries on sealed teeth in Thailand have been reported. At one year, the caries rate on sealed surfaces was 24% [16] and at two years 14.5-32.6% [11, 13-17]. In 2014, the 5-year caries on sealed surface rate was reported to be 13.4% [25].

In a follow-up study of sealant effectiveness in Thailand based on the Markov model [12], in which sealant was evaluated every 6 months for 30 months, the rate of sealant loss decreased with time. The first six months after application was the most vulnerable period of sealant retention, with a loss of 32.8% of teeth while caries incidence surged in the first year and also in the subsequent six months, the caries rates on sealed teeth were 10.2 % and 16.9 % in 1 and 1.5 years.

These data from the Markov model are in concordance with data presented in Tables 1 and 2, which show that school dental sealant in Thailand had relatively short-term retention and most of the caries on sealed teeth develops within 1-1.5 years after application.

4. Factors related to the school dental sealant effectiveness

Sealant retention depends on the time since application. For short-term retention, loss of sealant is related to application technique and saliva contamination. Long-term retention, on the other hand, is related to masticatory function and wear. However, a recent report of the strategy adopted to improve sealant effectiveness indicated that sealant policy also had an effect on sealant effectiveness [26]. Since, in Thailand, most of the studies have examined sealant effectiveness over the short term and have shown rather poor effectiveness, the related factors have included those dealing with basic techniques, sealant delivery conditions and strategies to improve dental sealant performance comprising attitude of the provider and sealant policy [8, 9, 26]. By contrast, international studies have dealt with more advance techniques and policy to increase coverage or access to sealant [27-32].

As mentioned above, loss of sealant in Thailand occurs within 6-12 months; such loss is related with techniques and factors of moisture control. In a study of factors related to short-term sealant retention in Thailand [8], the researcher controlled for sealant type, oral hygiene, child's cooperation and position of the teeth. After reviewing sealant procedure according to manufacturer's instruction, sealant was performed within the routine program, and after sealing for 6 months the sealant retention was examined. It was found that the checking procedure and the presence of an assistant were significant factors influencing full sealant retention. The odds of full sealant retention increased significantly, 2.8 times, when the providers checked for both occlusion and sealant retention compared with checking for sealant retention alone. The presence of an assistant increased the odds of full retention 2.3 times when compared to not having an assistant present. The shortage of dental assistants was also found to be a limitation in optimizing the mix of basic dental services (sealing, filling and extraction) for southern Thai schoolchildren [33]. This study identified the limited number of dental assistants as the crucial constraint for school dental service delivery.

The setting of the Thai school sealant program, i.e., school-based or mobile dental clinic and school-link or hospital-based dental clinic, has also been investigated as a potential factor in sealant effectiveness [9, 26], but with conflicting results. One study reported that the application of sealant in a school-based or mobile setting significantly increased the rate of sealant loss compared to that done in a hospital-based setting [26]. The other study reported a higher percentage of full sealant retention in school or mobile dental clinics than in hospital-based dental clinics [9]. However, the mobile dental conditions of two studies were different. The latter study employed a split mouth design with high power suction and the presence of a dental assistant. In each child, a dentist provided sealant on the two lower first permanent molars and restricted the number of children to be sealed in order to reduce the providers' stress from working. In this study, the percentage of full sealant retention was the highest among the studies of sealant effectiveness in Thailand (please see Table 1). On the other hand, the former study conducted in an actual situation, employing a mobile dental clinic with saliva ejector, and with no restriction on number of children or number of teeth to be sealed. Therefore, either hospital-based or school-based dental clinic could provide good results if optimal conditions for sealant – good moisture control and no tension of provider – are fulfilled. Moreover, the researcher [9] discussed that children felt more comfortable in school setting than hospital-based setting.

A recent study on strategies to improve sealant performance yielded an interesting result regarding providers' attitude and sealant policy [26]. The study examined whether audit and feedback could improve the quality of application of dental sealant in rural Thai school children. The design was a single-blind, cluster-randomized controlled trial. Sealant qualities (retention and caries), were examined prior to and after the intervention. The intervention consisted of confidential feedback of data and tailor-made problem-solving workshops. After the audit and feedback, focus group discussions (FGD) were conducted in 6 intervention clusters, including 22 dental nurses. The participating dental nurses were asked how they felt about the results from the audit and feedback and what they did when they received feedback indicating poor sealant quality. It became apparent that the participants had two distinct reactions to such feedback. The impression emerging from their direct statements was of a conflict between the quantity of children treated and the quality of service they received. On the other hand, their indirect statements indicated their wish to identify problems and to find ways of solving the problems identified by the data in the feedback. The dental nurses in all the clusters complained that the policy, which aims to maximize the number of cases in whom sealant is applied, has resulted in poor service quality because the goal of the policy does not take account of the actual situation in terms of the available manpower, overall workload, number of children needing to be treated and the condition of their teeth.

In the international perspective, more studies than in Thailand have been conducted on techniques to improve sealant effectiveness. Such studies have examined surface preparation before sealing [28, 29], four-handed sealant condition [30] and type of operator [22].

Gray et al. (2009) [28] conducted a study to review manufacturers' instructions for surface preparation in sealant use. Ten sealant products from five manufacturers which were commonly used in school sealant programs were included. The use of pumice, prophylaxis paste or prophylaxis brush was included in five products, implying handpiece use. The other five products were nonspecific. Seven products indicated that the use of fluoride-containing or oil-containing pastes should be avoided. None of the products mentioned that the operator should perform enameloplasty, fissureotomy, air abrasion or air polishing to clean the tooth surface before placing the sealant. However, one product directed the operator to remove minimal caries with a small round bur in a slow-speed handpiece after surface cleaning. In the same study, the authors conducted a review of studies comparing sealant effectiveness between mechanical preparation with pumice and using an air-water spray with sharp probe and found two studies of clinical design. Both studies reported retention rates greater than 96% at one year after sealing. Various modes of fissure preparation in combination with two filling levels were studied by Geiger (2000) [29]. In this *in vitro* study, fissure preparation was divided into three groups; no mechanical preparation, mechanical preparation with a round carbide bur, and mechanical preparation with a tapered fissure diamond bur. Then, sealant filling level in each preparation group was subdivided into minimal filling (just to the border of pit and fissure) or overfilled. The result showed that sealant penetration and retention were significantly improved in mechanically prepared compared to non-prepared fissures and preparation with a tapered fissure diamond bur was superior to that with a round carbide bur. Overfilled fissures caused significantly higher levels of micro leakage. However, nowadays, the sealant placement recommendation developed by an expert working group supported by the Centers for Disease Control and Prevention (CDC) does not recommended additional surface preparation methods, such as air abrasion or enameloplasty [27].

The effect of having a dental assistant or four-handed delivery for sealant application was reviewed after controlling for various factors, namely years since placement, tooth-surface cleaning method, isolation technique, and type of primary operator [30]. The review included 11 studies; eight studies using four-handed delivery and the other three using two-handed delivery. Summary retention rates in studies using four-handed delivery were higher than those in studies using two-handed delivery at 1, 2 and 3 years; 89.8% vs 84.8%, 83.0 % vs 72.4% and 83.0% vs 67.9%, respectively. Multivariate analysis indicated that four-handed delivery increased sealant retention by about 9 percentage points compared with two-handed delivery.

Most school dental sealant application in Thailand is implemented by dental nurses. From Tables 1 and 2, the sealant effectiveness does not obviously differ between dentists and dental nurses. In other countries sealant application in school programs is mostly done by dentists (Table 1 and 2). There was the review to identify the effect of operator and sealant effectiveness [30]. This review showed unexpected finding of the association between having a dentist as the primary operator and lower sealant retention rates. The authors suggested two possible reasons for unexpected results. First, many dentists likely had limited experience with sealant materials and/or placement techniques. And the studies in which dentists were the primary operators may have been less likely to provide training in sealant placement than the studies in which the primary operators were non dentists.

There has been an effort to distribute the simple task of sealant application to other dental personnel, i.e., dental assistants [22] or dental therapists [23]. Very high sealant was achieved when sealing was performed by a dental assistant [22]. In another study, conducted in Australia [23], it was difficult to evaluate the performance of dental therapists owing to variation of follow-up time of the sealant. It seems, therefore, that type of operator is not a critical factor influencing sealant effectiveness.

First author, year	Age, tooth	Number of children, teeth at baseline	Setting, Provider	Material	Full sealant retention rate (% of teeth)							
					Period of follow-up (years)							
					1	2	3	4	5	10	15	20
Thailand												
Tianviwat, 2011 [8]	Grade 1[s], M1	206, 347	M, DN with or without DA	Light-cured resin	67.7*							
Choomphupan, 2011 [9]	6-9, M1	212, 848	M, D / H, D	Light-cured Helioseal F	62.7 / 42.5		35.9 / 24.6					
Charnvanishporn, 2009 [10]	Grade 1[s], M1	175, 355	M, NA	NA			52.1					
Thamtadawiwat, 2008 [11]	6-8, M1	183, 349	H, DN	Light-cured Prevocare		41.8						
Tianviwat, 2008 [12]	Grade 1[s], M1	184, 332	M and H, DN	Light-cured resin	54.8		30.7[f]					
Obsuwan, 2008 [13]	6-8, M1	500, 2000	H, NA	NA	45.6*							
Kongtawelert, 2008 [14]	6-8, M1	865, 2193	H, DN without DA	Light-cured resin		36.0						
Kantamaturapoj, 2008 [15]	6-8, M1	320, 1280	H, NA	Resin (not specific)		33.2**						
Thipsoonthornchai, 2003 [16]	6-7, M1	107, 107	M, NA	Light-cured resin	19.6	8.9						
Tianviwat, 2001 [17]	6-7, M1	102, 260 / 20-21 months: 86 teeth / 32-33 months: 174 teeth	M, DN	NA		18.6**	0***					
Other countries												
Hsieh, 2014 Taiwan [18]	6-9, M1	122, 229	M, 1D:1DA	Light-cured 3M ESPE	86.0							
Muller-Bolla, 2013 France [19]	6-7, M1	253, 421	H, 1D:1DA	Light-cured Delton	52.7							
Francis, 2008 Kuwait [20]	6-8, M1	452, 1372	H, D	Light-cured Delton plus	79.8	75.0						
Wendt, 2001 Sweden [21]	NA, M1 / NA, M2	45, 153 / 45, 161	H, D / H, D	Self-cured Delton							65.0	65.0
Holst, 1998 Sweden [22]	6-10, M1 11-14, M2	976, 3218	H, DA	Light-cured Delton	91.0	85.0	81.0	76.0	69.0			
Messer, 1997 Australia [23]	6-12, All	774, 2875	H, 2DT: 1DA	NA Conceal	56.0 (1-48 months)							
Bravo, 1996 Spain [24]	6-8, M1	104, 416	M, 1D:1DA	Light-cured Delton	87.3	74.7	61.7					

[s] average 6-8 years old; * follow-up at 6 months; [f] follow-up at 30 months; ** follow-up at 20-21 months; *** follow-up at 32-33 months

M1 = first permanent molar; M2 = second permanent molar; All = permanent premolar and molar; NA = not available

M = mobile dental equipment or van; H = hospital or clinical dental equipment; DN = dental nurses; D = dentist; DT= dental therapist; DA= dental assistant

Table 1. Full sealant retention rates in Thailand and other countries by period of follow-up

First author, year	Age, tooth	Number of children, teeth at baseline	Setting, Provider	Material	Caries rate on sealed surfaces (% of teeth) Period of follow-up (years)							
					1	2	3	4	5	10	15	20
Thailand												
Plengsringam, 2014 [25]	Grade 1$, M1	473, 1795	NA, NA	NA					13.4			
Charnvanishporn, 2009 [10]	Grade 1$, M1	175, 355	M, NA	NA			21.5					
Thamtadawiwat, 2008 [11]	6-8, M1	183, 349	H, DN	Light-cured Prevocare		16.3						
Tianviwat, 2008 [12]	Grade 1$, M1	184, 332	M and H DN	Light-cured resin			26.1#					
Obsuwan, 2008 [13]	6-8, M1	500, 2000	H, NA	NA		32.6						
Kongtawelert, 2008 [14]	6-8, M1	865, 2193	H, DN without DA	Light-cured resin		14.5						
Kantamaturapoj, 2008 [15]	6-8, M1	320, 1280	H, NA	Resin (not specific)		29.7*						
Thipsoonthornchai, 2003 [16]	6-7, M1	107, 107	M, NA	Light-cured resin	24	25						
Tianviwat, 2001 [17]	6-7, M1	102, 260 20-21 months: 86 teeth 32-33 months: 174 teeth	M, DN	NA		22.1*	21.9**					
Other countries												
Hsieh, 2014 Taiwan [18]	6-9, M1	122, 229	M, 1D:1DA	Light-cured 3M ESPE	6.1							
Muller-Bolla, 2013 France [19]	6-7, M1	253, 421	H, 1D:1DA	Light-cured Delton	10.7							
Francis, 2008 Kuwait [20]	6-8, M1	452, 1372	H, D	Light-cured Delton plus	0.8	0.9						
Wendt, 2001 Sweden [21]	NA, M1 NA, M2	45, 153 45, 161	H, D H, D	Self-cured Delton							5.0	13.0
Holst, 1998 Sweden [22]	6-10, M1 11-14, M2	976, 3218	H, DA	Light-cured Delton					8			

$ average 6-8 years old; # follow-up at 30 months; * follow-up at 20-21 months; ** follow-up at 32-33 months
M1 = first permanent molar; M2 = second permanent molar; All = permanent premolar and molar; NA = not available
M = mobile dental equipment or van; H = hospital or clinical dental equipment; DN = dental nurses; D = dentist; DT= dental therapist; DA= dental assistant

Table 2. Caries rates on sealed surfaces in Thailand and other countries by period of follow-up

5. Critical findings and most common failures

Most studies of sealant effectiveness have reported sealant retention as full, partial or total loss, and reported caries or no caries on sealed surfaces. However, among these sealant failures, there were a few common or typical types of sealant loss, and these reflect the cause of failures and could suggest how to improve school dental sealant effectiveness [26]. The most common failure scenarios in the Thai context are presented below with illustrations. In each picture, a combination of failures might be seen; however, for explanation purposes the major failure is demonstrated. The causes of failure which were summarized from a problem-solving work-shop in the audit and feedback study [26] are also discussed.

5.1. Partial retention with ledge and caries present

The common characteristics of this type of loss are loss of some sealant and a pit/fissure with ledge exposed when exploring with a sharp probe. Caries is present with loss of tissue beyond the boundaries of the pits and fissures on occlusal surfaces and lesions contain demineralized dentine, usually light brown, and have a soft texture when explored with a blunt probe using gentle pressure (Figure 4). This common failure was present in 67.6% of the total caries on sealed surfaces at 6 months follow-up after a single sealant application [26] (data available from author). The same result was found in a long-term follow-up study in the context of high caries risk children in an inefficient school dental sealant program [12]. The effect of partial sealant retention with ledge present is to increase the risk of caries 3.1 times compared with total sealant loss [12]. A study in Scotland [34] confirmed the result: teeth with partially retained sealant at baseline were found to have a significantly higher percentage of caries (22.9%) than teeth with complete sealing (14.4%).

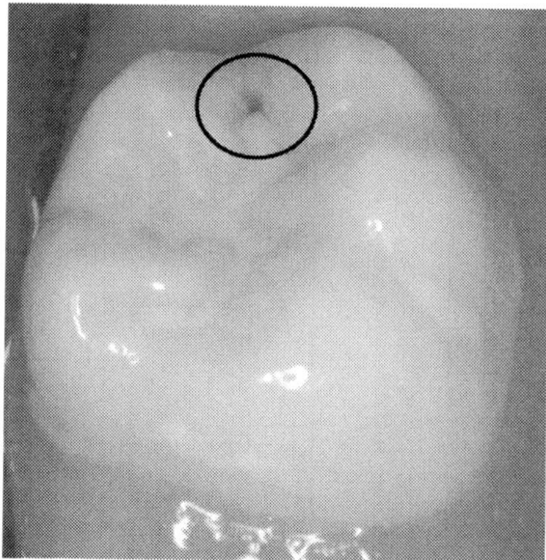

Figure 4. Partial retention with ledge and caries present

One review has addressed the controversy over the caries risk in formerly sealed teeth [35]. The authors examined the risk of caries development in teeth with partially or fully lost sealant relative to the risk in teeth that had never received sealants and concluded that teeth with fully or partially lost sealant were not at a higher risk of developing caries than teeth that had never been sealed. The studies included in the review were conducted in developed countries, where the risk of caries is quite low, the services are provided in well-equipped clinics and the sealant effectiveness is high.

It is obviously important that follow-up and repair of sealant loss should be promoted to increase the effectiveness of any school dental sealant program.

5.2. Loss of sealant at poor oral hygiene surfaces

From observational study, this type of loss accounts for approximately 60.7% of all failures of dental sealant [26]. Poor oral hygiene gauged by the presentation of soft debris covering more than 2/3 of the exposed tooth surface (Figure 5) based on the Debris index of Simplified Oral Hygiene Index [36]. The characteristics are partial or total loss of sealant and the presence of poor oral hygiene. This recent finding indicates a significant effect of poor oral hygiene on failure of sealant retention.

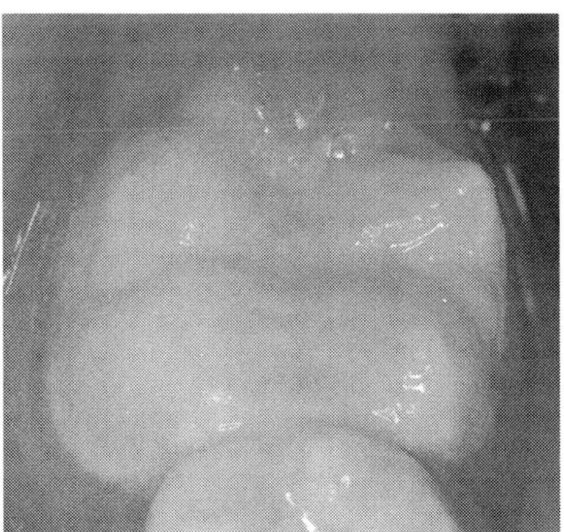

Figure 5. Loss of sealant at poor oral hygiene surfaces

5.3. Loss of sealant at cervical part of buccal pit and groove among lower first permanent molars.

In Thailand, lower first permanent molar is the first priority for the school dental sealant program among grade 1 schoolchildren as the first permanent molars present the highest percentage of caries: 51.4% in 12-year-old children [37]. Among all children, the lower first permanent molars comprised 36.4% and the upper first permanent molars 17.5% of all carious teeth [5]. The ratio of sealant service between lower teeth and upper teeth varied between 1.4:1 and 2.2:1 [8, 26]. This failure is characterized by a lack of sealant remaining at the lower end of the the buccal pit and groove (Figure 6) and was found in approximately 31.9% of sealed lower permanent molars. The significant concern of the scenario is the frequent presentation of caries development. The causes are related to tooth eruption and policy. Findings from focus group discussion in the sealant study [26] revealed that the policy of achieving 50% of first grade children being sealed placed a considerable burden on providers and had a negative impact on the quality of the program. A study of the eruption pattern in American children [38] found that only 57 % of first graders had all first permanent molars sufficiently erupted for sealing. In Taiwan [18], children aged 6-9 years presented only 46.9% (229 teeth among 488 teeth) of first permanent molars had erupted without decay, and eruption with decay or filling was present in 23.8% (116 teeth among 488 teeth). The loss of buccal surface was higher than that of occlusal surface among lower first permanent molars [23].

A study of eruption pattern of first permanent molar among Thai kindergarten level 2 and grade 1 and grade 2 schoolchildren [39] found that the percentages of at least one first permanent molar eruption were 6.0%, 75.1% and 98.5%, respectively. Among grade-1 children, who are the target group of the school dental sealant program in Thailand, the right lower first permanent molar had erupted 65.3% and caries was found 12.1%, whereas on the left side 64.3% had erupted and caries was present 9.1%. In the context of high caries prevalence, it is likely that the provider might seal teeth that are not in a suitable condition for sealing, such as being insufficiently erupted which more than half of the buccal surface covered by gingival tissue.

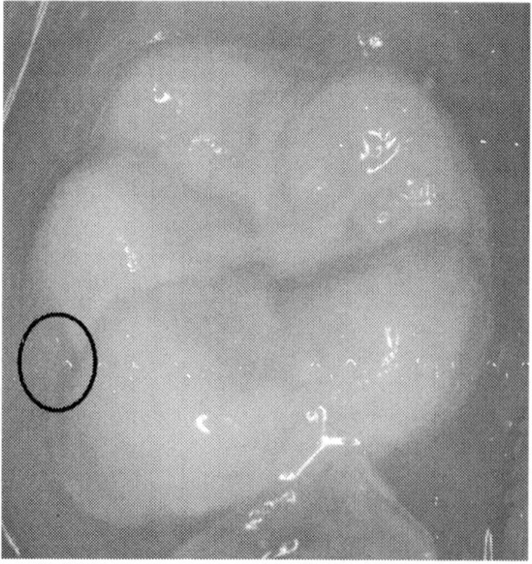

Figure 6. Loss of sealant at cervical part of buccal pit and groove among lower first permanent molars.

5.4. Loss of sealant at distal pit and groove of the occlusal surface of lower molars

The characteristics of this failure were no sealant remaining at the distal pit and groove of the occlusal surfaces of the lower molars and the presence of a ledge (Figure 7). The sealant was often was bulked or thick. This type of failure was seen in 16.3% of sealed lower permanent molars [26] (data available from author). The cause of failure, summarized from the problem-solving workshop, concerned the application technique. The provider used a brush to deliver sealant onto the tooth surface and the excess sealant flowed under gravity collecting in bulk and forming a thick layer at the distal end of the groove. When the children chewed, this area was at risk of fracture.

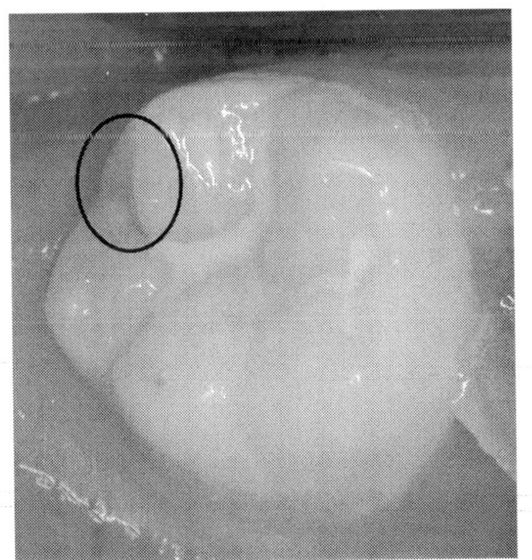

Figure 7. Loss of sealant at distal pit and groove of the occlusal surface of lower molars

There were other failures related with case selection and sealant technique; for instance, operculum covered on sealed surfaces (Figure 8), and void in sealant with or without caries (Figure 9). Most of the failures could be prevented by following the correct sealant procedure and instructions. The study of audit and feedback showed that these common failure scenarios and their own performance data as reflected in retention and caries rates could change the provider's attitude toward dental service quality [26]. The result from focus group discussion showed that they realized the poor quality of the dental service and felt they had to achieve a balance between quantity and quality of school dental sealant. They identified the means of solving their problems of service quality in terms of reallocating manpower, increasing their awareness, and improved equipment maintenance and sealant technique.

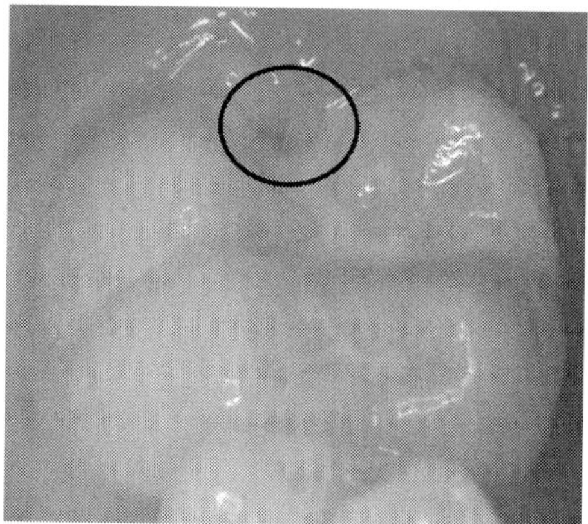

Figure 8. Operculum cover on sealed surface

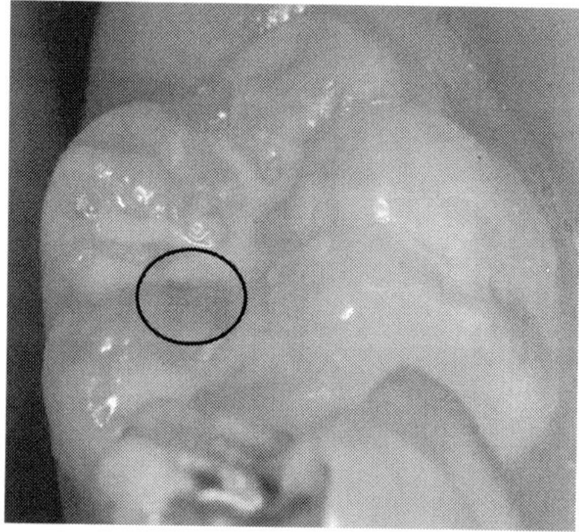

Figure 9. A void in sealant with caries

6. Impact of school dental sealant on oral health status

Evidence showing the effectiveness of dental sealant for caries prevention is drawn from several scientific papers [27, 40, 41]. Data from the evaluation of the school dental sealant program under the universal coverage of health care service in Thailand are presented. The macro scale data from Ministry of Public Health and data from each area and published in Thai journals are included. The impact of the program on the dental status of children as reflected in reports of the National Oral Health Survey before and after implementation of the school dental sealant program is also discussed.

As mentioned at the beginning of the chapter, the school As mentioned at the beginning of the chapter, the school sealant sealant program was first implemented in Thailand in 1996 on a small scale [17]. By 2001, the coverage of dental sealant was still very low; only 4.5% of 12-year-old children received dental sealant [42]. In 2005, the Oral Health Promotion and Prevention in School Children Project under National Health Security "Yim (smile) Sodsai (Bright), Dek Thai (Thai Children) Fun Dee (Health Teeth)", which was a joint project of the Dental health division, Department of health, and the National Health Security Organization was launched [5]. This project was managed as a vertical program by signing a contract between chief executive officers of the Provincial Health Office and the Department of Health. The project included prevention and promotion activities; full mouth examination of first grade and third grade students, sealant for the first grade students, and after-lunch tooth brushing for primary school children. Sealant activities of the project during 2005-2007 were evaluated based on monthly reports via a web-based system. After-lunch tooth brushing activity is an on-going activity which has been conducted since 1988 in the Oral Health Surveillance and Dental Health Promotion Program for primary school children [43].

The percentages of dental examination and sealant activities are presented in Table 3. The data were retrieved from 75 provinces in Thailand. Among first grade primary school children 35.9 – 48.8% had access to dental sealant in the period 2005-2007. In 2007, the number of sealed children was lower than in 2005-2006, partly explained by the diminished incentive for sealant service providers. However, the proportion of sealed children was still lower than that in other countries, for example, Slovenia with 62-100% (1988) [44], Ireland with 50-80% (1997) [45], and the United States with 51.1-88.0% and an extremely low coverage in one area of 41.0% (2002) [46].

The impact of the program was evaluated after two years of implementation based on the number of carious teeth among third grade children who had received sealant when they were in grade 1. Table 4 compares data between grade 3 sealed and unsealed children. Number of caries in first permanent molars among sealed children was 33.1% - much lower than that in unsealed children (66.9%). Nevertheless the number of caries in sealed group was quite high compared to other studies at the same follow-up period in Thai context (please see table 2). Evidence to support dental sealant effectiveness has been reported in several international publications. However, reports of the impact of the school dental sealant program at the macro level are few. In Slovenia, the most recent caries decline during 1987-1998; i.e. from 5.1 to 1.8 for 12-year-olds, and from 10.2 to 4.3 for 15-year-olds, was most likely due to supervised brushing with concentrated fluoride gel taking place several times a year in primary schools attended by children aged 7–15 years, improved oral hygiene, and a comprehensive program of applying fissure sealants, particularly on first molars. The Cochran database published a review of pit and fissure sealants for preventing dental decay in the permanent teeth of children and adolescents [40]. The review showed that the probability of sealed teeth remaining non-carious in patients who had received resin sealant at 24 months was 4.5 times less than that in the corresponding teeth of unsealed children (relative risk= 0.22; 95% confidence interval 0.34 to 0.22).

Activities	Educational year 2005		Educational year 2006		Educational year 2007	
	Number	Percent	Number	Percent	Number	Percent
Examination grade 1 and 3 (children)	1,299,959	81.3	1,257,486	78.6	941,968	58.9
Sealant grade 1 (children)	414,827	48.6	430,044	48.8	316,404	35.9
(teeth)	1,051,542	NA	1,212,398	NA	901,704	NA
Brushing (school)	28,647[s]	91.8	27,771[#]	94.1	27,432[#]	95.4
(children)	4,604,179[s]	87.5	4,190,561[#]	88.6	4,194,000[#]	92.5

NA = not available; [s] data from 75 provinces; [#] data from 70 provinces

Source: Modified from Jirapongsa W, Prasertsom P. [5]

Table 3. Percentage coverage of dental examination and dental sealant in the Oral Health Promotion and Prevention in School Children Project under National Health Security

Group	Number of examined children	Percent of children who had carious in first permanent molars
Children who receive sealant	149,837	33.1
Children who did not received sealant	303,023	66.9

Source: Jirapongsa W, Prasertsom P. [5]

Table 4. Number of children and percentage of carious first permanent molars classified by sealed and unsealed grade 3 primary school children

An area-based study in Thailand found a marginally significant impact of the program regarding the proportion of children in whom caries was prevented [13]. This was a cohort study comparing sealed and unsealed groups of children. Both groups were enrolled in after-lunch tooth brushing with fluoride toothpaste. Table 5 presents the frequency of caries on first permanent molars in the two groups. A high percentage of early sealant loss was found in this study; at 6 months only 45.6% had full sealant retention – a value that is quite low compared to the data for the same period in Thailand, 54.8-67.7 % (Table 1). Therefore, in the high and early sealant loss area, the caries preventive effect was difficult to reach.

Group	Number of children	Number of children with caries (%)		Carious teeth Mean (sd)
Children who receive sealant	500	163 (32.6)	p-value	p-value < .001
Children who did not received sealant	500	159 (31.8)	0.052	

Source: Obsuwan K. [13]

Table 5. Caries on first permanent molars at 24 months between sealed and unsealed group

The percentages of sealed and unsealed surfaces having caries have been compared in several cross-sectional studies using baseline data from the web-based system and examined caries at the end of the study. Table 6 summarizes the caries data from three studies comparing children who received dental sealant with others who did not. The differences were only marginally significant (rows 1 and 3) or non-significant (row 2). The sealant retention rates in these studies were quite low (please see Table 1). In two of the studies; 42% at 2 years [11] and 33.2% at 20 months [15], although somewhat higher in the third study, 52.1% at three years [10]. Thus, under low effectiveness conditions, caries preventive effect was low.

First author	Number of sealed children at last follow up	Number and percent of caries	Number of unsealed children at last follow up	Number and percent of caries	p-value
Charnvanishporn, 2009 [10]	130	28 (21.5%)	130	54 (41.5%)	0.038
Thamtadawiwat, 2008 [11]	183	57 (16.3%)*	215	56 (13.3 %)*	0.14
Kantamaturapoj, 2008 [15]	300	85 (28.3 %)	300	108 (36.0 %)	0.044

*only carious data at teeth level are available: 57 from 349 teeth (16.3%) among sealed group and 56 from 422 teeth (13.3%) among unsealed group

Table 6. Percentage of caries in sealed and unsealed children

In Thailand, the Dental Health Division, Department of Health, has conducted a National Oral Health Survey every 5 years, the most recent one was the 7th survey conducted in 2012. The data from 4 surveys were used to reveal the impact of dental sealant on the oral health status of children (Figure 10). As the target group of the school dental sealant project was grade 1 primary-school children, aged 6-8 years, the data of 12-year-olds were used. The number of examined children and caries experience in permanent teeth of each survey are shown in Table 7. The survey data did not report caries experience in first permanent molars (only the 4th survey reported caries by tooth), therefore the total caries experience in permanent teeth is present as proxy for caries experience of first permanent molars since 51.4% of caries teeth in 12 years old children were in first permanent molars [37].

The 4th, 6th and 7th surveys were conducted in 17 provinces, 4 provinces from each region (north, south, north-east and central) and Bangkok, the capital province. The sample size of the 5th survey was very large because the Dental Health Division expanded the survey from 17 to 48 provinces and increased the size of the sample for improved representativeness at the provincial level (Table 7). The 4th survey was conducted before the small scale implementation of school dental sealant activity, therefore the data from this survey together with other dental health programs could be used as baseline data. Data from the 5th survey were used to assess the impact of the small scale school dental sealant program. The 6th and 7th survey data were used to assess the impact of the large scale program. Caries experience of 12-year-old children from the four surveys is presented in Table 7. Coverage of dental sealant is shown in Table 8. Other dental health care programs implemented during 1994 to date are summarized in Table 9.

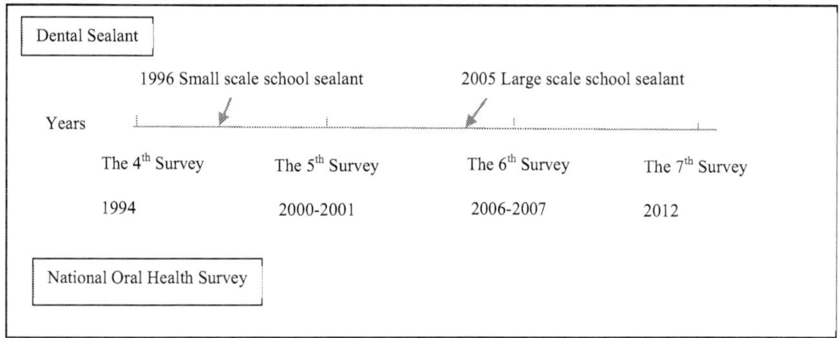

Figure 10. Summary of implementation timeline of National Oral Health Surveys and the dental sealant program

During the period 1994 to 2000/2001 [42, 47], the percentage of children affected by caries increased but the average caries experience in permanent teeth was quite stable (Table 7). The oral health program at that time comprised school dental sealant on a small scale, ongoing after-lunch tooth brushing and oral health education (Tables 8 and 9). However, from the 5th survey, the proportion of children who enrolled every day in the after-lunch tooth brushing program was low, only 26.3%. The proportion of children who brushed their teeth every day was 86.2% in the morning and 34.6% in the evening.

Between 2000/2001 and 2006/2007 [42, 6], caries experience in terms of percentage of children affected by caries and average carious teeth per child among 12-year-olds was slightly decreased (Table 7). Sealant service was increased 2.8 times from the 5th to the 6th survey. This period included the first phase of the large scale implementation of school dental sealant and the campaign to control of sugar consumption, which emphasized the creation of networks and activities in childcare centers. However, the number of sealed children was still low (Table 8). Other dental heath activities, such as after-lunch tooth brushing and oral health education, were ongoing. The proportion of children who brushed their teeth every day at school decreased to 21.7% and that of children who did not brush increased to 57.9%. Brushing at home seemed to increase slightly (Table 8).

During the 6th and 7th surveys [6, 7], the proportion of children having caries decreased approximately five percentage points and the average number of carious teeth decreased from 1.55 to 1.3 teeth per child. The percentage of children with sealant at 12 years of age increased from 12.7% to 35.2% (Table 8). The large scale dental sealant was implemented for nearly 7 years. The percentage of tooth brushing occasion continued on the rise. However, snack consumption also increased during the same period (Table 8).

	The 4th survey [47] (1994)	The 5th survey [42] (2000-2001)	The 6th Survey [6] (2006-2007)	The 7th Survey [7] (2012)
Number of children	2,801	35,623	2,208	2,618
Percent caries	53.9	57.3	56.9	52.3
Mean DMFT and SE	1.6± 0.04	1.64*	1.55*	1.30*

*SE data are not available

Table 7. Number of children, percentage and mean caries experience of 12-year-olds from four surveys

Activities	The 4th survey [47] (1994)#	The 5th survey [42] (2000-2001)	The 6th Survey [6] (2006-2007)	The 7th Survey [7] (2012)
Dental sealant''	NA	4.5	12.7	35.2
Daily tooth brushing after-lunch	NA	26.3	21.7	17.8$
Tooth brushing occation@	NA	Morning 86.2 Evening 34.6	Every day 89.6 Mean 2.2 times a day	Morning 97.7 Evening 71.5
Use Fluoride toothpaste	NA	94.1	89.9	91.4
Eating snack everyday	NA	28.2	38.8

NA = not available

* received dental sealant and dental sealant presence at 12 years old

Data of 12 years-old were not available since oral health care behavior interviewed in 17 years and older.

$ The question was not specific to after-lunch tooth brushing program at school

@ In each survey, different questions were applied - the 5th and 7th asked whether he/she brushed every day in the morning and evening, the 6th survey asked whether he/she brushed his/her teeth every day and how often

Table 8. Percentage of 12-year-old children enrolled in the oral health prevention and promotion activities

It is difficult to draw conclusion with certainty on the reasons explaining the decline of caries [44]. In Thailand, among 12-year-old children, the important factors related to caries decline seem to be the large scale school dental sealant and frequent tooth brushing with fluoride toothpaste [7]. Since the number of children with sealants in the survey was the number of children who received dental sealant and in whom the dental sealant was still present at 12 years of age, the actual coverage should be larger than the reported figures of 12.7% and 35.2% at the 6th and 7th surveys, respectively. The percentages of children having tooth-brushing behavior with fluoride toothpaste were high. The percentage with normal gingival condition also increased from 18.0% to 29.9% from the 6th to the 7th survey. This increase could be ascribed to the tooth brushing behavior [7]. However, the eating habit is a major problem that remains to be solved.

Period	Program	Brief activities
1988	Oral Health Surveillance and Dental Health Promotion Programme for primary school Children	Dental examination by school teachers After-lunch tooth brushing program Oral health education
1996	Small scale school dental sealant	Sealant in grade 1
1999	Health Promoting School (Oral health integrated in health promotion)	Key indicators for oral health; dental examination, no caries on permanent teeth (fillings are acceptable), no gingivitis After-lunch tooth brushing with fluoride toothpaste Healthy food in school
2003	Sweet enough project	Creating network and campaign to reduce sugar consumption
2005	Oral Health Promotion and Prevention in School Children Project under National Health Security (Large scale school dental sealant)	Full mouth examination grade 1 and 3 children Sealant grade 1 children After-lunch tooth brushing in primary school

Table 9. Dental health care programs implemented for school children in Thailand

7. Conclusion and suggestion

Although the effectiveness of school dental sealant program in Thailand has continuously improved, there is still much room for further improvement. This chapter has presented the findings on effectiveness and on failures in context of the actual school programs, where more factors are operating than in the context of experimental research. Looking at failures may provide valuable information. In this case, the types of failure could reflect their causes, and be used to improve performance. In the Thai context, short-term retention is still a problem. Improvement in the related factors such as equipment, application technique and presence of chair-side assistant might result in increased effectiveness. Important improvement measures may include adjusting the goal or key performance indicators of the sealant program based on actual workload, adding in some indicator to reflect the quality of the program and initiating evaluation by an external evaluator. The quality indicator must not place additional pressure on providers; evaluation should be reward-based rather than punishment-based. The guideline and recommendation on sealant application should be strictly followed and emphasized to providers.

A school dental sealant program alone could not have much impact on oral health status since its effect is only on pit and fissure surfaces. Comprehensive prevention and promotion should be strengthened, inclusive of dental sealant, tooth brushing with fluoride toothpaste and eating behavior.

Acknowledgements

I would like to acknowledge the Thailand Dental Public Health Society and the Lion Corporation (Thailand) Limited for the Lion award of Oral Health for School Sealant Project, which supported the publication of this chapter. I am also grateful to my respected PhD advisor, Professor Dr. Virasakdi Chongsuvivatwong, who gave me many valuable ideas; and I especially acknowledge Associate Professor Dr. Songchai Thitasomakul, Assistant Professor Dr. Janpim Hintao and Dr. Banyen Sirisakulveroj for their long time of friendship and great assistance. Special appreciation is expressed to Dr. Alan Geater and Mr. Sakda Pongcharoenyong for their kindness to review and edit this book chapter. I am also grateful to all the dental nurses and children who participated in the study.

Author details

Sukanya Tianviwat[1,2]

Address all correspondence to: Sukanya.ti@psu.ac.th

1 Faculty of Dentistry, Prince of Songkla University, Songkhla, Thailand

2 Common Oral Diseases and Epidemiology Research Center, Faculty of Dentistry, Prince of Songkla University, Songkhla, Thailand

References

[1] Guide to Community Preventive Services. Preventing Dental Caries: School-Based Dental Sealant Delivery Programs. www.thecommunityguide.org/oral/caries.html. (accessed 3 August 2013).

[2] Carter NL, with the American Association for Community Dental Programs and the National Maternal and Child Oral Health Resource Center. Seal America: The Prevention Invention (2nd ed., rev.). Washington DC: National Maternal and Child Oral Health Resource Center; 2011. http://www.mchoralhealth.org/seal/intro.html#school (accessed 12 May 2013).

[3] Tianviwat s, Hoerup NJ. Evaluation of an outreach oral health service and use of mobile dental equipment in Southern Thailand. Journal of Public Health 2002; 32(3): 167-177.

[4] Centers for Disease Control and Prevention. Infrastructure Development Tools Activity 5a: School-Based/School-Linked Dental Sealant Programs. http://www.cdc.gov/oralhealth/state_programs/infrastructure/activity5a.htm (accessed on 9 Sept 2014).

[5] Jirapongsa W, Prasertsom P. Evaluation of Oral Health promotion and Prevention in School Children Project under National Health Security "Yim (smile) Sodsai (Bright), Dek Thai (Thai Children) Fun Dee (Health Teeth)" 2005-2007. Thailand Journal of Dental Public Health 2008; 13(5): 85-96.

[6] Dental Division. The 6th Thailand National Oral Health Survey report 2006-2007. Bangkok: Health Department (Thailand), Ministry of Public Health; 2008.

[7] Dental Division. The 7th Thailand National Oral Health Survey report 2012. Bangkok: Health Department (Thailand), Ministry of Public Health; 2013.

[8] Tianviwat S, Hintao J, Chongsuvivatwong V, Thitasomakul S, Sirisakulveroj B. Factors related to short-term retention of sealant in permanent molar teeth provided in the school mobile dental clinic, Songkhla province, Southern Thailand. Journal of Public Health 2011; 41(1):50-58.

[9] Choomphupan V. Comparison of pit and fissure sealant retention rate between mobile dental unit in school and dental unit in health center at 6, 12, and 36 months in Minburi district, Bangkok. Thailand Journal of Dental Public Health 2011; 16(2): 33-42.

[10] Charnvanishporn S. The retention of sealed teeth of the students in third grade primary school, after 3 years of mobile sealant project in Ranong provinces, 2007. Thailand Journal of Dental Public Health 2009; 13(3): 63-70.

[11] Thamtadawiwat D. The effectiveness of dental pit and fissure sealant program for the student in Prathomsueksa 1 Cha-am district, Phetchaburi province. Thailand Journal of Dental Public Health 2008; 13(1): 25-36.

[12] Tianviwat S, Chongsuvivatwong V, Sirisakulveroj B. Loss of sealant retention and subsequent caries development. Community Dental Health 2008; 25(4): 216-220.

[13] Obsuwan K. The effectiveness of the pit and fissure sealant in the "Save our six" project Chiang Rai, Thailand. Thailand Journal of Dental Public Health 2008; 13(1): 52-62.

[14] Kongtawelert P. A two-year evaluation of pit and fissure sealant of first permanent molars in school-based program (Yim Sod Sai Dek Thai Fun Dee) in Sukhothai province during 2005-2007. Thailand Journal of Dental Public Health 2008; 12(3): 86-96.

[15] Kantamaturapoj K. The effectiveness of dental pit and fissure sealant program in primary school children in Kamphaengphet province. Thailand Journal of Dental Public Health 2008; 12(2): 7-16.

[16] Thipsoonthornchai J. The comparative study on retention rate and caries prevention between glass ionomer and resin using as pit and fissure sealant in mobile dental service, Buriram province. Thailand Journal of Dental Public Health 2003; 8(1-2): 62-77.

[17] Tianviwat S, Chukadee W, Sirisakunweroj B, Leewanant R, Larsen MJ. Retention of pit and fissure sealants under field conditions after nearly 2-3 years. Journal of the Dental Association of Thailand 2001; 51(2): 115-120.

[18] Hsieh H, Huang S, Tsai C, Chiou M, Liao C. Evaluation of a sealant intervention program among Taiwanese aboriginal schoolchildren. Journal of Dental Sciences 2014; 9 (2): 178-184.

[19] Muller-Bolla M, Lupi-Pe'gurier L, Bardakjian H, Velly AM. Effectiveness of school-based dental sealant programs among children from low-income backgrounds in France: a pragmatic randomized clinical trial. Community Dentistry and Oral Epidemiology 2013; 41(3): 232–241.

[20] Francis R, Mascarenhas AK, Soparkar P, Al-Mutawaa S. Retention and effectiveness of fissure sealants in Kuwaiti school children. Community Dental Health 2008; 25(4): 211-215

[21] Wendt LK, Koch G, Birkhed D. On the retention and effectiveness of fissure sealant in permanent molars after 15-20 years: a cohort study. Community Dentistry and Oral Epidemiology 2001; 29(4): 302-307.

[22] Holst A, Braune K, Sullivan A. A five-year evaluation of fissure sealants applied by dental assistants. Swedish Dental Journal 1998; 22(5-6): 195-201.

[23] Messer LB, Calache H, Morgan MV. The retention of pit and fissure sealants placed in primary school children by Dental Health Services, Victoria. Australian Dental Journal 1997; 42(4): 233-239.

[24] Bravo M, Osorio E, García-Anllo I, Llodra JC, Baca P. The influence of dft index on sealant success: a 48-month survival analysis. Journal of Dental Research 1996; 75(2): 768-774.

[25] Plengsringam N, Tharasombat S. Effectiveness of dental sealant in preventing dental caries among students in a school dental health program of Pranangklao hospital, Nonthaburi. Journal of Health Science 2014; 23(1): 91-98.

[26] Tianviwat S. Performance improvement of dental service quality in the school dental sealant program following the implementation of an audit and feedback system. Bangkok: Thailand Research Fund. 2012-2013.

[27] Gooch B, Griffin S, Gray S, Kohn W, Rozier R, et al. Preventing Dental Caries Through School-Based Sealant Programs: Updated Recommendations and Reviews of Evidence. Journal of the American Dental Association 2009; 140(11):1356-1365.

[28] Gray SK, Griffin SO, Malvitz DM, Gooch BF. A comparison of the effects of tooth brushing and handpiece prophylaxis on retention of sealants. Journal of the American Dental Association 2009; 140(1): 38-46.

[29] Geiger SB, Gulayev S, Weiss EI. Improving fissure sealants quality: mechanical preparation and filling level. Journal of Dentistry 2000; 28(6):407-412.

[30] Griffin SO, Jones K, Gray SK, Malvitz DM, Gooch BF. Exploring four-handed delivery and retention of resin-based sealants. Journal of the American Dental Association 2008; 139(3): 281-289.

[31] Albert DA, McManus JM, Mitchell DA. Models for delivering school-based dental care. Journal of School Health 2005; 75(5): 157-161.

[32] Jackson DM, Jahnke LR, Kerber L, Nyer G, Siemens K, et al. Creating a successful school-based mobile dental program. Journal of School Health 2007; 77(1): 1-6.

[33] Tianviwat S, Chongsuvivatwong V, Birch S. Optimizing the mix of basic dental services for Southern Thai schoolchildren based on resource consumption, service needs and parental preference. Community Dentistry and Oral Epidemiology 2009; 37(4): 372-380.

[34] Chestnutt I, Schafer F, Jacobson P, Stephen K. The prevalence and effectiveness of fissure sealants in Scottish adolescents. British Dental Journal 1994; 177(4): 125-129.

[35] Griffin S, Gray S, Malvitz D, Gooch B. Caries Risk in Formerly Sealed Teeth. The Journal of the American Dental Association 2009;140(4):415-423.

[36] Green JC, Vermillion JR. The simplified oral hygiene index. The Journal of the American Dental Association 1964; 68: 7-13.

[37] Dental Division. Oral Health Promotion and Prevention in School Children Project under National Health Security. http://www.anamai.ecgates.com/news/news_detail.php?id=323. (accessed 3 May 2014).

[38] Kuthy R, Ashton J. Eruption pattern of permanent molars: Implication for school-based dental sealant program. Journal of Public Health Dentistry 1989; 49(1):7-14.

[39] Muangmuen T. Permanent First Molar Eruption and Dental Caries in Children of Banklang Subdistrict, Lomsak District, Pethchabun Province. Thailand Journal of Dental Public Health 2014; 19(1): 9-20.

[40] Ahovuo-Saloranta A, Hiiri A, Nordblad A,MäkeläM,Worthington HV. Pit and fissure sealants for preventing dental decay in the permanent teeth of children and adolescents. Cochrane Database of Systematic Reviews 2008, Issue 4. Art. No.: CD001830. DOI:10.1002/14651858.CD001830.pub3.

[41] Ahovuo-Saloranta A, Forss H, Walsh T, Hiiri A, Nordblad A, et al. Sealants for preventing dental decay in the permanent teeth. Cochrane Database of Systematic Reviews 2013, Issue 3. Art. No.: CD001830. DOI: 10.1002/14651858.CD001830.pub4.

[42] Dental Division. The 5th Thailand National Oral Health Survey report 2000-2001. Bangkok: Health Department (Thailand), Ministry of Public Health; 2002.

[43] Dental Division. Manual of Dental Health Surveillance Project for Primary School Children. Bangkok: The War Veterans Organization of Thailand Publishing; 1988.

[44] Vrbic V. Reasons for caries decline in Slovenia. Community Dentistry and Oral Epidemiology 2000; 28(2):126-132.

[45] O'Mullane D, Clarke D, Daly F, McDermott S, Murphy B, et al. Use of fissure sealants in the Eastern Health Board in the Republic of Ireland. 45th ORCA Congress. Caries Research 1998; 32(4):267–317 (abstract no. 42).

[46] Kumar JV, Wadhawan S. Targeting dental sealants in school-based programs: evaluation of an approach. Community Dentistry and Oral Epidemiology 2002; 30(3): 210–215.

[47] Dental Division. The 4th Thailand National Oral Health Survey report 1994. Bangkok: Health Department (Thailand), Ministry of Public Health; 1995.

Prosthetics, Geiatric and Implant Dentistry

Chapter 9

Denture and Overdenture Complications

Elena Preoteasa, Cristina Teodora Preoteasa,
Laura Iosif, Catalina Murariu Magureanu and
Marina Imre

Additional information is available at the end of the chapter

http://dx.doi.org/10.5772/59250

1. Introduction

Dentures and overdentures, the most frequently used treatment options for the complete edentulism, can have local and systemic complications. For their prevention, treatment and reduction of their negative impact, it is necessary to understand their etiological context and to know their particularities of manifestation. Considering the relatively high rate of some complications of denture and overdenture treatment, knowing them is essential for ensuring a treatment that corresponds to the medical standards of care and patients' needs and expectations.

2. Context of denture and overdenture complications

All medical treatments should be approached with a holistic perspective in mind, due to the fact that there are numerous factors which, through interacting each other, have an impact on the final medical outcome. Understanding the problem and its realistic possible approaches, but also considering its treatment limitations and performing an analysis that evaluates the medium and long-term prognosis ensures the highest premises for obtaining a good result.

The previous also applies to the treatment of edentulism using dentures or overdentures. Some of the key aspects that might help understand better the denture and overdenture complications, as they define the etiological context, are mentioned in Table 1.

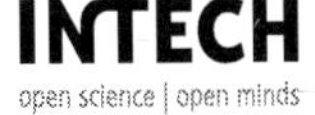

Context	General medical and social factors	Medical and social perception of edentulism
		Demographics of edentulism
	Denture and overdenture treatment factors	Treatment difficulty
		Treatment options overview
		Maintenance therapy
		Technical and biomechanical considerations
		Previous dental treatments
	Edentulous patient factors	Oral health status
		Systemic health status and medication use
		Age
		Health risk factors
		Patient need and preferences

Table 1. Context of denture and overdenture complications – key factors

2.1. Medical and social perception of edentulism

Edentulism is defined as the loss of all permanent teeth. Tooth loss is an outcome of a complex interaction between disease entities (e.g., caries and periodontal disease) and non-disease entities (e.g. economy, oral healthcare system, access to dental services, dental awareness, cultural tradition, education) [1]. Continuing exposure to risk factors after onset of edentulism (e.g., poor oral hygiene, smoking, deficient dental treatment) can have an etiological role in the occurrence of complication.

Edentulism is a chronic, severe, irreversible medical condition and is described as the final marker of disease burden for oral health [2,3]. It is common for elderly people, but it is not regarded any more as an inevitable phenomenon that comes with age [4].

Edentulism has several deleterious consequences on oral health (e.g., residual ridge resorption, impaired masticatory function, trouble speaking), general health (deficient nutritional status, increased risk for certain systemic diseases), mental and social well-being (dissatisfaction with appearance, avoidance of social contacts) and on quality of life [1,2,4]. The previous have impact on prosthetic treatment to be performed.

Thus, the current perception on edentulism is as non-fatal sequelae of diseases and injuries, which still represents a tremendous global health care burden [5,6]. It can be considered a physical impairment, because important body parts have been lost, a disability, because it associates functional limitations or a handicap, as it sometimes limits or prevents normal life or work activities [1,2,7-9].

Considering the impact and demographics of the edentulism, the health care barriers that older people face, the Active Ageing approach of the World Health Organization (keeping older people socially engaged and productive), intensive measures and new regulations regarding caring for the elderly population are needed. Consequently, implementation of gerodontology, as a new dental specialty, may be appropriate [10].

2.2. Demographics of edentulism

According to the current reports and predictions, edentulism is and will continue to represent a common disease for the elderly people segment.

There is a tendency for reduction of the edentulism prevalence, through the reduction of tooth loss. Thus, in the United States in the period of 1999-2004, the prevalence of tooth retention in seniors (65 years and older) significantly increased from 17.9 teeth to 18.9 teeth and the prevalence of edentulism significantly decreased from approximately 34% to 27% [11]. This phenomenon can be justified through the progress made in the dental field, the emphasis on prevention measures, improved access to dental care services and mass education for approaching a healthy behavior [4]. But, despite these efforts, complete edentulism continues to have a high prevalence, aspect associated mainly to the aging population phenomenon through growth of the life expectancy and thus the number of elderly people and the number of edentulous patients [12,13].

Estimates show that edentulism is found in 2.3% of the world's population regardless of age, respectively in 7-69% of adult populations internationally [5,14]. Considerably high disparities are noted between different countries, different regions, due to the important impact of the socio-economical and behavioral factors.

The prognoses show that edentulism is decreasing, but most probably will continue to be a condition with a significant prevalence, especially in elderly's people, which is estimated to be a growing category in the global population [15]. Douglas estimates that in the United States the population with one or two edentulous jaws will increase from 34 million in 1991 to 38 million in 2020 [1,12]. Felton considers that most probably the necessity for complete denture therapy will not disappear over the next 4 or 5 decades, and the economic conditions may even lead to a growing need [1,6].

2.3. Treatment difficulty

Edentulism is generally regarded as a clinical condition with a high degree of treatment difficulty, often being hard to achieve optimal functional parameters. The complexity of the edentulous condition derives from the extensive oral changes, both anatomical and functional, that sometimes require preprosthetic surgical intervention in order to optimize the biomechanical conditions, which are superimposed on general alterations (related to age, systemic disease, and psychosocial status). In order to support the differentiation of cases according to their treatment difficulty degree, the ACP (American College of Prosthodontists) has put together the Prosthodontic Diagnostic Index (PDI) Classification System for the complete edentulism [16]. Higher complexity of edentulism condition increase the risk of treatment complication (e.g., in cases with severe ridge resorption ill-fitting dentures are more frequently noticed), and complications can also contribute to increasing the degree of treatment difficulty (e.g., wearing unstable dentures accelerate the ridge resorption rate).

2.4. Treatment options overview

Complete denture used to be the only treatment option for the complete edentulism. Nowadays, this is still the most frequently used treatment option, but there can be seen a growing trend towards using implant prosthetic restorations fixed or removable. Each treatment option has the risk of specific complications, dependent on their manufacturing particularities and bio-mechanical features.

Dentures can have both local and systemic complications, such as gingival hyperplasia, denture stomatitis, loss of denture retention, fracture of the denture and functional impairment, mastication deficiencies having a negative impact on the nutritional status. Some patients cannot tolerate the dentures, aspect that can be connected to psychological factors, to patients' needs and expectations, but also to age, oral conditions, denture deficiencies and doctor-patient relationship.

Root supported overdentures, with or without attachment systems, have the advantage of improved retention and stability, with a positive impact on the oral functions and the accommodation with the future dentures. Their possible complications include the ones of the conventional dentures and, additionally, some modifications of the supporting teeth or the attachment system used.

Prosthetic implant restorations, either fixed or a removable, are alternatives that provide an improved functional integration and better treatment outcome, but are more complex and require preprosthetic interventions, with additional biological, financial and time costs. Using these treatment options involves the risk for additional complications, with regards to the higher complexity of the treatment –e.g., treatment plan related, surgical complications, technical complications.

2.5. Maintenance therapy

Maintenance is very important for the longevity of the treatment, having a positive impact in reducing the frequency and severity of its complications. Both type of procedures, those performed in the dental office, by the dentist and at home, by the patient, are relevant in this respect.

Periodical check-ups are essential, considering that there are some complications with a high prevalence rate both for dentures and implant overdentures (e.g., loss of denture stability due to progressive ridge resorption, denture adjustments and relinings, clip activations) [17]. Additionally, the edentulous patients are often elderly patients, and face access barriers to dental care services, in relation to aspects like lack of finances or transportation difficulties [18,19]. Due to this, it is recommended to keep in mind the possible complications and to take the appropriate preventive measures to limit them at the time the treatment is being planned and performed.

Informing and instructing the patient on how to take proper care of the oral care and prosthetic restorations are important aspects, since complications can be tightly related to this (e.g., the lack of appropriate cleaning of the denture, teeth or implants is associated with a higher risk for denture stomatitis, tooth or implant loss). Since we are frequently dealing with elderly people, who have less manual dexterity, it is recommended to choose simpler treatment option (e.g., if applicable, 2-implant overdentures are more appropriate than 4-implant overdenture [20].

2.6. Technical and biomechanical considerations

According to the current level of knowledge, treatment with dentures or implant/root overdentures must consider the risk for developing complications in relation to the technical and biomechanical features (e.g., design, attachment components, materials).

There are different types of design for dentures and overdentures, with different possible complications. Thus, using narrow-diameter implants associates a higher risk of implant fracture. Considering the occlusal scheme, there is evidence that patients prefer dentures with lingualized occlusion [21]. Metal or non-metal (glass and polyethylene fibers) inserts are recommended for denture base reinforcement when there is a high risk of denture fracture or when there are more than 2 teeth or implants supporting the denture [22].

Material used for denture/overdenture fabrication associates the risk of developing complications in relation to their physico-chemical properties and their biocompatibility. For example, polymethylmethacrylate (PMMA), the material mostly used for manufacturing of dentures or overdentures, through its features (porosity, increased wettability, low mechanical strength, monomer release after curing) facilitates the occurrence of complications such as microbial or contact denture stomatitis, fracture of the dentures, artificial teeth discoloration and wear [23].

2.7. Previous dental treatments

A key element in order to achieve a predictable outcome is the analysis of the previous dental and prosthetic treatments, by connecting patient's subjective complaints with prosthetic restoration's objective deficiencies. This gives important information that could be used for decision making in establishing the particularities of the future prosthetic treatment. For example, complete denture intolerance can be linked to personality traits, to objective patient's features that enhance the occurrence of functional deficiencies, or to some objective faults of the dentures. Differentiating between these three situations is the basis for selecting the optimal treatment option, with the possibility to prevent the complications that occurred in the past.

2.8. Oral health status

The complete edentulism cannot be regarded simply as the loss of teeth. It is accompanied by massive, progressive changes of the oral structures and functional alterations, which associates a high degree of treatment difficulty and the occurrence of specific complications. Impact of edentulism on oral health is mainly manifested in 3 directions: modifier of normal physiology; risk factor for impaired mastication; determinant of oral health [2]. Amongst the sequelae of treatment with complete dentures, as the most commonly used treatment option, there can be mentioned residual ridge resorption, mucosal reactions, burning mouth syndrome, denture stomatitis [24].

Considering the severe changes of the oral status in edentulous patients, the increasing elderly population and the relatively frequent barriers to oral health care of older people (e.g., financial hardship, transportation difficulties), Petersen et al. makes a series of recommendations among which are the incorporation of age related oral health concerns into the promotion of general health, that could ease the development of oral health care for older people [25].

2.9. Systemic health status and medication use

Between oral health and general health there are numerous interactions, that sometimes materializes as local or systemic complications.

The impact of complete edentulism on the general health status is manifested as an increased risk of conditions, such as nutritional deficiencies, inflammatory changes of the gastric mucosa, peptic or duodenal ulcers, obesity, noninsulin-dependent diabetes mellitus, hypertension, heart failure, ischemic heart disease, stroke, aortic valve sclerosis, chronic kidney disease, sleep-disordered breathing, including obstructive sleep apnea [2]. Additionally, functional limitations, mental and social well-being alterations that negatively impact the quality of life are more common in edentulous patients.

The impact of general health status and the medication used on the oral health of the edentulous patient is partially manifested through the occurrence of complications. Nutritional deficiencies increase the risk of occurrence of denture stomatitis, traumatic ulcer and burning mouth syndrome [25]. Patient's personality and psychological well-being influences treatment satisfaction and tolerance [10]. Decreased manual dexterity has a negative impact on care and maintenance of dentures/overdentures, which leads to negative effects on oral and systemic health [14].

2.10. Age

Patient's age is an important aspect to consider when planning the prosthetic treatment, being linked to particularities of oral and general health status, to specific needs and expectation towards the prosthetic rehabilitation, to particular medical approaches in order to ensure a good long-term prognosis. Prosthetic treatment of the edentulous patient should take into account the current situation, but also the most probable evolution and, if present, the inherent complications (e.g., preventive measures to reduce alveolar ridge resorption are recommended).

Young-elderly edentulous patients generally have more favorable clinical conditions for prosthetic rehabilitation, a better general health status, a faster adaptation to removable prosthesis if chosen and the ability to perform most accurately the necessary the maintenance procedures. They have higher expectations regarding the esthetics and functionality of the prosthetic rehabilitation and don't easily accept the removable treatment options.

Old-elderly edentulous patients generally register an increased treatment difficulty, as a consequence of numerous factors interacting. In previous ill-fitting complete denture wearers there is a severe ridge resorption [26,27]. The prevalence of co-morbidities is increased, such as physical or mental health problems that have a negative impact on oral health, systemic health, functioning and behavior. Most of the times the elderly people are not regular users of dental services since they overcome physical and psychological access treatment barriers (e.g., the cost of dental care services, transportation problems, doctor's attitudes-lack of responsiveness to patient's concerns, the lack of perceived need for care, fear), which are more significant for the functionally dependent elderly then for the independent elderly [28-30]. They have treatment expectations that target first the rehabilitation of the masticatory function, and second the esthetics. They usually prefer more simple medical procedures, that include limited surgical interventions and that demand easy maintenance procedures. The older completely edentulous patients show a more frequent rate of denture intolerance, probably due to less adaptability to new situations.

Demographic changes, namely population ageing and decreasing prevalence of tooth loss, have impact on the edentulous patient profile. There is an increasing of the age when edentulism occurs, aspects that associates an increased treatment difficulty. Considering the latter, additional measures are necessary to ensure adequate oral health for older edentulous patients e.g., access to and financing for dental services, an adequately trained workforce to provide dental care and appropriate education to edentulous individuals [30].

2.11. Health risk factors

Health risk factors should be assessed since they can explain some of the case particularities and may have a negative impact on the treatment outcome. Among them, there can be mentioned behavioral risk factors (e.g. tobacco and alcohol consumption, obesity related to physical activity and diet), social risk factors (e.g., socio-economical status, social networks and social support, occupational factors, social inequalities), inadequate disease screening practices, exposure to increased stress [31]. Their role is proven both as a cause of complete edentulism and also as a factor that impacts the treatment outcome, being risk factors for some complications.

2.12. Patient need and preferences

Health care decisions require integrating the patient's individual preferences and values, according to the ethical principle of respecting the patient's autonomy [32]. A good relation and communication between doctor and patient offers the best premises for reaching a consensus regarding the medical decision, with a positive effect on the treatment outcome.

Patient preferences are related to numerous variables, e.g., age, social status, personality type, education. Acknowledging them may be difficult, especially in elderly patients, sometimes in relation to objective reasons, as physical changes that affect the communication (e.g., loss of hearing or visual acuity). Additional efforts should be made in order to understand the patient's health needs and preferences, since they can have important consequences, such as rejection of the prosthetic treatment or even avoiding addressing for medical treatment.

3. Classification of denture and overdenture complications

The classification of denture and overdenture complications can enhance practitioner's understanding of them, with a positive effect on their management and prognosis.

Denture and overdenture complications can be classified considering their etiology, according to risk factor's nature and mechanism of action, as described in table 2, or in regarded to some descriptive criteria, as presented in table 3.

Classification of denture and overdenture complications, considering their etiology

A. According to the nature of the risk factor

Host or patient related factors
- *edentulism-related*, e.g., ridge resorption, impaired mastication;
- *oral health-related*, excluding the conditions linked to edentulism, e.g., reduced salivary flow increases the risk for denture stomatitis and denture intolerance;
- *systemic health-related*, including medication use, e.g., diabetes mellitus is a risk factor for denture stomatitis; the bisphosphonate treatment is a risk factor for osteonecrosis;
- *patient's behavior and other characteristics-related*, like income and social status, education, physical environment, e.g., poor financial status limits the access to dental treatment;

Dental treatment related factors
- *removable dental prosthesis-related*, considering the manufacturing accuracy, technical features and materials used, e.g., overextended dentures causes traumatic ulcers or hyperplasia; artificial teeth wear is linked to mastication deficiencies; allergic reactions to polymethylmethacrylate (PMMA);
- *teeth or dental implants-related*, e.g., periodontal disease of supporting roots causes denture instability; implant overdentures have additional surgical complications like nerve injury; treatment failure may appear consequently to tooth or dental implant loss;
- *attachment system-related*, e.g., ill-fitting overdenture due to loosening or loss of the matrix;

Dentist's intervention related factors [33]
- *inherent complications*, in which dentist's role is irrelevant, e.g., allergic reaction to polymethylmethacrylate (PMMA), when patients' history is inconclusive;
- *passive intervention*, as improper conduct regarding early signs of disease, e.g., implant loss due to excessive denture pressure or due to ignored early signs of peri-implantitis;
- *wrongful judgment*, as errors in conceiving and conducting the treatment, e.g., improper implant location or number; incorrect registration of maxillomandibular relationship, as an increased vertical dimension of occlusion.

B. According to the mechanism of action of the risk factor

Susceptibility factors increase the chance of complications occurrence, e.g., implant failure is frequenter in smokers and diseases like diabetes;
Initiation factors directly initiate the complication, e.g., overextended dentures cause traumatic lesions of the oral mucosa;
Progression factors cause worsening of a preexistent condition, e.g., ill-fitting dentures increase the rate of alveolar ridge resorption.

Table 2. Classifications of denture and overdenture complications, considering their etiology

Descriptive classification of denture and overdenture complications

A. According to localization

Host

- *oral*, e.g., oral soft and hard tissue complications, functional alterations; remaining teeth complications in case of root overdentures as caries, periodontal disease, root fracture;
- *facial*, e.g., aged prognathic appearance;
- *systemic*, e.g., malnutrition, gastro-intestinal disorders;

Dental restoration

- *removable dental prosthesis*, e.g., denture/overdenture fracture; retention loss; aging of the material, teeth wear
- *dental implants*, that are classified according to Berglundh et al. [34] as biological complications (functional disturbances that affect the tissues supporting the implant, e.g., peri-implantitis) or technical complications (mechanical damage of the implant, implant components and suprastructures)
- *attachment system*, e.g., loosening, loss, damage

B. According to modification type

Anatomical changes, e.g., alveolar ridge resorption; decrease of the muscular mass;
Functional changes, e.g., mastication or phonation deficiencies, protruded mandibular position;
Pathological changes, e.g., traumatic ulcers, atrophic stomatitis, candidiasis.

C. According to severity

Light – few clinical signs, whose treatment is simple, requires reduced costs in terms of biological, financial and clinical time and has a good prognosis, e.g., loosening of attachment system; ulcerations or irritations related to surplus material on denture's base;
Moderate – functional alterations are associated and treatment requires medium costs, e.g., denture base fracture; loss of stability and need for relining; artificial tooth wear;
Severe – associates important functional alterations, can lead to treatment failure, addressing them imply high costs, e.g., damage of inferior alveolar nerve, denture intolerance.

D. According to the moment of occurrence

During the preprosthetic procedures, e.g., pain during the surgical procedures for frenum plastia or reshaping of exostosis;
While manufacturing the removable prostheses, e.g., discomfort due to vomiting reflex;
During the surgical phase of implant placement, according to Misch & Wang [35] being encountered treatment plan-related complications (e.g., wrong angulation or improper implant location), anatomy-related complications (e.g., nerve injury, bleeding, cortical plate perforation, sinus membrane complication), procedure-related complications (e.g., mechanical complications, lack of primary stability, ingestion and aspiration) and others (e.g., iatrogenic damage and human error);
Immediately after inserting the denture/overdenture, e.g., traumatic ulcers;
During maintenance, e.g., root or implant complications, retention loss

Table 3. Classifications of denture and overdenture complications, considering descriptive criteria

4. Main complications of denture and overdenture

Some of the most common complications of the completely edentulous patient, treated by dentures or implant/root overdentures will be presented. Aspects related to their etiology, clinical features and management will be covered.

4.1. Alveolar ridge resorption

The residual ridge derives from the alveolar process after tooth loss. It registers the most significant changes and it supports the highest pressures during the worn of dentures or implant-retained overdentures. The ridge resorption is manifested as a continuous, cumulative and irreversible process, visible as the decrease of the quantity and quality of the bone [36].

Etiology. The ridge resorption is inherent after tooth loss and during denture wearing. It is a cronic plurifactorial condition as a joint result of physical, physiological and pathological factors.

The process of postextractive bone restructuring, after tooth loss, has variable rate and pattern, in relation to general physiological and pathological factors (age, menopause, systemic alterations), local factors (the edentulism and its cause, features of the jaws – volume, density). Also, the rate of bone resorption (the quantity of bone lost in a time period) varies in relation to the moment of tooth loss-it is maximum immediately after it in the first month, high in the first year after the tooth loss and decreases consequently. The pattern of bone resorption registers topographic differences – as for the maxilla and the mandible, for the anterior and posterior regions and in relation to anatomical features. The resorption is maximum at the top of the ridge and is lower at the base of the ridge, in the biostatical areas (maxillary tuberosity, retromolar pad), at the ligaments' insertion site (frenum) and in the region of the hard palate. The ridge resorption occurs from the top to the basis, and is centripetal in the maxilla and centrifugal in the mandible. The pattern of ridge resorption varies according to the anatomical features and the size of the jaws, e.g., in class II skeletal patients, brachicephals, with mandibular micrognathism the resorption is more severe in the mandible, and in class III skeletal patients, dolicocephals, with mandibular macrognathism the resorption is more severe in the maxilla. Also, ridge resorption is more pronounced in women (probably linked to smaller jaws and lower bone density, related to postmenopause osteoporosis), in patients who lost their teeth due to periodontal disease and in those with high occlusal forces (natural teeth as antagonists, bruxism). Systemic conditions, particularly diabetes mellitus and other metabolic disorders, can accelerate the rhythm of ridge resorption.

The dentures accelerate the rate of ridge resorption, mainly through the pressure exercised by them on the support structures during oral functions. The severity of ridge resorption is connected to the parameters of functional and parafunctional forces of occlusion and to biomechanical aspects related to the prosthesis-the support and stability of the denture, the positioning of artificial teeth, type of occlusion, antagonists (teeth, implants, edentulous), and correctness of the registration of maxillomandibular relationship. The support surface for occlusal forces is reduced in edentulous patients, compared to the dentulous ones, and through progressive ridge resorption, both in high and width, consequently the support surface decreases even more. The magnitude of occlusal forces are generally lower in the edentulous patients, but there are variations related to age, sex, parafunctions as bruxism, stress level, food consistency preferences, and also the correctness of prosthetic rehabilitation. Increased duration of occlusion contacts, as a risk factor for ridge resorption, is related to bruxism, ill-fitting dentures, unstable occlusion and increased vertical dimension of occlusion. Compared to maxillary edentulism, mandibular edentulism has greater risk of registering more severe ridge resorption, due to the decreased denture support surface and related higher magnitude of pressure beared. Also, denture wearing associates the risk of specific complications that favor the occurrence of an accelerated rate of ridge resorption, such as inflammatory lesions of the oral mucosa (e.g., denture stomatitis). Due to these factors, it is considered that ridge resorption is in tight relation with the period of wearing the dentures, but is also influenced by the quality of the treatment.

Clinical features. Ridge resorption is characterized by changes of the morphology of the alveolar ridges and of maxillomandibular relationship, with consequences on the prosthetic treatment and its outcome with time.

Ridge resorption implies a decrease in bone volume, as ridges' height (assessed as reduced, medium and severe resorption), ridge's width (assessed as wide, medium or thin "knife edge ridge") and ridge's surface layout (normal or abnormal morphology, with exostosis). The characteristics of the alveolar ridge influence treatment conduct and have impact on its outcome, e.g., severe ridge resorption (Figure 1) is more frequently associated with denture instability and reduced denture tolerance, difficulties in mounting the artificial teeth and esthetic deficiencies.

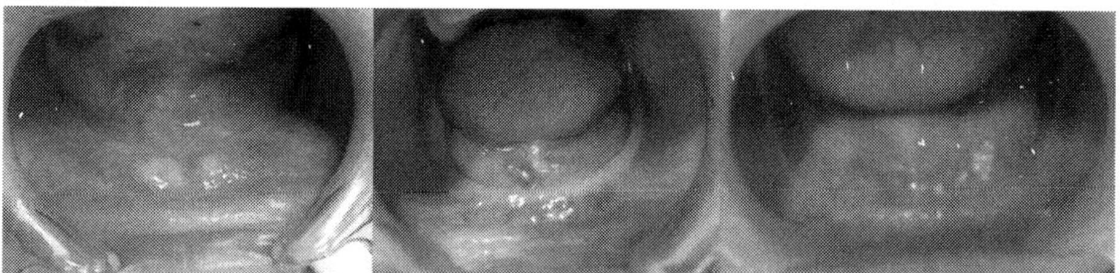

Figure 1. Severe ridge resorption, in long-term denture wearers

Associated to ridge resorption particular aspects of the maxillomandibular relationship can be noticed, as lack of parallelism between the ridges direction and anterior or/and posterior inverse ridge relationship (Figure 2). According to their skeletal jaw relations and in relation with the different patterns of jaws resorption, class III skeletal patients have the tendency to register an inverse ridge relationship, and class II skeletal patients an apparently normal relationship.

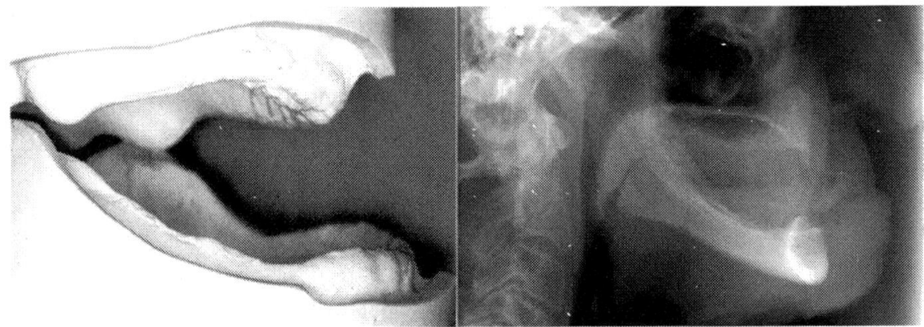

Figure 2. Inverse ridge relationship, related to skeletal class III and the pattern of bone resorption (centripetal in the maxilla and centrifugal in the mandible)

Through resorption and replacement of the bone with fibrous tissue, a floating ridge, usually named "flabby ridge" is noticed. This aspect is most commonly observed in the edentulous anterior maxilla, being related to the excessive pressure of the mandibular anterior teeth (Combination Syndrome). Flabby ridge can also be seen in other places, like maxillary tuberosity or retromolar pad, being linked to instability of the denture or excessive occlusal trauma.

Severe mandibular ridge resorption is accompanied by reduction of the area of the fixed mucosa, difficulties in acknowledgement of the extension of the denture base (due to the sublingual gland herniation through the mylohyoid muscle and modifications of the muscle and ligaments' insertion sites, which can get close to the ridge crest) and pain as a result of dental pressure in the mental foramen area and nerve exposure.

Denture wearing associates inherent ridge resorption, manifested as the occurrence of denture instability. Consequently, clinical procedures as relining or rebasing are required for readjustment of the dentures, in order to correspond to patient's need and to prevent worsening of the edentulous condition.

Management. The ridge resorption, due to its impact on the prosthetic treatment, is the first criteria for the classification of treatment difficulty level according to the Prosthodontic Diagnostic Index (PDI) for complete edentulism of ACP [16]. Thereby, a detailed analysis of the severity of ridge resorption and associated clinical signs is essential in the treatment planning. Useful data can be gained through clinical examination, analysis of the old dentures (when available, they are essential) and evaluation on panoramic and cephalometric radiographs. Computed tomography provides information that are most valuable when implant prosthetic restorations are used, as implant overdentures, especially in complex cases as those with severe ridge resorption or flabby ridge.

In edentulous patients, considering the irreversible and progressive character of bone resorption, preventive interventions should be taken towards reduction of resorption rate and its complications. In this respect, addressing the risk factors and correct management of the supporting tissue should be a priority. In order to limit the bone resorption it is recommended to preserve the tooth roots, to use dental implants, to realize immediate prosthetic rehabilitation, especially in cases with tooth lost due to periodontal disease since this conduct favors a more reduced guided bone resorption. Correctness of dentures manufacturing is essential and it should rely on the principles of retention, stability and support, with proper maintenance and on time replacement. Implant overdentures can be used both as a preventive solution, in order to reduce the bone resorption, and as a curative solution, for solving the cases with severe ridge resorption where conventional dentures did not succeed or were not tolerated.

Severe ridge resorption associates decreased denture stability, which is associated with complications such as pain, lesions of the mucosa, reduced denture tolerance, that need to be addressed. The surgical preprosthetic interventions (bone augmentation, frenectomy, excision of hyperplasic lesions, as in figure 3) and non-surgical interventions (tissue conditioning, antifungal medication, improvement of the nutrition) are preparative treatments that aim achieving better conditions for prosthetic rehabilitation. Taking into account edentulous patient's profile (aged, with systemic co-morbidities), stress related to the fear of surgical interventions and healing parameters (as time needed or remaining scar tissues), the non-surgical or less invasive surgical interventions are preferred. Soft lining materials are indicated since they facilitate the uniformly distribution of the functional stress and can reposition the abused tissues.

The prosthetic treatment of the edentulous patient can be performed using conventional or implant restorations, fixed or removable, with or without preprosthetic interventions, according to the clinical case's particularities and patient's needs. Treatment requirements include accurate physiological impression of the oral structures, correct registration of maxillomandibular relationship and teeth mounting and selection of appropriate occlusal scheme, in order to ensure dentures' stability and esthetic and functional rehabilitation.

Accurate establishment of the peripheral extension of the denture base, considering also the pressures supported by the denture-bearing area, is extremely important, being directly relate to denture's retention, stability and tolerance. In this respect, the correct 2-phase impression technique (primary and custom tray impression) is essential. In edentulous patients with severe ridge resorption, additional adjunctive procedures may be required as tissue conditioning, supplementary functional impressions or usage of neutral zone impression technique. In displaceable or "flabby ridges", the selective pressure impression technique (e.g., using a custom tray with a window opening over the mobile tissue) is more recommended, being at equal importance to other aspects as stable posterior occlusion. Thin mandibular "knife edge ridges", that are accompanied by pain related to denture pressure, needs special treatment conduct, with usage of soft liners, a selective pressure impression technique, preprosthetic surgery (some disagree because ridge reduction implies loss of potential stabilizing zone) and dental implants.

Registration of maxillomandibular relationship is essential for the treatment success. It implies establishing the functional vertical dimension of occlusion, in accordance with minimum speaking space and the freeway space, and respecting the coincidence of maximal intercuspal position and centric relation. The most recommended occlusal schemes for removable prosthesis are the lingualized occlusion, for the bimaxillary complete edentulous patient, in

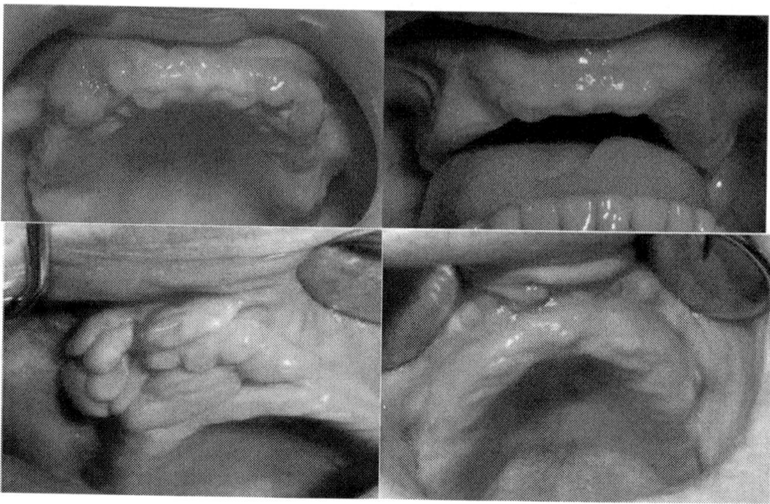

Figure 3. Preprosthetic surgical interventions for excision of hyperplastic lesions

skeletal class II patients or in severe mandibular ridge resorption or the linear occlusion, for mandibular overdentures, in patients with combination syndrome or skeletal class III pattern and severe maxillary ridge resorption.

Mandibular conventional dentures register frequently retention and stability deficiencies, mainly related to ridge resorption. These can be addressed through usage of implant prosthetic restorations, fixed or removable. There are multiple treatment options when considering usage of dental implants, as removable prosthesis (conventional or narrow dental implant overdenture, with different attachment systems as bars, ball, Locator) or fixed restorations (All an four, Fast & Fixed, conventional fixed implant restorations). Current perspective identifies 2 implant overdentures as the minimum standard for mandibular edentulism taking into account performance, patient satisfaction, cost and clinical time [37]. Selecting between them require acknowledgement of case futures and patient's need and preferences. For example, fixed restorations have better treatment outcome, but have limited usage due to aspects like cost and higher complexity of the interventions required (e.g., sometimes surgical procedures as bone augmentation or sinus lift cannot be avoided).

4.2. Traumatic ulcers

Traumatic ulcers are small, painful mucosal lesions that most commonly develop in the first days after insertion of a new denture [38].

Etiology. Traumatic ulcers are caused by dentures with overextended margins, unbalanced occlusion, small excess of material or related to some conditions of the denture bearing area, like exostosis or tori. Ill-fitting dentures can lead to soft tissue irritation or ulceration due to excessive movement of denture. Additional to the mechanical trauma, ulcers can appear due to chemical or thermal insults.

Clinical features. The painful mucosal ulcerations are tender, have a yellowish floor and red margins, with no hardening or thickening of mouth tissues. The irregularly shaped lesions are usually localized in the buccal and lingual sulcus, are covered by a grey necrotic membrane and surrounded by an inflammatory halo. It looks as a hyperemic area, covered or not with fibrin deposits..

Management. Traumatic ulcers usually heal fast, in about a week, after removal of the cause. Usually, denture base and occlusion adjustments are made. Additionally, benzamine hydrochloride 0.15% mouthwash or spray, to provide symptomatic relief, and chlorhexidine gluconate 0.2% mouthwash for oral rinses and soaking the dentures overnight, to prevent and treat infection, can be recommended [39]. Traumatic ulcer decreased in frequency as the length of denture use increased and occurred more frequently during the first 5 years of denture use [40]. Traumatic ulcers must be differentiated from squamous carcinoma, bacterial, fungal and viral diseases, and other oral mucosal diseases, through their clinical aspect, evolution, lack of response to treatment [39]. Patients with an ulcer of over three weeks' duration should be referred for biopsy or other investigations to exclude malignancy or other serious conditions such as chronic infections.

4.3. Denture related hyperplasia

Denture related hyperplasia is an enlargement of the oral mucosa, appeared in relation to the denture base. There are two main types of denture related hyperplasia, namely denture-related fibrous hyperplasia (epulis fissuratum) and inflammatory papillary hyperplasia.

Etiology. Denture-related fibrous hyperplasia occurs as a reaction to low-grade continuous chronic trauma induced by denture flanges, which have thin sharp edges. Other risk factors are ill-fitting unstable dentures, increased vertical dimension of occlusion and parafunctional habits [41]. Inflammatory papillary hyperplasia occurs in relation to wearing the denture continuously, poor oral and denture hygiene, severe ridge resorption, unstable dentures, smoking, age-related changes and some systemic conditions [42]. Denture related hyperplasia is more common in elderly due to oral mucosa changes and their decreased immune response to infection.

Clinical features. Denture-related fibrous hyperplasia appears as a reactive mucosal enlargement, corresponding to the denture flange, which is more common in the maxillary buccal sulcus. The pedunculated, sessile or nodular formations, single or multiple can be red, hyperemic or light pink, usually being asymptomatic. Microbial colonization can occur, most common being Candida species.

In inflammatory papillary hyperplasia the hard palatal mucosa has an erythematous aspect, with a pebbly or papillary surface [42]. According to its severity, we can see forms with limited localization or that cover the entire hard palatal mucosa. The previously described two types of denture related hyperplasia can be observed in figure 4.

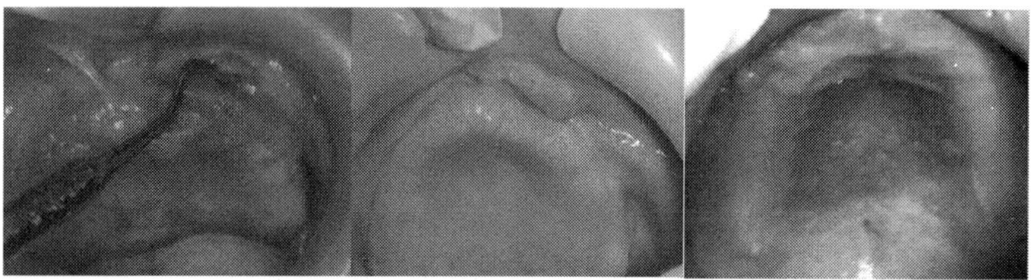

Figure 4. Denture related hyperplasia

Management. Denture-related fibrous hyperplasia usually diminishes considerably, almost entirely, after removal of the cause, correcting the denture flanges. Sometimes minor surgery is required.

The treatment of inflammatory papillary hyperplasia requires removal of the denture at night, improvement of the oral hygiene and denture hygiene. Antifungal therapy, surgical excision of the hyperplastic tissues and renewal of the denture can be recommended in some cases [42].

4.4. Denture stomatitis

Denture stomatitis is a chronic infectious inflammatory disease of the oral mucosa that is in direct contact with the base of the removable prosthesis, either conventional or implant-supported.

Etiology. It has a multifactorial etiology, it is primary related to denture wearing, but the dominant etiological factor is the microbial one-frequently fungal infection with Candida albicans and other sub-strains, but also bacteria such as Staphylococcus and Streptococcus species being identified [43]. Additionally, there are local and systemic and behavioral risk factors.

Acrylic dentures produce ecological changes that facilitate the accumulation of bacteria and yeasts and thus commensal organism may become pathogenic, denture stomatitis being considered an opportunistic infection [44]. A higher prevalence is noticed in cases with poor denture hygiene with denture plaque accumulation, continuous wear of the dentures (including at night) and in ill-fitting dentures. Other risk factors for denture stomatitis are related to the material characteristics, as their changes in time that favor plaque accumulation and microbial colonization (soft linings materials through their fast deterioration and difficulties of achieving proper hygiene; hard acrylic materials through their increased porosity that occurs in time) or as determining hypersensitivity reactions.

Host related risk factors for denture stomatitis include local factors (reduced salivary flow rate, low salivary pH, poor oral hygiene), general factors (physiological such as age, sex, nutritional status and associated medication) which act towards decreasing the resistance and defense mechanisms of the oral mucosa. The prevalence of denture stomatitis is higher among elderly denture users, women, smokers, alcohol consumers, vitamin A deficiency, diabetes and immune deficiency [44-47]. Changes in the salivary flow rate may be signs of a systemic disease, as in Sjögren or Mikulicz syndromes, or associated to medication use, as diuretics, antihypertensive, antipsychotic, anxiolytic, analgesic, anti-inflammatory, antihistaminic drugs. Also, incorrect antibiotic therapy, without fungal protection and broad spectrum antibiotics are seen as risk factors.

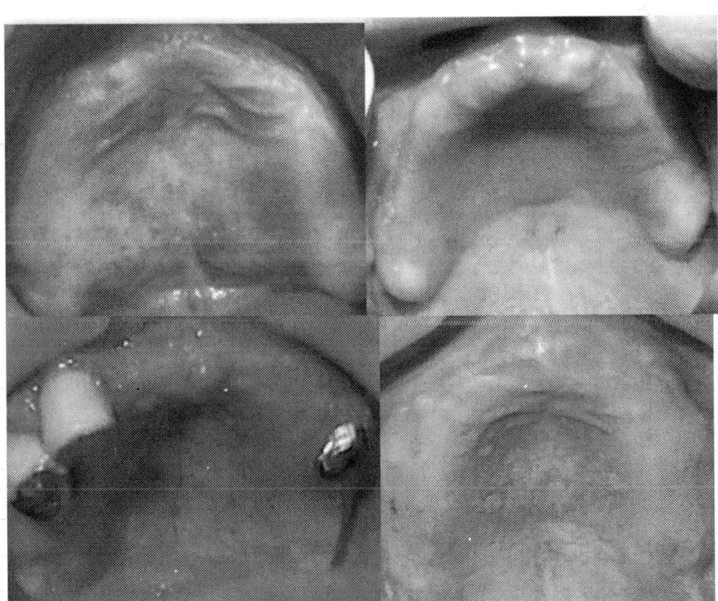

Figure 5. Denture stomatitis – clinical aspect

Clinical features. Denture stomatitis (Figure 5) is characterized by usually asymptomatic inflammatory lesions, with erythema and edema that are found in the denture bearing area, more frequently in the maxilla [44]. The reference classification for denture stomatitis is the one suggested by Newton in 1962, based exclusively on clinical criteria, including 3 types, namely type I (pin-point hyperemic lesions, as a localized simple inflammation), type II (diffuse erythema of the mucosa contacting the denture, as a generalized simple inflammation), and type III: (granular surface, as an inflammatory papillary hyperplasia) [43]. Denture stomatitis can be accompanied by other soft tissue lesions as angular cheilitis, median rhomboid glossitis or candidal leukoplakia.

Management. Considering the relatively high prevalence of denture stomatitis and its relapses, a preventive approach is recommended, by making the patient aware of this disease in order to motivate them to adopt the proper oral and denture hygiene methods, to remove the denture over nighttime and adopt a healthy life-style (quitting smoking, proper nutrition). Since most of the times the condition has no clinical signs, it is recommended to perform a routine basis screening for denture stomatitis. Additional tests may be useful, such as micro-biological exam and thermography –Figure 6 [14,43,48].

Treatment of denture stomatitis consists mainly in adopting strict methods for oral and denture hygiene, with removal of the denture overnight and soaking it in an antiseptic solution, such as chlorhexidine mouthwash. Considering the frequent Candida colonization, antifungal agents, usually as topical application, are recommended either when the yeasts have been isolated or in the absence of a favorable response to the previous interventions [14,44]. Additionally, denture deficiencies and other risk factors should be identified and addressed.

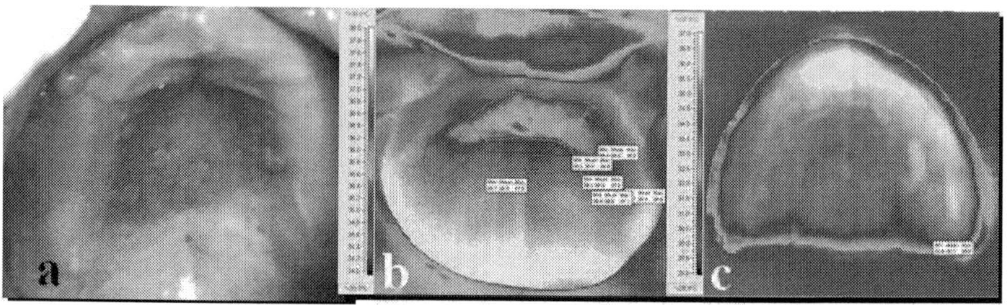

Figure 6. Denture stomatitis – clinical aspect (a); thermography of the oral mucosa (b); thermography of the maxillary denture (c)

4.5. Muscles changes

Edentulousness and dentures can lead to muscle changes, which are mainly an adaptation to the anatomical and functional changes. These can be encountered to the muscle that define the extension of the denture base and the neutral zone and play a role in the denture stability and retention (lips, cheeks and tongue), to masticatory muscles and to the muscles of facial expression.

Etiology. The muscle changes are linked to multiple interrelated factors. Aging associates loss of muscle tone and skin elasticity, decrease of the muscular mass and the force of contraction. The edentulism and the alveolar bone resorption induce major anatomical changes, with muscular consequences. Changing the support for the soft tissues causes the retraction of the lips and cheeks, and the muscular attachment changes in relation to the bone resorption. In severe forms of bone resorption, the muscles are inserted up to the ridge crest and the tongue, due to loss of the guiding offered by the teeth, changes gradually its shape, position and tonicity [49]. The patient's skeletal pattern associates muscular particularities also in the edentulous patient. In skeletal class II patients the tongue is hyperkinetic and has an elevated position that negatively influences the denture stability. In skeletal class III patients the tongue is less active and has a low position. An excessively large tongue, with a retracted position can be observed in edentulous patients that had not been treated for a long period of time. Patients with combination syndrome and skeletal class II with a retrognathic mandible show a tendency towards a protruded mandibular position. Certain systemic alterations, as degenerative and autoimmune conditions, vascular accidents, paresis, burns, traumatisms, nutritional status alterations as protein deficiencies, associate muscular changes.

Prosthetic treatment deficiencies favor abnormal muscular changes. Increased vertical dimension of occlusion and ill-fitting dentures cause muscle spasms, habitual and involuntary movements. Oversized anterior buccal flange of the maxillary denture associates the overextension of the upper lip, with possible anatomical and functional consequences. Association of posterior artificial tooth wear with over jet or lack of coincidence of maximal intercuspal position and centric relation leads to an abnormal protruded mandibular position, which makes difficult the registration of maxillomandibular relationship (centric relation).

Clinical features. Generally, the clinical aspects are the result of complex muscular changes, such as regarding the tone, volume and attachment of the muscle, combined with neuromuscular coordination and control deficiencies.

The changes in muscle tonus can be seen as hypertonia or hypotonia. Muscle hypertonia (Figure 7) is more obvious in lower lip orbicularis oris muscle and in tongue muscles, and causes instability of the mandibular denture. It occurs in the edentulous patients in relation to prosthetic factors as ill-fitting dentures, to patient's individual characteristics as hypodivergent skeletal class II pattern, to parafunctions as bruxism or some systemic conditions. Muscle hypotonia is more frequent for upper lip orbicularis oris muscle and the buccinator muscle, and it occurs related to ageing, to deficient nutritional status and various systemic conditions. Less favorable condition for denture retention and stability, decrease of the efficiency of self-cleaning and reduced visibility of the anterior maxillary teeth in phonation or smiling are some of the effects of muscle hypotonia.

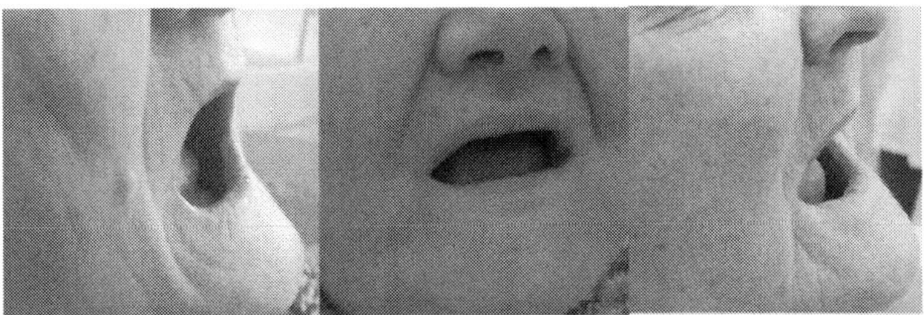

Figure 7. Lower lip orbicularis oris muscle hypertonia, that affects mandibular denture stability\

The changes in volume of the muscles is usually represented by muscular atrophy, which combined with muscular hypotonia, lead to the characteristic facial aspect of old people, with masseter muscle thickness and loose or sagging skin.

Buccinators, orbicularis oris and tongue muscles define the neutral zone, whose accurate limitation is difficult to identify in severe ridge resorption. Changes in the position of the muscle insertions occur, such as high muscle insertions, even on the ridge top (genioglossus and mentalis muscle), with detached oral mucosa. Considering that position of muscle attachments has a major impact to denture base stability and retention, through changes of the denture bearing area, severe ridge resorption with consecutive muscles changes increase the treatment difficulty degree, especially in the mandible.

Muscle force decreasing leads to decrease in the capacity of performing a voluntary act (such as mastication). This occurs in relation to ageing, paresis, depression, denture instability or pain caused by the dentures. Alterations in jaw movements can occur in relation to deficiencies of the prosthetic restorations, as unstable occlusion, denture instability, increased vertical dimension of occlusion or in bruxism. Muscular spasms are encountered in particular situations as in the jaw-closing muscles, related to an increased vertical dimension of occlusion or for jaw-opening muscles related to a decreased vertical dimension of occlusion.

Neuromuscular coordination and control deficiencies, which occur in relation to age and systemic alterations, can increase treatment difficulty and negatively influence the accommodation with the prosthesis. For example, in Parkinson disease a lack of neuromuscular coordination occurs, which leads to difficulties in registration of maxillomandibular relationship and in the insertion and removal of the denture or the overdenture. Abnormal, involuntary, patterned or stereotyped and purposeless orofacial movements (oral dyskinesia) can occur linked to ill-fitting unstable dentures, oral discomfort, and lack of sensory contacts [2]. Facial nerve paresis includes affected unilateral facial musculature movement with asymmetry of facial expression and functional disorders, taste alterations and salivary changes, all having impact on the prosthetic treatment – difficulties in impression taking and in registration of maxillomandibular relationship, reduced masticatory efficiency with unilateral mastication, increased risk of unstable dentures, aesthetic alterations and denture intolerance.

Management. Considering the importance of the muscle factor for the oral functioning, an accurate evaluation should be performed. In some cases, besides the clinical evaluation, additional tests are recommended, such as electromyography or kinesiography, and sometimes special treatment conduct is required [50].

If muscle changes have been identified, these should be taken into account in planning and performing the prosthodontic treatment. In muscle hypertonia, aspects like positioning the artificial teeth in the neutral zone, correct placement of the occlusal plane and correct occlusal relations are essential. In muscle hypotonia, it is recommended to design the buccal flange of the denture with a convex shape and usage of medium viscosity impression materials, in order to have a correct registration of the extension of the denture base and to use the muscle contractions for denture stabilization. Impression taking technique varies according to case's particularities – in patients with protruded tongue at rest, wider movement are required during impression taking, comparing to a retracted tongue, in order to adequately register functional movements (Figure 8).

Extension of denture or overdenture base is limited by the muscle insertions, their encroachment causing, during muscle contraction, movement of the prosthesis. In severe ridge

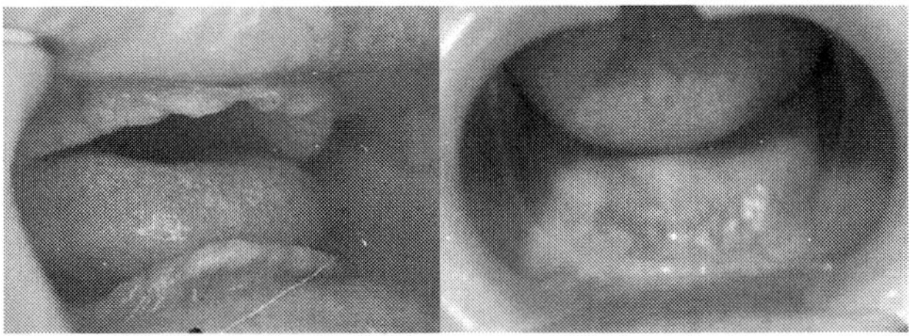

Figure 8. Tongue position at rest – anterior vs. posterior

resorption cases, as for those with muscle insertions on the ridge top, preprosthetic surgery for repositioning of muscle and mucosal attachments is indicated [51].

In neuromuscular coordination and control deficiencies, considering the severe functional alterations, conventional dentures usually don't respond to patient's need and implant overdenture should be chosen instead. Compared to conventional dentures, implant over-dentures provides better functional parameters – exertion of higher masticatory forces promotes better nutrition through the ability to chew harder foods.

Last but not least, manufacturing of a new prosthesis requires an adjustment period for the establishment of the new memory patterns for the masticatory muscles, of about 6 to 8 weeks, aspect that should be mentioned to the patient [52].

4.6. Facial alterations, including esthetic complications

The complete edentulism contributes greatly to the facial aspect known as the aged appearance. Prosthetic treatment needs to adequately address this consequence of edentulism, considering the fact that patients' complaints are frequently related to aesthetic reasons.

Etiology. The facial appearance of the edentulous patient is the result of factors related to complete edentulism and prosthetic treatment, combined with others such as ageing, local and general particularities and medical conditions.

Edentulism associates significant anatomical and functional changes that impact the facial appearance. Lip and cheek support is severely altered by tooth loss and bone resorption. A tendency of increasing the facial concavity occurs in relation to the different pattern of bone resorption of the jaws (centripetal in the maxilla and centrifugal in the mandible). In association with the loss of the occlusal contacts, a counter-clockwise rotation of the mandible, with a decreasing height of the lower third of the face, and sometimes a tendency to a more advanced protruded mandibular position occurs. Facial alterations that are directly linked to edentulism can be considered worsening factors of the esthetic appearance, since there are also preexistent changes in relation to other factors.

As a consequence of aging, there are changes related to the evolution of bones and soft tissues (muscles, fat and skin), in addition to noticeable effects of gravity, with effect on facial esthetics [53]. Systemic health, medication use and behavior (e.g., alcohol and tobacco use) can influence the facial appearance. For example, smoking causes changes particularly in the lower and middle third of the face, like hyperpigmentation and accentuated wrinkles-deeper nasolabial folds, upper lip wrinkles, lower lip vermillion wrinkles, lower lid hyperpigmentation [54]. Premature aged appearance occurs in some diseases like Cutis laxa or glomerulonephritis [55,56].

The prosthetic treatment of the edentulous patient addresses positively some of the previous mentioned facial alteration, but can also contribute to an aged appearance through its deficiencies, as in cases with a decreased vertical dimension of occlusion, a reverse smile line or darker, yellow artificial teeth.

Clinical features. Facial appearance of the edentulous patient registers changes compared to the dentate period, which are mostly found in the lower third of the face (Figure 9).

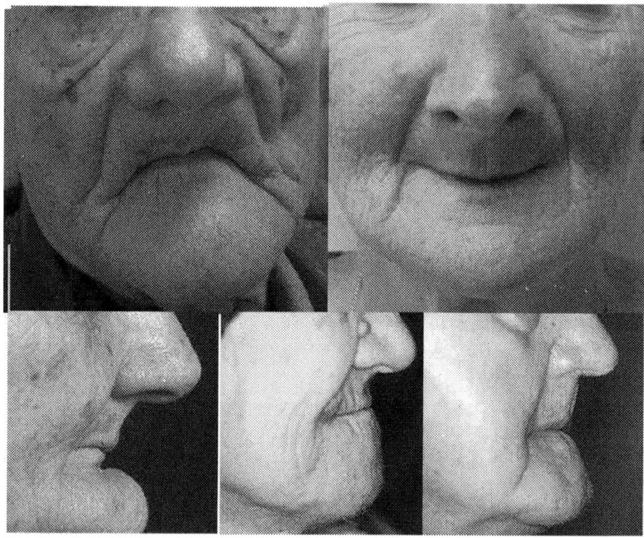

Figure 9. Facial appearance of edentulous patient, with severe bone resorption, without dentures

In edentulous patient, shape and vertical proportions of the face are modified compared to the dentate period. Frequently, edentulous patients have a short face morphotype, appeared in relation to the decrease in the facial lower and total height and the counter-clockwise rotation of the mandible.

Profile changes occur as decreasing its convexity compared to the dentate period. This aspect is due to the different pattern of bone resorption of the jaws and sometimes an advanced protruded mandibular position in the absence of stable occlusion. These changes are more obvious in the skeletal class III patients and are termed as pseudo-class III relation or the old man's prognathism. Profile changes include also modification of nasolabial angle related to nose tip lowering and loss of upper lip support.

Lips register great changes, as reduction of vermilion height and their volume, color modifications, retraction due to support loss, elongation (upper lip) and shortening (lower lip), straight or reversed lip line and low smile line, and reduced lips dynamics that contribute to a decreased teeth exposure during speaking and smiling, which associated a reduction of emotional display, as happiness or sadness [57].

Facial changes related to ageing mark the facial appearance. Lips and cheeks become less prominent and there can be noticed marked folds and wrinkles, loose or sagging skin, changes in the skin texture and hyperpigmentation. These are mainly connected to muscle changes, as hypotonia, and skin changes, as loss of skin elastic recoil.

The prosthetic treatment has a positive impact on the facial esthetics (Figure 10). Generally, it provides a support for the soft tissue, tries to compensate the tooth loss and bone resorption (through the artificial teeth and anterior buccal maxillary flange), ensures a functional vertical dimension of occlusion and give a natural look through exposure of the teeth during smiling or speaking. Some faulty prosthesis or some changes that occurs in time can have a negative impact on facial esthetic. Unpleasant facial appearance can be linked to errors in anterior artificial tooth mounting (too forward, too backward), shade selection (chosen incorrectly, too light, not matching the patient's age), to changes of the artificial teeth over time (through teeth wear the smile line can become reversed, or through aging of the material discolorations can appear). A decreased vertical dimension of occlusion leads to an aged appearance, with deeper perioral folds, and an increased vertical dimension of occlusion associate an unnatural, tensioned look. An overextended buccal flange, encountered more often in the maxillary dentures, leads to an over-supported lip with a tensioned unnatural look. Unstable dentures negatively influence facial appearance through movement while speaking and the facial changes related to protruded mandibular position that many times is associated.

Management. Facial esthetic evaluation must consider changes' severity and causes, in order to properly address them and respond to patients' need and expectations. In order to make an accurate analysis, regular clinical examination (from frontal and lateral view, with and without dentures, in rest and in maximal intercuspal position, during speech and smiling) can be supplemented by radiological examination (cephalometric radiographs) and records from the dentate period, as photos, dental casts, radiographs. The prosthetic rehabilitation of the completely edentulous patient must consider, from an aesthetic point of view, beside the general esthetic principles, also patient's features that are relatively obvious in the dentate period and rather difficult to assess in the edentulous one. The previous should be related to other patient's characteristics (e.g., age, sex, functional particularities, health status) and to prosthodontic biomechanical requirements in order to obtain a good treatment outcome.

4.7. Denture and overdenture biomechanical and technical complications

Removable dental prosthesis are described as having a series of complications in relation to the correctness and accuracy of their planning and execution (extension of the denture base,

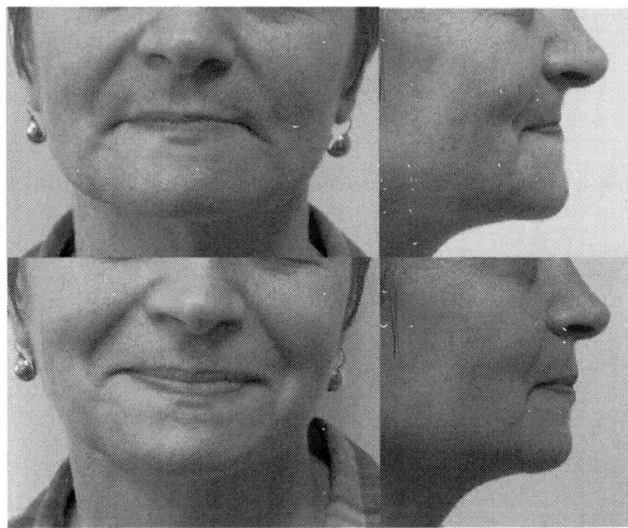

Figure 10. Facial appearance of a recently edentulous patient with and without the dentures

registration of maxillomandibular relationship, mounting of the artificial teeth, occlusal scheme), the technical and biomechanical features of the devices, the properties of the materials used, in conjunction with their evolution in time.

Considering the aims of medical treatments, not properly achieving the prosthodontic treatment goals (denture retention and stability, patient's satisfaction that is liked to aspects like the degree of esthetic and functional rehabilitations and absence of pain) may be considered treatment complications. Removable prosthesis instability can be caused by incorrect denture execution (e.g., overextended flanges, incorrect mounting of the artificial teeth, unstable occlusion), or can occur in time, as a consequence of bone resorption. This issue must be promptly addressed since it can lead to serious complications, such as the fracture of the prosthesis, abutment loss (teeth, implants) and intolerance of the prosthesis. In order to ensure good removable prosthesis stability, the primary aspect that should be consider is its correct execution, mainly regarding the extension of the denture base and artificial teeth mounting. Secondary, usage of denture adhesives, relinings and placement of dental implants should be considered.

The fracture of the removable prosthesis (Figure 11) is a relatively common complication, having numerous risk factors, such as poor denture design, denture instability, teeth or fixed restorations in the opposite jaw, increased mucosal resiliency, previous fractures, accidents (dropping the denture, associated to reduced dexterity), material properties and changes in time, flexural fatigue or other impact factors. Its management includes identifying the cause and the treatment can range from conventionally repairing procedures to reinforcement of the denture base with metal or non-metal products (as glass and polyethylene fibers or net), to changing the previous denture or even the treatment option [58].

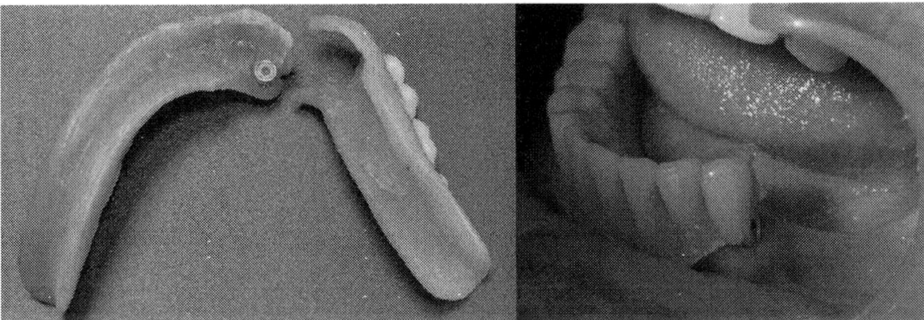

Figure 11. Overdenture fracture at the attachment site

The complications associated to the properties of the material used, mainly polymethylmethacrylate (PMMA), are linked to changes that appears during their evolution in time, as discolorations, artificial teeth wear, increased porosity and decrease flexural strength. Considering their functional and aesthetic impact, denture and overdenture treatment should be renewed at approximately every 5 years.

Additionally, signs of combination syndrome can appear when mandibular overdentures (supported or retained by roots or dental implants) are opposed by an edentulous maxilla. In this situation the masticatory field moves anteriorly, favoring the instability of the maxillary denture and the increased bone resorption rate in the anterior maxilla. This iatrogenic effect can be managed by using implants also in the maxilla, aiming to address or prevent this functional consequence and the destructive process of the oral structures [59].

4.8. Teeth complications, with root overdentures

The root overdentures can have teeth related complications, mainly due to primary or recurrent caries, periradicular lesions developed by vital teeth, endodontically lesions developed by endodontically treated teeth due to loss of the restoration sealing the root canal, periodontitis or root fracture [60]. Their management is dependent of the problem type, in most severe forms tooth loss and recurrent failure of prosthodontic treatment occurring. It is important to preserve the roots as a prevention factor for bone resorption and due their positive impact on the oral functioning [61]. Patients' awareness, instruction and motivation regarding maintaining a proper oral hygiene are essential considering that is the main factor for periodontal disease and caries control. When caries occur, it is important to identify them quickly in order to have high a high success rate for the treatment. Topical fluoridation or coverage with metallic caps can be performed preventively for patients with a high caries risk. For the periodontal disease it is recommended to use Chlorhexidine 0.12% mouthwash twice daily. Also, the removal of the denture overnight and maintenance of proper denture hygiene are recommended. If tooth mobility appears, it can be addressed by reducing the tooth height, which leads to an increase in the crown to root ratio. The risk of root fracture is higher in endodontically treated teeth and when the magnitude of occlusal forces is higher, as in denture instability, bruxism, increased vertical dimension of occlusion, when teeth or fixed prosthesis in the opposite jaw. Preventively, thimble crowns can be used.

4.9. Implants complications, with implant overdentures

For the implant overdenture, the implants complications can be related to the treatment planning (insufficient implant number), implant positioning (surgical complications can appear, such as nerve or blood vessel injuries, penetration of the maxillary sinus or the nasal cavity, hemorrhages or pain) and their evolution (post-insertion infections, compromised survival or implant loss associated deficient osseointegration, peri-implantitis, implant fracture) [62].

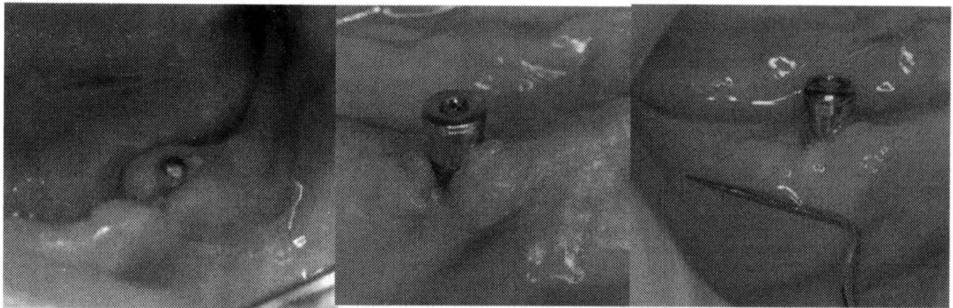

Figure 12. Peri-implant soft tissue lesions-clinical aspect

Therefore, treatment planning considering the fundamental principles of removable implant prosthodontics, overdenture design and execution, maintenance procedures, regular check-ups are all essential for prevention or adequate management of treatment complications. Implant problems are differently addressed according to their type and severity, ranging from simple denture adjustments and enhancing the oral hygiene, to denture relinings or replacement of the denture, to inserting new implants. An important aspect to consider is that implant failure is more common in the maxilla than the mandible, consequently being favorable to place more implants in the upper jaw.

Mandibular implant overdenture is generally considered as being a good predictable treatment, its major implant complication, namely implant loss usually occurring in the first year of function [63,64]. Therefore, regular check-ups are absolutely necessary in this period, for an early intervention that ensures the best prognosis. It is recommended that the dentists performs periodically an accurate evaluation of the implants and surrounding soft tissue regarding the peri-implant marginal bone loss, implant mobility, peri-implant soft tissue, peri-implant bleeding, implant sensitivity during function, result of implant percussion test, plaque accumulation. The overdentures must be verified regarding the overdenture base that is in direct contact with the implant, as risk factor for peri-implant soft tissue complications, regarding the occlusion and maxillomandibular relationship whose faults may be related to exerting increased pressure on implants, as risk factor for implant failure, as its stability and hygiene. Other aspects, like the prosthetic treatment on the opposite jaw (an unstable denture as antagonist can produce excessive forces on the implants) and parafunctions should be checked.

4.10. Attachment system complication, with overdentures

Attachment system complications can occur as a consequence of an incorrect treatment planning, improper treatment conduct (e.g., errors during placement of the retentive housing in the overdenture base) or related to their changes that occur in time, during functioning (e.g., loosening or damage). These vary according to the type of attachment system, e.g., bar, ball, Locator. Most frequent attachment system complications, with overdentures, are: decreased prosthesis retention due to deactivation, detachment, damage or loss of the retentive housing; abutment screw loosening or fracture; fracture of the attachment system components (e.g., bar or clip fracture); soft tissue lesions as hyperplasia under the bar or peri-implant mucositis.

The management of attachment system complications varies according to the attachment system used and the complication type. Technical complications are more common for bar than ball attachments, and both of them are more common compared to locator system [65,66]. Usually low severity complications occurs, such as loss of rubber ring and matrix deactivation, which need to be promptly addressed since they cause overdenture instability with possible negative impact on the dental implants. A more severe complication is bar fracture, that requires increased clinical time and expenses to be resolved, considering that usually the overdenture must be replaced. In elderly edentulous patients simpler prosthetic reconstructions, with complications that require decreased time and money are preferred. Thus, if the option of implant overdenture has been selected, the ball attachment system can be more appropriate than the bar attachment system, due to the more simple maintenance procedures and easier replacement of the implant if necessary.

4.11. Patient satisfaction and quality of life

The conventional dentures are the most common treatment option for the edentulous patients, and usually register good results in terms of patient's satisfaction. Dissatisfaction reasons most claimed by patients are related to denture instability, improper mastication, esthetic deficiency and phonation problems [67]. Denture intolerance is usually connected to subjective factors (the patient's needs and expectations, psychological type, misconceptions) or objective factors (denture instability, pain, functional deficiencies).

The root or implant overdenture have improved retention that contributes to physical and psychological comfort. According to the current evidence, mandibular implant overdentures provide a higher satisfaction and oral health related quality of life compared to conventional denture, but there is uncertainty about the true magnitude of difference between the two [68].

5. Conclusions

Dentures and overdentures, the most frequently used treatment options for the complete edentulism, have complications that are related to patient and prostheses features. Patient's general and local conditions and behavior must be acknowledged as their manifestations, interactions and impact on the prosthetic treatment. Removable implant prosthodontics principles should be well-known and respected during prosthesis execution. The previous, additional to regular check-ups, represent the basis of the prevention removable prosthesis complications.

Denture and overdenture complications are partially similar, differences being related to design particularities, biomechanical aspects and execution procedures. Addressing them depends on their nature and severity, requiring a specific medical conduct. Often simple clinical interventions are needed, but sometimes complex procedures with increased clinical, biological and financial costs must be considered in order to achieve a medical result that corresponds to the current medical standards and patient needs and expectations.

Author details

Elena Preoteasa[1*], Cristina Teodora Preoteasa[2], Laura Iosif[1], Catalina Murariu Magureanu[1] and Marina Imre[1]

*Address all correspondence to: dr_elena_preoteasa@yahoo.com

1 Department of Prosthodontics, Faculty of Dental Medicine, Carol Davila University of Medicine and Pharmacy, Bucharest, Romania

2 Department of Oral Diagnosis, Ergonomics, Scientific Research Methodology, Faculty of Dental Medicine, Carol Davila University of Medicine and Pharmacy, Bucharest, Romania

References

[1] Carlsson GE, Omar R. The Future of Complete Dentures in Oral Rehabilitation. A Critical Review. Journal of Oral Rehabilitation 2010;37(2): 143-156.

[2] Emami E, de Souza RF, Kabawat M, Feine JS. The Impact of Edentulism on Oral and General Health. International Journal of Dentistry 2013; 2013. DOI: 10.1155/2013/498305 (accesed 1 September 2014).

[3] Cunha-Cruz J, Hujoel PP, Nadanovsky P. Secular Trends in Socio-Economic Disparities in Edentulism: USA, 1972–2001. Journal of Dental Research 2007;86(2): 131–13.

[4]   Beltrán-Aguilar ED, Barker LK, Canto MT, Dye BA, Gooch BF, Griffin SO, Hyman J, Jaramillo F, Kingman A, Nowjack-Raymer R, Selwitz RH, Wu T. Surveillance for Dental Caries, Dental Sealants, Tooth Retention, Edentulism, and Enamel Fluorosis--United States, 1988-1994 and 1999-2002. Morbidity and Mortality Weekly Report. Surveillance Summaries 2005;54(3): 1-43.

[5]   Vos T, Flaxman AD, Naghavi M, Lozano R, Michaud C, Ezzati M, Shibuya K, et al. Years Lived with Disability (YLDs) for 1160 Sequelae of 289 Diseases and Injuries 1990-2010: A Systematic Analysis for the Global Burden of Disease Study 2010. Lancet 2012; 380(9859): 2163-96. DOI: 10.1016/S0140-6736(12)61729-2 (accesed 1 September 2014).

[6]   Felton DA. Edentulism and Comorbid Factors. Journal of Prosthodontics 2009;18(2): 88–96.

[7]   World Health Organization. International Classification of Functioning, Disability and Health. Geneva, Switzerland. World Health Organization; 2001.

[8]   O' Reilly E. Treatment Options for Our Edentulous Patients. http://www.burlington-dentalclinic.ie/wp-content/uploads/2012/10/Dr-Eddie-OReilly-Edentulous-Patients.pdf (accesed 1 September 2014).

[9]   Suarez-Sanchez OR. Evaluating Epidemiological Properties of the American College of Prosthodontists (ACP) Prosthodontic Diagnostic Index for Complete Edentulism (PDI-CE)(PDI-Study). Harvard School of Dental Medicine; 2007.

[10]   Papadaki E, Anastassiadou V. Elderly Complete Denture Wearers: A Social Approach to Tooth Loss. Gerodontology 2012; 29(2):e721-7. DOI: 10.1111/j.1741-2358.2011.00550.x. (accesed 14 September 2014).

[11]   Dye BA, Tan S, Smith V, Lewis BG, Barker LK, Thornton-Evans G, Eke PI, Beltrán-Aguilar ED, Horowitz AM, Li CH. Trends in Oral Health Status: United States, 1988-1994 and 1999-2004. Vital Health Stat 11. 2007;Apr. (248): 1-92.

[12]   Douglass CW, Shih A, Ostry L. Will There Be a Need for Complete Dentures in the United States in 2020? Journal of Prosthetic Dentistry 2002;87(1): 5–8.

[13]   Osterberg T, Carlsson GE. Dental State, Prosthodontic Treatment and Chewing Ability-a Study of Five cohorts of 70-Year-Old Subjects. Journal of Oral Rehabilitation 2007;34(8): 553-9.

[14]   Felton D, Cooper L, Duqum I, Minsley G, Guckes A, Haug S, Meredith P et al. Evidence-Based Guidelines for the Care and Maintenance of Complete Dentures: a Publication of the American College of Prosthodontists. Journal of the American Dental Association 2011;142(Suppl 1): 1S-20S.

[15]   Thompson GW, Kreisel PS. The Impact of the Demographics of Aging and the Edentulous Condition on Dental Care Services. Journal of Prosthetic Dentistry 1998;79(1): 56-9.

[16] American College of Prosthodontists (ACP). The Prosthodontic Diagnostic Index for Complete Edentulism (PDI-CE). http://ww-w.gotoapro.org/assets/1/7/Complete_Edentulism_Checklist.pdf (accesed 1 September 2014).

[17] Al-Zubeidi MI, Payne AG. Mandibular Overdentures: A Review of Treatment Philosophy and Prosthodontic Maintenance. New Zealand Dental Journal 2007;103(4): 88-97.

[18] Kiyak HA, Reichmuth M. Barriers to and Enablers of Older Adults' Use of Dental Services. Journal of Dental Education 2005; 69(9): 975-6.

[19] [19]. Montini T, Tseng TY, Patel H, Shelley D. Barriers to Dental Services for Older Adults. American Journal of Health Behaviour 2014;38(5): 781-8.

[20] Wismeijer D, Ten BC, Schulten EA. Notes Concerning an Overdenture on 2 Implants as the Standard for Treating an Edentulous Mandible. Nederlands Tijdschrift Voor Tandheelkunde 2011;118(12): 633-9.

[21] Sutton AF, Glenny AM, McCord JF. Interventions for Replacing Missing Teeth: Denture Chewing Surface Designs in Edentulous People. The Cochrane Database of Sysematic Reviews 2005;25(1). DOI: 10.1002/14651858.CD004941.pub2 (accesed 1 September 2014).

[22] Preoteasa CT, Nabil Sultan A, Popa L, Ionescu E, Iosif, L, Ghica, MV, Preoteasa E. Wettability of Some Dental Materials. Optoelectronics and Advanced Materials – Rapid Communications 2011; 5(8): 874-8.

[23] Preoteasa E, Imre M, Preoteasa CT. A 3-Year Follow-up Study of Overdentures Retained by Mini–Dental Implants. The International Journal of Oral & Maxillofacial Implants 2014; 29(5). 1034-41.

[24] Carlsson GE. Clinical Morbidity and Sequelae of Treatment with Complete Dentures. Journal of Prosthetic Dentistry 1998;79(1): 17-23.

[25] Petersen PE, Kandelman D, Arpin S, Ogawa H. Global Oral Health of Older People-Call for Public Health Action. Community Dental Health 2010;27(4 Suppl 2): 257-67.

[26] Hummel SK, Wilson MA, Marker VA, Nunn ME. Quality of Removable Partial Dentures Worn by the Adult U.S. Population. Journal of Prosthetic Dentistry 2002;88(1): 37-43.

[27] Pietrokovski J, Harfin J, Levy F. The Influence of Age and Denture Wear on the Size of Edentulous Structures. Gerodontology 2003;20(2): 100-5.

[28] Fitzpatrick AL, Powe NR, Cooper LS, Ives DG, Robbins JA. Barriers to Health Care Access Among the Elderly and Who Perceives Them. American Journal of Public Health 2004; 94(10):1788-94.

[29] Dolan TA, Atchison KA. Implications of Access, Utilization and Need for Oral Health Care by the Non-Institutionalized and Institutionalized Elderly on the Dental Delivery System. Journal of Dental Education 1993;57(12): 876-87.

[30] Dolan TA, Atchison K, Huynh TN. Access to Dental Care Among Older Adults in the United States. Journal of dental Education 2005; 69(9): 961-74.

[31] Health and Behavior. The Interplay of Biological, Behavioral, and Societal Influences. Institute of Medicine (US) Committee on Health and Behavior: Research, Practice, and Policy. Washington DC. National Academies Press (US); 2001. http://www.ncbi.nlm.nih.gov/books/NBK43743/ (accesed 1 September 2014).

[32] Barratt A. Evidence Based Medicine and Shared Decision Making: The Challenge of Getting Both Evidence and Preferences Into Health Care. Patient Education and Counseling 2008;73(3): 407-12.

[33] Graber T, Eliades T, Athanasiou AE. Risk Management in Orthodontics: Expers' Guide to Malpractice. Chicago: Quintessence Publishing Co; 2004.

[34] Berglundh T, Persson I., Klinge B. A Systematic Review of the Incidence of Biological and Technical Complications in Implant Dentistry Reported in Prospective Longitudinal Studies of at least 5 Years. Journal of Clinical Periodontology 2002;29 (Suppl 3): 197-212.

[35] Misch K, Wang H. Implant Surgery Complications: Etiology and Treatment. Implant Dentistry 2008; 17(2): 159-68.

[36] Atwood DA. Reduction of Residual Ridges: A Major Disease Entity. Journal of Prosthetic Dentistry 1971;26(3): 266-79.

[37] Thomason JM, Kelly SA, Bendkowski A, Ellis JS.Two implant retained overdentures--a review of the literature supporting the McGill and York consensus statements. Journal of Dentistry 2012;40(1):22-34.

[38] Budtz-Jörgensen E. Oral Mucosal Lesions Associated with the Wearing of Removable Dentures. Journal of Oral Pathology 1981; 10(2): 65-80.

[39] Dunlap CL, Barker CF. A Guide to Common Oral Lesions. http://dentistry.umkc.edu/Practicing_Communities/asset/OralLesions (accessed 23 July 2014).

[40] Coelho CM, Sousa YT, Daré AM. Denture-Related Oral Mucosal Lesions in a Brazilian School of Dentistry. Journal of Oral Rehabilitation 2004;31(2): 135-9.

[41] Sudarshan R, Sree Vijayabala G, Prem Kumar KS. Inflammatory Hyperplasia of the Oral Cavity. Archives Medical Review Journal. 2012; 21(4): 299-307.

[42] Canger EM, Celenk P, Kayipmaz S. Denture-Related Hyperplasia: A Clinical Study of a Turkish Population Group. Brazilian Dental Journal 2009; 20(3): 243-8.

[43] European Association of Oral Medicine (EAOM). Denture Related Stomatitis. http://www.eaom.eu/empty_24.html (accesed 1 September 2014).

[44] Gendreau L, Loewy ZG. Epidemiology and Etiology of Denture Stomatitis. Journal of Prosthodontics 2011; 20(4): 251-60.

[45] Petersen PE, Yamamoto T. Improving the Oral Health of Older People: The Approach of the WHO Global Oral Health Programme. Community Dentistry and Oral Epidemiology 2005;33(2): 81-92.

[46] Shulman JD, Rivera-Hidalgo F, Beach MM. Risk Factors Associated with Denture Stomatitis in the United States. Journal of Oral Pathology and Medicine 2005 34(6): 340-6.

[47] Lylajam S, Prasanath V. Denture Stomatitis-Etiological Factors and Management. Journal of Clinical Dentistry 2011;2(1): 9-11.

[48] Preoteasa E, Iosif L, Amza O, Preoteasa CT, Dumitrascu C. Thermography, an Imagistic Method in Investigation of the Oral Mucosa Status in Complete Denture Wearers. Journal of Optoelectronics and Advanced Materials 2010;12(11): 2333–4.

[49] Pietrokovski J, Kaffe I, Arensburg B. Retromolar Ridge in Edentulous Patients: Clinical Considerations. Journal of Prosthodontics 2007;16(6): 502-6.

[50] Melescanu Imre M, Preoteasa E, Tancu A, Preoteasa CT. Imaging Technique for the Complete Edentulous Patient Treated Conventionally or With Mini Implant Overdenture. Jornal of Medicine and Life 2013;6(1): 86-92.

[51] Cawood JI, Stoelinga PJ. International Research Group on Reconstructive Preprosthetic Surgery. Consensus Report. International Journal of Oral Maxillofacial Surgery 2000;29(3): 159-62.

[52] Goiato MC, Filho HG, Dos Santos DM, Barão VA, Júnior AC. Insertion and Follow-Up of Complete Dentures: A Literature Review. Gerodontology 2011;28(3): 197-204.

[53] Nkengne A, Bertin C. Aging and Facial Changes--Documenting Clinical Signs, Part 1: Clinical Changes of the Aging Face. Skinmed 2012;10(5): 284-289.

[54] Okada HC, Alleyne B, Varghai K, Kinder K, Guyuron B. Facial Changes Caused by Smoking: A Comparison Between Smoking and Nonsmoking Identical Twins. Plastic and Reconstructive Surgery 2013;132(5): 1085-92.

[55] Mataix J, Bañuls J, Lucas A, Pastor N, Betlloch I. Prematurely Aged Appearance. Clinical and Experimental Dermatology 2006;31(6): 833-4.

[56] Joss N, Boulton-Jones JM, More I. Premature Ageing and Glomerulonephritis. Nephrology Dialisis Transplantation 2001;16(3): 615-8.

[57] Tupac R, et al. Parameters of Care for the Speciality of Prosthodontics. Jornal of pros‐ thodontics. Implant, Esthetic, and Reconstructive Dentistry. Official Journal of The American College of Prosthodontists 2005;14(4)Suppl: 1-103.

[58] Preoteasa E, Murariu CM, Ionescu E, Preoteasa CT. Acrylic Resin Reinforcement With Metallic and Nonmetallic Inserts. Revista Medico-Chirurgicala a Societatii de Medici si Naturalisti din Iasi 2007; 111(2): 487-93.

[59] Kreisler M, Behneke N, Behneke A, d'Hoedt B. Residual Ridge Resorption in the Edentulous Maxila in Patients With Implant-Supported Mandibular Overdentures: An 8-Years Retrospective Study. International Journal of Prosthodontics 2003;16(3): 265-300.

[60] Ettinger RL, Qian F. Postprocedural Problems in An Overdenture Population: A Lon‐ gitudinal Study. Journal of Endodontics 2004; 30(5): 310-4.

[61] Crum RJ, Rooney GE Jr. Alveolar Boneloss in Overdentures: A 5-Years Study. Jour‐ nal of Prosthetic Dentistry 1978; 40(6): 610-3.

[62] Preoteasa E, Meleşcanu-Imre M, Preoteasa CT, Marin M, Lerner H. Aspects of Oral Morphology as decision factors in mini-implant supported overdenture. Romanian Journal of Morphoogy and Embryology 2010;51(2): 309-14.

[63] Burns DR. Mandibular Implant Overdenture Treatment: Consensus and Controver‐ sy. Journal of Prosthodontics 2000;9(1): 37-46.

[64] Eckert SE, Choi YG, Sánchez AR, Koka S. Comparison of Dental Implant Systems; Quality of Clinical Evidence and Prediction of 5-Year Survival. The International Journal of Oral & Maxillofacial Implants 2005; 20(3):406-15.

[65] Gotfredsen K1, Holm B. Implant-Supported Mandibular Overdentures Retained With Ball Or Bar Attachments: A Randomized Prospective 5-Year Study. Internation‐ al Journal of Prosthodontics 2000;13(2): 125-30.

[66] Cakarer S, Can T, Yaltirik M, Keskin C. Complications Associated with the Ball, Bar And Locator Attachments for Implant-Supported Overdentures. Medicina Oral, Pa‐ toogial Oral Y Cirurgia Bucal 2011;16(7): e953-9.

[67] Preoteasa E, Marin M, Imre M, Lerner H, Preoteasa CT. Patients' Satisfaction With Conventional Dentures and Mini Implant Anchored Overdentures. Revista Medico-Chirurgicala a Societatii de Medici si Naturisti din Iasi 2012;116(1): 310-16.

[68] Emami E, Heydecke G, Rompré PH, de Grandmont P, Feine JS. Impact of Implant Support for Mandibular Dentures on Satisfaction, Oral and General Health-Related Quality of Life: A Meta-Analysis of Randomized-Controlled Trials. Clinical Oral Im‐ plants Research 2009; 20(6): 533-44.

Chapter 10

Does the Demographic Transition Impact Health? The Oral Epidemiological Profile of the Elder Population

Javier de la Fuente Hernández,

Sergio Sánchez García,

Fátima del Carmen Aguilar Díaz,

Erika Heredia Ponce and

María del Carmen Villanueva Vilchis

Additional information is available at the end of the chapter

http://dx.doi.org/10.5772/59266

1. Introduction

The term "demographic transition" was introduced more than 70 years ago to refer the process of changing from a traditional demographic model identified with high levels of mortality and birthrate to another one characterized by a fall on these indicators.

Between these conditions two phases can be identified: during the first one the growth rate of the population increases like a consequence of the decrease of the mortality, and during the second phase a deceleration of the population growth can be observed because of the decrease of fertility. Among the causes of this change of profile in the population we can find the process of industrialization, economic modernization, urbanization and the social and cultural changes.

The increase on life expectancy and the exposition to unhealthy lifestyles have modified the main causes of the morbidity and mortality, increasing the prevalence of non transmissible diseases. The first causes of mortality now fall in chronic degenerative diseases like diabetes *mellitus*, cardiovascular diseases or respiratory diseases. This change has been reflected as well in the oral status, determined by the life course of the individuals and the exposition to different risk factors. Through this chapter some of the oral conditions on elderly will be analyzed as well as the relationship between oral status and quality of life.

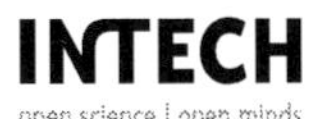

2. The demographic and epidemiologic transition

2.1. Demographic trends of the aging population — The international perspective

One of the best indicators of the improvement of the health of a population is ageing which is an intrinsic process of the demographic transition. The decline of the birthrate and the progressive rise of the life expectancy impact directly on the composition of the age groups of the population, reducing the number of persons in the younger age groups and expanding the segment of more advanced age groups.

The birthrate and mortality of the world population have decreased considerably particularly during the second half of the last century. The birthrate decreased between 1950-1955 and 2005-2010 from 37.0 to 20.0 births per 1000 persons [1]; while the mortality changed from 19.1 deaths per 1000 persons to 8.1 during the same period[2]. This transformation is known as demographic transition and has provoked a progressive increase of the size of the world population as well as its aging.

Migration can also affect aging in different ways, for example massive emigration due to circumstances like getting a better job, improving quality of life, or other motivations can reduce the number of young people, which can increase the ageing population [3].

The proportion of the world population over 60 years of age, of the most developed countries, will be increasing 1% per year before 2050 and it is expected to have increased 45% by mid-century, going from 287 millions in 2013 to 417 millions in 2050. In other words, 8% of the current population is 60 years old or more, but this proportion will be duplicated by 2050, reaching 19% that year[4].

The increase in life expectancy of the general population and particularly of the elderly around the world, should be considered like a success for humanity. The advance in preventive and curative technology of many diseases, coupled with the low exposure to risky conditions, increases the expectation to reach the elderly in better health conditions to live an adequate old age [3]. The increase in the life expectancy of the population poses a major challenge for public health, especially when we are going through a period in which poverty persists in those countries facing developing problems generating a bigger pressure on the already burdened health systems.

Aging is a continuous universal and irreversible process that can lead to a progressive lost of the ability to adapt. In healthy old individuals, many physiological functions are maintained, but when they are placed under stress, a loss of the functional reserve is revealed.

Aging is not a condition that is necessarily associated with disease and dependency, but it is a fact that the accumulative effect of multiple exposures and the unfavorable psychological, physical and social conditions increase the risk of older people to get sick [5]. It starts during the early years of the adult life, but it manifests some decades later, when people are called old. One unfair way to define elderness is to affirm that it starts with the age of retirement (60 or 65), but physiologically individuals get older in a different rate and some persons live more than 80 years. In developed countries, a person is considered old when he/she reaches the age of 65 years or more, but in developing countries 60 is considered as the starting point [6]

The countries with a more advanced stage of demographic transition recognize the need to evaluate the models for provision of health services for the elderly and achieve the mainte‐ nance of the pension systems and sanitary assistance despite all the requirements of the fast growing segment of older people in the population. However, the difficulties in the attention of the sanitary, social and economical needs may vary considerably by region. A common principle for the action is the need to focus on health promotion and the reduction of the dependency of elders.

Daily, seniors face risk situations that threaten their integrity and can alter the functions and structures of their body, if this happens, they face their environment in a different way and frequently the environmental and personal factors can force them to limit their activities. Therefore the functioning or disability of the individual must be seen as the result of the interaction between the health condition and the environment. Although different geographic, social or economical factors contribute to the functional dependency of seniors, chronic diseases are one of the main factors that impact this functioning and can even be its direct cause; this has been demonstrated in some previous studies in different populations. [7,8,9]

The aging process can affect the individual and social development, as well as the relative well‐ being of the younger persons. Among the factors with the greatest repercussion are the pension and retirement systems, the active population and its participation, the arrangements with the family and home, the intra-family transfers from one generation to other and the health condition of seniors. The importance of each one of these aspects can vary and depends of the demographic regimens and the institutional idiosyncrasy of every country. All countries in different levels and in different moments will have to include the topic of the repercussion of aging of the population in their priority issues on the health public and economic field.

3. Oral health problems in the elder population

The analysis of the oral health of elders has taken interest recently due to the accelerated changes on the demographic structure. Old people have poorer oral health, they seek oral health services less, and lose more teeth due to chronic conditions, they represent an important part of the health budget. [11, 12, 13].

The knowledge of the main problems of oral health of this population, is valuable in the planning of effective strategies that optimize the programs and has a positive effect in oral and general health. Among the main problems that affect the oral health there are:

3.1. Disorders of the oral mucosa

In the oral mucosa of old people there may be atrophy of the epithelium, decrease of the keratin and number of cells of the connective tissue, an increase of the intercellular substance and decrease in the oxygen consume. When there is a lack of elasticity of the mucosa with dryness and atrophy, hyperkeratosis can be found. The oral mucosa can present changes related to local factors that are acquired through the course of life like malnutrition, systemic diseases, the use of pharmacological drugs, unhealthy habits and others that can cause the thinning of the mucosa, making it smooth, dry and more permeable to harmful substances. Oral squamous cell carcinoma and pemphigoid carcinoma are almost exclusive of the elderly. [14,15]

3.2. Tooth loss

Complete or partial prosthesis is the most common treatment for tooth loss. Tooth loss has a deep emotional meaning; it symbolically reveals ageing and weakness. It is important to point out that in developing countries the oral care for the elderly has focused on dental extraction, and is the principal cause of the low number of remaining teeth. [16, 17]

Although the number of persons keeping their natural dentition has grown considerably during the last decades, the mean number of remaining teeth may vary according to the school level and the income. Thus it is pertinent to study tooth loss like a social issue according to the social determinants of health, since individuals with lowest school levels tend to a major loss of teeth [18].

3.3. Conditions related to the use of dentures

Denture stomatitis is one of the most frequent diseases that affect the oral tissues in denture wearers. [19] The prevalence of denture stomatitis is from 11 to 67% [20] and there are some factors involved like:

3.3.1. Hygiene of the prosthesis

The prevalence of denture stomatitis has been strongly correlated with hygiene [21,22]. The surface of the prosthesis can be a reservoir for plaque that conforms an ecosystem with a particular pH that can be influenced by the diet, saliva and other factors [23].

3.3.2. Prosthetic trauma

This is caused by maladjusted prosthetic devices and bad habits in their use [19, 20].

3.3.3. Candidiasis infection

The presence of plaque promotes the colonization of fungi species like candida on the prosthetic surface or the mucosa [19,20,22]. The Candida fungi, mainly the genre *Albicans* is a part of the normal flora of the oral cavity, but in some circumstances it is able to develop and produce infection, although some authors mention that there are other involved species [24, 25].

The typical lesions of oral candidiasis are white plaques that are easy to remove on the oral, oropharyngeal and palatal mucosa; in some cases there is angular cheilitis as well. The predisposing factors are xerostomy, treatment with broad-spectrum antibiotics, the use of inhaled corticosteroids and alterations of the cellular immunity [25,26].

When candidiasis infection is associated with old removable prosthetics or maladjusted devices, it can induce the formation of denture stomatitis [27,28]. The treatment for the condition is the eradication of the local factors and therefore the prosthetic devices must be removed a long period, good hygiene conditions should be kept as well as using mouth rinses and antifungal medication.

3.4. Dietetic factors

The diet of the elderly is characterized for being very limited since the lack of a denture in good conditions avoids eating fresh fruits and vegetables or raw food. The diet is regularly is composed of canned food, which can cause vitamin deficiencies and therefore hematological deficit [29]

3.5. Caries

Caries can be considered an infectious disease caused by multiple factors: biologic, social, economical, cultural and environmental. Its formation and development is conditioned by the lifestyle of the individual. It affects the crown and root of the teeth and in the absence of dental attention it can cause the loss of the tooth and it constitutes a source of infection for the organism.

This disease occurs on the dental structures in contact with the microbial deposits (biofilm) and due to the imbalance between the tooth substance and the plaque surrounding fluid, there is a loss of minerals on the dental surface which leads to located destruction of the hard tissues.

The prevalence of dental caries in developed countries has decreased because a high sector of the old population has access to dental services promoting a major use of dental prevention measures, this allows, that the individuals keep a higher number of functional teeth [18,30]

The other kind of caries, root caries, is very common in the elderly since it is a consequence of the gingival recession. The root surface, composed by cementum and dentin is more susceptible to the oral environment than the crown surface composed by enamel and dentin [31,32]

The reported prevalence of root caries is from 24 to 37% in some populations [33]. Almost all the published studies reporting incidence have included old people from public institutions, patients with periodontal disease, participants of some clinic studies and some communities, however they have reported to 10 to 40% incidence [32,34].

Loss of periodontal attachment, low salivary flow, presence of caries in the past, cognitive impairment, use of some kind of medication, low scholar level, high number of cariogenic microorganisms, and the lack of dental attention are among the most studied risk factors for root caries [35].

3.6. Periodontal disease

Periodontal disease constitutes one of the main causes of tooth loss [16]. Traditionally it was accepted that the loss of epithelial attachment and alveolar bone was caused by the periodontal changes related to the ageing process, however nowadays the theory indicates that is not like that.

The periodontum reacts to ageing in two ways: if there is low hygiene, the plaque accumulation affects the periodontal tissues causing gingivitis and in some susceptible patients the retraction of the gingival tissue, formation of gingival pockets and dental loss. However in some old patients there can be tissue recovery with a minimal change on the marginal gingival, narrowness of the periodontal ligament, firm adherence of the teeth, and accumulation of cementum [14,36]

3.7. Xerostomy or low salivary flow

Saliva is a complex exocrine secretion, important for the maintenance of the homeostasis of the oral cavity. The salivary functions in relation with the flow and molecular composition (proteins, glycoproteins and phosphoproteins) are well known: the protection of the oral tissues against desiccation and the environmental attacks, the modulation of the desmineralization-remineralization processes, the lubrication of the occlusal surfaces and the maintenance of the ecological balance [37].

The protection of the salivary flow in the elderly can be reduce because of the medical prescription of some drugs for the treatment of certain conditions in this age group like depression or other systemic conditions like hypertension [38,39].

Although it has not been well demonstrated, a physiological decrease of the salivary flow may occur with aging, however it seems that structural alterations may occur in some salivary glands, concretely submandibular and minor glands, however, despite all these conditions the global functioning and the salivary volume is not modified.

The cause of the xerostomy or the decrease on the salivary flow is more related to the existence of some diseases like hypertension, diabetes *mellitus*, Sjögren syndrome, rheumatoid conditions, cystic fibrosis, neurological conditions, depression and immune system dysfunction and their treatment, since most of them have a repercussion on the salivary glands [40,41].

3.8. Oral cancer

This disease is related with aging, since nearly 95% of the cases take place in people 40 years of age and older and the mean age of the diagnosis is around 60. It is estimated that half of the cases of cancer are in people 65 years of age. [42,43,44].

The etiology of oral cancer and precancerous lesions is multiple. The most common cited factors are: tobacco and alcohol consumption, genetics, nutrition, the presence of some virus, radiations and occupational risks in addition to use of maladjusted dental prostheses, destroyed teeth by caries or trauma and low oral hygiene.

Most of these factors have an accumulative effect with time, and due to this effect, many authors affirm that age is the main risk factor for the development of oral cancer [44,45]. The early detection of the malignant lesions is fundamental for providing the best prognosis of this disease.

3.9. Pain

Pain is often a manifestation of the oral problems reflected on other facial structures like the orbital frontal region that can be confounded with classic headache.

Sometimes, pain appears like a consequence of the degenerative phenomena of the structures that support the oral cavity (bones, joints muscles and others). Among these phenomena we can find osteoarthritis and osteoporosis of the jaw, or disorders on the temporomandibular jaw that can cause pain, snaps and the added locking of joint function like limitation to the mouth opening and difficulty for chewing [46].

The temporomandibular dysfunction is frequent in old people and it is characterized by constant pain on the periauricular area, otic pain that can increase while the patient is chewing, or in patients with bruxism, when they clench teeth consciously or unconsciously during stress [47,48].

4. Links between oral health and systemic diseases

It is clear that oral health problems affect the general condition of old people. Many systemic diseases have specific signs in the mouth that allow the diagnosis. Among them we can find genetic diseases, systemic infections, immune alterations, neoplasms, nutritional problems, connective tissue diseases, gastrointestinal diseases, renal diseases, cardiovascular diseases, endocrine diseases, dermatologic diseases, neurologic diseases and skeletal diseases. There are also some medications that can affect the consistency and characteristics of the saliva and that can alter the texture of the tongue, or affect the gingiva [36,37,48,49,50]

4.1. Periodontal disease related to systemic diseases

Among the conditions related to periodontal disease and the cardiovascular system we can find bacterial endocarditis, myocardial infarction, ischemic heart disease, thrombosis, coronary heart disease and varicose veins [51].

The links between periodontal disease and respiratory diseases can be established only if the defensive mechanisms fail. The most commonly associated conditions are the bacterial pneumonia, bronchitis, chronic obstructive pulmonary disease and lung abscesses [52,53,54].

The bacteria create their own ecological niches on different surfaces of the mouth like teeth, gingival sulcus, dorsal area of the tongue and oral and pharyngeal mucosa using the saliva and crevicular fluid like their main nutritional source, and through bacteremia, derive in systemic processes. The sepsis is the responsible for the beginning and progression of diverse inflammatory diseases like arthritis, peptic ulcers and appendicitis [54]

Pneumonia is the infection of the lung parenchyma caused by several infectious agents that include bacteria, fungi, parasites and viruses. Bacteria of the oral flora like *Actinobacillus actinomycetem-commitans*, *Actinomyces Israeli*, and the anaerobic *P gingivalis*, and *Fusobacteri-*

um, can be aspirated and taken to the lower airways and cause pneumonia [55,56]. The source can be from bacteria of the normal flora or from periodontal cases [56].

5. Oral health related quality of life in the elder population

The relationship between quality of life and oral health has been understood like a multidimensional concept that reports the aspects concerning to oral health including the functional, social and pshycological aspect of the individuals [57,58,59,60].

One of the major contributions of dentistry is to improve and maintain the quality of life of the person since most oral diseases and their consequences have an impact on the performance of daily activities [36].

The contemporary concepts of health suggest that oral health could be defined as the physical, psychological and social wellbeing in relation to the dental status as well as the hard and soft tissues of the oral cavity and not only absence of disease [36]. This definition proposes that the measure of oral health not only has to take into account oral indexes that measure the presence or severity of a pathology (physical well-being) but it must also complemented with social and pshycological measures [36,60,61].

Traditionally, the methods used to estimate oral health, have been limited to clinic indicators or oral indexes, and the presence or absence of disease. This view leaves out all the subjective measures, in other words the perception of the persons about their oral health status.

This view about oral health related quality of life (OHRQOL) promotes the knowledge of the origin and behavior of the oral diseases, largely because the social factors and the environment are the main causes of these diseases and some interventions can be applied [62,63,64]).

In elder people, the self-perception of oral health can be affected by the perception of other personal values, like the belief that some pains and disabilities are unavoidable because of the ageing. These ideas can lead to the over and under estimation of the oral health condition. The available information about self-perception is subjective, and for this reason the perception about how oral health affects the quality of life must be evaluated according to instruments that have been adapted and validated on specific populations.

The dental status in old people has a repercussion on their ability to perform daily activities affecting their quality of life with a bigger impact on some activities such as eating, speaking and pronunciation [61]

The existing subjective measures on oral health as well as the focus on oral health cannot provide data that helps the decision makers to allocate the resources related with improving the oral health of the elderly, however they can give an idea about the degree of affection for the individual and populations [62].

6. Conclusions

Oral health problems among old people are caused mainly by the accumulation of sequels that the null assistance to the dental services has left as well as the lack of self-care in this age group.

The most common affections are the tooth loss, coronal and root caries, periodontal diseases, lesions derivated from the use of defective prosthesis and temporomandibular joint pain. Besides, this group, can also present oral cancer and oral manifestations of other systemic diseases. These conditions are associated with pain when chewing, a frequent reason of consultation in primary care.

It is important to continue studying the convergence of sociodemographic information with the oral health diagnosis, to determine the therapeutic needs and the factors that make it difficult to access the dental services and to design adequate interventions to solve the most common oral health problems of this group of the population.

Public and private oral health services must prevent the onset of diseases that can produce serious effects on quality of life of the elderly.

Author details

Javier de la Fuente Hernández[1], Sergio Sánchez García[2,3], Fátima del Carmen Aguilar Díaz[1], Erika Heredia Ponce[3] and María del Carmen Villanueva Vilchis[1*]

*Address all correspondence to: vv.carmen@gmail.com

1 Escuela Nacional de Estudios Superiores, Unidad León. Universidad Nacional Autónoma de México, México

2 Unidad de Investigación en Epidemiología y Servicios de Salud. Área Envejecimiento. Centro Médico Nacional Siglo XXI. Instituto Mexicano del Seguro Social, México

3 Departamento de Salud Pública y Epidemiología Bucal. Facultad de Odontología. Universidad Nacional Autónoma de México, México

References

[1] United Nations, Department of Economic and Social Affairs. Worls Population Prospects: The 2012 Revision; Excel tables-Fertility Data "Crude Birth Rate". Available en: http://esa.un.org/wpp/Excel-Data/fertility.htm

[2] United Nations, Department of Economic and Social Affairs. Worls Population Prospects: The 2012 Revision; Excel tables-Mortality Data "Crude Death Rate". Available en: http://esa.un.org/wpp/excel-data/mortality.htm

[3] United Nations, Department of Economic and Social Affairs, Population Division (2013). World Population Ageing 2013. ST/ESA/SER.A/348.

[4] World Population Prospects: The 2012 Revision. Key Findings and Advance Tables. United Nations Department of Economic and Social Affairs/Population Division, Working Paper No. ESA/P/WP.227, June 13, 2013, 54 p.

[5] Gutiérrez Robledo LM, García Peña MC, Jiménez Bolón JE. Envejecimiento y dependencia. Realidades y previsión para los próximos años. México: Intersistemas Editores, 2014.

[6] Organización Panamericana de la Salud. Salud en las personas de edad. Envejecimiento y salud: un cambio de paradigma. E.U., Washington D.C., 1998.

[7] Sousa RM, Ferri CP, Acosta D, Guerra M, Huang Y, Jacob K, Jotheeswaran A, Hernandez MA, Liu Z, Pichardo GR, Rodriguez JJ, Salas A, Sosa AL, Williams J, Zuniga T, Prince M. The contribution of chronic diseases to the prevalence of dependence among older people in Latin America, China and India: a 10/66 Dementia Research Group population-based survey. BMC Geriatr. 2010;10:53.

[8] Daigo Yoshida, Toshiharu Ninomiya, Yasufumi Doi, Jun Hata, Masayo Fukuhara, Fumie Ikeda, Naoko Mukai, Yutaka Kiyohara. Prevalence and Causes of Functional Disability in an Elderly General Population of Japanese: The Hisayama Study. J Epidemiol. 2012; 22:222–229

[9] Wolff JL, Boult C, Boyd C, Anderson G. Newly reported chronic conditions and onset of functional dependency. J Am Geriatr Soc. 2005;53:851-5.

[10] Kalache, A. y Coombes, Y. Population aging and care of the elderly in Latin America and the Caribbean. Review of Clinical Gerontology, 1995; 5:347-355.

[11] Medina-Solís CE, Pérez-Núñez R, Maupomé G, Avila-Burgos L, Pontigo-Loyola AP, Patiño-Marín N, Villalobos-Rodelo JJ. National survey on edentulism and its geographic distribution, among Mexicans 18 years of age and older (with emphasis in WHO age groups). J Oral Rehabil 2008;35:237-244.

[12] Marino R. Oral health of the elderly: reality, myth, and perspective. Bull Pan Am Health Organ 1994;28:202-210.

[13] Sánchez-García S, Heredia-Ponce E, Cruz-Hervert P, Juárez-Cedillo T, Cárdenas-Bahena A, García-Peña C. Oral health status in older adults with social security in Mexico City: latent class analysis. J Clin Exp Dent. 2014;6(1):e29-35.

[14] Mckenna G, Burke FM. Age-related oral changes. Dent Update. 2010 Oct;37(8): 519-23.

[15] Silverman S Jr. Mucosal lesions in older adults. J Am Dent Assoc. 2007 Sep;138 Suppl:41S-46S.

[16] Renvert S, Persson RE, Persson GR. Tooth loss and periodontitis in older individuals: results from the Swedish National Study on Aging and Care. J Periodontol. 2013 Aug;84(8):1134-44.

[17] Dable RA, Yashwante BJ, Marathe SS, Gaikwad BS, Patil PB, Momin AA. Tooth loss--how emotional it is for the elderly in India? Oral Health Dent Manag. 2014 Jun;13(2): 305-10.

[18] Slade GD, Akinkugbe AA, Sanders AE. Projections of U.S. Edentulism Prevalence Following 5 Decades of Decline. J Dent Res. 2014 Aug 21. pii: 0022034514546165. [Epub ahead of print]

[19] Wilson J. The aetiology, diagnosis and management of denture stomatitis. Br Dent J. 1998 Oct 24;185(8):380-384.

[20] Jeganathan S, Lin CC. Denture stomatitis--a review of the aetiology, diagnosis and management. Aust Dent J. 1992 Apr;37(2):107-14.

[21] Vigild M. Oral mucosal lesions among institutionalized elderly in Denmark. Community Dent Oral Epidemiol, 1987; 15:309-313.

[22] Salerno C, Pascale M, Contaldo M, Esposito V, Busciolano M, Milillo L, Guida A, Petruzzi M, Serpico R. Candida-associated denture stomatitis. Med Oral Patol Oral Cir Bucal. 2011 Mar 1;16(2):e139-43.

[23] Catalan A, Herrera R, Martinez A. Denture plaque and palatal mucosa in denture stomatitis: scanning electron microscopic and microbiologic study. J Prosthet Dent. 1987 May;57(5):581-6.

[24] Morimoto K, Kihara A, Suetsugu T. Clinico-pathological study on denture stomatitis. J Oral Rehabil. 1987

[25] Guinea J. Global trends in the distribution of Candida species causing candidemia. Clin Microbiol Infect. 2014 Jun;20 Suppl 6:5-10.

[26] Kulak-Ozkan Y, Kazazoglu E, Arikan A. Oral hygiene habits, denture cleanliness, presence of yeasts and stomatitis in elderly people. J Oral Rehabil, 2002; 29:300-304.

[27] Marinoski J, Bokor-Bratić M, Canković M. Is denture stomatitis always related with candida infection? A case control study. Med Glas (Zenica). 2014 Aug;11(2):379-84.

[28] Peltola MK1, Raustia AM, Salonen MA. Effect of complete denture renewal on oral health--a survey of 42 patients. J Oral Rehabil. 1997 Jun;24(6):419-25.

[29] García-Arias MT, Villarino Rodríguez A, García-Linares MC, Rocandio AM, García-Fernández MC. Iron, folate and vitamins B12 & C dietary intake of an elderly institutionalized population in León, Spain. Nutr Hosp. 2003 Jul-Aug;18(4):222-5.

[30] Glass RL. The first international conference on the declining prevalence of dental caries Secular changes in caries prevalence in two Massachusetts towns. J Dent Res, 1982; 61 (Spec Issue):1301-1383.

[31] Papapanou PN, Wennström JL, Gröndahl K. Periodontal status in relation to age and tooth type. A cross-sectional radiographic study. J Clin Periodontol. 1988 Aug;15(7): 469-78.

[32] Bignozzi I, Crea A, Capri D, Littarru C, Lajolo C, Tatakis DN. Root caries: a periodontal perspective. J Periodontal Res. 2014 Apr;49(2):143-63. doi: 10.1111/jre.12094. Epub 2013 May 7.

[33] Beck, J. D. Indentification of risk factors. In: Bader, J. D., USA: ed. Risk assessment in dentistry. Chapel Hill, University of North Carolina Dental Ecology, 1990.

[34] Sánchez-García S, Reyes-Morales H, Juárez-Cedillo T, Espinel-Bermúdez C, Solórzano-Santos F, García-Peña C. A prediction model for root caries in an elderly population. Community Dentistry and Oral Epidemiology 2011 Feb;39(1):44-52.

[35] Saunders RH Jr, Meyerowitz C. Dental caries in older adults. Dent Clin North Am 2005; 49:293-308.

[36] Sánchez-García S, Juárez-Cedillo T, Heredia-Ponce E, García-Peña C. El envejecimiento de la población y la Salud Bucodental. Breviarios de Seguridad Social. México D.F.: Centro Interamericano de Estudios de Seguridad Social, Edito; 2013. ISBN: 978-607-8088-14-0.

[37] Sreebny LM. Saliva in health and disease: an appraisal and update. Int Dent J. 2000 Jun;50(3):140-61.

[38] Närhi TO, Vehkalahti MM, Siukosaari P, Ainamo A. Salivary findings, daily medication and root caries in the old elderly. Caries Res. 1998;32(1):5-9.

[39] Gerdin EW, Einarson S, Jonsson M, Aronsson K, Johansson I. Impact of dry mouth conditions on oral health-related quality of life in older people. Gerodontology. 2005 Dec;22(4):219-26.

[40] Sreebny L. Saliva: its role in health and disease. Int Dent J 1992; 42: 291–304.

[41] Sánchez-García S, Gutiérrez-Venegas G, Juárez-Cedillo T, Reyes-Morales H, Solórzano-Santos F, García-Peña C. A simplified caries risk bacteriologic test in stimulated saliva from elderly patients. Gerodontology 2008; 25: 26-33.

[42] Silverman S. Oral cancer. 3ªed. EUA, Atlanta: American Cancer Society, 1990.

[43] Canto MT, Devesa SS. Oral cavity and pharynx cancer incidence rates in the United States, 1975-1998. Oral Oncol. 2002 Sep;38(6):610-7.

[44] Sánchez-García S, Juárez Cedillo T, Espinel Bermudez MC, Mould Quevedo JF, Gómez Dantés H, de La Fuente Hernández J, Leyva Huerta ER, García Peña C. Egresos

Hospitalarios por cáncer bucal en el Instituto Mexicano del Seguro Social, 1991-2000. Rev Med Inst Mex Seguro Soc 2008; 46 (1): 101-108.

[45] Hunter KD, Yeoman CM. An update on the clinical pathology of oral precancer and cancer. Dent Update. 2013 Mar;40(2):120-2, 125-6.

[46] Serrano Garijo, P. y otros. La salud bucodental en los mayores. Prevención y cuidados para una prevención integral. En: Promoción de salud en los mayores, volumen 6. Madrid, Instituto de Salud Pública, 2003.

[47] Sánchez-García S, Heredia-Ponce E, Villanueva Vilchis M del C, Rabay Gánem C. Dolor para masticar. En García Peña M del C, Gutiérrez Robledo LM, Arango Lopera VE, Pérez-Zepeda MU. Geriatría para el médico familiar. Manual Moderno. Edito; 2012.

[48] Smith BJ, Valdez IH, Berkey DB. Oral problems. En: Ham RJ, Sloane PD, Warshaw GA, Bernard MA, Flaherty E. Primary care geriatrics: a case-based approach. 5th ed Mosby, 2007.

[49] Mariño R, Albala C, Sanchez H, Cea X, Fuentes A. Prevalence of Diseases and Conditions Which Impact on Oral Health and Oral Health Self-Care Among Older Chilean. J Aging Health. 2014 May 21.

[50] Gaffen SL, Herzberg MC, Taubman MA, Van Dyke TE. Recent advances in host defense mechanisms/therapies against oral infectious diseases and consequences for systemic disease. Adv Dent Res. 2014 May;26(1):30-7.

[51] Demmer RT, Kocher T, Schwahn C, Völzke H, Jacobs DR Jr, Desvarieux M. Refining exposure definitions for studies of periodontal disease and systemic disease associations. Community Dent Oral Epidemiol. 2008 Dec;36(6):493-502. doi: 10.1111/j. 1600-0528.2008.00435.x. Epub 2008 Apr 14.

[52] Papapanou Panos, N. Populations studies of microbial ecology periodontal health and diseases. Ann Periodontol 2003; 7:54-61.

[53] Bansal M, Rastogi S, Vineeth NS. Influence of periodontal disease on systemic disease: inversion of a paradigm: a review. J Med Life. 2013 Jun 15;6(2):126-30.

[54] Scannapieco, F. A. Position paper: periodontal disease as a potential risk factor for systemic diseases. J. Periodontol, 1998; 69:841-850.

[55] Reynolds MA. Modifiable risk factors in periodontitis: at the intersection of aging and disease. Periodontol 2000. 2014 Feb;64(1):7-19.

[56] Scannapieco, F. A., Papandonatos, G. y otros. Associations between oral conditions and respiratory disease in a national sample survey population. Ann. Periodontol, 1998; 3:251-256.

[57] Cohen, K. y Jago, J. D. Toward the formulation of socio-dental indicators. Int J Health Serv, 1976; 6:681-687.

[58] WHO definition of health. Fecha de consulta: 1 de septiembre de 2014: URL: www.who.int/about/definition/en/print.html.

[59] Engel, G. L. The clinical application of biopsychosocial model. Am J Psychiatry, 1980; 137:535-544.

[60] Sánchez-García S, Heredia-Ponce E, Juárez-Cedillo T, Gallegos-Carrillo K, Espinel-Bermúdez C, De la Fuente-Hernández J, García-Peña C. Psychometric properties of the General Oral Health Assessment Index (GOHAI) and their relationship in the state of dentition of an elderly Mexican population. Journal of Public Health Dentistry 2010;70(4):300-307.

[61] Sánchez-García S, Juárez-Cedillo T, Reyes-Morales H, De la Fuente-Hernández J, Solórzano-Santos F, García-Peña C. Estado de la dentición y sus efectos en la capacidad de los ancianos para desempeñar sus actividades habituales. Salud Pública Mex 2007;49 (3): 173-181.

[62] Petersen PE, Kandelman D, Arpin S, Ogawa H. Global oral health of older people–call for public health action. Community Dent Health 2010;27:257–267.

[63] Cushing, A. M., Sheiham, A. y otros. Developing socio-dental indicators – the social impact of dental disease. Community Dental Health 1986; 3:3-17.

[64] Locker, D. Measuring oral health: A conceptual framework. Community Dent Health, 1988; 5:3-18.

Chapter 11

Narrow Diameter and Mini Dental Implant Overdentures

Elena Preoteasa, Marina Imre, Henriette Lerner,
Ana Maria Tancu and Cristina Teodora Preoteasa

Additional information is available at the end of the chapter

http://dx.doi.org/10.5772/59514

1. Introduction

Complete dentures are most frequently a challenge for practitioners. The complexity of this disease is often associated with general health problems, but also with the physiological ageing phenomenon, that increases the treatment difficulty. Completely edentulous patients, usually elderly, often complain about the functionality of conventional dentures, especially the mandibular ones, claiming their instability, poor retention and discomfort during wear.

Following the development of public health programs, a beneficial effect was found in terms of percentage decrease in the number of completely edentulous patients, but this was partially offset by the increased life expectancy. Consequently, complete edentulism remains a frequent medical condition that needs to be addressed through treatment alternatives that meet the needs of modern man. This aspect is integrated in the current medical perception that highlights the importance of an active aging process, with preservation of elderly participation in social and economic activities [1]. Additionally to population aging as a demographic trend, changes in the dental field have also occurred, related to the use of dental implants and implant prosthesis, but also to patients' perception and expectations regarding the prosthetic rehabilitation, demanding more stable, functional and aesthetic prosthesis.

Complete maxillary and mandibular dentures have been for over 100 years the standard treatment of complete edentulism. If complete maxillary denture wearers tolerate better the complete dentures, given the better conditions for support, retention and stability, the tolerance of mandibular prosthesis is generally lower. The relatively frequent instability of the mandibular denture, poor retention and associated discomfort were the starting point for the

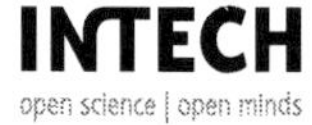

idea of setting the overdenture on 2 implants as first treatment alternative for the mandibular complete edentulism (according to McGill and York consensus) [2, 3, 4].

2. Concept of implant overdentures

Implant overdentures are inspired, as treatment concept, from the of the overdentures, the dental implants being used instead of tooth roots. If for teeth overdentures the attachment systems are optional, for the implant-supported ones they become mandatory. Therefore, the structural components of implant overdenture are the prosthesis (partial or complete overdenture), the dental implants and the attachment system. Using dental implants mainly aims to increase retention and/or to provide support for the prosthesis.

Considering the relation between the structural components of the implant overdentures, their interaction with the oral structures and functions, the biomechanical aspects, all with impact on implants survival and treatment success, numerous treatment options and concepts have been developped. These differ in various aspects, such as the design of the dental implants used (as diameter - conventional, narrow or mini dental implants, as length), as implant number, as technique of implant placement and loading, as attachment system, as prosthesis design and as their effect on the prosthesis balance, retention and patients satisfaction [5]. Regardless of their type, implant-supported overdentures bring a number of benefits compared to the conventional dentures, by increasing their stability and retention, improving the mastication and phonation, and ensuring a physical and psychological comfort.

Dental implants that are used for implant overdentures are made of high-strength alloy (Ti-Al-V), with good biocompatibility, with different designs and sizes that aim to address the prosthetic needs according to the oral particularities and clinical limitations of its execution. The first implants that were introduced in the dental practice were the ones with standard diameter, around 3.75mm. Later on, their diameter was increased and decreased (narrow), ranging between 3 and 6mm. Afterwards, the mini implants with one-piece design for implant overdentures appeared (IMTEC, later 3MESPE), with diameters of 1.8mm, 2.1mm and 2.4mm.

Using dental implants with a diameter under the conventional one has increased, aspect related to the extension of their clinical indications. These were firstly used for temporary retention of the interim prosthesis and for orthodontic anchorage. Nowadays there is an increased use of them for prosthesis stabilization.

Dental implants with a diameter below the conventional one, are classified mainly on their diameter, or design (i.e. one piece/two piece). Thus, implants with a diameter below the conventional one have been classified by some authors as narrow-diameter implants (3.0 to 3.5 mm) with smaller implants (3.0 to 3.25 mm), and mini-implants (<3.0mm) [6]. The mini-implants are sometimes divided in hybrid implants (2.7 to 2.9 mm) and mini implants (1.8 to 2.7mm).

Conventional Diameter Implant Overdentures (CDIO) use two-piece implants, with usually two-stage placement protocol, with larger diameters (over 3.5mm) and variable lengths

(8-16mm), in a number of minimum two for the mandibular overdenture. Its implementation requires wide ridges (over 5-6mm), condition that rather often is not met in the aged edentulous patients, therefore bone augmentation, supplemented sometimes by sinus lift being required. The protocol of conventional implant placement is with or without a flap, usually involves two phase surgery (one for implant placement and one for removal of the cover screw and abutment placement), with delayed implant loading, after the implants osseointegration (after 3-6 months). As prosthetic parameters and attachment selection, conventional implants have a wider spectrum of indications and treatment options. Implants can be splinted with bars as attachment systems, or be used unsplinted, with ball, locator, magnets and telescopes. When selecting the attachments, one must take into account the prosthetic space, as well as patient's manual dexterity and the degree of oral hygiene.

Narrow Diameter Implant Overdenture (NDIO) represents a category of implants that combines features from conventional implants and mini implants, with diameters between 3 and 3.5mm and variable lengths (10-18mm), comprising two distinctive subgroups, namely two-piece design (e.g. Seven Narrow Line implants, MIS Implants Technologies Inc. 18-00 Fair Lawn Ave. Fair Lawn, NJ 07410, UNITED STATES, mini Sky 2, Bredent Medical GmbH & Co, Germany, Straumann implant, Straumann Group SIX: STMN, Basel Switzerland) and one-piece design (e.g. uno line, MIS implants). Two-piece narrow implants can be used as the conventional implants (with delayed loading), or as one-piece mini implants (with immediate loading protocol). In relation to anatomical, functional and prosthetic case particularities, the number of dental implants used can be reduced, similar to that of the conventional implants (e.g., two narrow implants for the mandibular overdenture).

Mini Dental Implant Overdentures (MDIO) use mostly-one piece dental implants (miniSky1, Bredent, MDI 3MESPE) with diameters between 1,8mm and 3mm and variable lengths (10mm-18mm), that require one-stage surgery for implant placement, followed by prosthesis application in the same appointment, with soft material in the housing area (progressive loading) or fixation of the matrices in the denture base (immediate loading). Within the mini implants, those with a diameter between 2.7 and 3mm are classified as hybrid implants, these having sometimes a two-piece design and can be used as narrow dental implants (e.g., two narrow implants for the mandibular overdenture).

The main features of the overdentures on dental implants with a diameter below the conventional one, considering their three main categories according to their diameter, are synthesized in table 1.

The decision to use either a CDIO, NDIO or MDIO as treatment for complete edentulism, starts from the acknowledgment of patient's preferences and expectations, within the limitations of the systemic and oral health-status. In systemic alterations with indications of limited surgery or that negatively affects the healing process, NDIO and MDIO are more indicated than CDIO, due to their reduced invasiveness. Oral particularities, such as the anatomical conditions (bone quality and quantity, the shape of the alveolar ridge, skeletal class), thickness and health of the oral mucosa (e.g., denture stomatitis, candidiasis), available prosthetic restorative space (especially as vertical dimension, given the necessary space for abutment, attachments and prosthesis thickness, in order to prevent its fracture) should all be considered when choosing between the implant prosthesis alternatives.

	Conventional implant overdenture(CDIO)	Narrow diameter implant overdenture (NDIO)	Mini dental implant overdenture (MDIO)
Implant's diameter	>3.5mm	3.5 – 3.0 mm 3.0- 3.25 mm (smaller)	2.9-2.7mm (hybrid) 1.8mm – 2.7mm
Implant's length	> 8mm	> 10mm	> 10mm
Design	Two-piece implants	One- and two-piece implants	One-piece implants and two-piece (hybrid)
Number			
Maxilla	Minimum 4	Minimum 4	Minim 6 (minimum 4 for hybrid implants)
Mandible	Minimum 2	Minimum 2	Minimum 4 (minimum 2 for hybrid implants)
Surgery	Usually two-stage implant placement protocol	One- or two-stage implant placement protocol	One-stage implant placement protocol
Loading	Usually delayed loading	Immediate or delayed loading	Immediate loading
Overdenture support	Soft tissue and implant support	Soft tissue-support	Soft tissue-support
Overdenture design	Open palate maxillary denture	As a conventional complete denture	As a conventional complete denture
Attachment system	Splinted implants (bar) and unsplinted (ball, locator, magnets, telescope)	Unsplinted (ball, locator, magnets, telescope)	Unsplinted (Ball with O- ring)
Aim	improve overdenture retention, stability and support	improve overdenture retention and stability	improve overdenture retention and stability

Table 1. Main features of the overdentures on dental implants, in regard to their diameter

Patients with a high risk of developing implant or overdenture-related complications should be identified, and treatment personalized according to their nature. There are conditions with absolute contraindications of surgical procedures (e.g., recent myocardial infarction, stroke, cardiovascular surgery, and transplant; profound immunosuppression; bisphosphonate use, diabetes), but even in these cases the degree of disease-control is far more important than the nature of the systemic disorder itself [7, 8]. Behavioral aspects may increase some complication rates (e.g., implants are not indicated in heavy drinkers or smokers, more than 10 cigarettes per day). In patients with decreased manual dexterity or coordination deficiencies alternatives that promote simpler plaque control and easier overdenture placement and removal should be chosen (e.g. ball attachments are preferred to bars). Bruxism or other parafunctions with occlusal overloads associates high occlusal loading that increases the risk of implant failure, in this cases more frequent check-ups and sometimes the increase of the implant number are required. When more than two implants are used, there is a higher risk of overdenture fracture, and the reinforcement of the overdenture base is recommended [9].

The patient's expectations towards the prosthetic outcomes must be assessed in terms of functional restorations, esthetics and prosthesis retention. It is recommended to acknowledge the patient's perception and reasons of dissatisfaction toward the previous prosthesis, in order to correctly evaluate and inform him about the benefits of each particular type of implant overdenture. Additionally, financial aspects need to be explained to the patient, as comparative analysis of the additional costs of each treatment alternative, putting them in balance with the treatment benefits.

2.1. Concept of Mini Dental Implant Overdentures (MDIO)

Based on similar principles of overdentures with roots or conventional implants, using mini implants for overdenture has been suggested, as an alternative with advantages such as the less invasive surgical interventions with lower risks and lower costs, but with similar results [10, 11].

Implant overdentures are nowadays increasingly preferred to conventional dentures. Patients are more informed about the benefits of implant prosthesis, more frequently request and accept these treatment alternatives. The significant improvement in denture retention, with rapid regaining of functionality after implant placement, is an important motivating factor. The surgical and prosthetic techniques are significantly simplified, being more widely used one-stage implant placement protocol, with immediate loading, becoming a less invasive treatment that promotes rapid healing and has good treatment outcomes. MDIO fits this prosthetic treatment trend, and is seen as an appropriate option for the elderly edentulous, implants having a survival rate between 88.5% and 96%, higher in the mandible than in the maxilla [12, 6, 13]. Their use is increasing in relation to the relatively frequently reduced ridge width in the edentulous patient, that often limit using conventional implants without extensive surgical procedures for augmentation, that are usually not easily accepted, especially by the elderly patients [14].

Biomechanical studies support the use of narrow and mini implants, but draw attention to their increased risk of fracture, which should be considered. The decrease of implant diameter does not affect the implant osseointegration. Block et al. analyzed the effect of implant diameter on the pullout force required to extract the implant and proved that, after 15 weeks for osseointegration, no correlation was found to its diameter, but only with its length [15]. Clinical studies confirm that short implants were often accompanied by failure, but narrow implants have a good prognosis [16]. Therefore the narrow and mini implants used for overdenture should have at least 10mm length, in relation to their diameter, but also to the bone's height.

Given the good results obtained in vivo and in vitro, narrow and mini implants, seem to be the successors of conventional diameter implants in overdentures. Mini dental implants were originally designed by Victor Sendax [17]. At first they had diameters between 1.8- 2.4 mm, and were used for stabilization of interim prosthesis during implant osseointegration, stabilization of occlusion rims and for orthodontic anchorage. Afterwards, histological studies confirmed that these implants osseointegrate and clinical studies acknowledge a high survival rate, of about 83,9 to 97.5% [18]. Consequently, their usage expanded for definitive prosthesis both fixed (for single narrow edentulous spaces) and removable (for partial and complete denture stabilization). Mini implants, as endoosseous implants, are indicated to complete edentulous patients with narrow ridges, where the prosthetic treatment on implants is chosen, but reduced surgical invasiveness is beneficial, for example for those with general systemic risk factors [6]. It is particularly suitable for elderly patients, with multiple comorbidities and a low income, and who often do not accept complex and expensive dental interventions.

The mini implants have a number of features that have to be known and considered, both when it comes to selecting the implants, as well as during the treatment phases. Thus the mini dental implants are most commonly one-piece implants, with reduced diameter, conventional length, tapered, self-threading, made of biocompatible titan-based materials, with rough sandblasted surface treated by acid. IMTEC (currently part of 3M ESPE) developed mini dental implants with a diameter of 1.8mm to 2.4mm, supplemented recently by those with a diameter of 2.9mm (indicated especially in the maxilla), and with lengths of 10, 13, 15 and 18 mm. These implants have been designed differently, with 2.5mm transgingival collar (for thick gingiva) or without it (for thin gingiva). The upper surface of the endosteal dental implant may be polished and remain outside the bone within the mucosa, but the rough surface must be placed within the bone. Regarding the implant thread, it may be standard for D1 and D2 Misch bone densities (usually encountered in the mandible), or Max Thread, for D2 and D3 bone density (most frequently encountered in the maxilla) [19]. The implant prosthetic element, the abutment, has a spherical design like the ball attachment system, with an overall height of 4mm or 6 mm. Its gingival part has a square-profile section, with or without transgingival collar, which must remain outside the mucosa for at least half of its length. The attachment system is O-ring type, a resilient retention device composed of a metal matrix and a rubber ring, available in the following three options:

- standard: provides strong retention and tolerate a divergence of implants up to 30°;

- micro: has a 30% lower height than the standard matrix, offers an advantage for reduced prosthetic restorative spaces, provides a higher retention and compensates less for the implant divergence;

- O-Cap: provides extra-firm retention, mini-implants should be placed almost parallel, being used with delayed implant loading.

Therefore, the main coordinates of mini implant selection, according to the case particularities, are the following:

- Implant number: at least 4 in the mandible and at least 6 in the maxilla;

- Implant size, as diameter and length, is chosen according to ridge width, bone height and bone density. Usually, smaller diameter implants, of 1.8-2.1mm are used in the mandible, in bone with D1 and D2 Misch density, and mini implants with diameter of at least 2,4mm are recommended in D3 bone density in the maxilla. Implants should have a diameter with at least 2 mm less than the width of the ridge, which can be assessed using a clinical compass, or subtracting from the clinically measured width minimum 2mm corresponding to the mucosa thickness (Figure 1). The implants' length is chosen according to the bone height (at least 2 mm less than the bone height), which can be approximated by overlaying the specially designed grid on the panoramic radiography;

- Choosing between mini implants according to thread design is related to bone density (standard in the mandible and Max Thread in the maxilla);

- Choosing between mini implants with or without transgingival collar is related to the mucosa thickness.

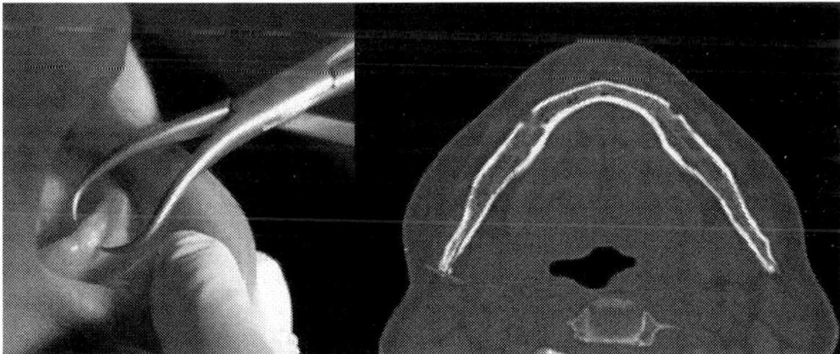

Figure 1. Clinical and radiological assessment of bone width

In case of MDIO, implants are placed without extensive augmentation procedure, through a less invasive surgical procedure, considering the anatomical limitation. In the mandible, mini implants are placed in the interforaminal region (7mm anterior to the mental foramen, to prevent damaging the inferior alveolar neurovascular bundle), and in the maxilla, anterior to the maxillary sinuses (protecting both the maxillary sinus and the nasal fosses). Within the mandible, when the mandibular canal is making a loop and the bone height allows it, implants can be placed behind the mental foramen. When placing the implants, it is recommended to keep a distance of at least 4.5 mm between them.

Most of the companies that produce implants are usually making available a line of implants with different diameters, and, for the same diameter, different corresponding implants lengths. Some of them, as mini Sky1 (Bredent Medical, Germany), that are hybrid implants, ensure a simpler implant selection and implant placement related to the implant options that differ only by implant length (10mm, 12mm and 14mm, and have the same diameter of 2.8mm, are identical as endosteal and abutment design) and have all the same simple implant placement protocol (only two drills are needed). Using hybrid implants allows, according to the bone quality and prosthetic needs, the reduction of the implant number (e.g., in the mandible only 2 mini Sky1 hybrid implants can be used instead of 4 mini implants with a diameter of 1,8-2,5 mm). Compared to the surgical implant kit of conventional denture, the one for mini implants is usually considerably simpler, containing fewer components (basically 1 or 2 drills for implant osteotomy and 2 ratchets), promoting a reduced time of the surgical phase, beneficial when considering this is a major stress for the patient.

Treatment with MDIO includes a surgical phase (implants placement) and a prosthetic phase (transformation of the denture in overdenture), both conducted in one clinical appointment.

Before implant placement some simple preoperative interventions are required, such as instruction and motivation on maintaining proper oral hygiene (antibacterial mouthwash as Chlorhexidine may be recommended), with prophylactic antibiotherapy and sedation.

For mini implant placement local anesthesia is sufficient, and a flap or flapless technique can be used, with or without a surgical guide (Figure 2).

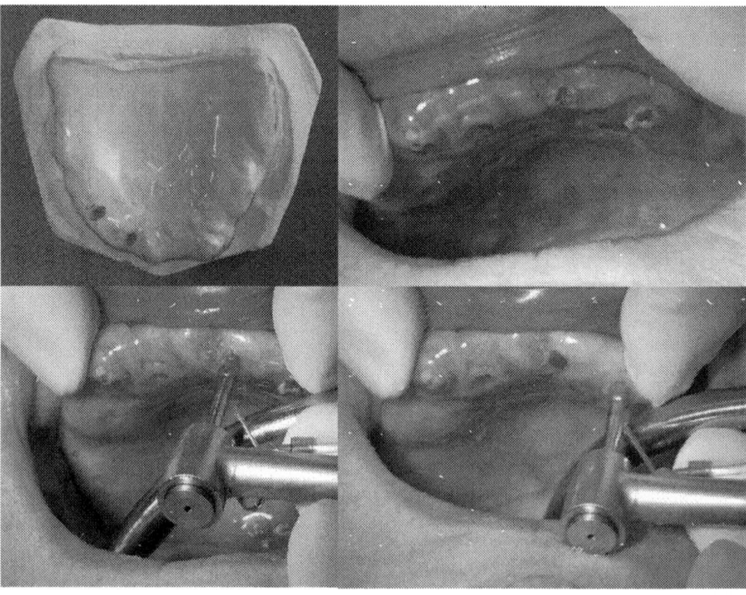

Figure 2. Implant placement using a surgical guide

For the flapless technique, the implant site is marked and the cortical bone is pierced with the same small size drill. Flap technique (Figure 3) is recommended in cases with thick mucosa or flabby ridge in order to properly asses bone offer, or in cases where 1.8 mm implants are to be placed into 3 mm narrow ridges. Initial implant osteotomy should be performed with a pilot drill with a diameter smaller than the one of the implant, in order to obtain bone condensation. Considering the positive effect of bone tapping on osseointegration, osteotomy depth varies according to bone density, about 2/3 of implant length for D1 bone density, about 1/2 of implant length for D2 bone density and about 1/3 of implant length for D3 bone density. Also, abundant irrigations with refrigerated sterile saline solution are mandatory. Implant placement should be done using slow movements, especially in high density bone, in order to avoid the heat trauma created by friction that may cause harmful effects in the bone (necrosis by heating) and also the implant fracture, which is more frequent in mini implants due to their decreased diameter. The self-tapped implant is placed and advanced into the bone by hand ratchet or headpiece and must be operated slowly, without extreme pressures. When screwing with the ratchet, the left hand finger is onto the ratchet in the mini implant's axis and the pressure is created with the right hand only on the ratchet arm, in the direction pointed by the arrow. The optimum value for the insertion torque is 35Ncm and should not exceed 45Ncm. If during the mini implant placement the torque exceeds 45Ncm it is recommended to unscrew the implant and expand the osteotomy, as depth or diameter. The implant body should be fully inserted into the bone.

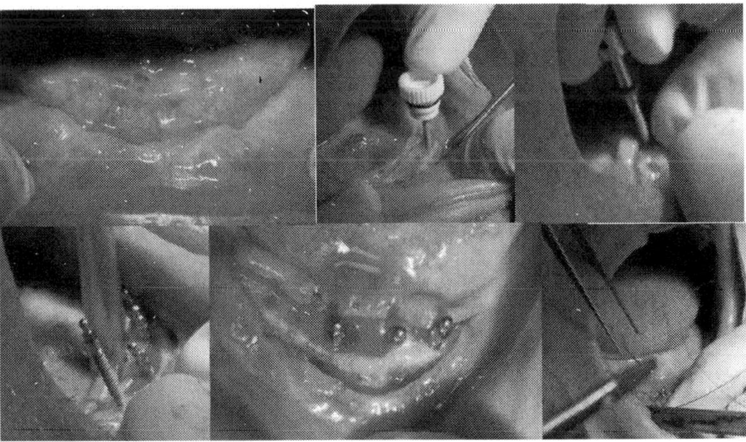

Figure 3. Mini implant placement, using a flap technique

In case of MDIO, for immediate loading, a good primary stability of the implants is required, which is related to the implant insertion torque (minimum 30 to 35 Ncm; in this respect, unfavorable situations are more frequently encountered in the maxilla, and are very rare in the mandible), bone compression and anchorage in the cortical bone. For immediate loading of the implants it is necessary to have a complete denture before the implants insertion that will be transformed into the overdenture, either as the old or newly manufactured prosthesis.

For immediate loading, the attachment caps, which contain rubber O-rings, are placed on the implants. The first clinical step is to remove the acrylic material from the inner part of the overdenture base, in the area corresponding to the implant site, quantitatively until the overdenture passive fits on the overdenture-bearing area. Fixing the housings can be done directly (by the dentist in the clinic) or indirectly (by the dental technician, in the laboratory). For housing fixing in the clinic, isolation of the gingival part of the implant abutment is done with latex materials (as piece of rubber dam or medical gloves), in order to prevent the acrylic material penetration under the O-ball head. Metal housings are placed combining rotational movements and pressure, until they fit passively. Preparing the prosthesis consists of repeatedly marking each matrix site accompanied by acrylic material removal from the corresponding denture base area. It is recommended to verify passive fit using soft silicone materials as Fit checker (GC Corporation). Afterwards, definitive metal housing fixation is done intraorally with acrylic materials, in centric occlusion. For a more accurate reproduction, before implant placement an occlusal registration can be taken and can be used during this treatment phase. Finally it is recommended to perform an accurate polishing of the denture around the metal matrices, in order to prevent plaque accumulation that favors occurence of peri-implant mucositis and peri-implantitis.

If the insertion torque is less than 35Ncm, the primary stability is not sufficient for immediate loading. Therefore, it is recommended to use progressive loading through the usage as soft lining material such as matrices during the osseointegration phase, and also to ensure weaker occlusal load in the area corresponding to the implant site. Metal housing fixation is recommended to be done after 3 to 6 months after implant placement.

A very important aspect is to verify, during the osseointegration period, the occlusion, the overdenture stability and the prosthesis of the antagonist jaw, as key elements for ensuring a good treatment prognosis.

Rubber O-rings are a part of the attachment system that wear-out over time and must be checked and periodically replaced in relation to loss of retention. Associated to the unavoidable alveolar bone resorption, denture relining or renewal are necessary over time. If overdenture renewal is desired, abutment analogues are used during impression.

MDIO has many advantages for older patients, often complete denture wearers that are dissatisfied with its retention and stability. Thus, through a reduced invasiveness surgical procedure, which requires less clinical time, with average costs, in a single session, a removable prosthesis with a good stability and with immediate functional integration can be achieved, providing the mental and physical comfort in order to carry out current social activities. At the same time, this treatment option has the advantage of an easy maintenance of oral and denture hygiene, through the unsplinted implants, an important aspect especially for elderly people, with frequent deficiencies when it comes to manual dexterity.

2.2. Concept of Narrow Diameter Implant Overdentures (NDIO)

The growing popularity of MDIO associated a general increase in the usage of implant overdentures among elderly completely edentulous patients. This is due to the clinical success of MDIO, the increase of its acceptability among edentulous patients, and the possibility for dentists to use it without extensive training in oral implantology (implant placement require one surgical intervention, relatively easy to perform. Within completely edentulous patients, narrow alveolar ridges are very common, mini and narrow implants being advantageous considering that they can be used without bone augmentations or other extensive surgical procedures, such as ridge splitting technique, being more easily accepted by elderly patients. At the same time, it is undeniable that the use of conventional diameter implants has numerous advantages, such as a reduced risk of implant fracture, reduced stress peaks at the implant-bone interface, the possibility to reduce the number of implants and the use of attachments according to the prosthetic needs, with different retention degrees [6]. Subsequently, the concept called NDIOhas developed, which uses implants with a diameter between the conventional and the mini dental implants, and is partially similar to both MDIO and CDIO. Narrow diameter implants with diameters between 3 and 3.5 mm, designed initially for fixed restorations of narrow edentulous spaces, expanded their use for implant overdentures. These can be found in different options, as size (implants with diameter between 3.0 and 3.25 are named sometimes small implants) and design (one- or two-piece implants, with different attachment systems).

NDIO, as treatment alternative has particularities common to both CDIO and MDIO, such as:

- Like the MDIO, it is mainly indicated in cases with narrow ridges (1.5-2 mm more than implant diameter) and resorbed ridges;

- Surgery is usually minimally invasive, similar to MDIO (without bone augmentation, possibility to use flapless implant insertion technique);

- The implant number can be reduced compared to MDIO, being similar to that of CDIO, due to the increased implant diameter;

- Narrow implants can be loaded immediately or delayed, depending on bone density, insertion torque, primary implant stability, being possible to use previous dentures or the ones manufactured after implant placement;

- Two-piece narrow implants allow insertion into bone with a lower density with delayed loading after 3 to 6 months, similar to CDIO;

- Two-piece narrow implants usually can be used with different attachment systems, with different retention degree, resiliency and possibility to compensate implant divergence (e.g., Locator can compensate up to 40° implant divergence);

- When compared to mini dental implants, narrow dental implants have a lower fracture risk, due to the larger diameter;

- NDIO, like MDIO, compared to CDIO, require reduced clinical time, reduced surgery (as number of appointments and complexity of the procedures), which favors a faster healing process and patient's comfort, reducing the biological and financial costs and overall being a more suitable treatment alternative for the elderly.

Narrow dental implants have diameters of 3 to 3.5 mm and are available in one- or two-piece design. Using the two-piece implants has the advantage of choosing to use either immediate or delayed loading, and for the latter either subgingival or transgingival healing. They may be placed flap or flapless, the latter the disadvantage of a less reliable assessment of the bone offer, but the advantage of promoting a faster healing. Usually, using a two-piece implant associates the possibility to choose from several attachment systems, and therefore a better treatment individualization, according to biomechanical and functional features, is available.

The increased interest towards implants designed for stabilization of the removable prosthesis is justified by the high prevalence of edentulism, which is usually treated by conventional complete dentures, alternatives that rather often have stability and retention deficiencies, problems that are more and more perceived as being unacceptable. In addition to this, more often cases with a high degree of treatment difficulty (mainly related to changes related to previous removable prosthetic treatment, as severe ridge resorption) are encountered and concerns are related to the increase of the age when edentulism occurs, that associates difficulties in generally adapting to new, and particularly to new prosthesis. Therefore, the increased use of narrow and mini implants is related to the reduced treatment invasiveness correlated to the functional benefits, which is a very important aspect for the elderly, population category in which most of the edentulous patients are encountered.

Treatment of edentulism with implant prosthesis is frequently accompanied by difficulties related to the limited bone offer – as a result of buccal or lingual bone resorption (narrow ridges) or as apical bone resorption (resorbed ridges). Narrow ridges are more often encountered in skeletal class II patients with a hypodivergent pattern. Conventional removable prostheses are barely tolerated by patients with sharp ridges (sometimes associated with irregularities such as exostosis, with thin covering mucosa, sensitive to pressures) or with severe ridge resorption and imprecise peripheral boundaries, situations which are encountered mainly in the mandible. Most of the completely edentulous patients that are denture wearers have severe ridge resorption, which associates difficulties both for conventional denture (through decreased support area) and CDIO (bone offer is insufficient for placement of conventional implants). Between these two treatment alternatives there are MDIO and NDIO, and when appropriate, the latter is preferred due to preserving the benefits of the first and having other important advantages (e.g., as stated before, a lower risk of implant fracture, possibility to use a reduced number of implants).

NDIO is found as a treatment option with indications similar to MDIO, in cases with narrow alveolar ridge, but it is a suitable treatment alternative also in cases of increased ridge resorption, associated with denture intolerance. Similar to MDIO, for NDIO implant diameter should be chosen according to ridge width (the ridge width should be at least 2 mm larger than the implant's diameter). NDIO are more indicated than MDIO in the maxilla, as a preventive mean, considering that the survival rate of implants is lower in the maxilla than in the mandible. NDIO versus MDIO has the advantage of the possibility to use a smaller number of implants, for example for the mandibular prosthesis 2 narrow implants can be used instead of 4 mini implants (Figure 4).

Implant placement is similar for the one-piece narrow implants to that of mini implants, and for the two-piece narrow implants to conventional implants. The surgical kit includes a reduced number of drills and ranches, which should be used according to the manufacturer's instructions. In two-piece implants a one- or two-stage protocol can be used, that depends

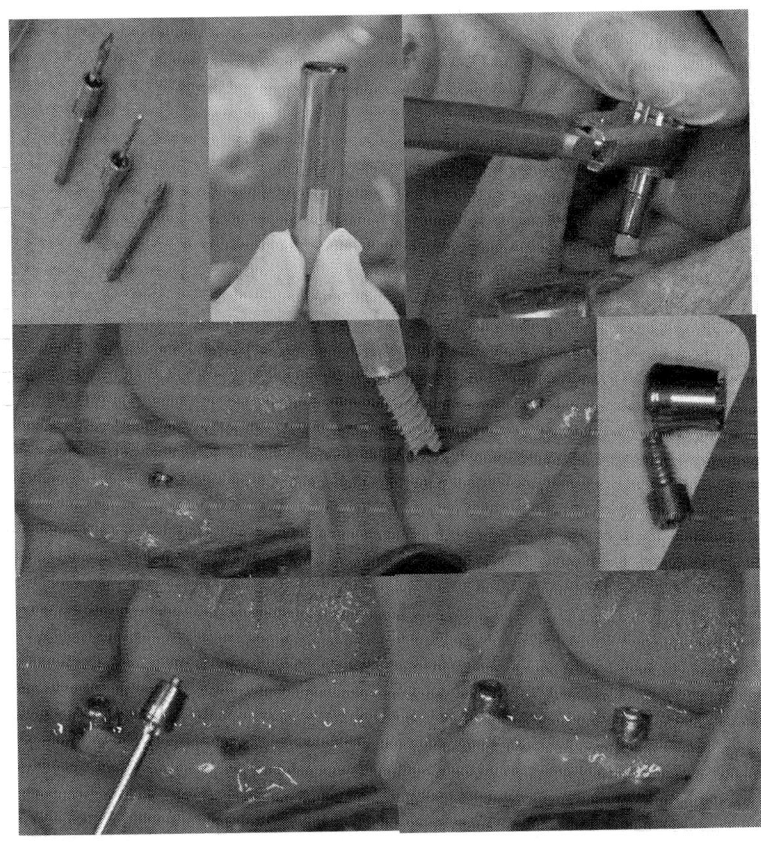

Figure 4. Narrow implant and Locator placement

mostly on the implant's primary stability. Therefore NDIO, compared to CDIO has the advantages of less surgical invasiveness and its associated benefits, overcoming some deficiencies of MDI, while preserving its advantages (good retention and stability of the overdenture, easy maintenance) [20].

Prosthesis execution differs according to the type of narrow implant used and coordination of treatment planning. Thus, when using one-piece narrow implants with one-stage surgery the process is similar to the one used for MDIO. When an attachment system with increased retention is used, like the Locator, it is recommended to use soft acrylic or silicone material as matrices during osseointegration. In this regard, silicone materials with different retention levels were developed, such as Retention.Sil (Bredent) that has 3 options according to the detachment force desired (200, 400, 600 gf). When using two-piece narrow implant with two-stage surgery, after osseointegration, the healing abutment is uncovered by a new surgical procedure, and replaced with the attachment, followed by the procedures needed in order to transform the denture into the overdenture.

3. Clinical phases of MDIO and NDIO

NDIO and MDIO are treatment options for complete edentulism, usually aiming the stabilization of the removable prosthesis. Alveolar ridge resorption, modifications of the muscle insertions and muscle tonus, neuromuscular coordination and control deficiencies increase treatment difficulties and favor occurrence of ill-fitting dentures, its retention and balance deficiencies being possible to be addressed through an implant overdenture. NDIO or MDIO have usually a mucosal support, not an implant one, the attachments only aiming to increase overdenture retention and stability. As clinical phases MDIO and NDIO are mostly similar, differences being encountered especially between one- and two-piece implants, when used with one or two-stage surgery.

Patient evaluation. Before implant placement, an accurate analysis of oral and systemic status is required. Although mini or narrow implant placement is done through surgical procedures with reduced invasiveness, the absolute contraindication should be accounted (e.g., recent myocardial infarction or stroke, profound immunosuppression, radiotherapy or bisphosphonate use) [7, 8]. Oral particularities should be accurately acknowledged through clinical and radiological examination, as anatomical and functional aspects. Considering the implant placement, ridge width should be evaluate by computed tomography or by clinical means (as using a clinical compass), the latter being sometimes confirmed by direct assessment during the surgical phase, after flap elevation. Bone height is best established using also computed tomography, but usually in the mandible only a panoramic radiography is used. Mucosa thickness is assessed by probing it with a periodontal probe.

The most commonly used radiological investigation is the panoramic radiography, which provides information on bone size and anatomical limitations (mandibular canal, mental foramen, maxillary sinus, nasal fossae). Computed tomography is indicated especially in cases with severe bone resorption, for an accurate bone offer evaluation and the establishment of implant site. Lateral cephalography can offer important data especially on skeletal relations, which associate anatomical and functional features relevant for treatment planning and prognosis.

Implants number and size. Implants are chosen according to the bone offer, the option with higher diameter and length being preferred. The higher the implant's diameter, the better it will resist to lateral forces, the longer it is, the better it will resist to vertical forces. Therefore, in order to compensate the decreased diameter of mini implants and to increase the resistance to lateral forces, a higher number of implants are placed. Usually, for mini implants 4 MDI in the mandible are placed between the mental foramens and 6 in the maxilla, anterior to the maxillary sinus. For hybrid and narrow implants their number may be reduced (2 in the mandible, 4 in the maxilla), related to the higher diameter. Bone density influences implant size selection. Therefore, 1.8 mm diameter implants can be placed in bone with D1 and D2 density, but an increased diameter, of 2.4 mm, is recommended for D3 bone density.

Implant placement. Mini- and narrow-implants are placed through a surgical procedure that is usually considered as having decreased invasiveness, and can be performed by a general dentist.

MDI and NDI insertion can be done with or without a surgical guide. The last option has the advantage of a more accurate positioning of the implants, in accordance with prosthetic aspects. Using a surgical radiological guide, manufactured based on the existing prosthesis, allows an accurate establishment of the most distal implant site, preventing the damage to anatomical proximity structures [21].

Mini and narrow diameter implants, by their design, associate bone condensation during implant placement, which favors a good primary stability. Screwing of the implant should be done slowly, with the ratchet, while performing manual control, in order to feel "the saturation point" and to avoid implant fracture.

Flap or a flapless technique may be used for mini and narrow implant placement. The flap technique, the most commonly used, has the advantage of directly visualizing the alveolar bone volume before the osteotomy, the possibility to reshape the bone and soft tissue. As a disadvantage, it is more invasive and prolongs the duration of the surgical phase, recovery and healing phase. Flapless technique is mostly done transmucosally, being a less invasive intervention, ensuring a more rapid healing, with a lower degree of patient discomfort (Figure 5). By not disturbing the periosteum layer, there is a higher chance, compared to the flap one, to maintain the alveolar bone levels [22, 23].

Last but not least, the decision to either use a flap or not is up to the practitioner, according to patient's particularities, but also to the clinician's surgical and prosthetic skills [24].The flap technique is recommended especially when interventions are needed in order to remodel the bone support (e.g., irregular alveolar bone; reduction of bone height needed due to insufficient prosthetic space) and when direct visual access is required (e.g. flabby ridge). The flapless technique is indicated when the bone width is adequate, the ridge shows no exostosis or alterations that require surgical correction, it is preferred when using immediate loading and in patients with systemic diseases that limit the extent of surgery or interfere in the healing process [24].

Implant loading protocol. Placement of mini- or narrow-dental implants can be followed by immediate-, progressive- or delayed-loading protocol, depending mainly on the implant primary stability

Immediate implant loading protocol is used when insertion torque is above 40Ncm, for D1 or D2 bone density, being a more commonly encountered in implants placed in the mandible, in the interforaminal area, especially when a flapless technique was used. In this regard previously made prosthesis are used, which are adjusted to the new situation, followed by the fixation of the matrix in the overdenture base. Occlusion analysis should be performed, considering these alterations can have a negative impact especially in the vulnerable period of osseointegration.

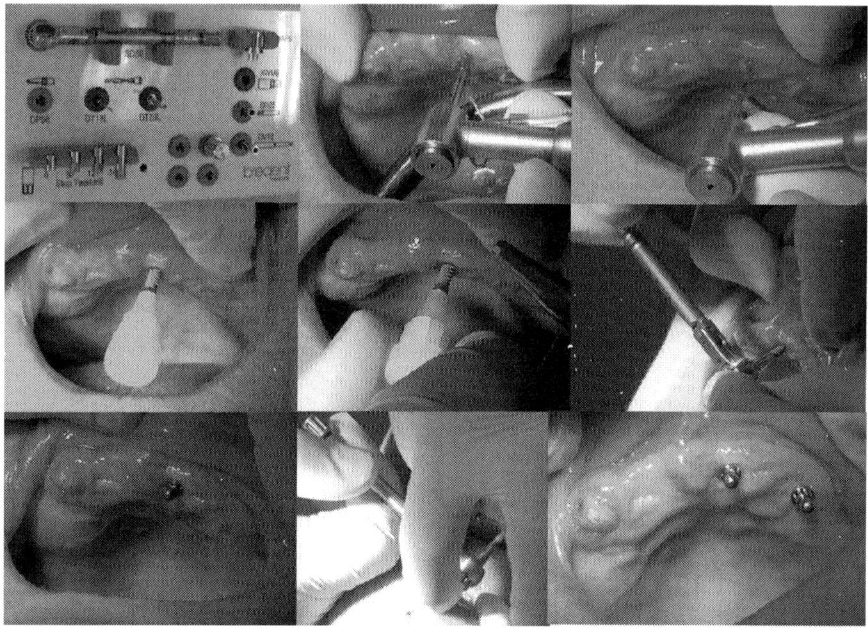

Figure 5. Hybrid implants placement, using a flapless technique

Progressive implant loading is recommended for D2 bone density and in cases with slower healing process after surgery, such as in flap techniques. Basically, for a period of 30 days postinsertion soft resilient acrylic or silicone materials are used as matrices, followed afterwards by the fixation of the matrices into the denture base.

In case of immediate and progressive loading, regular check-ups are at most importance during the osseointegration period. The overdenture must be verified in order not to exert direct pressure on the implants (only mucosal support should be noticed), as occlusal relations, as its stability and, if applicable, as the stability of the antagonist denture, as factors that may negatively influence the prognosis of the implant.

Delayed implant loading, performed at about 3 months, is indicated when the insertion torque is under 40Ncm and in patients with D3 bone density. In this case there is an additional surgical step in order to uncover the healing abutments.

Fixation of the matrices into the overdenture base. Fixing the prosthetic component of the attachment can be done in the dental office or in the dental laboratory, after verifying the denture correctness (e.g., as teeth mounting, occlusal relations, denture base extension, aesthetic and functional outcome, material status). One of the main advantages of NDIO and MDIO is related to the possibility of preserving the previous prostheses, this being related mainly to the denture correctness and patient preferences. Usually the dentures need to be renewal, most often due their deficiencies, occurred related to the improper execution or as changes in time. Even so, during the osseointegration period it is best to preserve the old denture, relined with resilient material, so that the patient can easily perceive modifications that may have a negative impact, such as the pressure on the implant.

Direct fixation of the prosthetic part of the attachment system, in the dental office, varies according to implant design, i.e. one- or two-piece implant. The clinical procedure for one-piece implants, which usually have O-ring as attachment system, is similar to that used for MDIO, previously described. For two-piece implants, applying the retention systems is different upon the implant placement protocol, i.e. one- or two-stage protocol. For one-stage protocol the procedures used are similar to those applied for one-piece implants, namely in the same clinical appointment with implant placement, the attachment abutment is applied (ball, locator, ferromagnetic metal keeper) and, depending on implant and prosthetic parameters (e.g., implant primary stability, insertion torque, bone density, occlusal loading) either a progressive implant loading (with soft material as matrices), or immediate implant loading (definitive fixation of the prosthetic attachment component, such as metal housing or ring, denture cap, magnet, in the denture base with self- or light-cured acrylic materials) is done. For two-stage protocol, after the osseointegration period, the endoosseous implants are surgically uncovered, the healing abutment are replaced by the attachment abutment, and followed by the fixation of the prosthetic attachment in the overdenture base (Figure 6).

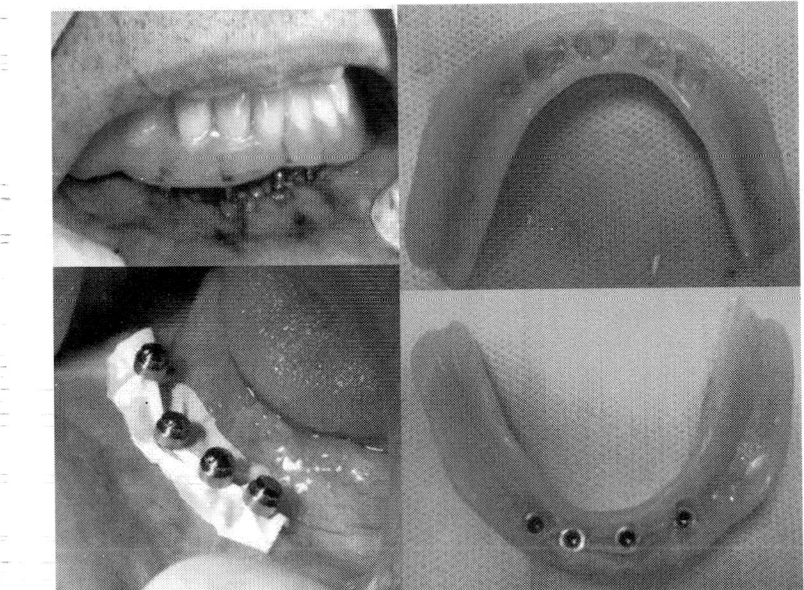

Figure 6. Direct metal housing fixing, in the dental office

Indirect fixation of the prosthetic part of the attachment system, in the dental laboratory, is mainly used when the overdenture renewal is desired. Correspondent, either impression transfer procedures after attaching the analogue, either impression taken with the prosthetic attachment component placed on the attachment abutment, can be used.

In all situations previously mentioned, overdenture adjustments and verifications are needed in order to achieve only mucosal support, passive fit on the implants and correct registrations of maxillomandibular relationship, without excessive occlusal loading. In the first 72 hours it is recommended to remove the denture only during oral and denture hygiene procedures, being highlighted to the patients the importance of a good plaque control in preventing treatment complications.

Considering that in case of MDIO and NDIO dental implants are applied in order to increase denture's retention and balance, overdenture execution should be done similar to that of conventional denture with a complete coverage of the support area, for ensuring proper retention, support and balance. Furthermore, choosing the occlusal scheme may be an important factor for treatment success, linear and lingualized occlusion being preferred for ensuring a more uniform distribution of the occlusal pressures over the bearing area, recommended especially for the mandibular overdenture. Key factors that ensure a good prognosis of conventional dentures should not be neglected in the case of MDIO and NDIO, such as the correct registration of maxillomandibular relations, at a correct vertical dimension of occlusion and centric relation.

Frequently used attachment systems for MDIO and NDIO. These types of implant prosthesis are usually retained by unsplinted implants, with attachment systems that only provide better denture retention and balance, while the prosthesis has only mucosal support. The most frequently used attachment systems are O-ring type, but also other alternatives are encountered, such as Locator, magnets, telescopes (especially double conical crowns, which are less rigid).

O-ring attachment system is used for both one- and two-piece narrow and mini dental implants. O-ring system is encountered in different designs, as the one of mini dental implant manufactured by 3M ESPE (spherical abutment with a metal matrix and rubber ring) or the one of miniSky 1 hybrid implants from Bredent Medical (spherical abutment with a metal ring and rubber ring). The metal matrix are made of Au or Ti, and can be activated, ensuring a different retention level. This attachment system has a resiliency degree, being a semi-rigid type, with positive effect on stress distribution. The system compensates for an implants divergence of about 20°-30°. Due to wearing over time, the rubber rings must be replaced periodically, when not ensuring the proper overdenture retention. This is encountered most frequently in cases with denture deficiencies that contribute to denture instability (e.g., overextended denture flanges, incorrect mounting of artificial teeth, unstable occlusal contacts).

Locator attachment systems, developed later, brought a number of advantages for NDIO. They can be used in cases with decreased vertical prosthetic space (at about 10 mm from the ridge crest to the height of the denture), generally having below 5 mm height with the denture cap in place, value that is below of that of O-ring attachment system. Also, it compensates for a higher angle of implant divergence, up to 40°. Even so, they are designed for ensuring an internal and external retention, but in order to use both, implants must be placed nearly parallel. If implants are placed under a divergent angle, only internal retention is preserved. Depending on the manufacturer, different alternatives are available according to the level of retention and gingiva thickness.

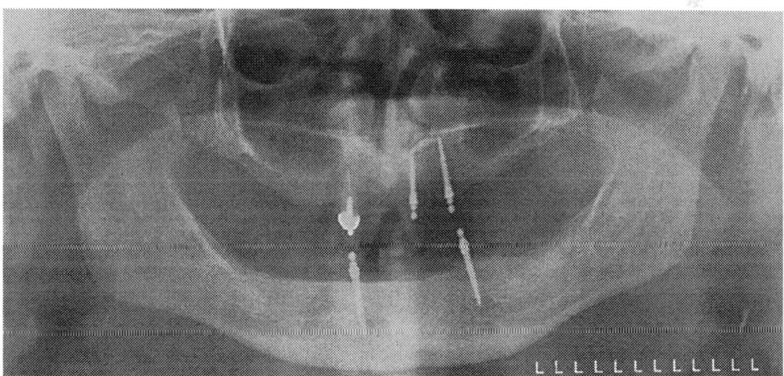

Figure 7. miniSky 1 implant overdentures – radiological examination 2 years after implant placement

4. Advantages and disadvantages of MDIO and NDIO

Implant overdentures, and especially MDIO and NDIO have registered an increased usage, which is probably related to its better treatment outcome, when compared to conventional complete denture. Among others, there can be mentioned beneficial aspects as the increased prosthesis balance and retention (especially for the mandibular denture), the improvement of oral functions (mastication, phonation) and self-confidence, with positive implications on the patient's physical and psychological comfort and on the quality of life.

MDIO and NDIO are particularly indicated in edentulous patients with an increased degree of treatment difficulty, unsatisfied by their conventional dentures (e.g., complaining about denture instability, pain and discomfort during wearing), with systemic alterations that limits the extent of the surgery or that refuse complex, prolonged, expensive medical interventions [25].

When compared to the fixed implant prosthesis, or even CDIO, MDIO and NDIO are simplified implant prosthetic treatment alternatives that have a satisfactory clinical success and are implemented through less invasive surgery, with reduced pain and trauma. These alternatives are well fitted to aged edentulous patients, who frequently have systemic comorbidities that associate a higher risk of complications, and generally have difficulties in accepting complex medical interventions in general, and implant treatment in particu-lar. For these patients, aspects like the reduced invasiveness of surgical procedures, of the clinical time needed, of postoperatory discomfort, additionally to the relatively reduced costs required, are arguments that may convince them to accept the implant restoration. Overall costs are generally rated as being lower for MDIO and NDIO than for CDIO, due to the price differences of mini and narrow implants, the reduced clinical time with avoidance of some procedures (e.g., bone augmentation), the possibility to use the previous complete denture, when it corresponds qualitatively, through complications that are in general relatively easy and cheaper to resolve (e.g., loss of an implant can be solved by applying another one, followed by adjusting procedures to the existing denture; at CDIO using bars, implant loss is usually accompanied by extensive interventions, which almost covers the whole implant-prosthetic treatment).

By improving the denture stability, mastication efficiency increases, promoting a better nutritional status, and the denture detachment during mastication and phonation is reduced, offering the patient a psychological comfort [26]. MDIO and NDIO may be considered preventive treatments for reducing the side effects of ill-fitting conventional dentures, as an accelerated ridge resorption rate [27]. Additionally, one-piece mini implants associate a decreased peri-implant bone resorption compared to two-piece conventional implants, that was linked to the absence of the microgap between the endoosseous implant and the abutment, as well as the less physical displacement [28].

MDIO and NDIO require usage of a reduced number of implants, starting with 2 narrow or hybrid implants in the mandible and 4 in the maxilla, placed in most predictable anatomic area (interforaminal area), by simple surgical techniques, which ensures, in case of immediate loading, rapid regaining of functionality. Mini and narrow diameter implants minimize, through their design, the soft tissue and bone damaging, compared to conventional implants, favoring a shorter and better healing and osseointegration [29]. Placing the implants in the anterior maxillary area is beneficial, considering the occlusal load is decreased when compared to the posterior maxillary area, and also the possibility to use bicortical implant stabilization. The survival rate of implants placed in the anterior area of the mandible is high, above 90%, similar to that of conventional implants [30, 31, 32].

Increased use of MDIO and NDIO may be related also to the extended usage of implants the dental field. Also, in the general dental practice an increased surgical placement of implants is observed, probably related to patient's demands. However, the cost for dental practitioners for conventional implants remains high, both in terms of education and equipment needs, but are affordable for mini- and narrow-dental implants.

Although the use of either MDIO or NDIO is accompanied by many advantages, it must be considered that the treatment and maintenance is more complex than the one for conventional prosthesis, that may be regarded as a disadvantage, when considering the barriers that elderly face (e.g., financial hardship, transportation difficulties). Therefore, simpler solutions must be chosen, with complications that can be easily resolved (e.g., in elderly, unsplinted implants with O-ball attachments are preferred to bars). Also, there are behavioral aspects or systemic conditions that associate a higher complication rate (e.g., smokers are at greater risk of implant failure compared to nonsmokers).

Specifically linked to the MDIO and NDIO is the disadvantage of not being recommended to be insert mini and narrow dental implant immediately after tooth extraction.

Also, when using mandibular MDIO or NDIO, opposed by an edentulous maxilla treated by conventional denture, signs similar to those of Combination Syndrome may appear, as instability of the conventional denture and increase bone resorption rate in the anterior maxilla. These are managed usually through using implant prosthesis also in the maxilla.

5. Conclusions

Stabilization of conventional denture with mini- or narrow-dental implants is beneficial especially for the elderly, considering the improvement achieved through a relatively easy surgical intervention, with moderate treatment costs. In this regard, for mandibular denture stabilization either 4 mini implants or 2 hybrid/narrow implants can be used. Treatment success is strongly related to acknowledgement of patient anatomical and functional particularities, rigorous planning and execution of prosthetic and surgical phase, as well as ensuring an adequate maintenance.

Considering that edentulism is and most probably will continue to remain a frequent medical condition mostly found in the elderly, MDIO and NDIO overdentures, through their specific parameters, may replace in time complete dentures and may be the most used treatment alternative.

Author details

Elena Preoteasa[1*], Marina Imre[1], Henriette Lerner[2], Ana Maria Tancu[1] and Cristina Teodora Preoteasa[3]

*Address all correspondence to: dr_elena_preoteasa@yahoo.com

1 Department of Prosthodontics, Faculty of Dental Medicine, Carol Davila University of Medicine and Pharmacy, Bucharest, Romania

2 Private Practice, Baden-Baden, Germany

3 Department of Oral Diagnosis, Ergonomics, Scientific Research Methodology, Faculty of Dental Medicine, Carol Davila University of Medicine and Pharmacy, Bucharest, Romania

References

[1] WHO. Active Aging. A Policy Framework. Madrid; 2002. http:// whqlibdoc.who.int/hq/2002/WHO_NMH_NPH_02.8.pdf?ua=1 (accessed 3 October 2014).

[2] Thomason JM, Kelly SA, Bendkowski A, Ellis JS. Two implant retained overdentures--a review of the literature supporting the McGill and York consensus statements. Journal of Dentistry 2012;40(1) 22-34.

[3] Feine JS, Carlsson GE, Awad MA, Chehade A, Duncan WJ, Gizani S, Head T et al. The McGill Consensus Statement on Overdentures. Montreal, Quebec, Canada. May 24-25, 2002. International Journal of Prosthodont 2002;15(4) 413-4.

[4] Melescanu Imre M, Marin M, Preoteasa E, Tancu AM, Preoteasa CT.Two implant overdenture--the first alternative treatment for patients with complete edentulous mandible. Journal of Medicine and Life 2011;4(2) 207-9.

[5] Preoteasa E, Marin M, Imre M, Lerner H, Preoteasa CT. Patients' Satisfaction With Conventional Dentures and Mini Implant Anchored Overdentures. Revista Medico-Chirurgicala a Societatii de Medici si Naturisti din Iasi 2012;116(1) 310-16.

[6] Klein MO, Schiegnitz E, Al-Nawas B. Systematic review on success of narrow-diameter dental implants. The International Journal of Oral & Maxillofacial Implants 2014;29 Supplement 43-54.

[7] Diz P, Scully C, Sanz M. Dental Implants in the Medically Compromised Patient. Journal of Dentistry 2013;41(3) 195-206.

[8] Gomez-de Diego R, Mang-de la Rosa M, Romero-Pérez MJ, Cutando-Soriano A, Lopez-Valverde-Centeno A. Indications and Contraindications of Dental Implants in Medically Compromised Patients: Update. Medicina Oral Patologia Oral y Cirugia Bucal 2014;19(5):e438, -9.

[9] Preoteasa E, Murariu CM, Ionescu E, Preoteasa CT. Acrylic Resin Reinforcement With Metallic and Nonmetallic Inserts. Revista Medico-Chirurgicala a Societatii de Medici si Naturalisti din Iasi 2007; 111(2) 487-93.

[10] Lerner H. Minimal invasive implantology with small diameter implants. Implant Practice 2009, 2(1) 30-5.

[11] Preoteasa E, Meleşcanu-Imre M, Preoteasa CT, Marin M, Lerner H. Aspects of oral morphology as decision factors in mini-implant supported overdenture. Romanian Journal of Morphology and Embryology 2010;51(2) 309-14.

[12] Shatkin TE, Shatkin S, Oppenheimer AJ, et al. A simplified approach to implant dentistry with mini dental implants. Alpha Omega. 2003; 96(3) 7-15.

[13] Preoteasa E, Imre M, Preoteasa CT. A 3-Year Follow-up Study of Overdentures Retained by Mini–Dental Implants. The International Journal of Oral & Maxillofacial Implants 2014; 29(5) 1034-41.

[14] Sohrabi K, Mushantat A, Esfandiari S, Feine J. How successful are small-diameter implants? A literature review. Clinical Oral Implants Research 2012;23 (5) 515–525.

[15] Block MS1, Delgado A, Fontenot MG.The effect of diameter and length of hydroxyla-patite - coated dental implants on ultimate pullout force in dog alveolar bone. Journal of Oral and Maxillofacial Surgery 1990;48(2) 174-8.

[16] Renouard F, Nisand D. Impact of implant length and diameter on survival rates. Clinical Oral Implants Research 2006;17 (2) Supplement 35-51.

[17] Singh RD, Ramashanker, Chand P. Management of atrophic mandibular ridge with mini dental implant system. National Journal of Maxillofacial Surgery 2010;1(2) 176-8.

[18] Griffitts TC, Collins CP, Collins PC. Mini dental implants: an adjunct for retention, stability, and comfort for the edentulous patient. Oral Surgery, Oral Medicine, Oral Pathology, Oral Radiology, and Endodontology 2005;100 (5) 81-4.

[19] Misch CE. Contemporary Implant Dentistry 2nd edition. St. Louis. Mosby Inc; 1999.

[20] Rossein KD. Alternative treatment plans: implant supported mandibular dentures. Inside Dentistry 2006; 2(6) 42-43.

[21] Melescanu Imre M, Preoteasa E, Tancu A, Preoteasa CT. Imaging Technique for the Complete Edentulous Patient Treated Conventionally or With Mini Implant Over-denture. Journal of Medicine and Life 2013;6(1) 86-92.

[22] Campelo LD, Camara JR. Flapless implant surgery: A 10-year clinical retro- spective analysis. International Journal Oral Maxillofacial Implants 2002;(17) 271–276.

[23] Sunitha RV, Sapthagiri E. Flapless implant surgery: A 2-year follow-up study of 40 implants. Oral Surgery, Oral Medicine, Oral Pathology and Oral Radiology 2013;116 (4) 237–243.

[24] Scherer MD, Ingel AP, Rathi N. Flapped or Flapless Surgery for Narrow-Diameter Implant Placement for Overdentures: Advantages, Disadvantages, Indications, and Clinical Rationale. The International Journal of Periodontics & Restorative Dentistry 2014;34(3) Supplement 89-95.

[25] Christensen GJ.The 'mini'-implant has arrived. The Journal of the American Dental Association 2006;137(3) 387-90.

[26] Preoteasa E, Iosif L, Amza O, Preoteasa CT, Dumitrascu C. Thermography, an Imag-istic Method in Investigation of the Oral Mucosa Status in Complete Denture Wear-ers. Journal of Optoelectronics and Advanced Materials 2010;12(11) 2333–4.

[27] Awad MA, Lund JP, Dufresne E, Feine JS. Comparing the efficacy of mandibular im-plant-retained overdentures and conventional dentures among middle-aged edentu-lous patients: satisfaction and functional assessment. The International Journal of Prosthodontics 2003;16, 117–22.

[28] Flanagan D, Mascolo A. The Mini Dental Implant in Fixed and Removable Prosthet-ics: A Review. Journal of Oral Implantology 2011;37 (1) 123-132

[29] Bulard RA. Mini implants. Part I. A solution for loose dentures. The Oklahoma Dental Association Journal. 2002;93.42-46.

[30] Dantas Ide S, Souza MB, Morais MH, Carreiro Ada F, Barbosa GA. Success and survival rates of mandibular overdentures supported by two or four implants: a systematic review, Brazilian Oral Research 2014;28(1) 74-80.

[31] Bergendal T, Engquist B. Implant-supported overdentures: a longitudinal prospective study. The International Journal of Oral & Maxillofacial Implants 1998;13 (2) 253–62.

[32] Klein MO, Schiegnitz E, Al-Nawas B. Systematic review on success of narrow-diameter dental implants. The International Journal of Oral & Maxillofacial Implants. 20

Chapter 12

Dental Implants

Dongliang Zhang and Lei Zheng

Additional information is available at the end of the chapter

http://dx.doi.org/10.5772/59258

1. Introduction

This chapter reviews the present and probable future need and demand for dental implants. A dental implant is defined as an artificial tooth root replacement and is used to support restorations that resemble a natural tooth or group of natural teeth.

2. The goal of modern dentistry

The goal of modern dentistry is to return patients to oral health in a predictable fashion. The partial and complete edentulous patient may be unable to recover normal function, esthetics, comfort, or speech with a traditional removable prosthesis. The patient's function when wearing a denture may be reduced to one sixth of that level formerly experienced with natural dentition; however, an implant prosthesis may return the function to near-normal limits. The esthetics of the edentulous patient are affected as a result of muscle and bone atrophy. Continued bone resorption leads to irreversible facial changes. An implant prosthesis allows normal muscle function, and the implant stimulates the bone and maintains its dimension in a manner similar to healthy natural teeth. As a result, the facial features are not compromised by lack of support as often required for removable prostheses. In addition, implant-supported restorations are positioned in relation to esthetics, function, and speech, not in neutral zones of soft tissue support. The soft tissues of the edentulous patients are tender from the effects of thinning mucosa, decreased salivary flow, and unstable or unretentive prostheses. The implant-retained restoration does not require soft tissue support and improves oral comfort. Speech is often compromised with soft tissue-borne prostheses because the tongue and perioral musculature may be compromised to limit the movement of the mandibular prosthesis. The implant prosthesis is stable and retentive without the efforts of the musculature. Implant prostheses often offer a more predictable treatment course than traditional restorations. Thus

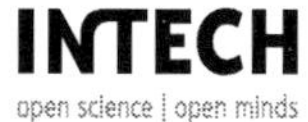

the profession and the public are becoming increasingly aware of this dental discipline. Manufacturers' sales have increased from a few million dollars to more than several hundred million dollars. Almost every professional journal now publishes refereed reports on dental implants. All U.S. dental schools now teach implant dentistry to all interfacing specialties. Implant dentistry to all interfacing specialties. Implant dentistry has finally been accepted by organized dentistry. The current trend to expand the use of implant dentistry will continue until every restorative practice uses this modality for abutment support of both fixed and removable prostheses on a regular basis as the primary option for all tooth replacement.

3. Options for replacement of lost teeth

Implants can be necessary when natural teeth are lost. When tooth loss occurs, masticatory function is diminished; when the underlying bone of the jaws is not under normal function it can slowly lose its mass and density, which can lead to fractures of the mandible and reduction of the vertical dimension of the middle face. Frequently, the physical appearance of the person is noticeably affected.

When a tooth is lost, the individual and dentist face two choices. The first choice is: should I replace the missing tooth? The second is: what is the best way to replace it? Although these decisions may seem sequential, they are interrelated in important ways. The technical options available can influence the decision to replace a tooth, and modern science has produced more and better options for tooth replacement in many circumstances. The age and general health of the patient are critical. The condition of the remaining dentition, its configuration in the mouth, and its periodontal support are very important aspects of the decision to replace. Finally, the relative cost of options can play a role, but should not be dispositive for a treatment plan. In making these decisions, the dentist and patient must evaluate all of these factors to reach the best treatment for a particular patient.

A number of restorative options for the treatment of missing teeth are recognized as accepted dental therapy, depending on particular circumstances the patient presents. These include:

1. Tissue-supported removable partial dentures (Figure 1)

2. Tooth-supported bridges

3. Implant-supported teeth (Figure 2)

Likewise, there are two basic options for replacing teeth in a completely edentulous arch:

1. Tissue-supported removable complete dentures

2. Implant-supported over-dentures

All these therapies have their indications for use.

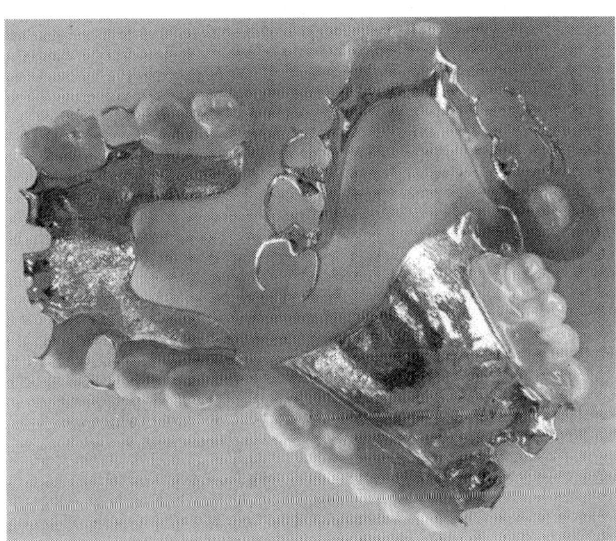

Figure 1. A typical collection of prosthetic devices, including flippers, removable partial dentures.

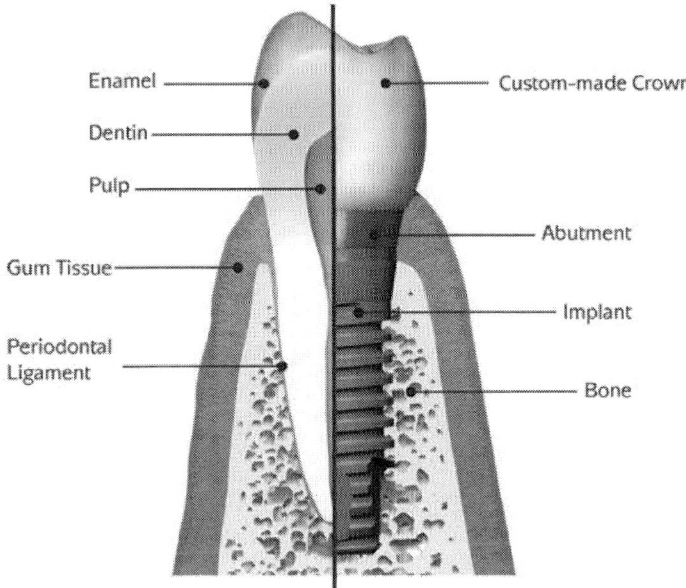

Figure 2. Comparison of natural tooth and crown with implant and crown.

4. Bone-supported prostheses

4.1. Dental implants

The implant is placed where the root of the missing tooth used to be. The replacement root is then used to attach a replacement tooth. Like the other options, dental implants are used to replace missing teeth and restore masticatory function to an individual's dentition.

The major types of dental implants are osseointegrated and fibrointegrated implants. Earlier implants, such as the subperiosteal implant and the blade implant, were usually fibrointegrated. The most widely accepted and successful implant today is the osseointegrated implant. Examples of endosseous implants (implants embedded into bone) date back over 1350 years. While excavating Mayan burial sites in Honduras in 1931, archaeologists found a fragment of mandible with an endosseous implant of Mayan origin, dating from about 600 AD.

Widespread use of osseointegrated dental implants is more recent. Modern dental implantology developed out of the landmark studies of bone healing and regeneration conducted in the 1950s and 1960s by Swedish orthopedic surgeon P.I. Brånemark. This therapy is based on the discover that titanium can be successfully fused with bone when osteoblasts grow on and into the rough surface of the implanted titanium. This forms a structural and functional connection between the living bone and the implant. A variation on the implant procedure is the implant-supported bridge, or implant-supported denture.

Today's dental implants are strong, durable, and natural in appearance. They offer a long-term solution to tooth loss. Dental implants are among the most successful procedures in dentistry. Studies have shown a 5-year success rate of 95% for lower jaw implants and 90% for upper jaw implants. The success rate for upper jaw implants is slightly lower because the upper jaw (especially the posterior section) is less dense than the lower jaw, making successful implantation and osseointegration potentially more difficult to achieve. Lower posterior implantation has the highest success rate of all dental implants.

Dental implants are less dependent than tooth-or tissue-supported prostheses on the configuration of the remaining natural teeth in the arch. They can be used to support prostheses for a completely edentulous arch, for an arch that does not have posterior tooth support, and for almost any configuration of partial edentulism with tooth support on both sides of the edentulous space.

Additionally, dental implants may be used in conjunction with other restorative procedures for maximum effectiveness. For example, a single implant can serve to support a crown replacing a single missing tooth. Implants also can be used to support a dental bridge for the replacement of multiple missing teeth, and can be used with dentures to increase stability and reduce gum tissue irritation. Another strategy for implant placement within narrow spaces is the incorporation of the mini-implant. Mini-implants may be used for small teeth and incisors.

Modern dental implants are virtually indistinguishable from natural teeth. They are typically placed in a single sitting require a period of osseointegration. This integration with the bone of the jaws takes anywhere from 3 to 6 months to anchor and heal. After that period of time a dentist places a permanent restoration for the missing crown of the tooth on the implant.

Although they demonstrate a very high success rate, dental implants may fail for a number of reasons, often related to a failure in the osseointegration process. For example, if the implant is placed in a poor position, osseointegration may not take place. Dental implants may break or become infected (like natural teeth) and crowns may become loose. Dental implants are not susceptible to caries attack, but poor oral hygiene can lead to the development of peri-implantitis around dental implants. This disease is tantamount to the development of perio-dontitis (severe gum disease) around a natural tooth.

Dental implant reconstruction may be indicated for tooth replacement any time after bone growth is complete. Certain medical conditions, such as active diabetes, cancer, or periodontal disease, may require additional treatment before the implant procedure can be performed. In some cases in which extensive bone loss has occurred in a jaw due to periodontal disease, implants may not be advised. Under proper circumstances, bone grafting may be used to augment the existing bone in a jaw prior to or in conjunction with placement.

5. Improvements in dental implant technology

New dental technology, materials, and designs have improved the dental implant procedure. Patients no longer have to wait to replace their missing teeth; the dental implant, abutment, and crown can be placed in just one visit. With immediate dental implants, the patient doesn't need to live with a space between teeth or wear a temporary crown while waiting for the dental implant to heal. With single-visit dental implants becoming more successful, more patients are inquiring about this procedure.

Using an ICAT cone beam CT scanner, a dentist can preplan dental implant surgery through 3-D imaging, creating a virtual mock-up of the mouth, which may eliminate an incision through the gums to find the bone. This, in turn, means less pain and healing time for the patient. During the planning stages, the prosthetic tooth can be fabricated by a dental labora-tory and can be ready at the time of surgery. This procedure bypasses the osseointegration period, in which the implant fuses to the bone. Although the implant still needs to heal, it can do so with the dental crown attached.

Mini-implants are a relatively recent implant technology. They are used primarily for dentures; a series of mini-implants are placed through the mucosa into the bone of the jaw. Posts are used to anchor the appliance into place. Mini-implants mean less pain and healing time, and normally cost less than traditional dental implants. These cutting-edge dental implants also eliminate the wait on the healing process for the final step. Patients can start wearing their replacement teeth right away.

Traditional dental implants meant that a new dental appliance was necessary, but some patients may be able to use existing dentures with mini-implants. Existing dentures can be fitted to attach to the posts implanted during surgery, enabling patients to return home with their repurposed dentures immediately after their surgery. Mini-implants are being used, in some indicated cases, to anchor dental crowns and dental bridges as well.

For the next 20 years the current elderly and baby-boom generations will be dominant factors in the demand for adult dental services. The former and a large portion of the latter did not experience the full benefits of modern preventive dentistry. They lost more teeth as children and young adults than the birth cohorts that follow them. Also, their dentitions suffered from greater caries attack, but they received substantial restorative care. Some of these restorations are likely to fail with time and a portion of those will require extraction, either due to the sequelae of previous restorative treatment or due to the advance of periodontal disease. Both generations have retained most of their natural teeth and are likely to want to replace those teeth they have already lost or will lose. Individuals aged 50 years and older today are likely to experience a substantial need for tooth replacement, and many of them will act on that need by choosing to have dental implants.

Over a longer time horizon, when today's young adults and children reach the age at which previous generations required substantial prosthetic replacement, their tooth loss is likely to be much less than those previous generations. That is good news. They will retain teeth, many of them sound. Hopefully, these groups will enjoy natural dentition throughout their life and will navigate old age with functioning, heal thy, natural teeth.

6. Generic prosthetic component terminology

A generic language for endosteal implants was developed by Misch and Misch in 1992. The order in which it is presented follows the chronology of insertion to restoration. In formulating the terminology, five commonly used implant system in the United States were referenced. Fifteen years later, the dramatic evolution of the U.S. implant market has resulted in changes in nearly all the implant lines and component designs. In 2000 the U.S. market alone ban to choose from more than 1300 different implant designs and 1500 abutments in various materials, shapes, sizes, diameters, lengths, surfaces, and connections. More than ever, a common language is needed. In pharmacology the variety of pharmaceutical components makes it impossible to list them all by proprietary names, but a list by category of drugs is useful. Likewise, implant components still can be classified into broad application categories, and the practitioner should be able to recognize a certain component category and know its indications and limitations.

This book incorporates a generic terminology, first introduced by Misch and Misch for endosteal implants, that blends a continuity and familiarity of many implant systems with established definitions from the terms of the Illustrated Dictionary of Dentistry and the glossaries from Terms of The Academy of Prosthodontics, American Implantologists.

7. Generic implant body terminology

Root from implant are a category of endosteal implants designed to use a vertical column of bone, similar to the root of a natural tooth. Although many names have been applied, the 1988 National Institutes of Health consensus statement on dental implants and the American Academy of Implant Dentistry recognized the term root form. The exponential growth of implant use over the last 20 years has been paralleled by an explosion of the implant manufacturing field. There are currently more than 90 implant body designs available, offering countless combinations of design features: screws, baskets, plateaus, ball, cylinders, diameters, lengths, prosthetic connections, and surface conditions.

The most common root form design combines a separate implant body and prosthodontic abutment abutment to permit only the implant body placement during bone healing. A second procedure is required to attach the implant abutment. The design and surgical philosophy is to achieve clinical rigid fixation that corresponds to a microscopic direct bone-to-implant interface without intervening fibrous tissue occurring over any significant portion of the implant body before the prosthetic phase of the procedure. Over the years, three different surgical approaches have been used for the two-piece implant systems: one stage, two stage, and immediate restoration.The two-stage surgical process places the implant body below the soft tissue, until the initial bone healing has occurred. During a second-stage surgery, the soft tissues are reflected to attach a permucosal element or abutment. During a one-stage surgical approach, the implant body and the permucosal abutment above the soft tissue are both placed until initial bone maturation has occurred. The abutment of the implant then replaces the permucosal element without the need for a secondary soft tissue surgery.

The immediate restoration approach places the implant body and the prosthetic abutment at the initial surgery. A restoration is then attached to the abutment (out of occlusal contacts in partially edentulous patients) at the appointment.

An implant body especially designed for one surgical method may also be selected. For example, a permucosal element may already be attached to the implant body by the manufacturer to facilitate a one-stage surgical approach. An implant body also may have a prosthetic abutment, which may be part of the inserted and restored at the initial surgery. This was the original concept first introduced by Strock in the 1930s.

There are three primary types of root form body endosteal implant based on design, cylinder, screw, or combination.

Cylinder (press-fit) root form implants depend on a coating or surface condition to provide microscopic retention to the bone. Most often the surface is either coated with a rough material (e.g., hydroxyapatite, titanium plasma spray) or a macro retentive design (e.g., sintered balls). Cylinder implant are usually pushed or tapped into a prepared bone site. They can be a paralleled wall cylinder or a tapered implant design. Screw root forms are threaded into a slightly smaller prepared bone site and have the macroscopic retentive elements of a thread for initial bone fixation. They may be machined, textured, or coated. There are three basic screw-thread geometries: V-thread, buttress (or reverse buttress) thread, and power (square) thread designs. Threaded implants are primarily available in a parallel cylinder or tapered cylinder design. Micro or macro thread features, variable thread pitch, depth, and angle, as well as self-tapping features, can be combined to create a myriad of implant designs. Combination root forms have macroscopic features from both the cylinder and screw root forms. The combination root form design also may benefit from microscopic retention to bone through varied surface treatments (machined, textured, and the addition of coatings).

Root forms also have been described by their means of insertion, healing, surgical requirements, surface characteristics, and interface.

8. Implant body regions

The implant body may be divided into a crest module (cervical geometry), a body, and an apex Each section of an implant has features that are of benefit in the surgical or prosthetic application of the implant

8.1. Implant body

An implant body is primarily designed for either surgical ease or prosthetic loading to the implant bone interface. Year ago, the implant body was the primary design feature. A round implant permits round surgical drills to prepare the bone. A smooth-walled cylinder implant allows the implant to be pressed or tapped into position, similar to a nail into a piece of wood. A tapered cylinder fits into the top of the osteotomy for further ease of placement.

A cylinder implant design system offers the advantage of ease of placement, even in difficult access locations. The cover screw of the implant also may be attached to the implant before implant placement. For example, in the very soft D4 bone the posterior regions of the maxilla, the surgeon must rotate a threaded implant design into place. Very soft bone may strip during threaded implant insertion. This may result in lack of initial fixation, and the implant will not be rigid. A tapered cylinder implant may be pressed by hand into soft bone and can be initially fixated more easily, The speed of implant rotation during insertion and the amount of apical force in implant insertion soft bone are less relevant for a press-fit cylinder. The cylinder system also presents some benefits for the single-tooth implant application, especially if adjacent to teeth with tall clinical crowns. Thread extenders are needed for the screw implant in these situations, as well as additional tools to insert the cover screw of the implant. In dense bone, cylinder systems also are easier and faster to place because bone tapping is not required

Most cylinder implants are essentially smooth-sided and bullet-shaped implants that require a bioactive or increased surface area coating for retention in the bone. When these materials are placed on an implant, the surface area of bone contact increases more than 30%. The greater the functional surface area of the bone implant contact, the better the support system for the prosthesis.

A solid screw implant body design is the most commonly reported in the literature. A solid screw body is defined as an implant of a circular cross section without penetrating any vents or holes. A number of manufactures provide this design (e.g., Nobel Biocare, Biomet, Zimmer, ITI, BioHorizons, LifeCroe, Bio-Lok). The thread may be V-shaped, buttress, reverse buttress, or square (power thread) in design. The V-shaped threaded screw has the longest history of clinical use. The most common outer thread diameter is 3.75mm, with 0.38-mm thread depth, and a 0.6-mm thread pitch (distance). The carious body lengths usually range from 7 to 16 mm, although lengths from 5 mm to 45 mm are available. Similar body designs are offered in a variety of diameters (narrow, standard, wide) to respond to the mechanical, esthetic, and anatomical requirements in different areas of the mouth.

A solid screw implant body permits the osteotomy and placement of the implant in dense cortical bone as well as in fine trabecular bone. The surgery may be easily modified to accommodate both extremes in bone density, The solid screw permits the implant removal at the time of surgery if placement is not ideal. It also permits implant removal at the Stage II surgery if angulation or crestal bony contours are not deemed adequate for long-term prosthesis success. The solid screw implant body may be machined or roughened to increase marginally the functional surface area or to take advantage of biochemical properties related to the surface coating (e, g., bone bonding or bone growth factors).

A threaded implant body is primarily designed to increase the bone-implant surface area and to decrease the stresses at the interface during occlusal loading. The functional surface area of a threaded implant is greater than a cylinder implant by a minimum of 30% and may exceed 500% depending on the thread geometry. This increase in functional implant surface area decreases the stress imposed on the implant-bone interface and is directly related to the thread geometry.

8.2. Crest module

The crest module of an implant body is that portion designed to retain the prosthetic component in a one-piece or two-piece implant system. It also represents the transition zone from the implant body design to the transosteal region of the implant at the crest of the ridge. The abutment connection area usually has a platform on which the abutment is seated; the platform offers physical resistance to axial occlusal loads. An antirotation feature also is included on the platform (external hex) or extends within the implant body (internal hex, octagon, Mores taper or cone screw, internal grooves or cam tube, and pin slots). The implant body has a design to transfer stress/strain to the bone during occlusal loads (e, g., threads or large spheres), whereas the crest module often is designed to reduce bacterial invasion. (e. g., smoother to impair plaque retention if crestal bone loss occurs). Its smoother dimension varies greatly from one system to another (0.5 to 0.5 mm). When the crest module is smooth, polished metal, it is often called a cervical collar.

A high-precision fit of the external or internal anti-rotational component (flat to flat dimension) is para-mount to the stability of the implant body/abutment connection. The prosthetic connection to the crest module is received by slip-fit or friction-fit with a butt or bevel joint. All prosthetic connections aim at providing a precise mating of the two components with minimal tolerance.

Another antirotational feature of an implant body may be flat sides or grooves along the body or apical region of the implant body. When bone grows against the flat or groove regions, the bone is placed in compression with rotational loads. The apical end of each implant should be flat rather than pointed. This allows for the entire length of the implant to incorporate design features that maximize desired strain profiles. Additionally, if an opposing cortical plate is perforated, a sharp, V-shaped apex may irritate or inflame the soft tissues if any movement occurs (e. g., the inferior border of the mandible).

9. Implant surgery

At the of insertion of a two-stage implant body (stage I surgery), a frost-stage cover screw is placed into the top of the implant to prevent bone, soft tissue, or debris from invading the abutment connection area during healing.

After a prescribed healing period sufficient to allow a supporting bone interface to develop, a second-stage procedure may be performed to expose the two-stage implant or to attach a transepithelial portion. This transepitthelial portions is termed a permucosal extension because it extends the implant above the soft tissue and results in the development of a permucosal seal around the implant. This implant component has also been called a healing abutment because stage II uncovery surgery often uses this device for initial soft tissue healing.

In the case of a one-stage procedure, the surgeon may have placed the permucosal extension at the time of implant insertion or may have selected an implant body design with a cervical collar of sufficient height to be supragingival. In the case of immediate load, the permucosal healing abutment may not be used at all if a temporary prosthesis is delivered on the day of surgery or may be sued until the suture removal appointment and the temporary teeth delivery. The permucosal extension is available in multiple heights to accommodate soft tissue variations. It also can be straight, flared, or anatomical to assist in the initial contour of the soft tissue healing.

9.1. Prosthetic attachments

The abutment is the portion of the implant that supports or retains a prosthesis or implant superstructure. A superstructure is defined as a metal framework that attaches to the implant abutment(s) and provides either retention for a removable prosthesis (e, g., a cast bar retaining an overdenture with attachments) or the framework for a fixed prosthesis. Three main categories of implant abutments are described, according to the method by which the pros-thesis or superstructure is retained to the abutment; (1) an abutment for screw retention uses a screw to retain the prosthesis or superstructure, (2) an abutment for cement retention uses dental cement to retain the prosthesis or superstructure, and (3) an abutment for attachment uses an attachment device to retain a removable prosthesis(such as an O-ring attachment).The abutment for cement/screw/attachment may be screwed or cemented into the implant body, but this aspect is not delineated within the generic terminology

Each of three abutment types may be further classified as straight or angled abutments, describing the axial relationship between the implant body and the abutment. An abutment for screw retention uses a hygiene cover screw placed over the abutment to prevent debris and calculus from invading the internally threaded portion of the abutment retention during prosthesis fabrication between prosthetic appointments.

The lack of abutment design of a decade ago has been replaced by a variety of options. The expansion of implant dentistry, is applications for esthetic dentistry, and the creativity of manufacturers in this very competitive market is responsible today. In the abutment for cement category, the doctor may choose from one-and two-piece abutments; UCLA type(plastic castable, machined/plastic castable, gold sleeve castable); two-piece esthetic; two-piece anatomical; two-piece shoulder; preangled (several angulations); or ceramic, Zirconia, or computer-assisted custom design. The abutment for screw category also has been enlarged with one-and two-piece overdenture abutments of different contours and heights.

Many manufacturers classify the prosthesis as fixed whenever cement retains the prostheses, fixed/removable when screws retain a fixed prosthesis, and removable when the restoration is removed by the patient. This description implies that only screw-retained description, because a fixed, cemented prosthesis also may be removed by the dentist (especially when a temporary cement is used). The generic language in this chapter separates prostheses into either fixed or removable in a method similar to traditional prosthetics.

9.2. Prosthesis fabrication

An impression is necessary to transfer the position and design of the implant or abutment to a master cast for prosthesis fabrication. A transfer coping is used in traditional prosthetics to position a die in an impression. Most implant manufacturers use the terms transfer and coping to describe the component used for the final impression. Therefore a transfer coping is used to position an analog in an impression and is defined by the portion of the implant it transfers to the master cast, either the implant body transfer or the abutment transfer coping.

Two basic implant restorative techniques are used to make a master impression, and each uses a different design transfer coping, based on the transfer technique performed. An indirect transfer coping uses an impression material requiring elastic properties. The indirect transfer coping is screw into the abutment or implant body and remains in place when a traditional "closed tray" impression is set and removed from the mouth. The indirect transfer coping is usually slightly tapered to allow ease in removal of the impression and often has flat sides or smooth undercuts to facilitate reorientation in the impression after it is removed.

A direct transfer, often square, and a long central screw to secure it to the abutment or implant body and may be used a pick-up implant coping. An "open tray" impression tray is used to permit direct access to the long central screw securing the indirect transfer coping. After the impression material is set, the direct transfer coping screw is unthreaded to allow removal of the impression from the mouth, direct transfer copings take advantage of impression materials having rigid properties and eliminate the error of permanent deformation because they remain within the impression until the master model is poured and separated.

9.3. Laboratory fabrication

An analog is defined as something that is analogous or similar to something else. An implant analog is used in the fabrication of the master cast to replicate the retentive portion of the implant body or abutment (implant body analog, implant abutment analog). After the master impression is obtained, the corresponding analog (e, g., implant body, abutment for screw) is attached to the transfer coping and the assembly is poured in stone to fabricate the master cast.

A prosthetic coping is a thin covering, usually designed to fit the implant abutment for screw retention. It serves as the connection between the abutment and the prosthesis or superstructure. A prefabricated coping usually is a metal component machined precisely to fit the abutment. A castable coping usually is a plastic pattern cast in the same metal as the superstructure or prosthesis. A screw-retained prosthesis or superstructure is secured to the implant body or abutment with a prosthetic screw.

10. Prosthetic options in implant dentistry

Implant dentistry is similar to all aspects of medicine in that treatment begins with a diagnosis of the patient's condition. Many treatment options stem from the diagnostic information. Traditional dentistry provides limited treatment options for the edentulous patient. Because the dentist cannot add abutments, the restoration design is directly related to the existing oral condition. On the other hand, implant dentistry can provide. On the other hand, implant dentistry can provide a range of additional abutment locations. Bone augmentation may further modify the existing edentulous condition in both the partial and total edentulous arch and therefore also affects the final prosthetic design. As a result, a number of treatment options are available to most partially and completely, the implant treatment plan of choice at a par particular moment is patient and problem based. Not all patients should be treated with the same restoration type or design.

Almost all man-made creations, whether art, building, or prostheses, require the end result to be visualized and precisely planned for optimal results. Blueprints indicate the finest details for buildings. The end result should be clearly identified before the project begins, yet implant dentist often forget this simple but fundamental axiom. Historically in implant dentistry, bone available for implant insertion dictated the number and locations of dental implants. The prosthesis then was often determined after the position and number of implants were selected.

The goals of implant dentistry are to replace a patient's missing teeth to normal contour, comfort, function, esthetics, speech, and health, regardless of the previous atrophy, disease, or injury of the stomatognathic system. It is the final restoration, not the implant, that accomplish these goals. In other words, patients are missing teeth, not implants. To satisfy predictably a patient's needs and desires, the prosthesis should first be designed. In the stress treatment theorem, the final restoration is first planned, similar to the architect designing a building before making the foundation foundation. Only after this is accomplished can the abutments necessary to support the specific predetermined restoration be designed.

11. Completely edentulous prosthesis design

The completely edentulous patient is too often treated as though cost were the primary factor in establishing a treatment plan. However, the doctor and staff should specifically ask about the patient's desires. Some patients have a strong psychologic need to have a fixed prosthesis as similar to natural teeth as possible. On the other hand, some patients do not express serious concerns whether the restoration is fixed or removable as long as prosthetic problems are addressed. To assess the ideal final prosthetic design, the existing anatomy is evaluated after restoration is desired.

An axiom of implant treatment is not provide the most predictable, most cost-effective treatment that will satisfy the patient's anatomical needs and personal desires. In the completely edentulous patient, a removable implant. Supported prosthesis offers several advantages over a fixed-implant restoration.(Box 1).

BOX 1. Advantages of Removable Implant-supported Prostheses in the Completely Edentulous Patient

*facial esthetics can be enhanced with labial flanges and denture teeth compared with customized metal or porcelain teeth. The labial contours of the removable restoration can replace lost bone width and height and support the labial soft tissues without hygienic compromise.

*The prosthesis can be removed at night to manage nocturnal parafunction.

*Fewer implants may be required.

*Less bone augmentation may be necessary before implant insertion.

*Shorter treatment if no bone augmentation is required.

*The treatment may be expensive for the patient.

*Long-term treatment of complications is facilitated.

*Daily home care is easier.

However, some completely edentulous patients require a fixed restoration because of desire or because their oral condition makes the fabrication of teeth difficult if a superstructure and removable prosthesis are planned. For example, when the patient has abundant bone and implants have already been placed, the lack of crown height space may not permit a removable prosthesis.

Too often, treatment plans for completely edentulous patients consist of a maxillary denture and a mandibular overdenture with two implants. However, in the long term, this treatment option may prove a disservice to the patient. The maxillary arch will continue to lose bone, and the bone loss may even be accelerated in the premaxilla. Once this dimension is lost, the patient will have much more difficulty with retention and stability of the restoration. In addition, the lack of posterior implant support in the mandible will allow posterior bone loss to continue. Paresthesia, facial changes, and reduced posterior occlusion on the maxillary prosthesis are to be expected. The doctor should diagnose the amount of bone loss and its consequences on facial esthetics, function, and the psychological and overall health. Patients should be made aware of future compromises in bone loss and its associated problems with minimal treatment options, which do not address the continued loss of bone in regions where implants are not inserted.

It is even more important to visualize the final restoration at the onset with a fixed-implant restoration. After this first important step, the individual areas of ideal or key abutment support are determined to assess whether it is possible to place the implants to support the intended prosthesis. The patient's force and bone density in the region of implant support are evaluated. The additional implants to support the expected forces on the prosthesis designed may then be determined with implant size and design selected to match force and area conditions. Only then is the available bone evaluated to assess whether it is possible to place the implants to support the intended prosthesis. In inadequate natural or implant abutment situations, the existing oral conditions or the needs and desires of the patient must be altered. In other words, either the mouth must be modified by augmentation to place implants in the correct anatomical positions, or the mind of the patient must be modified to accept a different prosthesis type and its limitations. A fixed-implant restoration may be indicated for either the partially or the completely edentulous patient. The psychological advantage of fixed teeth is a major benefit, and edentulous patients often feel the implant teeth are better than their own. The improvement over their removable restoration is significant.

BOX 2. Advantages of fixed Restorations in the Partially Edentulous patient

1. psychological (feels,more like natural teeth)

2. Less food entrapment

3. Less maintenance (no attachments to change of adjust)

4. Longevity (lasts the life of the implants)

5. Similar overhead cost as completely implant-supported overdentures

---

The completely implant-supported overdenture requires the same number of implants as a fixed-implant restoration. Thus the cost of implant surgery may be similar for fixed or removable restorations. Fixed prostheses often last longer than overdentures, because attachments do not require replacement and acrylic denture teeth wear faster than porcelain to metal. The chance of food entrapment under a removable overdenture is often greater than for a fixed restoration, as soft tissue extensions and support are often required in the latter. The laboratory fees for a fixed prosthesis may be similar to a bar, coping attachments, and over denture. Because the denture or partial denture fees are much less than fixed prostheses, many clinicians charge the patient a much lower fee for removable over dentures on implants. Yet chair time and laboratory fees are often similar for fixed or removable restorations that are completely implant supported. One should consider increasing the patient fees for over dentures to a level more in line with fixed restorations.

Type	Definition
FP-1	Fixed prosthesis; replaces only the crown; looks like a natural tooth
FP-2	Fixed prosthesis; replaces the crown and a portion of the root; crown contour appears normal in the occlusal half but is elongated or hypercontoured in the gingival half
FP-3	Fixed prosthesis; replaces missing crows and gingival color and poration of the edentulous site, prosthesis most often uses denture teeth and acrylic gingival, but may be porcelain to metal
RP-4	Removable prosthesis ; overdenture supported completely by implant
RP-5	Removable prosthesis; overdenture supported by both soft tissue and implant

Table 1. Prosthodontic classification

12. Partially edentulous prosthesis design

A common axiom in traditional prosthodontics for partial edentulism is to provide a fixed partial denture whenever applicable. The fewer natural teeth missing the better the indication for a fixed partial denture. This axiom also applies to implant prostheses in the partially edentulous patient. Ideally, the fixed partial denture is completely implant supported rather than joining implants in the treatment plan. Although this may be a cost disadvantage, it is outweighed by significant intraoral health benefits. The added implants in the edentulous site result in fewer pontics, more retentive units in the restoration, and less stress to the supporting bone. As a result complications are minimized and implant and prosthesis longevity are increased (BOX 2)

13. Prosthetic options

In 1989, Misch proposed five prosthetic options for implant dentistry (Table 1). The first three options are fixed prostheses (FPs). These three options may replace partial (one tooth or several) or total dentitions and may be cemented or screw retained. They are used to communicate the appearance of the final prosthesis to all the implant team members. These options depend and the aspects of the prosthesis in the esthetic zone. Common to all foxed options is the inability of the patient to remove the prosthesis. Two types of final implant restorations are removable prostheses (RPS); they depend on the amount of implant support, not the appearance of the prosthesis.

13.1. Fixed prostheses

13.1.1. FP-1

An FP-1 is a fixed restoration and appears to the patient to replace only the anatomical crowns of the missing natural teeth. To fabricate this restoration type, there must be minimal loss of hard and soft tissues. The volume and position of the residual bone must permit ideal placement of the implant in a location similar to the root of a natural tooth. The final restoration appears very similar in size and contour to most traditional fixed prostheses used to restore or replace natural crowns of teeth.

The FP-1 prosthesis is most often desired in the maxillary anterior region, especially in the esthetic zone during smiling or speaking. The final FP-1 restoration appears to the patient to be similar to a crown on a natural tooth. However, the implant abutment can rarely be treated as a natural tooth prepared for a full crown. The cervical diameter of a maxillary central incisor is approximately 6.5 mm with an oval to triangular cross section. However, the implant abutment is usually 4 mm in diameter and round in cross section. In addition, the placement of the implant rarely corresponds exactly to the crown-root position of the original tooth. The thin labial bone lying over the facial aspect of a maxillary anterior root remodels after tooth loss and the crest width shifts to the palate, decreasing 40% within the first 2 years. The occlusal table is also usually modified in unesthetic regions to conform to the implant size and position and to direct vertical forces to the implant body, For example, posterior mandibular implant –supported prostheses have narrower occlusal tables at the expense of the buccal contour, because the implant is smaller in diameter and placed in the central fossa region of the tooth.

Because the width or height of the crestal bone is frequently lacking after the loss of multiple adjacent natural teeth, bone augmentation is often required before implant placement to achieve natural-looking crowns in the cervical region. These are no interdental papillae in edentulous ridges; therefore soft tissue augmentation also is often required to improve the interproximal gingival contour. Ignoring this step causes open "black" triangular spaces (where papillae usually be present) when the patient smiles. FP-1 prostheses are especially difficult to achieve when more than two adjacent teeth are missing. The bone loss and lack of interdental soft tissue complete the final esthetic result, especially in the cervical region of the crowns.

The restorative material of choice for an FP-1 prosthesis is porcelain to noble to noble-metal alloy. A noble-metal substructure can easily be separated and soldered in case of a nonpassive fit at the metal try-in, and noble metals in contact with implants corrode less than nonprecious alloys. Any history of exudate around a subgingival base-metal margin will dramatically increase the corrosion effect between the implant and the base metal. A single tooth FP-1 crown may use aluminum oxide cores and porcelain crowns, or ceramic abutments and porcelain crowns. However, the risk of fracture ma increase with the latter scenario, as implant forces are greater on implants than natural teeth.

13.1.2. FP-2

An FP-2 fixed prosthesis appears to restore the anatomical crown and a portion of the root of the natural tooth. The volume and topography of the available bone is more apical compared with the ideal bone position of a natural root (1 to 2 mm below the cement-enamel junction) and dictate a more apical implant placement compared with the FP-1 prosthesis. As a result, the incisal edge is in the correct position, but the gingival third of the crown is overextended, usually apical and lingual to the position of the original tooth. These restorations are similar to teeth exhibiting periodontal bone loss and gingival recession.

The patient and the clinician should be aware from the onset of treatment that the final prosthetic teeth will appear longer than healthy natural teeth (without bone loss). The esthetic zone of a patient is established during smiling in the maxillary arch and during speech of sibilant sounds for the mandibular arch. If the high lip during smiling or the low lip line longer are usually of no esthetic consequence, provided that the patient has been informed before treatment.

As the patient becomes older, the maxillary esthetic zone is altered. Only 10% of younger patients do not show any soft tissue during smiling, whereas 30% of 60 year old and 50% of 80year olds do not display gingival regions during smiling. The low lip position during speech is not affected as much as the mandibular soft tissue during speech.

A multiple-unit Fp-2 restoration does not require as specific an implant position because the cervical contour is not displayed during function. The implant position may be chosen in relation to bone width, angulation, or hygienic considerations rather than purely esthetic demands (as compared with the FP-1 prosthesis). On occasion, the implant may even be placed in an embrasure between two teeth. This often occurs for mandibular anterior teeth for full-arch fixed restorations. If this occurs, the most esthetic area usually requires the incisal two thirds of the two crowns to be ideal in width, as though the implant were not present. Only the cervical region is compromised. Although the implant is not positioned in the correct facial-lingual position, it should be placed in the correct facial-lingual position to ensure that contour, hygiene, and direction of forces are not compromised.

The material of choice for an FP-2 prosthesis is precious metal to porcelain. The amount and contour of the metal work is different than for a FP-1 restoration and is more relevant in an FP-2 prosthesis, because the amount of additional volume of tooth replacement increases the risk of unsupported porcelain in the final prosthesis, then the metal work in undercontoured.

13.1.3. FP-3

The FP-3 fixed restoration appears to replace the natural teeth crowns and has pink-colored restorative materials to replace a portion of the soft tissue. As with the FP-2 prosthesis, the original available bone height has decreased by natural resorption or osteoplasty at the time of implant placement. To place the incisal edge of the teeth in proper position for esthetics, function, lip support, and speech, the excessive vertical dimension to be restored requires teeth that are unnatural in length. However, unlike the FP-2 prosthesis, the patient may have a normal to high maxillary lip line during smiling or a low mandibular lip line during speech. The ideal high smile line displays the interdental papilla of the maxillary anterior teeth but not the soft tissue above the midcervical regions. Approximately 7% of males and 14% of females have a high smile or "gummy" smile and display more than 2 mm of gingival above the free gingival margin of the teeth.

The patient may also have greater esthetic demands even when the teeth are out of the esthetic simile and speech zones. Patients complain that the display of longer teeth appears unnatural even though they must lift or move their lips in unnatural positions to see the covered regions of the teeth. As a result of the restored gingival color of the Fp-3, the teeth have a more natural appearance in size and shape and the pink restorative material mimics the interdental papillae and cervical emergence region. The addition of gingival-tone acrylic or porcelain for a more natural fixed prosthesis appearance is often indicated with multiple implant abutments because bone loss is common with these conditions.

There are basically two approaches of denture teeth and acrylic and metal substructure or a porcelain metal restoration. The primary factor that determines the restoration material is the amount of crown height space. An excessive crown height space means a traditional porcelain-metal restoration will have a large amount of metal in the substructure, so the porcelain thickness will not be greater than 2-mm thick. Otherwise there is an increase in porcelain fracture Precious metals are indicated for implant restorations to decrease the risk of corrosion 'and improve the accuracy of the casting, as nonprecious metals shrink more during the casing process. However, the large amount of metal in the substructure acts as a heat sink and complicates the application of porcelain during the fabrication of the prosthesis, In addition, as the metal cools after casting, the thinner regions of metal cool first and create porosities in the structure. This may lead to fracture of the framework after loading. Furthermore when the casting is reinserted into the oven bake the porcelain, the heat is maintained within the casting at different rates, thus the porcelain cool-down rate is variable, which increases the risk of porcelain fracture. In addition, the amount of precious metal in the casting adds to the weight and cost of the restoration. An FP-3 porcelain-to-metal restoration is more difficult to fabricate for the laboratory technician than an FP-2 prosthesis. The pink porcelain is harder to make appear as soft tissue and usually requires more baking cycles. This increases the risk of porosity or porcelain fracture.

An alternative to the traditional porcelain-metal fixed prosthesis is a hybrid restoration (see Table 2). This restoration design uses a smaller metal framework, with denture teeth and acrylic to join these elements together. This restoration is less expensive to fabricate and is highly esthetic because of the premade denture teeth and acrylic pink soft tissue replacements. In addition, the intermediary acrylic between the denture teeth and framework may reduce the impact force of dynamic occlusal loads. The hybrid prosthesis is easier to repair in porcelain fracture, as the denture tooth may be traditional porcelain-metal restoration. However, the fatigue of acrylic is greater than the traditional prosthesis; therefore repair of the restoration is more commonly needed.

The crown height space determination for a hybrid versus the traditional porcelain-metal restoration is 15 mm from the bone to the occlusal plane. When less than this dimension is available, a porcelain-to-metal is suggested. When a greater crown height space is present a hybrid restoration is often fabricated.

Consideration	Porcelain-metal	Hybrid
Occlusal Vertical Dimension	$\leq$15 mm	$\geq$15 mm
Technique	Same	Same
Retention	Cement or screw	Cement or Screw
Precision of fit	Same	Same
Esthetics	Same	Same
Soft tissue	Difficult	Easier
Teeh	Difficult	Easer (resin)
Time/Appointments	Same	Less
Weight	More	Less
Cost	More	Less
Impact forces	More	Less
Volume (bulk)	Same	Same
Lone term	Same	Same
Occlusion	Same	Same
Speech	Same	Same
Hygiene	Same	Same
Complications	Same	Same
Aging of materials	Less	More

Table 2. Comparison of Porcelain-to-Metal versus Hybrid Prostheses (FP-3)

Implants placed too facial, lingual, or in embrasures are easier to restore when vertical bone has been lost and an FP-2 or FP-3 prosthesis is fabricated, because even extremely high smile lip lines do not expose the implant abutments. The greater crown heights allow the correction of incisal edge positions. However, the FP-2 or FP-3 restoration has greater crown height compared with the FP-1 fixed types of prostheses; therefore a greater moment of force is placed on the implant cervical regions, especially during lateral forces(e.g., mandibular excursions or with cantilevered restorations). As a result, should be considered with these restorations.

An FP-2 or FP-3 prosthesis rarely has the patient's interdental papillae or ideal soft tissue contours around the emergence of the crown, because these restorations are used when there is more crown height space and the lip does not expose the soft tissue regions of the patient. In the maxillary arch, wide open embrasures between the implants may cause food impaction or speech problems. These complications may be solved by using a removable soft tissue replacement device or making overcontoured cervical restorations. The maxillary FP-2 or FP-3 prosthesis is often extended or juxtaposed to the maxillary soft tissue so that speech is not impaired. Hygiene is more difficult to control, although access next to each implant abutment is provided.

The mandibular restoration may be left above the tissue, similar to a sanitary pontic. This facilitates oral hygiene in the mandible, especially when the implant permucosal site is level with the floor of the mouth and the depth of the vestibule. However, if the space below the restoration is too great, the lower lip may lack support in the labiomental region.

13.2. Removable prostheses

There are two kinds of removable prostheses, based upon support of the restoration (see Table 1). Patients are able to remove the restoration, but not the implant. Supported superstructure attached to the abutments. The difference in the two categories of removable restorations is not in appearance (as it is in the fixed categories). Instead, the two removable categories are determined by the amount of implant support. The most common removable implant prostheses are over dentures for completely edentulous patients, Traditional removable partial dentures with clasps on implant abutment crowns have not been reported in the literature with any frequency. No long-term or short –term studies are currently available. On the other hand, complete removable overdentures have often been reported with predictability. As a result, the removable prosthetic options are primarily overdentures for the completely edentulous.

13.2.1. RP-4

RP-4 is a removable prosthesis completely supported be the implant, teeth, or both. the restoration is rigid when inserted: overdenture attachments usually connect the removable prosthesis to a low-profile tissue bar or superstructure that splints the implant abutments. Usually five or six implants in the mandible and six to eight implants in the maxilla are required to fabricate completely with favorable dental criteria.

The implant placement criteria for an RP-4 prosthesis is different than for a fixed prosthesis. Denture teeth more acrylic are required for the removable restoration. In addition, a super-structure and overdenture attachments must be added to the implant abutments. This requires a more lingual and apical implant placement in comparison with the implant position for a fixed prosthesis. The implants in an RP-4 prosthesis (and an FP-2 or FP-3 restoration) should be placed in the mesiodistal position for the best biomechanical and hygienic situation. On occasion, the position of an attachment on the superstructure or prosthesis may also affect the amount of spacing between the implants. For example, a Hader clip requires the implant spacing to be greater than 6 mm from edge to edge, and as a consequence reduces the number of implants that may be placed between the mental foramina. The RP-4 prosthesis may have the same appearance as an FP-1, FP-2, or FP-3 restoration. A porcelain-to-metal prosthesis with attachments in selected abutment crowns can be fabricated for patients with the cosmetic desire of a fixed prosthesis,. The overdenture attachments permit improved oral hygiene or allow the patient to sleep without the excess of nocturnal bruxism on the prosthesis.

13.2.2. RP-5

RP-5 is a removable prosthesis combining implant and soft tissue support. The amount of implant support is variable. The completely edentulous mandibular overdenture may have: (1) two anterior mandibular independent of each other; (2) splinted implants in the canine region to enhance retention; (3) three splinted implants in the premolar and central incisor areas to provide lateral stability; or (4) implants splined with a cantilevered bar to reduce soft tissue abrasions and to limit the amount of soft tissue coverage needed for prosthesis support. The primary advantage of an RP-5 restoration is the reduced cost. The prosthesis is very similar to traditional overdentures supported by natural teeth.

A preimplant treatment denture may be fabricated to ensure the patient's satisfaction. This technique is especially indicated for patients with demanding needs and desires regarding the final esthetic result. The implant dentist can also use the treatment denture as a guide for implant placement. The patient can wear the prosthesis during the healing stage. After the implants are uncovered, the superstructure is fabricated within the guidelines of the existing treatment restoration. Once this is achieved, the preimplant treatment prosthesis may be converted to the RP-4 or RP-5 restoration.

The clinician and the patient should realize that the bone will continue to resorb in the soft tissue-bone regions of the prosthesis of the prosthesis. Relines and occlusal adjustments every few years are common maintenance requirements of an RP-5 restoration. Bone resorption with RP-5restorations may occur two to three times faster than the resorption found with full dentures. This can be a factor when considering this type of treatment in young patients, despite the lesser cost and low failure rate.

Author details

Dongliang Zhang[1*] and Lei Zheng[2,3]

*Address all correspondence to: zhangdongliang@hotmail.com

1 Beijing Stomatology Hospital affiliated to Capital University of Medical science, Beijing City, P.R. China

2 Clinical director, Xinya dental, Changchun City, P.R. China

3 The department oral maxillofacial surgery, Jilin University, Chaoyang District, Changchun City, P.R. China

References

[1] Mish CE: Dental education: meeting the demands of implant dentistry, J Am Dent Assoc 121:334-338, 1990.

[2] Davarpanah M, Martinez H, Kebir M, Tecucianu JF, Lazzara RC, et al: Clinical manual of implant dentistry, London, 2003, Quintessence.

[3] Branemark PI, Hansson BO, Adell R, et al: Osseointegrated implants in the treatment of the deentulous jaw. Experience from a 10-year period, Scand J Plast Reconstr Surg 16(Suppl):1-132, 1977

[4] Misch EC, Misch CM: Generic terminology for endosseous implant prosthodontics, J Prosthet Dent 68:809-812, 1992.

[5] Strock AE: Experimental work on dental implantation in the alveolus, Am J Orthod Oral Surg 25:5, 1939.

[6] The glossary of prosthodontics terms, J Prosthet Dent 94: 10-92, 2005.

[7] Misch CE: Consideration of biomechanical stress in treatment with dental implants, Dent Today 25:80,82,84,85; quiz 85, 2006.

[8] Jacobs R, Schotte A, van Steenberghe D et al: Posterior jaw bone resorption in osseointegrated implant overdentures, Clin Oral Implants Res 2:63-70, 1992.

[9] Goodacre CJ, Bernal G, Rungcharassaeng K et al: Clinical complications with implants and implant prosthodontics, J Prosthet Dent 90:121-132, 2003.

[10] Misch CE: Posterior single tooth replacement. In Misch CE, editor: Dental implant prosthetics, St Louis, 2005, Mosby.

Chapter 13

Factors Associated with the Presence of Teeth in the Adult and Elderly Xukuru Indigenous Population in Ororubá, 2010

Cecilia Santiago Araujo de Lima and
Rafael da Silveira Moreira

Additional information is available at the end of the chapter

http://dx.doi.org/10.5772/59415

1. Introduction

Indigenous peoples in Brazil have particular configurations of customs, beliefs and language, forms of integration with the environment, history of interaction with the settlers and relationship with the Brazilian state. Thus insert the different ways in national society [1].

In Brazil, as in many other parts of the world, indigenous peoples are constitute as one of the most disadvantaged segments of the economic, housing, educational standpoint and health indicators, as revealed by the census and other surveys that measure conditions life of the population. In addition, for cultural or relationship with the environment reasons, require specific public policies [1].

The indigenous people Xukuru has the largest indigenous ethnic population group among the 10 ethnic groups of Pernambuco. Located in Pesqueira in the Sierra Ororubá, 216km from Recife (principal city of Pernambuco State) and has a population of approximately 10.000 indigenous [2].

The Xukuru suffered from the loss of traditional lands to allow their social and cultural reproduction and were the target of every source of discrimination, especially from the eighteenth century [3]. After the retaking of their lands the indigenous territory Xukuru now has 25 villages that are distributed in three environmentally bounded regions: the Ribeira, the Serra and the Agreste (Figure 1). The approval of the land in this population resulted in changes in the social context [4] that seems to have contributed in some way to changes in the mode of life of this population. These changes are called acculturation, which is perceived as a result

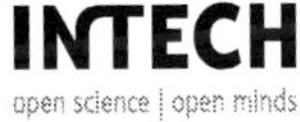

of an exchange process in which two cultures mutually absorb their characteristics and customs generating a new reference.

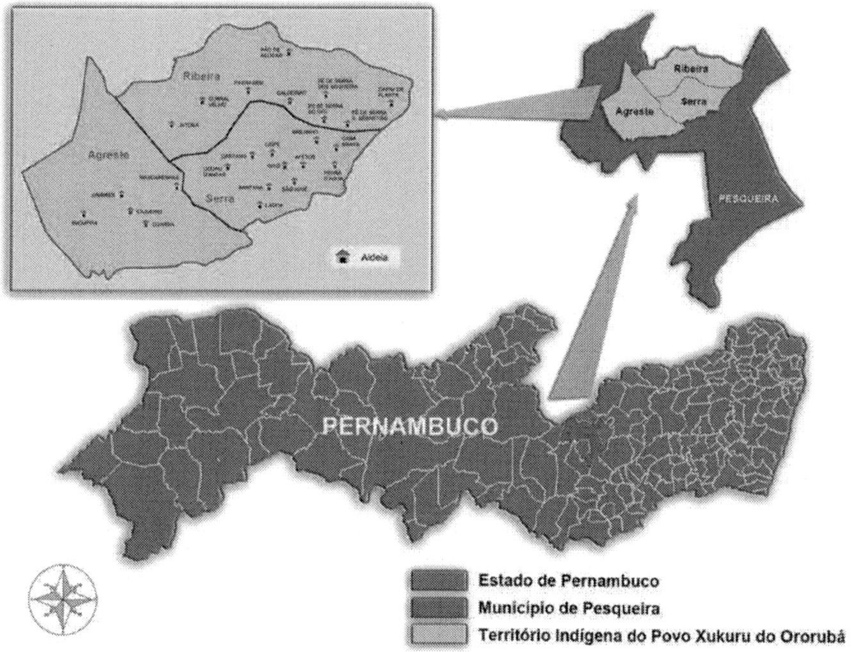

Figure 1. Geographical location of the Indian Territory Xukuru Ororubá and its division according to the socio-environmental regions and villages. Pesqueira, 2010 [5].

The health of indigenous peoples of Brazil presents complex and dynamic way. Is directly related to historical processes of social, economic and environmental changes, linked to the expansion and consolidation of demographic and economic fronts of society in various regions of the country [6].

The epidemiological profile of indigenous peoples is little known, which stems from the insufficiency of investigations, surveys and censuses, as well as the inaccessibility of information on morbidity and mortality systems. Any discussion of the health-disease process of indigenous peoples need to take into consideration, in addition to epidemiological and demographic dynamics, the enormous existing social diversity [7-11].

For proper understanding of the health-disease process on indigenous peoples it is necessary to appeal to the historical relations in which human societies are inserted [10]. Despite the fragmentation and lack of historical data on the history of contact between indigenous people and other population groups in Brazil records, it is known that the effects of this interaction on the profiles of illness and death were significant [12].

The epidemiology of oral health among indigenous peoples in Brazil is little known, which reflects a more general framework of ignorance about the health of these populations [7]. This perspective, intense socioeconomic and environmental changes that have been going these people, including subsistence and diet, are enablers of change in oral health status known aspects [10]. Main responsible for the deterioration in oral health are the changes in the traditional diet (especially intake of sugar and other processed products) and the economic system of this group, together with the lack of a preventive program [13].

From the 1960s, there was an increased incidence of caries, with the determining factor in changing dietary patterns and increased availability of fermentable carbohydrates in the diet. Although caries is a disease that has known and proven effective methods of prevention and control, precarious epidemiological profile found in indigenous populations illustrates the social exclusion of the latter from access to dental care groups and methods of oral health promotion [14].

Caries is the main cause of tooth loss. To a lesser degree are periodontal disease and dental injuries [15]. Tooth loss related to tooth extractions caused by preventable diseases, including, dental caries and periodontal diseases is very high and remains prevalent worldwide despite progress in prevention and early treatment of these diseases [16]. In addition to these diseases, tooth loss is due to attitudes of dental professionals and the public, accessibility and utilization of dental services, the type of financing of the health system and the way to provide dental care. Another primary cause or related of tooth extractions are the economic reasons [17-20].

Social conditions and dental practices hegemonic force the socioeconomically disadvantaged individuals to treat dental pain with extractions. Epidemiological data have shown significant increase of loss with age. In Brazil, the extraction mass begins at age 30 and is the most practical and economical solution for the accumulated oral health problems [16, 21].

The loss of teeth is the most common cause of impaired chewing, being related to the reduction of masticatory ability and perceptions of chewing ability. When associated with difficult access to prostheses result in functional and psychosocial disorders such as poor chewing, speech related problems, employment difficulties, dissatisfaction with appearance, among others. Little attention has been given to the impact that can cause tooth loss in chewing ability and changes in food thereon, which are determinants of nutritional status of these individuals as well as reduced self-esteem and social integration [21-25].

The variables related to tooth loss ranging from dental work (the increase in periodontal attachment loss, number of coronal and root surface caries, tooth mobility and fracture in restoration) to the individual level (the reporting dental pain, the need perceived dental treatment, frustration with dental care, preference for extraction instead of conservative treatment, older age group, black race and female) [26]. Early tooth loss should be considered a predictor of future tooth loss. There are significant correlations between early tooth loss and social variables, such as the human development index, ethnicity, education, income under the minimum wage, lack of fluoridated tap water and people living in cities with fewer than 10,000 inhabitants, which already were reported in other studies [27].

In Australia less than 2% of adults aged 35-54 years have complete tooth loss, but this increases to 36% for people aged 75 years or more [28]. The age distribution of edentulism for indigenous peoples is noticeably different from that of the total population. The level of edentulism is almost five times higher among people aged 35-54 years indigenous than among non-indigenous counterparts (7.6% compared with 1.6%). There is also a noticeable difference for those aged 55-74 years, 21% of indigenous peoples suffer from edentulism compared with 14% of non-Indians [29].

In general, lacking qualitative and quantitative information on the oral health status of indigenous peoples in Brazil, especially longitudinal studies to support an evolution of oral epidemiology. Particularly, in the northeast state of Pernambuco and the paucity of studies on the oral health status of indigenous peoples has become even more alarming which reflects the lack of information on the reality of these peoples and the consequent social exclusion which are submitted. This study aims to contribute to a better understanding of tooth loss in adults and elderly of this indigenous population, studying the factors associated with permanent teeth factors.

2. Methods

2.1. Location and study population

This study consists of a deepening of two studies entitled "Analysis of Living, Health and Vulnerability of Indigenous People Xukuru Ororubá as the tool for the Shares of Primary Health Care" [30] and "Health and Living Conditions of the Indigenous People Xukuru Ororubá of Pesqueira - PE "[31] that were developed in Pesqueira, Northeast Region of Brazil. The field work was developed with the participation of indigenous population only in the period January to March 2010.

2.2. Sampling plan

Due to the larger study have sought to analyze various health situations, the sample size was based on the condition of lower prevalence being studied which was equivalent to a third of the universe. This sampling strategy ensured the representativeness of the smaller study group, with the lowest prevalence being estimated. Consequently allowed the representation of the other study groups. It was found that the population of the ethnic group Xukuru is formed by 7,225 people, 1,896 households dwelling and socio-environmental distributed in 3 regions and 25 villages. From these census data, the sample consisted of 632 households (equivalent to a third of the universe).

The selection of households for the sample is given in a systematic random manner, ensuring all members of the population the same chance of being chosen. To systematize the sample, the following calculation was used: k = N (population) / n (sample). Then, the initial sampling unit was selected by lottery between 1 and k, ie, between the numbers one, two and three. With number three drawn, broke for the selection of households starting at home in 1001, ie, the first home of the village of number one. From there followed the systematization where every three households, the third was selected. This sampling was continued until the last possible home the last village. At the end, 632 households were randomly selected and all the inhabitants of these households who are aged 35-44 years and 60 years and older were included in the sample.

Those who were excluded during the visit had some temporary impossibility (as being hospitalized or sick) or a disability that prevented the completion of the oral clinical examination.

2.3. Instrument for data collection

The instruments for data collection were based on records proposed for the Project SB Brasil 2003 [32] and SB Brasil 2010[33]. The codes and criteria adopted are those proposed by the World Health Organization (WHO) publication *Oral health surveys: basic methods*, fourth edition [34].

Data collection was made up of eight teams formed by a dentist (examiner) and a annotator. Standardization was done as the criteria and approaches used to test intra-examiner and inter-examiner before and during the process of data collection. And were reexamined 5% of the sample that aimed to estimate the agreement of the main study findings.

The local and the organization of the examination areas were defined according to the availability of the site, with natural lighting, ventilation and proximity to a water source needed. The examiner, the annotator and the examined person sat for the exam. The tests were conducted using a combination of a dental mirror with handle, and a specific probe, developed by WHO, known as "CPI probe."

2.4. Description of variables

The dependent variable is being studied to tooth loss that represents the count of missing teeth (varying 0-32 teeth), is due to decay or other reasons.

The independent variables were collected through the questionnaire administered by a health survey and also by the census Xukuru be classified into three categories: Characterization of sociodemographic and socioeconomic profile (place of residence, income, age, sex, attends school, can read and write), Characterization of access to oral health care (dental visits, time of last dental appointment, place of last dental visit, reason for last dental visit) and characterization of self-perception and impact on oral health (dental appointment last assessment services, satisfaction with teeth / mouth, OIDP).

2.5. Processing of data

The data collected were criticized to correct fill failures and processed at the National School of Public Health - ENSP / FIOCRUZ, a partner institution of the Center Aggeu Magalhães - CPqAM / FIOCRUZ this health survey.

Before to the analysis, the database went through a cleansing process in which the entered data were compared with the information provided in the questionnaires. In case they found differences, the database was corrected.

2.6. Data analysis

The data were tabulated in EpiData (version 3.1). Data analysis was initially performed using the statistical package SPSS 13.0® with the distribution of frequencies and description of the measures of central tendency and dispersion. The analyzes were presented in tables.

Association analyzes/dependence were performed by means of parametric or non-parametric tests, depending on the type of distribution and the nature of the variables under study. Effect measures were calculated, emphasizing reason means (RM) and odds ratio (OR) simple and adjusted for confounding variables. For both, negative binomial regression models with inflated zero were adopted in order to check the direction and strength of the effect of independent variables on the outcome analyzed. This model is used when the variable is discrete with quantitative absence of normal distribution and when there is overdispersion of the data distribution [35]. Due to the large number of zeros present in the dependent variable (many adults and especially seniors had missing teeth, or teeth zero), it was recommended the use of this regression model. This model presents two regression coefficients, one for the non inflated zeros (whose measure of effect is the RM and is associated with increased number of teeth) and other coefficients for the part inflated zeros (whose measure is the OR and will be associated with the presence of teeth zero, ie the edentulous). The influence of the factors under study on tooth loss followed the hierarchical model proposed by Victora et al. [36] showed in the Figure 2.

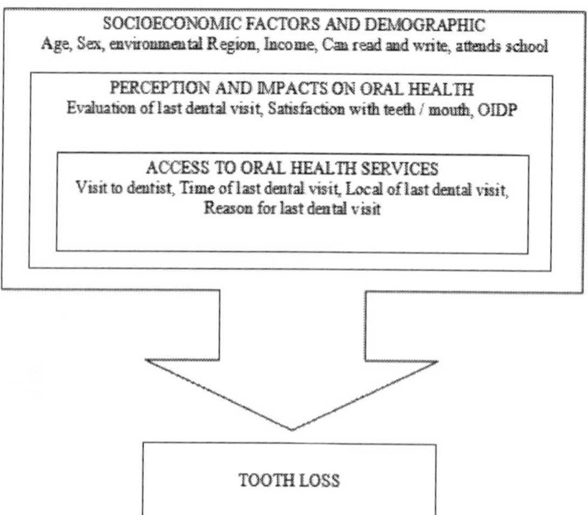

Figure 2. Theoretical Hierarchial Model of variables associated with the presence of permanent teeth. Pesqueira, 2010.

2.7. Ethical aspects

This study was based on "Health and Living Conditions of the Indigenous People Xukuru Ororubá the Pesqueira-PE" which was approved by the Ethics in Research-CEP (CPqAM / Fiocruz) and the National Committee for Research Ethics - CONEP / National Board of Health / Ministry of Health, through Opinion nº 34/2011. The study "Analysis of Living, Health and Vulnerability of Indigenous People Xukuru Ororubá as the tool for the Shares of Primary Health Care" that contains the census Xukuru also obtained approval of the CEP by Opinion nº 604/2009.

The project also received permission from FUNASA for this work, as well as the letter of consent from the ethnic Xukuru Ororubá signed by Cacique Marcos de Araújo Luidson after approval of the Local Council of Indigenous Health Xukuru was obtained and the Consent and Informed (IC) of the political leaders of each village existing in Indian Territory.

3. Results

A sample of the Survey of Health Xukuru the Ororubá constituted 632 selected households. Among these, 27 households were considered lost due to the absence of its residents in the three visits by field staff. Thus, the final sample consisted of 605 households.

The average of the presence of permanent teeth tooth was 10.43 (± 9.79). Table 1 shows the composition of the sample and the average of permanent teeth according to the independent variables. It was observed that 39.0% of individuals residing in the Agreste region of the Indigenous Territory and about 50.7% had an income between R$ 216,00 - 465,00.

The socio-demographic structure of the population studied was 45.6% of adults and 54.4% of elderly, composed mostly of males (50.7%). Among adults with an average age of 39.2 years and among older average age was 70.3 years. It was observed that 58.2% can not read and write and 56.1% have attended school.

Variable		N (%)	Average	±DP	CI 95%	Median	p-value *
Age group	Adults	195 (45,6%)	17,91	7,90	16,80-19,03	19,00	<0,001
	Elderly	233 (54,4%)	4,16	6,15	3,37-4,96	1,00	<0,001
Sex	Male	217 (50,7%)	11,49	9,97	10,15-12,82	10,00	0,010
	Female	211 (49,3%)	9,34	9,50	8,05-10,63	7,00	0,010
Enviromental region	Ribeira	131 (30,6%)	9,90	9,30	8,29-11,52	9,00	0,531
	Serra	130 (30,4%)	10,24	10,13	8,48-12,0	7,50	0,531
	Agreste	167 (39,0%)	11,16	9,95	9,61-12,72	11,00	0,531

	Variable	N (%)	Average	±DP	CI 95%	Median	p-value *
Income	Tertile 1 (R$ 0 - 215,00 reais)	140 (32,7%)	16,68	7,96	15,35-18,01	18,00	<0,001
	Tertile 2 (R$ 216,00 - 465,00)	217 (50,7%)	6,58	8,52	5,44-7,73	3,00	<0,001
	Tertile 3 (R$ 466,00 -1500,00)	62 (14,5%)	8,77	9,76	6,29-11,25	4,00	<0,001
	Missing	9 (2,1%)					
Can read and write	Yes	173 (40,4%)	13,47	9,89	11,98-14,95	13,00	<0,001
	No	249 (58,2%)	8,39	9,19	7,23-9,54	5,00	<0,001
	Missing	6 (1,4%)					
Attends school	Yes	25 (5,8%)	17,56	9,18	13,76-21,35	19,00	<0,001
	No, already attended	240 (56,1%)	11,76	9,74	10,52-13,0	11,00	<0,001
	No, never attended	154 (36,0%)	7,36	8,97	5,93-8,79	4,00	<0,001
	Missing	9 (2,1%)					
Satisfaction with teeth/mouth	Satisfied	235 (54,9%)	7,42	8,70	6,18-8,67	4,0	<0,001
	Neither satisfied nor dissatisfied	31 (7,2%)	12,28	8,35	9,04-15-52	11,50	<0,001
	Dissatisfied	158 (36,9%)	15,48	9,08	13,92-17,03	17,00	<0,001
	Missing	4 (0,9%)					
Review of last visit	Good	345 (80,6%)	10,58	9,66	9,51-11,65	9,00	0,424
	Regular	22 (5,1%)	12,94	8,82	8,69-17,19	14,00	0,424
	Bad	24 (5,6%)	10,81	9,60	6,55-15,07	9,00	0,424
	Missing	37 (8,6%)					
OIDP	No impact	155 (36,2%)	7,85	9,48	6,34-9,35	4,00	<0,001
	One or more impact	233 (54,4%)	13,07	9,40	11,85-14,28	13,00	<0,001
	Missing	40 (9,3%)					
Visit to dentist	Yes	397 (92,8%)	10,11	9,61	9,16-11,06	8,00	0,004
	No	28 (6,5%)	15,92	10,93	11,68-20,16	17,00	0,004
	Missing	3 (0,7%)					
Time of last visit	Less than 1 year	81 (18,9%)	15,37	8,40	13,51-17,22	17,00	<0,001
	1 to 2 years	84 (19,6%)	15,17	8,04	13,43-16,92	16,50	<0,001
	3 years and more	228 (53,3%)	6,62	8,90	5,44-7,79	2,00	<0,001
	Missing	35 (8,2%)					

Variable		N (%)	Average	±DP	CI 95%	Median	p-value *
Local of last visit	Public	241 (56,3%)	12,30	9,54	11,09-13,51	12,00	<0,001
	Particular, health plan, covenants	151 (35,3%)	7,02	8,79	5,58-8,45	3,00	<0,001
	Missing	36 (8,4%)					
Reason for last visit	Review, prevention, treatment and other	71 (16,6%)	13,91	10,42	11,44-16,38	16,00	<0,001
	Pain	47 (11,0%)	12,82	9,25	10,11-15,54	14,00	<0,001
	Extraction	278 (65,0%)	8,71	9,12	7,64-9,79	6,00	<0,001
	Missing	32 (7,5%)					
Total		**428 (100%)**	**10,43**	**9,79**		**9,0**	

*P-value from Mann-Whitney e Kruskall Wallis test.

Table 1. Description of average indigenous Xukuru permanent teeth in adults and the elderly. Pesqueira, 2010.

Regarding the perception and impact on oral health, 235 individuals (54.9%) say they are satisfied with their teeth / mouth, 80.6% rated the last query as good and 54.4% reported one or more impacts on oral health in daily life. Regarding access to dental services, 28 individuals (6.5%) had never been to the dentist, 53.3% had a dental appointment last three years and over and 56.3% held in the public service. The main reason for consultation to 65.0% of the subjects was to perform extraction.

Table 2 shows the results of a single regression model. The average ratio (RM) presented considers the variance present in each level and shown as a measure of effect corrected to factors associated presence of teeth.

Individuals of adult age group showed less tooth loss and RM 2.29. But women showed greater chance of tooth loss (OR = 1.99). Regarding environmental region and income were not significant for tooth loss. Reading and writing (RM = 1.27) is negatively associated to tooth loss as well as those attending (RM = 1.55) or have attended school at some time in life (RM = 1.26).

With regard to the variables of block 2, who says satisfied with teeth / mouth has greater tooth loss (RM = 0.74) and those with a greater number of teeth present in the mouth has more impact on oral health (RM = 1.23). Regarding the last consultation, evaluation dictates how fair and poor is related to having more teeth.

Among the variables in block 3 is important to note that anyone who has ever been to the dentist in life has more chance of not having teeth, or going to the dentist increases by 160% tooth loss than those who have never been. For people who performed the last visit for more than three years average of teeth present was lower (RM = 0.68). Having performed consulting in public service decreased the chance of tooth loss (OR = 0.36) and who was motivated to consultation with the purpose of extracting has fewer teeth (RM = 0.67).

Demographic variables Block 1		Not inflated			Inflated		
		RM	CI 95%	p-value	OR	CI 95%	p-value
Age group	Adults	2,29	2,02-2,59	<0,001	0,05	0,02-0,11	<0,001
	Elderly	1,00			1,00		
Sex	Male	1,00			1,00		
	Female	0,99	0,85-1,15	0.902	1,99	1,29-3,06	0,002
Can read and write	Yes	1,27	1,09-1,47	0,001	0,40	0,25-0,65	<0,001
	No	1,00			1,00		
Attends school	Yes	1,55	1,16-2,07	0,003	0,27	0,02-0,58	0,008
	No, already attended.	1,26	1,08-1,49	0,004	0,48	0,31-0,75	0.001
	No, never attended.	1,00			1,00		
Perception variables Block 2		Not inflated			Inflated		
		RM	CI 95%	p-value	OR	CI 95%	p-value
Satisfaction with teeth/mouth	Satisfied	0,74	0,63-0,86	<0,001	5,73	3,25-10,09	<0,001
	Neither satisfied nor dissatisfied	0,84	0,64-1,11	0,24	2,28	0,84-6,17	0,103
	Dissatisfied	1,00			1,00		
Review of last visit	Good	1,00			1,00		
	Regular	1,02	0,75-1,39	0,878	0,48	0,15-1,49	0,207
	Bad	0,86	0,64-1,17	0,348	0,42	0,13-1,33	0,143
OIDP	No impact	1,00			1,00		
	One or more impact	1,23	1,05-1,44	0,009	0,33	0,21-0,54	<0,001
Acess variables Block 3		Not inflated			Inflated		
		RM	CI 95%	p-value	OR	CI 95%	p-value
Visit to dentist	Yes	0,77	0,59-1,01	0,066	2,60	0,86-7,84	0,088
	No	1,00			1,00		
Time of last visit	Less than 1 year	1,00			1,00		
	1 to 2 years	0,92	0,75-1,12	0,421	0,37	0,10-1,39	0.143
	3 years and more	0,68	0,56-0,82	<0,001	6,78	3,17-14,47	<0,001
Local of last visit	Public	1,29	1,09-1,53	0,002	0,36	0,23-0,57	<0,001
	Particular, health plan, covenants	1,00			1,00		

| Demographic variables | Not inflated | | | Inflated | | |
Block 1	RM	CI 95%	p-value	OR	CI 95%	p-value
Reason for last visit — Review, prevention, treatment and other	1,00			1,00		
Pain	0,85	0,65-1,11	0,251	0,73	0,30-1,77	0,49
Extraction	0,67	0,55-0,81	<0,001	1,29	0,72-2,32	0,38

RM: Ratio of average

OR: Odds Ratio

CI 95%: confidence interval of 95%

Table 2. Average Ratio (RM) and odds ratio (OR) of teeth present estimates of the simple model of zero-inflated negative binomial regression. Pesqueira, 2010.

Table 3 presents the results of multiple hierarchical model, according to the theoretical model presented in Figure 2. Was observed that among the variables in block 1 only age and sex were statistically significant. Being female is an increased likelihood of tooth loss (OR = 2.68). In block 2 only satisfaction variable in the final model and their effects were controlled for block 1.

In block 3 variables time of last visit and reason for last visit remained the final model. A higher probability of not having teeth was related to having made the last visit for more than 3 years (OR = 2.65).

| Demographic variables | Not inflated | | | Inflated | | |
Block 1	RM	CI 95%	p-value	OR	CI 95%	p-value
Age Group — Adults	2,29	2,02-2,59	<0,001	0,04	0,02-0,09	<0,001
Elderly	1,00			1,00		
Sex — Male				1,00		
Female				2,68	1,63-4,43	<0,001
Perception variables	**Not inflated**			**Inflated**		
Block 2	RM	CI 95%	p-value	OR	CI 95%	p-value
Satisfaction with teeth/mouth — Satisfied	0,88	0,78-1,00	0,05	3,40	1,81-6,36	<0,001
Neither satisfied nor dissatisfied	0,95	0,76-1,19	0,69	1,83	0,59-5,63	0,287
Dissatisfied	1,00			1,00		
Acess variables	**Not inflated**			**Inflated**		
Block 3						

Demographic variables Block 1		Not inflated			Inflated		
		RM	CI 95%	p-value	OR	CI 95%	p-value
		RM	CI 95%	p-value	OR	CI 95%	p-value
Time of last visit	Less than 1 year				1,00		
	1 to 2 years				0,33	0,08-1,33	0,118
	3 years and more				2,65	1,05-6,70	0,038
Reason for last visit	Review, prevention, treatment and other	1,00			1,00		
	Pain	0,92	0,75-1,12	0,424	0,19	0,05-0,70	0,012
	Extraction	0,79	0,68-0,92	0,003	0,36	0,15-0,85	0,020

* Adjusted for variables in block 1.

* Adjusted for variables in block 1 and 2.

* Adjusted for variables in block 1, 2 and 3.

RM· Ratio of average

OR: Odds Ratio

CI 95%: confidence interval of 95%

Table 3. Average Ratio (RM) and Odds Ratio (OR) of teeth according to estimates from multiple hierarchical multilevel model of zero-inflated negative binomial regression. Pesqueira, 2010.

4. Discussion

The average number of permanent teeth found in this study was lower than that found by [37]. Adults in this study had an average of 17.91 permanent teeth ($\pm$ 7.90) and older had an average of 4.16 permanent teeth ($\pm$ 6.15). Early tooth loss is considered a predictor of future tooth loss and grows with increasing age. In studies carried out by [37-39] confirmed an increase in the loss of teeth with increasing age.

The increase in edentulism with age seems to be a universal trend, creating the social imaginary figure of the old toothless elderly and the acceptance of tooth loss as a natural evolution of the human dentition, more or less in the sense of "we are born without teeth and die without teeth" [40].

Females had increased likelihood of tooth loss. This finding corroborates the results found in the study done by Indians of the Guarani tribe [39] and in studies of the general population [21, 41, 42]. A possible explanation would be the increased use of dental services by women, resulting in overtreatment would cause the loss of the tooth.

According to [43], increased tooth loss in women reveals some phenomena related to gender differences in health. Among these phenomena, we have the longest life expectancy of women who would be prolonging exposure to determinants of edentulism or the greatest care that the woman spends with their health.

Although the social and environmental areas of study have been insignificant to tooth loss, studies are needed to better understand the influence of acculturation on tooth loss among indigenous.

Although in distinct and involving other human, social, economic and environmental factors timescale, contemporary indigenous groups, once in contact with national societies also experience socio-economic and ecological changes with strong potential to change oral health conditions [10, 44].

When related tooth loss and income observed insignificance, but the study shows that those who have a higher income have less teeth in the mouth. This is due to the elderly who have a higher income than adults and they have fewer teeth than adults. In our study, those who can read and write and who attends or has attended school any time in life, proved to be less chances of tooth loss. These conditions influence the pattern and type of use of oral health services. This model is reaffirmed by [39], where low education is strongly associated with greater tooth loss.

There are significant correlations between early tooth loss and social variables, such as the human development index, ethnicity, education, income under the minimum wage, lack of fluoridation of city water and living in cities with fewer than 10,000 inhabitants, which have already been reported in other studies [27].

However, it is difficult to compare studies of tooth loss among Indians and the general population because of the few relevant studies, different methodologies and different age groups.

Individuals who said they were satisfied with their oral health have fewer teeth. This result is related to the elderly, given the absence of teeth does not seem to impact on daily life. The adults in the study expressed dissatisfaction with oral health, but reported no problems related to functional activity and/or social.

Regarding the visit to the dentist was possible to observe an increased risk of tooth loss. According to[45], considering that the only way to experience tooth loss is to enter the dental care system (with the small exception of the self-extraction), since having access people have increased risk of tooth loss.

The main reason for the last visit was extraction. There are two hypotheses for [26]: firstly, those first decide to remove a tooth due to a specific problem and will extract it to the dentist or, on the other hand, decide to see a dentist first because of a problem specific and go to the dentist to see what can be done. In the first case, the specific symptoms and problems determine the loss of teeth. In the second case, the dental care determines tooth loss and problems and symptoms would have a direct effect on the use of dental services and indirect about losing teeth.

This latter fact reveals the importance of the function of the dentist in maintaining oral health, yet there to highlight all the influence of hegemonic paradigms and dominant ideology contained in the dental practice of a particular historical moment [40]. This is one of the reasons why teeth are extracted could be recovered, since this alternative is considered the most convenient and also the most economical [18, 46].

In the daily routine of the people, the alterations produced by the loss of teeth should be the object of concern of the dental profession [47]. However, the approach of professionals, most often only considers the biological and restorative perspectives, ie, the restoration of teeth should be done according to the best principles of the technique, neglecting the effects of tooth loss in quality of life patients [48, 49].

Considering the results in multilevel analysis, it was possible to contemplate some of the complexity inherent in the health-disease process. This possibility ensured the simultaneous approach of contextual and individual factors in the analysis.

5. Conclusion

This study showed that: the average permanent teeth decreases considerably with advancing age, male sex is what has more teeth, self-perception is a satisfactory condition when there is tooth loss and oral health impacts are mainly perceived on who has more teeth. Access to services reveals a high proportion of the population that has already been to the dentist in public service for over three years and the reason for the visit was tooth extraction.

The differences between the oral health status of indigenous and non-indigenous constitute a framework of inequality between these two populations. It is necessary to rethink the routine visits to the dentist, since the factors associated with the presence of teeth are different for both individuals of the same age group, as different age groups. As well as the services of dental care does not have adequate infrastructure is sufficient to absorb the demand of the indigenous population, especially in adult and elderly.

Considering the epidemiological profile of the indigenous ethnic groups is important to highlight that are developed and put into public policies, in order to seek intervention strategies in oral health care.
Aknowledgements

Aknowledgements to facepe and CNPQ for the financial support.

Author details

Cecilia Santiago Araujo de Lima and Rafael da Silveira Moreira[*]

*Address all correspondence to: moreirars@cpqam.fiocruz.br

Department of Public Health. Oswaldo Cruz Foundation. Aggeu Magalhães Research Center. Recife. Pernambuco, Brazil

References

[1] Instituto Brasileiro de Geografia e Estatística. Censo Demográfico 2010. Característi-cas Gerais dos Indígenas. Resultados do Universo. Rio de Janeiro, p. 1-245, 2010. ftp://ftp.ibge.gov.br/Censos/Censo_Demografico_2010/Caracteristi-cas_Gerais_dos_Indigenas/pdf/Publicacao_completa.pdf (Acesso 26 fev. 2013).

[2] Fundação Nacional de Saúde. Sistema de Informação da Atenção à Saúde Indígena de Pernambuco. Distrito Sanitário Especial Indígena de Pernambuco. Dados demo-gráficos dos índios de Pernambuco. Recife, 2008.

[3] Souza LC. "Doença que rezador cura" e "doença que médico cura": modelo etiológico Xukuru a partir de seus especialistas de cura. [Dissertação de Mestrado em Antropo-logia]. Recife: Universidade Federal de Pernambuco, 2004.

[4] Fundação Nacional do Índio. Atualização do levantamento fundiário do TI Xukuru: relatório GT PP nº 374. Brasília, DF, 2007.

[5] Maurício, H.A. A Saúde Bucal do Povo Indígena Xukuru do Ororubá na Faixa Etária de 10 a 14 anos. [Dissertação Mestrado em Saúde Pública]. Recife: Centro de Pesqui-sas Aggeu Magalhães, Fundação Oswaldo Cruz, 2012.

[6] Leite MS. Transformações e persistência: antropologia da alimentação e nutrição em uma sociedade indígena amazônica. Rio de Janeiro: Editora Fiocruz, 2007.

[7] Coimbra Jr CEA, Santos RV. Saúde, minorias e desigualdade: Algumas teias de inter-relações, com ênfase nos povos indígenas no Brasil. Ciência & Saúde Coletiva, 2000; 5:125-132.

[8] Coimbra Jr CEA, Flowers NM, Santos RV, Salzano FM. The Xavánte in Transition: Health, Ecology, and Bioanthropology in Central Brazil. Ann Arbor: University of Michigan Press; 2002.

[9] Fundação Nacional de Saúde. Política Nacional de Atenção à Saúde dos Povos Indí-genas, 2a Edição, Brasília:FUNASA/Ministério da Saúde; 2002.

[10] Santos RV, Coimbra Jr CEA. Saúde e Povos Indígenas. Rio de Janeiro: Editora Fioc-ruz; 1994. p. 545-566.

[11] Santos RV, Escobar AL. (eds.), 2001. Saúde dos povos indígenas no Brasil: Perspecti-vas atuais. Cadernos de Saúde Pública, 17(2) (número temático).

[12] Basta PC, Orellana, JDY. Arantes R. Perfil epidemiológico dos povos indígenas no Brasil: notas sobre agravos selecionados.In: Garnelo L, Pontes AL. Saúde Indígena: uma introdução ao tema. Brasília: MEC-SECADI, 280 p., 2012.

[13] Arantes R. Saúde oral de uma comunidade indígena Xavante do Brasil central: uma abordagem epidemiológica e bioantropológica. Dissertação (Mestrado em Saúde Pública) - Escola Nacional de Saúde Pública. Rio de Janeiro, 1998.

[14] Arantes R. Saúde bucal dos povos indígenas no Brasil: panorama atual e perspectivas. In: Coimbra Jr CEA, Santos RV, Escobar AL (organizadores). Epidemiologia e saúde dos povos indígenas do Brasil. Rio de Janeiro: Abrasco/Fiocruz; 2003. p. 49-72.

[15] Jovino-Silveira RC, Caldas Jr. AF, Souza EH, Gusmão ES. Primary reason for tooth extraction in a Brazilian adult population. Oral Health Prev Dent 2005; 3:151-7.

[16] Pinto VG. Epidemiologia das doenças bucais no Brasil. In: Kriger L. (Org.) Promoção da saúde bucal. São Paulo: Artes Médicas-Aboprev; 1997.

[17] Burt BA, Eklund AS. Dentistry, dental practice and the community. 4th Ed. Philadelphia: W.B. Saunders Company; 1992.

[18] Pinto VG. Saúde bucal coletiva. 4a Ed. São Paulo: Editora Santos; 2000.

[19] Barros AJD, Bertoldi AD. Desigualdades na utilização e no acesso a serviços odontológicos: uma avaliação em nível nacional. Ciência Saúde Coletiva 2002; 7:709-17.

[20] Cabral ED, Caldas Jr. AF, Cabral HA. Influence of the patient's race on the dentist's decision to extract or retain a decayed tooth. Community Dent Oral Epidemiol 2005; 33:461-6.

[21] Barbato PR, Nagano HCM, Zanchet FM, Boing AF, Peres MA. Perdas dentárias e fatores sociais demográficos e de serviços associados em adultos brasileiros: uma análise dos dados do Estudo Epidemiológico Nacional (Projeto SB Brasil 2002-2003). Cad Saúde Pública. 2007; 23(8):1803-14.

[22] Moyniham P. Bradbury J. Compromised Dental Function and Nutricion. Nutricion, United States, 2001 feb; 17(2): 177-178.

[23] N'Gom PI, Woda A. Influence of impaired mastication on nutricion. J. Prosthet Dent, United States, 2002 feb; 87(6): 667-673.

[24] Marcenes W, Steele JG, Sheiham A, Walls AWG. The relationship between dental status, food selection, nutrient intake, nutricional status, and body mass index in older people. Cad Saúde Pública, Rio de Janeiro, 2003 mai-jun; 19: 809-816.

[25] Musacchio E, Perissinotto E, Binotto P, Sartori L, Silva-Netto F, Zambon S, et al. Tooth loss in the elderly and its association with nutritional status, socio-economic and lifestyle factors. Acta Odontol Scand 2007; 65:78-86.

[26] Gilbert GH, Miller MK., Duncan RP, Ringelberg ML, Dolan TA, Foerster U. Tooth-specific and person level predictors of 24-month tooth loss among older adults. Community Dent Oral Epidemiol 1999; 27:372-85.

[27] Frazão P, Antunes JLF, Narvai PC. Perda dentária precoce em adulto de 35 a 44 anos de idade. Estado de São Paulo, Brasil, 1998. Rev Bras Epidemiol. 2003; 6(1): 49-57.

[28] Slade GD, Spencer AJ, Roberts-Thomson KF. Australia's dental generations: the national survey of adult oral health 2004-06. Canberra: Australian Institute of Health and Welfare 2007.

[29] Williams S, Jamieson L, MacRae A, Gray C. Review of Indigenous oral health. 2011. http://www.healthinfonet.ecu.edu.au/oral_review (Acesso 20 jan. 2013).

[30] Costa AM *et al.* Projeto de pesquisa: Análise das condições de vida, saúde e vulnerabilidade do povo indígena Xukuru do Ororubá como ferramenta para as ações de atenção primária de saúde. Projeto submetido ao edital FACEPE 09/2008 - Pesquisa para o SUS: Gestão compartilhada em saúde PPSUS – Pernambuco MS/CNPQ/ FACEPE/SES. Recife: CPqAM/FIOCRUZ, 2009.

[31] Costa AM *et al.* Projeto de pesquisa: Saúde e condições de vida do povo indígena Xukuru do Ororubá, Pesqueira – PE. Projeto submetido ao Edital CNPq – Chamada: Edital MCT/CNPq Nº 014/2008 – Universal. Recife: CPqAM/FIOCRUZ, 2009.

[32] Brasil. Ministério da Saúde. Projeto SB Brasil 2003: Condições de saúde bucal da população brasileira 2002-2003: resultados principais. Brasília: Ministério da Saúde; 2004.

[33] Brasil. Ministério da Saúde. Projeto SB Brasil 2010 – Manual da Equipe de Campo. Brasília – DF: 2009. www.saude.gov.br/bucal (Acesso 15 jan. 2013).

[34] World Health Organization. Oral health surveys: basic methods. 4 ed. Geneva; 1997.

[35] Gschlößl S, Czado C. Modelling count data with overdispersion and spatial effects. Statistical papers, 2008; 49(3): 531-532.

[36] Victora CG, Huttly SR, Fuchs SC, Olinto MT. The role of conceptual frameworks in epidemiological analysis: a hierarchical approach. Int J Epidemiol 1997; 26: 224–227.

[37] Ulhôa Netto, E.; Ferreira, T. F. L.; Drummond, M. M.; Sanchez, H. F.; Tooth loss and need of denture in Pataxó Natives. Rev Gaúcha Odontol., 2012 abr./jun; 60(2): 195-201.

[38] Arantes R, Santos RV, Coimbra Jr CEA. Saúde bucal na população indígena Xavante de Pimentel Barbosa, Mato Grossso, Brasil. Cad. Saúde Pública, 2001 mar.-abr; 17(2): 375-384.

[39] Alves Filho P, Santos RV, Vettore M V. Saúde bucal dos índios Guarani no Estado do Rio de Janeiro, Brasil. Cad. Saúde Pública, 2009 jan; 25(1): 37-46.

[40] Moreira RS, Nico LS, Tomita NE. O risco espacial e fatores associados ao edentulismo em idosos em município do Sudeste do Brasil. Cad. Saúde Pública, 2011 out; 27(10): 2041-2053.

[41] Susin C, Oppermann RV, Haugejorden O, Albandar JM. Tooth loss and associated risk indicators in an adult urban population from south Brazil. Acta Odontol Scand 2005; 63:85-93.

[42] Silva DD, Rihs LB. Sousa M LR. Fatores associados à presença de dentes em adultos de São Paulo, Brasil. Cad. Saúde Pública, Rio de Janeiro, 2009 nov; 25(11): 2407-2418.

[43] Moreira RS. Perda dentária em adultos e idosos no Brasil: a influência de aspectos individuais, contextuais e geográficos. [Tese Mestrado Acadêmico em Saúde Pública]. São Paulo: Faculdade de Saúde Pública, Universidade de São Paulo, 2009.

[44] Wirsing R. The health of traditional societies and effects of acculturation. Current Anthropology 1985; 26: 303-322.

[45] Gilbert GH, Duncan RP, Shelton BJ. Social determinants of tooth loss. Health Service Research 2003; 38: 1843-1862.

[46] Guimarães MM, Marcus B. Expectativa de perda de dente em diferentes classes sociais. REVCROMG 1996; 2(1): 16-20.

[47] Chianca TK, Deus MR, Dourado AS, Leão AT, Vianna RBC. El impacto de la salud bucal en calidad de vida. Rev Fola/oral 1999; 16: 96-102.

[48] Wolf SMR. O significado da perda dos dentes em sujeitos adultos. Rev Assoc Paul Cir Dent. 1998; 52(4): 307-315.

[49] Vargas AMD, Paixão HH. Perda dentária e seu significado na qualidade de via de adultos usuários de serviço público de saúde bucal do Centro de Boa Vista, em Belo Horizonte. Cien Saude Colet 2005; 10(4): 1015-1024.

like influenza and pneumonia are the fifth leading cause of death among elderly persons. Among the many infections to which the elderly are prone, some can be prevented by administration of suitable vaccines. Vaccination of the elderly can be one of the most effective and economic methods means of prevention of long term disease, disability, or death resulting from communicable illnesses [22].

There is an urgent need to train the entire oral health team to meet the needs (including oral health promotion) of older people [19]. A multidisciplinary team approach is needed, involving a complete team of oral health specialists & other primary health care providers (medical and allied health). The poor oral health status of people in residential aged care hospices is clear evidence that the requisite objectives are not achieved with current health planning. There is a need for a fresh approach to ensure that appropriate medical and oral health treatment needs are met within residential facilities for geriatric individuals [23 – 25].

7. Conclusion

Oral health while being important at all stages of life assumes greater value at extreme old age. Worldwide, people are living longer lives as a result of better understanding of disease processes, health concerns, and imprcvements in overall standards of hygiene and living conditions. Paradoxically, this does not signify that they are necessarily living healthier lives- chronic systemic diseases including oral diseases are on the rise. A decline in oral health is manifested as higher numbers of missing teeth, rise in caries index, and an increase in the prevalence rates of periodontal disease, xerostomia and oral pre-cancer/cancer. Non-communicable diseases are fast becoming the leading causes of disability and mortality, and in the near future health and social policy-makers will face tremendous challenges posed by the rapidly increasing burden of chronic diseases in old age.

The negative impact of poor oral conditions on the quality of life of older adults is an important public health issue, that must be addressed by health care planners at all levels. The need of the hour is to translate knowledge into action programmes for the oral health of older people. It is the responsibility of National health planners to develop policies and set priorities and targets for satisfactory oral health. National public health programmes should incorporate oral health promotion and disease prevention based on the common risk factors approach. In developing countries the challenges to provision of effective oral health care are predominantly high because of a variety of factors related to vast populations and the resultant disparity between the rich and the poor. In developed countries too, oral health services need to be revised to take a preventive approach when considering the oral care needs of older people. Funding for better research for optimum oral health should focus beyond just the biomedical and clinical aspects of oral disease. Private-Public partnerships must be encouraged to allow research and efforts to translate science into practice. Education and continuous training must ensure that oral health care providers have the requisite skills and a thorough understanding of the biomedical and psychosocial aspects of care for geriatric group of patients. It is imperative for all of us to undertake whatever we can do to ensure that the oral health care needs of the aged are met before it is too late. A sustainable plan to mitigate the spread of oral disease and illness in older adults should be strengthened by means of an organized, affordable, comprehensive oral health service which can be easily accessed by all.

Author details

Derek S J D'Souza*

Address all correspondence to: dsjdsouza@gmail.com

Pune, India

References

[1] Improving oral health amongst the elderly. World Health Organization Geneva. http://www.who.int/oral_health/action/groups/en/index1.html

[2] Shah N. Oral health care system for elderly in India. Geriatrics and Gerontology International 2004; 4: S162– S164.

[3] Bagg J. The oral micro flora and dental plaque. Essentials of microbiology for dental students. Oxford: Oxford University Press: 1999; 229 – 310

[4] Bhaskar SN. Oral pathology in the dental office: study of 20,575 biopsy specimens. JADA 1968; 76:761-71.

[5] Avlund K, Holm-Pedersen P, Schroll M. Functional ability and oral health among older people: A longitudinal study from age 75 to 80. J Am Geriatr Soc 2001; 49:954-62

[6] Marshall TA, Warren JJ, Hand JS, Xie X-J, Stumbo PJ. Oral health, nutrient intake and dietary quality in the very old. J Am Dent Assoc 2002; 133:1369-79.

[7] Atwood DA. Reduction of residual ridge: a major oral disease entity. J Prosthet Dent 1971; 26(3):266-79.

[8] Tallgren A. The continuing reduction of alveolar residual ridges in complete denture wearers: A mixed-longitudinal study covering 25 years. J Prosth Dent 1972; 27:120-32

[9] Nishimura I, Atwood DA. Knife-edge residual ridge: a clinical report. J Prosthet Dent 1994 Mar; 71(3):231-4.

[10] Bernier S, Shotwell J, Razzoog M. Clinical evaluation of complete dentures therapy: Examiner consistency. J Prosthet Dent 1984; 51(5):703-08.

[11] Langer A, Michman J, Seifert I. Factors influencing satisfaction with complete dentures in geriatric patients. J Prosthet Dent 1961; 11:1019-31.

[12] Vermeulen AH, Keltjens HM, Van't Hof MA, Kayser AF. Ten-year evaluation of removable partial dentures: survival rates based on retreatment, not wearing and replacement. J Prosthet Dent 1996 Sep; 76(3):267-72.

[13] Ritchie GM. A report of dental findings in a survey of geriatric patients. Journal of Dentistry 1973; 1:106-12.

[14] Budtz-Jörgensen E. Clinical aspects of Candida infection in denture wearers. J Am Dent Assoc 1978; 42: 619-23.

[15] Ettinger RL. The aetiology of inflammatory papillary hyperplasia. J Prosthet Dent 1975; 34:254-61.

[16] Bastiaan RJ. Denture sore mouth Aetiological aspects and treatment. Aust Dent J 1976; 21:375-82.

[17] Chalmers JM. Oral diseases in older adults. In: Chalmers JM et al. Ageing and Dental Health. AIHW Dental Statistics and Research Series No. 19. Adelaide: The University of Adelaide. 1999.

[18] Chalmers JM. Oral health promotion for our ageing Australian population. Australian Dental Journal 2003; 48(1): 2-9.

[19] Hopcraft MS, Morgan MV, Satur JG, Wright FA. Utilizing dental hygienists to undertake dental examination and referral in residential aged care facilities. Community Dent Oral Epidemiol. 2011 Aug; 39(4):378-84.

[20] Adachi M, Ishihara K, Abe S, Okuda K, Ishikawa T. Effect of professional oral health care on the elderly living in nursing homes. Oral Surg Oral Med Oral Pathol Oral Radiol Endod. 2002 Aug; 94(2):191-5.

[21] Kokubu K, Senpuku H, Tada A, Saotome Y, Uematsu H. Impact of routine oral care on opportunistic pathogens in the institutionalized elderly. J Med Dent Sci. 2008 Mar; 55(1):7-13.

[22] Verma R, Khanna P, Chawla S. Vaccines for the elderly need to be introduced into the immunization program in India. Hum Vaccin Immunother. 2014 Jun 23; 10(8). [Epub ahead of print]

[23] Morino T, Ookawa K, Haruta N, Hagiwara Y, Seki M. Effects of professional oral health care on elderly: randomized trial. Int J Dent Hyg. 2014 Nov; 12(4): 291- 7.

[24] Ishikawa A, Yoneyama T, Hirota K, Miyake Y, Miyatake K. Professional oral health care reduces the number of oropharyngeal bacteria. J Dent Res. 2008 Jun; 87(6):594-8.

[25] Petersen PE, Kandelman D, Arpin S and Ogawa H. Global oral health of older people – Call for public health action. Community Dental Health (2010) 27, (Supplement 2) 257–268.

Orthodontics

Chapter 15

White Spots Lesions in Orthodontic Treatment and Fluoride — Clinical Evidence

Hakima Aghoutan, Sana Alami, Farid El Quars, Samir Diouny and Farid Bourzgui

Additional information is available at the end of the chapter

http://dx.doi.org/10.5772/59265

1. Introduction

Orthodontic treatment aims to improve functions and facial aesthetics by ensuring harmonious occlusal and jaw relationship; with beneficial effects on the oral health and quality of life of patients. However, it also associates risks and complications. Enamel surface demineralization or white spots lesions (WSL) remain by far one of the major adverse sequelae of fixed ortho‐dontic appliance therapy, despite techniques and materials advances in preventive dentistry and orthodontics. They appear during and sometimes persist after orthodontic treatment; they can compromise the successful outcome of the treatment and result in the early termination of treatment. In severe cases of WSL, invasive interventions can be required and clinician responsibility may also be engaged.

WSL seem to be related to the interaction of several factors including inadequate elimination of dental plaque due to intrabuccal appliances that limit the self-cleansing mechanism of the oral musculature and saliva, patient's modifying factors and change in bacterial flora during fixed appliances wear. [1, 2]

Considering how quickly these lesions can develop, prevention, early diagnosis and treatment remain one of the greatest challenges facing orthodontists and requires a thorough knowledge of the caries disease and the risk factors specific to each patient. These risk factors should be accurately evaluated before and during any orthodontic treatment in order to minimize tooth decay and discoloration that could compromise the aesthetic of smile. Early detection of WSL during orthodontic treatment would allow clinicians to implement preventive measures to control the demineralization process before lesions progress.

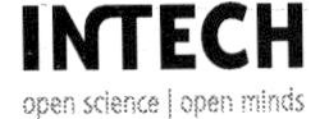

The non-invasive prophylactic techniques are of critical importance during orthodontic treatment in order to decrease the incidence of demineralization. They involve either decreasing the amount of plaque by maintaining good dietary and oral hygiene, or tackling the susceptibility of enamel to demineralization [3]. Among suitable caries preventative agents, fluoride agents are usually used to reduce enamel decalcification and enhance its mineralization since fluoride contains bactericide and bacteriostatic properties.

The aim of this chapter is to outline the evidence regarding the effectiveness of fluoride administration in the prevention and management of WSL during orthodontic treatment.

2. White spot lesions in orthodontic treatment

WSLs have been defined as "subsurface enamel porosity from carious demineralization" that is located on smooth surfaces and presents as "a milky white opacity" [4] due to consequential changes in the optical properties of the enamel [1]. Various risk factors can contribute to the development of these incipient lesions. Poor oral hygiene, low salivary volume and a sugary diet promote the proliferation and activity of the microbial biofilm for a period of time. Orthodontic treatments are known as non-negligible factors and equal susceptibility has been reported whether teeth are banded or bonded.

The levels of oral bacteria have been reported to increase five folds upon the application of fixed bonds [5]. So orthodontic patients develop significantly more WSLs than non-orthodontic patients [1, 4]. The fitting of fixed orthodontic appliances (figure 1) (brackets, bands, arch wires, springs, elastomeric modules…) makes oral hygiene very difficult, restricts salivary self-cleaning and creates more stagnation areas for plaque; encouraging a lowering of plaque pH in the presence of carbohydrates and forming a physical barrier prevent remineralization by calcium and phosphate ions from the saliva. All these changes in the oral ecosystem favor colonization of aciduric bacteria, resulting in a rise in the levels of mutans streptococci and lactobacilli, mainly around the bonding adhesives [6, 7]. This can disrupt balance between the processes of demineralization and remineralization in favor of demineralization, and would lead to the permanent formation of white spot lesions. To these conditions, one must add the duration of orthodontic treatment: the longer the time of oral appliances' wearing is; the most prolonged the caries risk is. WSLs can develop into cavities and can no longer be reversed even in smooth surfaces that would normally have a low risk of caries [5, 8]. Tipping the balance back toward remineralization is the basis of WSL treatment although they can remain as cosmetic scars. However, even if high levels of mutans streptococci and lactobacilli in plaque indicate an increased risk of caries, the prediction of caries development based on bacterial counts is uncertain and it is of minor clinical significance [1, 9].

On the other hand, resting salivary flow rate rises during fixed appliance therapy; which increases salivary pH and buffer capacity and thus counteract the tendency for demineralization to occur around orthodontic appliances in some patients despite moderate plaque scores. This is especially true in individuals with good dietary regimen [5, 9]. Therefore, an assessment of patients' susceptibility In order to identify those most at risk of demineralization prior to

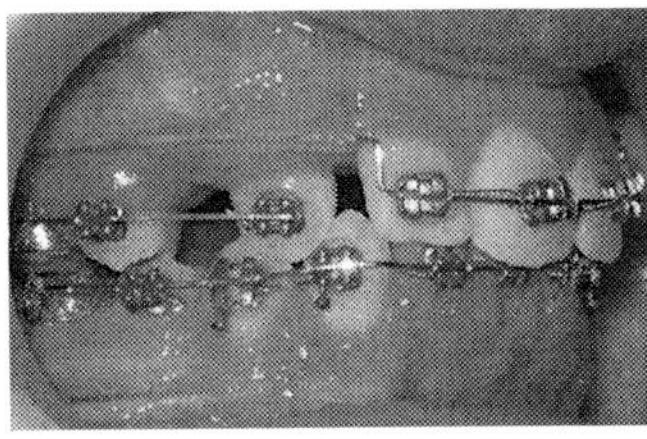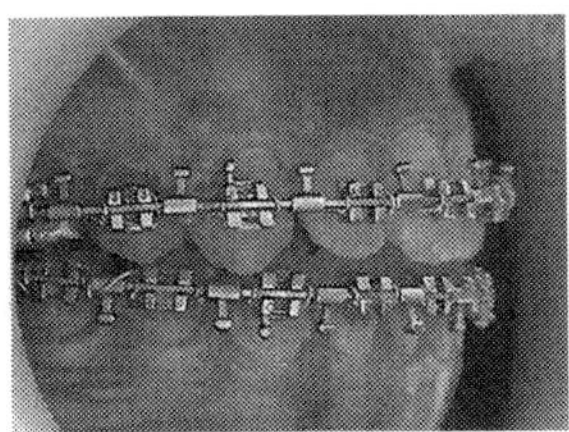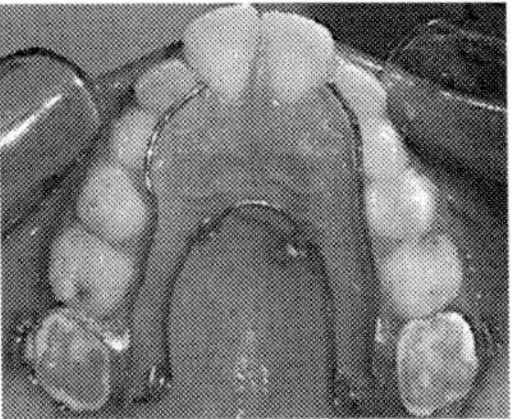

Figure 1. Fixed oral appliances increase stagnation areas of plaque and make oral hygiene difficult to carry out.

orthodontic treatment seems decisive. It was shown that subclinical demineralization before treatment may be a factor in the incidence of WSL during fixed appliance treatment [8].

In addition, orthodontic treatment is most often applied during adolescence, when the permanent teeth, recently erupted, are more vulnerable to caries because of their young enamel. Consequently, orthodontic treatment at this age will favor the formation of carious lesions in particular with the lack of cooperation encountered more frequently in this age group [10].

Commonly identified when the teeth are dry, WSL appears clinically as an opaque whitish or greyish halo under loose bands and around the bracket base periphery generally at the junction between the cement and the enamel, and at the gum level at the base of the half moon bracket (Figure 2). Studies show that these lesions can appear within a span of 4 weeks [11], which is even shorter than the time between two sessions of orthodontic appointments. Caries lesions may also develop after debonding in association with bonded retainer [1]. Furthermore, appliances' removing and tooth polishing cause a loss of the superficial enamel layer, rich in fluorine. This favors plaque retention due to porous enamel surface and thus decalcification. However, these alterations can gradually fade with natural abrasion and hygiene measures.

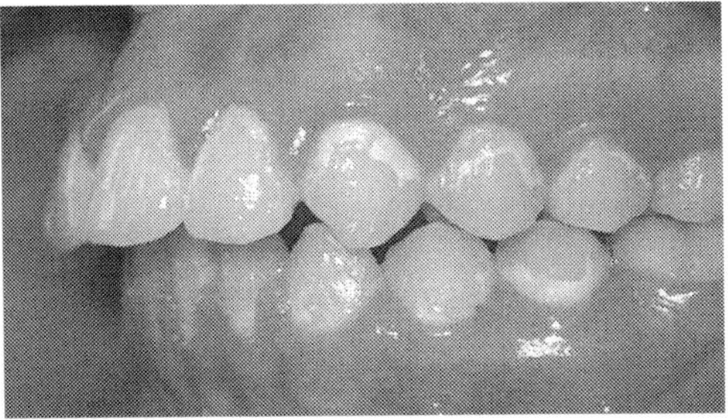

Figure 2. White spot lesions after orthodontic treatment localized at the gingival areas of teeth.

Since Zachrisson and Zachrisson (1971), WSL has been reported as a clinical observation [12]. Over the years, quantitative studies on decalcification incidence and prevalence have been reported. Depending on the examination technique used, the prevalence of WSL varies widely in the literature. It ranges from 23% and 89% when the teeth have been inspected using visual scales and photographic evaluation [8, 13-16].

Boersma et al. [16], using quantitative light fluoroscopy, investigated the prevalence of WSLs at the end of orthodontic treatment and reported that 97% of subjects had one or more lesions and on average, 30% of the buccal surfaces in a person were affected.

The large variation in reported prevalence may also be due to sample size disparity, the use or otherwise of a fluoride regimen during treatment and whether developmental or not other idiopathic enamel lesions, which artificially increases the prevalence quoted, are included or excluded [18].

Clinical studies [8, 13, 15, 19] have showed a sharp increase in the number of WSL during the first 6 months of treatment that continued to rise at a slower rate to 12 months; supporting the idea that the presence of fixed orthodontic appliances and greater treatment lengths serve as a risk factor for WSL formation. Hence, oral hygiene status of patients should be evaluated during the initial months of treatment and, if necessary, measures to prevent demineralization should be implemented.

With regard to the location of these lesions, studies have shown a significant increase in the prevalence on the cervical and middle thirds of the crowns. But they can broadly extend over the teeth surface and sometimes involve proximal extensions. The teeth most vulnerable to demineralization are the first permanent molars, the maxillary incisors, the mandibular lateral incisors and canines [1, 16, 18]. Premolars have also been reported to have greater frequency of WSL [8], and the lowest incidence was in the maxillary posterior segment. According to Samawi 2005 [In 18], upper anterior teeth showed larger mean demineralization surface area than anterior teeth in the lower arch; and the distogingival quadrant was particularly more affected than the mesiogingival quadrant in the upper lateral incisor teeth.

In a study conducted by Arneberg and coworkers [20], the bonded upper incisors have presented the lowest levels of total plaque fluoride and the lowest PH (as low as 4) during resting and fermenting conditions. This can be explained by both a prolonged retention of acids in plaque due to the slow salivary clearance at these sites, and also by loss of fluoride reservoirs associated with limited cariostatic effect of fluoride under low PH.

Regardless of WSL treatment approach, these conditions are difficult to treat and recover to some extent depending on the degree of their severity. Currently, there is a lack of conclusive long-term studies on WSL modifications after orthodontic treatment, but some clinical data can be stated. Once the orthodontic appliances have been removed and oral hygiene is restored, the area of WS was shown to decrease markedly during the first and second years following treatment [21, 22]. The most likely reason for this clinical healing can be explained by removal of the primary etiologic factor which is the cariogenic plaque adhered to fixed orthodontic elements, combined with enamel surface wear during tooth brushing and also by remineralization [1, 22]. However, some spots secondary to debonding can last from 6 to 12 years [22, 23] and ddo not not reach the pre-treatment level even 12 years after debonding [22]. Natural remineralization through saliva, involving mineral gain in the surface layer of WSL, has little improvement on the aesthetics and structural properties of the deeper lesions [24]. Evidence of success is characterized clinically by the recuperation of hardness and shine, whereas translucency is not always recovered. Indeed, WSL can take up stain and become discolored after many years. Therefore, it is necessary to apply remineralizing agents as early as possible for better aesthetic results.

3. Fluoride in management of orthodontic-related white spot lesions

Patients wearing orthodontic appliances are considered as patients at risk, for whom a preventive approach should be implemented before, during and after orthodontic treatment. Controlling risk factors, in addition to awareness of bucco-dental hygiene, and early diagnosis of WSL are key elements of success to reduce their prevalence and incidence during orthodontic treatment.

Both office-applied and self-care programs have been described for preventive and curative approaches of WSL. In self-administered programs, compliance has been identified as a significant problem.

Little information is available about measures that are really used in orthodontic practices to prevent and treat demineralization. But several procedures have been described in association with oral-hygiene instructions and patients' motivation. Reducing enamel susceptibility to demineralization by periodical professional fluoride application and varnishing reside at the bottom of the intervention hierarchy, and therefore represents the frontline of incipient caries treatment.

Actually, it has been known for many years that fluoride reduces the incidence of dental caries by maintaining the plaque fluoride supersaturated with respect to Fluor apatite, hence tipping the balance of the caries process in favor of remineralization. While full mineral recovery might be achieved through fluoride measures in the case of shallow enamel lesions in both children and adults, long-existing white spot lesions have demonstrated negligible remineralization after further contact with fluorides [25]. Upon failure of remineralization measures by fluoride agents in active lesions, other conservative procedures, such as resin sealing, have been advocated as alternative measures to prevent demineralization progression and cavitation.

There are two main methods of fluoride administration. However, there is little evidence about which fluoride supplement provides the greatest decrease in decalcification: In topical form, active ingredients are supplied in forms such as a toothpaste, mouth rinse, gel, varnish, mousse, pastille, or by adding it to chewing gum. Professionals usually apply gels and varnishes, particularly if they contain a high concentration of fluoride, whereas the other means of topical application can be self-administered. The second way is the use of materials containing the active ingredient fluoride as part of the appliance, either as a bonding or banding material, or an auxiliary such as a glass bead or elastic [3].

When topical fluoride is applied, a calcium fluoride-like material (CaF2) builds up in plaque, on the tooth surface or in incipient lesions. The CaF2 acts as a reservoir of fluoride ions for release when pH is lowered during a carious attack. When associated with phosphate ions,

CaF2 becomes more soluble and release fluoride at higher rate than the pure substance [1]. The preventive effect of fluoride can be illustrated using the Stephan curve (Figure 3). The limit of the fluoride effect is reached when pH drops below 4.5 so the solubility product of pure Fluor apatite is exceeded and no remineralization occurs. In old, acidic plaque a dose response to fluoride may not be apparent against lesion progression due to the low pH [26].

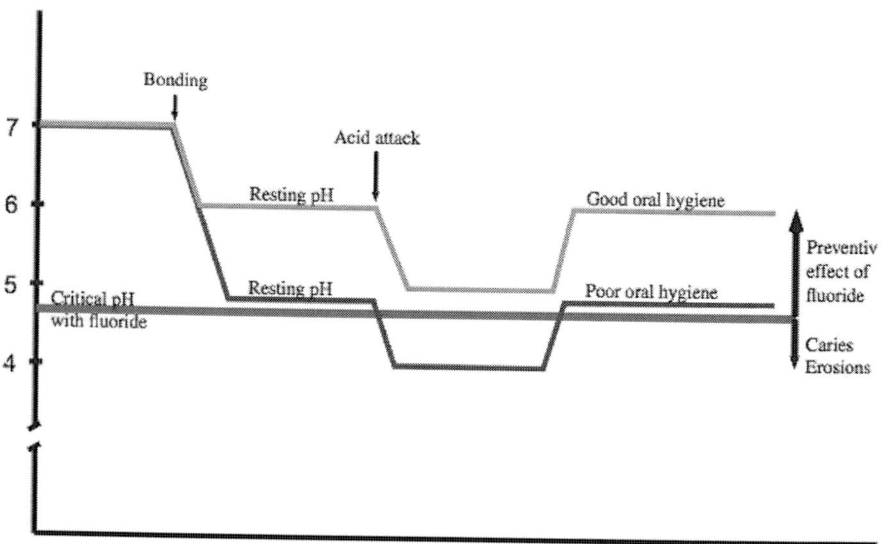

Figure 3. The Stephan curves in orthodontic patients with good or bad oral hygiene. After bonding, resting pH is lowered. An acid attack lowers the pH in the patient with bad oral hygiene below the critical pH of enamel. Assuming fluoride is frequently used, the critical pH of enamel is around 4.5 compared with 5.5 in the absence of fluoride. In the patient with good oral hygiene, fluoride is able to prevent lesions to develop. [1]

All these findings make optimal oral hygiene a crucial element that should be associated with fluoride prevention against WSL. Orthodontist must be cautious to create more favorable conditions to implement good oral hygiene by patients. Hence, the close fitting of bands on teeth is recommended and all excess bonging material around the attachment base should be eliminated. Also excessive surplus orthodontic etching of the complete labial enamel surface, instead of the bracket bases only, must be avoided to prevent iatrogenic white spot lesions [27], and steel ligatures or self-ligating brackets must be preferable to elastic ligatures [28]. (Figure 4)

According to Øgaard [1, 26], it is logical to differentiate between prevention of caries lesion development during orthodontic treatment and treatment of lesions present on labial surfaces at debonding. Clinical approaches differ in the two situations.

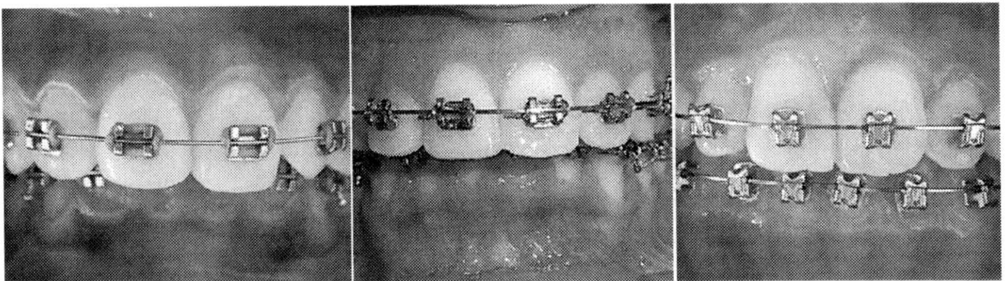

Figure 4. Different styles of ligatures: elastic ligatures (left) tend to discolor and increase the risk of plaque aggregation.

3.1. Fluoride prevention during orthodontic treatment

3.1.1. Oral-hygiene instructions

Clinical maintenance by elimination of plaque and food debris is essential throughout any orthodontic treatment as there is a much stronger relationship between oral hygiene and caries incidence in orthodontic patients than in non-treated individuals [26]. Therefore satisfactory level of oral hygiene should be successfully maintained despite the hindrance of the appliance.

Among the self-applied fluoride products available, toothpaste used in tooth brushing is thought to be the most important. Fluoridated toothpaste exerts a cariostatic effect. It increases fluoride levels in the biofilm, where it acts as an inhibitor of bacterial enzymes, and can reduce the frequency of caries by 15–30% [29]. Authors [30] have emphasized the need for at least two daily brushings in order to favor a continuous exchange of fluoride ions between the salivary and the enamel surface. The availability of fluoride from toothpaste is influenced by several factors, such as the concentration of fluoride, the amount of toothpaste used, and the post-brushing behavior (Davies and Davies, 2008; Zero et al., 2010 (In [31]). The fluoride concentration in toothpaste has traditionally been limited to 1450 ppm F; but in multicenter randomized controlled trial [31], authors have reported that daily use of high-fluoride (5000ppm) toothpaste may be recommended to prevent WSL during fixed oral appliances. This corroborates with other studies [32] that stipulate that the relative caries preventive effects of fluoride toothpastes of different concentrations increase with higher fluoride concentration. Fluoride concentrations below 0.1% should not to be recommended for orthodontic patients [1].

The daily use of a fluoride mouth rinse throughout brace treatment to prevent WSL is also highly recommended [33-34]. It was demonstrated that the daily use of a 0.05% sodium fluoride rinse during orthodontic treatment resulted in a statistically significant reduction of enamel white spot lesions. The more closely patients adhered to this rinsing regimen the more likely they exhibited a decrease in the occurrence of white spot lesions. The dose response effect between the frequency of rinsing and the incidence of white spots was evident regardless of oral hygiene status [34]. Besides self-controlled oral hygiene, professional prophylactic cleaning using fluoridated pastes is designed to reduce bacterial load and enhance the efficacy of brushing mainly in difficult areas around appliances [35].

3.1.2. In office-applied topical fluorotherapy

Use of additional topical fluorides designed to deliver additional fluoride to the tooth surface at-risk area near orthodontic brackets is likely to reduce the risk of DWL development. In a review conducted in 2103 [36], the authors found some moderate evidence that fluoride varnish applied every six weeks at the time of orthodontic review during treatment is effective. It has also been reported that the application of a fluoride varnish resulted in a 44.3% reduction in enamel demineralization in orthodontic patients [37], and there were significantly fewer new demineralized white lesions in the patients that had the application of the fluoride varnish at each visit compared with the placebo varnish [38].

Additionally, with in office-applied fluoride varnishes, the amounts of fluoride exposure can be controlled better and does not depend on patients' compliance. However, there is a limitation on the frequency of fluoride exposures received since the application occurs in the clinician's office only. In addition, the repeated varnish applications may lead to the temporary discoloration of the teeth and gingival tissue, and increase costs to the patient and/or chair time to the clinician [4]. In order to enhance the cariostatic potential of current fluoride agents and procedures for orthodontic purposes, substance like titanium fluoride or stannous fluoride has been described to reduce lesion depths and total mineral loss when compared to conventional fluoride preparations. The acid resistant coating deposited from these solutions can protect the enamel surface against severe acid challenges from plaque with low pH [1, 39, 40] (Figure 5).

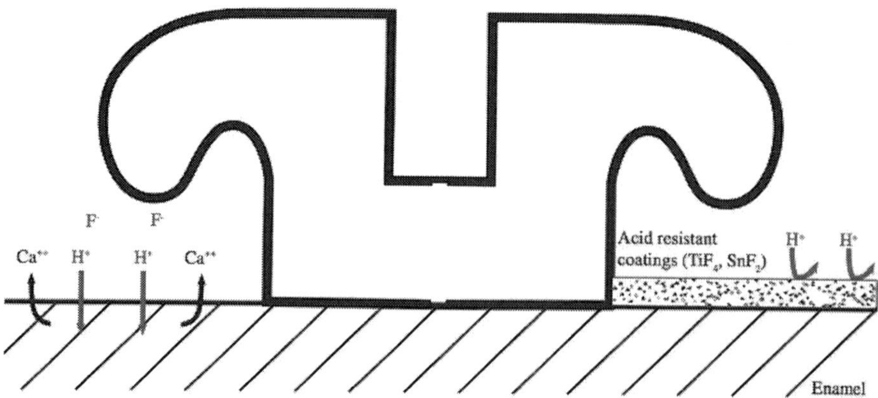

Figure 5. Acid resistant coating deposited from titanium fluoride or stannous fluoride, protect the enamel surface against severe acid challenges (H^+ions under the right bracket wing). Conventional fluoride preparations have a reduced cariostatic effect in plaque with low pH (under the left bracket wing). Ca^{2+}loss illustrates the caries process [1].

The use of antimicrobials like Chlorhexidene, as a complement to fluoride therapy, has also demonstrated demineralization-inhibiting tendencies in patients with fixed orthodontic appliances to reduce WSL at the time of debonding when compared with a control group [1, 4, 23, 26]. Chlorhexidene varnishes for long-term use may reduce the cariogenic challenge sufficiently to improve the fluoride effect on WSL instead daily Chlorhexidene rinsing, which is a well-known cause of teeth and tongue discoloration [23]. In this context, the use of products combining fluorides and antimicrobial agents should be seriously considered, especially among patients with a lack of motivation to maintain optimal oral hygiene, provided that such products do not significantly decrease mechanical properties of the adhesive system used [4].

On the other hand, if fluoride use may be beneficial for WSL prevention during orthodontic treatment, it can have conversely unwanted effects on properties of orthodontic alloys. In the presence of fluoride, β titanium, currently used for his elasticity and corrosion resistance, can undergo a degradation process and be affected in terms of biological and mechanical features. Thus, coating with TiAlN (deposing thin films of titanium aluminium nitride) has been recommended [41] in order to reduce the corrosive effects of fluorides on β titanium ortho‐ dontic archwires. Likewise, fluoride attacks the protective oxide surface film on Nickel-Titanium wires causing corrosion and nickel release, which increases with increasing fluoride concentration [42]. Some authors have recommended diamond-like carbon (DLC) coatings onto nickel-titanium wires to reduce fluoride-induced corrosion and improve orthodontic friction [43].

3.1.3. Fluoride-releasing materials used in orthodontic practice

While compliance with preventive protocols at home is the most frequently difficult to obtain [44], it would be an advantage if bonding materials could inhibit demineralization near the brackets. Presently, it seems impossible to make recommendations on the use of fluoride-containing orthodontic materials during fixed orthodontic treatment. However, it is advanta‐ geous to report some studies outcomes.

Using fluoride containing sealants and adhesives to bond brackets has been attempted. Glass ionomer cements (GIC) were initially introduced as orthodontic bonding adhesives for their ability to chemically bond to tooth structure and their sustained fluoride release following bonding. Resin particles were added to their formulation to create Resin-modified glass ionomer cements (RMGIC). These bonding systems have been developed to combine the desirable properties of composite resin bond strength and glass ionomer fluoride release. Studies have shown that RMGIC is more effective than an acrylic-bonding agent in preventing white spot formation, but weak evidence was reported [22, 45]. It has been suggested that these adhesives should be more widely used in bonding orthodontic brackets [46] particularly on the maxillary incisors that represent a significant aesthetic challenge to both the patient and the orthodontist.

Additionally, filled and fluoride releasing sealant may offer more enamel protection next to orthodontic brackets exposed to cariogenic conditions, mainly in patients with poor oral hygiene [47, 48]. Their application has been shown to not affect the shear bond strength (SBS) of orthodontic adhesives, and they are able to produce a sustained fluoride release [4, 42]. It was also found out that using the combination of an antimicrobial self-etching primer and a fluoride-releasing adhesive had acceptable bond strength for clinical use [49]. However, the clinical effectiveness of the fluoride release may be questionable, as the amount of fluoride required from a bonding material to be caries preventive is still unknown [50].

Resin composite bonding system with the ability of fluoride release was also developed for bracket bonding. An in-vitro study using nano-indentation test to evaluate the nano-mechanical properties of the enamel around and beneath orthodontic brackets, has showed that use of these product may reduce demineralization during orthodontic treatment [51].

3.2. Fluoride use after orthodontic treatment

The best treatment of WSL begins with a preventive approach, as they are difficult to recover especially in severe cases. In addition, White spot lesions treatment after appliance removal to produce a sound and aesthetically pleasing enamel surface is still a question to be fully answered. As patients respond differently to the presence of WSL, the course of treatment will likely be unique to each patient [4].

Debonding the orthodontic appliances eliminates an important cariogenic environment. However, the removal of stagnant plaque alone is not enough to achieve complete repair of WSL, and some spots secondary to debonding can last from 5 to 12 years [22, 52]. Evaluation of lesions that have developed during appliance therapy in the different sites of the dentition represents a clinical challenge for orthodontists [1]. Initial surface-softened lesions appear to remineralize quickly in saliva even without fluoride [53]. Resolution is thought to occur via the redisposition of various minerals soluble in saliva, particularly calcium, phosphate, and fluoride, but also and primarily via surface wear exposing the underlying enamel crystals, which are tightly packed and thus provide proper light reflection [54]. When arrested, they may exhibit a white color or may become yellowish or dark brown due to exogenous uptake of stains.

In general, treatment of WSL should begin with the most conservative approaches. If such approaches do not resolve the problem to the clinician's satisfaction, more aggressive treatment modalities can be pursued if the patient is interested (micro-abrasion, composite restorations, tooth whitening, porcelain veneers….)

Although the treatment of post-orthodontic WSL differs from their prevention, topical fluoride is thought to be the first step in WSL management. Based on the literature, and compared with the evidence on the WSL forestalling during orthodontic treatment, there is a lack of reliable evidence to support the effectiveness of remineralizing agents for the treatment of post-orthodontic white spot lesions [52, 55-56]. Nevertheless, for mild WSL, application of lower concentrations of fluorides can be used in an attempt to arrest their progression with successful and more aesthetic treatment results since hypermineralization maintains the whiteness of the lesions. Indeed, direct application of a high concentration of fluoride is not recommended as it causes rapid remineralization of the enamel surface, which restricts the passage of ions into the deeper, more affected layers, and limits their complete recovery [4, 57].

Finally, it has been suggested that acid etching of WSLs may increase the surface porosity and hence remineralization [1]. However, a study by Al-Khateeb et al (2000) [58] has shown lack of complete remineralization, and the etched lesions retained a porous structure of their surface layer even after a long period of remineralization in vitro.

4. Experience of Casablanca Dental School in fluoride use during orthodontic treatment

A clinical study was conducted for 10 months and 3 days in the Department of Dento Facial Orthopedics at the Faculty of Dentistry in Casablanca to determine the incidence of WSL in orthodontic population and to evaluate the fluoride varnish effect on the prevention and remineralization of carious lesions generated by orthodontic treatment.

5. Method framework

All patients starting treatment at the Dentofacial Orthopedics Unit from December 2010 to April 2011 were selected. The survey included healthy patients aged from 12 to 27 years old, and for whom treatment duration was estimated at more than 6 months. Patients with anterior restorations (composite, glass ionomer, endodontic treatment) or prosthetic devices, those displaying tooth tissue abnormalities (fluorosis, amelogenesis imperfecta, WSL....) or following preventive fluoride regimens (except toothpaste) and those with orthodontic treatment history were excluded. A total of 68 consecutive orthodontic patients fulfilled the eligibility criteria and were approached to participate.

This was a prospective study that has been made in the form of Crossover, which exposes teeth to the same factors: Oral hygiene, saliva composition, and enamel's structure. All patients were fitted with multi-bracket appliance and the same bonding system. The right side, from the central incisor to the first molar, has received a fluoride varnish (Fluor Protector 0, 1% F, Ivoclar Vivadent, Schaan, Liechtenstein) while the left side was taken as control. Before applying the varnish, an evaluation of oral hygiene status was recorded via plaque quantification for each tooth in both lower and upper arch. WSL were evaluated by naked eye after teeth brushing and drying with air spray, and scored depending on their severity and location according to the modified White spot lesion index (WSL-Index) by Gorelick et al. (1982) [59]. The visual evaluation of the individual teeth was based on a labial surface examination assessing the presence or absence of WSL. The severity of WSL was scored as follows: (Figure 6, 7)

(0)=No white spot lesion formation

(1)=Slight white spot or line formation

(2)=Excessive white spot formation

(3)=White spot formation with cavitations

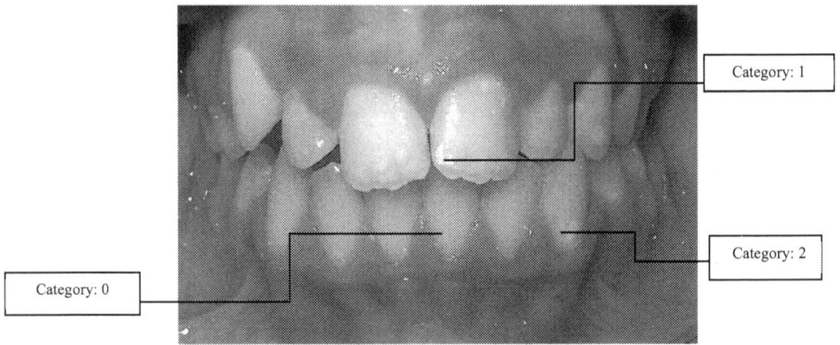

Figure 6. Evaluation of WSL 0, 1 and 2

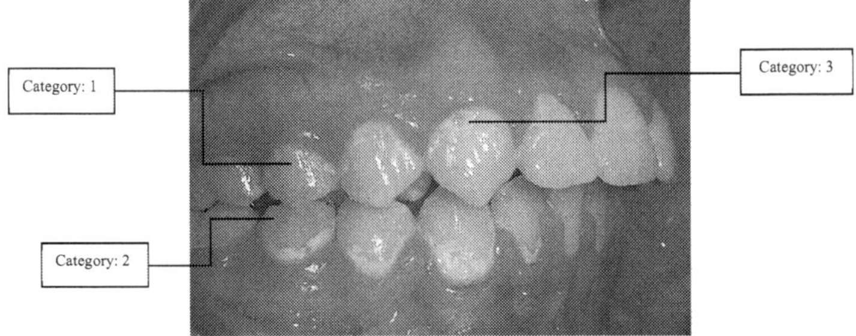

Figure 7. Evaluation of WSL 1, 2 and 3

Patients were notified about the importance of complying with the recommendations advocated by the manufacturer: Avoid eating and brushing teeth for 45 min after the application of fluoride varnish. The varnish was applied every 6 weeks for a six-month period. After every 6 weeks, the plaque index and the WSL formation have been evaluated for all the teeth in two arches.

In total, we conducted 5 applications of fluoride varnish during the 6 months of the study. The statistical analysis of the data was performed using the software Epi6.0 fr.

6. Results

From 68 selected, only 30 patients have been recruited for the study. 38 were excluded from the study because they did not respect their periodic appointments, they did not show up

The sample study was distributed as follows: (figure 8-10)

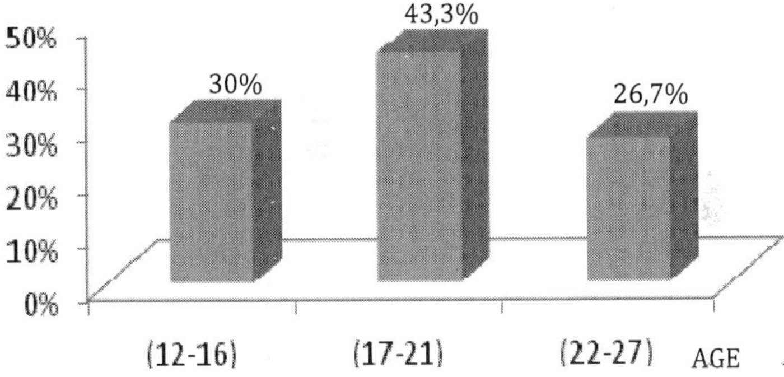

Figure 8. Sample distribution by age

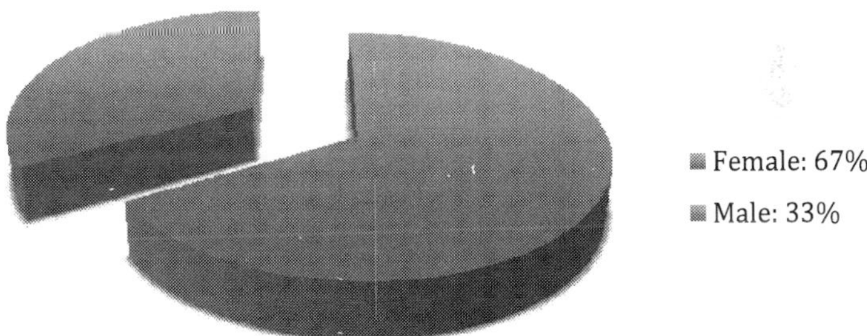

Figure 9. Sample distribution by sex

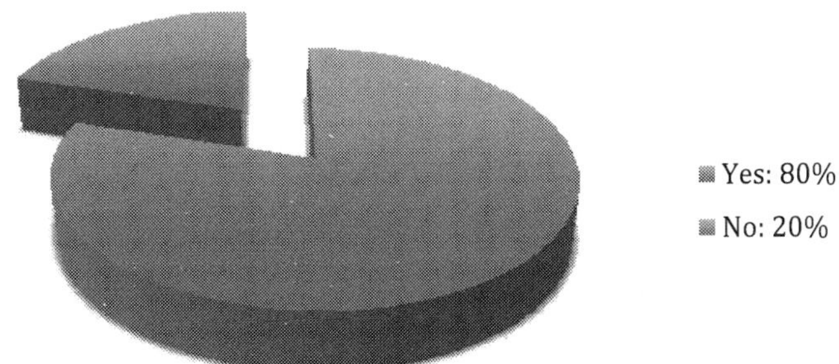

Figure 10. Sample distribution according to the sugary diet

Oral hygiene was evaluated by the frequency and method of brushing as well as the amount of plaque (table 1). The vertical brushing method was the most used by study's patients, and 73, 3% used no way adjuvant for their daily tooth brushing. According to the saliva parameters, 76, 7% of patients had a normal salivation and 63, 3% had fluid saliva.

Plaque	Appointment n°1		Appointment n°2		Appointment n°3		Appointment n°4		Appointment n°5	
	Number	%	Number	%	Number	%	Number	%	Number	%
0≤P<1	15	50, 0	15	50, 0	18	60, 0	20	66, 7	21	70, 0
1≤P<2	12	40, 0	11	36, 7	12	40, 0	9	30, 0	9	30, 0
P≥2	3	10, 0	4	13, 3	0	0, 0	1	3, 3	0	0, 0
Total	30	100	30	100	30	100	30	100	30	100

Table 1. Distribution of the study's sample according to the plaque amount

In the test group of teeth, the incidence of WSL was 60% versus 66.7% in the control group. In addition, 55.5% of female patients and 44.5% of male patients have developed WSL against 56, 5% and 43, 5% respectively in the control group.

On the other hand, 73.7% patients with snacking habit have developed at least one WSL versus 72, 7% in those without this practice. No association was found between the habit of snacking and the appearance of WSL. The frequency of people who had at least one WSL increases according to the number of snack, but the difference was not significant (table 2). Likewise and paradoxically, there was more WSL among those without sugary diet compared with those who consumed more sweet foods, but the difference was not significant. The saliva parameters have also been considered. The X^2 test (P=0. 71) has shown no association between the quality and the quantity of saliva and the appearance of WSL (table 3-4).

Both in the group of teeth test than in the control group, there was at baseline more of WSL among patients with mediocre and average oral hygiene compared with those who had good hygiene. By the end of the study, the opposite was observed. But in both cases, the difference was not significant.

As for varnish effect, there were fewer WSL in the teeth having benefited from fluoride varnish compared with the contralateral, but the difference was not significant. The relative risk was 0.73 with a confidence interval of [0.49-1.09]. It was < 1, which seems to be in favor of fluoride varnish. This reflects that fluoride is a protective factor, but we cannot draw any conclusions conclude on the basis of the results of the confidence interval of the relative risk (table 5).

Snacks number	0		1		2		3	
	Number	%	Number	%	Number	%	Number	%
WSL presence	8	72.7%	8	72.7%	6	85.7%	0	0, 0%
WSL absence	3	27.3%	3	27.3%	1	14.3%	1	100, 0%
$X^2 = 3, 30$		p = 0, 34				No significant difference		

Table 2. Association between snacks number and WSL formation

	Hyper salivation		Normal salivation	
	Number	%	Number	%
WSL presence	5	71.4%	17	73.9%
WSL absence	2	28.6%	6	26.1%
$X^2 = 0,02$	$p = 0,62$		No significant difference	

Table 3. Association between saliva quantity and WSL formation

	Viscous Saliva		Fluid Saliva	
	Number	%	Number	%
WSL presence	8	72.7%	14	73.7%
WSL absence	3	27.3%	5	26.3%
$X^2 = 0,14$	$p = 0,71$		No significant difference	

Table 4. Association between saliva quality and WSL formation

	WSL presence	WSL absence	Total
Test group	33	172	205
Control group	46	163	209
$X^2 = 0,92$	$p = 0,12$	No significant difference	

Table 5. Evaluation of the occurrence of WSL

7. Discussion

During this investigation, we have tried to avoid bias in order to obtain valid results and overcome some difficulties regarding:

- The lack of cooperation and refusal of participation of some patients.

- The lack of reliability concerning oral hygiene and dietary habits.

- The non-respect of appointments

- Gingival inflammation of the maxillary premolars after the brackets location and poor hygiene. So the cervical zone was often weakly induced by fluoride varnish.

7.1. Discussion of the findings

As discussed above, identification of risk factors of carious lesions is a necessary step before any orthodontic treatment is undertaken. In this respect, dietary habits are of great importance.

Beyond the amount of sugar ingested, the frequency of the daily ingestion maintains oral PH in critical levels, and thus, leads to the development of the caries process.

A study conducted on 155 patients in the Department of Dentofacial Orthopedics at Casablanca Dental Schoolto evaluate the prevalence of dental caries and associated risk factors in orthodontics (Bourzgui et al, 2010) [60], showed that 31, 6% of patients had an excessive sugary diet and 45, 8% had a snack habit. In the present investigation, this estimation was 80% and 63, 3%, respectively. However, the association between WSL formation and the dietary habits (number of meals, snacking and consumption of sugary diets)was not significant.

The fitting of orthodontic appliances causes adverse changes in the composition of the bacterial plaque increasing radically periodontal and caries risk. Adolescents following orthodontic treatment are considered to be high-risk patients and they need more motivation, hygiene control and use of topical fluoride [61]. Good individual control of dental plaque associated with a daily use of topical fluoride per toothpaste remains the most effective way. Patients with good oral hygiene during fixed orthodontic treatment have less prevalence of enamel decalcification. Simple daily oral hygiene procedures have shown a reduction in these decalcifications. Four factors influence the effectiveness of oral brushing: The frequency of brushing, brushing length, the concentration of fluoride and rinse after brushing. Oral brushing should be done at least twice a day and for a longer duration. The high fluoride concentration toothpaste is recommended. The use of fluoride supplementation (fluoride mouthrinse, varnishes, gel...) is of great interest to prevent WSL and reduce their severity [62]. Our study has shown a slight improvement in the frequency of brushing (43.3% brushed three times per day at the beginning of the investigation versus 53.3% at the end) with a non-significant difference between the WSL occurrence and the brushing frequency.

Additionally, all teeth have presented at least one demineralization except the first right upper Premolar. However, some patients presented a total lack of demineralization. The previous study conducted in the same Dental Clinic [60] showed that 7.7% of patients developed whit spots during their orthodontic treatment, with a similar distribution between front and posterior areas of the arches. Our study has shown that the most affected tooth in the control group was the first molar, followed by upper lateral incisor, upper cuspid, and then premolar group. While in the experimental group, the lateral incisor was the most affected, followed by canines, and the premolar group (Figures 11-12). The lateral incisors in some cases had a palatine position at the base, and they thereby were subject concurrently to the fastest accumulation of plaque due to the cleaning difficulty.

In the literature, all the studies conducted so far have used different fluoride concentration with different application frequencies (Table 6). The findings consolidated the use of topical fluorides in addition to fluoride toothpaste as the best evidence-based way to forestall these incipient lesions. Regular high fluoride varnish application around the brackets is the most effective topical method. It is a quick and easy professional application with conservation and a slow-release fluoride for an extended time period. Also, it is usefully independent of patients' compliance [63]. In our study, the incidence of whit lesions in the control group was slightly higher than the test group. However, the chi-2 test was not significant, so according to our study, there was no association between the application of fluoride varnish and the appearance of whitish lesions; this could be explained by the fact that our sample was small and the duration of our study was short. In this study, fluoride varnish reduced the severity of lesions, but it did not prevent their appearance.

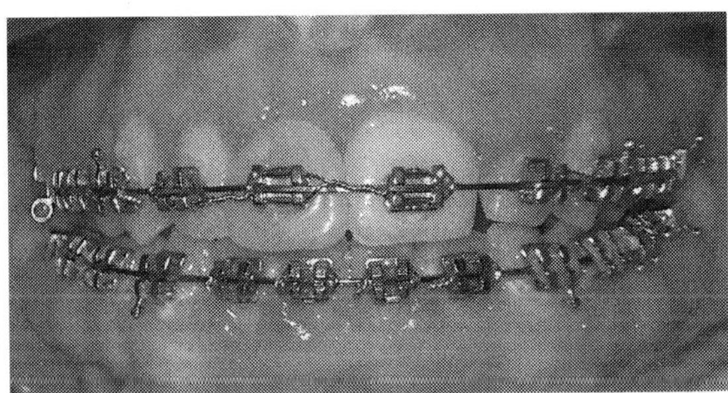

Figure 11. WSL on cervical area on lower and upper incisors and cupids during orthodontic treatment.

Authors (year)	Sample	Fluoride varnish	Frequency	Results	Incidence Test/ control
Gontijo (2007)	16 teeth	Duraphat 22600 ppm	One application	Significant Difference in the composition of enamel	-
Farhadian (2008)	15 patients	Bifluoride: 12, 6% of calcium fluorideand 6% of sodiumfluoride	One application	Significant difference	57/93
Stecksén-Blicks (2004)	273 patients	Fluor Protector 1000ppm	Every 6 weeks	Significant difference	7/26
Vivaldi-Rodrigues (2006)	10 patients	-	Every 3 months	Significant difference	0, 34/0, 51*

*Index of decalcification

Table 6. Examples of in vivo studies about WSL prevention

The secondary prevention, that is the control and treatment of existing WSL after debonding, has gained interest, too. Treatment of post-orthodontic WSL, with a remineralizing cream with casein phosphopeptide-stabilized amorphous calcium phosphate (CPP-ACP) as adjunct to fluoride toothpaste seemed to be beneficial with some mineral and aesthetic improvements compared with fluoride applications [63].

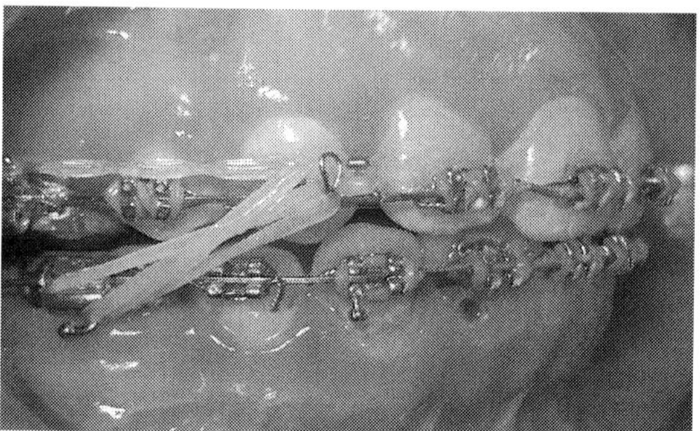

Figure 12. Development of a cavity in cervical zone of the 43 during orthodontic treatment

While the findings of the different studies areequivocal, further research with standardized protocols, is needed before practice guidelines on the fluoride/non-fluoride therapies can be recommended.

8. Conclusion

Even with the advances in material and techniques, demineralization around brackets during orthodontic treatment remains problematic. The literature points to the need for more evidence to clarify the most recent opinions, on which orthodontists can base their clinical practice. Developing a practice and standardized guideline for the prevention and the treatment of enamel demineralizations at the start of, during, and after orthodontic treatment is highly recommended to improve outcomes quality and manage unplanned debondings.

There are a number of products containing fluoride available to clinicians and their patients. Unfortunately, the evidence for the effectiveness of these products is weak. However, to date, using fluoride varnish in high concentration and with regular applications is the most effective way to avoid WSL appearance. This should be implemented in close association with the control of caries risk factors. Indeed, It is still crucial to emphasize that prevention of these lesions is the furthermost desirable outcome aesthetically and also the least costly for patients.

As for treatment of WSL already installed, the concerns are more complicated. It is expected that the majority of slight or mild the WSL will improve during the retention period if good oral hygiene is maintained. For more advanced cases, total recovery remains unsystematic. The lesions may induce aesthetic consequences and require more invasive approaches. However, current evidence supports the use of topical application of fluoride in low concentration or better the use of CPP-ACP to obtain a reduction in the severity of these lesions.

Author details

Hakima Aghoutan[1], Sana Alami[1], Farid El Quars[1], Samir Diouny[2] and Farid Bourzgui[1*]

*Address all correspondence to: faridbourzgui@gmail.com

1 Department of Dento-facial Orthopedic, Faculty of Dental Medicine, Hassan II University of Casablanca, Morocco

2 Chouaib Doukkali University, Faculty of Letters & Human Sciences, El Jadida, Morocco

References

[1] Øgaard B. White spot lesions during orthodontic treatment: mechanisms and fluoride preventive aspects. Seminars in Orthod. 2008; 14(3): 183-93.

[2] Hadler-Olsen S, Sandvik K., El-Agroudi MA et al. The incidence of caries and white spot lesions in orthodontically treated adolescents with a comprehensive caries prophylactic regimena prospective study. Eur J Orth 2012; 314 : 633-39

[3] Benson PE. Prevention of Demineralization during orthodontic treatment with fluoride-containing materials or casein phosphopeptide-amorphous calcium phosphate. In Huang GJ, Richmond S, Vig KWL.(eds) Evidence-Based Orthodontics. Blackwell Publishing, Ltd 2011 p149-65

[4] Bishara SE, Ostby AW. White Spot Lesions: Formation, Prevention, and Treatment. Semin Orthod 2008;14:174-82

[5] Chang HS, Walsh LJ, Freer TJ. Enamel demineralization during orthodontic treatment. Aetiology and prevention. Aust Dent J. 1997; 42(5): 322-7.

[6] Jung WS, Kim H, Park SY, et al. Quantitative analysis of changes in salivary mutans streptococci after orthodontic treatment. Am J Orthod Dentofacial Orthop. 2014; 145(5): 603-9.

[7] Lim BS, Lee SJ, Lee JW et al. Quantitative analysis of adhesion of cariogenic streptococci to orthodontic raw materials. Am J Orthod Dentofacial Orthop. 2008; 133(6): 882-8.

[8] Chapman JA, Roberts WE, Eckert GJ et al. Risk factors for incidence and severity of white spot lesions during treatment with fixed orthodontic appliances. Am J Orthod Dentofacial Orthop. 2010; 138(2): 188-94.

[9] Van Palenstein Helderman WH, Matee MI, van der Hoeven JS, et al. Cariogenicity depends more on diet than the prevailing mutans streptococcal species. Dent Res. 1996; 75(1): 535-45.

[10] Kukleva M P, Shetkova D G, Beev V H: Compara-tive age study of the risk of demin-eralization during orthodontic treatment with brackets. Folia Med 2002; 44: 56-9.

[11] Øgaard B, Rølla G, Arends J: Orthodontic appliances and enamel demineralization. Part 1. Lesion development. Am J Orthod Dentofacial Orthop 1988; 94: 68-73.

[12] Zachrisson BU, Zachrisson S. Caries incidence and orthodontic treatment with fixed appliances. Scand J Dent Res 1971; 79: 183-92.

[13] Julien KC, Buschang PH, Campbell PM. Prevalence of white spot lesion formation during orthodontic treatment. Angle Orthod. 2013; 83: 641-47.

[14] Lovrov S, Hertrich K, Hirschfelder U. Enamel demineralization during fixed ortho-dontic treatment—incidence and correlation to various oral-hygiene parameters. J Orofac Orthop. 2007; 68: 353-63.

[15] Tufekci E, Dixon JS, Gunsolley JC, Lindauer SJ. Prevalence of white spot lesions dur-ing orthodontic treatment with fixed appliances. Angle Orthod. 2011; 2: 206-10.

[16] Khalaf K. Factors affecting the formation, severity and location of white spot lesions during orthodontic treatment with fixed appliances. J Oral Maxillofac Res 2014; 5(1): e4. 10.5037/jomr.2014.5104

[17] Boersma JG, van der Veen MH, Lagerweij MD, et al. Caries prevalence measured with QLF after treatment; with fixed orthodontic appliances: influenc-ing factors. Ca-ries Res. 2005; 39: 41-7.

[18] Willmot D. White Spot Lesions After Orthodontic Treatment. Semin Orthod 2008;14: 209-19.

[19] Lucchese A, Gherlone E. Prevalence of white-spot lesions before and during ortho-dontic treatment with fixed appliances. Eur J Orthod. 2013; 35(5): 664-8.

[20] Arneberg P, Giertsen E, Emberland H, et al: Intra-oral variations in total plaque fluo-ride related to plaque pH. A study in orthodontic patients. Caries Res 1997; 31: 451-56.

[21] Mattousch TJ, van der Veen MH, Zentner A. Caries lesions after orthodontic treat-ment followed by quantitative light-induced fluorescence: a 2-year follow-up. Eur J Orthod 2007; 29: 294-8.

[22] Shungin D, Olsson AI, Persson M. Orthodontic treatment-related white spot lesions: a 14-year prospective quantitative follow-up, including bonding material assessment. Am J Orthod Dentofacial Orthop 2010; 138: 136-7.

[23] Øgaard B, Larsson E, Henriksson T, et al: Effects of combined application of antimi-crobial and a fluoride varnishes in orthodontic patients. Am J Orthod Dento-facial Orthop 2001; 120: 28-35.

[24] Cochrane NJ, Cai F, Huq NL, et al. New approaches to enhanced remineralization of tooth enamel. J Dent Res 2010; 89: 1187-97.

[25] Belli R, Rahiotis C, Schubert EW, Baratieri LN et al. Wear and morphology of infiltrated white spot lesions. J dentistry 2011; 39: 376–85

[26] Øgaard B: Oral microbiological changes, long-term enamel alterations due to decalcification, and caries prophylactic aspects, in Brantley WA, Eliades T, eds: Orthodontic Materials. Scientific and Clinical Aspects. Stuttgart, Thieme, 2001, p123-142

[27] Knösel M, Bojes M, Jung K, et al. Increased susceptibility for white spot lesions by surplus orthodontic etching exceeding bracket base area. Am J Orthod Dentofacial Orthop 2012;141:574-82.

[28] Garcez AS, Suzuki SS, Ribeiro MS, et al. Biofilm retention by 3 methods of ligation on orthodontic brackets: a microbiologic and optical coherence tomography analysis. Am J Orthod Dentofacial Orthop. 2011; 140 (4): e193-8.

[29] Derks A, Katsaros C, Frencken JE, et al. Caries-inhibiting effect of preventive measures during orthodontic treatment with fixed appliances: a systematic review. Caries Res 2004; 38: 413-20.

[30] Farhadian N, Miresmaeili A, Eslami B, at al. Effect of fluoride varnish on enamel demineralization around brackets: an in-vivo study. Am. J. Orthod. Dentofacial Orthop. 2008; 133: S95-98.

[31] Sonesson M, Twetman S, Bondmark L. Effectiveness of high-fluoride toothpaste on enamel demineralization during orthodontic treatment: a multicenter randomized controlled trail. Eur J Orth. 2013; Dec 28 doi: 10.1093/ejo/cjt096.

[32] Walsh T1, Worthington HV, Glenny AM, et al. Fluoride toothpastes of different concentrations for preventing dental caries in children and adolescents. Cochrane Database Syst Rev. 2010; 20(1):CD007868. doi: 10.1002/14651858.CD007868.pub2.

[33] Geiger AM, Gorelick L, Gwinnett AJ, Benson BJ. Reducing white spot lesions in orthodontic populations with fluoride rinsing. Am J Orthod Dentofacial Orthop 1992; 101: 403-7

[34] Kerbusch AE, Kuijpers-Jagtman AM, Mulder J, Sanden WJ. Methods used for prevention of white spot lesion development during orthodontic treatment with fixed appliances. Acta Odontologica Scandinavica 2012; 70(6): 564–8.

[35] Arnold WH, Dorow A, Langenhorst S et al. Effect of fluoride toothpastes on enamel demineralization. BMC Oral Health 2006; 6(8): 1-6.

[36] Benson PE, Parkin N, Dyer F, et al. Fluorides for the prevention of early tooth decay (demineralised white lesions) during fixed brace treatment. Cochrane Database of Systematic Reviews 2013 (12). Art. No.: CD003809. DOI: 10.1002/14651858.CD003809.pub3.

[37] Vivaldi-Rodrigues G, Demito CF, Bowman SJ, et al: The effectiveness of a fluoride varnish in preventing the development of white spot lesions. World J Orthod. 2006; 7:138-44.

[38] Stecksen-Blicks C, Renfors G, Oscarson ND. et al. Caries-preventive effectiveness of a fluoride varnish: a randomized controlled trial in adolescents with fixed orthodontic appliances. Caries Research 2007; 41: 455-59

[39] Buyukyilmaz T, Tangugsorn V, Øgaard B, et al: The effect of titanium tetrafluoride (TiF4) application around orthodontic brackets. Am J Orthod Dentofacial Orthop, 1994; 105: 293-96.

[40] Hove L, Holme B, Øgaard B, et al: The protective effect of TiF4, SnF2 and NaF on erosion of enamel by hydro-chloric acid in vitro measured by white light interferometry. Caries Res 2006; 40: 440-43.

[41] Krishnan V, Krishnan A, Remya R, et al. Development and evaluation of two PVD-coated ß-titanium orthodontic archwires for fluoride-induced corrosion protection. Acta Biomater. 2011; 7(4): 1913-27

[42] Brantley WA. Wires used in orthodontic practice. In Miles PG, Rinchuse DJ, Rinchuse DJ (Eds) Evidence-based clinical orthodontics. 2012 Quintessence Publishing Co Inc

[43] Huang SY, Huang JJ, Kang T, et al. Coating NiTi archwires with diamond-like carbon films: reducing fluoride-induced corrosion and improving frictional properties. J Mater Sci Mater Med. 2013; 24 (10): 2287-92.

[44] Geiger AM, Gorelick L, Gwinnett AJ, et al. Reducing white spot lesions in orthodontic populations with fluoride rinsing. Am J Orthod Dentofacial Orthop 1992; 101: 403-7.

[45] Rogers S, Chadwick B, Treasure E. Fluoride-containing orthodontic adhesives and decalcification in patients with fixed appliances: a systematic review. Am J Orthod Dentofacial Orthop. 2010; 138(4): 390.e1-8

[46] Eliades T: Orthodontic materials research and applica-tions: Part 1. Current status and projected future devel-opments in bonding and adhesives. Am J Orthod Dentofacial Orthop 2006; 130:445-51

[47] Hu W, Featherstone JD. Prevention of enamel demineralization: an in-vitro study using light-cured filled sealant. Am J Orthod Dentofacial Orthop. 2005; 128(5): 592-600

[48] Behnan SM, Arruda AO, Gonzàlez-Cabezas C, et al. In-vitro evaluation of various treatments to prevent demineralization next to orthodontic brackets. Am J Orthod Dentofacial Orthop 2010; 138: 712.e1-712.e7.

[49] Korbmacher HM, Huck L, Kahl-Nieke B: Fluoride-releasing adhesive and antimicrobial self-etching primer effects on shear bond strength of orthodontic brackets. Angle Orthod. 2006; 76:845-50.

[50] Pseiner BC, Freudenthaler J, Jonke E, et al. Shear bond strength of fluoride-releasing orthodontic bonding and composite materials. Eur J Orthod. 2010; 32(3): 268-73.

[51] Raji SH, Banimostafaee H, Hajizadeh F. Effects of fluoride release from orthodontic bonding materials on nanomechanical properties of the enamel around orthodontic brackets. Dent Res J. 2014; 11(1): 67–73.

[52] Chen H, Liu X, Dai J, et al. Effect of remineralizing agents on white spot lesions after orthodontic treatment: A systematic review. Am J Orthod Dentofacial Orthop. 2013; 143(3): 376-82.e3.

[53] Øgaard B, ten Bosch JJ: Regression of white spot enamel lesions. A new optical method for quantitative longitudinal evaluation in vivo. Am J Orthod Dentofacial Orthop 1994; 106 : 238-42.

[54] Artun J, Thylstrup A. A 3-year clinical and SEM study of surface changes of carious lesions after inactivation. Am J Orthod Dento-facial Orthop 1989; 95: 327-33.

[55] Kalha AS. Lack of reliable evidence of the effectiveness of remineralising agents for the treatment of post orthodontic white spot lesions. Evid Based Dent. 2013; 14(3): 76-7.

[56] Ballard RW, Hagan JL, Phaup AN, et al. Evaluation of 3 commercially available materials for resolution of white spot lesions Am J Orthod Dentofacial Orthop. 2013; 143: S78-84.

[57] Artun J, Thylstrup A. Clinical and scanning electron microscopic study of surface changes of incipient caries lesions after debonding. Scand J Dent Res 1986; 94: 193-201.

[58] Al-Khateeb S, Exterkate RAM, Angmar-Månsson B, et al: Effect of acid-etching on remineralization of enamel white spot lesions. Acta Odontol Scand 2000; 58:31-6.

[59] Gorelick L, Geiger AM, Gwinnett AJ. Incidence of white spot formation after bonding and banding. Am J Orthod. 1982; 81: 93-8.

[60] Bourzgui F, Sebbar M, Hamza M. Risk of caries in orthodontics: descriptive study on 155 patients. Rev Stomatol Chir Maxillofac. 2010; 111: 276-79.

[61] Chaussain C, Opsahl Vital S, Viallon V, et al. Interest in a new test for caries risk in adolescents undergoing orthodontic treatment. Clin Oral Investig. 2010; 14: 177–85

[62] Al Mulla AH, Kharsa SA, Birkhed D. Modified fluoride toothpaste technique reduces caries in orthodontic patients: A longitudinal, randomized clinical trial. Am J Orthod Dentofac Orthop. 2010; 138: 285-91

[63] Bergstrand F, Twetman S. A review on prevention and treatment of post-orthodontic white spot lesions–evidence based methods and emerging technologie. Open Dent J. 2011; 5: 158-62.

Chapter 16

Early Treatment of Anterior Crossbite Relating to Functional Class III

Sanaa Alami, Hakima Aghoutan, Farid El Quars,
Samir Diouny and Farid Bourzgui

Additional information is available at the end of the chapter

http://dx.doi.org/10.5772/59251

1. Introduction

Anterior crossbite is one of the most common orthodontic problems observed in children's growth, in both skeletal and functional Class III malocclusion. The latter presents an apparent imbalance in jaw size, considered to be essentially the result of a mesial thrust of the mandible. Its origins are multiple, ranging from abnormal eruption of deciduous or definitive incisors to lingual dysfunction (low position of the tongue) [1].

Functional Class III has long-term effects on the growth and development of the teeth. This widely justifies the need for early treatment to normalize the occlusion and create conditions for normal jaws development. An accurate diagnosis is required for successful treatment and stability.

Orthodontists must distinguish pseudo Class III crossbites from skeletal Class III. Thorough clinical assessment and accurate diagnosis must be performed in order to plan proper treatment strategies and appliance design during the early stages of dental development. In this respect, various modes of treatment have been suggested for anterior crossbite correction [2, 3, 4, 5]; early interceptive treatment is one mode of treatment, which has been suggested because of its diverse benefits.

This chapter aims (1) to define functional mandibular prognathism and its etiopathogeny, (2) to highlight the needs to manage earlier anterior crossbites, and finally (3) to illustrate the impact of interceptive approach with the use of a simple fixed appliance.

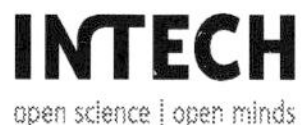

2. Functional mandibular prognathism

The functional mandibular prognathism referred as mandibular pseudo-prognathism, or pseudo-Class III, is a mandibular abnormal function belonging to the class III malocclusion according to the terminology of Angle [1, 6]. The aforementioned is an anomaly of occlusal origin, which develops into a skeletal anomaly (true Class III). Indeed, the functional disorder translates into a normal closure until the premature contact [7].

Anterior crossbite is defined as a situation in which one or more permanent mandibular incisors occlude labially to their antagonists [4], which can be associated or not to a mandibular lateral-deviation [7].

2.1. Etiopathogeny

Pseudo-Class III malocclusion is identified as an anterior crossbite as a result of mandibular displacement. The reported prevalence of anterior crossbites varies between 2.2% and 12%, depending on children's age and their ethnicity [2, 8, 9, 10].

Moyers suggested that pseudo-Class III malocclusion was a positional relationship related to an acquired neutomuscular reflex. The anterior crossbite that results is established in the mixed dentition. Different etiological factors are involved; they can be classified in dental, functional and skeletal factors [4, 8, 9].

Dental factors:

- Palatal eruption of the maxillary central incisors,

- Proclination of the lower incisors due to low thrust lingual or supernumerary anterior teeth in mandible,

- Premature loss of the the primary upper incisors following a dental trauma,

- Over-retained primary maxillary incisors due to odontomas,

- Crowding in the incisor region, and inadequate arch length

Functional factors:

- Tongue position anomalies

- Nasorespiratory problems

Skeletal factors:

- Minor transverse maxillary discrepancy.

Premature contact between the maxillary and mandibular incisors results in a forward displacement of the mandible to permit a comfortably occlusion [4, 9, 11].

2.2. Prognosis

Functional mandibular prognathism in the early mixed dentition can have long-term effects on the growth and development of the teeth and jaws (McNamara, 2002). Anterior crossbite may lead to abnormal enamel abrasion or proclination of the mandibular incisors, which, in turn, leads to gingival recession. Abnormal mandibular shift caused by lack of incisal guide may have adverse effects on the temporo-mandibular joints and masticatory system [4, 12].

What is most to be feared is that a functional anomaly becomes a skeletal prognathism. Indeed, spontaneous correction of such malocclusion has been reported to be too low to justify non-intervention. Therefore, interceptive treatment is often advised to normalize the occlusion and create conditions for normal occlusal development [4].

3. Diagnostic approach

Class III malocclusion has been divided into two subtypes: Skeletal and pseudo-Class III [5]. The early management of the pseudo-class III presents no real difficulties. Timing and modalities of treatment depend on the differential diagnosis which aims to determine whether the crossbite is dental or skeletal in nature. An essential aspect of the differential diagnosis in Class III malocclusion is the assessment of dental compensations and the presence of functional slide via a thorough clinical and radiographic analysis [13].

3.1. Clinical analysis

3.1.1. Exobuccal evaluation

Exobuccal signs are practically the same for both types of dysmorphia (skeletal and functional Class III) which are, most of the time, misleading. There is usually a concave profile, characterized by an inversion of the labial relationship as well as a projection at the front of the mandible (Figure 1). Usually, soft tissues tend to camouflage skeletal discrepancy so that the patient's profile appears normal or slightly concave in centric occlusion (Figure 2) [10].

It is important to note that although skeletal Class III is mandibular or maxillary, there is some degree of maxillary deficiency. Skeletal Class III, therefore, differs by a retrusive nasomaxillary area, and an important protrusive lower face and lip (Figure 3) [14].

The clinical assessment of profile changes from postural rest position to habitual occlusion is an additional criterion to be evaluated. The skeletal Class III profile remains concave in both positions, whereas the pseudo-class III profile is usually straight, but becomes concave as the mandible shifts forward into habitual occlusion position [9]. As many signs, which could mislead to a true Class III diagnosis.

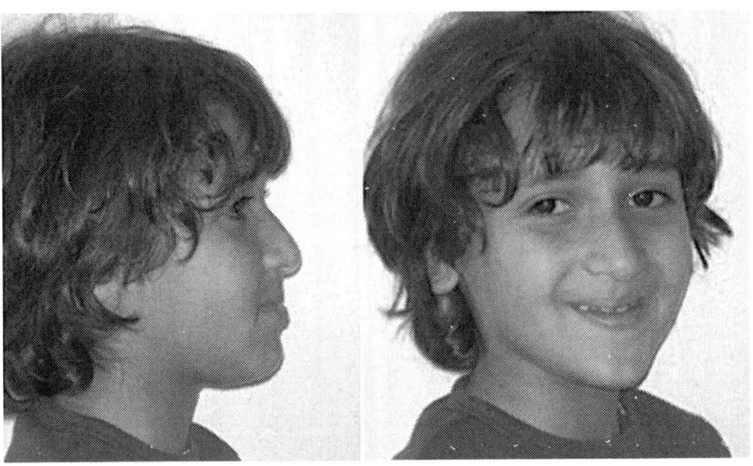

Figure 1. A patient, aged 8, presents pseudo-Class III malocclusion characterized by retrusion of the upper lip relative to the lower lip; smile betrays an anterior crossbite

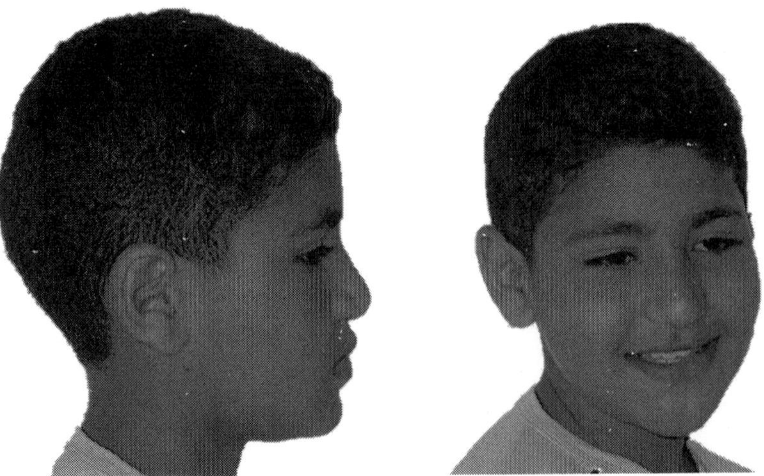

Figure 2. A patient, aged 9, presents pseudo-Class III malocclusion and a convex soft-tissue profile; labial relationships appear normal. Anterior cross-bite is revealed only on the views of smiling face and ¾.

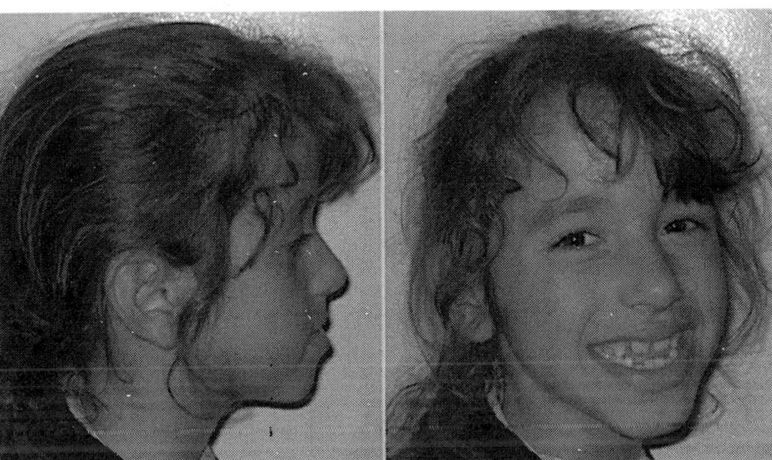

Figure 3. A patient, aged 8, presents skeletal Class III malocclusion characterized by concave profile and retrusive nasomaxillary area.

3.1.2. Endobuccal evaluation

Endobuccal exam allows the practician to identify his patient as a class I case. In skeletal Class III, dento-alveolar components compensations occur in the form of proclined maxillary incisors and retroclined mandibular incisors [9]. This is in contrast with pseudo-Class III cases, where anterior crossbite occlusion and Angle's Class III molars and canines are associated with dental compensations of class II malocclusion (Figure 4).

The assessment of dental relations must always be done with the mandible in centric relation. (Figure 5) It is important at this stage to proceed to the unique gesture, which allows making the differential diagnosis: It is the De Nevreze procedure, which consists in obtaining a more retrusive position of the mandible to minimize the dental relations in pseudo-prognathsm cases. Conversely, in true mesiocclusion, the maneuver does not succeed. The mandible cannot be retruded, and there is no modification of the dental reports [1, 15].

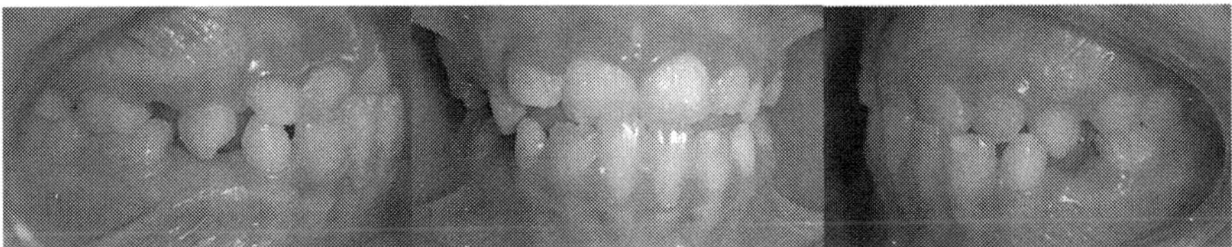

Figure 4. Pre-treatment intra-oral photographs in habitual occlusion showing characteristics of Angle's Class III molars and canines, vertical axis of the maxillary incisors, and the presence of anterior crossbite occlusion.

When the anterior crossbite exhibit a functional shift; that is, interincisal contact is possible in centric relationship, implying a pseudo Class III malocclusion with no inherent skeletal Class III discrepancy [8]. We find Characteristics of Angle's Class I molars and canines (Figure 5).

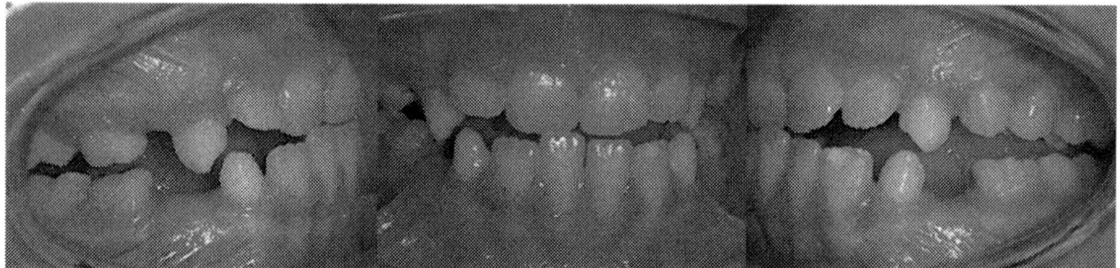

Figure 5. Pre-treatment intra-oral photographs in centric occlusion showing edge-to-edge occlusion and Angle's Class I molars and canines relationship.

3.2. Radiographic analysis

Lateral cephalogram largely contributes to establishing the diagnostic of a skeletal Class I. To evaluate the amount of mandibular shift, two lateral cephalograms, one at maximum intercuspation and one at the point of initial contact, are compared. (Figures 6)

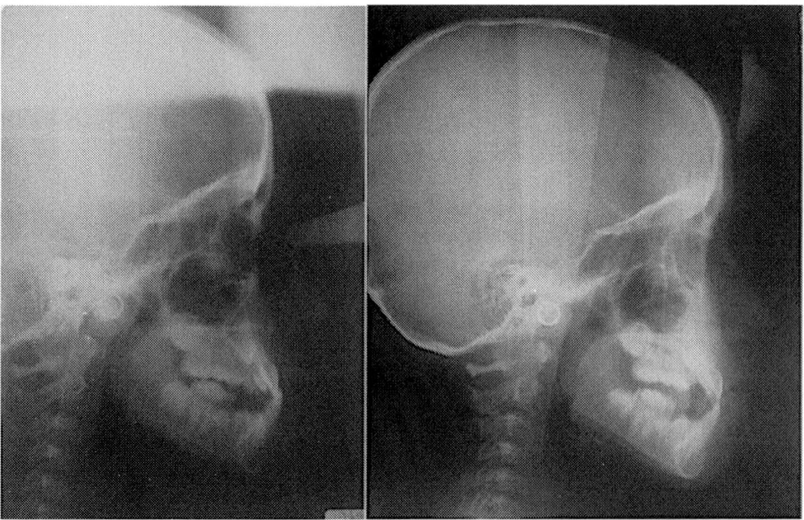

Figure 6. Pretreatment lateral cephalogram in maximum intercuspation position (AOBO=-7mm) and in position of initial contact with anterior edge to edge (AOBO=-4mm), showing that cephalometric values are in favor of a middle Class I.

In true Class III, the skeletal components are characterized by an underdeveloped maxilla, overdeveloped mandible or a combination of both. Dento-alveolar compensations are revealed by cephalometric values for proclined maxillary incisors and retroclined mandibular incisors.

Tweed defined a pseudo Class III malocclusion as having a conventionally shaped mandible. The sagittal jaw relation's show a Class I or a mild Class III pattern in centric relation. The upper incisors are often retroclined, whereas lower incisors are normally inclined or proclined [9].

4. Interceptive treatment

4.1. Timing

Optimum treatment timing for orthodontic problems continues to be one of the most controversial topics in orthodontics; this is especially true for the correction of Class III malocclusion [16].

However, spontaneous worsening during transition from deciduous to permanent dentition has been reported. For this reason, pseudo Class III malocclusion should be treated as early as possible to reduce the functional shift of the mandible and increase maxillary arch length [3, 5].

Several clinicians believe that early intervention has many advantages; they have suggested a number of reasons for early correction of anterior crossbite even in the deciduous dentition. The optimum period suggested for treatment is between 6 years and 9 years; intervention at this period permits normal growth [10].

4.2. Objectives

Generally, interceptive orthodontic treatment during mixed dentition is more effective to improve malocclusions than no treatment. Early intervention is, therefore, recommended preventing adverse effects on growth and development of the jaws and disturbance of temporal and masseter muscle activity, which would increase the risk of craniomandibular disorders during adolescence. A pseudo Class III malocclusion should be treated as early as possible to reduce the functional shift of the mandible and increase maxillary arch length [2, 3, 5].

In addition to its effectiveness and efficiency, early orthodontic treatment may have positive effects on the quality of life for both children and their families (self-esteem, social acceptance) [3].

The management of a pseudo-class III malocclusion via the proclination of upper incisors and/ or retroclination of lower incisors aims to correct anterior crossbite and eliminate mandibular displacement. Obtaining a front stop to lock the occlusion allows creating conditions for normal occlusal development [4, 9].

4.3. Modalities of treatment

Various appliances have been devised for early treatment of a pseudo Class III ; these include removable plates, fixed or removable inclined planes, functional appliances, face mask, and simple fixed appliances. Each device has its specific indication, its advantages and disadvantages [6, 10, 15].

4.3.1. Removable appliances

Hawley appliance with auxiliary springs is one of the earliest appliances introduced to produce proclination of upper incisors. The plate stabilization is provided by Adams clasp and the heightening of occlusion is strongly required to resolve an anterior crossbite (Figure 7 and 8).

A modified Hawley appliance with inverted labial bow is a simple way to manage pseudo Class III. The appliance is easy to construct and require trasferring the bite by guiding the mandible distally in an edge to edge (Figure 9) [15].

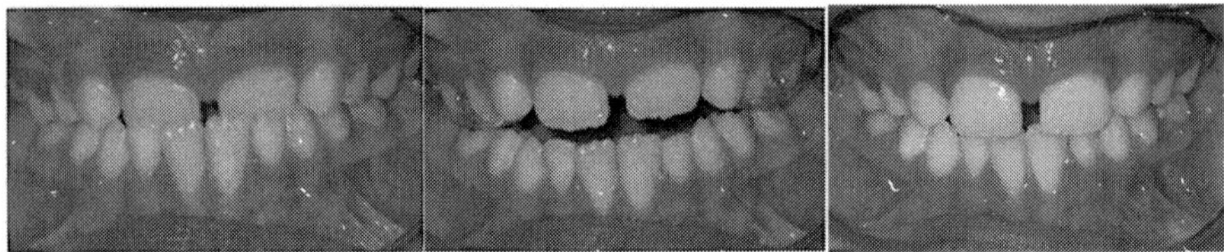

Figure 7. Correction of anterior crossbite by Hawley appliance with auxiliary springs

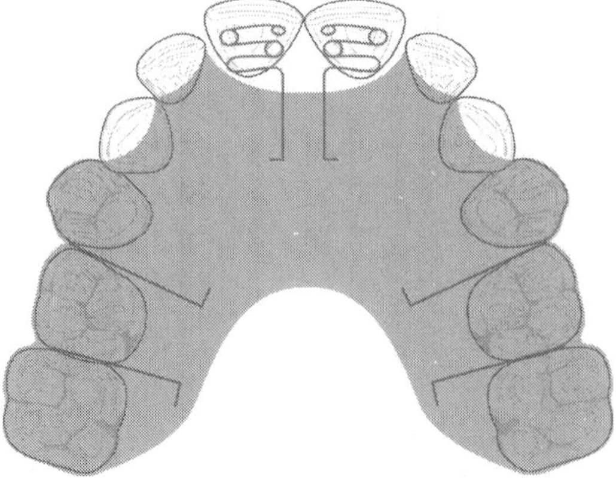

Figure 8. illustrating components of Hawley appliance with springs.

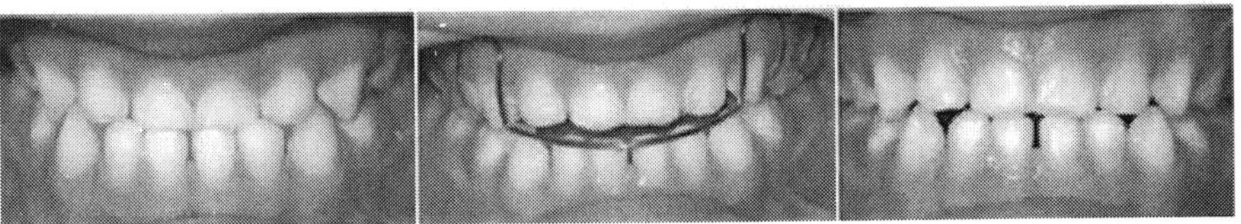

Figure 9. Correction of anterior crossbite, in deciduous dentition, by Hawley appliance with inverted labial bow

4.3.2. A modified quad helix appliance

This is one of the earliest appliances introduced for posterior expansion, it is made of 0.036 Blue Elgiloy and soldered to the bands on the first permanent maxillary molars. It can be modified by addition of an anterior extension arm. The appliance is expanded and cemented. The occlusion must be relieved by posterior bite-blocks to permit crossbite correction [9]. The gradually activation of both arms allows proclination maxillary incisors. The major indication of such device is the combination of anterior and posterior crossbites (Figure 10).

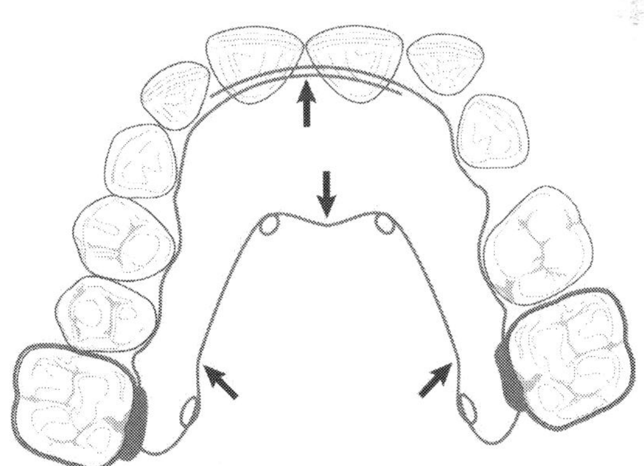

Figure 10. Illustrating activation of modified quad helix

4.3.3. Inclined plane

Some modalities for anterior crossbite correction include fixed or removable acrylic inclined planes (Croll, 1984), bonded resin-composite slopes (Bayrak and Tunc, 2008) [4, 12].

These are simple functional appliances placed on the lower arch; they allow quicker results. One of the identified advantages of removable appliance is that it can also be used as retention appliance after active treatment as well as it is possible to add acrylic teeth if necessary (Figure 11) [12].

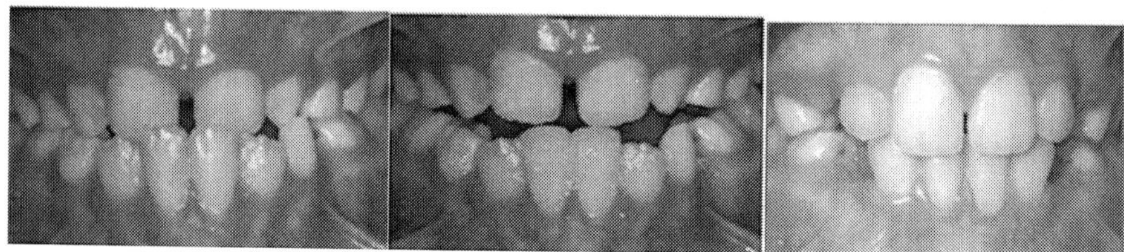

Figure 11. Correction of anterior crossbite by bonded resin-composite plane on mandibular incisors. The ramps should be progressively reduced.

4.3.4. Fixed appliance

The earlier treatment of pseudo-prognathism was feasible from a simple fixed appliance (partial bonding of brackets) simultaneously with elastics.

The most common pattern is to bond the brackets on the labial surfaces of the lower incisors and the palatal surfaces of the upper incisors. Intermaxillary elastics are then used to create an earlier proclination maxillary incisors and retroclination mandibular incisors.

This can also be composed of bands or tubes on the first permanent maxillary molars, brackets on the maxillary, and a wire with open coil springs. Brackets are also bonded on the mandibular incisors and the anterior cross-bite is simultaneously managed with Class III elastics (Figure 12) [17].

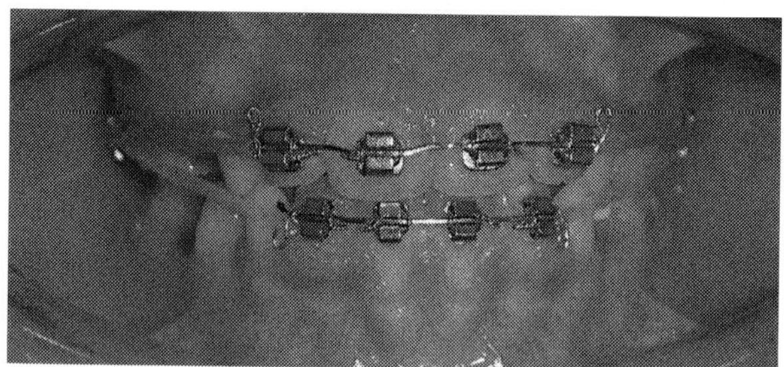

Figure 12. The components of standard edgewise appliance to resolve an anterior crossbite.

5. Case reports

5.1. Case N° 1

A 8 year-old girl was referred by her pediatric dentist for an orthodontic consultation regarding her anterior bite. Extra orally, she had a balanced face, *a slight retrusion of the upper lip while excessive mandibular anterior displacement is revealed to smile view. She presented in the early mixed dentition stage with* Class III left molar relationships. The anterior crossbite was expressed as a result of functional shift of the mandible in the sagittal plane due to lingually-inclined maxillary incisors and supernumerary anterior teeth in mandible. (Figure 13) When the mandible is manipulated into a terminal hinge-axis position, the incisors come into edge-to-edge contact, requiring the patient to move the mandible forward to achieve posterior occlusion. The panoramic radiograph showed presumptive signs of crowding in the maxilla. The cephalometric values confirmed retroclined maxillary incisors, proclined mandibular incisors, and normal vertical development. (Figure 14)

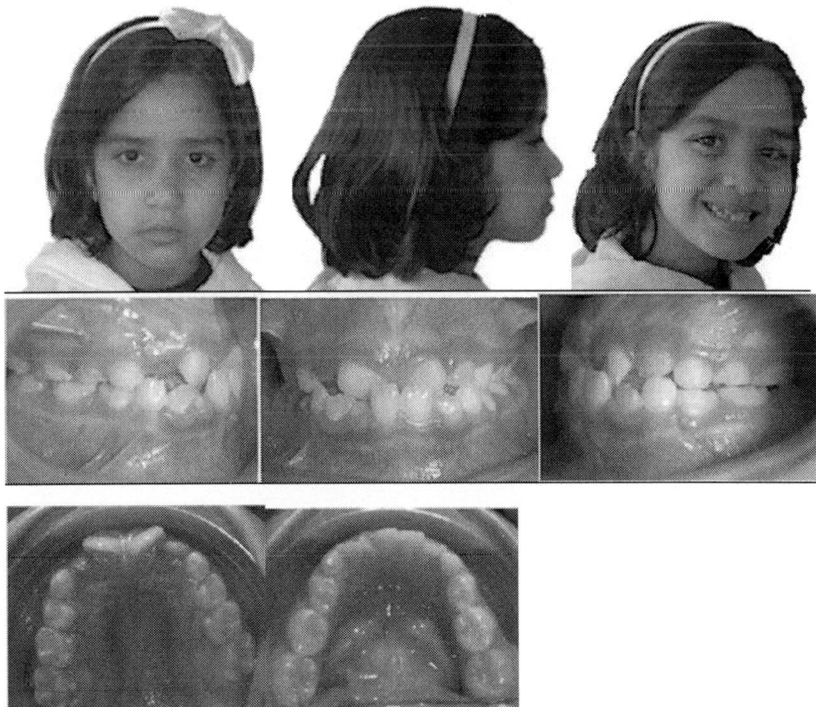

Figure 13. Pre-treatment extraoral and intraoral photographs.

The treatment aims to reduce the functional shift of the mandible and increase maxillary arch length, thus permitting eruption of the permanent canines and premolars into a Class I relationship. Bonding brackets to the two maxillary permanent central incisors in combination with banding the two maxillary permanent first molars was used. The device consists, in the first stage, of a round stainless steel arch wire to achieve alignment of upper incisors; an elevation of the occlusion was provided by resin-composite bite plane bonded to lingual side of the lower incisors. Then, an open-coil spring was compressed against the molar tube to push the incisors labially. So, the supernumerary incisor was extracted for the recovery of the lower incisor. (Figure 15)

The total active treatment period was about 6 months and follow-up appointments were scheduled every 4 weeks. Upon completion of treatment, the anterior crossbite was corrected, the molar relationships were restored to Class I. Advancing the maxillary incisors labially normalized the overjet and allow the mandible to close into a Class I without the anterior shift. Finally the treatment improved maxillary lip posture and facial appearance (Figure 16) Both skeletal and dento-alveolar effects of interceptive treatment are illustrated in Figure 15; the wits appraisal is a leading indicator of re-equilibation of maxillomandibular relationship (AOBO=0mm). (Figure 17)

The case was followed up out of retention 6 months later. Stable anterior and posterior relationships were evident, and continued spontaneous alignment of the mandibular incisors was noticed. (Figure 18)

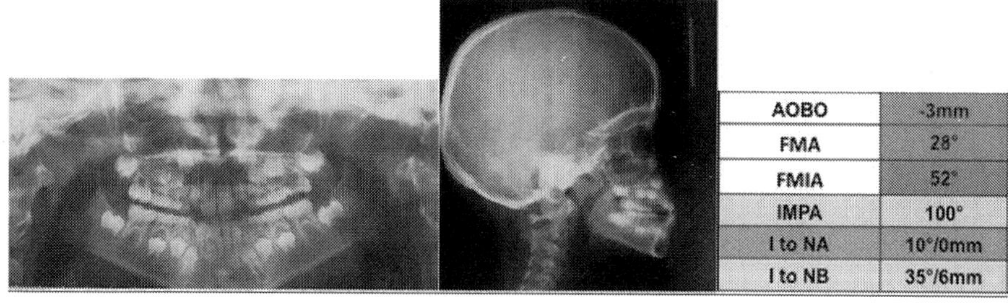

Figure 14. Pre-treatment radiographs.

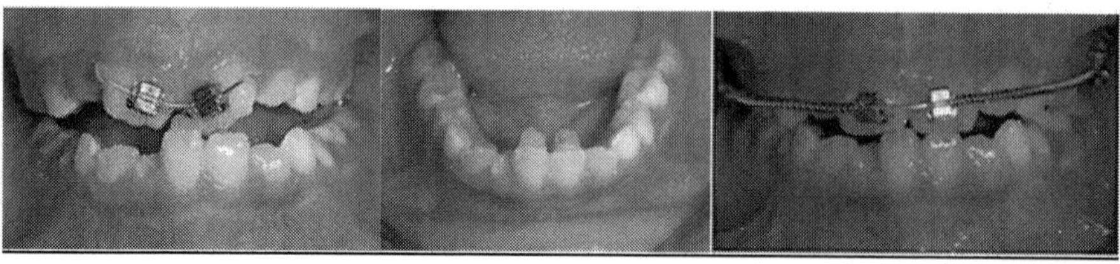

Figure 15. Treatment progress.

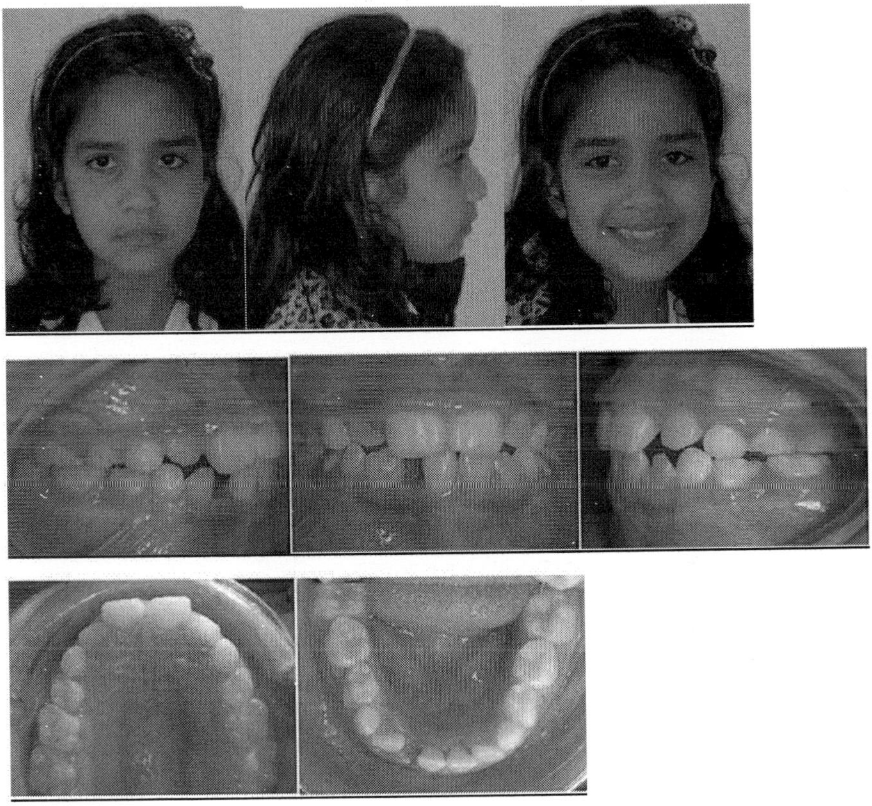

Figure 16. Extraoral and intraoral photographs after anterior crossbite correction.

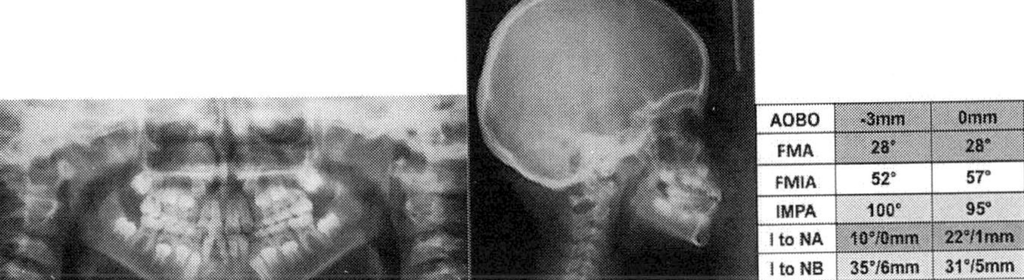

AOBO	-3mm	0mm
FMA	28°	28°
FMIA	52°	57°
IMPA	100°	95°
I to NA	10°/0mm	22°/1mm
I to NB	35°/6mm	31°/5mm

Figure 17. post-treatment radiographs.

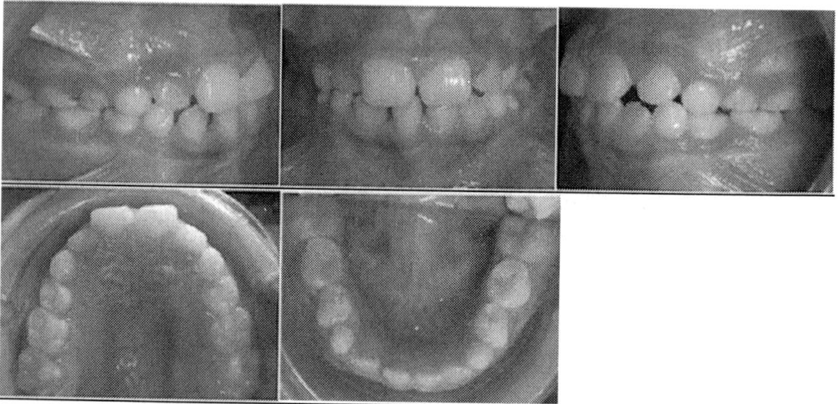

Figure 18. Six months post-treatment intraoral photographs.

5.2. Case N° 2

A 9-year-old boy consulted regarding his anterior bite that causes a concern for his parents. On extraoral examination, a slight retrusion of the upper lip was noticed, and smile betrays the anterior reversed occlusion. Intraoral examination revealed a mixed dentition stage, with erupted upper and lower permanent incisors and first molars. All maxillary incisors were in crossbite with the mandibular incisors. The molar relation on both sides was developing class III malocclusion (Figure 19). There was no family history of class III malocclusion. On assessment guidance of the mandible on closure, a functional shift of the mandible was seen. An occlusal prematurity in relation to erupting 41 and retroclination of maxillary incisors appeared to be responsible for the present functional shift [Figure 20]. Based on the above findings, a diagnosis of pseudo class III malocclusion was made and the treatment aimed at eliminating the anterior interlock. It was expected to position the mandible backward and promote maxillary growth with standard edgewise appliance.

Bite opening and bracket and tube bonding to the four maxillary incisors and the two maxillary permanent first molars (2 * 4 fixed appliance) were used to resolve an anterior crossbite in combination with open coil spring and Class III elastics (Figure 21). After leveling and alignment stage, crossbite was corrected in 4 months. After six months of treatment, significant improvement in the patient's profile and smile was noted. An increase in upper incisor inclination was obtained, and reduction in lower incisor inclination resulted in normalized overbite and overjet. So, for more security, we opted for a bonded maxillary retainer (Figure 22). The effects observed were attributed to the correction of interlocking and also to the guidance of the mandible in a normal backward position. The intraoral examination after a 1-year follow-up revealed a normal overjet and overbite relation [Figure 23].

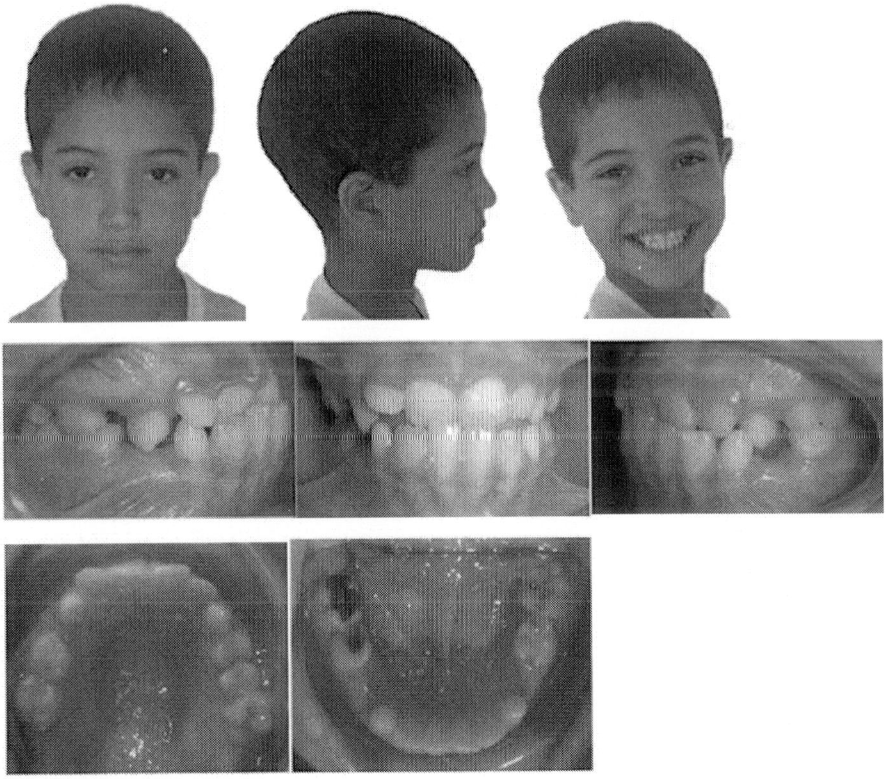

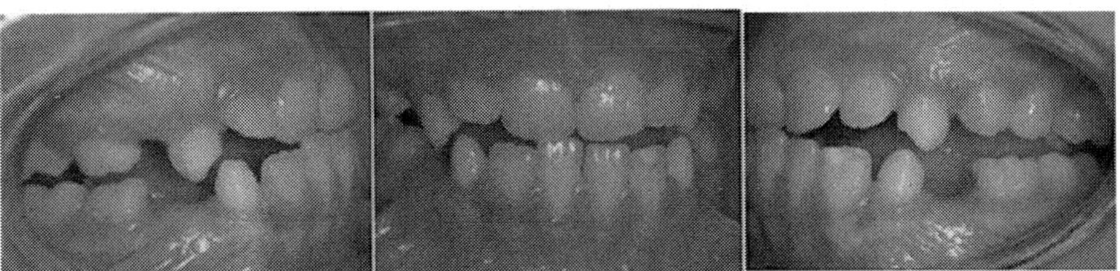

Figure 19. Pre-treatment extraoral and intraoral photographs.

Figure 20. Pre-treatment intra-oral photographs in centric occlusion.

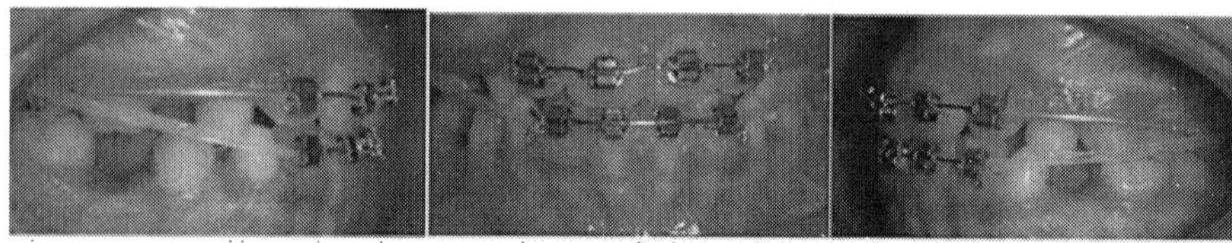

Figure 21. Upper and lower 2*4 appliances in combination with Class III elastics, used for advancing maxillary incisors into desired overjet.

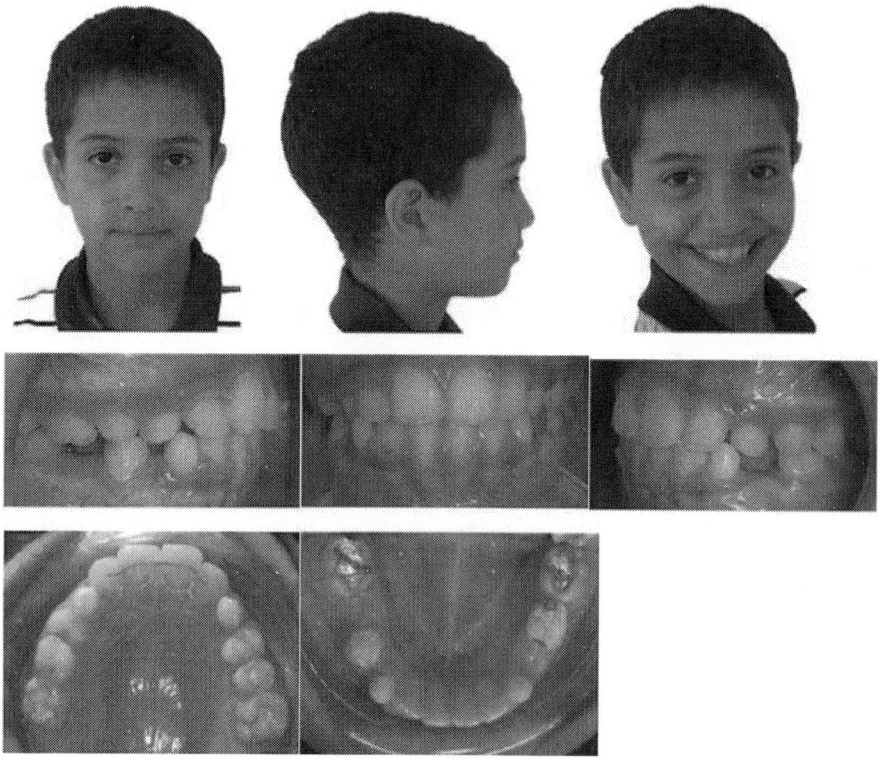

Figure 22. Extraoral and intraoral photographs after anterior crossbite correction.

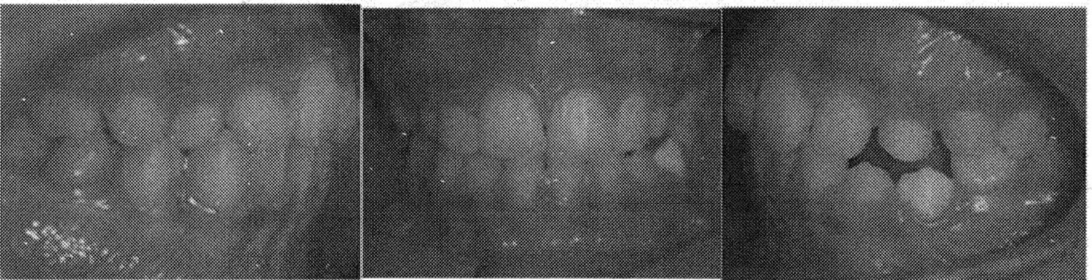

Figure 23. Year-follow-up

6. Discussion

Anterior crossbite is a major concern for both parents and clinicians. It requires early intervention to achieve a normal occlusion that is morphologically stable in the long term and functionally and esthetically acceptable. However the fundamental goal of interceptive approach is to improve the growth.

The pseudo-Class III malocclusion involves both permanent teeth and deciduous dentition. Some practitioners prefer to wait for the permanent maxillary incisors to erupt before initiating therapy due to the natural tendency of teeth to erupt in a lingual position during dental arch development. And the possible spontaneous correction of functional deciduous anterior crossbites occasionally corrects themselves spontaneously. However, the optimum period for successful treatment suggested being between the ages 6–9 years [10].

Interceptive orthodontic procedures must be relatively simple and inexpensive treatment approaches that target developing malocclusions during the mixed dentition. In cases of pseudo-Class III malocclusion, early intervention has a highly favorable cost-benefit ratio, and treatment usually takes less time [18]. So, it was suggested that early management of anterior crossbite in these kind of case be successful in 100% of treated young patients [17].

The various treatments suggested in the literature for correction of anterior crossbite include different appliances, both fixed and/or removable with heavy intermittent forces (inclined bite plane, tongue blade) or light-continuous forces (removable appliance with auxiliary springs). A recent systematic review disclosed a wide variety of treatment modalities, more than 12 methods, in use for anterior crossbite correction [19]. However, strong evidence in support of any treatment technique is lacking [8].

Removable appliances have been shown to be effective in the correction of anterior crossbite and elimination of mandibular displacement. Nonetheless, the major inconvenience of these tools is the necessity of an absolute cooperation on the part of the patient due to a high risk of loss or repetitive fractures.

A modified quad helix appliance has proved to be an economical alternative, which is easy to fabricate and causes minimal patient discomfort [9].

Other alternative therapies that may correct skeletal problems in young patients have been shown to be effective in functional Class III, with significant changes in the craniofacial complex, including the use of protraction headgear, chin cup, and Frankel III [10, 15].

The face mask should be advised during the deciduous dentition phase in cases of minor skeletal component. This produces protrusive forces to the maxilla and maxillary dentition.

The literature demonstrates that functional appliances are effective in anterior crossbite correction. This approach prevents unfavourable growth especially mandibular protrusion, and eliminates traumatic occlusion. Giancotti suggested the therapeutic use of a Balters' Bionator appliance. The patients wore the bionator approximately 15 hours daily for a period of 60-90 days. However, the cooperation of the patient is essential for the success of this approach [10].

Bonding brackets to the four maxillary incisors in combination with banding or bonding the two maxillary permanent first molars is one of the methods used for the correction of anterior crossbite with fixed appliances. It has been reported to effectively manage anterior crossbite in the mixed dentition [20]. For some authors, the main reason for using the fixed appliance treatment seems to be misalignment, [17] For others, this method has the advantages of requiring little or no patient compliance or alteration of speech [4].

One of the benefits claimed for early treatment with fixed appliance is that space is provided for the eruption of the canines and premolars in the upper arch, allowing the erupting dentition to be guided into a Class I relationship in centric relation [17].

There is disagreement about the need for a second phase of treatment during adolescence, A retrospective cohort study of interceptive orthodontic treatment indicate that interceptive orthodontic treatment is effective for improving malocclusion, but does not produce finished-quality results without a second phase of treatment in the permanent dentition [3]. Several studies have suggested that systematically planned interceptive treatment in the mixed dentition might contribute to a significant reduction in treatment need between the ages of 8 and 12 years, In a Finnish study, the need was reduced significantly from 8 to 12. However, Only 25% of these patients required a second stage of treatment after eruption of the remaining permanent teeth [21].

With respect to stability of such approach, it was reported, in follow-up study, that in young patients diagnosed with pseudo Class III malocclusion and treated early with a fixed appliance, the overjet was corrected, and the treatment result was maintained in the long term (for mor than 5 years after active treatment) [17]. So, it was suggested that either fixed or removable appliances with similar long-term stability could successfully correct anterior crossbite [22].

A systematic review of early correction of anterior crossbite has highlighted the lack of high quality evidence, and concludes that despite the low level of evidence, there is similarity in the length of time it took to successfully treat anterior crossbites using similar treatment modalities [19].

The therapeutic use of a fixed appliance is suggested in two case reports of subjects with anterior crossbite in mixed dentition. Careful clinical evaluation of Class III malocclusion checked anterior and posterior dental relationships with the mandible in centric relation. The prognosis was favorable for the treatment and post-retention results to be stable in the future. The two patients achieved a positive and often slightly overcorrected overjet during the active treatment after six months of treatment.

As early correction of anterior crossbite was undertaken in the growing child, it is important to evaluate post-treatment changes. The overjet remained stable because the corrected upper incisors were kept in place by normalizing the overjet and overbite.

7. Conclusion

Interceptive orthodontic treatment aims to recognize and eliminate potential irregularities and malpositions in the developing dento-facial complex. Early treatment of Class III malocclusion is one of the most challenging problems confronting orthodontists. The treatment should be carried out as early as possible with the aim of permitting normal growth, and improving facial attractiveness and psychosocial well being of children.

In spite of its weak prevalence, functional Class III must be prematurely detected and treated to prevent a functional anomaly from becoming a skeletal anomaly. A well-conducted clinical and radiographic examination, highlighting skeletal Class I, allows judicious and appropriate therapeutic choices.

The optimum treatment timing and the treatment modalities influence therapy. It is believed to have many benefits, including a better use of the patient's growth potential, a lower risk of progression to a true Class III malocclusion, and more stable results.

Author details

Sanaa Alami[1*], Hakima Aghoutan[1], Farid El Quars[1], Samir Diouny[2] and Farid Bourzgui[1]

*Address all correspondence to: alamisana89@gmail.com

1 Department of Dento-facial Orthopedic, Faculty of Dental Medicine, Hassan II University of Casablanca, Morocco

2 Chouaib Doukkali University, Faculty of Letters & Human Sciences, El Jadida, Morocco

References

[1] Le Gall M, Philip C, Bandon D. The functional mandibular prognathism. Archives de pédiatrie. 2009; 16; 77–83.

[2]   Keski-Nisula K, Lehto R, Lusa V, Keski-Nisula L, Varrela J. Occurrence of malocclusion and need of orthodontic treatment in early mixed dentition. Am J Orthod Dentofacial Orthop. 2003; 124:631-8.

[3]   King GJ, Brudvik P. Effectiveness of interceptive orthodontic treatment in reducing malocclusions. Am J Orthod Dentofacial Orthop. 2010;137;18-25.

[4]   Bindayel NA. Simple removable appliances to correct anterior and posterior crossbite in mixed dentition: Case report. The Saudi Dental Journal. 2012; 24, 105–13.

[5]   Kumar A, Tandon P, Singh GP. Management of pseudo Class III malocclusion-synergistic approach with fixed and functional appliance. Int J Orthod Milwaukee. 2013; 24 (2) 41-4.

[6]   Randrianarimanarivo HM, Rasoanirina MO, Andriambololo-Nivo RD, Ralison G, Rakotovao JD. Interception de la pseudo-prognathie mandibulaire: comparaison de la plaque en "V" et du plan incliné antéro-inférieur. Revue d'odontostomatologie malgache en ligne. 2011; 3; 29-38.

[7]   Langlade M. Diagnostic orthodontique, Paris : Maloine ;1981.

[8]   Wiedel AP, Bondemark L. Stability of anterior crossbite correction: A randomized controlled trial with a 2-year follow-up. Angle Orthod. 2014.

[9]   Kumar A, SA, Shetty KS, Prakash AT. Pseudo-Class III: Diagnosis and Simplistic Treatment. J Ind Orthod Soc. 2011; 45 (4) 198-201.

[10]   Giancotti A, Maselli A, Mampieri G, Spanò E. Pseudo-Class III malocclusion treatment with Balters' Bionator. Journal of Orthodontics. 2003; 30; 203–15.

[11]   Ngan P1, Hu AM, Fields HW Jr. Treatment of Class III problems begins with differential diagnosis of anterior crossbites. Pediatr Dent. 1997 Sep-Oct;19(6):386-95.

[12]   Jirgensone I, Liepa A, Abeltins A. Anterior crossbite correction in primary and mixed dentition with removable inclined plane (Bruckl appliance). Stomatologija. 2008;10 (4):140-4.

[13]   Park JH. Orthodontic correction of Class III malocclusion in a young patient with the use of a simple fixed appliance. Int J Orthod Milwaukee. 2012 ; 23 (3 43-8.

[14]   Arman A, Ufuk Toygar T, Abuhijleh E. Profile Changes Associated with Different Orthopedic Treatment Approaches in Class III Malocclusions Angle Orthodontist. 2004; 74 (6) 733-40.

[15]   Negi KS, Sharma KR. Treatment of pseudo Class III malocclusion by modified Hawleys appliance with inverted labial bow. Journal of Indian Society of Pedodontics and Preventive Dentistry. 2011; 29 (1) 57-61.

[16]   Le Gall M, Philip C, Salvadori A. Early treatment of Class III malocclusion. Orthod Fr. 2011;82 (3) 241-52.

[17] Hägg U, DDS, Tse A, Bendeus M, Rabie ABM. A Follow-up Study of Early Treatment of Pseudo Class III Malocclusion. Angle Orthodontist, Vol 74, No 4, 2004.

[18] Bowman SJ. A Quick Fix for Pseudo-Class III Correction. J. clin Ortho. 2008; 42(10) 1-7.

[19] Borrie F1, Bearn D. Early correction of anterior crossbites: a systematic review. J Orthod. 2011; 38(3) 175-84.

[20] Dowsing P1, Sandler PJ. How to effectively use a 2 x 4 appliance. J Orthod. 2004; 31(3) 248-58.

[21] Gu, Y.; Rabie, A.B.; and Hägg, U.Treatment effects of simple fixed appliance and reverse headgear in correction of anterior crossbites, Am. J. Orthod. 2000.117:691-99,

[22] Wiedel AP, Bondemark L. Stability of anterior crossbite correction: A randomized controlled trial with a 2-year follow-up. Angle Orthodontist. 2014.

Chapter 17

Fränkel Functional Regulator in Early Treatment of Skeletal Distal and Mesial Bite

Zorana Stamenković and Vanja Raičković

Additional information is available at the end of the chapter

http://dx.doi.org/10.5772/59228

1. Introduction

Skeletal distal and mesial bite are irregularities in sagittal direction. During treatment of these malocclusions we want to achieve correct occlusion and morphology, right implementation of all orofacial functions and good facial aesthetics. If we start with orthodontic treatment in early mixed dentition we can expect good and stabile therapeutic results and we can prevent later developmental problems. This way, we avoid treatment with fixed appliances in permanent dentition and orthognatic surgery after the end of growth. It is important given the fact that orthodontic treatment is very expensive.

Etiology of skeletal distal and mesial bite are heredity and some exogenous etiologic factors. These malocclusions are inherited polygenically. Skeletal distal bite is often present among the members of the same family and among twins. Other general etiological factors are Pierre Robin syndrome, syndrome of hemifacial microsomia and endocrine disorders. Local etiological factors, are, mostly, bad habits, in the age after the third year of life. The most important bad habit is thumb sucking, which causes protrusion of the upper and retrusion of the lower incisors and increasing of overjet. Skelatal distal bite is one of symptoms in CMD, as a result of ankylosis and trauma of TMJ. Dodic [1] found that 79.9% patients with skeletal class II has positive index of CMD. Etiology of skeletal mesial bite are heredity, some specific factors, functional effects, trauma and environmental factors [2]. Previously it was thought that this malocclusion was inherited as an autosomal dominant trait. Accordingly there is the existence of the so-called Habsburgs mandible. Many members of the Habsburg monarchy had a typical large lower jaw and skeletal mesial bite [3]. If in a family exists severe skeletal Class III in 33% of their children will appear Class III and in 17% of their siblings. Some scientific studies find that there is a gene which is related to mandibular prognathism. There is different expressivity of genes in specific types

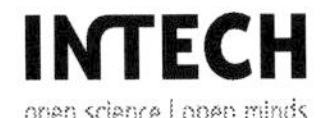

of progeny. Different genetic locus are responsible for the definitive form of the lower jaw. Other local etiologic factors are enlarged tonsils, breathing through the mouth and early extraction of deciduous molars. Patients with cleft lip and palate and some syndromes (Apert, Crouzon) often have mesial bite due to insufficient growth of the upper jaw.

Skeletal distal bite is most common in white population (38%), two times more frequent than in members of black race(20%), while frequency of this malloclusion in yellow race is 10-15%. The frequency of skeletal distal bite decreases with age, from 25-30% in mixed dentition, 20-25% in early permanent dentition to 15-20% in adult population [4]. Mesial bite commonly occurs among members of the yellow race with a frequency of 4% to 14% because they have underdeveloped nasomaxillary complex and deficient growth of the upper jaw. In the black population frequency of mesial bite is between 5% and 8%, while in the white population frequency of this malocclusion is from 1% to 4%. Frequency of malocclusion increases during the time. Skeletal mesial bite occurs in 23% in deciduous dentition, 30% in mixed dentition and 34% in permanent dentition.

2. Aim

The aim of this investigation was to compare clinical effects of different mobile orthodontic appliances (active and functional) in early treatment of skeletal distal (Class II division 1) and mesial (pseudo Class III) bite.

3. Material and method

In this study 60 patients were included with skeletal distal bite caused by mandibular retrognatism. All patients with this malocclusion had increasing value of angle ANB (>4°), due to the decrease of angle SNB (<80°). Main clinical characteristics of skeletal distal bite caused by mandibular retrognatism are: convexity of facial profile with distal position of the lower lip and chin and protrusion of the upper lip, distal relationship of dental arch and jaw bases, protrusion of the upper incisors and retrusion of the lower incisors with increasing value of overjet, inserting of the lower lip between upper and lower incisors, passing of the upper and lower incisors during eruption and their supraposition, traumatic deep bite, short mandibular corpus and lower dental arch, narrow and elongated upper dental arch, expressed mentolabial and nasolabial sulcus, shortened lower third of face and retroinclination of the lower jaw. Clinical effects were analysed on 60 patients with skeletal distal bite, without earlier orthodontic treatment. Patients were divided in three groups, with 20 patients in each. First group was treated with FR-I, second with bionator by Balters type I and the third group with Hotz mobile appliance. Effects were determined on study casts and lateral cephalometrics before and after treatment, and during functional clinical examinations and analysis of facial aesthetics.

Also, in this study were included 40 patients with skeletal Class III caused by maxillary retrognatism. They have typical changes in facial aesthetic and profile. All patients had decreasing value of angle ANB (<2°), due do decrease of angle SNA (<82°). Main clinical characteristics of pseudo Class III (caused by maxillary retrognatism) are: concavity of the facial profile with distal position of the upper lip and correct position of the lower lip and chin, mesial relationship of dental arches and jaw bases, normoinclination of upper and lower incisors, narrow and short upper dental arch, reverse overjet, lateral cross bite, underdeveloped nasomaxillary complex, crowding in upper dental arch, anteinclination of the upper jaw and changes in vertical direction. In this group of patients, also, study casts and profile teleradiograms have been analysed before and after orthodontic treatment.

Growth modification is possible if we start with orthodontic treatment early enough, before pubertal growth acceleration. Ideal period for growth modification is early mixed dentition. In this period we can affect the size and position of upper and lower jaw and their relationship. In girls treatment should be initiated at an earlier age than in boys, approximately two years. In girls "juvenile acceleration" starts 1-2 years before pubertal growth acceleration. Overall growth is affected by age, constitution, seasonal and cultural factors. Before orthodontic treatment it is necessary to determine skeletal maturity of our patients [5] Treatment with growth modification is possible when patient is in one of three first stage of skeletal maturation (Fig. 1).

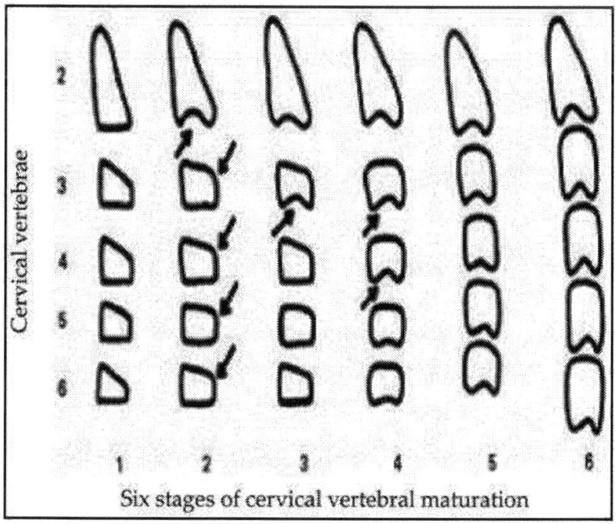

Figure 1. Six stages of cervical vertebral maturation (O'Relly & Yanneillo, 1988).

When we make decisions about growth modification treatment we need to know the degree of discrepancy between viscerocranium and neurocranium, age and sex of the patient, external and internal motivation, which appliances we want to use, at what stage of skeletal maturation is patient and how much growth left to the end of maturity [6, 7].

4. Treatment of skeletal distal bite

In modern orthodontics treatment of skeletal distal bite can be performed using many dental worn functional appliances, such as activator, bionator by Balters, twin block, Herbst appliance, Hotz appliance and vestibular plate. These appliances rest on teeth and they stimulate growth of the lower jaw due to changes in activity of orofacial muscles.

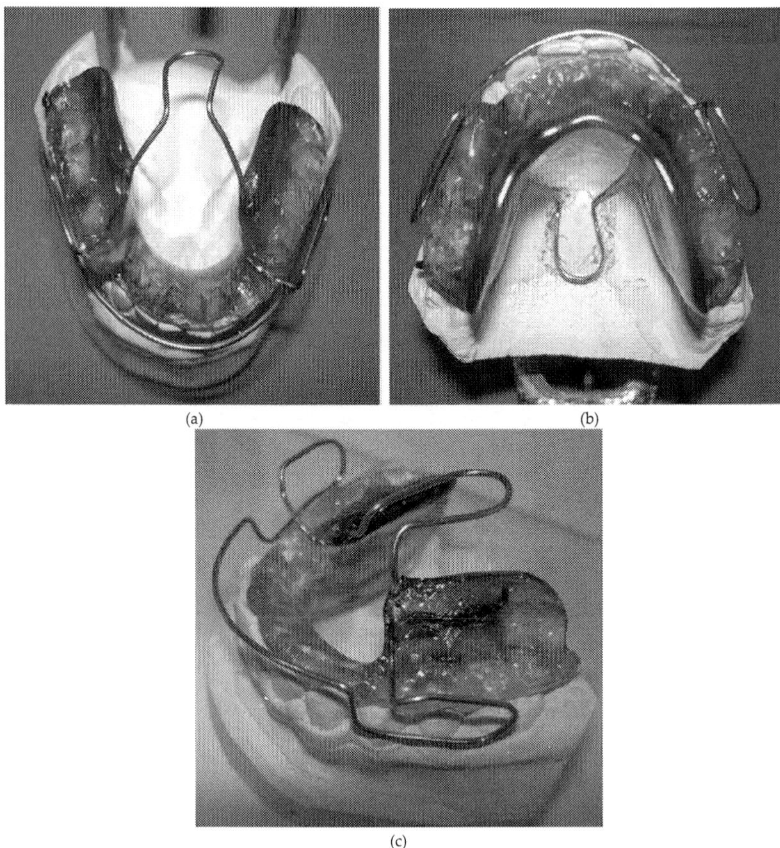

Figure 2. a.,b.,c. Balters bionator type I

To Balters opinion distrurbed function, size and tone of tongue are the main cause of all malocclusions. Bionator was designed and used in orthodontic practice by Balters in Germany (1950.). Bionator by Balters type I or the standard form is used in treatment of skeletal distal bite. This appliance is known in literature as reduced activator with interoclusal acrylic.

Components of this appliance are palatal arch directed pharyngeal, vestibular arch above upper incisors and buccal loops in the area of canines (Fig 2.a.,2.b.,2.c.). Construction bite is determined and taken in incisal relationship of incisors without activation in vertical direction. Skeletal effects are increasing of mandibular corpus and ramus, anterior displacement of the lower jaw, increasing value of angle SNB and decreasing value of angle ANB [8, 9, 10].

Hotz appliance is modified active mobile orthodontic appliance. This appliance in orthodontic practice was introduced by Hötz (1966.) in Germany. Appliance has angular frontal bite plane (Fig.3.). This appliance causes growth modification and anterior growth of the lower jaw in patients with forward facial rotation. It is necessary that inclined frontal bite plane has sufficient length for anterior movement and sliding of the lower jaw [11]. Skeletal effects are stimulation of saggital growth of the lower jaw and anterior displacement. Dental effects are retrusion of the upper and protrusion of the lower incisors and extrusion of the posterior teeth [12].

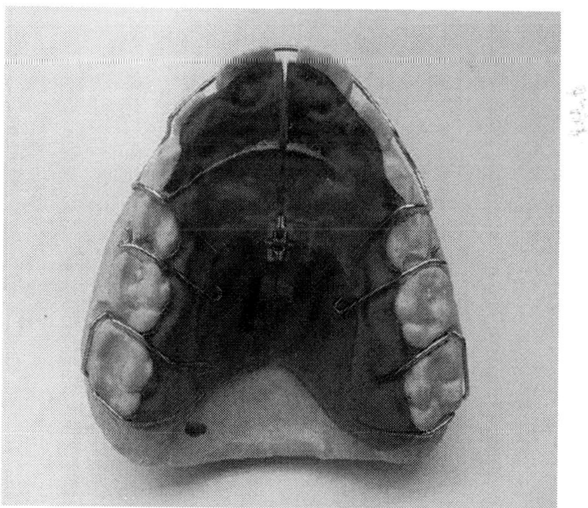

Figure 3. Hotz appliance

5. Fränkel appliance type I (FR-I)

Fränkel functional regulator (FR) is only mounted functional appliance which can effectively correct morphological (skeletal and dental) and functional irregularities. It works by pressure application at skeletal and dental structures, elimination of the pressure surrounding perioral musculature and causing tensile stress in the area of mucosal fornix, where exist bone apposition. Construction of this appliance was suggested by Rölf Fränkel in Germany (1966.)

[13]. During time the position of the lower jaw permanently changed without affecting the position of the teeth. The essential changes are tissue changes at the articular zone of growth. This appliance significantly changed muscles activity and whole physiological state of orofacial complex. There are early and late treatment of skeletal distal bite using FR-I. Early treatment begins in the age of 7-8 years, in early mixed dentition, after eruption of first permanent molars and incisors. Late treatmen starts in the age of 12 years (average) after eruption of canines and premolars [14]. Whole treatment contains active and retention period. Active period lasts an average of 18 to 24 months. During this period patient wears appliance continuously during the day, except during meals. Retention period lasts, also, 24 months. During this period patient wears appliance only at night. After 6 months of treatment sagittal relationship was corrected for half a molar width.

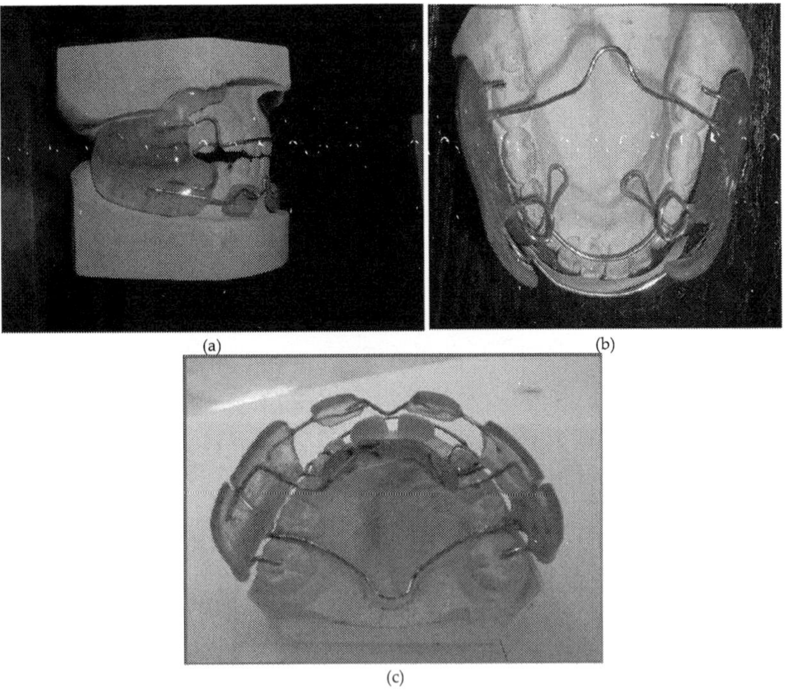

Figure 4. a.,b.,c. Fränkel appliance type I (FR-I)

In treatment of skeletal Class II we use three type of FR-I (Ia, Ib, Ic). FR-Ia is indicated for use in cases with: skeletal Class I with deep bite, skeletal Class I with protrusion of the upper and retrusion of the lower incisors, skeletal Class I with apical crowding, bilateral crossbite, skeletal Class II division 1 with overjet less than 5mm, skeletal Class II divison 1 with deep bite and retrusion of the lower incisors. FR-Ib is indicated in patients with skelelat Class II divison 1 and overjet between 5mm and 7mm and skeletal Class II divison 1. with deep bite. FR-Ic is indicated for use in cases with severe skeletal Class II divison 1 and overjet over 7mm, skeletal Class II with deep bite and difficulties to establish contact between lips during anterior movement of the lower jaw. Components of this appliance (FR-Ia) are: lateral acrilyc shields, pelotas for lower lip, labial arch, linqual arch, palatal arch with anchorage on the upper first molars and loops for upper canines (Fig. 4a.,b.,c.). For construction and making of this appliance is necessary construction bite in incisal relation of incisors without activation in vertical direction (Fig.5.). FR-Ib besides these elements includes linqual shield with linqual arch and additional arch for protrusion of the lower incisors. For FR-Ic we determine and take construction bite in relation of Class I on posterior teeth. This appliance has screw for compensatory anterior movement of the lower jaw. Construction and design of this appliance is very gentle, so patients should be very careful during manipulation with it [15].

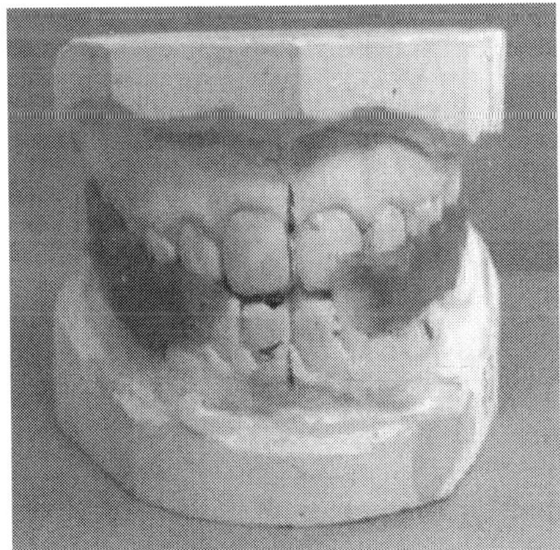

Figure 5. Construction bite for FR-I

6. Treatment of skeletal Class III

Skeletal Class III can be treated by many different dental worn functional appliances. Representatives of this group of appliances are activator, bionator by Balters type III, orthopedic bionator, chin cup, Y appliance, appliance with Bertoni screw and facial mask. The only representative of tissue worn appliances is FR-III. In older age surgical treatment is indicated in combination with fixed appliances [16].

Clinical effects were determined on 40 patients with skeletal Class III caused by maxillary retrognatism (angle SNA<82°, angle ANB<2°). None of the patients have previously had an orthodontic treatment, all of them were in period of early mixed dentition, after eruption of first permanent molars. These patients were divided in two groups, with 20 patients in each. Patients in the first group were treated by FR-III, while patients in the second group were treated by Y appliance. Clinical effects were analyzed on study casts, lateral cephalometric and facial aesthetic before and after treatment. Separately were analyzed and interpreted parameters of position and development of the upper and lower jaw, parameters of intermaxillary relations, parameters of the facial growth, the cranial base parameters, parameters of the position of the incisors, parameters of TMJ, soft tissue profile parameters, parameters of skeletal and dental changes during the treatment and methods of investigation of orofacial functions.

Y appliance is active, mobile orthodontic appliance. This appliance has acrylic plate cut to shape letter Y with two screws in the area of canine (Fig.6.). Patients turn both screws in the same time, that way the appliance causes protrusion of the upper incisors. Y appliance is useful in patients with pseudo Class III [12]. With this appliance we correct reverse overjet and eliminate premature contact with stabile treatment result. Ideal time for treatment is period of mixed dentition. Patients turn screws once in 7 days, with biological movement less than 1mm during one month. During retention period patient wear appliance only during the night, without turning the screws.

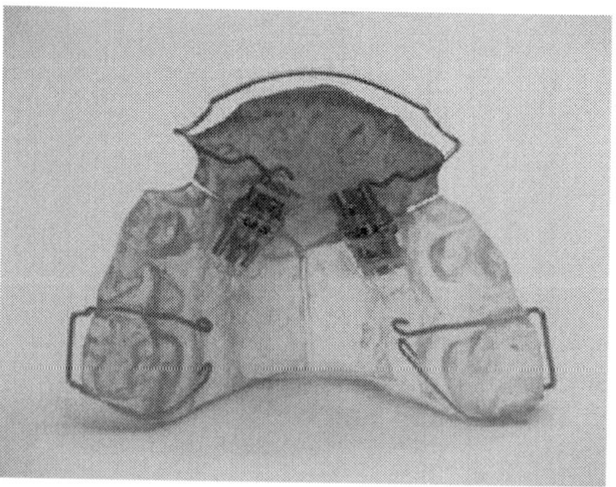

Figure 6. Y appliance

7. Fränkel appliance type III — (FR-III)

Fränkel functional regulator (FR) is passive, mobile functional appliance. At the same time it is the only tissue worn functional appliance. With FR we can correct both occlusal (dental and skeletal) and functional irregularities. Three main mechanisms of action of this device are: aplication of pressure, elimination of pressure and application of pulling force. Rölf Fränkel presented this appliance to orthodontic public in Germany in 1966. Application of pressure prevents excessive growth of the lower jaw in sagittal direction. Elimination of pressure separates the soft tissues of the lips and cheeks and prevents their contact with dentoalveolar structures. FR-III contributes to the proper formation of dentoalveolar structures of the upper and lower jaw. Application of pulling force increases the activity of osteoblasts in the periost, that way appliance contributes to the creation of new bone tissue in the upper jaw [17]. Acrylic pelotas are located in the upper vestibule and stimulate the sagittal growth of the upper jaw. FR-III causes tissue changes in the articular zone of growth. During wearing of appliance there is a continual activation of the muscles of the orofacial region to change their tone and activity. Optimal time for treatment with this appliance is early mixed dentition, immediately after eruption of all upper permanent molars, at an age of about seven years of age. The best therapeutic results are expected in patients with reverse overjet (4-5mm). The whole thera-peutic procedure contains active and retention phase. Active phase lasts 24 to 30 months. During this active period, patients wear FR-III continuosly during the day and night, except during meals. Retention phase lasts about 24 months. During retention period, patients wear appliance only at night. This phase is important to preserve the stabile therapeutic results. From this we can conclude that the total duration of therapy is quite long. Patients can easily get used to this appliance, it is comfortable to use, they are motivated for treatment and we expect full cooperation with them and their parents. In treatment of skeletal Class III we use Fränkel functional regulator type III (FR-III). There are two different types, type FR-IIIa and type FR-IIIb. Type FR-IIIa is indicated in early mixed dentition in patients with pseudo mesial byte and deep reverse overjet. Type FR-IIIb is indicated in early mixed dentition in patients with pseudo mesial byte, but without deep reverse overjet. Contraindications for treatment with FR-III are: late age of patients, skeletal Class III caused by mandibular prognatism, severe teeth rotation and malpositions and coronary crowding. FR-IIIa consists of: two lateral vestibular acrylic shields, pelotas for upper lip, lower labial arch, bilatteral posterior acrylic plate on teeth, wire anchorage on the lower first permanent molars, palatal arch with protru-sion arch in the upper jaw and wire elements between pelotas and shileds (Fig. 7a.,b.,c.). FR-IIIb has simillar construction. The only difference is that FR-III does not have bilatteral posterior acrylic plate on teeth, because it is indicated in cases without deep reverse overjet, and in this situation desarticulation is not necessary. Construction and design of this appliance are very delicate. That is why patients must be very careful and patient during wearing and manipulation with FR-III. The most important phase in the development of this device is taking an accurate construction bite. Construction bite determines the position of the lower jaw in all directions. For this appliance construction bite is taken in maximal retrusion of the lower jaw, with proper midline alignment of the upper and lower jaw. The ideal would be to provide edge to edge contacts between upper and lower incisors in sagittal direction. Activation in vertical direction depends of depth of reverse overjet. In cases with deep reverse overjet, construction bite is taken with vertical activation of 2 4mm above the physiologic rest position. If patients do not have deep reverse overjet, construction bite is taken without activation in vertical direction, at physiologic rest position. Design of appliance enables correct teeth eruption with elimination of irregular muscle activity. It is said that appliance causes oral gymnastics. Pelotas stimulate growth of the upper jaw and cause increase of the width of apical base. Pelotas have triple effect: elimination of the pressure of the upper lip to the sagittal underdeveloped upper jaw, creating tensile stress in the vestibule and stimulate osteoblasts activity at the level of the periost and directing the force of the upper lip to the lower jaw over the lower vestibular arch, thus resulting in retrusion Acrylic lateral shields are in contact with lower teeth and apical base, while settle 3mm of dentoalveolar structures of the upper jaw. Appliance then stimulates both, transversal and sagittal growth of underdevolped maxilla. Fränkel suggests that functional disorder is result of malocclusion, and rarely is the primary cause of the irregularities. Appliance stimulates proper orofacial functions and achieves a balance between the muscles of tongue and buccal muscles. It eliminates the disturbed functions due to activation and adaptation of muscles. It is important to wear the appliance during the day because it achieves a constant muscle activity, while the activity is significantly reduced during the night. It is necessary to examine the relationship between form and function if we want a successful therapeutic result. FR-III regulates the function of swallowing due to buccal shields. These shields eliminate the pressure of buccal muscles and allow extension of dentoalveolar structures by changing the position and functions of tongue during swallowing. This provides a transition from infantile to mature swallowing. In some patients function of tongue is changed due to adaptation to the existing malocclusion, while in other groups of patients that is the primary cause of malocclusion. FR-III significantly increases anterior and posterior width in the upper and lower jaw and length of the upper dental arch. Appliance decreases buccal inclination of the upper first permanent molar. With FR-III dental arch can expand for 6mm and alveolar base for 5mm. Palatal arch allows expansion of lateral shields, gives support to appliance and contributes to transverse anchorage of appliance. Palatal arch is 0.5mm from the mucosae. Protrusion arch has function to cause protrusion of the upper frontal teeth. Active arch is in contact with palatal surfaces of upper incisors, close to incisal edge. Therefore, arch causes protrusion of incisors without influencing their vertical eruption. Pelotas have a parallelogram shape with rounded corners. Lower edge of pelotas is located deeply in the vestibule, 2.5-3mm from mucosa and 7-8mm from gingival edge. Upper edge of pelotas is 5mm from marginal gingival edge. The appliance does not rely on the posterior teeth in the upper jaw, because in that case pelotas cause distal movement of upper posterior teeth [13, 14]. Phases in treatment and creating of FR-III are: clinical examination, functional analysis, impressions of upper and lower jaw for study casts, analysis of lateral cephalograms and orthopantomograms, construction bite, preparation of study casts, definite preparation in the laboratory, giving the appliance to the patient and regular check-ups every four to six weeks. Phase of adaptation to FR-III is longer than with the other functional appliances. A common protocol is that patient wears the appliance for 2 hours a day for first two weeks of therapy. Next two weeks the appliance is worn for 4 hours a day. At the next check-up the appliance wearing time extends to 6 hours a day in combination with speech exercise. After the third control check-up, it is recommended to wear the appliance at all times for 24 hours, except during meals. After three months of properly wearing of appliance changes in sagittal, vertical and transversal direction are observed. Generally, after six months of treatment, skeletal Class III is corrected for half a premolar width. If there is lateral open bite it is a sign of good cooperation of the patient, because the changes in the vertical plane are more slowly than in the transversal and vertical direction, and eruption of the lower posterior teeth happens later.

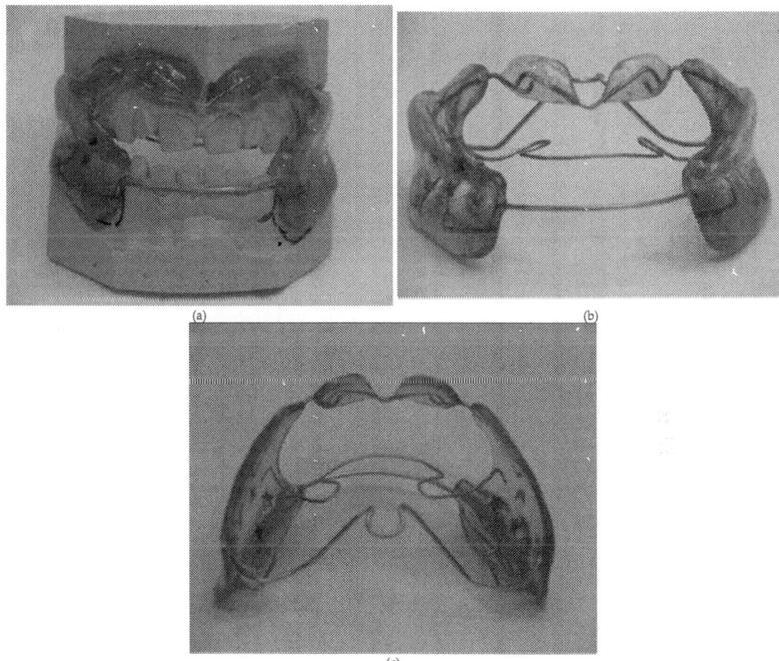

Figure 7. a.,b.,c. Fränkel appliance type III (FR-III)

8. Results and discusion

8.1. Comparative analysis of the FR-I appliance, bionator by Balters and Hotz appliance treatment effects

Position and development of the upper jaw were analyzed using values of angles SNA, SN/SpP and J and linear distance which determines length of maxillary corpus. All used appliances didn't have significant impact on position of the upper jaw. Their effects were directed to the lower jaw. Changes on the lower jaw were determined using values of angles SNB, SN/MP and SNPg and linear distances of length of mandibular corpus, total length of lower jaw, height and width of mandibular ramus. All appliances significantly changed sagittal position of the lower jaw [18]. The most pronounced increase of angle SNB causes FR-

I from 74.70° to 77.65° (p=0.001*). FR-I and bionator by Balters type I cause reducing of vertical inclination of the lower jaw to the anterior cranial base, while Hotz appliance causes increasing of vertical inclination of the lower jaw. Analysis of linear parameters showed mandibular growth in all directions, especially during the application of FR-I. Length of mandibular corpus increased from 71.22mm to 73.20mm. Malocclusion was corrected due to the joint effect of the pubertal growth process and appliances effects. All effects of appliances resulting in anterior displacement of the lower jaw and chin, with increasing value of angle SNB, without affecting the total amount of growth. In some cases existed inhibition of sagittal growth of the upper jaw, resulting in better relation between jaw bases [19, 20, 21].

Interjaw relationship was analyzed using values of angles ANB (sagittal interjaw angle), B (basal angle-vertical interjaw angle), SpP/OcCP (inclination between upper jaw and occlusal plane) and MP/OcCP (inclination between lower jaw and occlusal plane). All appliances caused the correction of skeletal Class II with decreasing values of ANB angle from 6.60° to 3.60° (p<0.001 FR-I), 5.90° na 4.90° (p=0.001 bionator by Balters type I), 5.80° to 5.10° (p=0.032 Hotz appliance). Skeletal effect was greater in the younger age. After that age, in permanent dentition, dental effects were dominant. FR-I changed function and activity of orofacial muscles and caused their transformation [22].When appliance is in the mouth vestibular pelotas provide anterior movement of the lower jaw. "U" loop prevents distal movement of the lower jaw in initial position. It is necessary to provide at the same time growth stimulation of the lower jaw and adaptation of soft tissues. This is the only way therapeutic result can be stabile and long-term. It is suggested to provide neutroocclusion through several phases, with gradually mesial movement of the lower jaw, using construction bite.

FR-I decreased basal angle, while bionator by Balters type I and Hotz appliance (p=0.044) increased value of this angle. These appliances are contraindicated in patients with backward facial rotation, because the use of this appliance would result in opening of the bite and divergent growth of jaw bases [23]. All used appliances increased vertical inclination of the upper jaw to the occlusal plane, without statistical significance. FR-I indicated anteinclination of the lower jaw to the occlusal plane, while Hotz appliance and bionator by Balters type I caused retroinclination of the lower jaw. Hotz appliance caused extrusion of posterior teeth, which reduced overbite and contributed to the opening of the bite. These changes are consequence of movement of fossa glenoidalis during growth.

All used appliances increased values of angles NSAr and ArGoMe, while FR-I and Hotz appliance increased value of angle SArGo, but bionator by Balters type I decreased value of this angle. Sum of angles of Björk polygon were increased, most evident when using FR-I, from 393.55° to 395.70°. Mostly, patients in this sample had forward rotation before beginning of the orthodontic treatment. It was good prognostic sign for patients with skeletal Class II, while vertical growth was not significant in cases with mandibular retrognathism. If we start with orthodontic treatment early enough (in early mixed dentition) we can change type of facial growth [24, 25]. FR-I and bionator by Balters mostly didn't change type of facial growth, while Hotz appliance caused backward rotation and vertical facial growth. During therapeutic procedure anterior and posterior facial height were decreased, partially as a consequence of intensive growth in this age and as a result of used appliances. Simillar changes were registred on both, anterior and posterior facial height, but facial growth in total was not changed during this period. Both methods, Björk and Jarabak, are metric, static and they show type of facial growth in one moment. That's why these methods are not reliable for long-term research.

Changes on the cranial base were analyzed by linear distances N-S (length of anterior cranial base), S-Ba (length of posterior cranial base) and N-Ba (total length of cranial base) and angle of cranial base NSBa. All parameters were increased during orthodontic treatment. Changes in linear distances were not statistically significant during this period. Thereby distance N-Se can be used as a reference plane for superposition of lateral cephalometrics for longitudinal studies. Changes in linear distances were primarily consequence of intensive facial growth in this period, not as a effect of used appliances [26]. Angle NSBa was increased during treatment with FR-I and Hotz appliance, while bionator by Balters type I caused decreasing value of angle NSBa. Size, form and structure of cranial base are under genetic control, with some specific characteristics of race and gender. Bones of cranial base are primarily in cartilage. After that enhondral ossification and bone formation begins. Whole cranial base was elongated due to the growth of synhondrosis. We cannot affect the cranial base the same way as the facial bones. Between bones of cranial base are immobile joints, so the whole cranial base appears as one long bone. When we plan orthodontic treatment we can not expect severe changes in morphology and size of cranial base. Present changes were result of intensive displacement and bone remodelation and growth on synhondrosis.

Inclination of upper incisors was changed during orthodontic treatment, angle I/SpP was increased in whole sample. All used appliances caused retrusion of upper incisors, the most visible during treatment with bionator by Balters type I (angle I/SpP was changed from 69.35° to 71.15°). Retrusion of upper incisors is one of the most important dental effects during orthodontic treatment with these appliances. In the beginnig of treatment lower incisors were, mostly retruded or had normoinclination. Position of lower incisors is important information when planning orthodontic treatment. Correct relation between lower incisors and bone jaw base is necessary for stabile therapeutic result [27, 28]. During orthodontic treatment all appliances caused protrusion of lower incisors with decreasing values of angle i/MP. FR-I caused change of this angle from 89.75° to 88.30°, Hotz appliance from 89.75° to 87.00°, with statistical significance p<0.001, while bionator by Balters type I decreased value of angle i/MP from 89.15° to 89.00°, without statistical significance. Balance between retrusion of the upper and protrusion of the lower incisors provides decreasing of overjet.

During orthodontic treatment changes on TMJ were made in two dimensions, the change in a height of TMJ (vertical direction) and anteroposterior position of TMJ (sagittal direction). TMJ is one of growth zones during this period. "Answer" of TMJ to orthodontic treatment is one of the most important facts for final therapeutic result. During orthodontic tretmant the height of TMJ was decreased, without statistical significance. Sagittal position of TMJ was analyzed by distance S-E. This distance was increased during orthodontic treatment, statistically significant during treatment with FR-I (from 22mm to 23mm) and bionator by Balters type I (p=0.042). These changes are consequence of used functional appliances and their effects to upper and lower jaw [29, 30].

Harmonious facial aesthetics means a balance between skeletal and dentoalveolar structures from one side and structures of soft tissue profile, from the other side. All structures of orofacial complex constitute one indivisible whole. Changes on soft tissue profile were determined using analysis of angles T and H, position of the upper and lower lip to aesthetic line and height of upper lip. Effects on soft tissue structures are necessary for stabile therapeutic result and good facial aesthetics. During period of growth changes on soft tissues are much more pronounced than on skeletal structures. Upper and lower lip and other soft tissues move down a function of time [31]. As a result of increasing values of angles SNB and SNPg changes in values of angles T and H appear. Angle T is in correlation with angle J and it was significantly decreased during treatment, from 21.60° to 17.15° with FR-I. Angle H is in correlation with angle ANB. With decreasing of angle ANB decreases the value of angle H. This angle was significantly decreased, most evident when using FR-I from 16.45° to 13.40°, p<0.001. Patients with skeletal distal bite have convex profile, with irregular position of the upper and lower lip. During orthodontic treatment upper lip had smaller distance to aesthetic line, when using FR-I from 0.77mm to 0.12mm. Lower lip had, also, smaller distance to aesthetic line, except when using Hotz appliance. During orthodontic treatment height of the upper lip was decreased, when using FR-I from 26.15mm to 25.85mm, while Hotz appliance and bionator by Balters increased height of the upper lip. Decreasing of profile convexity appears as a consequence of movement of the upper and lower lip to Ricketts aesthetic line [32, 33, 34].

Patients with Class II divison 1 often have disturbed orofacial functions, especially swallowing and speech. These patients have infantile swallowing with tongue insertion between upper and lower frontal teeth. FR-I has the greatest impact on correction of orofacial functions [35]. This appliance provides the transition from infantile to mature swallowing. Design of FR-I prevents insertion of lower lip and tongue between upper and lower incisors. It creates conditions for correct articulation of interdental consonants. FR-I causes continuous muscle activation and changes in tone and muscle activity [36, 37, 38].

Pancherz's analysis defines skeletal and dentoalveolar changes during orthodontic treatment. Measurements have been done in the area of upper and lower first permanent molars and incisors and skeletal points pg and ss [39, 40]. FR-I changed molar relation for 1.45mm, Hotz appliance for 2.12mm and bionator by Balters type I 1.15mm. Relation between incisors was changed for 2.05mm when using FR-I, 1.85mm with Hotz appliance and 1.40mm with bionator by Balters type I. Skeletal correction was the most evident when using FR-I 3.35mm, bionator by Balters type I changed it for 2.80mm and Hotz appliance for 2.40mm.

8.2. Review of clinical effects using FR-III and Y appliance in treatment of skeletal Class III

Dimensions, position and development of the upper jaw were analyzed using values of angles SNA (angle of maxillary prognatism), SN/SpP (vertical position of the upper jaw to anterior cranial base) and J (angle of facial inclination), and linear distances Cmax which determines the length of the upper jaw. Both appliances had significant effect to the upper jaw, causing her anterior movement in relation to the anterior cranial base and increase the value of the angle SNA, with statistical significance p<0.001*. FR-III caused increasing of SNA angle from 76.65° to 79.85°, while Y appliance increased this angle from 76.60° to 77.90° Both appliances caused increasing of vertical inclination of the upper jaw to the anterior cranial base. This has resulted in increasing values of angle SN/SpP, with FR-III from 10.20° to 10.50° and with Y appliance from 11.75° to 12.75°. Y appliance caused significant increasing of angle J, from 80.45° to 81.90°. FR-III, also, caused, an increase in the angle J, but to a much lesser extent, from 83.10° to 83.35°. In the whole sample there was a significant increase in the value of the upper jaw length corpus, with FR-III from 43.24mm to 46.15mm and with Y appliance from 46.87mm to 48.35mm. Increasing of maxillary corpus length is a result of simultaneously intensive growth and effect of orthodontic appliance [41, 42, 43]. Position, development and dimension of the lower jaw vere analyzed by angles SNB (angle of mandibular prognatism), SN/MP (angle of vertical position of the lower jaw to the anterior cranial base) and SNPg (sagittal position of chin to the anterior cranial base) and linear parameters: length of mandibular corpus, total length of the lower jaw, height and width of mandibular ramus. Changes in the lower jaw are low, which is in accordance with the design of the appliances, and design of the appliances, and mainly the upper jaw. FR-III increased value of angle SNB from 78.55° to 78.60°, while Y appliance increased this angle from 79.00° to 79.45°. Both appliances caused retroinclination of the lower jaw and increasing of angle SN/SpP. FR-III caused changes of SN/MP angle from 35.40° to 36.65° and Y appliance from 36.85°to 38.90°. Angle SNPg was increased during the treatment, in correlation with increasing of SNB angle. Y appliance caused major changes from 79.45° to 80.05°, while FR-III increased this angle from 78.80° to 79.30°. Appliances caused retroinclination of the lower jaw to the anterior cranial base and inhibiting the growth of the lower jaw. All linear parameters were increased, mostly as a result of facial growth. Length of mandibular corpus was increased from 68.85mm to 70.00mm using FR-III, while Y appliance caused change from 73.55mm to 74.75mm. Total length of the upper jaw was increased with FR-III from 104.05mm to 105.60mm and with Y appliance from 118.10mm to 118.55mm. FR-III increased height of mandibular ramus from 52.77mm to 53.70mm, while Y appliance changed this parameter from 54.15mm to 54.95mm. Both appliances increased width of the mandibular ramus, FR-III from 11.55mm to 12.55mm and Y appliance from 11.15mm to 12.10mm. All effects of appliances resulted in anterior movement of the upper jaw and stimulation of maxillary sagittal and transversal growth [44, 45, 46, 47].

Relationship between upper and lower jaw was determined by values of angles ANB (sagittal interjaw angle, skeletal Class), B or SpP/MP (basal angle – vertical interjaw angle), SpP/OcCP (vertical postion of the upper jaw to occlusal plane) and MP/OcCP (vertical position of the lower jaw to occlusal plane). Both appliances caused significant increasing value of ANB angle. It allows correction of skeletal Class III to skeletal Class I. FR-III changed angle ANB from-1.90° to 1.25°, while Y appliance changed this angle from-2.40° to-1.55°, with statistical significance on the level p=0.001*. FR-III primarily affects the skeletal structures due to pelotas which stimulate the growth of the upper jaw, increasing its length and raise the value of ANB angle. Increasing value of ANB angle is a consequence of increasing the value of the angle SNA. Mobile, active appliances mostly affect dentoalveolar structures and skeletal changes are minimal. During the treatment, both appliances increased value of basal angle (B). It can contribute to opening bite. FR-III increased value of angle B from 25.20° to 26.30° and Y appliance changed angle B from 25.05° to 26.15°. Angle SpP/MP was increased during treatment, with FR-III from 10.30° to 11.45° and with Y appliance from 10.40° to 11.55°. At the same time value of angle MP/OcCp was decreased, without statistical significance, with FR-III from 14.90° to 14.85° and with Y appliance from 14.65° to 14.60°. Changes in basal angle were mostly result of increasing angle between upper jaw and occlusal plane [48, 49]. Appliances are contraindicated in patients with backward facial rotation, because their use can contribute to the bite opening and divergent growth of the bases of upper and lower jaw.

Facial growth and rotation are determined by Björk and Jarabak method. FR-III increased angle NSAr from 122.80° to 123.87° and Y appliance from 127.35° to 128.65°. Also, both appliances increased value of gonial angle-ArGoMe, FR-III from 131.10° to 131.85° and Y appliance from 131.75° to 132.15°. FR-III increased value of articular angle-SArGo from 141.50° to 142.17°, while Y appliance decreased tih angle from 134.95° to 134.25°. As a result there is an increase in values of sum of angles of Björks polygon, with FR-III from 395.40° to 396.90° and with Y appliance from 394.05° to 395.05°. Linear distances, N-Me and S-Go, were increased during this period. This increase was a consequence of pubertal facial growth in this age and use of orthodontic appliances. Relation between anterior and posterior facial height was slightly changed, without influence to total facial growth during the treatment. Relation was changed by FR-III from 64.34% to 63.35% and with Y appliance from 63.73% to 64.30%. If we start with orthodontic treatment early enough we can change the type of facial growth. Generally, FR-III caused slight backward rotation and tendency to the vertical facial growth [50, 51, 52].

FR-III and Y appliance caused increasing of length of anterior cranial base, FR-III from 68.70mm to 69.50mm, Y appliance from 71.55mm to 72.85mm. Also, both appliances increased value of total length of cranial base, FR-III from 101.30mm to 103.85mm, Y appliance from 106.85mm to 107.45mm. FR-III caused decreasing of posterior cranial base from 44.55mm to 42.70mm, while Y appliances increased this distance from 47.25mm to 47.40mm. All changes did not have statistically significance. Both appliances caused increase of angle NSBa. Increase was significant during treatment with Y appliance, which changed this angle from 130.15° to 131.35°, with statistical significance on the level p=0.003*. Dimension and structure of the cranial base are genetically determined. Changes on the cranial base are not a consequence of orthodontic treatment. Usually changes are results of displacement and remodelation of bones and growth of cranial base [53]. When we plan orthodontic treatment we can not expect severe changes in structures of cranial base.

Position of the upper incisors was analyzed by angle I/SpP. Usually patients with skeletal Class III (except severe mandibular prognatism) have normoinclination of the upper incisors. Both appliances significantly changed value of angle I/Spp, FR-III from 72.70° to 70.80° and Y appliance from 71.30° to 68.70°, with significance on the level p<0.001*. Y appliance caused, as a mobile active appliance, major changes in dentoalveolar structures. Inclination of the lower incisors was analysed by angle i/MP. FR-III increased value of angle i/MP from 89.50° to 90.60°, with statistical significance p<0.001*. Y appliance had no significant effect on the change of value of the angle i/MP (from 90.15° to 90.05°). It was consequence of design of appliance, which is located only on the upper jaw. Protrusion of the upper incisors and retrusion of the lower incisors created conditions for correct overjet [54, 55].

Orthodontic treatment can change vertical position (height of TMJ) and sagittal position of TMJ. TMJ is one of the growth zone during period of puberty. For stable therapeutic results changes on the TMJ structures are very important and their answer to applied force [56]. Both appliances did not have big influence to vertical position of TMJ. FR-III changed height of TMJ from 6.15mm to 5.75mm, while Y appliance caused change from 4.55mm to 4.60mm. S-E distance was increased during treatment, which is related to the distal movement of TMJ. Y appliance caused greater increasing of S-E distance from 21.90mm to 22.65mm, with statistical significance p=0.012*. FR-III changed S-E distance from 20.40mm to 21.25mm. All changes on TMJ structures are consequence of changes on the upper and lower jaw.

Changes on soft tissue structures were analysed by angles T and H, position of the upper and lower lip to aesthetic line and height of the upper lip. Angle T is in correlation with angle J. Changes of angle J during the treatment caused increasing value of angle T in patients with skeletal Class III. FR-III increased angle T from 7.05° to 10.50°, while Y appliance increased this angle from 8.80° to 10.70°. Angle H (Holdaway) is in positive correlation with angle ANB. Patients with skeletal Class III have angle ANB<2°. Orthodontic treatment increase value of ANB angle and, at the same time, increase of angle H. FR-III changed angle H from 5.35° to 8.25° and Y appliance from 6.60° to 7.85°, both with statistical significance p<0.001*. Patients with pseudo skeletal Class III have typical concave profile, with back position of the upper jaw. That is why upper lip is significantly posteriorly moved to the aesthetic line. FR-III approach upper lip to the aestetic line and changed distance from-5.15mm to-1.80mm. Y appliance, also, change sagittal position of the upper lip and decreased distance to the aesthetic line from-4.85mm to-3.45mm. In the whole sample lower lip was significantly back to the aesthetic line. Both appliances affect the movement of the lower lip to the aesthetic line. Y appliance changed position of the lower lip from-0.80mm to 0.30mm and FR-III changed distance of the lower lip to the aesthetic line from-1.25mm to-0.80mm. Patients with pseudo Class III have underdeveloped upper jaw and reduced height of the upper lip. Orthodontic treatment stimulated sagittal growth of the upper jaw. This allows changes in soft tissue profile and increasing the height of the upper lip. FR-III caused increasing of height of the upper lip from 21.75mm to 23.45mm, while Y appliance increased this parameter from 21.60mm to 22.30mm. Changes of position of the upper and lower lip and increasing of height of the upper lip contributes to the reduction of profile concavity [57, 58, 59]. During the period of puberty growth, changes on soft tissues are much more pronounced than on skeletal structures. Upper and lower lip and other soft tissues move down a function of time. It is important to choose the best possible treatment procedure if we want to achieve a good relationship between soft tissue and bone structures. It is important to analyse value of nasolabial angle. In patients with decreased nasolabial angle orthodontic treatment has to achieve posterior movement of the upper jaw. In cases with increased value of nasolabial angle, it is necessary to move nasomax-illary complex forward during orthodontic treatment. Orthodontic treatment caused decrease of profile concavity, increasing of height and thickness of the upper lip and anterior movement of the upper lip to the aesthetic line [60].

Patients with skeletal Class III often have infantile swalowing with anterior tongue position and oral respiration. Speech is orofacial function which last develops during individual maturation. Patients with skeletal Class III have reverse overjet. That is why articulation of interdental and labial consonants is incorrect. FR-III equally successfully corrects morphological and functional differences and contributes the correct performance of orofacial functions. FR-III significantly affects the function of swallowing and contributes to the transition from infantile to mature swallowing. In this sample (treated with FR-III) before treatment 12 patients had infantile swallowing, while 8 patients had mature swallowing. After orthodontic treatment with FR-III 13 patients had mature swallowing, while 7 had infantile swallowing. Design of FR-III prevents tongue insertion between upper and lower incisors. FR-III change activity and tongue position and it contributes changes in the function of swallowing [61]. Y appliance did not have influence on changing of swallowing function. FR-III improves articulation of interdental cionsonants, due to activity of lip muscles and changing of upper incisors inclination. Before orthodontic treatment 8 patients had correct speech and 12 patients had incorrect speech. After orthodontic treatment with FR-III 14 patients had correct speech, while 6 patients had incorrect speech. FR-III changes activity of muscles and eliminates incorrect relation between upper and lower lip.

Pancherz's analysis explained changes on dental and skeletal structures. FR-III corrected molar relation for 3.25mm and Y appliance for 2.35mm. Relations between incisors were changed for 2.40mm when using FR-III and for 2.10mm when using Y appliance. Skeletal correction was more effective when using FR-III, for 3.30mm, while Y appliance caused skeletal correction for 1.40mm. FR-III caused skeletal correction according to stimulating of osteoblasts in periost and intensive sagittal growth of the upper jaw [62, 63, 64]. Mobile appliance caused primarily dental correction, while skeletal changes were irrelevant. Dental effects were manifested as correction of reverse overjet due to protrusion of the upper and retrusion of the lower frontal teeth.

9. Conclusion

FR-I is the most effective functional appliance in early treatment of skeletal distal bite. This appliance corrects occlusal morphology, orofacial functions and facial aesthetics. Main skeletal effects of FR-I are:

- anterior displacement and stimulation of sagittal growth of the lower jaw

- suppression of the sagittal growth of the upper jaw

- significantly increasing of length of mandibular corpus and ramus

- decreasing value of ANB angle and correction of skeletal Class II to Class I

- decreasing of vertical interjaw angle

- elimination of the pressure, application of pressure, application of pulling force and continuous activation of orofacial muscles

- increasing of sum of angles of Björk polygon and moderate backward rotation

The main dental effects of FR-I are:

- retrusion of the upper incisors

* protrusion of the lower incisors

* rotation of the occlusal plane

* mesial movement of lower posterior teeth

* distal movement of upper posterior teeth

This appliance is very comfortable for wearing, does not affect the function of speech, patients are motivated to cooperate. Treatment is very efficient, therapeutic results are stabile and tendency to relapse is minimal. That's why FR-I is the most appropriate appliance for success-ful early treatment of Class II divison 1 malocclusion.

Also, FR-III is one of the best choice for early orthodontic treatment of skeletal Class III caused by maxillary retrognatism. This functional appliance affects occlusal morphology, orofacial functions and facial aesthetics. In all segments FR-III is much more efficient in comparing with Y mobile appliance. Effects of this appliance are the result of stimulating of sagittal and transversal growth of the upper jaw, inhibition of growth of the lower jaw, elimination of the pressure, aplication of the pressure, tensile stress force and continuous activation of orofacial muscles. Pseudo Class III is severe skeletal problem which is transferred from the deciduous dentition to mixed and permanent dentition. If we use FR-III in early mixed dentition we avoid the use of other functional appliances during puberty growth. First therapeutic results appear after 3 to 6 months from the beginning of treatment, results are stabile, without signs of relapse, with correct protocol of wearing. The main disadvantages of this appliance are complicated preparation in dental laboratory, gracile structure, inability to repair appliance and a long duration of orthodontic therapy. The main advantages of this appliance are the possibilities of application at an early age, correction of functional and occlusal irregularities at the same time, the patient's motivation, good cooperation and comfort.

The main skeletal effects of FR-III are:

* stimulation of sagittal growth of the upper jaw

* increasing of vertical angle between upper jaw and anterior cranial base

* significant increase of length of maxilarry corpus

* inhibition of sagittal growth of the lower jaw

* increasing of vertical angle between lower jaw and anterior cranial base

* increasing value of ANB angle and correction skeletal Class III to Class I

* increasing of basal angle (B)

* increasing of sum of angles of Björk polygon and moderate backward rotation

The main dental effects of FR-III are:

* protrusion of the upper incisors

* retrusion of the lower incisors

- rotation of the occlusal plane

- distal movement of lower posterior teeth

- mesial movement of upper posterior teeth

Dental effects allow correction of reverse overjet and achieve proper overjet and correction of molar relations.

FR-III significantly alters the activity of orofacial muscles and affects the correction of swallowing and speech functions. Treatment with FR-III contributes to achieving better facial aesthetics and establishing harmony between the soft and hard tissues of the craniofacial complex.

We can recommend this functional appliance for everyday clinical practice and successful early treatment in patients with skeletal distal and mesial (pseudo Class III) bite.

Author details

Zorana Stamenković* and Vanja Raičković

*Address all correspondence to: zzokac@yahoo.com

Department of Orthodontics, Faculty of Dentisty, University of Belgrade, Serbia

References

[1] Dodić S.: Analiza morfologije i funkcije orofacijalnog kompleksa u adolescenata sa kraniomandibularnim disfunkcijama. Doktorska teza. Beograd, 2003.

[2] Battagel J.: The aetological factors in Class III malocclusion. Eur. J. Orthod. 1993; 15: 347-370.

[3] Mc Guigan D. G.: The Hapsburgs. London. WH Allen. 1966.

[4] Bishara SE. Textbook of orthodontics. W. B. Saunders; Philadelphia, 2001.

[5] O'Relly T., Yanneillo G.: Mandibular growth changes and maturation of cervical vertebrae – A longitudinal cephalometric study. Angle Orthod. 1988; 4: 179-184.

[6] Ball G, Woodside D, Tompson B, Hunter WS, Posluns J. Relationship between cervical vertebral maturation and mandibular growth. Am J Orthod Dent Orthop 2011; 139 (5): 455-461.

[7] Proffit W.B. Fields H. W., Sarver D. M.: Contemporary orthodontics. The Mosby Co. St: Louis, 2007.

[8]   Almeida M. R., Henriques J. F. C., Almeida R. R., Almeida-Pedrin R. R., Ursi W.: Treatment effects produced by the Bionator appliance. Comparison with an untreated Class II sample. Eur. J. Orthod. 2004; 26: 65-72.

[9]   Carlos Flores-Mir and Paul W. Major: A systematic review of cephalometric facial soft tissue changes with the Activator and Bionator appliances in Class II division 1 subjects. Eur. J. Orthod. 2006; 28: 586-593.

[10]   Faltin K. J., Faltin R. M., Baccetti T., Franchi L., Ghiozzi B., McNamara J. A. Jr.: Long-term effectiveness and treatment timing for Bionator therapy. Angle Orthod. 2003; 73 (3): 221-230.

[11]   Hotz R.: Orthodontics in daily practice. Bern, Switzerland, Huber. 1974.

[12]   Isaacson K. G., Muir J. D., Reed R. T. Removable orthodontic Appliances, Oxford, 2002.

[13]   Fränkel R., Fränkel Ch.: Orofacial Orthopaedics with the Function Regulator. Karger, Basel – Munchen –Paris – London – New York – New Delhi – Singapore – Tokyo – Sydney, 1989

[14]   Fränkel R.: Funktionskieferorthopadie und der Mundvorhof als Papparatus Basis, VEB Verl., Berlin, 1967.

[15]   Fränkel R.: A functional approach to orofacial orthopaedics. Br. J. Orthod. 1980; 7: 41-51

[16]   Kanas R. J., Carapezza L., Kanas S. J.: Treatment Clasification of Class III Malocclusion. The Journal of Clinical Pediatric Dentistry. 2008; 33(2): 175-186.

[17]   Baik H. S., Jee S. H., Lee K. J., Oh T. K.: Treatment effect of Frankel functional regulator III in children with class III malocclusions. Am. J. Orthod. Dentofacial Orthop. 2004; 125: 294-301.

[18]   Stamenković Z.: Klinički efekti primene Fränkel-ovih regulatora funkcije u terapiji distalnog i mezijalnog zagrižaja. Doktorska disertacija. Beograd, 2011.

[19]   Almeida M. R., Henriques J. F. C. and Ursi W.: Comparative study of the Frankel (FR-2) and bionator appliances in the treatment of Class II malocclusion. Am. J. Orthod. Dentofacial Orthop. 2002; 121: 458-466.

[20]   Araujo A. M., Buschang P. H., Melo A. C. M.: Adaptive condylar growth and mandibular remodeling changes with bionator therapy – an implant study. Eur. J. Orthod. 2004; 26: 515-522.

[21]   Chen J. Y., Will L., Neiderman R.: Analysis of efficacy of functional appliances on mandibular growth. Am. J. Orthod. Dentofacial orthop. 2002; 122: 470-476.

[22] Yamin-Lacouture C., Woodside D.G., Sectakof P.A., Sessle B.J.: The action of three types of functional appliances on the activity of the masticatory muscles. Am. J. Orthod. Dentofacial Orthop. 1997; 112: 560-572.

[23] Martins R. P., Martin J. C., Martins L. P., Buschang P. H.: Skeletal and dental components of Class II correction with the bionator and removable headgear splint appliances. Am. J. Orthod. Dentofacial Orthop. 2008; 134: 732-741.

[24] Chadwick S.M., Aird C., Taylor S., Bearn D.R.: Functional regulator treatment of Class II division 1 malocclusions. Eur. J. Orthod. 2001; 23: 495-505.

[25] Barton S., Cook P. A.: Predicting functional appliance treatment outcome in Class II malocclusions – a rewiew. Am. J. Orthod. Dentofacial Orthop. 1997; 112: 282-286.

[26] Cevidanes L. et al: Clinical outcomes of Fränkel appliance therapy assessed with a counterpart analysis. Am. J. orthod. Dentofacial Orthop. 2003; 123: 379-387.

[27] Moreira Melo A. C., dos Santos-Pinto A., da Rosa Martins J. C., Martins L. P., Sakima M. T.: Orthopedic and orthodontic components of Class II, division 1 malocclusion correction with Balters Bionator: A cephalometric study with metallic implants. World J. Orthod. 2003; 4: 273-242.

[28] Rodrigues de Almeida M., Castanha Henriques J. F., Rodrigues de Almeida R., Ursi W.: Treatment effects produced bz Fränkel appliance in patients with Class II, division 1 malocclusion. Angle Orthod. 2002; 72 (5): 418-425.

[29] Falck F., Fränkel R.: Clinical relevance of step-by-step mandibular advancement in the treatment of mandibular retrusion using the Fränkel appliance. Am. J. Orthod. Dentofacial Orthop. 1989; 96: 333-341.

[30] Thieme KM, Nägerl H, Hahn W, Ihlow D, Kubein D. Variations in cyclic mandibular movements during treatment of Class II malocclusions with removable functional appliances. Eur J Orthod 2011: 33(6): 628-635.

[31] Patel H. P., Moseley H. C., Noar J. H.: Cephalometric determinants of successful functional appliance therapy. Angle Orthod. 2002; 72: 410-417.

[32] Battagel J. M.: Profile changes in Class II, division 1 malocclusions: a comparison of the effects of Edgewise and Fränkel appliance therapy. Eur. J. Orthod. 1989; 11: 243-253.

[33] Battagel J. M.: The relationship between hard and soft tissue changes following treatment og Class II division 1 malocclusions using Edgewise and Fränkel appliance techniques, Eur. J. Orthod. 1990; 12: 154-165.

[34] [34]Quintao C., Helena I., Brunharo V. P., Menezes R. C., Almeida M. A. O: Soft tissue facial profile changes following functional appliance therapy. Eur. J. Orthod. 2006; 28: 35-41.

[35] Creekmore T. D., Radney L.J.: Frankel appliance therapy: orthopedic or orthodontic? Am. J. Orthod. 1983; 83:89-108.

[36] Janson G.R.P., Alegria Toruno J.L., Rodrigez Martins D., Henriques J.F.C., de Freitas M.R.: Class II treatment effects of the Fränkel appliance. Eur. J. Orthod. 2003; 25: 301-309.

[37] Read M. J. F.: The integration of functional and fixed appliance treatment. Am. J. Orthod. 2001; 28 (1): 13-18.

[38] Woodside D. G.: Do functional appliances have an orthopedic effect? Am. J. Orthod. Dentofacial Orthop. 1998; 113:11.

[39] Pancherz H., Zieber K., Hoyer B.: Cephalometric characteristics of Class II division 1 and Class II division 2 malocclusions: a comparative study in children, Angle Orthod. 1997; 67: 111-120.

[40] Rushforth C. D., Gordon P. H., Aird J. C.: Skeletal and dental changes following the use of the Frankel funkcional regulator. Br. J. Orthod. 1999; 26:127-134.

[41] Bacetti T. et al.: Skeletal effects of early treatment of Class III malocclusion. Am. J. Orthod. Dentofac. Orthop. 1998; 113: 333 – 343.

[42] Levin A. S., McNamara J. A. Jr., Franchi L., Baccetti T., Frankel C.: Short-term and long-term treatment outcomes with the FR-3 appliance of Frankel. Am. J. Orthod. Dentofacial Orthop. 2008; 134: 513-524.

[43] Miethke R. R., Lindenau S., Dietrich K.: The effect of Fränkel's function regulator type III on the apical base. Eur. J. Orthod.2003; 25: 311-318.

[44] Negi A., Singla A., Mahajan V.: Effects of Maxilarry Protraction And Frankel Appliance Therapy On Craniofacial Structures And Pharyngeal Airway. Indian Journal of Dental Sciences. 2013; 5(5): 30-33.

[45] Pangrazio-Kulbersh V., Berger J., Kersten G.: Effects of protraction mechanics on the midface. Am. J. Orthod. Dentofacial Orthop. 1998; 114: 484-491.

[46] Seehra J., Fleming P. S., Mandall N., DiBiase A. T.: A comparison of two different techniques for early correction of Class III malocclusion. The Angle Orthodontist. 2012; 82(1): 96-101.

[47] Fränkel R: Maxillary retrusion in Class III and treatment with the functional corrector III. Trans. Eur. Orthod. Soc. 1970; 46: 249-259.

[48] Almeida M. R., Almeida R. R., Oltramari-Navarro P. V., Conti A. C., Navarro R de L, Camacho J. G.: Early treatment of Class III malocclusion: 10-year clinical follow-up. J Appl Oral Sci.: 2011; 19: 431-439.

[49] Zentner A., Doll G. M., Peylo S. M.: Morphological parameters as predictors of successful correction of Class III malocclusion. Eur. J. Orthod. 2001; 23: 383-392.

[50] Santos-Pinto A. D., Paulin R. F., Moreira Melo A. C.: Pseudo-Class III treatment with reverse traction: case report. Journal of Clinical Pediatric Dentistry. 2001; 25 (4): 264-274.

[51] Ulgen M., Firatli S.: The effects of Fränkel's function regulator on the Class III malocclusions. Am. J. Orthod. 1994; 105: 561-567.

[52] Oltramari-Navarro P. V. P., Almeida R. R., Conti A. C., Navaro R de L. et al: Early treatment Protocol for Skeletal Class III Malocclusion. Brazilian Dental Journal. 2013; 24(2): 167-173.

[53] Toffol L. D., Pavoni C., Bacceti T., Franchi L. and Cozza P.: Orthopedic treatment outcomes in Class III malocclusion. The Angle Orthod. 2008; 78: 561-573.

[54] Giancotti A., Maselli A., Mampieri G. and Spano E.: Pseudo-Class III malocclusion treatment with Balters´ bionator. Br. Orthodontic Soc. 2003; 30 (3): 203-215.

[55] Loh M. K., Kerr W. J. S.: The function regulator III: effects and indications for use. Br. J. Orthod. 1985; 12: 153-157.

[56] Kapur A., Chawla H. S., Utreja A., Goyla A.: Early Class III occlusal tendency in children and its selective management, Journal of the Indian Society of Pedodontics and Preventive Dentistry. 2008; 26 (3): 107-113.

[57] Stamenković Z., Nedeljković N.: Karakteristike mekotkivnog profila kod pacijenata sa III skeletnom klasom. Stomatološki glasnik Srbije, 2006. Vol. 53, 166-173.

[58] Zhao G., Sha L., Chang B.: Soft tissue profile changes by Frankel-III appliance on correcting Angle Class III malocclusion in mixed dentition. Shanghai Journal of Stomatology. 2011; 20(2): 201-203.

[59] Kerr W. J., Ten Have T. R.: Changes in soft tissue profile during the treatment of Class III malocclusion. Br. J. Orthod. 1987; 14(4): 243-249.

[60] Prashanth C. S., Dinesh M. R., Akshai Shetty K. R.: Class III – Three way approach, a review of contemporary treatment modalities. Journal of International Oral Health. 2010; 2(1): 27-30.

[61] Robertson N. R. E.: An examination of treatment changes in children treated with the function regulator of Frankel. Am. J. Orthod. 1983; 83: 299-310.

[62] Chen F., Terada K., Wu L., Saito I.: Longitudinal evaluation of the intermaxilarry relationship in Class III malocclusions. Angle Orthod. 2006; 76: 955-961.

[63] Standt C. B., Kiliaridis S.: Different skeletal types underlying Class III malocclusion in a random population. Am J Orthod Dentofacial Orthop. 2009; 136: 715-721.

[64] Zentner A., Doll G. M.: Size discrepancy of apical bases and treatment success in Angle Class III malocclusion. Journal of Orofacial Orthopedics 2001; 62: 97-106.

Chapter 18

Interceptive Orthodontics — Current Evidence

Maen H. Zreaqat

Additional information is available at the end of the chapter

http://dx.doi.org/10.5772/59256

1. Introduction

From evidence found in human skulls, crooked teeth have been around since the time of Neanderthal man (about 50,000 BC), but it was not until about 3000 years ago that we had the first written record of attempts to correct crowded or protruding teeth. Long before braces, long before the word orthodontics" was coined, it was known that teeth moved in response to pressure. Primitive (and surprisingly well-designed) orthodontic appliances have been found with Greek and Etruscan artifacts. Archaeologists have discovered Egyptian mummies with crude metal bands wrapped around individual teeth. It is speculated that catgut was used to close the gaps [1]. The earliest description of irregularities of the teeth was given about 400 BC by Hippocrates (460-377 BC). The first treatment of an irregular tooth was recorded by Celsus (25 BC-50 AD), a Roman writer, who said, "If a second tooth should happen to grow in children before the first has fallen out, that which ought to be shed is to be drawn out and the new one daily pushed toward its place by means of the finger until it arrives at its just proportion." A clear mechanical treatment was advocated by Pliny the Elder (23-79 AD), who suggested filing elongated teeth to bring them into proper alignment. This method remained in practice until the 1800s [2].

Dentistry entered a period of marked decline during middle ages (5th to 15th centuries), as did all sciences. After the 16th century, considerable progress was made. Matthaeus Gottfried Purmann (1692) was the first to report taking wax impressions. In 1756, Phillip Pfaff used plaster of Paris impressions. Malocclusions were called "irregularities" of the teeth, and their correction was termed "regulating." It remained for the Enlightenment to reawaken the spirit of scientific thought necessary to advance dentistry and other disciplines. Beginning in the 18th century, Pierre Fauchard (1678-1761) was leading efforts in the field of dentistry. He has been called the "Father of Orthodontia." He was the first to remove dentistry from the bonds of empiricism and put it on a scientific foundation. In 1728, he published the first general work on dentistry, a 2-volume opus entitled "The Surgeon Dentist: A Treatise on the Teeth".

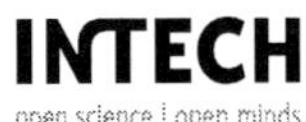

Fauchard described for first time the bandeau, an expansion arch consisting of a horseshoe-shaped strip of precious metal to which the teeth were ligated (Fig 1). This became the basis for Angle's E-arch, and even today its principles are used in unraveling a crowded dentition. He also "repositioned" teeth with a forceps, called a "pelican" because of its resemblance to the beak of that bird, and ligated the tooth to its neighbors until healing took place. At that time, little attention was paid to anything other than the alignment of teeth and then almost exclusively to the maxilla. moreover, he was the first to recommend serial extraction by extracting premolars to relieve crowding [3].

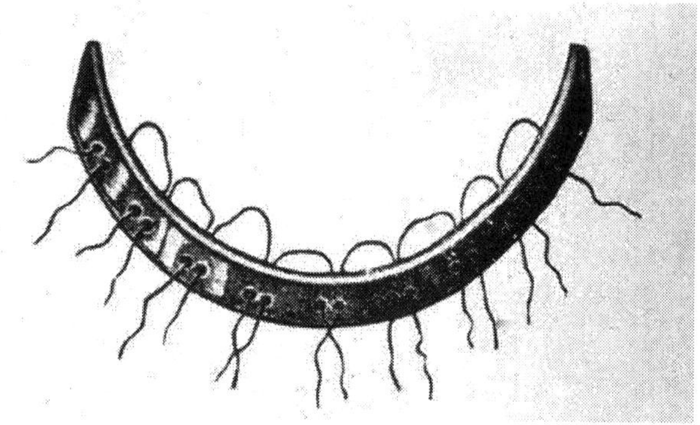

Figure 1. Fauchard's bandeau

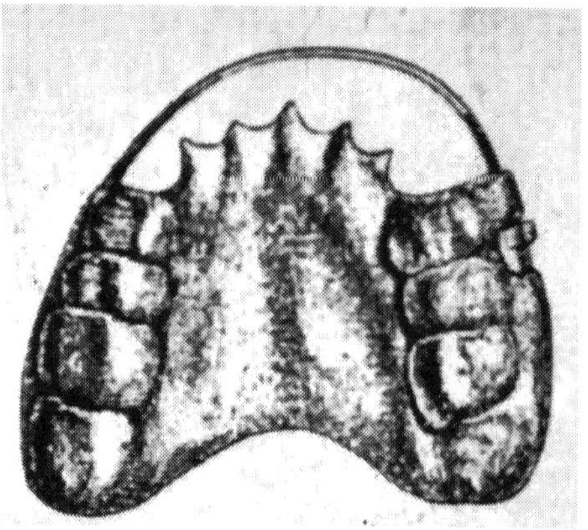

Figure 2. Removable "plate" used by Friedrich Christoph

Friedrich Christoph Kneisel (1797-1847), a German dentist, was the first to use plaster models to record malocclusion and removable appliance to fit prognathic teeth with a chin strap (Fig.

2). However, before the time of Edward Angle, the treatment of malocclusions was chaotic, with little understanding of normal occlusion and even less understanding of the development of the dentition. Appliances were primitive, not only in design but also in the metals and materials used. There was no rational basis for diagnosis and case analysis. It was Edward Hartley Angle (1855 –1930), early in the 20th century, who dominated the emergence of "orthodontia as a science and a specialty". He also created the first educational program to train specialists in orthodonticsand he developed the first prefabricated orthodontic appliance system. Angle is considered the father' of modern orthodontics [4].

2. The development of the occlusion of the teeth

The primary dentition begins to erupt at the age of about 6 months, and is normally completely in occlusion by about 3 years of age. Details of mean age of eruption and the range of variation have been reported by Van der Linden (1983) for Swedish children and by Sato and Ogiwara (1971) for Japanese children. There appear to be no significant differences between the sexes for the age of primary tooth eruption. The first teeth to erupt and to form occlusal contacts are the incisors, which ideally take up occlusal positions that are more vertical than the permanent incisors, with a deeper incisal overbite. The lower incisors in this condition will contact the cingulum area of the upper incisors in centric occlusion. Spaces are present between the primary incisor teeth. Following eruption of the incisors, the first primary molars erupt into occlusion. These teeth take up occlusal contacts so that the lower molars are slightly forward in relation to the upper molar. The last teeth to erupt into occlusion in the primary dentition are the second molars. These teeth erupt slightly spaced from the first molars, but the space quickly closes by forward movement of the second molars which take up a position so that the distal surfaces of the upper and lower second molars are in the same vertical plane in occlusion. Thus certain features of the 'ideal' occlusion of the primary dentition when fully erupted can be described as following:

1. Spacing of incisor teeth.

2. Anthropoid spaces mesial to upper canine and distal to lower canine, into which the opposing canine interdigitates.

3. Vertical position of incisor teeth, with lower incisor touching the cingulum of upper incisor.

4. The distal surfaces of the upper and lower second primary molars in the same vertical plane.

From the age of about 6 years onwards the primary dentition is replaced by the permanent dentition. The primary incisors, canines and molars are replaced by the permanent incisors, canines and premolars, and the permanent molars erupt as additional teeth. There is some difference in size between the primary teeth and the permanent teeth which directly replace them. The permanent incisors and canines are usually larger than the corresponding primary teeth, and the premolars are usually smaller than the corresponding primary molars. Studies reported by Van der Linden (1983), have shown that the overall difference in size between the two dentitions is not large, amounting on average to about 3 mm in the upper teeth and less than 1 mm in the lower teeth. There is, however, not a strong correlation between the sizes of the primary dentition and the permanent teeth. The relationship of the jaws to each other will have a large influence on the relationship of the dental arches. The relationship of the jaws to each other can also vary in all three planes of space, and variation in any plane can affect the occlusion of the teeth. The antero-posterior positional relationship of the basal parts of the upper and lower jaws to each other, with the teeth in occlusion, is known as the skeletal relationship. This is sometimes called the dental base relationship, or the skeletal pattern. A classification of the skeletal relationship is in common use, namely:

1. Skeletal Class 1—in which the jaws are in their ideal antero-posterior relationship in occlusion.

2. Skeletal Class 2—in which the lower jaw in occlusion is positioned further back in relation to the upper jaw than in skeletal Class 1.

3. Skeletal Class 3—in which the lower jaw in occlusion is positioned further forward than in skeletal Class 1.

In addition, the teeth erupt into an environment of functional activity governed by the muscles of mastication, of the tongue and of the face. The muscles of the tongue, lips and cheeks are of particular importance in guiding the teeth into their final position, and variation in muscle form and function can affect the position and occlusion of the teeth. Moreover, some dental and local factors can affect the development of occlusion. These include: alterations in size of the dentition in relation to jaw size, crossbite, aberrant developmental position of individual teeth, presence of supernumerary teeth, developmental hypodontia, labial frenum, thumb or finger sucking. Early interference and modification of these basic etiological features can help to avoid malocclusion or reduce the need for treatment in some cases. Consequently interceptive orthodontic treatment has been set as an important aspect of orthodontic care [5].

3. Interceptive orthodontics: Definition of the concept

The concept and the necessity of interceptive orthodontic treatment, so called early, have been controversial. Some define it as removable or fixed appliance intervention in the deciduous, early mixed, or midmixed dentition. Others place it in the late mixed dentition stage of development (before emergence of the second premolars and the permanent maxillary canines). The American Association of Orthodontists' Council of Orthodontic Education defines interceptive orthodontics as "that phase of the science and art of orthodontics employed to recognize and eliminate potential irregularities and malpositions in the developing dentofacial complex." [6]. While some profession's leaders advocate that early treatment is always desirable because tissue tolerance and their power of adjustment are at or near their maximum, others warn that there is no assurance that the results of early treatment will be sustained, and that several-phased treatment will always lengthen overall treatment time.

Early treatment not only may do some damage or prolong therapy, it may exhaust the child's spirit of cooperation and compliance [7]. Joseph Fox (1776-1816, English), in his "Natural History of the Human Teeth" (London, 1803), recommended that treatment be started "before 13 or 14 years of age, and as much earlier as possible." Angle advocated the institution of orthodontic treatment "as near the beginning of the variation from the normal in the process of the development of the dental apparatus as possible". Although Nance advocated that "active treatment in the mixed dentition period is desirable only in Class III cases, crossbites, and Class II cases wherein facial appearance is markedly affected," he freed orthodontists from their hesitancy to treat patients before the development of the adult dentition [8].

4. Orthodontic interceptive measures during primary and mixed dentition

4.1. Space maintainers

The primary dentition plays a very important role in the child's growth and development, not only in terms of speech, chewing, appearance and the prevention of bad habits but also in the guidance and eruption of permanent teeth. Exfoliation of primary teeth and eruption of permanent teeth is a normal physiological process. When this normal process is disrupted, due to factors like premature loss of primary teeth, proximal carious lesions etc, it may lead to mesial migration of teeth resulting in loss of the arch length which may manifest as malocclusion in permanent dentition in the form of crowding, impaction of permanent teeth, supraeruption of opposing teeth etc. The best way to avoid these problems is to preserve the primary teeth in the arch till their normal time of exfoliation is attained. Hence it is rightly quoted that primary teeth serve as best space maintainers for permanent dentition. However, if premature extraction or loss of tooth is unavoidable due to extensive caries or other reasons, the safest option to maintain arch space is by placing a space maintainer. The fixed space maintainers are usually indicated to maintain the space created by unilateral/bilateral premature loss of primary teeth in either of the arches. Of the various fixed space maintainers, Band and Loop type of space maintainers are one of the most frequently used appliances with good high success rates [9]. Cemented lower lingual bars, transpalatal arches, crowns with distal extensions are other forms of space maintainers utilizing similar mechanisms (Fig. 3) Nevertheless, disintegration of cement, solder failure, caries formation along the margins of the band and long construction time are some of the disadvantages associated with them [10].

Considering this, there has been many pilot studies that explain the use of newer adhesive directly bonded splints. They are glass fiber reinforced composite resins (e.g. Ribbond, Everstick) as fixed space maintainers [11, 12]. Ribbond is a biocompatible esthetic material made from high strength polyethylene fibers (Fig. 4). The various advantages of this material includes its ease of adhesion to the dental contours, fast technique of application and good strength, well tolerated by the patient [13]. However there is limited literature is available in terms of efficacy and longevity [14].

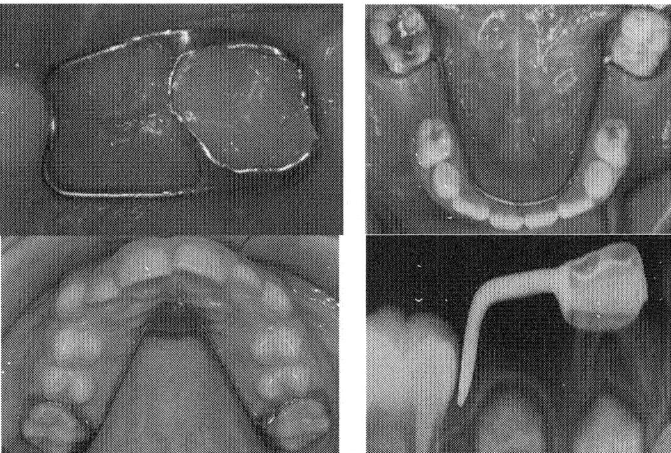

Figure 3. Various space maintainers

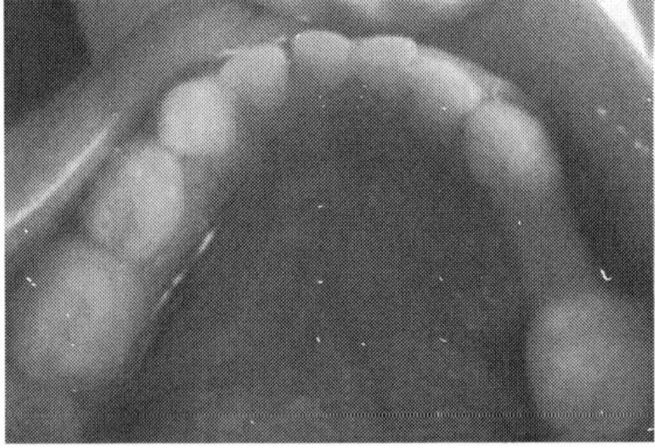

Figure 4. Ribbond space maintainer

5. Elimination of oral habits

Oral habits are learned patterns of muscle contraction and have a very complex nature. They are associated with anger, hunger, sleep, tooth eruption and fear. Some children even display oral habits for release of mental tension. These habits might be non-nutritive sucking (thumb, finger, pacifier and/or tongue), lip biting and bruxism events. These habits can result in damage to dentoalveolar structure; hence, dentists play a crucial role in giving necessary information to parents. This information includes relevant changes in the dentoalveolar structure and the method to stop oral habits. Also, a dentist is required to treat the ensuring malocclusion. The prevalence of oral habits in high school girls and primary school students has been reported to be 87.9 and 30%, respectively [15].

Oral habits could be divided into 2 main groups:

1. Acquired oral habits: Include those behaviors which are learned and could be stopped easily and when the child grows up, he or she can give up that behavior and start another one.

2. Compulsive oral habits: Consist of those behaviors which are fixed in child and when emotional pressures are intolerable for the child, he or she can feel safety with this habit, and preventing the child from these habits make him or her anxious and worried.

5.1. Thumb sucking

Thumb sucking is the most common oral habit and it is reported that its prevalence is between 13 to 60% in some societies [16]. Basically, sucking is one of an infant's natural reflexes. They begin to suck on their thumbs or other fingers while they are in the womb. Infants and young children may suck on thumbs, other fingers, pacifiers or other objects. It makes them feel secure and happy, and it helps them learn about their world. The prevalence of this habit is decreased as age increases, and mostly, it is stopped by 4 years of age. There is a relationship between the level of education in parents, the child nutrition and the sucking habit [17]. If the child chooses this habit in the first year of his or her life, the parents should move away his or her thumb smoothly and attract the child's attention to other things such as toys. After the second years of age, thumb sucking will decrease and will be appear just in child's bed or when he/she is tired. Some of children who do not stop this habit, will give it up when their permanent teeth erupt, but there is a tendency for continuing the sucking habit even until adult life. According to a study in 1973, millions of kids do not give up this habit before the eruption of teeth [18]. Nowadays, the level of stress is higher than the time of that study, and as stress is a powerful stimulus in sucking habit, it is probable to find more kids with long-term sucking habit if we do a research exactly like the one which was done in 1973.

Thumb sucking has 2 types:

1. Active: In this type, there is a heavy force by the muscles during the sucking and if this habit continues for a long period, the position of permanent teeth and the shape of mandible will be affected.

2. Passive: In this type, the child puts his/her finger in mouth, but because there is no force on teeth and mandible, so this habit is not associated with skeletal changes.

In the case of active thumb sucking habit, it is better for a child not to be blamed, teased, offended, humiliated and punished, because these methods will increase the anxiety and consequently increase the incidence of the habit. Long-term finger sucking habit has harmful effects on dentition and speech. In 1870s decade, Camble and Jander reported for the first time that long-term finger sucking has harmful effects on dentition [19].

The side effects of finger sucking are: Anterior open bite, increased overjet, lingual inclination lower incisor and labial inclination upper incisor, posterior cross bite, compensatory tongue thrust, deep palate, speech defect, and finger defects (Eczema of the finger due to alternate dryness and moisture that occurs and even angulations of the finger). The severity of changes in dentition due to finger sucking is related to the duration and times of doing the habit. Also, the position of finger in mouth, dental arches relation and child's health affect the severity of changes [20].

Dental changes due to finger sucking do not need any treatment if the habit stopped before the 5 years of age and as soon as giving up the habit, dental changes will be corrected spontaneously [21]. At the time of permanent anterior teeth eruption and if the child is motivated to stop the sucking habit, it is time to start the treatment as follows:

1.   Direct interview with child if he/she is mature enough to understand

2.   Encouragement: This can give the child more pride and self-confidence

3.   Reward system

4.   Reminder therapy

5.   Orthodontic appliance: The final stage in treatment is the use of orthodontic appliance whether fixed or removable, which can play the role of reminder and can reduce the willing of finger sucking. For long-term habits or unwilling patient, the fixed intra oral appliance is the most effective inhibitor. In the case of using fixed or removable appliance, we should alarm the parents about potential problems in speaking or eating during the first 24 to 48 h, which are usual and self correcting. After active phase of treatment, the appliance should remain in place for more 3 to 6 month to minimize the relapse potential [22, 23].

5.2. Use of pacifier

The use of pacifier is common in most countries and it will not cause permanent changes in dentition if it is stopped at the age of 2 or 3 years. After that, the use of pacifier has harmful effects on dentition development, and if it is used more than 5 years old, these effects would be more severe [24]. The children who use pacifier are not willing to suck their fingers. pacifier has the following negative effects:

1.   Anterior open bite

2.   Shallow palate

3.   Increased width of lower arch

4.   Posterior cross bite.

5.   Median otitis

It is suggested that pacifier should be replaced in children who have the habit of finger sucking, because the harmful effects of sucking pacifier are less than finger. In comparison between different pacifiers, despite the claims, it has been shown that there is no significant advantage for physiologic pacifiers over conventional ones [25].

5.3. Nail biting or onychophagia

Nail biting is a common and untreated medical problem among children. This habit starts after 3 to 4 years of age and is in its peak in 10 years of age. Its rate increases in adolescency, while it declines later. This problem is not gender dependent in children less than 10 years of age, but its incidence in boys is more than girls among adolescents [26]. This problem is a reaction in response to psychological disorders and some children will shift their habits from thumb sucking to nail biting. Complications caused by nail biting include malocclusion of the anterior teeth, teeth root resorption, bacterial infection and alveolar destruction. Moreover, about one forth of patients with temporo-mandibular joint pain and dysfunction have been shown to suffer from nail biting habit [27]. It is seen in clinic that boys with nail biting have a kind of psychological disorder especially attention deficient hyperactivity disorder (ADHD) more than girls. This habit in higher ages will be replaced with some habits such as lip chewing, gum chewing or smoking (Finn, 1998). Children with nail biting should be evaluated for emotional problems. In addition, putting nail polish or distasteful liquids on nails may be a therapeutic choice.

5.4. Tongue thrust

Tongue Thrust refers to a swallowing pattern in which the tongue is placed in the front of the mouth to begin the swallow (Fig. 5). Forward position of the tongue may also be seen at rest (mouth breathers). Normal swallowing patterns after infancy involve a coordinated smooth movement of the tongue toward the back of the mouth. This consistent forward movement of the tongue may cause speech errors and misaligned teeth. Forward positioning of the tongue during rest has the most influence on misaligning the teeth due to duration of the pressure. The speech disorder most commonly associated with tongue thrust is a frontal lisp, in which the tongue is place between the teeth for the sounds s and z, and sometimes for sh, ch, j, and soft g.

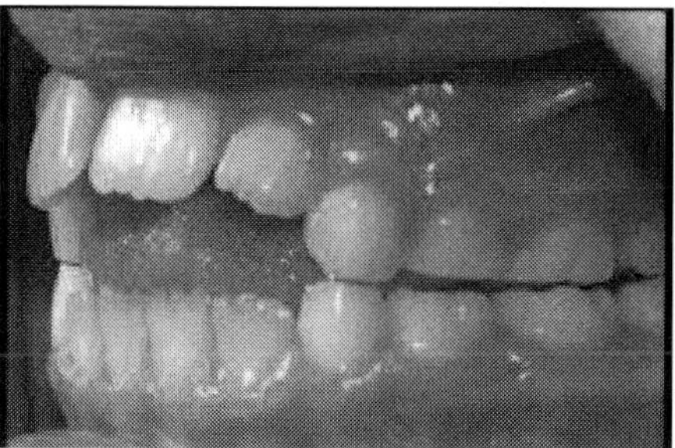

Figure 5. Tongue thrust

The line of treatment for these habits includes removal of the etiology, retraining exercises, and use of mechanical restraining appliances. Tongue bead appliances are commonly used as retraining exercise devices. In severe tongue thrusting cases and in cases with anterior open bite, a bead appliance alone may not be effective in restricting the habit. Tongue crib appliances (Fig. 6) are extremely effective in breaking the tongue thrust habit [28]. They create a mechanical barrier and prevent the tongue from thrusting between the incisors. In most of the cases with severe thumb/digit sucking habit, an anterior open bite develops. This will result in the development of a secondary tongue thrust habit. Hence, in cases with severe prolonged thumb or digit sucking, an appliance which can eliminate both of these habits. The Hybrid Habit Correcting Appliance (HHCA) can be used to effectively restrain and correct tongue thrusting as well as thumb sucking habit (Fig.7). HHCA incorporates a tongue bead, a palatal crib and a U-loop which is attached to the molar bands on either sides. The tongue bead consists of a spinnable acrylic bead of 3mm diameter. The appliance is designed to position the acrylic bead over the posterior one-third of the incisive papilla. The bead acts as a tongue retrainer. The patient is asked to constantly pull the bead towards the posterior region of the mouth. The palatal crib and the U-loop are made of 0.9mm stainless steel wire. Three to four spurs are bent on either sides of the bead, starting from the canine region on one side, running anteriorly as a smooth curve (in conventional crib appliances, the cribs run obliquely from one canine to the other side canine) and lying 1mm lingual to the cervical margin of the maxillary anterior teeth. In the region of the incisive papilla, the acrylic bead is incorporated in such a way that it lies over the posterior one-third of the incisive papilla. The tip of the crib should be almost in line with the incisor tip of the maxillary central incisor or 2 mm longer without interfering with the lower incisors when in occlusion. In cases with anterior open bite, the crib should be longer and can be up to 3/4th of the interincisal distance between the upper and lower central incisors. This is to avoid the tongue from thrusting over the tip of the crib. The palatal crib acts as a barrier against the thrusting tongue and works as a mechanical restrainer. The U-loop is incorporated in the second premolar region and it helps to reposition the appliance posteriorly during the retraction phase, when it is used along with fixed orthodontic appliances.

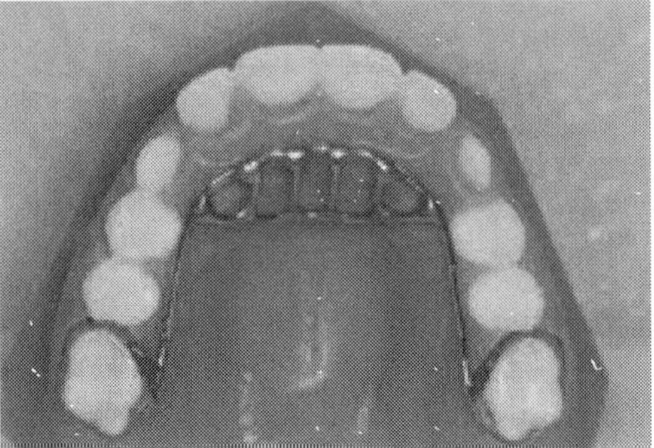

Figure 6. Tongue crib appliances

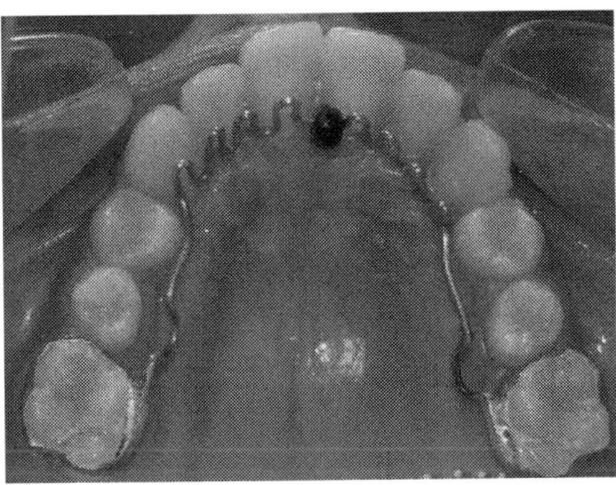

Figure 7. Hybrid Habit Correcting Appliance (HHCA).

5.5. Bruxism

The actions of masticatory system are divided into 2 groups. Functional actions such as mastication, speaking and swallowing, and parafunctional actions such as teeth impacting (clenching) and bruxism.

Functional activities are controllable and occurred daily. Parafunctional actions may be conscious or unconscious and are normally without sound. However, bruxism in nights is unconscious and mostly it is with sound production. Sleep bruxism occurs during stages first and second of non rapid eye movement (REM) sleep and REM sleep. These people do not have any complaint about bruxism, and it would not affect their quality of sleep. But in the old and people with sleep apnea, bruxism can reduce the quality of sleep [29]. Sleep bruxism has 2 types: Primary or idiopathic and secondary or iatrogenic. The first type is without any medical reason and the secondary type is whether with use of drug or without the use of drug. Risk factors are as follows: Genetics: 20 to 50% of patients with sleep bruxism have positive family history [30]; age: The prevalence of this habit decrease with age; cigarette smoking: The prevalence of sleep bruxism in smokers is 1.9 times more than non-smokers; use of alcohol and caffeine [31]; tension and stresses. Clinical findings of sleep bruxism include; report of grinding or impacting sounds of teeth; erosion of the teeth occlusal surfaces and breakdown of repairs; hypertrophy of masticatory muscles; hypersensitivity of teeth to cold air, and joint sounds. The treatment includes no special recommended regimen, but increasing awareness of the patient, intra oral appliances, behavioral treatment and drugs like diazepam and clonazepam have been reported to be effective [32,33].

6. Anterior cross bite correction

Anterior crossbite is defined as a malocclusion resulting from the lingual positioning of the maxillary anterior teeth in relationship to the mandibular anterior teeth. An anterior crossbite is present when one or more of the upper incisors are in linguo-occlusion (reverse over jet). This may involve just a single tooth or could include all four upper incisors. Anterior dental crossbite has a reported incidence of 4-5% and usually becomes evident during the early mixed-dentition phase [34]. Anterior crossbite correction in early mixed dentition is highly recommended as this kind of malocclusion does not diminish with age. Uncorrected anterior crossbite may lead to abnormal wear of the lower incisors, dental compensation of mandibular incisors leading to thinning of labial alveolar plate and/or gingival recession. However early treatment does not always eliminates orthodontic treatment need in permanent occlusion. The aim of early treatment of this type of malocclusion is to correct anterior crossbite, as otherwise often can lead to very serious Class III mallocclusion which would be possible to treat only with combined orthodontic and orthognatic method.

A variety of factors has been reported to cause anterior dental crossbite, including a palatal eruption path of the maxillary anterior incisors; trauma to the primary incisor resulting in lingual displacement of the permanent tooth germ; supernumerary anterior teeth; an over-retained necrotic or pulpless deciduous tooth or root; odontomas; crowding in the incisor region; inadequate arch length; and a habit of biting the upper lip. Various treatment methods have been proposed to correct anterior dental crossbite, such as tongue blades, reversed stainless steel crowns, fixed acrylic planes, bonded resin-composite slopes, and removable acrylic appliances with finger springs.

Bayraka and Tunca, 2008, described the use of bonded resin-composite slopes for the management of anterior crossbite in children in early mixed dentition. Dental crossbite was corrected by applying a 3-4 mm bonded resin-composite slope to the incisal edge of the mandibular incisor with an angle 45° to the longitudinal axis of the tooth (Fig. 8). Correction was achieved within 1-2 weeks with no damage to either the tooth or the marginal periodontal tissue. The procedure was a simple and effective method for treating anterior dental crossbite [35].

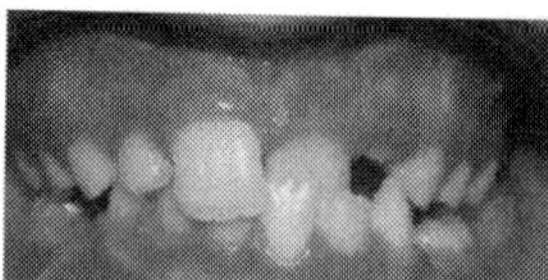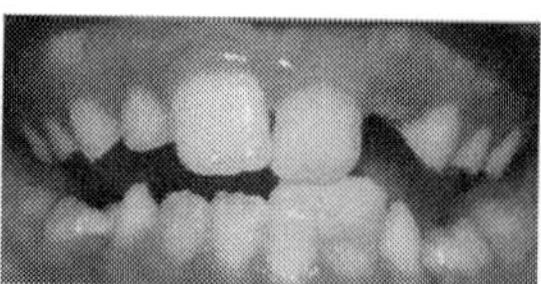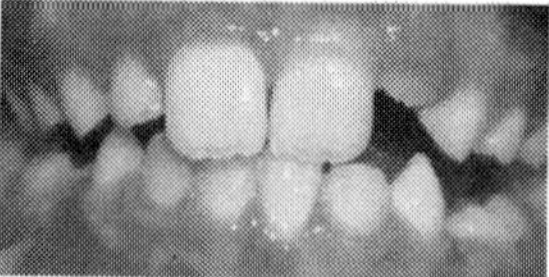

Figure 8. Anterior crossbite correction with bonded resin-composite slope

Some authors believe that removable appliances are not preferred in anterior crossbite correction as they tend to get displaced as the turning frequency decreases following activation. Moreover, poor patient compliance with removable appliance can cause relapse of the case and poor success rate. Therefore, a fixed appliance was proposed as a more sound therapy. Yaseen and Acharya, 2012, described the use of hexa helix, a modified version of quad helix for the management of anterior crossbite and bilateral posterior crossbite in early mixed dentition (Fig. 9). Correction was achieved within 15 weeks with no damage to the tooth or the marginal periodontal tissue. The procedure is a simple and effective method for treating anterior and bilateral posterior crossbite simultaneously. it provides advantages such as minimal discomfort, reduces need for patient cooperation, and better control of tooth movements [36].

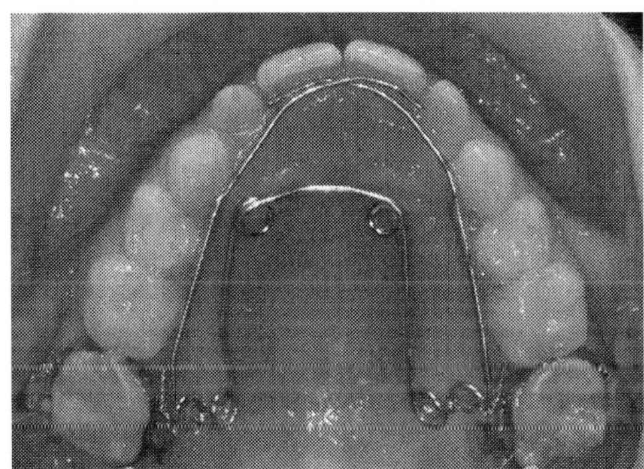

Figure 9. Hexa helix appliance.

In a recent study, Wiedel and Bondemark, 2014, evaluated and compared the stability of correction of anterior crossbite in the mixed dentition by fixed or removable appliance therapy. The study comprised 64 consecutive patients who met the following inclusion criteria: early to late mixed dentition, anterior crossbite affecting one or more incisors, no inherent skeletal Class III discrepancy, moderate space deficiency, a nonextraction treatment plan, and no previous orthodontic treatment. The study was designed as a randomized controlled trial with two parallel arms. The patients were randomized for treatment with a removable appliance with protruding springs or with a fixed appliance with multi-brackets. The outcome measures were success rates for crossbite correction, overjet, overbite, and arch length. Measurements were made on study casts before treatment (T0), at the end of the retention period (T1), and 2 years after retention (T2). Results showed that at T1 the anterior crossbite had been corrected in all patients in the fixed appliance group and all except one in the removable appliance group. At T2, almost all treatment results remained stable and equal in both groups. From T0 to T1, minor differences were observed between the fixed and removable appliance groups with respect to changes in overjet, overbite, and arch length measurements. These changes had no clinical implications and remained unaltered at T2. It was concluded that in the mixed dentition, anterior crossbite affecting one or more incisors can be successfully corrected by either fixed or removable appliances with similar long-term stability [37].

7. Anterior diastema and abnormal labial fraenum

Angle described the midline diastema as a common form of incomplete occlusion character-ized by a space between the maxillary and, less frequently, mandibular central incisors. In his classical article, Andrews stated that interdental diastemas should not exist and all contacts should be tight so that the patient has 'straight and attractive teeth as well as a correct overall dental occlusion'.

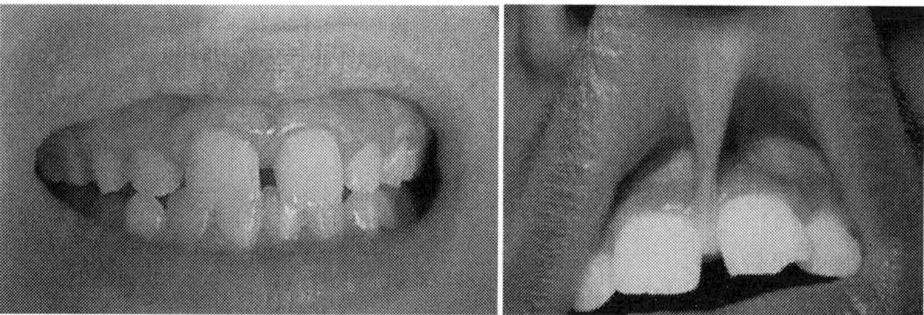

Figure 10. Midline diastema

Sanin et al., developed a method that could predict whether the space would close spontaneously in the developing dentition. This method is based on millimeter measurements in the early mixed dentition and is claimed to have an accuracy of 88%. As the size of the diastema increases the possibility of space closure without treatment reduces. Sanin's prediction is as follows:

- For a 1 mm space in the early mixed dentition the possibility of spontaneous space closure is 99%.

- For a 1.5 mm space the possibility is 85%.

- For a 1.85 mm diastema it is 50%.

- For a 2.7 mm space the possibility of closure without treatment is only 1%.

The measurement should be made after the eruption of the lateral incisors. Hence it is advisable to intervene early if the midline diastema is more than 1.85 mm after the eruption of the permanent lateral incisors [38].

To treat the midline diastema effectively, an accurate diagnosis of the etiology and an intervention relevant to the specific etiology is necessary. Timing of the treatment is important to achieve satisfactory results. Most of the researchers do not recommend tooth movement until the eruption of the permanent canines, but in certain cases, where very large diastemas exist, treatment can be initiated early [39].

Nainar and Gnanasundaram noted in their study of midline diastemas on 9774 Southern Indian individuals, that there was a relatively increased frequency of familial occurrence and hence proposed the presence of a genetic factor in the expression of midline diastema. Treatment methods include orthodontic correction with a fixed or removable appliance and prosthetic correction with composites and crowns. If the diastema is large, it is advisable to close the space using orthodontic appliances. In most cases, simple removable appliances incorporating finger springs or a split labial bow can give good results [40].

A hypertrophic labial frenum may be considered as a major etiological factor for midline diastema. In a thick and fleshy labial frenum, the fibro-elastic band crosses the alveolus and inserts into the incisive papilli, preventing the approximation of the maxillary central incisors. The blanching test is a simple diagnostic test to predict whether a normal tight contact between the central incisors. Most of the researchers, like Angle, Sicher, and Edwards, [41-43] are of the opinion that superior labial frenum causes midline diastema. Some researchers, like Popovich et al, believe that there is an inverse relationship between high frenal attachment and midline diastema. According to them, labial frenum persists owing to the existing diastema and, as the dentition applies little or no pressure on the tissues, here is little or no atrophy of the frenum [44]. However, most of the researchers agree that removal of the high bulbous labial frenum is important for the stability after the closure of the midline diastema.

Excessive anterior overbite is another major contributing factor for midline diastema. As a result of trauma to the maxillary anterior teeth from the mandibular incisors, the maxillary incisors procline. This results in an increase of the upper arch circumference, leading to a diastema. Practitioners should not fail to identify deep bite as an aetiology for the diastema. Any attempt to close the midline spacing without correcting the deep bite and anterior traumatic bite will lead to a speedy relapse of the condition.

Oral habits such as tongue thrusting and finger sucking can be other etiological factors for the appearance of the midline diastema. According to Proffit and Fields, tongue position at rest may have a greater impact on tooth position than tongue pressure, as the tongue only briefly contacts the lingual surface of the anterior teeth during thrusting [45]. The tongue pushes the anterior teeth to a forward position, increasing the circumference which results in spacing. An abnormal habit of the tongue can be detected by the tip of the tongue popping out through the anterior spacing when the patient is asked to swallow. In cases of anterior open bite, the tongue may be seen thrusting between incisal edges of the maxillary and mandibular incisors. Patients with tongue thrust often produce a snap sound on swallowing and also have hyperactivity of the orbicularis oris muscle.Deleterious habits have to be corrected by using habit-breaking appliances and by psychological approaches. The use of fixed tongue cribs are found to be effective in breaking the tongue-thrusting habit.

Peg-shaped laterals Supernumerary teeth/mesiodens, missing teeth, pathologic migration of teeth Tooth size, arch size discrepancy, angulation of teeth, odontomas occurring in the maxillary midline, developmental cysts in the orofacial midline, and flaccid lips are other proposed etiological factors leading to midline diastema. Relapse is a major concern in the correction of midline diastema. However, exact diagnosis and removal of the etiology is the key to obtaining a stable result. Long-term use of retainers or even permanent bonded lingual retainers are advocated, especially in cases with large diastema. Large pretreatment diastema presence of at least one family member with a similar condition increases the risk of relapse [46,47].

8. Serial extraction

The term serial extraction describes an orthodontic treatment procedure that involves the orderly removal of selected deciduous and permanent teeth in a predetermined sequence (Dewel, 1969). Serial extraction can be defined as the correctly timed, planned removal of certain deciduous and permanent teeth in mixed dentition cases with dento-alveolar disproportion in order to: Alleviate crowding of incisor teeth and to allow unerupted teeth to guide themselves into improved positions (canines in particular), and to lessen (or eliminate) the period of active appliance therapy. Thus, it is one of the positive interceptive orthodontic procedure generally applied in most discrepancy cases where supporting bone is less than the total tooth material [48].

Serial extraction has been of interest to dentist for many years. Throughout the history of dentistry it has been recognized that the removal of one or more irregular teeth would improve the appearance of the reminder. Nance presented clinics on his technique of progressive extraction in 1940 and has been called as the father of serial extraction philosophy in the United States. Kjellgren in 1940 termed this extraction procedure as planned or progressive extraction procedure of teeth. Hotz, 1970, named the same procedure on "Guidance of eruption". According to him the term guidance of eruption is comprehensive and encompasses all measures available for influencing tooth eruption [49]. Widespread adoption of serial extraction as a corrective treatment procedure continues to be a source of concern to all pedodontists who are aware of its limitations as well as of its possibilities. The principle reason is that its application involves growth prediction. Every serial extraction diagnosis is based on the promise that future growth will be inadequate to accommodate all of the teeth in a normal alignment.

If primary teeth are extracted prematurely, this will influence the eruption rate and position of the permanent successors. In general, the eruption will be delayed if the primary tooth overlying the permanent tooth is extracted 1 ½ years or more from the time the primary tooth would normally exfoliate. Conversely, the eruption rate can be accelerated if the primary tooth overlying the permanent tooth is extracted less than a year before the primary tooth would normally exfoliate. Biologic variation in eruption rates will affect these time tables, as will periapical inflammation of the primary tooth. Another useful principle is that crowded teeth adjacent to an extraction site tend to align themselves [50].

Normal dental, skeletal and profile development – influences the rationale for serial extraction. The work of Moorrees et al on arch dimensions and serial extractions indicates that there is minimal increase in mandibular intercanine width between 8 and 18 years, occurring usually around the time the permanent mandibular canines erupt. The maxillary intercanine width increases slightly more and over a longer time. The dental arch perimeter from the distal of the mandibular primary second molar to its antimere is less in the permanent dentition than in the primary. Also the principles of leeway space, interrelationship of overjet, overbite, axial inclinations, and mesial shift, and arch-length analysis must be considered in determining whether to institute a serial extraction procedure. The skeletal and profile factors that influence serial extractions are the another-posterior, vertical, and transverse relationships as well as the developmental pattern. Specifically the relation of the maxilla to the mandible and of the both to the cranial base must be determined to identify protrusions, retrusions, hyperdivergences, hypodivergences, crossbites, and asymmetries. Also rotational, vertical, and transverse growth patterns need to be integrated into the decision-making process [51].

The idea of serial extraction started when Pedodontist sees a child 5 or 6 years of age with all the deciduous teeth present in a slightly crowded state or with no spaces between them, he can predict, with a fair degree of certainly, that there will not be enough space in the jaws to accommodate all the permanent teeth in their proper alignment. As Nance (1940), Dewel (1954), and others have pointed out, after the eruption of the first permanent molars at 6 years of age, there is probably no increase in the distance from the mesial aspect of the first molar on one side around the arch to the mesial aspect of the first molar on the opposite side. If there is any change, it may be an actual reduction of the molar-to-molar arch length, as the "leeway" space is lost through the mesial migration of the first permanent molars during the tooth-exchange process and correction of the flush terminal plane relationship. At that time, a list of possible clinical clues for serial extraction were proposed: Premature loss of deciduous teeth, arch-length deficiency and tooth size discrepancies, lingual eruption of lateral incisors, unilateral deciduous canine loss and shift to the same side, mesial eruption of canines overlateral incisors, mesial drift of buccal segments, abnormal eruption direction and eruption sequence, flaring of incisors, ectopic eruption of mandibular first deciduous molar, abnormal resorption of II deciduous molar, ankylosis, labial stripping, and gingival recession, usually of lower incisor. However, a number of contraindications for serial extractions were addressed: Congenital absence of teeth providing space, mild to moderate crowding, deep or open bites, severe Class II, III of dental/skeletal origin, cleft lip and palate, spaced dentition, anodontia / oligodontia, Midline diastemia, dilacerations extensive caries, disportion between arc length and tooth material.

9. Considerations in serial extraction

1. Extracting primary canines will produce maximum amounts of self improvement in crowding with greatest inter-ception of lingual cross bite.

2. Extracting primary first molars produces earliest eruption of first premolars but reduces speed and amount of improvement in permanent central and lateral incisors crowding and position due to retention of C that it has limited application.

3. Extracting primary canines and first molars is a compromise between rapid improvement in and desired early eruption of permanent central and lateral incisors due to simultaneous eruption of first premolars with this extraction sequence.

There is no single technique for Serial Extraction. It is a long-range guidance program and it may be necessary to reevaluate and change tentative decisions several times. Usually the child is 7-8 years of age when he/she brought to the pedodontist. At this time the maxillary and mandibular central incisors are usually erupted, but there is inadequate space in anterior segments to allow normal eruption and positioning of lateral incisors. In some cases, mandibular lateral incisors have already erupted but they are usually lingually positioned and rotated. The same is with the maxillary lateral incisors.

9.1. Dewel's method

There are 3 stages in Serial Extraction Therapy:

First: Removal of deciduous canines : to permit eruption and optimal alignment of lateral incisors. There is some amount of improvement in position of central incisors also.

Second: Removal of first deciduous molars: to accelerate eruption of first premolars ahead of canine if possible.

Third: Removal of erupting first premolars: Before the first premolars are extracted, all the diagnostic criteria must again be evaluated. The status of developing third molars must be evaluated, because if the third molars are congenitally missing then extraction of 1st premolars would be unnecessary because there would be enough space. So in short, Dewel's method is:

$$\text{Step I} \longrightarrow \text{II} \longrightarrow \text{III}$$

$$\frac{C \mid C}{C \mid C} \qquad \frac{D \mid D}{D \mid D} \qquad \frac{4 \mid 4}{4 \mid 4}$$

9.2. Tweed's method

According to Tweed, if diagnosis shows the discrepancy exists between teeth and basal bone structures and if patient is between 7 ½ to 8 ½ years, Serial Extraction program is should be carried out. Sequence is:

First: At approximately 8 years all deciduous molars are extracted. It is preferable to maintain in deciduous canines to retard eruption of permanent canines.

Second: extract of first premolar and deciduous canines should he done 4-6 months prior to eruption of permanent canines when they erupt they migrate posteriorly into good position. Any irregularities in mandibular incisors if not too severe, get corrected themselves and they are also tipped lingually due to normal muscular forces.

9.3. Moyers method

Proposed when crowding seen in central incisor region. Fairly eruption of lateral incisors.

Stage I (Extraction of all deciduous lateral incisors). It helps in alignment of central incisors.

Stage II (Extraction of all deciduous canines after 7-8 months). It helps in alignment of lateral incisors and provides space for lateral incisors.

Stage III (Extraction of all deciduous first molars). It stimulates eruption of all first premolars.

Stage IV (Extraction of all first premolars after 7-8 months). It provides space for canines and stimulates eruption of canines.

$$\text{Step I} \text{-----------} \rightarrow \text{II} \text{-----------} \rightarrow \text{III} \text{-----------} \rightarrow \text{IV}$$

$$\frac{B \mid B}{B \mid B} \qquad \frac{C \mid C}{C \mid C} \qquad \frac{D \mid D}{D \mid D} \qquad \frac{4 \mid 4}{4 \mid 4}$$

The technique of serial extraction was biologically sound proven, and was not considered a compromise. with continuous observation and study, the sight has changed. conventional orthodontic therapy is required to complete the alignment of teeth, to parallel the roots on either side, of the extraction space, to eliminate overbite, and to effect residual space closure. With advances in fixed orthodontics, less damage and more stable results are obtained. Moreover, it must be remembered that, once teeth have been extracted, they cannot be replaced if an error in judgment must be made, it is more expedient to error in a conservative manner without extraction as teeth can always be extracted at a later date. To summarize the limitations a and side effects of serial extraction:

First: Tendency of bite to close following loss of posterior teeth. A normal overbite depends on adequate vertical growth and Serial Extraction involves removal of strategically located deciduous and permanent teeth. Vertical and horizontal growth depends great part on normal proximal and occlusal function in maintaining arch length and normal overjet and overbite.

Second: Failure of premolars that fail to reach their normal occlusal level. In normally developing dentition, the premolars are ready to emerge soon after the loss of the deciduous molars and then proceed occlusally with no delay. But in Serial Extraction cases the premolars have to travel a long way before penetrating the gingival tissues. Prolonged absence of teeth in the posterior segment of arches permits the tongue to flow into remaining spaces and this may remain as a tongue thrusting habit. This in turn prevents premolars from attaining full eruption.

Third: Effect of serial extraction on facial esthetics. Most of us over emphasize on straight profile which has led to extraction of teeth in mixed dentition because the lips appear to be prominent. Its normal for lip line to have greater convexity during early transitional stages than it will have in mature dentition. Lip fullness is not a reliable criterion for extraction in early mixed dentition. The straight profile must be viewed with greater concern because early removal of premolars is likely to cause a concave profile.

Fourth: Nasal development is another unpredictable hazard. The nose is one structure that continues to grow long after other facial parts have reached maturity. Unrestrained extraction will accentuate its prominence by reducing skeletal development in dental area. Moreover growth of chin is unpredictable. If growth in nose and chin exceeds normal range a concave profile is obtained.

In conclusion, one team of clinicians and practioners demonstrate that undertaking a serial extraction protocol can afforded an improvement of the patient's self-esteem, resulting in a positive social impact due to esthetic enhancement. Furthermore, the low cost of this protocol permits the use of this therapy in underprivileged communities provided the diagnosis is certain and the post extraction movement of teeth is controlled by mechanical means. The other team suggest that serial extraction is counter-productive. The early extraction of primary cuspids will invariably result in crowding of the permanent cuspids region. In reality, they adopt the idea that the problem is maintained and the crowding shifts to involve the permanent cuspids. They remind us with the most basic canon of the health profession which is "first do no harm" [52].

10. Interceptive functional therapy

There is little doubt that functional appliances produce tooth movement and in many cases can correct occlusal discrepancies. The controversy over their use relates mainly to their mode of action, and in particular to two aspects. The first is the question of modification of growth of the basal parts of the jaws. Many authorities believe that basal jaw growth can be altered by functional means. The temporo-mandibular joint area has been thought to be a reactive growth site, i.e. any prolonged change in the position of the mandible during the growth period, such as is induced by wearing the appliance, results in bone apposition on the mandibular and temporal surfaces of the enlarged joint cavity. Baume, (1969) quotes histological evidence to support this concept, and ample clinical evidence has been produced in attempts to show that the use of functional appliances can alter the skeletal relationship of the jaws [53]. On the other hand, this clinical evidence does not always take into account the effects of normal growth. As functional appliances are normally used during the mixed dentition stage a considerable amount of normal growth must occur which could alter jaw size and relationships. Several investigators have failed to find evidence of altered growth with functional appliances, but instead have found the main effects to be tipping of the incisors and an opening rotation of the mandible [54,55].

The first practitioner to use functional jaw orthopedics to treat a malocclusion was Pierre Robin (1902).

His appliance influenced muscular activity by changing the spatial relationship of the jaws. Robin's monoloc was actually a modification of Kingsley's maxillary plate. It extended all along the lingual surfaces of the mandibular teeth, but it had sharp lingual imprints of the crown surfaces of both maxillary and mandibular teeth. It incorporated an expansion screw in the palate to expand the dental arches. In 1909, Viggo Andresen, a Danish dentist, used lingual horseshoe flange that guides the mandible forward to eliminate Class II malocclusion cases. The original Andresen activator was a tooth-borne, loosely fitting passive appliance consisting of a block of plastic covering the palate and the teeth of both arches, designed to advance the mandible several millimeters for Class II correction and open the bite 3 to 4 mm. The original design had facets incorporated into the body of the appliance to direct erupting posterior teeth mesially or distally, so, despite the simple design, dental relationships in all 3 planes of space could be changed.

The Herbst appliance (Dentaurum, Newtown, Pa) is suitable for slightly older children whose cooperation might not be dependable, because it is a fixed appliance worn 24 hours a day. The Herbst was introduced in 1905 by Emil Herbst, but his findings were not published until 1935. Little more was published on the appliance until the late 1970s, when Hans Pancherz, recognizing its possibilities for mandibular growth stimulation, revived interest. The typical Herbst consists of a telescoping mechanism connected to the maxillary first molars at one end and a cantilevered arm attached to the mandibular first molars at the other end; it forces the mandible forward (Fig. 11).

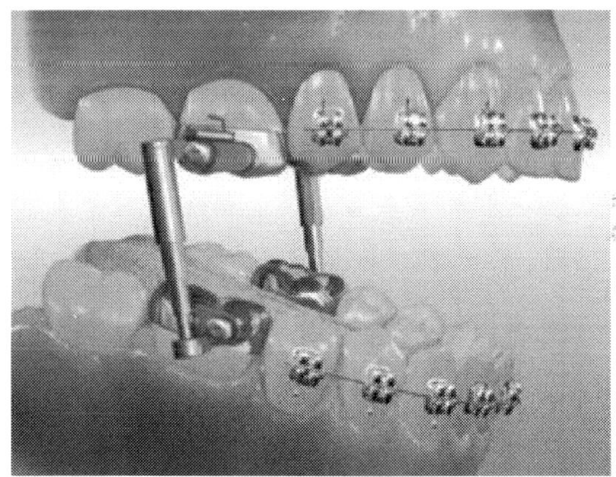

Figure 11. Herbst Appliance

In 1950, Wilhelm Balters (1893-1973), in an effort to treat Class II malocclusions characterized by deficient mandibles, began to modify Andresen's activator. He gave it the name bionator. It is indicated for patients with favorable facial growth patterns and is designed to produce forward positioning of the mandible. As with the function regulator, the bionator is available in 3 designs. Consisting of 2 halves connected by a Coffin spring, it is less restrictive of speech than Andresen's appliance. However, the treatment also highly depends on patient compliance, especially with regard to exercising

The Clark twin-block (Clark 1988) consists of separate upper and lower removable appliances, each with a 45° posterior bite plane designed to induce a mandibular posture of the desired amount and direction (Fig. 12) One or both sections may incorporate a mid-line screw to effect arch expansion(Fig. 13), and there is provision for the addition of extraoral traction.

Many clinical studies have been done on skeletal and dentoalveolar changes associated with functional appliances therapy in Class II malocclusions, but the scientific data are still controversial. Concerning skeletal effects induced by the functional appliances some authors

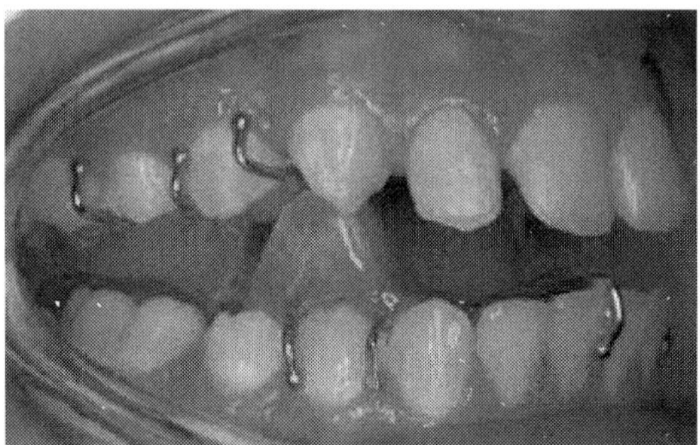

Figure 12. Twin-block appliance

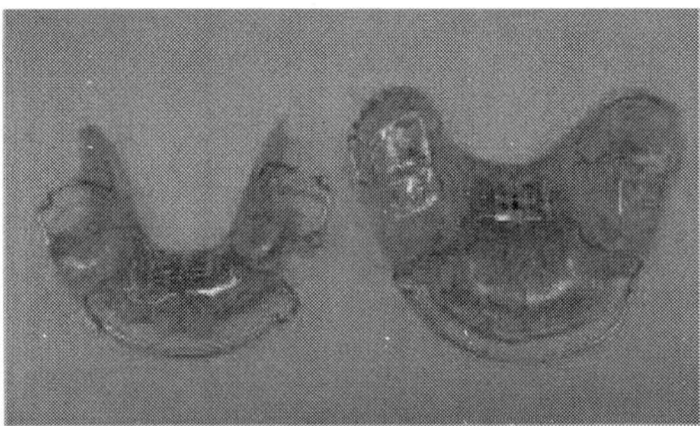

Figure 13. Expansion screw within Twin block appliance

demonstrate significant influences on mandibular growth [56], the others claim that it may be induced only small skeletal changes by this type of treatment [57]. The latter group of researchers found that the main changes occurred with functional appliance therapy were dentoalveolar distalization of the buccal and retroclination of the frontal upper teeth, along with mesial movement of the lower buccal segments and proclination of the lower labial segments[58]. Such diversity of results on skeletal changes might be related first of all to difficulties in applying treatment at the maximum growth spurt time. Another reason for the inconsistence in assessment of treatment results might be the use of not reliable reference lines and/or structures for cephalometric analysis before and after treatment. This makes difficult to assess real contribution of skeletal and dental components to occlusal changes [59]. A new paradigm for successful treatment presents a philosophical challenge to combine the benefits of orthodontic and orthopedic techniques to extend our horizons in the treatment of malocclusion that requires dental and skeletal correction.

The prefabricated myofunctional appliances are a series of prefabricated appliances produced by myoresearch company, Queensland, Australia. These appliances were also called "Trainers™" which include T4K™ and T4F™ appliances (Fig.14,15). The idea of prefabricated functional appliances was recently introduced to the orthodontic field and it becomes more practical with the new customizable functional appliance T4F™. The T4F™ appliance is a prefabricated re-mouldable appliance when immersed in very hot water so it can be customized to accommodate the patient's dentition in the mouth and increase the retention. This new functional appliance has the advantage of the immediate issuing and the direct fitting of the appliance in the patient's mouth and it is also a better choice in terms of the cost for the private practitioners. The prefabricated appliances were claimed to be effective for class II Div.1 management but there was no evidence except for T4K™ type which is designed for young children.

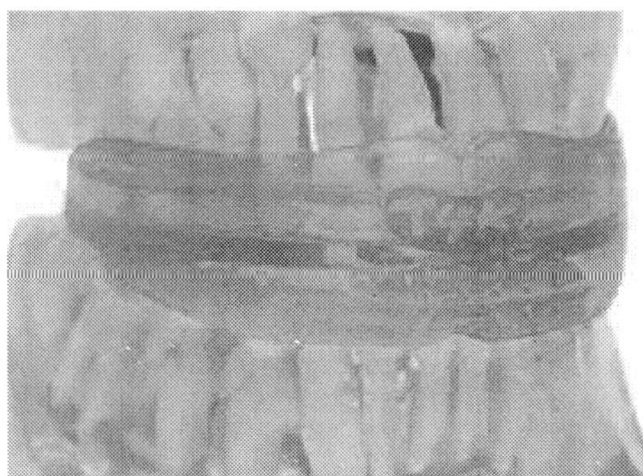

Figure 14. T4K™ The Pre-Orthodontic Trainer

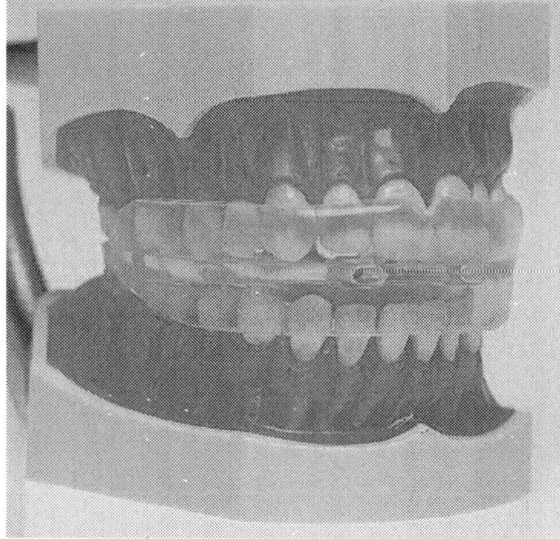

Figure 15. T4F™ The Pre-Orthodontic Trainer

Uysal et al., 2012, evaluated the effects of Pre-Orthodontic Trainer (T4F™) appliance on the anterior temporal, mental, orbicularis oris, and masseter muscles through electromyography (EMG) evaluations in subjects with Class II division 1 malocclusion and incompetent lips. Twenty patients (mean age: 9.8 ± 2.2 years) with a Class II division 1 malocclusion were treated with T4F™ (Myofunctional Research Co., Queensland, Australia). A group of 15 subjects (mean age: 9.2 ± 0.9 years) with untreated Class II division 1 malocclusions was used as a control. EMG recordings of treatment group were taken at the beginning and at the end of the T4F™ therapy (mean treatment period: 7.43 ± 1.06 months). Follow-up records of the control group were taken after 8 months of the first records. Recordings were taken during different oral functions: clenching, sucking, and swallowing. Statistical analyses were undertaken with Wilcoxon and Mann-Whitney U-tests. During the T4F™ treatment, activity of anterior temporal, mental, and masseter muscles was decreased and orbicularis oris activity was increased during clenching and these differences were found statistically significant when compared to control. Orbicularis oris activity during sucking was increased in the treatment group (P < 0.05). In the control group, significant changes were determined for anterior temporal (P < 0.05) and masseter (P < 0.01) muscle at clenching and orbicularis oris muscle at swallowing during observation period (P< 0.05). Findings indicated that treatment with T4F™ appliance showed a positive influence on the masticatory and perioral musculature [60].

Usumez et al., 2004, evaluated the dentoskeletal treatment effects induced by a preorthodontic trainer appliance (T4K™) treatment on Class II, division 1 cases. Twenty patients (10 girls and 10 boys, mean age 9.6+/-1.3 years) with a Class II, division 1 malocclusion were treated with T4K™ (Myofunctional Research Co., Queensland, Australia). The patients were instructed to use the trainer every day for one hour and overnight while they slept. A control group of 20 patients (mean age 10.2+/-0.8 years) with untreated Class II, division 1 malocclusions was used to eliminate possible growth effects. Lateral cephalograms were taken at the start and end of treatment. Final cephalograms were taken 13.1+/-1.8 months after trainer application, compared with a mean of 11.2+/-2.4 months later for the control group. The mean and standard deviations for cephalometric measurements were analyzed by paired-samples t-test and independent-samples t-tests. At the end of the study period, the trainer group subjects showed significant changes including anterior rotation and sagittal growth of the mandible, increased SNB and facial height, reduced ANB, increased lower incisor proclination, retroclination of upper incisors, and overjet reduction. However, only total facial height increase, lower incisor proclination, and overjet reduction were significantly higher when compared with the changes observed in the control group. This study was the first that demonstrated that the preorthodontic trainer application induces basically dentoalveolar changes that result in significant reduction of overjet and can be used with appropriate patient selection [61].

In a very recent study, Dr. Hanoun and his colleagues evaluated the effectiveness of the pre-fabricated myofunctional appliance T4F™ (compared to Twin Block appliance) in the treatment of Class II Div.1 malocclusion. The study was a prospective randomized clinical trial. All subjects were growing patients aged 11 -14 years old with Class II Div.1 malocclusion based on Class II skeletal relationship with overjet of 7 mm or more. Those subjects who had anterior open bite or previous orthodontic therapy or craniofacial anomalies or history of facial trauma were all excluded from the trial. The overjet was reduced more favourably in the Twin Block group than in the T4F™ group with a mean difference between the two groups of 2.14 mm (p <0.01). Moreover, there was a significant difference between both groups in terms of horizontal skeletal linear dimensions of the mandible with more favourable increase in the Twin Block group (p < 0.05).

11. Conclusion

Interceptive orthodontics is employed to recognize and eliminate potential irregularities and malposition in the developing dentofacial complex. These procedures are directed to lessen or to eliminate the severity of developing malocclusion. The early assessment of the child, followed by regular review, and treatment at the appropriate time if necessary, will do much to reduce malocclusion to the basic non-preventable level. The key to prevention of this kind is awareness. This part examines the key areas relating to interceptive orthodontics with the available evidence to support the clinical management of common problems presenting in the mixed dentition.

Acknowledgements

I offer my sincerest gratitude to my wife, Mrs. Huda Zurigat who has supported me throughout my project with a lot of patience and enthusiasm. Her assistance in typing and organizing words and figures in this article was indispensible.

Author details

Maen H. Zreaqat*

Address all correspondence to: maenzreqat@yahoo.com

Al-Ogaly Medical Group, Saudi Arabia

References

[1] Weinberger BW. Historical résumé of the evolution and growth of orthodontia. J Am Dent Assoc 1934;21:201-221.

[2] Asbell MB. A brief history of orthodontics. Am J Orthod Dentofacial Orthop 1990;98:176-83.

[3]   Casto FM. A historical sketch of orthodontia. Dent Cosmos 1934;76:111-35.

[4]   Brodie AG. Orthodontic history and what it teaches. Angle Orthod 1934;4:85-97.

[5]   Irurita J, Alemán I, López-Lázaro S, Viciano J, Botella MC. Chronology of the development of the deciduous dentition in Mediterranean population. Forensic Sci Int. 2014;240:95-103.

[6]   Borrie F, Bonetti D, Bearn D. What influences the implementation of interceptive orthodontics in primary care? Br Dent J. 2014;216(12):687-91.

[7]   Kerosuo H1, Väkiparta M, Nyström M, Heikinheimo K. The seven-year outcome of an early orthodontic treatment strategy. J Dent Res. 2008;87(6):584-8.

[8]   Norman W. Orthodontics in 3 millennia. Chapter 12: Two controversies: Early treatment and occlusion Am J Orthod Dentofacial Orthop. 2006;130(6):799-804.

[9]   Baroni C; Franchini A; Rimondini L: Survival of different types of space maintainers. Pediatr Dent. 1994;16:360-61.

[10]   Kirzioglu Z, Ozay MS Z, Ozay MS. Success of reinforced fibre material space maintainers. J Dent Child. 2004;71;2:158-62.

[11]   Kargul B, Caglar E, Kabalay U. Glass fibre reinforced composite resin as fixed space maintainer in children 12 month clinical follow up. J Dent Child. 2005; 72(3):109-12

[12]   Kargul B, Çaglar E, Kabalay U. Glass fiber-reinforced composite resin space maintainer: case reports. J Dent Child. 2003;71:258-61.

[13]   Goldberg AJ, Frelich MA. Tooth splinting and stabilisation Dent Clin North Am. 1999; 43 (1) :127-33.

[14]   Setia V, Pandit IK, Srivastava N, Gugnani N, Sekhon HK. Space maintainers in dentistry: past to present. J Clin Diagn Res. 2013;7(10):2402-5.

[15]   Kharbanda O. P, Sidhu S. S, Sundaram K, Shukla D. K, "Oral habits in school going children of Delhi: a prevalence study," Journal of the Indian Society of Pedodontics and Preventive Dentistry. 2003; 21 (3): 120–124.

[16]   Larson EF. The prevalence and etiology of prolonged dumy and finger sucking habit. Am. J. Orthod., 1985; 87(5):172-174.

[17]   Farsi NM, Salama FS.. Sucking habits in Saudi children: prevalence, contributing factors and effects on the primary dentition. Pediatr. Dent. 1997; 19(1):28-33.

[18]   N. L. Villa, "Changes in the dentition secondary to palatal crib therapy in digit-suckers: a preliminary study," Pediatric Dentistry, vol. 19, no. 5, pp. 323–326, 1997.

[19]   B. S. Haskell and J. R. Mink, "An aid to stop thumb sucking: the "Bluegrass" appliance," Pediatric Dentistry. 1991; 13 (2): 83– 85.

[20] Van Norman RA (1997). Digit-sucking: A review of the literature, clinical observations and treatment recommendations. Int. J. Orofacial Myol., 23: 14-34

[21] Warren JJ, Bishara SE (2002). Duration of nutritive and nonnutritive sucking behavior and their effects on the dental arches in the primary dentition. Am. J. Orthod., 121: 347-356.

[22] Moimaz SA, Garbin AJ, Lima AM, Lolli LF, Saliba O, Garbin CA. Longitudinal study of habits leading to malocclusion development in childhood. BMC Oral Health. 2014; (4):14-96.

[23] Maia-Nader M, Silva de Araujo Figueiredo C, Pinheiro de Figueiredo F, Moura da Silva AA, Thomaz EB, Saraiva MC, Barbieri MA, Bettiol H. Factors associated with prolonged non-nutritive sucking habits in two cohorts of Brazilian children. BMC Public Health. 2014;14:14-17.

[24] Fleming PJ, Blaive PS Pacifier use an sudden infant death syndrome. Arch. Dis. Children. 1999; 81(2): 112-116.

[25] Lopes TS, Moura Lde F, Lima MC. Breastfeeding and sucking habits in children enrolled in a mother-child health program. BMC Res Notes. 2014;14(7): 23-38.

[26] Tanaka OM, Vitral RW, Tanaka GY, Guerrero AP, Camargo ES. (. Nailbiting, or onychophagia: A special habit. Am. J. Orthod. Dentofacial Orthop. 2008;134(2): 305-308.

[27] Saheeb D. Prevalence of oral and parafunctional habits in Nigerian patients suffering temporomandibular joint pain and dysfunftion. J. Med. Biomed. Res., (2005; 4(1): 59-64

[28] Feu D1, Menezes LM, Quintão AP, Quintão CC. A customized method for palatal crib fabrication. J Clin Orthod. 2013 Jul;47(7):406-12.

[29] Kato T, Thein NMR, Montplaisir JY, Lavigne GJ. Bruxism and orofacial movements during sleep. Dent. Clin. North Am. 2001;45(4):651-676.

[30] Hublin C, Kaprio J, Partinen M, Koskenvuo M. Sleep bruxism based on self – report in a nationwide twin cohort. Sleep Res. 1998;7(1): 61-68

[31] Dahan JS, Lelong BA, Celant S, Leysen V. Oral perception in tounge thrust and other oral habits. Am. J. Orthod. Dentofacial Orthop., 2000;118:385-91.

[32] Pierce CJ, Gale EN. A comparison of different treatments for nocturnal bruxism. J. Dent. Res., 1988;67: 597-601.

[33] Ferreira NM, Dos Santos JF, Dos Santos MB, Marchini L. Sleep bruxism associated with obstructive sleep apnea syndrome in children. Cranio. 2014 Sep [Epub ahead of print].

[34] Major PW, Glover K. Treatment of anterior cross-bites in the early mixed dentition. Journal of the Canadian Dental Association. 1992;58(7):574–578.

[35] Bayrak S1, Tunc ES. Treatment of anterior dental crossbite using bonded resin-composite slopes: case reports. Eur J Dent. 2008;2(4):303-6.

[36] Yaseen SM, Acharya R. Hexa Helix:Modified Quad Helix Appliance to Correct Anterior and Posterior Crossbites in Mixed Dentition. Case Reports in Dentistry. 2012: 1-5.

[37] Wiedel AP1, Bondemark L. Stability of anterior crossbite correction: A randomized controlled trial with a 2-year follow-up. Angle Orthod. 2014 Jul 8. [Epub ahead of print]

[38] Sanin C, Sekiguchi T, Savara BS. A clinical method for the prediction of closure of the central diastema. ASDC J Dent Child 1969; 36: 415–418.

[39] Baum AT. The midline diastema. J Oral Med 1966; 21: 30–39.

[40] Nainar SM, Gnanasundaram N. Incidence and etiology of midlinediastema in a population in southIndia (Madras). Angle Orthod 1989; 59: 277–282.

[41] Angle EH. Treatment of Malocclusion of the Teeth 7th edn. Philadelphia: SS White Dental Manufacturing Company, 1907: p167.

[42] Sicher H. Oral Anatomy 2nd edn. St Louis: CV Mosby Co, 1952: pp272–273.

[43] Edwards JG. The diastema, the frenum, the frenectomy: a clinical study. Am J Orthod 1977; 71:489–508.

[44] Popovich F, Thompson GW, Main PA. Persisting maxillary diastema: indications for treatment. Am JOrthod 1979; 75(4): 399–404.

[45] Proffit WR, Fields HW. Contemporary Orthodontics 2nd edn. St Louis: Mosby Yearbook, 1993: p467

[46] Shashua D, Artun J. Relapse afterorthodontic correction of maxillarymedian diastema: a follow-up evaluation of consecutive cases. Angle Orthod 1999; 69: 257–263.

[47] Nagalakshmi S, Sathish R, Priya K, Dhayanithi D. Changes in quality of life during orthodontic correction of midline diastema. J Pharm Bioallied Sci. 2014 (Suppl 1): 162-4

[48] Almeida RR, Almeida MR, Oltramari-Navarro PV, Conti AC, Navarro Rde L, Souza KR. Serial extraction: 20 years of follow-up. J Appl Oral Sci. 2012; 20(4):486-92.

[49] Hotz P.R. Guidance of eruption versus serial extraction. Am. J. Orthod, 1970; 58(1): 1-20.

[50] Nagalakshmi S, Sathish R, Priya K, Dhayanithi D. Changes in quality of life during orthodontic correction of midline diastema. J Pharm Bioallied Sci. 2014; 6 (Suppl 1):. [Epub ahead of print]

[51] Lee KP. The fallacy of serial extractions. Aust Orthod J. 2013;29(2):217-21.

[52] Almeida RR, Almeida MR, Oltramari-Navarro PV, Conti AC, Navarro Rde L, Souza KR. Serial extraction: 20 years of follow-up. J Appl Oral Sci. 2012 Jul-Aug;20(4): 486-92.

[53] Baume, L. J. Cephalo-facial growth patterns and the functional adaptation of the tem‐poro-mandibular joint structures. Eur Orthod Soc Trans, 1969: 79—98.

[54] Calvert, F. J. () An assessment of Andresen therapy on Class II Division I malocclu‐sion. Br J Orthodk 1982; 9: 149-153.

[55] Hamilton, S. D., Sinclair, P. M. & Hamilton, R. H. A cephalometric, tomographic and dental cast evaluation of Frankei therapy. Am J Orthod. 1987; 92: 427-434.

[56] Pancherz H. A cephalometric analysis of skeletal and dental changes contributing to Class II correction in activator treatment. Am J Orthod 1984;85:125-134

[57] Mills C, McCulloch K. Treatment effects of the Twin-block appliance: a cephalomet‐ric study. Am J Orthod 1998;114:15-24.

[58] Windmiller EC. Acrylic splint Herbst appliance: cephalometric evaluation. Am J Or‐thod Dentofac Orthop 1993;104:73-84.

[59] Baccetti T. et al. Treatment timing for Twin-block therapy. Am J Orthod dentofacial Orhop 2000;118:159-70.

[60] Usumez S, Uysal T, Sari Z, Basciftci FA, Karaman AI, Guray E. The effects of early preorthodontic trainer treatment on Class II, division 1 patients. Angle Orthod. 2004 Oct;74(5):605-9.

[61] Uysal T1, Yagci A, Kara S, Okkesim S. Influence of pre-orthodontic trainer treatment on the perioral and masticatory muscles in patients with Class II division 1 malocclu‐sion. Eur J Orthod. 2012 34(1):96-101

[62] Hanoun AB, Khamis MF Mokhtar N. The effectiveness of the prefabricated myofunc‐tional appliance T4FTM in comparison with Twin Block (TB) appliance in the treat‐ment of Class II Div.1 malocclusion. A randomized clinical trial. Master thesis. School of Dental Sciences, University Science Malaysia, 2014.

Chapter 19

Pain Evaluation Between Stainless Steel and Nickel Titanium Arches in Orthodontic Treatment — A Comparative Study

M. Larrea, N. Zamora, R. Cibrian, J.L. Gandia and V. Paredes

Additional information is available at the end of the chapter

http://dx.doi.org/10.5772/59125

1. Introduction

The pain has traditionally been one of the most common side effects in orthodontic treatment. Orthodontic movement causes an inflammatory reaction in the periodontium and the pulp, which stimulates the production of biochemical mediators that cause the sensation of pain [1].

Different factors such as gender, personality and previous experience with other dental treatments may influence the concrete experience that each patient experiences with a particular orthodontic treatment [2].

It has been described by several authors [3-10] that pain begins at 4 hours after application of the force, after 24 hours, it descends, maintaining a plateau of lower intensity for two or three days, to continue descending from the fifth and sixth day until it disappears.

In the beginning, the pain was evaluated in a subjective manner, though in recent decades, numerous studies [11-12] have focused on the composition of crevicular fluid and changes that occur in it during orthodontic treatment as a more objective assessment of pain.

The application of mechanical forces moves the tooth and induces an inflammatory reaction by compression of the periodontal ligament. As a result, a variety of mediators are produced within the periodontal space, spread out at the crevicular fluid and reflecting the biological processes taking place. Several in vivo studies have used crevicular fluid analysis to monitor changes.

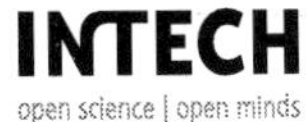

Crevicular fluid analysis is a noninvasive study of the cellular responses of the periodontal ligament during orthodontic treatment [13]. There are a variety of substances involved in the bone remodeling, produced in the cells of the periodontal ligament, that are spread out in the crevicular fluid [14].

Three substances, interleuquin 1β (IL-1β), prostaglandin E2 (PG-E2) and substance P (SP) were independently associated with pain [15-17], and are expressed during initial tooth movement in sufficient amounts to be detected in the crevicular fluid [18].

2. Problem statement

95% patients perceive pain during orthodontic treatment [6, 19], this pain being an important factor in rejecting treatment [20] or in interrupting it [21]. The pain involved has been described by various authors [3-10], there being different factors that modify it; gender, personality and previous experience with other dental treatments [2].

Ogura *et al.* [22] found a relationship between the magnitude of the force applied on the tooth and pain response, although other authors did not [23-25]. Additionally, the type of force (continuous or non-continuous) is also important. High and non-continuous forces [11,26,27] tend to significantly reduce the levels of IL1β at 168 hours from applying the force, which suggests the need for reactivation in order to maintain a sufficient production of IL1β. These types of forces not only increase the risk of radicular resorption on raising the hyalinization of the periodontal tissue [28,29], but also induce very sharp peaks of rises and falls in cytokine levels of which lead to undesirable results on the tissular level and the need for reactivating the forces. Light and continuous forces, however, tend to maintain high levels of IL1β so the need for reactivation is diminished [30-32]. These forces keep cytokine levels, which are necessary for continuous periodontal remodelling, high for a longer time.

The efficiency of orthodontic forces with different intensity and different duration has long been a major problem in the orthodontic clinic. In this study, to evaluate the efficacy and duration of each type of orthodontic force inducing initial tissue reaction two potent mediators of pain and bone resorption were measured; Prostaglandin E2 (PGE2) and substance P (SP).

Lastly, the material of the archwires that are fitted in the mouths of patients stailess-steel (SS) and nickel-titanium (Ni-Ti) exercise the force that may have an influence on pain, although there is controversy on this point [33]. There are few studies that compare pain depending on the type of archwire employed.

The aims of this work were, therefore:

- To compare pain during the initial stages of orthodontic treatment depending on the type of archwire employed; stainless steel (SS) or nickel-titanium (Ni-Ti).

- To determine a mathematical equation for predicting the level of pain depending on the time elapsed from fitting the archwire and that, therefore, would allow us to obtain the moment of peak of pain and to establish the moment when pain begins and ends depending on the type of archwire.

- To determine the difference in pain between time intervals.

- To analyse the crevicular fluid samples taken from patients to whom it has been performed the subjective study of pain.

3. Application area

A comparative, prospective clinical study was carried out at the Orthodontics Teaching Unit of the University of Valencia, Spain from January to April 2010. The study had previously been approved by the Ethics Committee of the University of Valencia. Rights have been protected by an appropriate Institutional Review Board and written informed consent was granted from all subjects. The Helsinki declaration was considered and its guidelines were followed in our investigation. All patients agreed to participate in the study, even though the diagnosis material was gathered as part of their treatment protocol.

4. Material and methods

4.1. Sample

A total of 150 patients who presented themselves at the Master in Orthodontics in order to receive Orthodontic treatment were selected.

The following inclusion criteria were established:

Patients who were to undergo a fitted Orthodontic treatment without dental extractions.

The presence of bracket cementing throughout the upper and/or lower arch.

The presence of good oral and periodontal health.

Whereas the exclusion criteria were:

The taking of any drug during the study.

The presence of active two band dental appliances during the treatment that would cause additional pain.

The presence of extra-oral appliances during the treatment that would cause additional pain.

On applying all these criteria, we obtained a total of 112 patients with a mean age of 19.8 years, ranging from between 9.5 and 64 years old. The sample comprised 37 males and 75 females.

The sample was divided according to the type of archwire that each of the patients wear: 49 patients with stainless-steel (SS) archwires and 63 patients with nickel-titanium (Ni-Ti) archwires. Of the 49 patients with SS archwires, 31 were females and 18 males and of the 63 patients with Ni-Ti archwires, 44 were females and 19 males.

Table 1 shows the distribution of the sample depending on age, gender, archwire type and according to where their archwires were fitted (upper, lower or both arches).

Archwire type	Female	Male	Arch upper	Arch lower	Both arches	Age (mean)
Ni-Ti Archwire (N =63)	44	19	38	25	4	22.6
Stainless-Steel Archwire (N=49)	31	18	31	18	2	17.2

Table 1. Sample distribution according to gender, the arch on which the archwire was fitted, age and archwire type used.

4.2. Method

After completing the appropriate orthodontic diagnosis, bracket bonding, which was carried out by 8 previously trained students of the Master of Orthodontics, Faculty of Medicine and Dentistry, University of Valencia, was scheduled.

Once the bonding of the brackets was performed, a 0.12"(diameter) Ni-Ti or SS arches were placed ramdomly in the patients enrolled in the study in order to compare the difference between groups in relationship with pain. In order to standardize the protocol, o elastomeric ligatures were used in all patients to hold the arches into the bracket system. The placement of the selected type of archwires did not alter the treatment of each patient.

5. Subjective assessment of pain — Patient questionnaire

First of all, a questionnaire was designed in order to assess the subjective level of pain. Having fitted the orthodontic appliance and the different archwires (SS and Ni-Ti), the patients filled in a pain questionnaire especially designed for this study, specifying the amount of pain (0=No pain; 1=discomfort; 2=slight pain; 3=intense pain) they experienced each day (from day 1 to day 14) and the time of day (morning, afternoon and night) they felt it. They were instructed to stop filling in this questionnaire after two consecutive days with an absence of pain. By doing so, the subjective values were obtained on an arbitrary scale. The appraisal of the questionnaire allowed us to assess both the subjective level of pain at each moment after the archwire was fitted and the total pain level experienced during the entire process of adapting to the archwire, obtained as the sum of the reported pain.

6. Objective assessment of pain — Crevicular fluid analysis

Secondly, an objective evaluation of pain was performed by analyzing the biochemical pain mediators in the crevicular fluid, in the laboratory.

The crevicular fluid samples were taken at the following stages of orthodontic treatment:

Before bracket bonding.

After 24 hours of placement of the archwire (Stainless Steel or Nickel Titanium).

A week after the archwire and bracket placement.

One month after the positioning of the initial archwire.

Crevicular fluid, using sterile paper strips (Periopaper Strip®. Proflow Incorporated. New York), was collected. Each sample was collected according to the technique described by Ottenbacher et al. [34] and later modified by Uematsu et al. [11], without removing the plaque of the tooth in order to not alter the outcome of the study. However, efforts were made to collect the sample in the absence of plaque. The collection of all the crevicular fluid samples was taken by the same observer.

The technique used for sample collection was made by: firstly, drying of the mouth with suction; after that, isolating the area with cotton rolls;thirdly, looking for drying places where the paper strip is placed; and then, taking the sample of crevicular fluid by placing the Periopaper ® in the binding groove between the tooth and gum. The paper strip is kept in this position within 30 seconds; and finally, the samples are placed between the sensors of the Periotron® 8000 (Proflow Incorporated. New York. USA) in order to obtain the crevicular fluid collection in Periotron units (Figures 1 and 2).

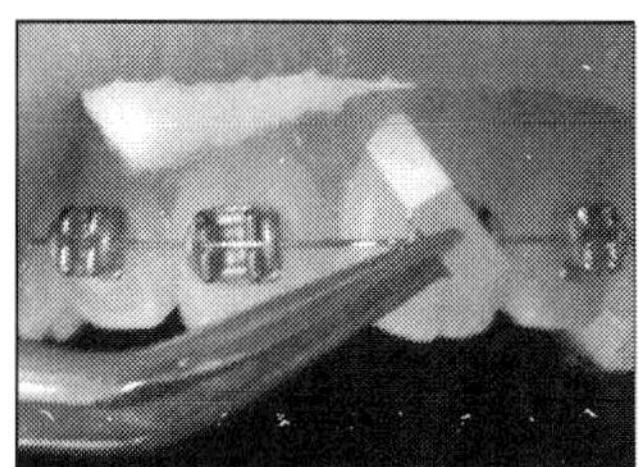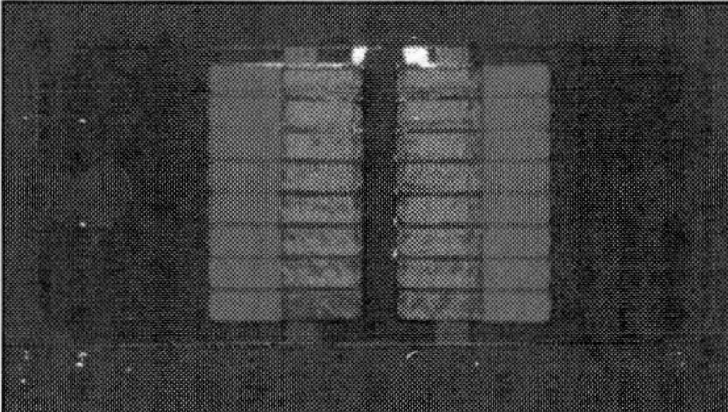

Figure 1. Sample collection of crevicular fluid with Periopaper®.

The extracted samples obtained were measured by ELISA immunofluorescence technique. To quantify the levels of substance P and PGE2, all samples were measured in duplicate. In our case, kits of high purity of the R & D Systems (Inc Minneapolis brand, USA) were used.

The spectrophotometer UV.vis shown in Figure 3 was used for the sample analysis. The spectrometer is an instrument used in biochemical analysis that measures, as a function of

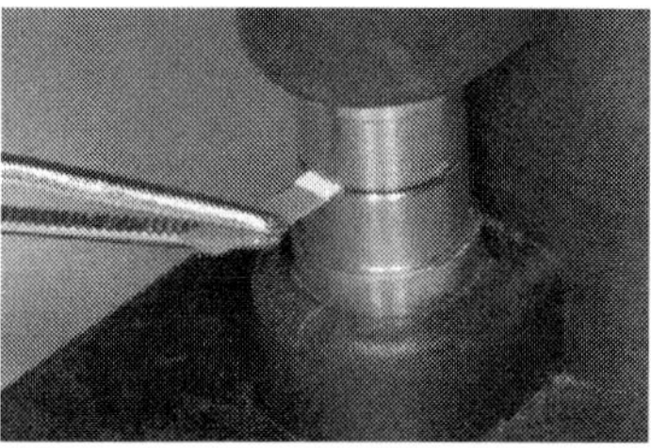

Figure 2. Crevicular fluid sample placement between Periotron® sensors.

wavelength, the relationship between the values of the same photometric magnitude related to two beams of radiation and the concentration and chemical reactions that are measured in a sample.

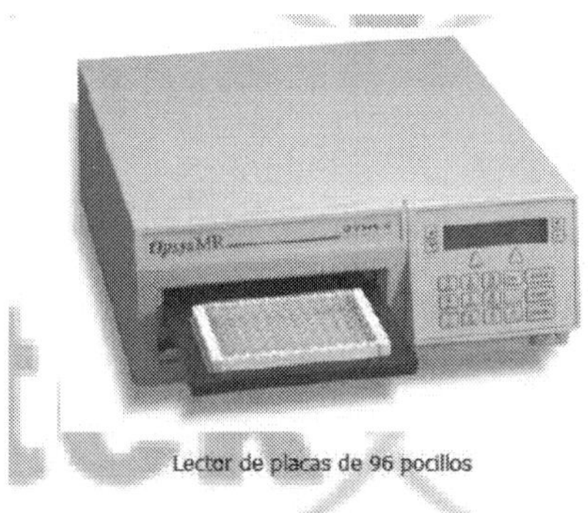

Figure 3. Spectrophotometer UV. vis

The Periotron® (Figure 4), must be properly calibrated before its use. It consists in a device for measuring the volume of the gingival crevicular fluid, collected by the paper strips (Periopaper®). Usually, a number, defined as Periotron unit, appears on the screen; constructing calibration graphs is required to obtain microliters, by using known amounts of fluid.

Once the device is switched on, it should be heated for 10 minutes. Then, it should be set to zero. After that, a dry paper strip must to be placed inside and the dial has to be adjusted until the zero value appears on the digital screen. A Hamilton microsyringe is then used (maximum volume 2µl, with 0'02µl gradations) to dispense known volumes of calibration liquid (human serum, being similar to the gingival crevicular fluid viscosity and composition) in the paper strips.

In our study, the paper strips were transferred to the Periotron® sensors (2-3 seconds) quickly to avoid evaporation errors. These paper strips were positioned in a standardized way, with the orange tips off the sensors.

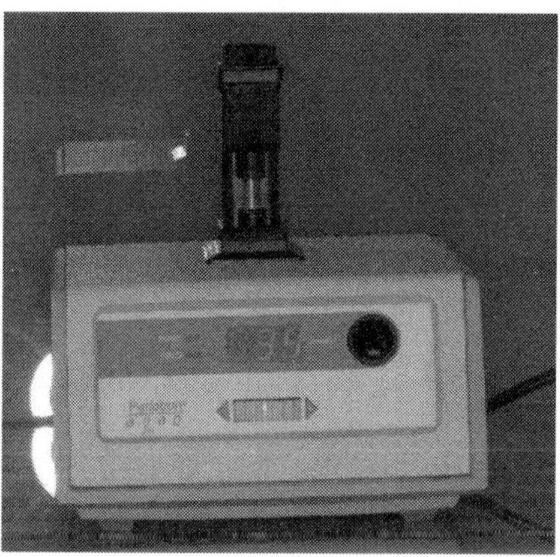

Figure 4. Periotron® machine.

After about 16 seconds, the Periotron Unit of each of the samples analysed was obtained. This occurred when the screen went from position I to position II in the frontal side of the device. Using moistened gauze with alcohol, the Periotron® sensors were cleaned between each sample.

Each volume was measured at least three times and the machine was set after each sample to zero.

In this way two variables were obtained:

1. The volume (in µl) of serum dispensed with Hamilton microsyringe (Figure 5).

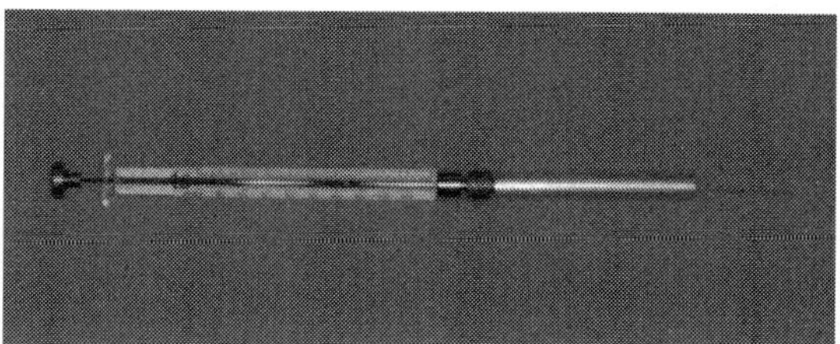

Figure 5. Hamilton Microjsyringe.

2. The Periotron Unit values of each of the parameters of the sample (average of the measurements made three times).

With these measurements, a linear regression curve was performed, obtaining a formula of the type y=ax+b, where "a" is the slope of the curve, "b" the intersection of the axis, and "x" in the crevicular fluid in Periotron Units.

6.1. Statistical method

The normality of the total pain (TP) distribution experienced by the patients throughout the treatment was checked using the Kolmogorov-Smirnovtest, which allows us to compare the means of independent samples using Student's t-test.

A two-factor (time and archwire type) ANOVA was applied with the Scheffé test for multiple comparisons.

The χ^2 test was used to analyse factor dependence.

Non-linear regression was used for the variables, PL: pain level and T: time elapsed from fitting the dental archwire, with an estimation of best-fit parameters and quality assessment of the same through R^2, which indicates the percentage of variation of one variable that can be explained by the variation of the other.

7. Results

The total pain (TP) experienced throughout treatment, the pain level (PL) associated with each time section (morning, afternoon, night) and, therefore, the time elapsed from the beginning of treatment and the peak of maximum pain experienced have all been analysed.

7.1. Subjective study of pain

7.1.1. Total pain associated with treatment

From the data provided by the patients in the questionnaire, the total subjective pain (TP) reported by each patient throughout the study was determined as the sum of pain level at each time of the day.

With both types of archwires, there was no case of pain after the tenth day onwards so, in the study that follows, we are only going to consider the data up until that moment, which amounts to 232 hours following the fitting of the initial archwires. With these considerations, the maximum TP possible would be 90 points, even though the maximum value suffered was 48 points for the SS archwires and 36 points for Ni-Ti archwires.

TP data distribution for each type of archwire (Ni-Ti and SS) corresponded to a normal distribution with p>0.850 and p>0.150, respectively. Data on level, mean, standard deviation and percentiles of 25% and 75% for each type of archwire and for the total of the sample are presented in Table 2.

It could then be confirmed that the mean pain value for SS archwires was greater than for Ni-Ti archwires with p<0.007.

Using the percentile values of the total group, the pain suffered throughout the treatment can be classified as: "slight" for under 10 points; "moderate" for between 10 to 20 points; and

Treatment	mean	SD	Minimum	Maximum	Percentile 25%	Percentile 75%
Ni-Ti	14.6	7.2	0	36	10	19
SS	19.8	11.5	3	48	11	29
TOTAL	16.8	9.5	0	48	10	21

Table 2. Total pain (TP) over the 10 days following the beginning of treatment with Ni-Ti or SS archwires regardless of the archwire used. Mean and standard deviation (SD), minimum and maximum values and the percentiles of 25 and 75% were also presented.

"intense" for over 21 points. Applying this criterion, figure 6 shows the percentage of TP suffered using the two types of archwire in the study.

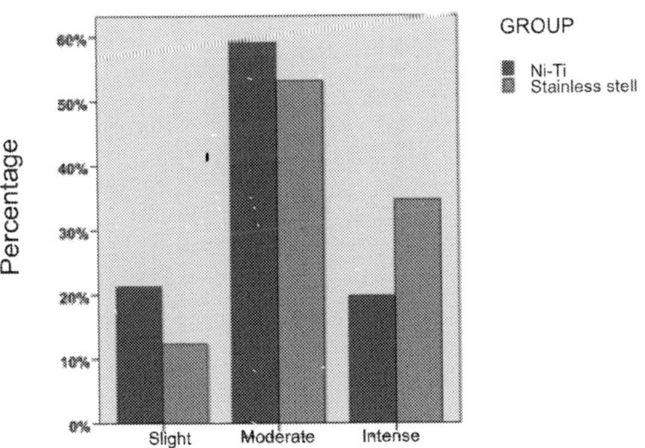

Figure 6. Percentage of total pain, slight (less than 10 points), moderate (between 10 and 20 points) and intense (over 20 points) for the two types of archwire studied (SS and Ni-Ti).

Dependence between the pain level and type of archwire was found to be p<0.006. It can be observed that the percentage of cases with intense pain in the SS group, 34.7%, is greater than in that of the Ni-Ti group, 19.7%, whereas in the case of slight pain, the percentage is the other way around being greater in that of the Ni-Ti group with 21.2% than the 12.2% of the SS group, although, in this case, without statistically significant difference.

Furthermore, the mean of the days that the patients experienced pain was 4.84 days in general, with 4.5 of mean for patients with Ni-Ti archwires as opposed to 5.4 days of mean for the group with SS archwires, with a statistically significant difference of p<0.04.

7.1.2. Pain level depending on the time elapsed from beginning of treatment

The subjective pain level (PL) for each time period was analysed according to the pain experienced during those same periods. As has been indicated in Material and Methods section, the possible evaluation in this case ranges from 0-3 points. The experimental results for each type of archwire are shown in figure 7.

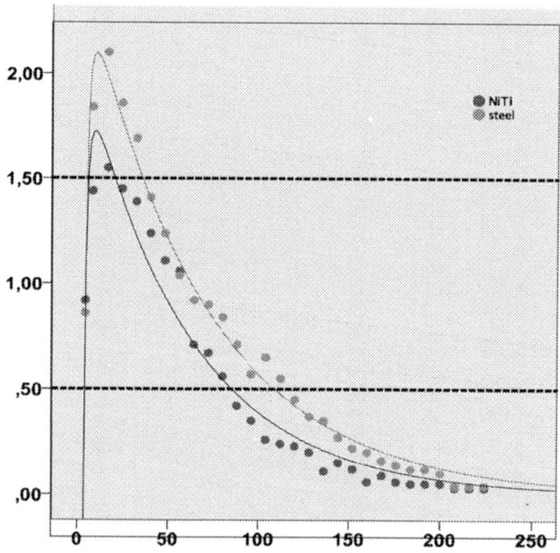

Figure 7. Experimental results and fit to the proposed curve PL=a* T⁻³+c * exp (-b*T) for the two types of archwires studied. PL values have been categorized as slight: less than 0.5; moderate from 0.5 to 1.5; and high: greater than 1.5.

It can be observed that, in general, the shape of the curve is similar for both types of archwires, pain appearing after a few hours and decreasing gradually. This similarity in pain behaviour encouraged us to look for a mathematical function that would fit the points of the curve in order to evaluate pain depending on time and that, therefore, would provide a predictive study of the pain associated with the archwire or with the physiological characteristics of the process them self.

Given that the representation of pain level (PL) with the time period, regardless of the archwire used, also had a similar shape to that shown in figure 7, we then analysed this situation, as here the number of cases was higher and the fitting of the mathematical function would have more statistical validity and offer information on the evolution of pain in general. The points were fitted using non-linear regression curves of different types, the maximum fit being found to be a curve of the form: PL=a* T⁻³+c * exp (-b*T), where PL, is pain level, T is the time elapsed in hours and the values "a", "b" and "c" correspond to the best-fit parameters that could differ or not depending on the type of archwire. The curve chosen for fitting consists of two terms: a decreasing exponential in which the parameters "b" and "c" are related, respectively, to the fall in the exponential and to PL in each time period, and a potential term that becomes insignificant for long times, but which modulates the growth of the exponential for low times, being responsible for the height that the peak of the curve reaches and is characterized by the "a" parameter. In this way, the first term of the equation and, therefore, the "a" coefficient is important in the first hours following the fitting of the archwire and represents the higher or lower PL corresponding to the "peak". The "b" parameter indicates the greater or lesser speed in the reduction of pain and value "c" represents the higher or lower PL throughout the treatment.

The parameters of fit for the 3 cases considered (pain in general regardless of the type of archwire, pain due to Ni-Ti archwire and pain due to SS archwire) are shown in Table 3. The goodness of fit for the three cases analysed is provided by the correlation coefficient R^2, which is very high, 0.983, 0.964 and 0.987, for the total group, the SS archwires group and the Ni-Ti group respectively.

	Parameter	Estimation	Typical error	IC 95%		R^2 value
				Lower limit	Upper limit	
	a	-83.1	6.4	-96.2	-70.0	
Total	b	0.016	0.001	0.015	0.017	0.983
	c	2.31	0.07	2.17	2.45	
	a	-70.4	8.8	-88.5	-52.4	
SS archwires	b	0.017	0.001	0.015	0.019	0.964
	c	2.12	0.09	1.93	2.32	
	a	-100.8	6.1	-113.3	-88.2	
Ni-Ti archwires	b	0.015	4.8 E-4	0.014	0.016	0.987
	c	2.56	0.06	2.43	2.68	

Table 3. Values of parameters (a,b,c) and IC95% of the same corresponding to the non-linear fit of pain level (ND) depending on time in hours (T) elapsed since the beginning of treatment for the two types of archwires used and for the set of all cases. The non-linear fit corresponds to the expression $PL = a * T^{-3} + c * \exp(-b * T)$

The values of the best-fit parameters indicate that: patients with SS archwires have a higher pain level at first than Ni-Ti patients (statistically significant difference in parameter a); a parallel reduction in pain level takes place (statistical equality in parameter b); but during the entire treatment patients with SS archwires experience more pain (statistically significant difference in parameter c).

Figure 7 also shows that after the tenth day no patient reported any pain, which is why our study ended at that point, 232 hours from the fitting of the archwire. The moment of the pain disappearing was practically the same for the two types of archwires, but it is interesting to calculate the average time that pain may be considered as high, moderate or slight. To do so, the PL experienced during the treatment was categorized on these three levels. The criterion was established that under 0.5 points (approximately 30% of the maximum PL experienced) pain could be considered as slight, between 0.5 and 1.5 as moderate, and above 1.5 (approximately 70% of the maximum PL experienced) as high. These stratification values are shown in figure 7. Using this categorization we can consider that the Ni-Ti archwires cease to hurt from 85h (3.5 days) from beginning of treatment as opposed to 109 hours (4.5 days) for SS archwires.

7.1.3. Peak of maximum pain

It is interesting to analyse the moment at which the peak of maximum pain intensity is reached. In our experimental data, the maximum pain is reached in the morning of the day after fitting the archwires, both for Ni-Ti and SS archwires. More specifically, if we observe the fits made (figure 7), maximum pain arrives at between 10 to 12 hours after fitting either of the types of archwire. However, if we consider the peak of the pain when the PL≥ 1.5, as we commented earlier, we can see that that the peak takes place between 8-36 hours in SS and 8-20 hours in Ni-Ti, being, therefore, longer in patients with SS archwires.

7.1.4. Comparison of pain between time periods

Figure 8 represents the average PL for each time period and it can be observed that there are no "pain peaks" associated with night time, although in the first 5 days, during the night time period a slight increase in pain or a lower decrease than that which would correspond to the 8 hours elapsed from the previous afternoon is noted. This has no statistical significance as the increase or decrease in pain is associated more with the number of hours elapsed since fitting the appliance. Indeed, the AVOVA carried out on the PL values for morning, afternoon and night, the results of which can be seen in Table 4, shows that there is no difference between the mean values with p>0.999, although a very slightly higher mean value of PL can be appreciated for the night period.

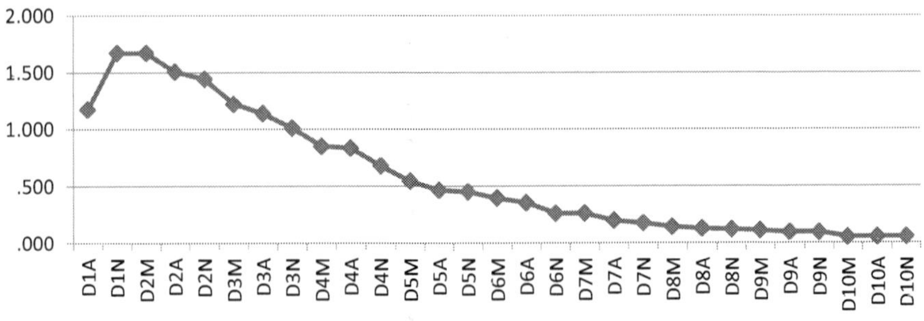

Figure 8. Pain level (PL) for each time period, regardless of the archwire used. The points in red correspond to the PL of night time periods.

	Mean PL	SD	IC95%	Minimum	Maximum
Morning	.58	.56	0.15 - 1.01	.06	1.67
Afternoon	.59	.53	0.27 - 0.97	.06	1.51
Night	.60	.59	0.17 - 1.02	.06	1.67

Table 4. Mean values and standard deviation (SD) of pain level (PL), confidence interval for the mean of PL at 95% (IC95%) and minimum and maximum values of each time period (morning, afternoon and night), regardless of the type of archwire used.

7.2. Subjective study of pain

7.2.1. Biochemical mediators analysis

To complete the study of pain, an objective assessment was performed. Two biochemical mediators of pain (Prostaglandin E2 (PGE2) and Substance P (SP)) were determined for each patient during treatment in four time intervals: prior to bracket bonding, 24 hours after bonding, a week and a month after bonding. In all cases, direct measurements were not considered but the proportion to the amount of crevicular fluid collected.

It was analyzed the possible correlations between the subjective pain reported by the patient with the levels of these mediators in the crevicular fluid for all the times studied.

7.2.2. Prostaglandin E2 (PGE2).

Correlations have been found between the concentration of PGE2 (PC) in the 4 times in which the determinations of this mediator were taken (PCT1: start, PCT2: 24 hours, PCT3: 7 days and PCT4: 30 days) and the subjective pain level of each individual in each interval analyzed, taking into account the 10 days in which there was existence of subjective pain. The results are shown in Table 5.

		D6N	D7M	D7T	D7N	D8M	D8T
P_Ct1	r-Pearson	0,102	0,274*	,280*	0,288*	,303**	0,140
	Sig. (bilateral)	0,386	0,017	,015	0,012	0,008	0,231
P_Ct2	r-Pearson	-0,032	0,053	,064	0,020	0,029	0,001
	Sig. (bilateral)	0,787	0,650	,583	0,862	0,803	0,993
P_Ct3	r-Pearson	0,010	0,161	,122	0,139	0,273*	0,173
	Sig. (bilateral)	0,931	0,167	,296	0,234	0,018	0,137
P_Ct4	r-Pearson	0,242*	0,326**	0,420**	0,442**	0,252*	0,295*
	Sig. (bilateral)	0,037	0,004	0,000	0,000	0,029	0,010

Table 5. Study of the correlation between the level of concentration of PGE2 (PC) in the 4 time times analyzed (PCT1 correspond to the time prior to bracket bonding, PCT2 to 24 hours after, PCT3 a week after and PCT4 a month after) and the level of pain reported by each patient. Values with * correspond to the times when correlation was found between the two measures of pain.

It can be seen that, in general, individuals with initially high values of PC mediator have a correlation with higher levels of pain one week after the archwire placement. This situation is also shown with PCT3 values and with those of PCT4, with no significant correlation with PCT1.

If the correlation of this mediator is analysed, not with the level of pain but with the total pain experienced by the subjects during the first 10 days, we find that high values of PC are correlated with subjects having more total level of pain throughout the treatment (Table 6). This finding does not happen with this marker in the other periods of time.

		P_Ct1	P_Ct2	P_Ct3	P_Ct4
Total Pain	r- Pearson	0,229*	0,059	0,025	0,166
	Sig. (bilateral)	0,048	0,616	0,831	0,156

Table 6. Study of the correlation between the level of PGE2 concentration (PC) and total pain level.

Furthermore, we analyzed whether there was correlation between the values of PGE2 in the four times studied. The results are shown in Table 7 and confirm that initially high values of this mediator are correlated to high values along the entire treatment.

		Total Sum	P_Ct1	P_Ct2	P_Ct3	P_Ct4
P_Ct1	CP	-0,042	1	0,484**	0,352*	0,365*
	SG	0,797		0,002	0,026	0,021
	N	40	40	40	40	40
P_Ct2	CP	-0,037	0,484**	1	0,120	0,297
	SG	0,821	0,002		0,462	0,063
	N	40	40	40	40	40
P_Ct3	CP	-0,268	0,352*	0,120	1	0,318*
	SG	0,094	0,026	0,462		0,046
	N	40	40	40	40	40
P_Ct4	CP	-0,004	0,365*	0,297	0,318*	1
	SG	0,978	0,021	0,063	0,046	
	N		40	40	40	40

Table 7. Study of the correlation between the values of prostaglandin PGE2 in the four times tested. CP (Pearson Correlation) and SG (Sig. Bilateral) ** significant correlation at the 0.01 level and * at the 0.05 level (bilateral).

7.2.3. Substance P (SP)

In orther to analyse this biochemical mediator, 86 cases were taken into account. The mean values of SP in the four times analysed of the study are shown in Table 8 and Figure 9.

Factor 1	Mean	Error	IC 95%	
			Lower limit	Upper limit
SPC1	173,165	21,470	130,469	215,860
SPC2	139,728	20,928	98,111	181,345
SPC3	190,621	26,825	137,278	243,965
SPC4	230,510	45,338	140,351	320,670

Table 8. Mean values of SP for each of the times studied.

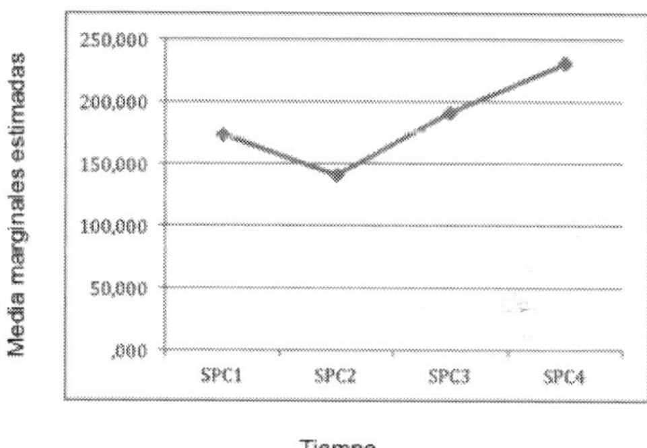

Figure 9. SP concentration at each time for each of the times studied.

According to these data, no statistical difference was found between the objective pain (SP crevicular fluid analysis) with the SS or Ni-Ti archwires, and the total subjective pain experienced according to the questionnaire.

8. Further research

In the literature, we have found few studies that compare pain depending on the type of archwire used [5, 32, 35] and none that introduces a mathematical equation for predicting pain level or peak of pain.

8.1. Subjective study of pain

8.1.1. Pain level

Our results coincide with those of Lee *et al.* [32] in stating that there is less pain in the group of patients treated with Ni-Ti archwires than in the group treated with SS archwires. However, neither our results nor the previously mentioned ones coincide with those of Jones and Chan

[5], who did not find differences in the pain experienced by patients between Ni-Ti archwires or SS archwires. Moreover, despite being a quite different study, Fernandes et al. [35] also did not find any difference on comparing conventional Ni-Ti archwires with super elastic Ni-Ti archwires.

In our results, pain receded at 4.5 days in cases treated with SS archwires, whereas it receded one day earlier (at 3.5 days) in those cases treated with Ni-Ti archwires. Moreover, the pain level was lower in the group with Ni-Ti archwires than in those with SS archwires.

If we analyse the results of the subjective study of pain recorded by the patients, we observe how 38.2% of patients felt discomfort and 43.1% felt slight pain, whereas only 18.6% experienced intense pain. These results do not coincide with those of Kaneko et al. [36], where only 10.3% felt discomfort and the great majority (72.4%) felt only slight pain. However, their results are in line with ours in stating that 17.2% experienced intense pain.

8.1.2. Peak of maximum pain

If we analyse when the peak of maximum pain takes place, the results of our study show that the peak occurs 15 hours after fitting the archwires into the mouth of the patient, both in the Ni-Ti group and the SS archwire group, results that are similar but not identical to those of other authors [1, 3, 6,18, 25, 37] who observed a maximum peak of pain 24 hours after fitting the archwire in the patient's mouth.

In contrast, our results and those mentioned above do not coincide with the results of the work of Jones and Chan [5] who found the maximum peak of pain to be on the same morning when fitting the archwire in the mouth, or the results of Jones and Richmond [38] who found the maximum peak of pain in the afternoon or night of the same day that the archwire was fitted.

8.1.3. Duration of pain

On studying how long pain lasts, the results of our study show that pain ceased at 3.5 days in the Ni-Ti group, whereas, in the SS group, it ceased at 4.5 days, the decrease in pain taking place earlier in the Ni-Ti group than in the SS group. These results do not coincide with those of Jones and Richmond [38], Jones and Chan [5], Ngan et al. [4] or Scheurer et al. [6] in whose studies, the pain caused by the fitting of the archwires was observed to last for approximately 5 days.

Our results show how both groups of patients, both the patients fitted with SS archwires and those fitted with Ni-Ti archwires, began to experience pain at 4 hours, results similar to those of Jones and Richmond [38] with the same intensity of pain.

However, SS and Ni-Ti metals do not have the same stress deformation curve and it can be observed that in order to achieve the same deformation, the stress that has to be applied in the case of steel is greater than in the case of Ni-Ti, which would account for the greater initial pain of the patient in cases treated with SS archwires. Nevertheless, as the teeth adapt to the forces applied and, therefore, the stress applied on the archwire material diminishes, these two materials behave differently, SS maintains a residual deformation, whereas Ni-Ti returns to practically its original dimensions, meaning that its effect on the tooth is more continuous and produces a sensation of pain over a longer time, so evening out the total time of pain duration for both types of archwire.

8.1.4. Comparison of pain between time periods

In our study, we did not find pain peaks associated with night time, unlike those shown in the results of Kaneko et al. [36] but that the increase or decrease of pain was similar in the morning or afternoon and was only associated with the number of hours following the fitting of the appliance. These results coincide with those of Scheurer et al. [6] who found that pain increased as the day elapsed.

8.2. Objective study of pain

Authors like Erdinic and Dincer [8] or Awawdeh et al. [39] have observed that the perception of pain during orthodontic movement is related to substance P. Substance P is involved in the nervous system signals required to perceive pain [40] also influencing the concentration of other pain mediators associated with dental pain like the metalloproteinase 8 [41], and in the secretion of IL-1β from the monocytes. These three substances (IL-1β, PG-E2 and SP) were independently associated with pain [15-17] and are expressed during initial tooth movement in sufficient amounts to be detected in the crevicular fluid [18].

Then we will discuss some variables affecting the collection of this sample.

8.2.1. Sources of error in the collection of the crevicular fluid

Before taking the samples, one have to keep in mind that the most frequent sources of contamination of the crevicular fluid samples are blood, saliva and plaque. Respect to the presence of plaque, its presence in the paper strips used for collecting the sample has a considerable effect on the volume of the sample, thus being a source of bias [42-44].These considerations have been supported also by other authors, who demonstrate that the non-removal of the plaque has a bad effect on the determination of the volume [43,45].

In order to avoid these problems of contamination prior to bracket bonding, scaling was performed to all patients of the study, thus reducing the possibility of bleeding and contamination by plaque.

Also, in our study, in order to reduce saliva contamination, a good insulation protocol was carried out by placing the aspiration system and cotton rolls in each patient. Saliva contamination is a problem when the sample is collected with paper strips, as it can alter the volume of the sample collected [46].

8.2.2. Sample recording time

The first authors who described the use of Periotron® [43] recommended a sample recording time of five seconds. However, to increase the volume of the sample in order to subsequently analyze it sometimes it is necessary to increase the sample time.

Therefore, in our work, a sample time of 30 seconds was established following the recommendations from other authors [32, 47-50]. For the analysis of the crevicular fluid, the collection should be made in such way that minimum groove environment deterioration occurs in the shortest time possible. By doing so, correct protein concentrations are maintained and also sufficient time is achieved to collect the required sample volume.

8.2.3. Methods of collection of crevicular fluid

There are many ways to collect the crevicular fluid; gingival washing, micropipettes and paper strips. Gingival washing method is suitable for obtaining cells of the gingival groove. It is a complex method and has limited applications since it can only be used in the maxillary arch due to the complexity of the technique. On the other hand, samples cannot be analyzed later in the laboratory and all the fluid cannot be recovered during aspiration and re-aspiration.

With micropipettes is difficult to collect a necessary amount of fluid in a short period of time unless there is gingival inflammation, resulting in more volume of crevicular fluid. It can cost up to 30 minutes to collect the amount of fluid necessary and this makes this technique traumatic [51].

The crevicular fluid analysis it is a useful and advantageous method, especially for in vivo studies, it is not invasive, and the sample can be split as many times as necessary. This allows the perfect monitor development in a given area for a certain period of time. Therefore and because of the complications mentioned above with the two methods described, in our work we decided to take the sample by this method, using paper strips, like other authors [32, 47-50] because it is a simple, rapid and non-traumatic method and can be applied to isolated areas.

Crevicular fluid samples of each patient who also had filled the subjective pain questionnaire were collected, in order to later compare the subjective data of pain with the objective values obtained from the analysis of the biochemical mediators.

8.3. Biochemical mediators analysis

8.3.1. Prostaglandin E2 (PGE2)

In our study, PGE2 production reached its maximum peak at 24 hours, coinciding with the results found by Bergius et al. [37], Giannopoulou et al. [18] and Grieve et al. [52]. In another study by Lee et al. [32], initial measurements of IL-1 β and PGE2 showed little variation, however, once force is applied, the individual variation became large enough to estimate the overall response.

Lee et al. [32] observed an increase in the levels of interleukins in patients during the third week, even without the revive forces, causing an increase in the average concentration but without statistical significance. Iwasaki et al. [30] found that IL-1β levels fluctuate with a period of 28 days when a force is applied continuously.

Interestingly, when a discontinuous force (equivalent to steel arches) is reactivated after a week, a significant increase in the levels of IL-1β, 24 hours after reactivation was found, compared with the results found 24 hours after the initial activation. This finding implies that timely reactivating discontinuous forces might be more effectively in the regulation of IL-1β than the continuous application of forces. Instead, they did not found any increased after a second reactivation. This could be due to a refractory period or excessive applied pressure. Since excessive pressure causes a large area of hyalinization in the pressure side and a wide acellular area, which produces impairment in cytokine secretion and its spread to the periodontal space. These results suggest that the application of a suitable pressure force intermittent and timely recovery may be effective to promote secretion of IL-1 β. However, authors like Yamaguchi et al. [26], Tian et al. [27] or Uematsu et al. [11], argue that the intense and discontinuous forces tend to significantly reduce levels of IL1β suggesting the need for reactivation to maintain sufficient production of IL1β. Such forces not only increase the risk of root resorption but also increase the hyalinization of periodontal tissue [28,29] which also induce very pronounced rise and fall peaks in the levels of cytokines, leading to undesirable tissue level and the need for the reactivation of the forces.

On the contrary, continuous light forces [30-32] tend to maintain high levels of IL1β so the need for reactivation is reduced. These forces maintain, high longer, cytokine levels, which are necessary for continuous periodontal remodeling.

The efficiency on the recovery is shown in a series of experiments in rats done by King et al. [53] where the reactivation during the end of the cycle stimulates bone resorbing osteoclasts and reduce root resorption.

In the study by Lee et al. [32], changes in the levels of PGE2 to mechanical stress and the interactions between the IL-1β and PGE2 in vivo were investigated. The mechanical loads applied to the periodontal ligament cells are known to induce the expression of cyclooxygenase-2 (COX-2), which facilitates the formation PGE2 [54]. In the study of Saito et al. [55], a significant increase in PGE2 was observed when IL-1β was applied to periodontal ligament cells alone or in combination with mechanical stress. The synergistic action of IL-1β and mechanical stress on the production of PGE prove the hypothesis that mechanical stress provides more substrate for cyclooxygenase by activation of phospholipase A2, while IL-1β formation increases cyclooxygenase.

PGE2 levels in this initial study showed significant peaks at 24 hours (T2) of the application of force, compared to the control site. This appears to be a direct effect of mechanical stress. By applying continuous force, high levels of PGE2 was observed only temporarily, compared to the control site, even though the average concentration is maintained at a high level during the experiment. With discontinuous forces, significantly higher levels of PGE2 for 1 week were observed. This regulation is an example of the synergistic effect of the mechanical stresses sustained and secreted IL-1β.

In this study we found that, if the total pain recorded by the subjects is determined and their correlation is sought with the values of this mediator, patients with high values of PC1 have more total level of pain during the treatment. Furthermore, PC3 high values are related with high values one week after the archwire placement. We did not find association between patients who had elevated levels of PC4 with high levels of pain between the 6th and 8th day.

These results cannot be compared with other authors as there are no studies reported in the literature.

8.3.2. Substance P (SP)

The results of the substance P values were inconsistent with what would be expected of a biochemical mediator of pain as, in the initial time of the study, when no level of pain exists (and therefore this substance should have a baseline), we found higher values, both overall levels and concentrations, than in the rest of study for 56 of the 86 patients analyzed.

The apparently anomalous behavior of this marker with a decrease at 24 hours and a later increased tendency to grow up is not statistically significant because, due to the high variability of the data. However, other authors as Giannopoulou et al. [18], found more predictable values in the levels of these biochemical mediators after insertion of ligatures.

The experience of pain has its peak 1 day after starting treatment and is reduced to normal levels at 7 days. The IL-1β, SP, PGE2 mediators are expressed during initial tooth movement. The initial perception of pain (1h) is related to the levels of PGE2, the IL-1β is related to pain at 24 hours and the SP has its peak at 24 hours. This is possible because of the relationship that has with PGE2 as an indicator of periodontal inflammation [56].

On the other hand, Yao et al. [57], did not find relationship between pain intensity and PGE2 at 12, 24 and 72 hours of the beginning of tooth movement. Another authors, though [26], found no relationship between IL-1β and substance P. Indirectly, this finding also has an association between IL-1β and pain.

9. Conclusions

This paper has analyzed the pain associated with the placement of the first archwire in the beginning of the orthodontic treatment, analyzing the influence that several variables have (such as the type of wire used) on pain.

A questionnaire for the subjective assessment of pain has been designed, registering the pain indicated by the patient at each time interval (morning, afternoon and evening), from the time of placing the archwire for the first time until it disappears. Furthermore, the objective assessment of pain has been determined in the crevicular fluid through the different biochemical mediators of pain, such as prostaglandin 2 (PGE2) and substance P (SP).

- Total pain (TP) and the maximum level of pain (PL) are lower in the group of patients fitted with Ni-Ti archwires than in the group fitted with SS archwires, although pain for both groups recedes at the same time.

- Pain level (PL) is determined by the mathematical equation:

PL=a* T^{-3}+c * exp (-b*T) where parameters a, b and c represent: "a" coefficient represents the higher or lower PL corresponding to the "peak". The "b" parameter indicates the greater or lesser speed in the reduction of pain and value "c" represents the higher or lower PL throughout the treatment.

- Both the patients with SS archwires and those with Ni-Ti archwires began to feel pain after 4 hours of the placement of the archwires. The maximum peak of pain is established generally within the first hours of the placement of the archwire (10 hours) and lasts for about 20 hours. The pain becomes moderate and mild, respectively, about one and a half (30 hours) and 4 days (100 hours) after the beginning of the treatment. Pain disappears generally before 10 days after the placement of the archwire. There is no difference in the time when pain is greatest for both types of archwire, being situated at between 15 and 20 hours following the fitting of the archwire in the mouth.

- Biochemical mediators (prostaglandin E2 (PGE2) and substance P (SP)) have not reported generally good correlation with the subjective pain reported by the patient. Only it should be noted that high values of PGE2 before treatment (PCT1), correlate with higher levels of subjective pain a week after the archwire is placed. This situation is also shown in the values determined after one week (PCT3) and after a month (PCT4).

Author details

M. Larrea[1], N. Zamora[1*], R. Cibrian[2], J.L. Gandia[1] and V. Paredes[1]

*Address all correspondence to: natalia.zamora@uv.es

1 Department of Orthodontics. Faculty of Medicine and Dentistry, University of Valencia, Spain

2 Department of Physiology. Faculty of Medicine and Dentistry, University of Valencia, Spain

References

[1] Krishnan V. Orthodontic pain: from causes to management-a review. European Journal of Orthodontics. 2007; 29:170–9.

[2] Williams JM, Murray JJ, Lund CA, De Franco A. Anxiety in the child dental clinic. Journal of Child Psychology and Psychiatry. 1985; 26:305-10.

[3] Ngan P, Kess B, Wilson S 1989. Perception of discomfort by patients undergoing orthodontic treatment. American Journal of Orthodontics and DentofacialOrthopedics 96:47-53.

[4] Ngan P, Wilson S, Shanfeld J, Amini H 1994 The effect of ibuprofen on the level of discomfort in patients undergoing orthodontic treatment. American Journal of Orthodontics and DentofacialOrthopedics106: 88-95

[5] Jones M, Chan C 1992 The pain and discomfort experienced during orthodontic treatment. A randomized controlled clinical trial of two initial aligning arch wires. American Journal of Orthodontics and DentofacialOrthopedics 102: 373-381.

[6] Scheurer PA, Firestone AR, Burgin WB 1996 Perception of pain as a result of Orthodontic treatment with fixed appliances. European Journal of Orthodontics 18:349-357

[7] Firestone A R, Scheurer P A, Bürgin W B 1999 Patient's anticipation of pain and pain-related side effects, and their perception of pain as a result of orthodontic treatment with fixed appliances. European Journal of Orthodontics 21: 387-396

[8] Erdinç A M E, Dinçer B 2004 Perception of pain during orthodontic treatment with fixed appliances. European Journal of Orthodontics 26:79-85

[9] Polat O, Karaman A 2005 Pain control during fixed appliance therapy. Angle Orthodontist 75: 214-219

[10] Jones ML 1984 An investigation into the initial discomfort caused by placement of an archwire. European Journal of Orthodontics 6:48-54.

[11] Uematsu S, Mogi M, Deguchi T 1996 Interleukin (IL)-1 beta, IL-6, tumor necrosis factor-alpha, epidermal growth factor, and beta 2-microglobulin levels are elevated in gingival crevicular fluid during human orthodontic tooth movement. Journalof Dental Research75: 562-567

[12] Hofbauer LC, Lacey DL, Dunstan CR, Spelsperg TC, Riggs BL, Khosla S. (1999) Interleukin-1beta and tumor necrosis factoralpha, but not interleukin-6 stimulate osteoprotegerin ligand gene expression in human osteoblastic cells. Bone. 25: 255-259.

[13] Ren Y, Maltha JC, Van't Hof MA, Von den Hoff JW, Kuijpers-Jagtman AM, Zhang D. (2002) Cytokine levels in crevicular fluid are less responsive to orthodontic force in adults than in juveniles. J Clin Periodontol. 29:757-762.

[14] Kavadia-Tsatala S, Kaklamanos E, Tsalikis L. (2002) Effects of orthodontic treatment on gingival crevicular fluid flow rate and composition: Clinical implications and applications. Int J Adult Orthod Orthog Surg. 17;191-205.

[15] Hori T, Oka T, Hosoi M, Aou S. (1998) Pain modulatory actions of cytokines and prostaglandin E2 in the brain. Ann NY Acad Sci. 840:269-281.

[16] Lundy FT, Linden GJ. (2004) Neuropeptides and neurogenic mechanisms in oral and periodontal inflammation. Crit Rev Oral Biol Med. 15;82-98.

[17] Sommer C, Kress M. (2004) Recent findings of how proinflammatory cytokines cause pain: peripheral mechanisms in inflammatory and neuropathic hyperalgesia. Neurosci Lett. 361:184-187.

[18] Giannopoulou C, Dudic A, Kiliaridis S 2006 Pain discomfort and crevicular fluid changes induced by Orthodontic elastic separators in children. Journal of Pain7: 367-76

[19]   Kvam E, Gjerdet N, Bondevik O 1987 Traumatic ulcers and pain during orthodontic treatment. Community Dentistry and Oral Epidemiology 15:104-110

[20]   Oliver R G, Knapman Y M 1985 Attitudes to Orthodontic treatment. BritishJournal of Orthodontics 12: 179-188

[21]   Patel V 1992 Non-completion of active orthodontic treatment. British Journal of Orthodontics 19: 47-54

[22]   Ogura M,Kamimura H, Al-KalalyA, Nagayama K, Taira K, Nagata J, MiyawakiS2009 Pain intensity during the first 7 days following the application of light and heavy continuous forces. European Journal of Orthodontics 31: 314-319

[23]   Dubner R 1968 Neurophysiology of pain. Dental Clinics of North America 22: 11-30

[24]   Brown D F, Moerenhout R G 1991 The pain experience and psychological adjustments to orthodontics treatment of preadolescents, adolescents and adults. American Journal of Orthodontics and DentofacialOrthopedics 100: 349-356

[25]   Bergius M, Kiliardis S, Berggren U 2000 Pain in orthodontics: a review and discussion of the literature. Journal of OrofacialOrthopedics 61:125-137

[26]   Yamaguchi M, Yoshii M, Kasai K 2006 Relationship between substance P and interleukin-1beta in gingival crevicular fluid during orthodontic tooth movement in adults. European Journal of Orthodontics 28: 241-246

[27]   Tian YL, Xie JC, Zhao ZJ, Zhang Y 2006 Changes of interlukin-1beta and tumor necrosis factor-alpha levels in gingival crevicular fluid during orthodontic tooth movement.Hua Xi Kou Qiang Yi XueZaZhi 24: 243-245

[28]   Maltha JC, Van Leeuwen EJ, Dijkman GE, Kuijpers-Jagtman AM 2004 Incidence and severity of root resorption in orthodontically moved premolars in dogs. Orthodontics and Craniofacial Research 7:115-121

[29]   Von Bohl M, Maltha JC, Von Den Hoff JW, Kuijpers-Jagtman AM 1986 Focal hyalinization during experimental tooth. American Journal of Orthodontics and DentofacialOrthopedics 125:615-623

[30]   Iwasaki LR, Haack JE, Nickel JC, Reinhardt RA, Petro TM 2001 Human interleukin-1 beta and interleukin-1 receptor antagonist secretion and velocity of tooth movement. Archives of Oral Biology46: 185-189

[31]   Iwasaki LR, Crouch LD, Tutor A, Gibson S, Hukmani N, Marx DB, Nickel JC 2005 Tooth movement and cytokines in gingival crevicular fluid and whole blood in growing and adult subjects. American Journal of Orthodontics and DentofacialOrthopedics128: 483-491

[32]   Lee KJ, Park YC, Yu HS, Choi SH, Yoo YJ 2004 Effects of continuous and interrupted orthodontic force on interleukin-1beta and prostaglandin E2 production in gingival

crevicular fluid. American Journal of Orthodontics and DentofacialOrthopedics 125:168-177

[33] Fuck LM, Drescher D2006 Force systems in the initial phase of orthodontic treatment-a comparison of different leveling arch wires.Journal of OrofacialOrthopedics 67(1): 6-18

[34] Offenbacher S, Farr DH, Goodson JM. (1981) Measurement of prostaglandin E in crevicular fluid. J Clin Periodontol. 8:359-367.

[35] Fernandes LM, Ogaard B, Skoglund L 1998 Pain and discomfort experienced after placement of a conventional or a super-elastic NiTi aligning archwire. Journal of OrofacialOrthopedics 59:331-339

[36] Kaneko K, Kawai S, Tokuda T, Kamogashira K, Kawagoe H, Itoh T, Matasumoto M 1990 On the pain experience of the tooth caused by placement of initial archwire. Fukuoka ShikaDaigakuGakkaiZasshi17(1): 22-27

[37] Bergius M, Berggren U, Kiliaridis S 2002 Experience of pain during an orthodontic procedure. European Journal of Oral Sciences 110: 92-98

[38] Jones M, Richmond S 1985 Initial tooth movement: force application and pain. A relationship? American Journal of Orthodontics 88: 111-116

[39] Awawdeh LA, Lundy FT, Linden GJ, Shaw C, Kennedy JG, Lamey PJ. (2002) Quantitative analysis of substance P, neurokinin A and calcitonin gene–related peptide in gingival crevicular fluid associated with painful human teeth. Eur J Oral Sci. 110:185-191.

[40] Cerveró F. (1998) El papel de la sustancia P en el dolor. Rev SocEsp Dolor. 5, N.º 4, Julio-Agosto.

[41] Avellán NL, Sorsa T, Tervahartiala T, Forster C, Kemppainen P.(2008) Experimental tooth pain elevates substance P and matrix metalloproteinase-8 levels in human gingival crevice fluid. Acta Odontol Scand.66:18-22.

[42] Stoller NH, Karras DC, Johnson LR. (1990) Reliability of crevicular fluid measurements taken in the presence of supragingival plaque. J Periodontol. 61:670-673.

[43] Griffiths GS, Wilton JM, Curtis MA. (1992) Contamination of human gingival crevicular fluid by plaque and saliva. Arch Oral Biol. 37:559-564.

[44] Hanschke M, Splieth C, Kramer A. (1999) Activities of lysozyme and salivary peroxidase in unstimulated whole saliva in relation to plaque and gingivitis scores in healthy young males. Clin Oral Investig. 3:133-137.

[45] Martin P, D'Aoust P, Landry RG, Valois M. (1994) The reliability of the Periotron 6000 in the presence of plaque. J Can Dent Assoc. 60: 895-898.

[46] Nakashima K, Demeurisse C, Cimasoni G. (1994) The recovery efficiency of various materials for sampling enzymes and polymorphonuclear leukocytes from gingival crevices. J Clin Periodontol. 21:479-483.

[47] Reinhardt RA, Masada MP, Kaldahl WB, DuBois IM, Kornman KS, Choi JI, Kalkwarf KL, Allison AC. (1993) Gingival fluid IL-1, and IL-6 levels in refractory periodontitis. J Clin Periodontol. 20:225-231.

[48] Rossomando EF, Kennedy JE, Hadjimichael J. (1990) Tumor necrosis factor alpha in gingival crevicular fluid as a possible indicator of periodontal disease in humans. Arch Oral Biol.35:431-434.

[49] Atilla G, Kütükçüler N. (1998) Crevicular fluid interleukin-β tumor necrosis factor-α and interleukin-6 levels in renal transplant patients receiving cyclosporine. Am J Periodontol. 69:784-790.

[50] Ataoglu H, Alptekin NÖ, Haliloglu S, Gürsel M, Ataoglu T, Serpek B, Durmus E. (2002) Interleukin-1β tumor necrosis factor-α levels and neutrophil elastase activity in peri-implant crevicular fluid. Clin Oral Implants Res.13:470 476.

[51] Sueda T, Bang J, Cimasoni G. (1969) Collection of gingival fluid for quantitative analysis. J Dent Res.48: 159.

[52] Grieve III WG, Johnson GK, Moore RN, Reinhardt RA, DuBois LM. (1994) Prostaglandin E (PGE) and interleukin-1 beta (IL-1β) levels in gingival crevicular fluid during human orthodontic tooth movement. Am J Orthod Dentofacial Orthop.105: 369-374.

[53] King GJ, Archer L, Zhou D. (1998) Later orthodontic appliance reacti-vation stimulates immediate appearance of osteoclasts and linear tooth movement. Am J Orthod Dentofacial Orthop. 114; 692-697.

[54] Kanzaki H, Chiba M, Shimizu Y, Mitani H. (2002) Periodontal ligament cells under mechanical stress induce osteoclastogenesis by re-ceptor activator of nuclear factor kB ligand up-regulation via prostaglandin E2 synthesis. J Bone Miner Res. 17; 210-220.

[55] Saito S, Ngan P, Saito MJ, Lanese R, Shanfeld J, Davidovitch Z. (1990) Interactive effects between cytokines on PGE production by human periodontal ligament fibroblasts in vitro. J Dent Res. 69:1456-1462.

[56] Hanioka T, Takaya K, Matsumori Y, Matsuse R, Shizukusihi S. (2000) Relationship of the substance P to indicators of host response in human gingival crevicular fluid. J Clin Periodontol. 27: 262-266.

[57] Yao YL, Feng XP, Jing XZ. (2003) The correlation between tooth pain and bioactivators changes in gingival crevicular fluid after applying orthodontic stress. Shanghai Kou Qiang Yi Xue. 12: 331-333.

Chapter 20

Non-Surgical Treatment of Class III with Multiloop Edgewise Arch-Wire (MEAW) Therapy

Paulo Beltrão

Additional information is available at the end of the chapter

http://dx.doi.org/10.5772/59257

1. Introduction

The incidence of class III malocclusion among the western population is low, but in Japan and South Korea is high and since many patients don`t accept orthognatic surgery, a conservative/ camouflage treatment is often necessary. The MEAW (multiloop edgewise arch wire) was developed in 1967 by Dr. Young H. Kim to correct open bite malocclusions and was found to be extremely effective. Further development of Meaw technique extends its application to treat any type of malocclusion, especially Class III malocclusion.

The MEAWs are constructed with 0.016 x 0.022stainless steel (bracket 0.018 inch slot) or 0.017x0.025 stainless steel (bracket 0.022– inch slot). The arches have ideal arch form with five loops on each side of the arch.

Prof. Sadao Sato developed the use of MEAW and introduced different concepts about the etiology of malocclusions. According to Sato genetics may not be the only reason to class III malocclusion, the posterior discrepancy may be the major contributing factor to class III malocclusion.

The degree of basicranial flexion differs in the various types of malocclusion. According to Hooper (1986) the spheno-basilar articulation is the most important among the cranial bones and it is where the movement of flexion-extension occurs. The cranial base angles (Na-S-Ar) comes to approximately 124,2 ° in class I patterns.

From this average value a more obtuse (extension) angle indicates skeletal Class II and a more acute (flexion) angle means skeletal Class III.The rotating movement of the cranial base (flexion/extension) occurs at the spheno-occipital articulation and it is transmitted to the maxilla through the Vomer. This dynamic mechanism has a great influence on the growth pattern of an individual during the growth period.

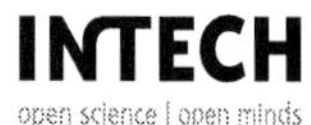

When the sphenoid makes flexion the rotating force of the vomer is postero-inferior and the maxilla is strongly pushed down. This causes vertical elongation of the maxillary complex, short anteroposterior dimension and posterior crowding. This is related to the development of a class III skeletal frame (Sato 2001).

The posterior discrepancy increases the probability of wisdom teeth impaction and once their impaction occurs a "squeezing-out "effect may occur, causing an over-eruption of the adjacent teeth, flatten the posterior occlusal plane and an increase in the posterior occlusal vertical dimension. The over-erupted molars produce occlusal interferences that act as a fulcrum causing a mandibular forward adaptation with subluxation of the mandibular condyles and active remodeling of the condylar cartilage. The result is a mandibular prognathism.

The skeletal Class III relationships may be due to a lack of sagital development of maxillary or mandibular overdevelopment, or a combination of both.

Skeletal class III malocclusion is usually characterized by a steep mandibular plane angle, obtuse gonial angle, a small cranial base angle which may displace the glenoid fossa anteriorely to cause a forward positioning of the mandible, flat occlusal plane, short antero posterior diameter of the maxilla, increased vertical growth of the maxilla, labial tipping of the maxillary teeth, lingual tipping of the mandibular teeth.

In adults patients,without growing ability, orthognatic surgery is indicated for severe skeletal class III malocclusion, but moderate class III cases (borderline cases) can be treated orthodontically if the patients refuse surgery. The MEAW is often used in skeletal class III treatment without orthognatic surgery or extraction of intermediate teeth.

The objectives of the treatment are: a) to eliminate posterior discrepancy, b) to intrude the posterior teeth and to upright them, c) reconstruction the occlusal plane (steepning the occlusal plane) which induces mandibular backward adaption. The entire lower dentition is moved distally and uprighted using a MEAW with short class III elastics after extraction of the third molars. The skeletal features of the class III malocclusions are closely related to the deviation in the vertical aspect of the occlusion. According to this correcting the occlusal plane by controlling the vertical dimension is extremely important in the treatment of class III malocclusion.

To eliminate the posterior discrepancy, the upper and lower third molars should be extracted prior to the onset of treatment. The upper second molars can be extracted, if the patient is young and if the the upper third molars have quality in terms of size, shape and direction of eruption. This approach will allow steepen the occlusal plane with the elimination of the "squeezing-out effect "at the upper molars. The treatment mechanics use tip back bend activations of the MEAW and vertical or short class III elastics (3/16 inch – 6 oz) on the anterior teeth.

The steps of treatment of the class III malocclusion are: a) Levelling, b) elimination of occlusal interference,,c) establishing mandibular position d) reconstruction of the occlusal plane, e) achieving a physiological occlusion.

Sassouni and Nanda (1964) proved the vertical disproportion were, in many cases, at the origin of anteroposterior dysplasias. Therefore, treatment strategies should focus on vertical control in order to correct anteroposterior disharmony.

Angle(1899) – The class III malocclusion occurred when lower teeth occluded mesial to their normal relationship by the width of one premolar or even more in extreme cases.The class III can be defined as a skeletal facial deformity characterized by a forward mandibular position with respect to the cranial base and/or maxilla.

2. The etiology of class III malocclusion

- Genetics-an example is the famous mandibular prognathism of Habsburg family.

- Syndromes

- Crouzon syndrome

- Acromegaly

- Gorlin and Goltz syndrome Hypertrophy

- Cleido cranial dysplasia

- Achondroplasia

- Environmental factors-ex : thyroid deficiency cause large tongue, causing mandibular prognathism

- Functional factors

- Naso-respiratory diseases and enlarged tonsils

- Mental diseases-compulsive habits of protruding the mandible

- Posterior crowding – "The posterior squeezing out effect "

3. Classification of class III malocclusion

Moyers classified the class III malocclusion according the cause: osseous; muscular; dental.According to him, it was necessary to determine whether the mandible on closure was in centric relation or "convenient" anterior position.

In 1966 Charles Tweed divided class III malocclusion in pseudoclass III and skeletal class III. Tweed also divided the class III onto two distinct categories : The category A-the FMA ranges between 10° and 22°,with a large mandible ; underdeveloped maxilla and a ANB between 7° to 10° and the category B – FMA ranges between 30° to 50° with an obtuse gonial angle and a lower lip overactive.

The characteristics of Pseudoclass III are the following: normal mandible and underdeveloped maxilla, concave straight profile, skeletal pattern is class I, normal gonial angle and the retrusion of the mandible is possible.

The skeletal class III discrepancy may be the result of a large mandible, a small maxilla, a distally positioned maxilla or a combination of the three. Vertically the class III can be divided in high angle, average and low angle.

The class III subdivision is characterized by a class I molar relation on one side and a class III on the other side.

4. The differential diagnosis of skeletal class III malocclusion

The diagnostic criteria for pseudo class III according to Rabie and Yan Gu (AJODO 2000) is the following : a) 72 % showed no family history; b) molar class I in CR and class III at habitual occlusion ; c)decreased midface length ; d) forward mandibular position with normal length ; e) retroclined upper incisors with normal lower incisors; f) presence of mandibular anterior sliding into a edge-to-edge or crossbite relationship due to premature tooth contact (with CO–CR discrepancy), absence of skeletal signs of class III malocclusion. The differential diagnosis of skeletal class III malocclusion with skeletal class I include the following differences:

- In class III the SNA is lower

- The SNB is greater in class III

- The mean ANB angle in class III is negative

- The gonial angle is more open in class III

- The lower anterior facial height is increased

- Cranial base angle is smaller in class III patients

The dentoalveolar class III malocclusion present a normal ANB angle and a lingual tipping of upper incisors and labial tipping of lower incisors. The skeletal class III malocclusion show a maxillary retrusion or mandibular protrusion, or both with negative ANB, increased mandibular length, increased gonial angle, labial tipping of upper incisors and lingual tipping of lower incisors.

There are three important diagnostic principles of class III such as:

- To determine whether the mandible on closure is in centric relation or in a "convenient " anterior position

- Identify the nature of skeletal discrepancy

- To evaluate the potential growth and development of a patient with a class III malocclusion

5. Treatment of pseudo class III malocclusion

The ideal age to treat pseudo class III is between 6 to 9 years, because treating the pseudo class III during the mixed dentition has some advantages such as : the stability of correction is better, prevent unfavourable growth of skeletal frame,prevent deleterious habits.There are many options to treat the pseudo class III malocclusion such as : equilibration of occlusion, bionator appliance, fixed appliance, acrylic crowns, acrylic inclined planes, functional appliance therapy, and orthopaedic appliances.

6. Treatment of skeletal class III malocclusiom in growing patients

During the primary, mixed and permanent dentition the growth is present and the treatment is different from when the growth is finished. The first step is to distinguish if the class III is due to maxillary undergrowth, mandibular overgrowth or both or a skeletal class I with anterior cross bite. When the class III is due to mandibular overgrowth the options of treatment are : chin cap therapy, reverse class III activator (to produce retrusive force on the mandible), low or high pull head gear (HPHG) to control posterior eruption.

When class III is due to maxillary undergrowth and/or retrognatic maxillary with a orthognatic mandible, it is necessary to promote the growth and protact the maxillary using a face mask (Delaire or Petit) or a functional appliance therapy (activator or Frankel III regulator).

7. Treatment of skeletal class III malocclusion in non growing patients

The treatment of class III in adults and non growing patients can be a surgical treatment or a camouflage treatment. When a non growing patient is diagnosed as a class III malocclusion and has a strong skeletal component, the treatment of choice is usually orthodontic/orthognatic surgery. After determined that the surgery will be necessary the surgeon usually waits until the growth is finished. Maxillary growth may be completed at age 14-15 years, but mandibular growth may continue until 20 years. Then the orthodontist will decompensate the incisors and after that the surgery will be done.

8. Camouflage treatment of class III malocclusion

Beyond the adolescent growth spurt, to correct a mild skeletal class III, teeth must be displaced relative to their supporting bone to mask the underlying class III discrepancy by dental compensation. This is termed camouflage treatment. A patient with class III malocclusion, with the growth completed, a slight skeletal class III, acceptable alignment of teeth and acceptable facial proportions is a good candidate for a camouflage treatment. Since 1967 the MEAW technique has proved to be an effective treatment camouflage and a non-surgical treatment of class III malocclusion. The extraction theraphy of premolars may have limited applicability in class III treatment, for example extractions in the lower arch will increase the lingual inclination of the incisors which were already inclined. Another contraindication to extract is the cases that combine orthodontics and surgery.

9. Non-surgical treatment of class III with multiloop edgewise archwire(MEAW) therapy

Many times during the diagnosis process the etiology of the malocclusion and the mechanism of its development are depreciated. The cephalometric analysis doesn`t clearly shows the cause of malocclusion, it only localizes the site of skeletal malocclusion and shows the degree of deviation. This means that current orthodontics many times identifies and treats symptoms rather than aiming the cause. Hence there is a need for the insertion of a new treatment philosophy based on the function rather than esthetic needs of the patient. It is necessary to understand the dynamic mechanism of development of malocclusion and to know the treatment technique for orthodontic occlusal reconstruction.

9.1. The dynamic mechanism of the development of class III malocclusion

During the human evolution the cranial base was modified with the bipedalism and erect posture, producing a flexion of the cranial base and a displacement of the foramen occipitale magnum from one end to the middle of the skull. The result of this displacement, is a vertical growth pattern rather than horizontal. The degree of basicranial flexion is different according to the type of malocclusion. Thus a cranial base angle (Na-S-Ar) about 124,2 degrees is characteristic of class I pattern. When the angle is closed to 130 degrees (extension of cranial base) indicates a class II malocclusion and a more acute angle closer to 120 degrees (flexion) indicates a skeletal class III. If more severe is the class III pattern, more pronounced is the flexion of the cranial base and greater is the tendency of vertical growth. Thus the vertical component of class III malocclusion is very important, contrary to be considered just a sagital problem. According to this the use of chin cap, long class III elastics, premolar extraction, surgery are treatment approaches of skeletal class III malocclusion in the sagital direction, neglecting the vertical component. When the angle of cranial base presents a flexion, the rotating movement occurs at the spheno-occipital synchondrosis and it is transmitted to the maxillary through the vomer. This dynamic mechanism affects the growth pattern of the growing patients. With the flexion of the sphenoid, the rotating force of the vomer is posteroinferior and the maxillary is pushed dowm. This produce vertical elongation, undersized sagital dimension and posterior crowding of the maxillary. The lack of maxillary translation creates a deficit of space in the tuberosity, and a posterior crowding, that causes the "squeezing out effect ". The squeezing out effect is an over-eruption of the molars and modifies the inclination of the occlusal plane, making it flatter. Once the over-eruption of the molars occurs, then occlusal interferences appear and in order to avoid them, the mandible adapts forward.This mandibular forward movement, produces a distraction of the mandibular condyles and active reformulation of the condylar cartilage, resulting in mandibular prognathism.

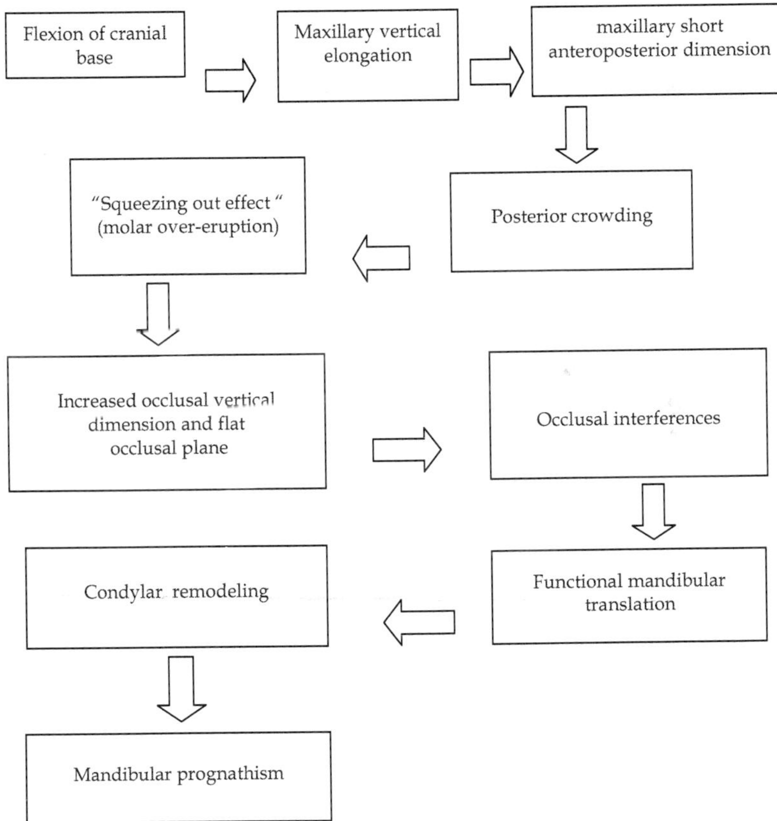

Figure 1. The dynamic mechanism of the development of class III malocclusion

9.2. General characterization of class III malocclusion

The class III malocclusion has the following characteristics:

- Increased vertical dimension
- short maxillary length
- posterior crowding
- Increased FH-MP angle

- Labial tipping of maxillary teeth

- lower anterior teeth are inclined lingually (dento-alveolar compensation)

- ANB angle is negative

- flexion of the cranial base

- Skeletal frame is class III (APDI is more than 85)

9.3. Non-surgical treatment of class III malocclusion

It is very important to understand the dynamic mechanism of the development of class III malocclusion to establish a correct treatment plan. In the development of class III malocclusion the key point is the molar over-eruption (due to the posterior crowding) which is responsible for the flatness of the upper posterior occlusal plane.The upper posterior flat occlusal plane produces a forward mandibular adaptation. According to this there are two significant goals to attain with the treatement of class III:

- Elimination of the posterior crowding

- To Rebuilt the occlusal plane (to steepen the upper posterior occlusal plane)

The posterior crowding is usually solved, by extraction of third molars prior to the onset of the treatment. The upper second molars can be extracted if the patient is young and the third molars are too high in the tuberosity. Before the decision to extract the upper second molars, the third molars should be radiographically evaluated to check if they have correct size and shape as well as appropriate position and inclination to erupt properly, replacing the extracted second molars. Another significant goal to attain with the treatment of class III is the reconstruction of the occlusal plane, because the class III malocclusion requires a steeper occlusal plane for backward adaptation of the mandible. The tip back bends of the MEAW correct the premolars and molars to an upright position and intrude the molars. The correct treatment mechanics used are progressive tip back bends activations of 3° to 5° from the premolars teeth to molar area along with short class III elastics 3/16 inch, 6 oz) on the anterior teeth.

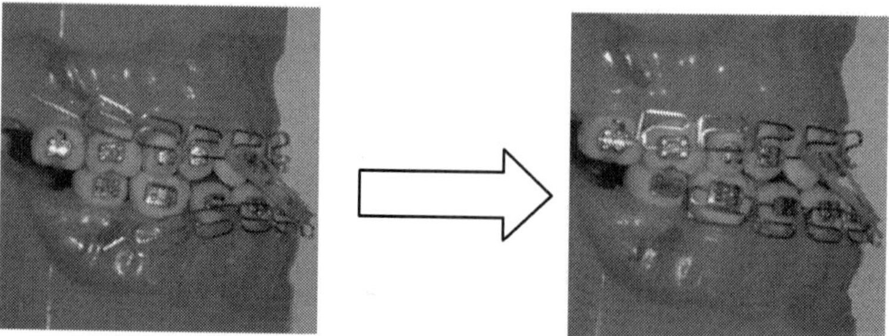

Figure 2. The tip back bends of MEAW

9.3.1. treatment steps of class III malocclusion

- Levelling

- Elimination of occlusal interferences

- Establishig mandibular position

- Occlusal plane reconstruction

- Obtain a physiologic occlusion

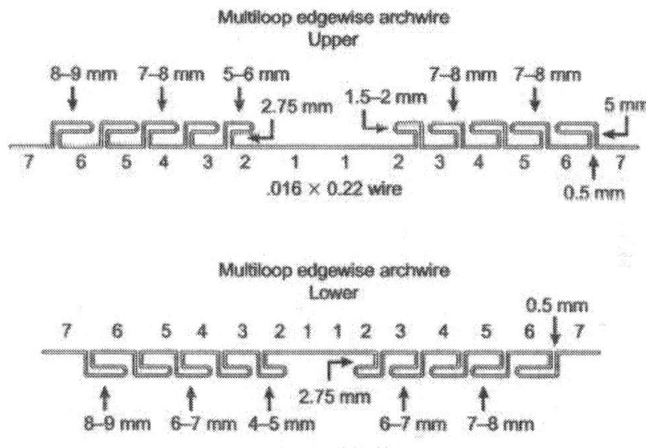

Figure 3. The MEAW's are constructed with.016x.022 stainless steel (bracket 0.018 – inch slot) or.017x.025 ss (bracket 0.022 – inch slot).

The arches have ideal arch form with five loops on each side of the arch.

10. Case report 1

Patient female 13 years old and 3 months of age, with skeletal class III and dental class III on a normodivergent face pattern, mandibular prognathism, overbite (0 mm), overjet (0 mm), flat occlusal plane in the upper molar area producing interference in the posterior area. The patient began the treatment with 13 years old and 3 months and the duration of the treatment was 18 months. The type of appliance was an edgewise multi-bracket 0,022x0,028 slot, 0° torque, 0° angulation and MEAWs arch wires. The appliance was removed in January 2013 (14Y+11M).

The purpose of the treatment for this patient with class III malocclusion was to provide a steep occlusal plane in order to achive a posterior adaptative repositioning of the mandible, to correct the crowding and improve the occlusion by uprighting and alignment the dentition. First the impacted upper and lower third molars should be removed, but she refused. It was explained to the patient and the parents, that without the extractions the probability of relapse was high. It was then accepted to extract the teeth later, after the end of treatment.During the last control visit (one year after the end of treatment) the patient was informed that she should extract the third molars and she agreed.

The steps of the treatment:

a-Leveling; b-Elimination of occlusal interferences ; c-Establishing mandibular position ; d-Reconstruction of the occlusal plane; e-Achieving a physiological occlusion.

Step one-Levelling – The levelling was performed using 0.016 SS wire arches.

Step two-Elimination of occlusal interferences-0,017x0,025 multiloop edgewise archs wire (MEAW) were incorporated in both dental arches. The alignment and intrusion began through progressive tipback of 3° to 5°,from premolars to the molar area along with the use of short class III (3/16 inch, 6oz) elastics on both sides.

Step three-Establishing mandibular position: At the end of this phase the molar occlusion was in class one.

Step four/five-Reconstruction of the occlusal plane and achieving a physiological occlusion: In this step the tipback in molar area was removed and the occlusal plane in the molar area was steepen. A stable occlusion was obtained after 18 months of treatment the retention phase was done with maxillary Hawley plate for night time use (6months) and bonded lingual wire from 33 to 43.

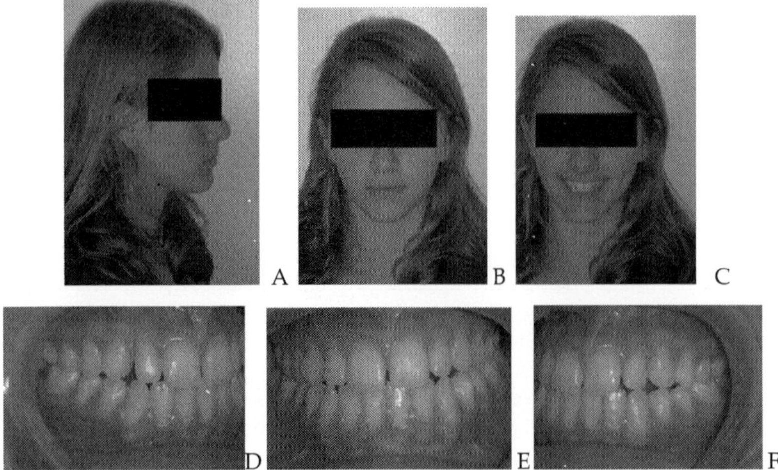

Figure 4. Pre-treatment extraoral (A-C) and intraoral (D-F) photographs

Post-treatment results show an improved profile, occlusion and a pleasant smile. The intra-oral photos show a class I molar relationship and a correct overbite and overjet. The mandibular superposition shows a slight mandibular posterior shift.

	Range	Beginning	End of treatment	End of retention
FMIA	67º+- 3	71	77	75
FMA	25º+- 3	27	28	28
IMPA	88º+- 3	82	75	77
SNA	82º+- 2	85	86	86
SNB	80º+- 2	85	84	84
ANB	2º-+ 2	0	2	2
Ao-Bo	2mm	-2mm	3mm	3mm
OP	10º-14º	6	5	5
Z	75º+-5	91	88	88
PFH	45mm	45	46	46
AFH	65mm	62	64	66
INDEX	0,69	0,73	0,72	0,70

Table 1. Cephalometric analysis (Tweed-Merrifield)

	Beginning		End of treatment		End of retention	
ODI	MP/AB 60	60	60	60	60	60
	FH/PP 0		0		0	
APDI	HF/FP 95	93	94	87	92	87
	FP/AB -02		-05		-05	
	HF/PP 0		-2		0	
CF	ODI+APDI	153		147		147

Table 2. Cephalometric analysis (Kim)

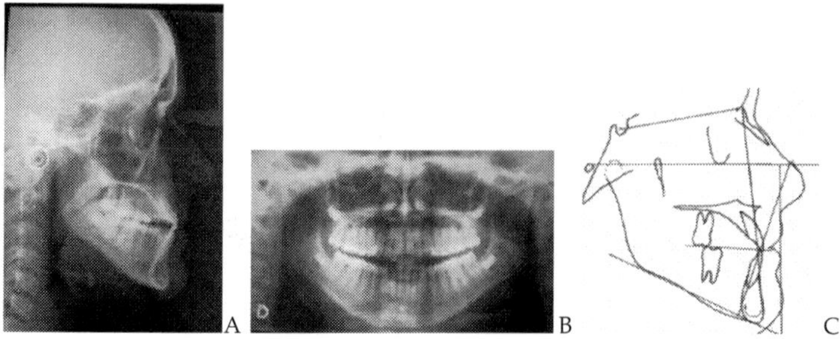

Figure 5. pre-treatment records (A-C)

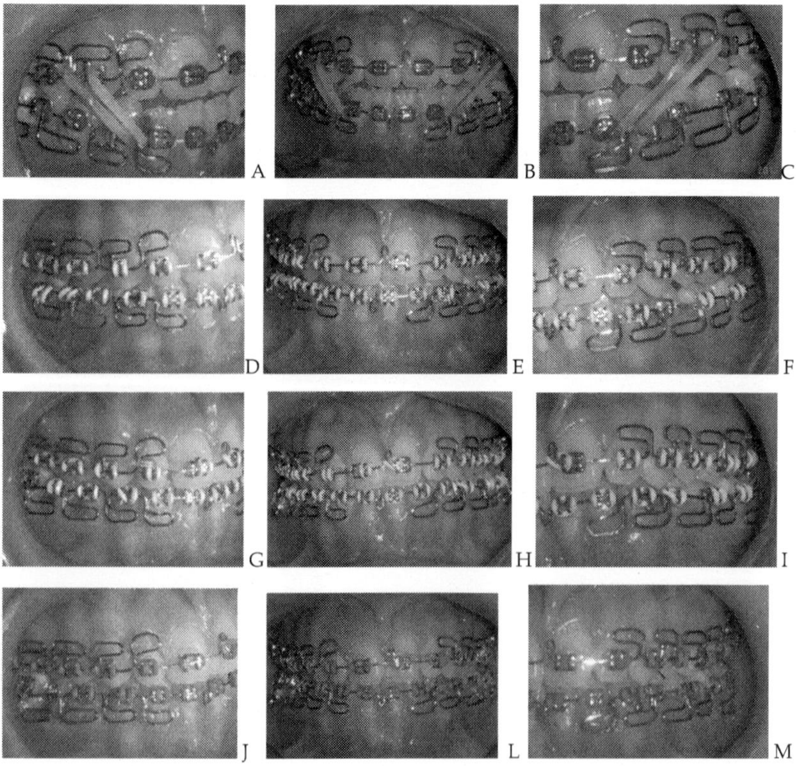

Figure 6. Photos during the treatment (A –M)

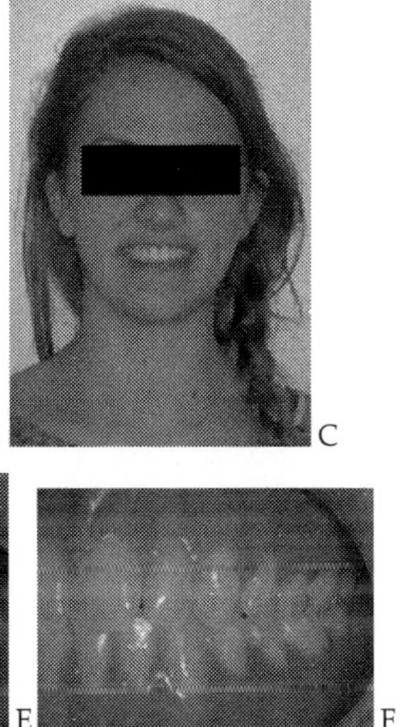

Figure 7. post-treatment extraoral (A-C) and intraoral (D-F) photos

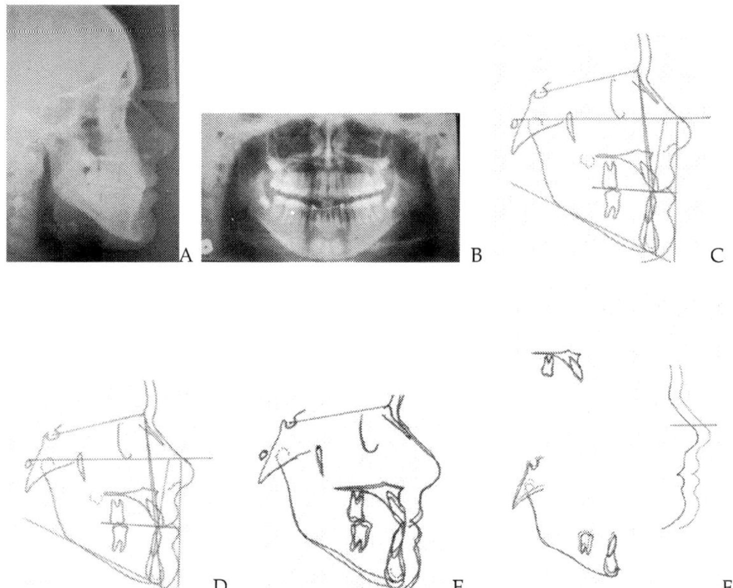

Figure 8. Post-treatment records (A-D),superimpositions (E-F)

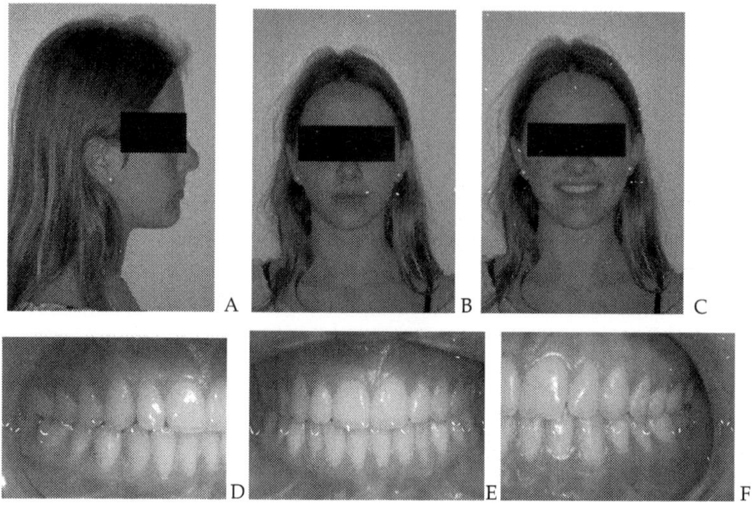

Figure 9. post-retention extra oral photos (A-C) and intraoral photos (D-F)

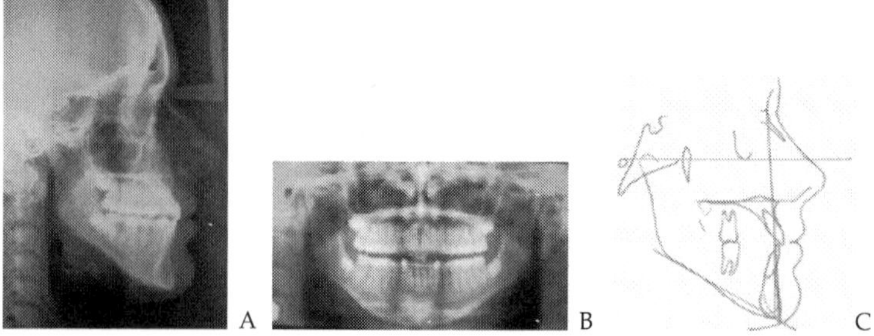

Figure 10. post-retention records (A – C)

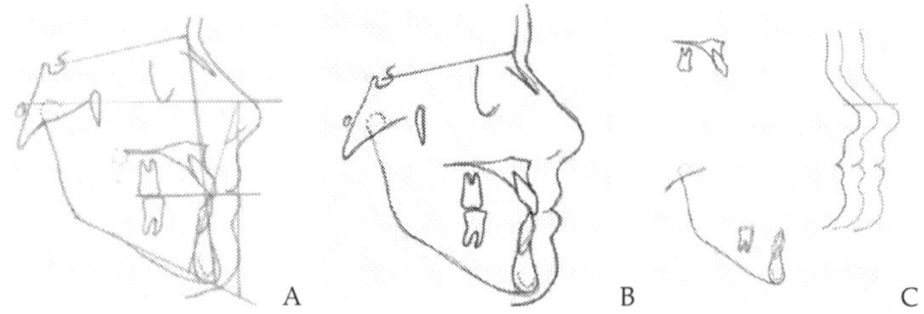

Figure 11. superimpositions (A-C)

11. Case Report 2

Patient female (15 years old/10 months), with skeletal class III (ANB-2°, APDI 91)and dental class III on a hypodivergent face pattern (FMA 22°), mandibular prognathism, open bite tendency (ODI 55); overjet (0 mm), flat occlusal plane in the molar area producing interference in the posterior area.

The z angle of 85° confirms an unbalanced face which is based on a prognathic chin.

According to Kym's analysis, the ODI (55°) indicates a openbite skeletal pattern. The APDI (91°).indicates a class III skeletal pattern and the CF (combination factor of 146) indicates a skeletal pattern requiring extraction of permanent teeth (third molars). The posterior crowding was solved by extraction of third lower molars and upper second molars prior to the onset of the treatment. The upper second molars were extracted because the third molars were too high in the tuberosity. Before the decision to extract the upper second molars, the third molars were radiographically evaluated to check if they had correct size and shape as well as appropriate position and inclination to erupt properly, replacing the second molars.

Treatment began with age (15/10), 0.016 ss arch wires were inserted for levelling and alignment of both dental arches.

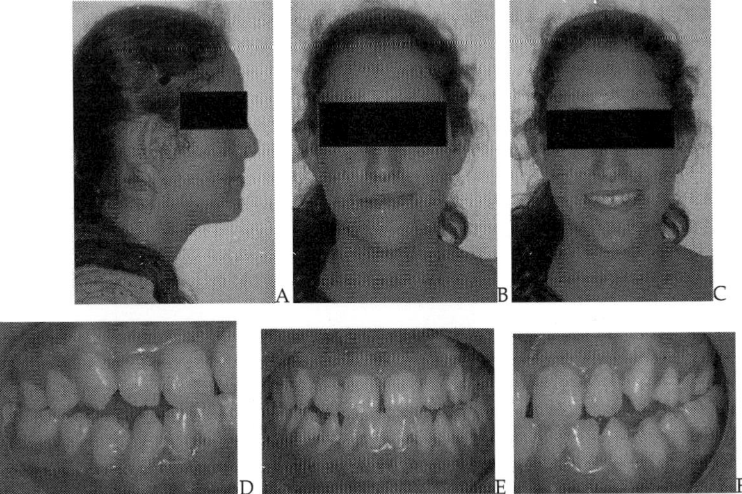

Figure 12. Pre-treatment extraoral(A-B-C) and intraoral (D-E-F) photos

After 2 months, the use of MEAW and short class III elastics (3/16 inch, 6 oz) started. The elastics were used 24 hours per day and were removed only for brushing the teeth and to eat. The correct treatment mechanic used was progressive tip back bends activations of 3° to 5° from the premolars teeth to molar area along with short class III elastics (3/16 inch, 6 oz) on the anterior teeth.

This treatment lasted 18 months. At the end of the treatment, the maxillofacial disharmony and the profile were improved. The patient displayed a pleasant smile, a normal canine and molar class I relationship, the overbite and overjet were corrected.

The lower incisors were lingually tipped (IMPA 85°) and the lower molars were moved distally.

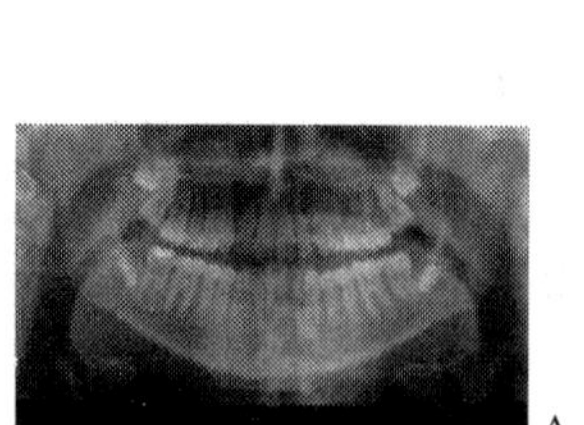 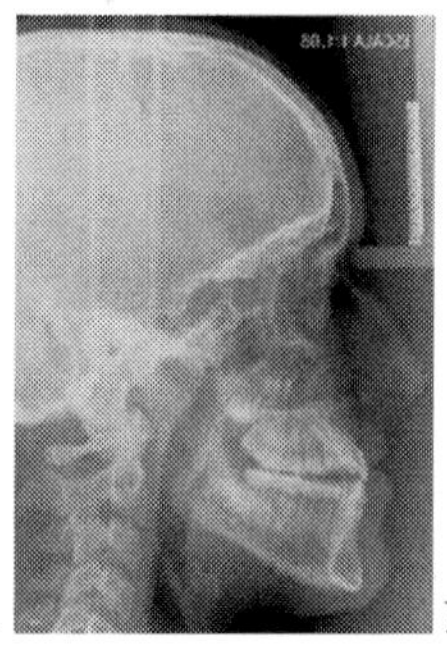 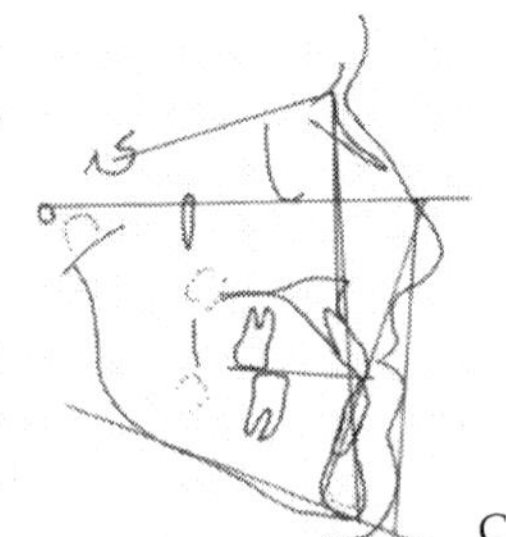

Figure 13. Pre-treatment records (A-C)

	Range	Beginning	End of treatment	End of retention
FMIA	67º+- 3	68	74	74
FMA	25º+- 3	22	21	22
IMPA	88º+- 3	90	85	84
SNA	82º+- 2	73	75	75
SNB	80º+- 2	75	74	74
ANB	2º-+ 2	-2	1	1
Ao-Bo	2mm	-7mm	-2mm	-2mm
OP	10º-14º	3	3	3
Z	75º+-5	85	80	81
PFH	45mm			
AFH	65mm			
INDEX	0,69			

Table 3. Cephalometric analysis (Tweed-Merrifield)

The general superimposition shows that the entire lower dental arch was moved distally and uprighted.

The final ODI of 63° show that the vertical aspect of the occlusion (open bite tendency) was improved. This case shows a successful orthodontic treatment of a skeletal class III malocclusion, eliminating the posterior crowding and reconstructing the occlusal plane using the MEAW technique.

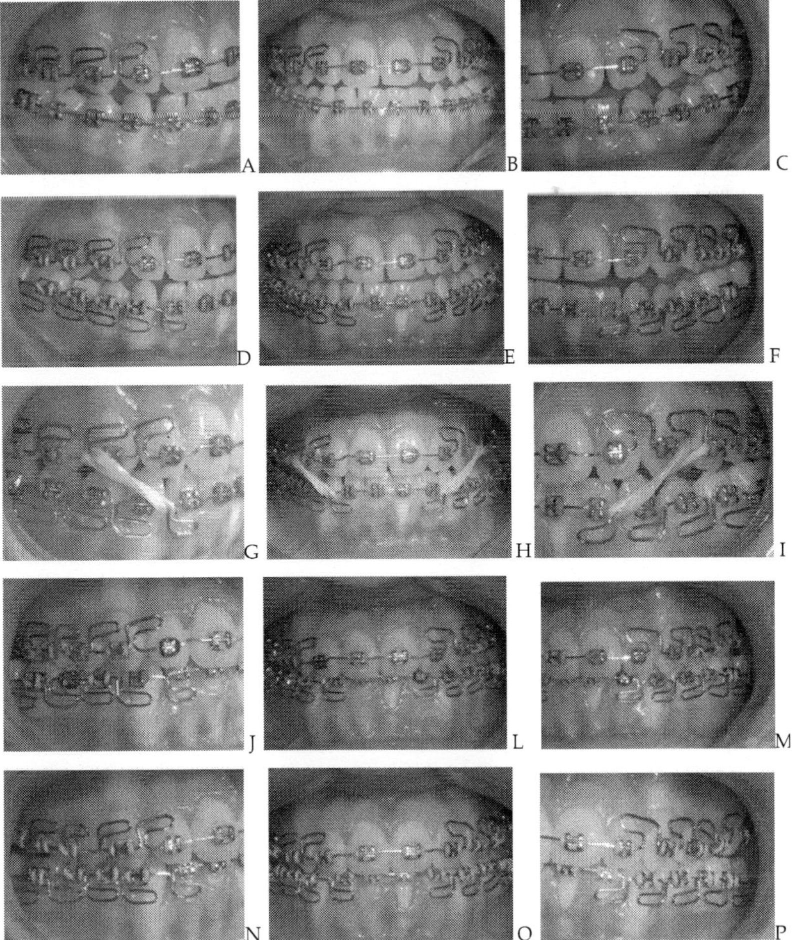

Figure 14. Photos during the treatment.(A-P) with MEAW upper and lower and short class III elastics (6 oz, 3/16 inch).

	Beginning		End of treatment		End of retention	
ODI	MP/AB 60	55	67	63	67	63
	FH/PP -5		-4		-4	
APDI	HF/FP 92	91	92	90	92	90
	FP/AB 4		2		2	
	HF/PP -5		-4		-4	
CF	ODI+APDI	146		153		153

Table 4. cephalometric analysis (Kim)

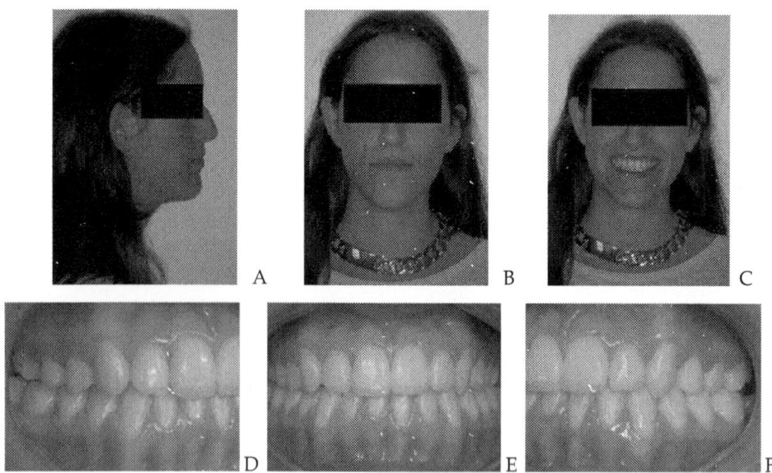

Figure 15. Post-treatment extraoral photos (A-C) and intraoral photos (D-F)

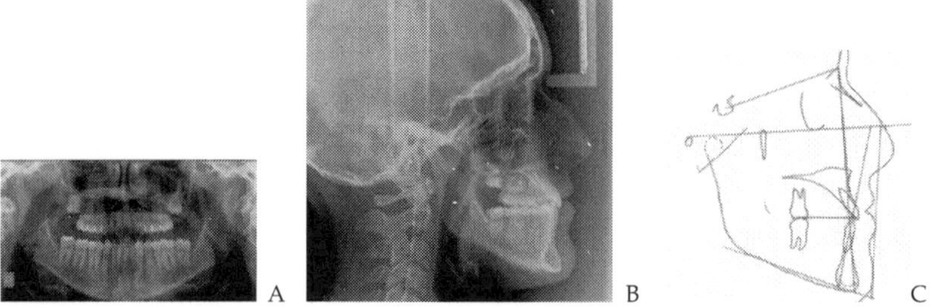

Figure 16. Post-treatment records

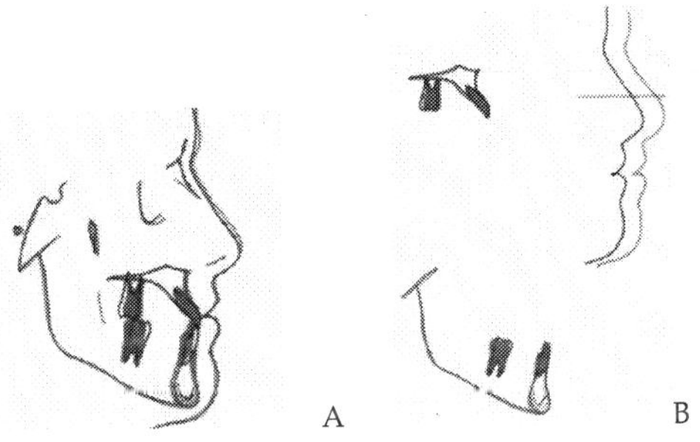

Figure 17. superimpositions (D – E)

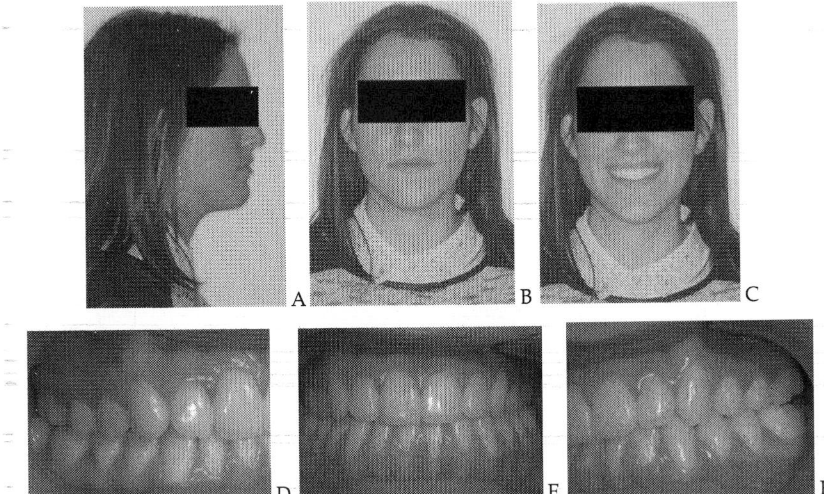

Figure 18. Post-retention extraoral photos (A-C) and intraoral photos (D-F)

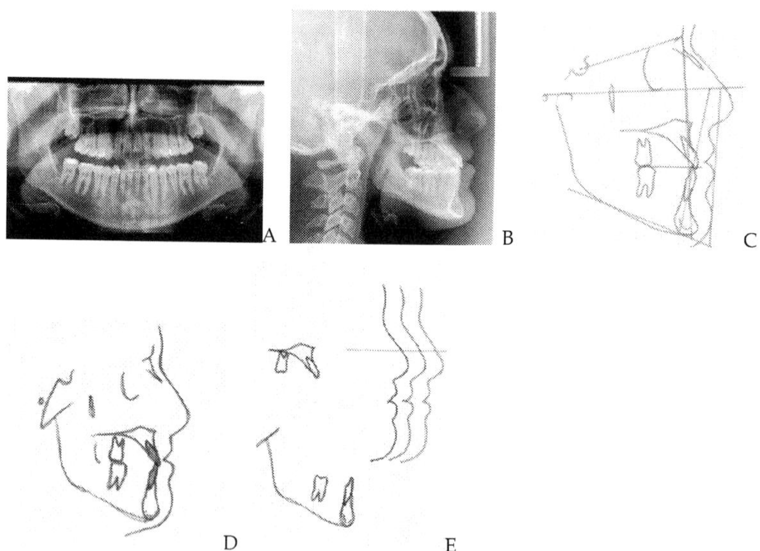

Figure 19. post-retention records (A –E)

12. Conclusion

The MEAW technique proved to be effective in the treatment of class III malocclusion. The MEAW is a valid alternative in the treatment of class III malocclusion, when patients refuse surgery and when the disharmony of the skeletal structure is not harsh. The MEAW used correctly can properly reconstruct the occlusal plane, allowing toachieve a correct and stable occlusion, improving the profil and facial balance.

Author details

Paulo Beltrão*

Address all correspondence to: paulobeltrao@sapo.pt

French Board Of Orthodontics, Portugal

References

[1] Beltrão, Paulo (2011) Treatment of class II deep Overbite with multiloop edgewise arch-wire(MEAW) therapy; Principles in contemporary orthodontics (Edited by Silvano Naretto),Intech

[2] Dawson,P.E.(1989) *Evaluation, diagnosis and treatment of occlusal problems, Dawson,P.E. (ed),*The C.V. Mosby company

[3] Fushima, K ; Kitamura,Y; Mita,H ; Sato,S; Kim,Y (1996).The significance of the cant of occlusal plane in class II/1 malocclusion. *European journal of orthodontics*, 18,27-40

[4] Hyun-Sook Kim,Seon-Young Kim (2004).Compensatory changes of a occlusal plane angles in relation to a skeletal factors; *Korea journal of orthodontics:*34 (3) :229-40

[5] Kim, YH,(1979),ODI/APDI combination factor, Angle orthodontics,49:77-84

[6] Kim, YH;(1999);Treatment of anterior openbite and deepbite malocclusions with MEAW therapy; The enigma of vertical dimension-craniofacial growth series vol 36 Ann Arbor (edited by James McNamara Jr): center for Human growth and development-University of Michigan

[7] Knierim, RW (1999).diagnosis of openbite and deepbite problems: a clinician`s perspective on the Kim approach; ; The enigma of vertical dimension-craniofacial growth series vol 36 Ann Arbor (edited by James McNamara Jr): center for Human growth and development-Univ.Michigan

[8] Mc Namara,J.A. jr and Carlson,D.S. (1979)Quantitative analysis of temporomandibular joint adaptations to protrusive function; American journal of orthodontics, 76,593-611

[9] Merrifield,LL.(1966)The profile line as an aid to critical evaluation of facial esthetics; American journal of orthodontics,804-822

[10] Ortial,J.P(1989),Les modifications faciales par l`orthodontie, journal de l`edgewise, vol.20,53-86

[11] Petrovic,A.G. and Stutzaman,J.(1975) Control process in the postnatal growth of the condylar cartilage,in McNamara J.A.jr,ed.determinants of mandibular growth,monograph 4:craniofacial growth series,Ann Arbor-Center for Human growth and development,University of Michigan

[12] Sassouni,V,(1969)A classification of skeletal facial types,AJODO,55,109-123

[13] Sato, Sadao (1994)-Case report: developmental characterization of skeletal class III malocclusion,the Angle orthodontics, vol.64,n°2-1994

[14] Sato,Sadao; Akimoto (2007)-Development and orthodontic treatment of skeletal class III malocclusion without surgical intervention, The bulletin of kanagawa dental college,vol,35,n°1, March 2007

[15] Sato, Sadao(2001) –A treatment approach to malocclusions under the consideration of craniofacial dynamics,Grace printing press, inc

[16] Sato,Sadao (2008),orthodontic marathon course at Kanagawa dental college-Japan

Chapter 21

Clinical Consideration and Management of Impacted Maxillary Canine Teeth

Belma Işık Aslan and Neslihan Üçüncü

Additional information is available at the end of the chapter

http://dx.doi.org/10.5772/59324

1. Introduction

Impaction is a retardation or halt in the normal process of tooth. There are various terminology in literature to define impaction including delayed eruption, primary retention, submerged teeth, impacted teeth ets. A canine is considered as being impacted if it is interrupted after complete root development or the contralateral tooth is erupted for at least 6 months with complete root formation [1].

Impaction of maxillary canines is a frequently encountered clinical problem. The cause of canine impaction can be the result of localized, systemic or genetic factor(s). There are a number of possible sequelae to canine impactions. The diagnosis and localization of the impacted canines is the most important step in the management of impacted canines based on clinical and radiographic examinations. Treatment of impacted maxillary canines usually requires an interdisciplinary approach. Treatment options include no treatment, interseptive approach, extraction, autotransplantation and surgical exposure and orthodontic alignment of the impacted canine. The most desirable treatment approach is early diagnosis and interception of potential impaction. However, in the absence of prevention, surgical exposure and orthodontic alignment should be considered. Surgical treatment techniques and orthodontic considerations depend on the location of the impacted canine in the dental arch.

2. Incidance of impacted canines

Maxillary canines are the second-most frequently impacted teeth after the third molars [2] with prevalence from 0.8-5.2 % depending on the population examined [3,4]. The incidence of maxillary canine impaction is about 20 times more than mandibular canine impaction [5].

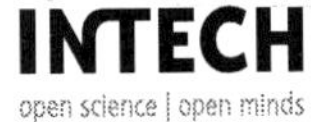

Approximately one third of impacted maxillary canines are positioned labially or within the alveolus, and two thirds are located palatally [6]. In another study [7], Ericson and Kurol reported that, 50% of the 156 ectopically positioned canines were in a palatal or distopalatal position, 39% in a buccal or distobuccal position, and 11% apical to the adjacent incisor or between the roots of the central and lateral incisors. Maxillary canine impactions occur twice as often in females than in males [8] and only 8% of canine impactions are bilateral [9].

3. Developmental considerations

Maxillary canines develop lateral to the priform fossa and have a longer and difficult path of eruption than any other tooth through they reach their final position in occlusion. Coulter and Richardson [10] stated that in three planes of space, maxillary canines travel almost 22 mm from their position at the age of 5 years to their position at 15 years. At the age of 3 maxillary canine is high in the maxilla, with its crown directed mesially and lingually. At the age of 8 it angulates medially with its crown lying distal and slightly buccal to the lateral incisor [11]. Also at this stage the canine normally migrates buccally from a position lingual to the root apex of its deciduous precursor, however, if it cannot make this transition from the palatal to the buccal side, it remains palatally impacted [12]. Maxillary canines follow a mesial path until it reaches the distal aspect of the lateral incisor root and gradually uprights to a more vertical position by moving towards the occlusal plane guided by the lateral incisor root. However, maxillary canines often erupt into the oral cavity with a marked mesial inclination [13]. If the lateral incisors are congenitally missing, the canine may erupt in a mesial direction until it comes into contact with the distal aspect of the central incisor root and erupts into the lateral incisor space [14]. Consequently, the roots of the lateral incisors play an important role in the guidance of upper permanent canines [15].

Table 1 shows the calcification and eruption timing of the maxillary canines according to Brand and Isselhard [16].

Calcification begins	4 months
Enamel complete	6-7 years
Eruption	11-12 years
Root completed	13-15 years

Table 1. Calcification and eruption timing of the maxillary canines

The mean eruption age for the maxillary canine is approximately 1 year earlier in females (10.98 years) than in males (11.69 years) [17]. Hurme [17] suggested that if maxillary canine has not appeared by the age of 13.1 in males or by 12.3 in females, the eruption may be considered late.

4. Etiology of impacted canines

Eruption is a tightly coordinated process, regulated by a series of signaling effects between the dental follicle and the osteoblast and osteoclast cells found in the alveolar bone [18]. A wide variety of localized, systemic and genetic reasons may cause disruption in eruption process, ranging from delayed eruption to a complete failure of eruption [19]. Systemic reasons include endocrine deficiencies, febrile diseases, and irradiation. There is not only one etiology to explain the occurrence of a majority of impactions or either the localization of impaction occuring labially or palatally [20]. Environmental factors may cause impaction during the long, tortuous eruption path of a canine. The primary causes of impacted canines are localized conditions and result of one or a combination of following factors [21]:

1. tooth size, arch length discrepancies,

2. prolonged retention or early loss of the deciduous canine,

3. apical periodontitis of deciduous teeth [22],

4. abnormal position of the tooth bud,

5. presence of an alveolar cleft,

6. ankylosis,

7. premature root closure [23],

8. cystic or neoplastic formation,

9. dilesaration of the root,

10. disturbances in tooth eruption sequence,

11. mucosal barriers-scar tissue: trauma/surgery [24],

12. gingival fibromatosis/ gingival hyperplasia [25],

13. supernumerary teeth [26],

14. iatrogenic,

15. idiopathic including primary failure of eruption [27].

If no physical barrier can be identified, the cessation of eruption of a normally placed and developed tooth germ before emergence is described as primary retention [28]. Generally genetic etiology is related with primary retention [29]. If the teeth becomes impacted due to an obstruction of the eruption pathway such as crowded dental arch, it is defined as secondary retention [28].

The etiology of impacted teeth may depend upon the location of impacted tooth. The exact etiology of palatally displaced maxillary canines is unknown yet hypothesized to be both multifactorial and genetic in origin [30]. Where as buccal canine impaction is result of ectopic migration of the canine crown over the root of the lateral incisor due to crowding or shifting of the maxillary dental midline, causing insufficient space for the canine to erupt [31].

Two main theories have been associated with the occurrence of palatally impacted maxillary canines: the "guidance theory" and the "genetic theory" [2]. According to the guidance theory, the presence of the lateral incisor root with right length and formed at the right time are important variables needed to guide the mesially erupting canine in a more favorable distal and incisal direction. If excessive space exists due to malformed or absent lateral incisor the canine would cross back from the buccal to the palatal side behind the buds of the other teeth [3]. In the clinical observation of Jacoby [32], he stated that 85% of the 40 palatally impacted canines had sufficient space for eruption in the dental arch. He claimed that labially impacted maxillary canine could only be due to arch length deficiency where as palatal impaction due to excessive space in the canine area. In accordance, Al-Nimri and Gharaibeh [33] stated that the presence of an excess palatal width and anomalous lateral incisor may contribute to the etiology of palatal canine impaction. They have also found that palatal canine impaction occurred most frequently in subjects with a Class II division 2 malocclusion. Conversely, McConnell [34] found transverse maxillary deficiency in palatally impacted canine cases. On the other hand, Langberg and Peck [35] observed no statistically significant difference in the anterior and posterior maxillary arch widths between subjects with palatally displaced canines and a comparison sample.

The genetic theory assigns genetic factors as the primary origin of the eruption anomaly of maxillary permanent canines. Palatally impacted canines, such as familial and bilateral occurrence, sex differences, are genetically associated with dental anomalies such as ectopic eruption of first molars, infraocclusion of primary molars, aplasia of premolars and one third molar [36]. Sacerdoti and Baccetti [38] showed that unilateral palatal canine displacement was associated with missing upper lateral incisors where as bilateral canine displacement with agenesis of third molars, indicating the genetic etiology of palatal canine displacement. Peck et al., [37] also found a positive correlation between palatally displaced canines and third molar agenesis.

5. Sequelae of canine impaction

Careful observation of the development and eruption of canines during periodic dental examination of the growing child is essential to prevent potential complications. Shafer et al. [39] suggested the following sequelae for canine impaction:

1. labial or lingual malpositioning of the impacted tooth,

2. migration of the neighboring teeth and loss of arch length,

3. internal resorption,

4. dentigerous cyst formation,

5. external root resorption of the impacted tooth, as well as the neighboring teeth,

6. infection particularly with partial eruption, and

7. referred pain and combinations of the above sequelae.

6. Diagnosis of impacted canines

The diagnosis and localization of the impacted canines is the most important step in the management of impacted canines based on clinical and radiographic examinations.

6.1. Clinical evaluation

In clinical evaluation firstly patient's age and dentition should be examined to detemine whether there is a delayed eruption or not. Secondly, the presence or absence of a factor such as certain diseases that may cause tooth structure, size, shape, and color defects adversely affecting tooth development should be searched [40]. Subsequently the amount of space in the arch for the unerupted canine, the morphology and position of the adjacent teeth, the contours of the bone, the mobility of teeth should be considered through clinical evaluation [41].

Indicative clinical signs of canine impaction may be listed as following: [20]

1. delayed eruption of the permanent canine or prolonged retention of the deciduous canine beyond 14 to 15 years of age,

2. the presence of an asymmetry in the canine bulge or absence of a normal labial canine bulge observed during alveolar palpation,

3. presence of a palatal bulge, and

4. distal tipping, or migration of the lateral incisor

During normal eruption of the maxillary canine, usually a labial bulge is noted on the mucosa superior to the maxillary primary canine. When such a bulge is not visible, an intraoral palpation is required to provide a clear localization of the permanent canine. Also mobility of all present teeth should be assessed during palpation. Mobile deciduous canines may indicate normal resorption of the roots by the permanent canines where as mobility of the permanent lateral incisor may be the potential result of root resorption by the impacted canine [20].

According to Ericson and Kurol [42] the absence of the "canine bulge" at earlier ages should not be considered as indicative of canine impaction. In their evaluation of 505 schoolchildren between 8 and 12 years of age, they found that at 10 years, 29% of the children had nonpalpable canines, but only 5% at 11 years of age, whereas at later ages only 3% had nonpalpable canines. They found that many of the children under 10 years of age whose canines initially were determined by palpation to be potentially abnormal, actually later developed and erupted normally. Thus they found radiographic examination impractical and unnecessary for children under 10 years of age [43].

In contrast, examination of intrabony movement of the canines between the dental age of 8 to 10 years was advised by Williams [44]. If permanent canine bulges are not palpable, he offered to examine lateral and frontal radiographs specifically for Class I malocclusions, even with minimal arch length loss. He suggested removing the deciduous canine when a position apparently lingual to the anterior teeth on the lateral radiograph and a medial tilt of the long axis of the canine in relation to the lateral wall of the nasal cavity on the frontal radiograph are observed.

6.2. Radiographic verification

The accurate location of impacted canines and determining their relationship to adjacent incisors and anatomical structures is the part of the diagnostic process and is essential for successful treatment. This required information can be partially obtained from conventional two-dimensional radiographs as the first step which includes periapical radiographs, occlusal films, panoramic views, and lateral cephalograms [45].

In most cases analysis should begin with routine periapical films. A single periapical film would relate the canine with the neighboring teeth both mesiodistally and superoinferiorly. In order to estimate the buccolingual position of the canine, a second periapical film is obtained by using [46]: (1) Tube-shift technique or Clark's rule, (2) buccal-object rule.

In tube-shift technique two adjacent periapical radiographs of the impacted tooth are taken at slightly different horizontal angles. The object that moves in the same direction as the cone, is palatally impacted. If the impacted canine is located buccally, the crown of the tooth moves in the opposite direction as the x-ray beam. Consequently the object closest to the film will move in the same direction as the tube head.

In the buccal-object rule two periapical films are taken of the same area, with approximately 20° vertical angulation of the cone changed when the second film is taken. The buccal object will move in opposite direction to the source of radiation.

Occlusal films also aid to detect the buccolingual position of the impacted canine in conjunction with the periapical films especially when treating an uncooperative child, a child with very small oral aperture. However, alone, this type of radiograph provides no information relative to the vertical position of the impacted tooth [47].

Frontal and lateral cephalograms can sometimes be useful in determining the position of the impacted canine, particularly its relationship to other facial structures, such as the maxillary sinus and the floor of the nose.

Panoramic radiography has also been utilized as a diagnostic tool for determination of unerupted canine positions [48]. Radiographic variables on panoramic x-rays: α-angle (angle measured between the long axis of the impacted canine and the midline), d-distance (distance between the canine cusp tip and the occlusal plane), and s-sector where the cusp of the impacted canine is located (sector 1, between the midline and the axis of the central incisor; sector 2, between the axes of the central incisor and the lateral incisor; or sector 3, between the axes of the lateral incisor and the first premolar) have been shown to be predictive factors for prediction of eventual impaction, the durations of orthodontic traction and comprehensive orthodontic treatment to reposition the impacted tooth. However these features are not valid predictors of the final periodontal status of orthodontically-repositioned impacted canines [49]. The more severely displaced the canine with regard to the adjacent maxillary incisors, the longer the orthodontic treatment.

Medical computerized tomography (CT) was an improvement which overcomes the limitations of conventional two-dimensional (2D) imaging however, radiation exposure of CT scans limits its clinical utility [50]. The advent of 3D cone beam computed tomography (CBCT) has reduced the radiation dose, making it an advantageous tool in dentistry [51]. CBCT images have been proven to be useful for the accurate diagnosis of the impacted canines, treatment planning and the identification of associated complications, such as root resorption in adjacent incisors. In addition it was found that CBCT reduces the treatment duration and increases the success of treatment in difficult cases to a similar level of simpler cases [52]. Small volume CBCT may be indicated as a supplement to a routine panoramic X-ray in the following cases if: [53]

- canine inclination in the panoramic X-ray exceeds 30°

- root resorption of adjacent teeth is suspected

- the canine apex is not clearly discernible in the panoramic X-ray, implying dilaceration of the canine root.

6.3. Root resorption and radiographic evaluation

The ability to evaluate the condition of the lateral incisor root is of great importance to the clinician because 80% of the teeth resorbed by the ectopically erupting canines were found to be lateral incisors [21]. Lateral incisor image could only be evaluated in 37% of the cases with the use of periapical films [47]. However CBCT provides more detailed information about the location and extent of the resorbed roots and may notably alter the prevalence of root resorption [54].

Ericson and Kurol [7] found the incidance of lateral resorption as 38%, in a study of 156 ectopically impacted maxillary canines with using CT. In a more recent study, Oberoi and Knueppel [55] determined no root resorption in 40.4%, slight root resorption in 35.7%, moderate resorption in 14.2% and severe root resorption in 4% of the adjacent lateral incisor evaluated by CBCT.

7. Treatment planning considerations

Maxillary canines play an important role in creating good facial and smile esthetics, since they are positioned at the corners of the dental arch, forming the canine eminence for support of the alar base and the upper lip. Moreover, when the maxillary canines are properly aligned and have good shape and size, pleasing anterior dental proportions and correct smile lines are achieved. Functionally, they support the dentition, contributing to disarticulation during lateral movements in certain persons [56]. Treatment of impacted maxillary canines usually requires an interdisciplinary approach involving oral surgical, restorative, periodontic as well as orthodontic components. Prudent treatment planning is necessary to achieve the various treatment goals [21].

The patient with an impacted maxillary canine initially must undergo a comprehensive clinical and radiographic evalution of the malocclusion to localize the impacted canine and decide on its prognosis for alignment. Patient's cooperation, age, general oral health, skeletal variation and presence of spacing or crowding in the arch are important agents affecting prognosis [57]. Any root resorption of the adjacent teeth should also be considered. Orthoontist should also be aware of the normal development and eruption pattern in order to conduct interceptive treatment if appropriate, which provides cost benefit than other more invasive prosedures. Patient and parent counselling on the treatment options and informed constent is essential to avoid any medicolegal problems [58].

8. Treatment options

The clinician should consider the various treatment options available for the patient, including: [21]

1. No treatment

2. Interseptive treatment

3. Extraction of the impacted canine

4. Autotransplantation of the canine

5. Surgical exposure and orthodontic alignment

1. No treatment

No active treatment could be recommended when: [59]

- the patient does not request treatment

- there is no sign of resorption of adjacent teeth or other pathology

- there is a severely displaced canine with no evidence of pathology, if it is remote from the dentition ideally there is a good contact between lateral incisor and first premolar or good esthetics/prognosis for deciduous canine

In this instance, the unerupted canine should be periodically monitored with respect to cystic degeneration, root resorption and the other possible complications. The optimal time interval between radiographs is not known to reduce the radiation dosage. In most cases, long-term prognosis of retained deciduous canine is poor, regardless of its root length and crown shape since the root of retained deciduous canine will eventually resorb and it will have to be extracted [21].

2.   Interseptive treatment

Early diagnosis and intervention is very important for it could save the time, expense, and more complex treatment in the permanent dentition. If early signs of ectopic eruption of the canines is determined, the clinician should made an attempt to prevent their impaction and its potential sequalae. Frequently, primary canines are extracted as an interceptive measure to facilite the permanent canine eruption or at least provide changes to a more favorable position [12]. The extraction of the primary canine is recommended when:

- the patient is aged 10-13 years.

- the maxillary canine is not palpable in its normal position and radiographic examination exhibites palatal canine ectopia. If the permanent canine is located in a more medial position or the patient is older than the ideal age group, extraction of the primary canine may provide less favourable results [60].

Clinical re-evaluation and follow-up radiographs should normally be taken at 6-month intervals. If there is no improvement in canine position within 12 months on panaromic films after the extraction of primary canines, an alternative treatment is indicated [61].

The severity of the angulation of the impacted canine is an important factor in the prognosis. The more inclined the tooth is, the less is the probability that it will spontaneously erupt [61]. Power and Short [62] predicted the chances of canine impaction based on orthopantomographs between the years of 10-13 and claimed that eruption chance of the impacted tooth will decrease even after deciduous extraction is performed if the permanent canine is angled more than 31° to the midline.

Ericson and Kurol [61] stated that the removal of the deciduous canine before 11 years of age will normalize the position of the ectopically erupting permanent canines up to 91% if the permanent canine crown is distal to the midline of the lateral incisor. However the success rate decreases to 64% when the canine crown overlaps medially to the long axis midline of the lateral incisor.

Williams [44] suggested the extraction of the maxillary deciduous canine as early as 8 or 9 years of age to enhance the eruption and self-correction of a labial or intra-alveolar maxillary canine impaction in Class I uncrowded cases.

Extraction of deciduous canines in conjunction with the use of cervical pull headgear, and rapid maxillary expansion have been reported to be effective procedures in the interceptive treatment of maxillary canine impaction [2]. Baccetti et al. [63] found that 65 percent of palatally displaced cases that underwent the removal of the deciduous canine resulted in successful eruption of permanent canines without any other treatment. The prevalence rate could be improved significantly up to 88 percent by preventing mesial migration of the upper posterior teeth after extraction of the deciduous canine, such as with the use of cervical-pull headgear [63]. Also Olive [64] stated that opening space for the canine crown with routine orthodontic mechanics might allow for spontaneous eruption of an impacted canine. However early correction of the flared and distally tipped lateral incisors is not recommended in order not to cause impaction of the canines or the resorption of lateral incisor roots [65].

Another randomized clinical trial performed by Bagetti et al. [66] reported that TPA and deciduous canine extraction alone was as effective as rapid maxillary expansion followed by a TPA coupled with the extraction of deciduous canines, as an interceptive treatment option for patients from 9 years 5 months to 13 years of age with palatally displaced canines. The use of these protocols in late mixed dentition subjects increased the eruption rate significantly more than only extraction and untreated groups.

3.   Extraction of impacted canines

The surgical removal of impacted canines although seldom considered might be a viable option in the following situations: [29]

- patient declines active treatment and/or is happy with apperance.
- there is evidence of early resorption of adjacent teeth.
- the patient is too old for interseption.
- there is a good contact for lateral incisor and first premolar or the patient is willing to undergo orthodontic treatment to substitute first premolar for the canine
- if the impacted canine is ankylosed and cannot be transplanted
- if the root of impacted canine is severely dilacerated
- if the impaction is severe and the degree of malocclusion is too great for surgical repositioning/transplantation.

Especially extraction of the labially erupting and crowded canine is contraindicated. Such an extraction might temporarily improve the aesthetics however may complicate and compromise the orthodontic treatment results.

If removal of the impacted canine is required, the orthodontist should decide whether to replace the premolar into the canine position or restore the missing canine space with a prosthesis or an implant. If the canine space is going to be closed orthodontically, the posterior segment has to be protracted. Before the extraction decision is made, factors such as linguai cusp interferences, tooth size discrepancy, and the difficulties encountered when employing unilateral mechanics should also be considered [21].

When an extraction is performed, it often leaves a critical alveolar defect of difficult management. Puricelli et al. [67] recommended maxillary partial osteotomy as an efficient resolution for the correction of bone defects within the dental arches which is performed by mobilizing an alveolar bone segment. They have indicated this technique within the concept of individual and multiple sustenance of integrity in occlusion and of the dental arches, especially in young patients, where the indication for fixed prosthetics or osseointegrated implants might be precocious. They stated that this technique offers a superior time efficient solution for the loss of the maxillary canines compared to the osseointegrated implant rehabilitation or orthodontic space closure.

Surgical extraction of impacted canines and their substitution by first premolars eliminates all the risks and uncertainty related to orthodontic extrusion of an impacted canine. Good functional and esthetic results can be achieved, if an accurate and detailed anterior tooth position is managed during orthodontic finishing [68]. Smile esthetics of maxillary premolar substitution can be improved by intruding the first premolars to a higher gingival margin with respect to the maxillary lateral incisors and restoring the premolars with composite resin buildups or porcelain veneers to produce natural canines [69]. Otherwise slightly extrusion of the maxillary first premolars is also acceptable if premolar crowns are long, with prominent buccal cusps. Also, slight negative crown torque and a mesiopalatal rotation is recommended to resemble a natural canine as possible [68]. Additionally it is reported that there is no scientific evidence that one occlusal scheme is better than the other. Hence canine guidance can well be constructed by premolar guidance or a group function, by slightly extruding the maxillary first premolar [70].

4. Autotransplantation of the canine

Autotransplantation could be performed as a treatment option when: [59]

- interceptive treatment is inconvenient or has failed,

- the degree of malocclusion is too severe to achieve orthodontic alignment,(crown tip mesial to the mid-line of the lateral incisor or mesial angulation greater than 55° [47],

- adequate space is available for the canine

- the prognosis is good for the tooth to be transplanted and it can be removed atraumatically.

- patient refuses a conventional orthodontic therapy

- failure of orthodontic alignment due to immobility

Successful prognosis of transplanted teeth depends on the following factors: the condition of the remaining periodontal ligament attached to the extracted donor tooth [72], the adaptation of the donor tooth to the socket [73], the duration and the method of splinting after transplantation [74], and the timing of endodontic treatment of the transplanted teeth [75].

Recent studies of autotransplantation of canines have reported success rates of 38–58% over more than 10 years [76, 77]. In another recent study, Huth et al. [71] found that the success rate of autotransplanted teeth was 74%, along with a high patient satisfaction [37]. They recommended autotransplantation especially in adolescent patients in whom alternative treatments, such as dental implants, are not yet indicated since autotransplanted teeth increase or at least maintain the bone level and facilitate a later dental implant supply.

The most relevant complications in autotransplantation of teeth that affect the success rate are inflammatory or replacement resorption [78]. Periodontal healing is responsible for root resorption after autotransplantation. At a later stage of development the root is fully formed and the chances of pulpal and periodontal healing is reduced [79, 80]. The optimal developmental stage for autotransplantation is when the root is 50-75 percent is formed [81].

In some clinical studies it was suggested that the preapplication of mechanical stimuli to the donor teeth might stimulate the periodontal ligament, prevent ankylosis, reduce the damage to the periodontal ligament, and prevent root resorption after replantation [82,83]. Recently,

Ru and Bai [84] reported a maxillary canine autotransplantation case where the extraction site of deciduous canine was preserved with a titanium prosthesis and a bioresorbable membrane to prevent root resorption and anyklosis.

The prognosis of ectopic canine autotransplantation in adults is poor. In the research of Schatz and Joho [85] on 20 transplanted maxillary canines, they determined that pulp vitality remained in 80% of the patients aged 13 to 20 years group however all impacted canines required root canal therapy in the 20-to 48-year age-group.

Endodontic treatment of autotransplanted teeth with closed apices is considered as mandatory analog of traumatically avulsed teeth with closed apices [86]. If the toot has a open apice, a wait-and-see strategy is accepted due to the considerable potential of revascularization [87], which occurs in up to 100% of these teeth [81]. In such a case, endodontic treatment is performed only if signs of pulp necrosis or root resorption are detected [87]. On the other hand, some authors suggested a wait-and-see strategy even in cases with closed apices [88, 89]. In the study by Ahlberg et al. [89], 30% of 33 maxillary canines with complete root formation required no endodontic treatment after an average of 6 years. (Figure 1)

5.   Surgical exposure of teeth and orthodontic treatment

The most desirable treatment approach for the management of impacted maxillary canines is early diagnosis and interception of potential impaction. However, in the absence of prevention, clinicians should consider surgical exposure and orthodontic alignment.

This treatment option is recommended when: [59]

a.   the patient tends to wear orthodontic appliances

b.   the patient is well motivated and has general good dental health

c.   the long axis of the ectopic canine is not too horizontal or oblique. The closer the crown is to the midline and the root to the mid-palatal suture, the poorer pronosis for alignment [60]

d.   any evidence of root resorption or other pathology is such that it is more desirable to preserve the canine. For instance if the adjacent lateral incisor is resorbed and have a very poor prognosis, it would be advantageous to attempt alignment of impacted canine to replace the lateral incisor [59].

Two approaches could be followed after surgical exposure: [21]

1.   surgical exposure to allow for natural eruption to occur

2.   surgical exposure with the placement of an auxiliary

8.1. Surgical exposure to allow for natural eruption to occur

This method is often used when:

- the canine has an appropriate axial inclination and does not need to be uprighted during its eruption,

- the root development has not been completed yet, therefore patient' s age is important

The progress of canine eruption should be monitored with roentgenograms, using reference points such as an adjacent tooth or the arch wire. If the tooth fails to erupt, removal of any cicatricial tissue surrounding the crown is recommended. The main disadvantages of this approach are the spontaneous but slow canine eruption, the increased treatment time, and the inability to influence the path of eruption and the risk of ankylosing [21].

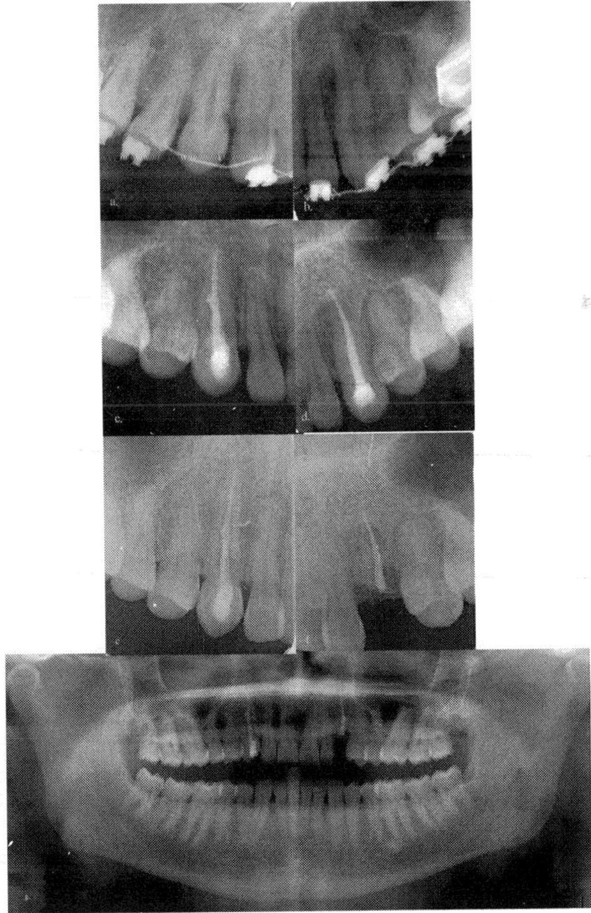

Figure 1. Bilateral impacted canines were treated with autotransplantation in a 22 year old adult patient. A wait and see strategy was followed and canal therapy was applied after seven months from autotransplantation as external root resorption was detected. 10 years after treatment the patient came with the left canine broken due to external root resorption, however no difference was observed in the contralateral canine.

8.2. Surgical exposure with the placement of an auxiliary

Surgically assisted orthodontic guidance is required when all possibilities of its natural eruption have been failed. It is preffered to be performed at least 6 months after root apex completion [10]. The duration of this orthodontic treatment varies from 12–36 months depending on a number of factors including the patient's age, crowding, the angulation and bucco-palatal position of the tooth, its distance from the occlusal plane and the periodontal health [8]. If the inclination of the canine is greater than 45 degrees in relation to the midline then the prognosis for alignment worsens. The further the canine needs to be moved then the poorer the diagnosis for a successful outcome. Either the tooth should not be anyklosed or the root not be dilaserated [60]. Correct root positioning and a good buccal overlap is necessary for a stable result [90]. The prognosis is worse in older patients than in young patients, thus early diagnosis is essential [42]. The upper age limits suggested for successful alignment of an unerupted canine are 16 and 20 years [57]. In contrast Nieri et al. [8] found the position of the impacted canines closer to the physiologic position of the dental arch in older subjects which affected the treatment duration positively.

Combined forced eruption treatment approach is performed at three phases [8].

- surgical exposure of the impacted tooth

- placement of an attachment to the tooth

- application of orthodontic mechanics to align the impacted teeth

Mostly two approaches are recommended in regards to the timing of attachment placement: [21]

1. The first method is a two-step approach. Firstly the canine is surgically uncovered and the area is packed with a surgical dressing in order to avoid filling in of tissues around the tooth. After wound healing within 3-8 weeks, the pack is removed, then an attachment is bonded on the impacted tooth [91]. This approach is preferred when bleeding compromises attachment bonding [92].

2. The second method is a one-step approach, in which, the attachment is placed on the tooth at the time of surgical exposure. This method is especially recommended for palatally impacted teeth which aids the clinician to visualize and better control the direction of tooth movement when traction force is applied.

8.3. Surgical exposure of the impacted tooth

During surgical exposure of an impacted tooth, only enough bone should be removed for the placement of a bonded bracket [21]. Excision of tissues must be carefully performed and the cementoenamel junction (CEJ) should not be intentionally exposed. If done incorrectly, the unerupted tooth may be left with inadequate keratinized tissue. Therefore the use of electrosurgical or laser techniques is contraindicated for surgical exposure. These instruments are designed for removal of hard and soft tissues, the contact of the instrument to the tooth may lead to permanent damage of either type of tissue and/or devitalization of the tooth [20].

Main indicator of the treatment success of impacted maxillary canines is related with the final periodontal outcome [49]. In earlier methods, radical bone was removed during surgical exposure and all bony obstacles were removed to provide an easier path for tooth eruption. Literature shows that the most serious periodontal damage is loss of supporting bone which is associated with more heavy surgical procedures involving exposure of the tooth underneath the cementoenamel junction (CEJ) [93]. Therefore exposure of the CEJ was a critical variable and special attention has to be given during surgery or when placing a wire lasso with or without a gold chain.

Classification and treatment techniques will be presented in detail according to the position of impacted maxillary canines:

8.4. Palatal versus labial impactions

The incidence rate of palatal impaction is at least 3:1 [94] and up to 6:l when compared to labial impaction [95]. Labial impactions generally have a more favorable vertical angulation whereas palatally impacted canines are more often inclined in a horizontal/oblique direction [21]. Jacoby [32] determined that 85% of palatally impacted canines had enough space in the dental arch where as only 17% of the labially unerupted maxillary canines appeared to have sufficient space for eruption. Consequently he claimed arch length deficiency as a primary causative factor for labially impacted canines.

Ectopic labially positioned canines may erupt frequently high in the sulcus or alveolar ridge on their own without either surgical exposure or orthodontic treatment. Contrarily, palatally impacted canines seldom erupt without intervention due to the thickness of the palatal cortical bone and also the dense, thick, and resistant palatal mucosa [21].

8.5. Management of labially impacted canines

Labially impacted maxillary canine is often positioned high in the alveolar bone and erupts through the alveolar mucosa. It has been emphasized that labially impacted canines are more challenging to manage without the occurrence of adverse periodontal problems. Therefore, special attention has to be given to surgical technique, marginal gingival placement, control of inflammation, magnitude of force, atraumatic surgery, and proper gingival attachment [96].

Generally 3 techniques are used for uncovering a labially impacted maxillary canine [31]:

i.   excisional uncovering (gingivectomy)

ii.   apically positioned flap

iii.   closed eruption techniques

The orthodontist should guide the surgeon properly to select an appropriate technique. If the correct uncovering technique is chosen, the eruption process can be simplified, resulting in a predictably stable and esthetic result. Four criteria should be evaluated by the orthodontist in order to determine the appropriate method for uncovering the tooth before referring a patient for surgical exposure. First, the labiolingual position of the impacted canine crown should be determined. If the tooth is impacted labially, then any of the 3 techniques could be performed, since there is usually little or any bone covering the crown of the impacted canine. However, if the tooth is impacted in the center of the alveolus, an excisional approach and an apically positioned flap are usually more difficult to perform, for large amount of bone removal might be required from the labial surface of the crown.

The second criterion to evaluate is the vertical position of the tooth relative to the mucogingival junction. Any of the 3 techniques can be chosen to uncover the tooth, if most of the canine crown is positioned coronal to the mucogingival junction. (Figure 2)

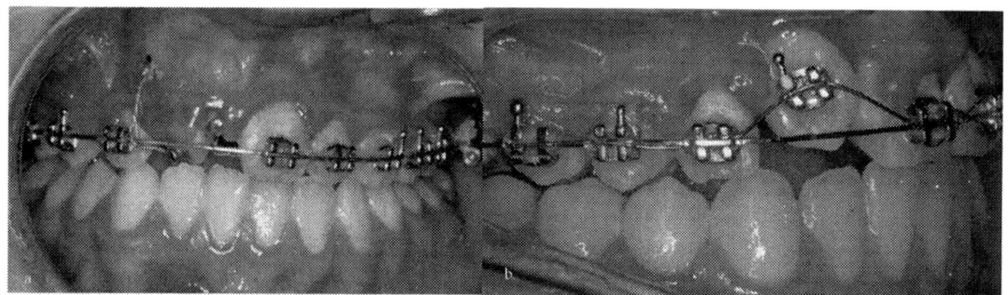

Figure 2. Closed flap technique was performed for the maxillary canine to erupt and orthodontic traction was applied to align the canine into the lateral position.

When the canine crown is positioned apical to the mucogingival junction, the most appropriate approach is the closed eruption technique for it would provide adequate gingiva over the crown and prevent reintrusion of the tooth in the long term [97]. Excisional technique would be inappropriate, because it would result in no gingiva over the labial surface of the tooth after eruption has completed. An apically positioned flap would either be inappropriate since it would cause possible reintrusion and instability of the crown of the tooth after orthodontic treatment [98].

The third criterion to evaluate is the amount of attached gingiva in the area of the impacted canine. The creation and preservation of the band of attached gingiva is very critical for periodontal health in the management of labially impacted teeth [12]. The only technique that predictably would produce more gingiva is an apically positioned flap, if there were insufficient gingiva in the area of the canine. Otherwise, mucogingival recession and alveolar bone loss may occur. Any of the 3 techniques could be selected, if there were sufficient gingiva to provide at least 2 to 3 mm of attached gingiva over the canine crown after it had been erupted [31].

The final criterion to evaluate is the mesiodistal position of the canine crown. An apically positioned flap should be preferred if the crown were positioned mesially and over the root of the lateral incisor, since it could be difficult to move the tooth through the alveolus unless it was completely exposed. In this situation, closed eruption or excisional uncovering generally would not be recommended [31].

There are conflicting reports in the literature regarding apically positioned flap technique and closed eruption technique [64,98-100]. Unfortunately, some reports and studies have failed to differentiate that the "open" technique is different from an apically positioned flap approach [96]. There is conclusive evidence that an open eruption approach through nonkeratinized gingival should be avoided [98]. The absence of an adequate band of attached gingiva around the erupting canine may cause inflammation of the periodontium. Vanarsdall and Corn [99] emphasized that it is risky to move teeth in the presence of inflammation. In addition Caprioglio et al. [101] stated that it is necessary to use conservative surgical techniques and orthodontic systems mimicking the natural pattern of eruption in order to achieve adequate periodontal status.

An apically repositioned flap or closed eruption techniques through keratinized gingival tissue are recommended [102]. If the tissue is too thin to be dissected as a partial thickness graft, laterally repositioned pedicle graft, a free gingival graft can be performed initially to increase the thickness of keratinized gingiva. After approximately 30 to 60 days or complete healing of the grafted tissue, the tooth may be exposed, bonded, and orthodontic traction might be applied.

Vernette et al. [98] compared the esthetic and periodontal results between the apically repositioned flap and the closed eruption techniques of surgically uncovering labially impacted maxillary teeth (incisors and canines). They have concluded that periodontal attachment differences between uncovered and contralateral teeth were not clinically significant in either the apically positioned flap or closed-eruption groups. However labially impacted maxillary anterior teeth uncovered with an apically positioned flap technique have more unesthetic sequalae than those with closed-eruption technique. Also adverse effects were detected treated with apically positioned flap technique such as increased clinical crown length, width of attached tissue, gingival scarring, and intrusive relapse since the mucosal attachment tends to pull the crown of the tooth apically.

However in literature the disadvantages of closed eruption technique were reported as increase in treatment time, additional surgical procedures, diminished control of tooth movement, as well as adverse periodontal responses [21,96]. Advantages of the apically positioned graft are that it is minimally invasive, provides controlled tooth movement (even high in the vestibular depth), prevents cystic follicles, decreases treatment time. Also it prevents ankylosis if bonding is delayed for 1 week [96]. It was reported that only 4 to 5 months was enough to erupt labially impacted teeth into the arch with apically positioned grafts even in severe cases [103].

In the review article of Vanarshdal [96] it was concluded that adverse responses have not been determined with labially uncovered teeth with grafts that have been left open and activated a week later. Surgical exposure with careful attention to the periodontal tissues and proper orthodontic alignment without intentional closing over with soft tissue could provide a more predictable result for patients. It was also emphasized that the pedicle graft is necessary on the labial of the maxilla. The gingivally repositioned procedure as described earlier [99] didn' t create a compromised periodontal outcome, and treated teeth were indistinguishable from untreated sides Vanarshdal [96] stated that closed eruption technique was not superior to apically repositioned flap technique as a result of this evidence based data.

Apart from these comman used three techniques explained above, the application of tunnel technique might be indicated in the following situations: [8]

i.   if persistent deciduous canines exists with impacted canines or space available in the dental arch and

ii.   feasibility of direct traction of the impacted canine to the center of the alveolar ridge as assessed on the diagnostic radiographic records to reproduce the physiologic eruption pattern of the canine.

8.6. Management of the palatally impacted canines

The most common impaction encountered by orthodontists is the palatal impaction of maxillary canines (95-Stellzig et al., 1994). With palatal impactions it is critical to recognize that the entire palate is covered with specialized mucosa and a graft is not necessary [104]. The most commonly used surgical methods for exposing the impacted canine are: [59]

1. open surgical exposure and allowing for natural eruption

2. open surgical exposure and packing with subsequent bonding of an auxillary

3. closed surgical exposure with the placement of an auxiliary attachment intraoperatively.

The first method is most appropriate if the canine has the correct inclination and will then erupt spontaneously. Schmidt [105] suggested to uncover palatally impacted canines early, during the mixed dentition in order to encourage autonomous eruption, without orthodontic intervention. They have reported that the overall treatment time is reduced with superior periodontal and aesthetic results since the bone levels and attachment levels improved on the canine and lateral incisor and also little to no root resorption occured on the lateral incisors.

Kokich and Mathews [100] also recommended earlier timing for uncovering palatally impacted canines before starting orthodontic treatment. In some cases, surgical exposure could be performed during the late mixed dentition. First a full-thickness mucoperiosteal flap is elevated, then all bone over the crown is removed down to the cementoenamel junction. Following the flap is returned, and a hole is made through the gingival flap. If the tooth is highly positioned in the palate a dressing might be placed over the exposed area in the flap. Although it has been noted that autonomous eruption occurs within 6 to 9 months postoperatively, there is currently no report in the literature to support this statement [106]. After the canines erupt to the occlusal level an attachment could be bonded for the further orthodontic treatment.

The second approach is the "open window" eruption technique in which a flap is elevated and enough amount of bone is removed to expose the tip of the impacted crown to be bonded. The flap is then repositoned and sutured with a small "window" cut into the flap of the palatal soft tissue, covering the embedded crown packed with surgical dressing. To provide a good periodontal prognosis, a special attention should be given in maintaining the attached gingiva on the impacted tooth. One week later postoperatively the pack is removed and an attachment is bonded with subsequent traction using a fixed appliance. There is some evidence that the periodontal status may be compromized [107]. (Figure 3)

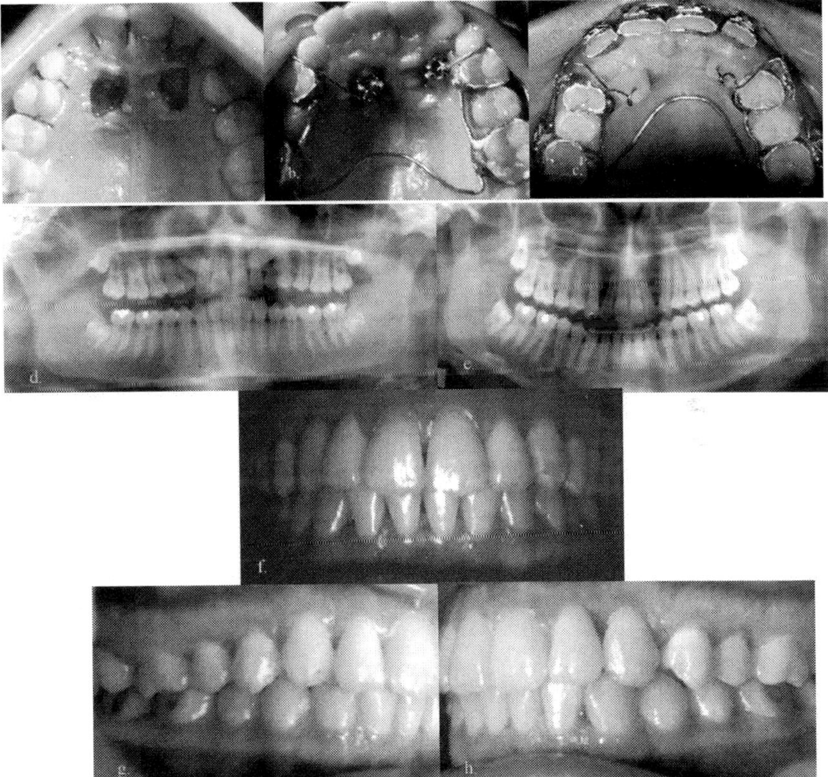

Figure 3. Bilateral palatally impacted maxillary canines were uncovered by open surgical technique, orthodontic traction was performed by ballista springs. Alignment of bilateral maxillary canines lasted 4,5 years.

The third option is the closed eruption technique. If a canine is associated with severe resorption of the root of the incisor, an open exposure is not indicated since it endangers the vitality and existence of the incisor. In such a case a closed eruption technique would provide both teeth a vital state [108]. In this technique sufficient space should be created before the surgical exposure. Usually uncovering a palatally impacted canine occurs after the first 6 to 9 months of orthodontic alignment of the maxillary dentition. In this technique firstly a mucoperiostal flap is reflected and a minimum of bone is removed to reveal the follicle,which is opened at the most superficial point only. Bone is not cleared away from the neck of the tooth, nor more of the follicular tissue than is essential for bonding, and certainly not down to the cementoenamel junction [109]. A small eyelet, threaded with soft twisted ligature wire of 0.012-in gauge, is then bonded while hemostasis is maintained. The flap is then sutured fully back to cover the entire wound and exposed area, with the twisted ligature wire drawn through the flap at a point strategically placed to permit traction in the direction that will have been confirmed when the orthodontist actually sees the tooth in situ. Generally, orthodontic traction begins soon after the surgery towards to the edentulous site [109].

On the other hand if not enough bone is removed then the tooth will not move and orthodontist might suspect from anyklosis. However the incidence of ankylosed maxillary canines is low [100]. In the case of insufficient bone removal over the impacted tooth, the tooth will not be able to resorb the bone over the crown efficiently for the dental follicle is deflated and removed. When a force is applied the enamel of the impacted crown comes into contact with the bone however there are no cells in the enamel to resorb the bone. Therefore resorption will eventually occur slowly through pressure necrosis [31].

Closed eruption technique is a more conservative approach however if bond failure occurs then re-exposure is required. Also direct bonding of the impacted canine during surgery may cause soft tissue injury due to the acid etching contamination. Becker et al. [108] suggested the use of an eyelet bonded in a mid-buccal position on the crown of the impacted tooth at surgery as these have the highest success rate. Becker and Chausu [109] stated that morbidity is lower in closed eruption approach than for open procedures since healing is faster, postoperative pain is considerably reduced, and postsurgical bleeding is virtually eliminated.

There is a controversy in the literature regarding the periodontal outcome of open or closed surgical exposure and subsequent orthodontic alignment of the palatally displaced canines [110]. It is believed that periodontal health is compromised when the palatal mucosa is excised with open technique [93].) However in a systematic review Parkin et al. [111] found no robust evidence to support one surgical technique over the other.

Also in recent studies [112, 113] evaluating the differences in the periodontal outcomes of palatally displaced canines (PDC) exposed with either an open or a closed surgical technique, no significant differences in post-treatment periodontal status of the canines and adjacent teeth were determined between the techniques. Both treatment methods were found acceptable for treatment of the palatally impacted canine. In addition Smailine et al., [113] 2013 concluded that post-treatment periodontal status and the level of bone support were not dependent on the patients' age at the start of treatment, the duration of treatment, or the initial horizontal and vertical localization of impacted canine.

9. Orthodontic considerations

Orthodontic treatment methodology for impacted canines depends on various factors, such as location of the impacted canine in the dental arch relative to adjacent incisors, the distance from the occlusal plane, canine crown overlaps, canine angulations, the possible presence of ankylosis, root resorption, or dilaceration [100]. Generally, horizontally impacted or ankylosed canines are the most hazardous to manage and have the poorest prognosis [114]. Some of these teeth may need to be extracted. These variables are also used as predictors of the orthodontic treatment duration [100].

Frequently, when the palatally impacted canine is surgically uncovered, only the lingual surface of the tooth is available for bonding attachments. However Becker and coworkers [107] stated that the palatal surface as the poorest bonding surface. The orthodontic force to be applied to the bonded attachment requires careful planning because if an orthodontic force is applied from the adjacent maxillary teeth, it will tend to embed the buccal surface of the crown and may create periodontal problems. In order to prevent this problem, first the tooth should be erupted vertically and once a facial attachment can be bonded, forces should direct the tooth facially [115].

When removal of premolars is planned for the orthodontic treatment, it is advised to delay their extractions until the canine is surgically uncovered and feasibility of moving the impacted canine is insured. However, the premolar has to be removed initially prior to any attempt to move the canine in severely crowded cases. In such a case, the patient or parents should be made aware of the possible complications [21].

During closed-eruption technique, the orthodontist should select mechanics that erupt the tooth through the center of the alveolar ridge. The eruption of the tooth between the alveolar cortical plates prevents bone dehiscence and unfavorable orthodontic and esthetic consequences [49]. The mechanics that draw the tooth labially should be avoided, in order not to produce a bony dehiscence or labial recession of gingival magrin [31].

The impacted tooth under orthodontic traction forces should be periodically checked for excessive mobility or bleeding from gingiva around the tooth. It is important to ensure that periodontal attachment is following the tooth as it is guided into the arch [116]. Furthermore correction of torque, labio-palatal root angulation of the impacted canine should be considered to achieve proper functional occlusion. The bracket on the labial aspect of the canine can be inverted to correct the torque or a mandibular premolar bracket can bonded to the ectopic canine to produce a more negative torque [117].

9.1. Methods of attachment

Wire ligatures, a bracket, a hook, button or an eyelet directly may be attached to the enamel surface after the surgical exposure of the impacted tooth crown [29]. (Figure 2,3) If the canines are deeply impacted, a gold chain may be used that can pass through a long tunnel created between the impacted tooth and the empty socket of the extracted primary canine [118]. A circumferential, dead soft, ligature wire (lasso) passing around the cervical area of the tooth shouldn' t be used as an attachment since too much bone removal is required. This "heavy exposure," may provoke the risk of injuring the adjacent teeth, external root resorption and ankylosis [119]. Celli et al. [120] advocated bonding of two attachments to the impacted canine instead of the classic single one for closed eruption of palatally impacted canines in order to reduce the potential risk of a second surgical operation when the traction attachment comes off.

9.2. Traction methods

Various methods have been used for moving the canine into proper alignment. These include the use of light wires (Figure 2) or springs soldered to a heavy labial or palatal base wire, mousetrap loops, K-9 spring, ballista loops (Figure 3c), Kilroy I, II springs [31, 121, 122]. Vardimon et al. [123] recommended the use of magnets to treat impacted canines on the basis of a less invasive surgical procedure, effective forces at short distances, and controlled spatial guidance. (Figure 4) With the introduction of new orthodontic materials such as elastic threads, elastometric chains, and nickeltitanium springs, the orthodontist has a wider choice of materials and also greater control of the force magnitude and direction.

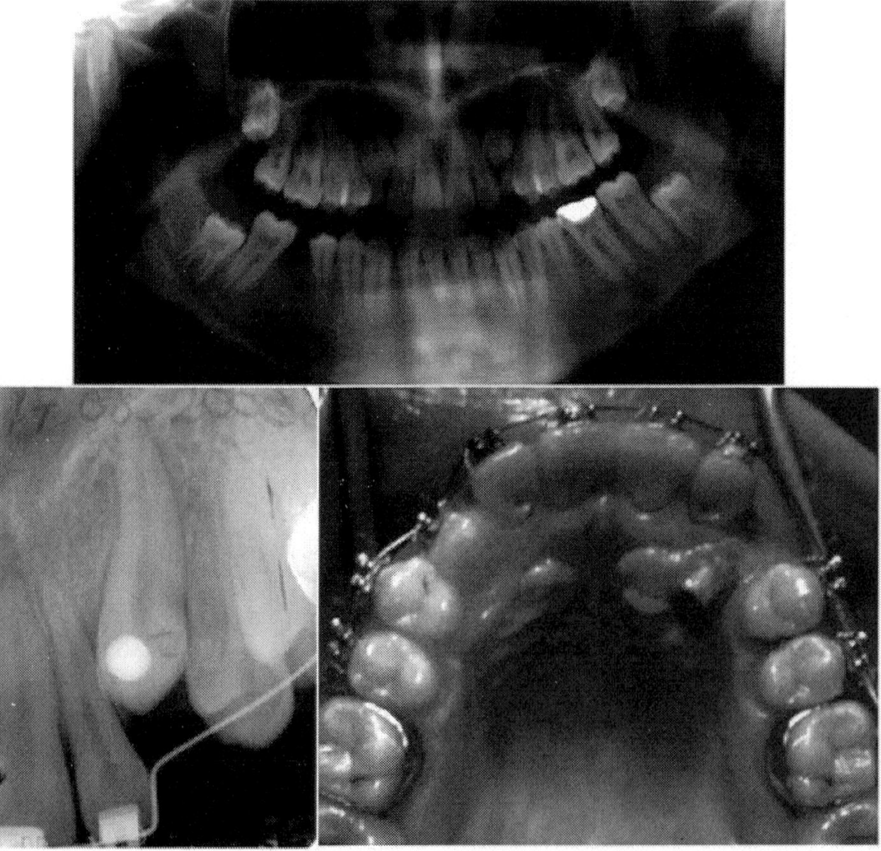

Figure 4. Orthodontic traction of bilateral impacted canines with the use of magnets. Right maxillary canine closer to the surface could be erupted with magnets. The left canine also moved closer along the top of the arch, however the patient discontinued his treatment.

An efficient way to make impacted canines erupt is to use closed-coil springs with eyelets, as long as no obstacles impede the path of the canine. If the canine is in close proximity to the incisor roots and a buccally directed force is applied, then it will contact the roots of adjacent teeth and may cause damage. (Figure 5) In addition, the canine position may not improve due to the root obstacle. Therefore regardless of the material used, the direction of the applied force should initially move the impacted tooth away from the roots of the neighboring teeth. In addition, the following is recommended: [21]

1. Initially maxillary arch should be levelled and aligned until a rigid rectangular arch can be inserted prior to the surgical exposure of the impacted tooth and application of traction forces [115].

2. Enough space should either be available in the arch or should be created for the impacted tooth;

3. In order to preserve the space created, either continuously tie the teeth mesially and distally to the canine or place a close coiled spring on the arch wire;

4. The eruption path might require the fabrication of auxiliaries numerous times due to anatomic obstructions during the traction process to redirect forces [115].

5. The use of light forces to move the impacted tooth, no more than 2 oz (60 g);

6. The arch wire should have enough stiffness, such as.018 ×.022, to resist deformation against traction forces during canine extrusion (Figure 2). The added stiffness of the arch wire will diminsh the undesirable "rollercoaster" effect caused by intrusion of the neighboring anchor teeth as a reaction to the deflection of a lighter and hence more flexible arch wire. Therefore, the magnitude of the force applied should not deflect the arch wire.

Orthodontic traction on the impacted tooth should be applied with light forces (20 to 30 g). In most of the cases, the root tip of the impacted canine is usually in a good position, so a tipping movement (light movement) is appropriate to move the crown toward the dental arch. The combined effects of "light" surgical exposure, "light" orthodontic movements, and "light" orthodontic forces are beneficial to the future periodontal health of the tooth since they minimize the loss of alveolar bone support and potential injury to the tooth during traction. However "heavy movement" such as torque during the traction cause more bone loss [21].

Fixed or removable appliances can be used for the traction of impacted tooth. However there are certain disadvantages of removable appliances such as the need for patient cooperation, limited control of tooth movement, and the inability to treat complex malocclusions [21] therefore only in cases with multiple missing teeth Hawley-type appliances might be used which transfer anchorage demands to the palatal vault and the alveolar ridge [124].

Most techniques have used the maxillary arch as anchorage for traction, which may be unsuitable in many clinical situations [94]. In cases in which the impacted canine is situated palatal to the lateral incisor, firstly an attempt should be made to move the canine away from lateral incisor before moving the impacted tooth toward the dental arch. In this situation if the desired forces cannot be applied from within the maxillary arch, mandibular arch might be

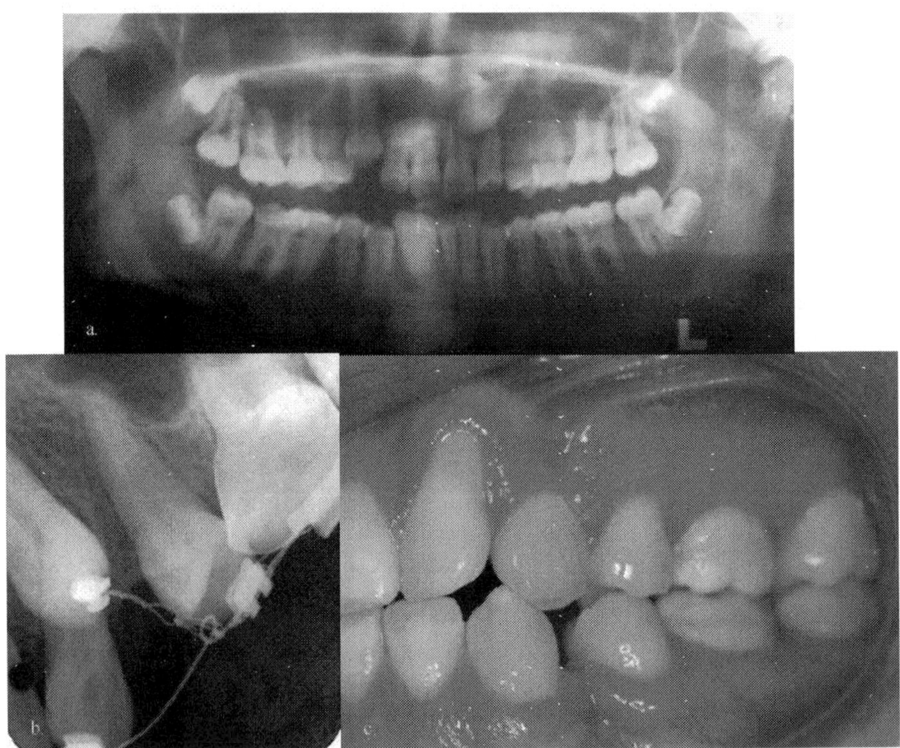

Figure 5. A buccally directed traction of a palatally impacted maxillary canine resulted in the buccal movement of the adjacent lateral root due to the close approximity and gingival recession was observed 10 years after treatment.

used as a source of anchorage. A mandibular fixed lingual arch with a vertical hook can be used for this purpose. Elastics are engaged in these vertical hooks and to the attachment on the impacted teeth for the required traction. In addition directional forces can be used by applying elastics. The main disadvantege of mandibular anchorage is the difficulty encountered in controlling the magnitude and direction of the applied forces because of the mobile mandibular arch [115].

Recently mini-screws have been proved to be reliable and convenient skeletal anchorage devices in the management of unerupted canines. Their mechanical resistance was found suitable for the initial orthodontic traction of these teeth. Mini-screws are placed in the alveolar process to improve the initial angulation of impacted canine teeth. Following soft tissue healing around the exposed tooth, mechanical traction can be activated with a nickel-titanium closed-coil spring exerting gentle forces 0.5–0.8 N (50–80 g) of force. The main advantage of this method is that the maxillary arch should not be bracketed until the canine has begun to move and ankylosis can be ruled out [125].

Poggio et al. [126] studied the interradicular anatomy of 25 patients with volumetric tomographic imaging. On the palatal side, the most available bone was determined between the second premolar and first molar whereas on the buccal side between the two premolars. These areas were found convenient for the clinical application of a mini-screw if extrusion of a palatally impacted canine is planned. On the buccal side less bone was determined between the second premolar and first molar. On the palatal side, the interseptal distance between the two molars was either less, yet still sufficient.

Impacted teeth tend to respond much later in adults than do those in children. Chaushu et al. [127] advised the placement of a temporary anchorage device in the palate at the time of closed exposure and the immediate application of elastic traction for several months since they have experienced failure of teeth to erupt despite the application of traction in patients in their fourth and fifth decades of life. They place orthodontic appliances if positive signs of movement are observed.

9.3. Retention considerations and long term follow-up of impacted canines

Treatment of impacted tooth is almost always a clinical challenge. Holistic treatment planning, prudent flap design, coupled with forced eruption using light extrusive forces, periodontal health and functional occlusion are central to achieving the desired long-term results.

Becker et al. [128] evaluated the posttreatment alignment of the impacted canines in patients who had completed their orthodontic treatment. They observed an increased incidence of rotations or spacings on the "impacted" side in 17.4% of the cases, whereas on the control side the incidence was only 8.7%. The control side had ideal alignment twice as often as did the impacted side.

Capriogli et al. [101] evaluated the long-term (4.6 years) periodontal response of palatally impacted maxillary canines aligned using a closed-flap surgical technique in association with a codified orthodontic traction system. No damage to periodontium was detected in the long-term.

Woloshyn et al. [129] evaluated the posttreatment changes nearly 4 years after treatment and compared the differences in the periodontal and pulpal status, root length, and tooth alignment between the side of the forced-erupted ectopically canine and the contralateral side. The probing attachment level was found lower on the mesial and distal aspect of the previously impacted canines, also the roots of the adjacent teeth were found shorter. The incidance of pulpal obliteration was 21% in the previously impacted canines. Significant posttreatment changes such as intrusion, lingual displacement, rotation, and discoloration was determined in 40% of the previously impacted teeth where as 91% had a normal appearance on the contralateral side.

A fiberotomy or a bonded fixed retainer is suggested to prevent rotational relapse, after the completion of the desired movements and often before the appliances are removed. Removing a "halfmoon-shaped wedge" of tissue from the lingual side of the canine might intercept lingual drift after correction of palatally impacted canines [130].

D'Amico et al. [131] reported the adverse effects of the orthodontic-surgical treatment for impacted maxillary canines in the long term conducted in a sample of 61 cases. 6.5% of the patients were dissatisfied with the esthetic results, whereas the orthodontist estimated the results as good in only 57% of the cases. Canine guidance was detected less frequently on the working side during lateral movements in previously impacted canines due to the significant difference in their inclination compared to normally erupted ones.

9.4. Frequent complications observed with unerupted teeth

Surgical exposure of the impacted tooth and the complex orthodontic mechanisms that are applied to align the impacted tooth into the arch may lead to deleterious consequences for the supporting structures of the tooth, such as displacement and devitalization, ankylosis or loss of vitality, recurrent pain, cystic degeneration, invasive servical root resorption, external root resorption of the canine and adjacent teeth. Furthermore loss of periodontal bone support, gingival recession, sensitivity problems or combinations of these factors may be observed [129].(Figure 5) Most of these risks can be prevented with proper management of periodontal tissues and timing of care. These problems can result in prolonged treatment time, esthetic deformities and often the loss of teeth.

If no movement of the impacted canine is observed, this may be as a result of single or combination of the following reasons: [132]

- inappropriate positional diagnosis of the impacted teeth and its relationship with the roots of the adjacent teeth which leads to incorrect direction of traction

- a lack of considerably anchorage requirement will lead to inefficient mechanotherapy and unnecassarily longer treatment

- anyklosis might have afflicted the impacted tooth either a priori or as the result of the earlier surgical or the orthodontic maneuers.

- scar tissue might have blocked the wire chain, [133]

If, the tooth does not show clear evidence of movement after six months of orthodontic force application, a re-evaluation is necessary. Ankylosis, one of the major complications associated with impacted canines, can rarely be detected based on clinical and conventional radiographic examinations however CBCT provides a better diagnosis of the area of ankylosis [134].

In the recent study of Koutzoglou and Kostaki [135] evidence of an association between exposure technique and ankylosis was determined. The percentage of ankylosis was 3.5% in the open technique and 14.5% in the closed technique. They have defined anyklosis as impacted canines being immobilized a priori or during traction, due to all the possible causes that could contribute to immobilization, such as all types of external tooth resorption and other known or unknown factors. Additionally, they found a evidence that the grade of impaction and the patient's age are significant predictors of ankylosis.

Traditionally, once a tooth becomes ankylosed, surgical luxation has been the treatment of choice [136]. Although orthodontic light forces are applied immediately after luxation to prevent reankylosis, ankylosis often occurs again [137]. Another viable treatment option for ankylosed or dilacerated maxillary canines is apicotomy proposed by Puricelli [138] in 1987. An apicotomy is a guided fracture of a canine root apex performed with a small chisel followed by orthodontic traction of the canine crown. Puricelli's data [138, 139] showed that in 29 patients who had the procedure, 26 procedures were successful and 3 failed.

Becker and Chausu [109] stated that invasive cervical root resorption is the cause of many failed impacted teeth, rather than the knee-jerk and usually unproven application of the label "ankylosis." It is difficult to diagnose on a radiograph, yet, as the lesion grows, bone is usually deposited in the depth of the resorption lacunae, and then the tooth will no longer respond to extrusive traction [140]. Radical surgery extending down to the cementoenamel junction is likelihood of this possible sequel.

Becker et al. [132] reported that repeat surgery was required for 62.9% of the impacted canines in which corrective treatment was started, mostly to redirect the ligature wires with the guidance of the 3-dimensional imaging. If orthodontic traction fails other treatment options should be considered. Prosthetic replacement might be performed yet preparation of the adjacent, usually healthy teeth for a conventional fixed bridge is far from ideal. Implant placement would be another option that generally requires extraction of the impacted tooth. However this causes a bony defect which must be bone-grafted. Orthodontic closure of the gap might also be considered but it results in asymmetry in unilateral cases [125].

10. Conclusions

The management of impacted canines is important in terms of esthetics and function and, requires a qualified experience of a number of clinicians. If patients are evaluated and treated appropriately, then the frequency of ectopic eruption and subsequent impaction of the maxillary canine can be reduced. Various surgical and orthodontic techniques may be used to uncover impacted maxillary canines related to its position. Accurate localization, conservative management of the soft tissues, selection of appropriate surgical approach, rigid anchorage unit, and the direction of the orthodontic traction are the important factors for the successful management of impacted canines.

Author details

Belma Işık Aslan* and Neslihan Üçüncü

*Address all correspondence to: belmaslan2003@yahoo.com

Gazi University, Faculty of Dentistry, Department of Orthodontics, Ankara, Turkey

References

[1] Lindauer SJ, Rubenstein LK, Hang WM, Andersen WC, Isaacson RJ. Canine Impaction Identified Early with Panoramic Radiographs. The Journal of American Dental Association 1992;123(3) 91–92.

[2] Litsas G, Acar A. A Review of Early Displaced Maxillary Canines: Etiology, Diagnosis and Interceptive Treatment. The Open Dentistry Journal 2011; 5: 39-47.

[3] Brin I, Becker A, Shalhav M. Position of the Maxillary Permanent Canine in Relation to Anomalous or Missing Lateral Incisors: a Population Study. European Journal of Orthodontics 1986; 8(1) 12-16.

[4] Chu FC, Li TK, Lui VK, Newsome PR, Chow RL, Cheung LK. Prevalence of Impacted Teeth and Associated Pathologies-a Radiographic Study of the Hong Kong Chinese Population. Hong Kong Medical Journal 2003; 9(3) 158-163.

[5] Thilander B, Myrberg N. The Prevalence of Malocclusion in Swedish School Children. Scandinavian Journal of Dental Research 1973; 81(1) 12-21.

[6] Johnston WD. Treatment of Palatally Impacted Canine Teeth. American Journal of Orthodontics 1969; 56(6) 589-596.

[7] Ericson S, Kurol J. Resorption of Incisors After Ectopic Eruption of Maxillary Canines. A CT study. Angle Orthodontist 2000; 70(6) 415-423.

[8] Nieri M, Crescini A, Rotundo R, Baccetti T, Cortellini P, Pini Prato GP. Factors Affecting the Clinical Approach to Impacted Maxillary Canines: a Bayesian Network Analysis. American Journal of Orthodontics and Dentofacial Orthopedics 2010; 137(6) 755-762.

[9] Ericson S, Kurol J. Radiographic Examination of Ectopically Erupting Maxillary Canines. American Journal of Orthodontics and Dentofacial Orthopedics 1988; 91(6) 483-492.

[10] Coulter J, Richardson A. Normal Eruption of the Maxillary Canine Quantified in Three Dimensions. European Journal of Orthodontics 1997; 19(2) 171–183.

[11] Van Der Linden PGM. Transition of the Human Dentition. Monograph, Craniofacial Growth Series. Ann Arbor, MI, Center For Human Growth And Development: University Of Michigan;1982

[12] Becker A. The Orthodontic Treatment Of Impacted Teeth 2nd Ed. Jerusalem: Informa Healthcare; 2007.

[13] Moyers RE, Van Der Linden FP, Riolo ML, Mcnamara Jr. Standards of Human Occlusal Development. Monograph 5, Craniofacial Growth Series. Ann Arbor, MI, Center For Human Growth And Development: The University Of Michigan; 1976.

[14] Nanda SK. The Developmental Basis of Occlusion And Malocclusion. Chicago, IL: Quintessence Publishing; 1983.

[15] Roberts-Harry D, Sandy J. Orthodontics. Part 10: Impacted Teeth. British Dental Journal 2004; 196(6) 319–327.

[16] Brand RW, Isselhard DE. Anatomy of Orofacial Structures. 3rd Ed. St. Louis, MO: CV Mosby; 1986.

[17] Hurme VO. Ranges of Normalcy in the Eruption of Permanent Teeth. Jounal of Dentistry for Children 1949; 16(2) 11-15.

[18] Wise GE, King GJ. Mechanisms of Tooth Eruption and Orthodontic Tooth Movement. Journal of Dental Research 2008; 87(5) 414-434.

[19] Suri L, Gagari E, Vastardis H. Delayed Tooth Eruption: Pathogenesis, Diagnosis, and Treatment. A Literature Review. American Journal of Orthodontics and Dentofacial Orthopedics 2004; 126(4) 432-445.

[20] Ngan P, Hornbrook R, Weaver B. Early Timely Management of Ectopically Erupting Maxillary Canines. Seminars in Orthodontics 2005; 11: 152–163.

[21] Bishara SE. Clinical Management of Impacted Maxillary Canines. Seminars in Orthodontics 1998; 4(2) 87-98.

[22] Yawaka Y, Kaga M, Osanai M, Fukui A, Oguchi H. Delayed Eruption of Premolars with Periodontitis of Primary Predecessors and a Cystic Lesion: A Case Report. International Journal of Paediatric Dentistry 2002; 12(1) 53-60.

[23] Acquavella FJ. Delayed Eruption. Why? The New York State Dental Journal 1965; 31(10) 448-449.

[24] Tomizawa M, Yonemochi H, Kohno M, Noda T. Unilateral Delayed Eruption of Maxillary Permanent First Molars: Four Case Reports. Pediatric Dentistry 1998; 20(1) : 53-56.

[25] Katz J, Guelmann M, Barak S. Hereditary Gingival Fibromatosis with Distinct Dental, Skeletal and Developmental Abnormalities.Pediatric Dentistry 2002; 24(3) 253-256.

[26] Sekletov GA. Supercomplect Retained Tooth is the Cause of Delayed Eruption of the Upper Central Left Incisor. Therapy Stomatologiia 2001; 80(4) 66-68.

[27] Proffit WR, Vig KWL. Primary Failure of Eruption: A Possible Cause of Posterior Open-Bite. American Journal of Orthodontics and Dentofacial Orthopedics 1981;80(2) 173-190.

[28] Raghoebar GM, Boering G, Vissink A, Stegenga B. Eruption Disturbances of Permanent Molars: A Review. Journal of Oral Pathology & Medicine 1991; 20(4) 159-166.

[29] Bishara SE. Impacted Maxillary Canines: A Review. American Journal of Orthodontics and Dentofacial Orthopedics 1992; 101(2) 159-171.

[30] Pirinen S, Arte S, Apajalahti S. Palatal Displacement of Canine is Genetic and Related to Congenital Absence of Teeth. Journal of Dental Research 1996; 75(10) 1742-1746.

[31] Kokich VG. Surgical and Orthodontic Management of Impacted Maxillary Canines. American Journal of Orthodontics and Dentofacial Orthopedics 2004; 126(3) 278-283.

[32] Jacoby H. The Etiology Of Maxillary Canine Impactions. American Journal of Orthodontics 1983; 84(2) 125–132.

[33] Al-Nimri K, Gharaibeh T. Space Conditions and Dental and Occlusal Features in Patients with Palatally Impacted Maxillary Canines: An Aetiological Study. European Journal of Orthodontics 2005; 27(5) 461–465.

[34] Mcconnell TL, Hoffman DL, Forbes DP, Jensen EK, Wientraub NH. Maxillary Canine Impaction in Patients With Transverse Maxillary Deficiency. Journal of Dentistry for Children 1996; 63(3) 190–195.

[35] Langberg BJ, Peck S. Adequacy of Maxillary Dental Arch Width In Patients with Palatally Displaced Canines. American Journal of Orthodontics and Dentofacial Orthopedics 2000; 118(2) 220–223.

[36] Peck S, Peck L, Kataja M. Site-Specificity of Tooth Maxillary Agenesis in Subjects with Canine Malpositions. Angle Orthodontist 1996; 66(6) 473-476.

[37] Peck S, Peck L, Kataja M. Concomitant Occurrence of Canine Malposition and Tooth Agenesis: Evidence of Orofacial Genetic Fields. American Journal of Orthodontics and Dentofacial Orthopedics 2002; 122(6) 657-660.

[38] Sacerdoti R, Baccetti T. Dentoskeletal Features Associated With Unilateral Or Bilateral Palatal Displacement Of Maxillary Canines. Angle Orthodontist 2004; 74(6) 725-32.

[39] Shafer WG, Hine MK, Levy BM, Editors. A Textbook Of Oral Pathology. 2nd Ed. Philadelphia: WB Saunders; 1963.

[40] Suri L, Gagari E, Vastardis H. Delayed Tooth Eruption: Pathogenesis, Diagnosis, and Treatment. A Literature Review. American Journal of Orthodontics and Dentofacial Orthopedics 2004; 126(4) 432-445.

[41] Moss JP. The Unerupted Canine. The Dental Practitioner and Dental Record 1972; 22(6) 241-248.

[42] Ericson S, Kurol J. Longitudinal Study and Analysis of Clinical Supervision of Maxillary Canine Eruption. Community Dent Oral Epidemiol Community Dentistry and Oral Epidemiology 1986; 14(3) 172-176.

[43] Ericson S, Kurol J: Radiographic Assessment Of Maxillary Canine Eruption In Children with Clinical Signs of Eruption Disturbances. European Journal of Orthodontics 1981; 8(3) 133-140.

[44] Williams BHJ. Diagnosis and Prevention of Maxillary Cuspid Impaction. Angle Orthodontist 1981; 51(1) 30-40.

[45] Bishara SE. Clinical Management of Impacted Maxillary Canines. Seminars in Orthodontics 1998; 4(2) 87-98.

[46] Langland OE, Francis SH, Langlois RD. Atlas Of Special Technics in Dental Radiology. In: Textbook of Dental Radiology. Springfield, IL: Charles C. Thomas Publishes; 1984.

[47] Ericson S, Kurol J. Radiographic Examination of Ectopically Erupting Maxillary Canines. American Journal of Orthodontics and Dentofacial Orthopedics 1987; 91(6) 483-492.

[48] Turk MH, Katzenell J. Panoramic Localization. Oral Surgery, Oral Medicine and Oral Pathology 1970; 29(2) 212-215.

[49] Crescini A, Nieri M, Buti J, Baccetti T, Pini Prato GP. Pre-Treatment Radiographic Features for the Periodontal Prognosis of Treated Impacted Canines. Journal of Clinical Periodontology 2007; 34(7) 581-587.

[50] Liu DG, Zhang WL, Zhang ZY, Wu YT, Ma XC. Localization of Impacted Maxillary Canines and Observation of Adjacent Incisor Resorption with Cone-Beam Computed Tomography. Oral Surgery, Oral Medicine and Oral Pathology, Oral Radiology and Endodontics 2008; 105(1) 91-98.

[51] Boeddinghaus R, Whyte A. Current Concepts In Maxillofacial Imaging. European Journal of Radiology 2008; 66(3) 396-418.

[52] Alqerban A, Jacobs R, Keirsbilck P, Aly M, Swinnen S, Fieuws S, Willems G. The Effect of Using CBCT In the Diagnosis of Canine Impaction and Its Impact on the Orthodontic Treatment Outcome. Journal of Orthodontic Science. 2014; 3(2) 34–40.

[53] Wriedt S, Jaklin J, Al-Nawas B, Wehrbein H. Impacted Upper Canines: Examination and Treatment Proposal Based On 3D Versus 2D Diagnosis. Journal of Orofacial Orthopedics 2011; 73(1) 28-40.

[54] Alqerban A, Jacobs R, Lambrechts P, Loozen G, Willems G. Root Resorption of the Maxillary Lateral Incisor Caused by Impacted Canine: A Literature Review. Clinical Oral Investigations 2009; 13(3) 247-255.

[55] Oberoi S, Knueppel S. Three-Dimensional Assessment of Impacted Canines and Root Resorption Using Cone Beam Computed Tomography. Oral Surgery Oral Medicine Oral Pathology and Oral Radiology 2012; 113(2) 260-267.

[56] Taylor RW. Eruptive Abnormalities In Orthodontic Treatment. Seminars in Orthodontics 1998; 4(2) 79-86.

[57] Mc Sherry PF. The Assessment of and Treatment Options for the Burried Maxillary Canine. Dental Update 1996; 23(1) 7-10.

[58] Machen DE. Legal Aspects of Orthodontic Practice:Risk Management Concepts. The Impacted Canine. American Journal of Orthodontics and Dentofacial Orthopedics 1989; 96(3) 270-271.

[59] Mc Sherry PF. The Ectopic Maxillary Canine: A Review. British Journal of Orthodontics 1998; 25(3) 209-216.

[60] Kurol J, Ericson S, Andreasen JO. The Impacted Maxillary Canine. In: Andreasen JO, Kølsen Petersen J, Laskin D (eds.) Textbook And Color Atlas Of Tooth Impactions. Copenhagen: Munksgaard; 1997. p124-164.

[61] Ericson S, Kurol J. Early Treatment of Palatally Erupting Maxillary Canines by Extraction of the Primary Canines. European Journal of Orthodontics 1988; 10(4) 283-295.

[62] Power SM, Short MB. An Investigation into the Response of Palatally Displaced Canines to the Removal of Deciduous Canines and an Assessment of Factors Contributing to a Favourable Eruption. British Journal of Orthodontics 1993; 20(3) 215-223.

[63] Baccetti T, Leonardi M, Armi P. A Randomized Clinical Study of Two Interceptive Approaches to Palatally Displaced Canines. European Journal of Orthodontics 2008; 30(4) 381–385.

[64] Olive RJ. Orthodontic Treatment of Palatally Impacted Maxillary Canines. Australian Journal of Orthodontics 2002; 18(2) 64-70.

[65] Broadbent BH. Ontogenic Development of Occlusion. Angle Orthodontist 1941; 11(4) 223-241.

[66] Baccetti T, Sigler LM, Mcnamara JA. An RCT on Treatment of Palatally Displaced Canines with RME and/or a Transpalatal Arch. European Journal of Orthodontics 2011; 33(6) 601–607.

[67] Puricelli E, Morganti MA, Azambuja HV, Ponzoni D, Friedrisch CC. Partial Maxillary Osteotomy Following an Unsuccessful Forced Eruption of an Impacted Maxillary Canine-10 Year Follow-Up. Review and Case Report. Journal of Applied Oral Science 2012; 20(6) 667-72.

[68] Mirabella D, Giunta G, Lombardol. Substitution of Impacted Canines by Maxillary First Premolars: A Valid Alternative to Traditional Orthodontic Treatment. American Journal of Orthodontics and Dentofacial Orthopedics 2013; 143(1) 125-33.

[69] Rosa M, Zachrisson B. Integrating Space Closure and Esthetic Dentistry In Patients with Missing Maxillary Lateral Incisors. Journal of Clinical Orthodontics 2007; 41(9) 563-573.

[70] Thoraton L. Anterior Guidance: Group Function/Canine Guidance. A Literature Review. The Journal of Prosthetic Dentistry 1990; 64(4) 479-482.

[71] Huth KC, Nazet M, Paschos E, Linsenmann R, Hickel R, Nolte D. Autotransplantation and Surgical Uprighting of Impacted or Retained Teeth: A Retrospective Clinical

Study and Evaluation of Patient Satisfaction. Acta Odontologica Scandinavica 2013; 71(6) 1538–1546.

[72] Blomlof L, Lindskog S, Andersson L, Hedstrom KG, Hammarstrom L. Storage of Experimentally Avulsed Teeth In Milk Prior to Replantation. Journal of Dental Research 1983; 62(8) 912-916.

[73] Oswald RJ, Harrington GW, Van Hassel HJ. Replantation 1: The Role of the Socket. Journal of Endodontics 1980; 6(3) 479-484.

[74] Andersson L, Lindskog S, Blomlof L, Hedstrom KG, Hammarstrom L. Effect of Masticatory Stimulation on Dentoalveolar Ankylosis After Experimental Tooth Replantation. Endodontics Dental Traumatology 1985; 1(1) 13-6.

[75] Andreasen JO. The Effect of Pulp Extirpation or Root Canal Treatment on Periodontal Healing After Replantation of Permanent Incisors in Monkeys. Journal of Endodontics 1981; 7(6) 245-252.

[76] Gonnissen H, Politis C, Schepers S, Lambrichts I, Vrielinck L, Sun Y, et al. Long-Term Success and Survival Rates of Autogenously Transplanted Canines. Oral Surgery Oral Medicine Oral Pathology Oral Radiology and Endodontics 2010; 110(5) 570–578.

[77] Patel S, Fanshawe T, Bister D, Cobourne MT. Survival and Success of Maxillary Canine Autotransplantation: A Retrospective Investigation. European Journal of Orthodontics 2011; 33(3) 298–304.

[78] Hall GM, Reade PC. Root Resorption Associated with Autotransplanted Maxillary Canine Teeth. The British Journal of Oral Surgery 1983; 21(3) 179-191.

[79] Andreasen JO. Ectopic Eruption of Permanent Canines Eliciting Resorption of Incisors. Tandlaegebladet 1987; 91(11) 487-492.

[80] Shatz JP, Byloff F, Bernhard JP, Joho JP. Severely Impacted Canines: Autotransplantation as an Alternative. International Journal of Adult Orthodontics and Orthognathic Surgery 1992; 7(1) 45-52.

[81] Kristerson L. Autotransplantation of Human Premolars. International Journal of Oral Surgery 1985; 14(2) 200-213.

[82] Oshimi H. Nemawashi Jiggling and Gingival Muffler in Autogenous Tooth Transplantation. Nippon Dental Review 1993; 607: 65-74.

[83] Suzaki Y, Matsumoto Y, Kanno Z, Soma K. Preapplication of Orthodontic Forces to the Donor Teeth Affects Periodontal Healing of Transplanted Teeth. Angle Orthodontist 2008; 78(3) 495-501.

[84] Ru N, Bai Y. Canine Autotransplantation: Effect of Extraction Site Preservation with a Titanium Prosthesis and a Bioresorbable Membrane. American Journal of Orthodontics and Dentofacial Orthopedics 2013; 143(5) 724-734.

[85] Schatz JR, Joho JR. A Clinical and Radiographic Study of Autotransplanted Impacted Canines. International Journal of Oral and Maxillofacial Surgery 1993; 22(6) 342-346.

[86] Arikan F, Nizam N, Sonmez S. 5-Year Longitudinal Study of Survival Rate and Periodontal Parameter Changes at Sites of Maxillary Canine Autotransplantation. Journal of Periodontology 2008; 79(4) 595–602.

[87] Gonnissen H, Politis C, Schepers S, Lambrichts I, Vrielinck L, Sun Y, et al. Long-Term Success and Survival Rates of Autogenously Transplanted Canines. Oral Surgery Oral Medicine Oral Pathology Oral Radiology and Endodontics 2010; 110(5) 570–578

[88] Pogrel MA. Evaluation of Over 400 Autogenous Tooth Transplants. Journal of Oral and Maxillofacial Surgery 1987; 45(3) 205–211.

[89] Ahlberg K, Bystedt H, Eliasson S, Odenrick L. Long-Term Evaluation of Autotransplanted Maxillary Canines with Completed Root Formation. Acta Odontologica Scandinavica 1983; 41(1) 23–31.

[90] Zachrisson BU, Thilander B. Introduction to Orthodontics, 5th Edn. Stockholm: Tandlakaförlaget; 1985.

[91] Lewis PD. Preorthodontic Surgery in the Treatment of Impacted Canines. American Journal of Orthodontics 1971; 60(4) 383-397.

[92] Nordenvall KJ. Glass Ionomer Cement Used as Surgical Dressing After Radical Surgical Exposure of Impacted Teeth. Swedish Dental Journal 1992(3) 16: 87-92.

[93] Kohavi D, Becker A, Zilberman Y. Surgical Exposure, Orthodontic Movement, and Final Tooth Position as Factors in Periodontal Breakdown of Treated Palatally Impacted Canines. American Journal of Orthodontics 1984; 85(1) 72-77.

[94] Fournier A, Turcottej, Bernard C. Orthodontic Considerations in the Treatment of Maxillary Impacted Canines. American Journal of Orthodontics 1982; 81(3) 236-239.

[95] Stellzig A, Basdra EK, Kourposch G. The Etiology of Canine Tooth Impaction: A Space Analysis. Fortschritte Der Kieferorthopadie 1994; 55(3) 97-103.

[96] Vanarsdall RL Jr. Efficient Management of Unerupted Teeth: A Time-Tested Treatment Modality. Seminars in Orthodontics 2010; 16(3) 212-221.

[97] Becker A, Brin I, Ben-Bassat Y, Zilberman Y, Chaushu S. Closed-Eruption Surgical Technique for Impacted Maxillary Incisors: A Postorthodontic Periodontal Evaluation. American Journal of Orthodontics and Dentofacial Orthopedics 2002; 122(1) 9-14.

[98] Vermette M, Kokich V, Kennedy D. Uncovering Labially Impacted Teeth: Closed Eruption and Apically Positioned Flap Techniques. Angle Orthodontist 1995; 65(1) 23-32.

[99] Vanarsdall R, Corn H. Soft Tissue Management of Labially Positioned Unerupted Teeth. American Journal of Orthodontics 1977; 72(1) 53-64.

[100] Kokich VG, Mathews DA. Impacted Teeth: Surgical and Orthodontic Considerations. In: JA McNamara Jr. (ed.) Orthodontics and Dentofacial Orthopedics. Ann Arbor, Michigan: Needham Press; 2001.

[101] Caprioglio A, Vanni A, Bolamperti L. Long-Term Periodontal Response to Orthodontic Treatment of Palatally Impacted Maxillary Canines. European Journal of Orthodontics 2013; 35(3) 323–328.

[102] Kuftinec MM, Stom D, Shapira Y. The Impacted Maxillary Canine: I. Review of Concepts. ASDS Journal of Dentistry for Children 1995; 62(5) 317-324.

[103] Tulcan T. An Evaluation of Treatment Outcomes of Labially Impacted Maxillary Canines. PhD Thesis, Department of Orthodontics, Philadelphia; 1997.

[104] Graber TM, Vanarsdall RL Jr. Orthodontics Current Principles and Techniques 3rd Ed. St Louis: Mosby; 2000.

[105] Schmidt A. Periodontal Reaction to Early Uncovering, Autonomous Eruption, and Orthodontic Alignment of Palatally Impacted Maxillary Canines. PhD Thesis. University of Washington, Seattle; 2004.

[106] Schmidt AD, Kokich VG. Periodontal Response to Early Uncovering, Autonomous Eruption, and Orthodontic Alignment of Palatally Impacted Maxillary Canines. American Journal of Orthodontics and Dentofacial Orthopedics 2007; 131(4) 449-455.

[107] Becker A, Shpack N, Shteyer A. Attachment Bonding to Impacted Teeth at the Time of Surgical Exposure. European Journal of Orthodontics 1996; 18(5) 457-463.

[108] Becker A. The Orthodontic Treatment of Impacted Teeth. Oxford, London: Wiley-Blackwell; 2012.

[109] Becker A, Chaushu S. Palatally Impacted Canines: The Case for Closed Surgical Exposure And Immediate Orthodontic Traction 2013; 143(4) 451-459.

[110] Burden DJ, Mullally BH, Robinson SN. Palatally Ectopic Canines: Closed Eruption Versus Open Eruption. American Journal of Orthodontics and Dentofacial Orthopedics 1999; 115(6) 640-644.

[111] Parkin NA, Milner RS, Deery C, Tinsley, Smith AM, Germain P, Freeman JV, Bell SJ, Benson PE. Periodontal Health of Palatally Displaced Canines Treated with Open Or Closed Surgical Technique: A Multicenter, Randomized Controlled Trial. American Journal of Orthodontics and Dentofacial Orthopedics 2013; 144(2) 176-184.

[112] Parkin N, Benson PE, Thind B, Shah A. Open Versus Closed Surgical Exposure of Canine Teeth That are Displaced in the Roof of the Mouth. The Cochrane Database of Systematic Reviews 2008; 8(4) CD006966

[113] Smailiene D, Kavaliauskiene A, Pacauskiene I, Zasciurinskiene E, Bjerklin K. Palatally Impacted Maxillary Canines: Choice of Surgical Orthodontic Treatment Method Does not Influence Post-Treatment Periodontal Status. A Controlled Prospective Study. European Journal Of Orthodontics 2013; 35(6) 803–810.

[114] Kuftinec MM, Shapiray. The Impacted Maxillary Canine: II. Surgical Consideration and Management. Quintessence International Dental Digest 1984; 15(9): 895-897.

[115] Sinha PK, Nanda RS. Management of Impacted Maxillary Canines Using Mandibular Anchorage. American Journal of Orthodontics and Dentofacial Orthopedics 1999; 115(3) 254-257.

[116] Goodsell JF. Surgical Exposure And Orthodontic Guidance of the Impacted Tooth. Dental Clinics of North America 1979; 23(3) 385–392.

[117] Mclaughlin R, Bennett C, Trevisi HJ. Systemized Orthodontic Treatment Mechanics 1st Ed. Barcelona, Spain: Mosby; 2002.

[118] Crescini A, Clauser C, Giorgetti R, Cortelini P, Pini Prato GP. Tunnel Traction of Infra-Osseous Maxillary Canines: A Three Year Periodontal Follow-Up. American Journal of Orthodontics and Dentofacial Orthopedics 1994; 105(1) 61-72.

[119] Shapira Y, Kuftinec MM. Treatment of Impacted Cuspids the Hazard Lasso. Angle Orthodontist 1981 ; 51(3) 203-207.

[120] Celi D, Catalfamo L, Deli R. Palatally Impacted Canines:The Double Traction Technique. Progress in Orthodontics 2007; 8(1) 16-26.

[121] Bowman SJ, Carano A. The Kilroy Spring for Impacted Teeth. Journal of Clinical Orthodontics 2003; 37(12) 683-688.

[122] Shastri D, Nagar A, Tandon P. Alignment of Palatally Impacted Canine with Open Window Technique and Modified K-9 Spring. Contemporary Clinical Dentistry 2014; 5(2) 272–274.

[123] Vardimon AD, Graber TM, Drescher D, Bourauel C. Rare Earth Magnets and Impaction. American Journal of Orthodontics and Dentofacial Orthopedics 1991; 100(6) 494-512.

[124] Mcdonald E Yap WL. The Surgical Exposure and Application of Direct Traction of Unerupted Teeth. American Jounal of Orthodontics 1982; 89(4) 331-340.

[125] Kocsis A, Seres L. Orthodontic Screws to Extrude Impacted Maxillary Canines. Journal of Orofacial Orthopedics 2011; 73(1) 19-27.

[126] Poggio PM, Incorvati C, Velo S, Carano A. "Safe Zones": A Guide for Miniscrew Positioning in the Maxillary and Mandibular Arch. Angle Orthodontist 2006; 76(2)191–197.

[127] Chaushu S, Chaushu G. Skeletal Implant Anchorage in the Treatment of Impacted Teeth—A Review of the State of the Art. Seminars in Orthodontics 2010; 16: 234-241.

[128] Becker A, Kohavi D, Zilberman. Periodontal Status Following the Alignment of Palatally Impacted Canine Teeth. American Journal of Orthodontics 1983; 84(4) 332-336.

[129] Woloshyn H, Årtun J, Kennedy DB, Joondeph DR. Pulpal and Periodontal Reactions to Orthodontic Alignment of Palatally Impacted Canines. Angle Orthodontist 1994; 64(4) 257-264.

[130] Clark D. The Management of Impacted Canines: Free Physiologic Eruption. Journal of the American Dental Association 1971; 82(4) 836-840.

[131] D'Amico RM, Bjerklin K, Kurol J, Falahat B. Long-Term Results of Orthodontic Treatment of Impacted Maxillary Canines. Angle Orthodontist 2003; 73(3) 231-238.

[132] Becker A, Chaushu G, Chaushu S. Analysis of Failure in the Treatment of Impacted Maxillary Canines. American Journal of Orthodontics and Dentofacial Orthopedics 2010; 137(6) 743-754.

[133] Becker A, Chaushu S. Success Rate and Duration of Orthodontic Treatment for Adult Patients with Palatally Impacted Canines. American Journal of Orthodontics and Dentofacial Orthopedics 2003; 124(5) 509–514.

[134] Haney E, Gansky SA, Lee JS, Johnson E, Maki K, Miller AJ, Huang JC. Comparative Analysis of Traditional Radiographs and Cone-Beam Computed Tomography Volumetric Images in the Diagnosis and Treatment Planning of Maxillary Impacted Canines. American Journal of Orthodontics and Dentofacial Orthopedics 2010; 137(5) 590-597.

[135] Koutzoglou SI Kostaki A. Effect of Surgical Exposure Technique, Age, and Grade of Impaction on Ankylosis of an Impacted Canine, and the Effect of Rapid Palatal Expansion on Eruption: A Prospective Clinical Study. American Journal of Orthodontics and Dentofacial Orthopedics 2013; 143(3) 342-352.

[136] Pithon MM, Bernardes LA. Treatment of Ankylosis of the Mandibular First Molar with Orthodontic Traction Immediately After Surgical Luxation. American Journal of Orthodontics and Dentofacial Orthopedics 2011; 140(3) 396-403.

[137] Turley PK, Crawford LB, Carrington KW. Traumatically Intruded Teeth. Angle Orthodontist 1987; 57(3) 234-244.

[138] Puricelli E. Treatment of Retained Canines by Apicotomy. RGO 1987; 35(4) 326-330.

[139] Puricelli E. Apicotomy: A Root Apical Fracture for Surgical Treatment of Impacted Upper Canines. Head Face Med 2007; 6(3) 33.

[140] Becker A, Abramovitz I, Chaushu S. Failure of Treatment of Impacted Canines Associated with Invasive Cervical Root Resorption. Angle Orthodontist 2013; 83(5) 870-876.

Periodontics, Oral Medicine and Diagnosis

Oral Fluid Biomarkers in Smoking Periodontitis Patients and Systemic Inflammation

Anna Maria Heikkinen, Päivi Mäntylä,
Jussi Leppilahti, Nilminie Rathnayake,
Jukka Meurman and Timo Sorsa

Additional information is available at the end of the chapter

http://dx.doi.org/10.5772/59813

1. Introduction

Periodontitis is a chronic destructive condition caused by periodontopathogenic bacteria and inflammatory response combined with immune system effects characterized by gingival inflammation and loss of periodontal attachment and alveolar bone (Irfan et al. 2001). Host response is modified by genetic and environmental factors such as smoking (Seymour and Taylor, 2004), which has proven to be the very important risk factor for chronic periodontitis in adults (Genco and Borgnakke, 2013) as well for adolescents (Heikkinen et al. 2008, Heikkinen 2011). In periodontitis host response indeed plays an important role in the destruction of connective tissue and bone (Graves 2008). Smoking affects the immune system and impairs host response by several mechanisms both systemically and locally in saliva and gingival crevicular fluid (GCF). Systemically smoking increases the number of neutrophils in peripheral blood but their ability to migrate through capillary walls is impaired (Hind et al. 1991).

Several types of inflammatory biomarkers associating both with oral diseases and systemic diseases have been detected in saliva and GCF. These include interleukins-1β, -6 and -8 (IL-1β, -6 and -8), tumor necrosis factor-α (TNF-α) and matrix metalloproteinases (MMP)-8 and -9 (Fox 1993, Kaufman and Lamster 2000, Seymour and Gemmell 2001, Kaufman and Lamster 2002, Miller et al. 2006, Rathanayake et al. 2012 and 2013), and tissue inhibitors (TIMP)-1 of metalloproteinase (Seymour & Gemmel, 2001). Several studies have shown the association between increased MMP-8 levels and chronic periodontitis (Mäntylä et al. 2006, Kraft-Neumärker et al. 2012, Leppilahti et al. 2011). Matrix metalloproteinases (MMPs) and TIMP-1 might be candidates for monitoring periodontal status in smokers and non-smokers from oral fluids, such as GCF and saliva. GCF has a particular role in site specific diagnosis. However,

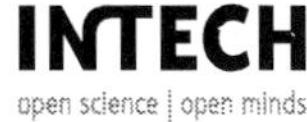

saliva is easy to collect and thus more practical. Saliva is mainly composed of water (98%), and other compounds (2%) are electrolytes, glycoproteins, antibacterial compounds, and various enzymes. This unique biological fluid has multiple functions, such as rinsing, solubilisation of food substances, food and bacterial clearance, lubrication of soft tissues, bolus formation, dilution of detritus, swallowing, speech and facilitation of mastication, all of which are related to its fluid characteristics and specific components. In addition, saliva components contribute to mucosal coating, digestion and antibacterial defence (Lee & Wong, 2009).

Periodontits is a major health problem involving 10% to 60% of population depending on definition (Albandar and Rams 2002) and it is traditionally diagnosed clinically and by radiographical examinations. New methods based on oral fluid inflammatory markers have been suggested for diagnosing oral diseases and inflammation associated with systemic diseases. However, smoking has an effect on levels of several possible diagnostic biomarker candidates. Thus the aim of this chapter is to clarify the diagnostic meaning of oral fluid inflammatory biomarkers in periodontitis in smoking adolescents and adults. We also discuss systemic inflammation and possibilities to analyze it with specific biomarkers in saliva.

2. Smoking as a modifier of the host defense

Cigarette smoking is a principal modifiable environmental risk factor for periodontitis (Palmer et al. 2005). It affects the immune system by impairing host defense by inhibiting granulocyte function (Söder et al. 2002) and by neutrophil respiratory burst which causes oxidative stress in tissues (Chapple and Matthews 2007). According to previous study results by Matthews et al. (2011) cigarette smoking seems to have two-sided effect on periodontal inflammation: on one hand smoking has an effect on oxygen depletion with tissue damage and on the other hand it impairs the ability of neutrophils to response to subgingival periodontal bacteria.

Smoking decreases both the inflammatory infiltrate and number of dendritic cells (DCs) in chronic gingivitis (Souto et al., 2011). In addition it seems that smoking decreases CC chemo-kine ligand (CCL)3 and CXC chemokine ligand (CXCL)8, while CC chemokine ligand (CCL)5 seems to be increased in chronic periodontitis (Souto et al., 2014). Impaired neutrophil chemotaxis is observed in smokers compared to nonsmokers too (Srinivas et al. 2012). Mature DCs are involved in the production of inflammatory cytokines and Th1/Th2/Th17 immune responses in periodontal disease (Cutler and Jotwani, 2004; Allam et al., 2011). Nicotine seems to play an important role in host immune modulation. DCs differentiated in the presence of nicotine and stimulated by lipopolysaccharide induced a differentiation of naive CD4 T cells into Th2 cells. However, DCs differentiated without nicotine and stimulated by lipopolysac-charide induced Th1 immune responses (Yanagita et al. 2014).

3. Effects of smoking on oral inflammatory biomarkers

Reduced neutrophil chemotaxis and impaired phagocytosis in smokers have been shown in several studies suggesting that smokers' periodontal defence is defective compared with non-smokers (Johannsen et al. 2014). This may also be reflected in GCF and salivary content of biomarkers in smokers, which is relevant when possible point-of care diagnostic application is considered. However, the intensity and duration of smoking may also have an effect on GCF biomarker levels, but studies which take into consideration different smoking history are lacking.

In a study of Stein et al. (2006), where GCF proteins were profiled by a protein chip technology, spectral fingerprints were significantly different between smokers and non-smokers. Several spectral peaks were detected only from GCF of smokers suggesting that some proteins are there over-expressed and could potentially serve as biomarkers (Stein et al. 2006). Several studies have reported that smoking either inhibits or intensifies individual biomarkers in GCF, but contradictory findings do exist concerning some biomarkers. This underlines the effect of differences in GCF sampling and analysing methods and other study specific factors, which may lead to inter-study variation in detected biomarker levels

MMP-8, MMP-8/TIMP-1 ratio, IL-1B, myeloperoxidase (MPO), elastase, OPG and some bacterial biomarkers, so called red complex species *Tannerella forsythia, Porphyromonas gingivalis, Treponema denticola,* and *Aggregatibacter actinomycetemcomitans* have proven diagnostic properties to differentiate periodontitis from healthy sites in multiple independent studies. This has been shown both at site level in GCF samples and at patient level in saliva or mouthrinse samples (Hernandez et al. 2010, Kraft-Neumärker et al. 2012, Leppilahti et al. 2011, Leppilahti et al. 2014a,b, Mantyla et al. 2003, Nwhator et al. 2014, Ramseier et al. 2009, Rathnayake et al., 2013; Sexton et al., 2011). Analyzing of multiple biomarkers simultaneously can give even better diagnostic performance (Gursoy et al. 2011, Ramseier et al. 2009).

Nevertheless, biomarkers mentioned above have clear diagnostic properties for periodontal diseases, but many oral fluid biomarkers exhibit large variation of detected levels in both healthy and diseased sites ((Kraft-Neumärker et al 2012, Leppilahti et al. 2014, Mantyla et al. 2003, 2006). Modifying factors, such as smoking, may have an effect on the GCF biomarker levels and disturb the diagnostic interpretation, if these factors are not taken into account (Heikkinen et al. 2010, Heikkinen et al. 2012, Leppilahti et al. 2014a,b). Another reason for large variation is caused by the nature of the periodontititis itself. Progression of periodontitis is regarded to consist of quiescent periods followed by randomly occurring bursts of activity (Goodson et al. 1982, Socransky et al. 1984). Large variation of levels of inflammatory bio-markers can also be an indication of the fluctuating characteristic of peridontitis. Inflammatory GCF biomarker levels can be low in periodontitis sites during the quiet period, but levels can multiply exponentially during the burst of activity (Leppilahti et al. 2014a,b, Sorsa et al. 2010, Mäntyla et al. 2006). This means that most of GCF biomarkers do not associate with perio-dontitis in a linear and deterministic way, and it is the dynamics between the bursts and quiet periods that matters (Papantonopoulos et al. 2013, Papantonopoulos et al. 2014). In addition possible biomarker candidates may have a role in normal physiologic tissue regeneration. Thus, biomarkers can be used as diagnostic tool only if we can define the range of physiological levels and the cutoff for pathological bursts. One definite cutoff for a biomarker is not realistic, however, and modifying factors should be taken into account. For example, even in stable periodontitis sites after successful treatment MMP-8 levels are higher compared to healthy controls (Mäntyla et al. 200, Sorsa et al. 2010). In addition, modifying factors, such as smoking and pregnancy, has to be taken into account (Gürsoy et al. 2008, 2010, Heikkinen et al. 2010, Leppilahti et al. 2014).

Saliva would be a non-invasive sample material for oral and periodontal diagnostics. However, it is less specific than GCF and should be regarded to give a more general picture of oral health. As an example of potential diagnostic capacity of whole saliva is a study where whole saliva periodontitis associated proteome was analysed (Salazar et al. 2013). Twenty proteins were present in different abundance levels in the periodontally healthy subjects and periodontitis patients. And further, nineteen out of these 20 proteins showed higher intensities in periodontitis saliva, and eight were previously reported potential periodontitis biomarkers, among others MMP-8. Also specific protein signatures displayed characteristics of chronic periodontitis. However, effect of smoking should also be considered when salivary or oral rinse sample biomarker levels are analysed.

3.1. Matrix Metalloproteinase (MMP) -8

MMP-8 is the major collagenase in GCF, and point-of-care diagnostic tests have been developed based on analysing it (Sorsa et al. 1999; Prescher et al. 2007, Mäntylä et al. 2003, 2006, Sorsa et al. 2010). The tendency to lower MMP-8 concentrations in GCF of smokers compared to non-smokers has been observed (Persson et al. 2003) as well as lower salivary levels of MMP-8 in current smokers (Liede et al. 1999). This should be noticed when diagnostic use of MMP-8 is being considered. However, the effect of smoking on GCF MMP-8 levels seems to be two-fold. While overall MMP-8 mean level tends to be lower in GCF of smokers when compared with non-smokers, in progressing attachment loss during the maintenance phase the MMP-8 concentrations of smokers are at the same level as in non-smokers (Mäntylä et al. 2006; Leppilahti et al. 2014a). In these studies, when sites were explored in respect of repeatedly substantially elevated MMP-8 concentrations during the maintenance phase, in part of smokers' sites MMP-8 concentrations reached the highest levels of all sampled sites. Thus, lower level of MMP-8 in smokers' GCF does not relate to all sites or to all smoking periodontitis patients. For this reason when MMP-8 is considered as target for point-of-care diagnostic test different cut-off levels for MMP-8 detection should be considered for smokers and non-smokers (Leppilahti et al. 2014a). When biomarkers in saliva samples were detected and compared with periodontal health status regarding smoking as dichotomous yes-no parameter, in smokers' saliva concentration of IL-8 and MMP-8/TIMP-1 ratio were lower than in non-smokers, and salivary MMP-8 had a borderline p-value significantly lower in smokers (Rathnayake et al. 2013a). Possible explanation was considered to be the lower GCF flow of smokers, but also that the effect of smoking on periodontal inflammatory cells is reflected in saliva. In another study salivary concentration of MMP-8 differentiated periodontitis patients from controls, but in periodontitis patients who were smokers this difference was lost; however, the combination of MMP-8 and ICTP and the MMP-8/TIMP-1 ratio differentiated periodontitis cases from controls suggesting, that a combination of biomarkers could be useful when saliva is used as diagnostic sample material (Gursoy et al. 2010).

3.2. Smoking, MMP-8 and elastase levels in early periodontitis and their clinical relevance

In the study of adolescents Heikkinen et al. (2010) observed that smoking associated the lower
levels of MMP-8 and PMN-leukocyte elastase (figure 1. and 2.) and the effect was strengthened
by increased pack-years. However, 15% of adolescents in this birth cohort study seemed to
have signs of early periodontitis (Heikkinen 2011). Salivary MMP-8 values were associated
with BOP and suggestively with deep pockets in the non-smoking teenage boys. In adults
MMP-8 has shown to be a key biomarker during early stages of periodontal diseases (Ramseier
et al. 2009). Clinically smoking reduces the signs of gingivitis (Kumar and Faizuddin, 2011)
masking periodontal diseases, and thus smokers have less observed signs of gingival inflammation, in adolescents as well as in adults, aggravating the diagnostics of periodontal disease.
It is important that patients receive a proper periodontal diagnosing as part of their regular
dental examination. Early diagnosis of periodontal disease could enable a successful therapeutic outcome, by reduction of etiologic factors such as smoking and by establishing periodontal therapy and maintenance protocol. Further, this might prevent the recurrence and
progression of disease and reduce the incidence of tooth loss (Kumar et al. 2012). Recently
Nhawator et al. (2014) demonstrated that neutrophil collagenase-2 lateral flow chair-side
(point-of-care) immunoassay analysed from mouth rinse had a high sensitivity for at least two
sites with BOP and two sites with periodontal pockets but a lower relationship for single-site
pockets and BOP. Further studies are needed to find out the clinical relevance for this test as
a screening tool in adolescents finding early periodontitis as well as for adults taking account
the effect of confounders such as smoking into inflammatory biomarkers.

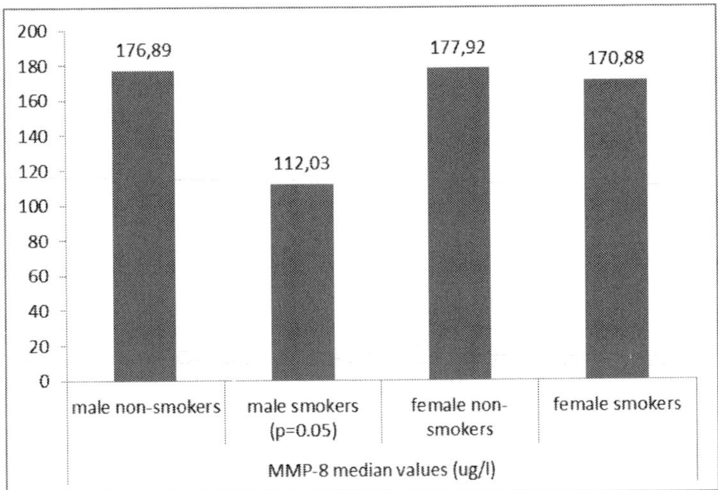

Figure 1. Salivary MMP-8 median values corresponding smoking and sex in adolescents. CI 95%s for male non-smokers, male smokers, female non-smokers and female smokers are 135.08-220.20 ug/l, 86.20-173.22 ug/l, 145.16-215.33
ug/l, 136.72-230.68 ug/l, respectively.

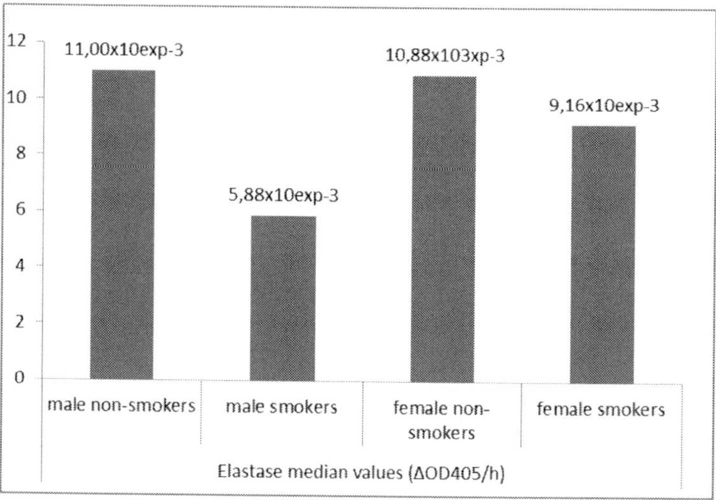

Figure 2. Salivary elastase median values corresponding smoking and sex in adolescents. CI 95%s for male non-smokers, male smokers, female non-smokers and female smokers are 8.75-13.63 x 10 exp-3 ΔOD405/h, 4.75-9.25 x 10exp-3 ΔOD405/h, 8.75-15.25 x10exp-3 ΔOD405/h, 6.63 -17.25 x10exp-3 ΔOD405/h, respectively

3.3. Predictive value of oral fluid MMP-8

It should be noted that MMP-8 levels in oral fluid possess a predictive value (Sorsa et al. 2010, Munjal et al. 2007, Prescher et al. 2007, Kraft-Neumärker et al. 2012, Leppilahti et al. 2014a,b). In this context, periodontitis patients were examined and followed over a course of 12 months at 2 month intervals. In these patients it was possible to clearly differentiate "stable sites" from "unstable" sites.

- "Stable sites": Improvement in pocket depth (PD) and attachment loss (AL) were continuously preserved after treatment, similarly the GCF MMP-8 values were and remained consistently low.

- "Unstable sites": No improvement or only temporary improvement in PD and AL were found, in parallel GCF MMP-8 values only improved shortly after treatment, followed by an immediate re-increase in the MMP-8 values.

Furthermore, Reinhardt et al. (2010) and Leppilahti et al. (2014a) demonstrated that increases in GCF MMP-8 during the periodontal maintenance are associated with increased odds of subsequent periodontal attachment loss and compromised treatment outcome. Overall, these authors concluded that elevated biomarkers of inflammation and bone resorption identify patients vulnerable to progressive periodontitis.

3.4. Elastase, protease inhibitors and sICAM-1

Elastase is another important neutrophil originating proteolytic enzyme. Contradicting findings about elastase activity in GCF of smokers compared with non-smokers with periodontitis have been reported, however: significantly higher mean levels of neutrophil elastase activity in smokers' than non-smokers' sites with matching PD has been detected (Söder 1999), but on the other hand lower concentrations of functional elastase in smokers' than in non-smokers' GCF has also been found (Alavi et al. 1995). This finding led Alavi et al. (1995) to the hypothesis that smokers' neutrophils may release elastase prior to reaching the periodontal tissues for example during passing through the lungs, or possibly a greater proportion of the elastase is bound to substrate and remains undetected which may complicate the diagnostic value of GCF elastase in smokers.

Smoking possibly intervenes in the levels of protease inhibitors α2-macroglobulin (α2-MG) and α1-antitrypsin (α1-AT), which may be one mechanism by which smoking can affect the inflammatory process. In severe periodontal lesions of smokers significantly lower concentrations and total amounts of GCF α2-MG as well as significantly lower total amounts of α1-AT were found. These findings lead to conclusion that decreased local levels of these inhibitors may result in increased tissue damage due to increased activity of elastase and collagenase (Persson et al. 2001).

A soluble form of intercellular molecule-1 (sICAM-1) is known to be elevated in smokers' blood compared with non-smokers (Koundouros et al. 1996). Conversely, in smokers with periodontitis GCF sICAM-1 is significantly lower compared with non-smokers (Fraser et al. 2001). Based on this finding Fraser et al. (2001) hypothesised that sICAM-1 molecules possibly bind to sequestrated neutrophils in periodontal microvasculature and provoke an inappropriate endogenous protease release contributing to periodontal destruction in the vicinity of the gingival microvasculature.

3.5. Cytokines

Bacterial products stimulate monocytes, macrophages and lymphocytes as well as resident fibroblasts and endothelial cells to secrete pro-inflammatory and immunoregulatory cytokines, which control cell growth and differentiation. Bacteria further stimulate chemokines and pro-inflammatory cytokines or subdue with anti-inflammatory cytokines and interferons the inflammation and regulate the development of the antimicrobial immunity in cooperation with antigen presenting cells (Julkunen et al. 2003). Smoking appears to affect normal balance of several cytokines, which are described as local hormones or cell-to-cell messengers. Especially the reduction of chemokines in smokers has been regarded to contribute to weakened neutrophil chemotaxis and migration to the site of inflammation in spite of the existing leukocytosis (Palmer et al. 2005).

In earlier studies increased levels of tumour necrosis factor (TNF) -α but decreased levels of IL-6 and IL-1β were detected in GCF of smoking periodontitis patients compared with non-smokers especially with tendency towards higher TNF-α levels in sites with an inferior treatment outcome (Boström et al. 1998a, 1999, 2000). Former smokers have also been reported to exhibit significantly higher GCF levels of TNF-α than non-smokers (Boström et al. 1998b). Parallel effect of smoking has been detected on GCF IL-10 both prior to as well as after periodontal treatment compared with non-smokers (Goutoudi et al. 2004).

Smoking seems to decrease the mean levels of GCF IL-1α concentrations significantly but does not affect mean total protein concentration (Petropoulos et al. 2004). In this study by Pertropulos et al. (2004) neutrophil numbers were not significantly different between smokers and non-smokers suggesting that the reduced IL-1α concentration of smokers may be independent of any effect of smoking on neutrophil chemotaxis, and smoking may directly inhibit IL-1α production. Thus GCF IL-1α may be derived from the inflamed tissues rather than being locally produced by neutrophils in pocket.

Recently multiplex immunoassays have been used to analyse simultaneously multiple GCF cytokines. A comprehensive investigation by a multi-bead array assay facilitated the characterization of 22 GCF cytokines, which were studied with respect to possible alterations in host response caused by smoking (Tymkiw et al. 2011). Quantities of pro-inflammatory cytokines, chemokines and regulators of T-cells and NK cells were found to be affected by smoking. Healthy sites of smoking periodontitis patients showed significantly less IL-6 and IL-12 than similar sites of non-smoking patients. In addition to these, smokers' periodontitis sites showed also significantly lower quantity of IL-1α. Of chemokines IL-8, IL-10, monocyte chemoattractant protein (MCP)-1, macrophage inflammatory protein (MIP) -1α and RANTES were detected in lower amounts both from healthy and diseased sites of smoking periodontitis patients compared with similar sites in non-smokers suggesting that low chemokine response leads to inability to recruit inflammatory and immune cells and further to ineffective defence. This may have a major role in the pathogenesis of periodontitis in smokers. Also IL-7 and IL-15, regulators of T-cells and NK cells, showed a decrease in smokers compared with non-smokers (Tymkiw et al. 2011).

However, another study also utilizing a multiplex immunoassay concluded that there were no correlations between GCF levels of MIP-1α and RANTES and the smoking status suggesting that at the local level smoking is not a major determinant of the CC group chemokine concentrations in GCF, and that the determinant is the level of local inflammation (Haytural et al. 2014). Another contradicting finding was detected by analysing MCP-1 with enzyme linked immunosorbent assay (ELISA), where MCP levels in GCF were highest in smokers with periodontitis when compared with non-smoking periodontitis patients and healthy controls (Anil et al. 2013), showing the possible effect of the analyse method on the results.

3.6. sRANKL and OPG

Soluble receptor activator of nuclear factor κ B ligand (sRANKL), its cellular receptor RANK and osteoprotegerin (OPG), a protein, which binds to RANKL blocking its interaction with RANK, are the regulators of bone formation and resorption (Tang et al. 2009). Periodontitis patients compared with healthy controls exhibit higher expression of RANKL in gingival tissues and GCF, which associates especially with active sites (Vernal et al. 2004). RANKL:OPG ratios may be increased in GCF of periodontitis patients (Bostanci et al. 2007). In current and former smoking periodontitis patients GCF OPG concentrations were lower compared with never smokers, and finding was opposite concerning the sRANKL concentration (Tang et al. 2009). Consequently, the sRANKL:OPG ratio also appeared to be higher in current and former smokers but the finding was not statistically significant. Interestingly, when pack-years were included in the analysis, OPG concentration decreased with increasing pack years and also the sRANKL:OPG ratio was significantly higher in the high pack-years group being significant also in the multivariate analysis (Tang et al. 2009). An increased lifetime exposure above a minimum threshold of cigarette smoking was required for this pattern. This finding is supported by earlier results where the combination of lipopolysaccharide and nicotine were shown to decrease OPG production in osteoblasts in a dose dependent manner (Tanaka et al. 2006) and where periodontal ligament fibroblasts and epithelial cells directly exposed to nicotine decreased their overall protein synthesis (Giannopoulou et al. 2001; Chang et al. 2002). This may lead to increased sRANKL:OPG ratio in smokers and further cause imbalanced tissue homeostasis and consequent tissue degradation (Tang et al. 2009).

4. Systemic inflammation and salivary biomarkers

Analyzing and utilization of inflammatory and disease specific biomarkers in saliva could offer an attractive solution for the diagnosis of different systemic diseases (Rathanayake et al. 2013b). The composition of saliva mainly originates from blood but in the salivary glands active transport and secretion mechanisms may change the saliva composition as the organic components of glandular specific saliva are derived from protein synthesis and are stored within the acinar cells (Kaufman & Lamster (2002), Malamud 1992). Nevertheless, saliva could be an alternative to blood as a biological fluid for analysis in diagnostic and prognosis purposes since the collection of saliva is non-invasive and is a plausible method. Systemic inflammation leads to the relief of pro-inflammatory mediators from immune cells, and the activation of the innate immune system. An increasing number of specific molecular markers for different conditions, such as cancer, cardiovascular disease (CVD), rheumatoid arthritis (RA), diabetes and human immunodeficiency virus has been identified (Boyle et al. 1994, Hu et al. 2008, Zhang et al. 2010).

4.1. Cardiovascular disease

High sensitive methods for biomarker detection have been developed since year 2000. There are certain biomarkers released due to a myocardial injury caused by myocardial ischemia- and necrosis, such as cardiac troponins I (TnI) and T (TnT), creatine kinase-MB (CK-MB), total creatine kinase, myoglobin, and lactate dehydrogenase (Mueller et al. 2013, Tiwari et al. 2012). Analysis of cardiac TnI and TnT are considered as the golden standard for diagnosis of acute myocardial infarction (AMI) as they are tissue specific for the myocardium (Tiwari et al. 2012). There are few earlier publications that have revealed correlations between serum and salivary biomarkers of CVD (Mirzaii-Dizgah et al. 2012, Quellet-Morin et al. 2011). The Tn I levels reaches its peak within 10–14 hours followed to an AMI, and according to the previous studies Tn I levels could be detected in saliva within 24 hours of onset of AMI (Mirzaii-Dizgah & Riahi 2013). A bedside saliva-based Nano-Biochip test together with electrocardiogram could provide prompt screening method for AMI patients in prehospital stage and the investigators of this study were able to detect elevated salivary levels of creatine kinase-MB, myoglobin, TnI and TnT, C-reactive proteins (CRP), TNF-α, MMP-9 and myeloperoxidase from AMI patients (Floriano et al. 2009).

In the study of Palm et al. (2013) on patients with acute ischemic stroke, systemic and local inflammatory markers were analysed of patients saliva. In this study, controls had enhanced levels of salivary MMP-8, MPO and IL-1β compared to the patients, since the control group was suffering from ongoing periodontal disease and the patients more often had evidence of end-stage periodontitis with edentulism and missing teeth. They also had higher levels of serum MMP-8 and MPO. Additional longitudinal studies are needed, however, to check the potential of salivary biomarkers associated in ischemic stroke.

4.2. Diabetes

There are a few studies concerning the detection of inflammatory biomarkers in saliva of patients with diabetes. Goodson and co-authors reported that in a child population unstimulated saliva samples were analysed and the salivary levels of CRP, insulin and leptin were remarkably higher in obese children compared with healthy normal weight children (Goodson et al. 2014). In a cross sectional study on 451 patients elevated salivary levels of MMP-8 were found among diabetes patients (Rathnayake et al. 2013). Salivary N-acetyl-β-D-hexosaminidase (HEX) which is associated with type I diabetes was found to be significantly increased in children with type 1 diabetes compared with healthy children (Zalewska-Szajda et al. 2013a).

4.3. Rheumatoid arthritis

The disease pattern of RA is similar to periodontal disease. Systemic inflammatory biomarkers from different chronic inflammatory conditions, such as RA could thus appear in saliva. There are few studies in this area, but when conducting an exploration of inflammatory biomarkers in RA patients, the periodontal status and the anti-TNF-α therapy taken by these patients need to take in to consideration. Salivary IL-1β was found to be significantly higher in the RA patients who were not on anti-TNF-α therapy compared with RA patients receiving anti-TNF-α therapy (Zalewska-Szajda et al. 2013b). Salivary exoglycosidases for detection of salivary gland involvement in RA patients were studied, in xerostomic RA group salivary β-glucuronidase was found to be significantly higher compared with healthy controls but the activity of salivary N-acetyl-β-hexosaminidase and β-glucuronidase was significantly lower than in xerostomic hyposalivary RA patients (Zalewska-Szajda et al. 2013b).

4.4. Cancer

To use salivary biomarkers to detect on / monitor all types of cancer is a growing research field in salivary diagnostics. The most common malignant neoplasm of the oral cavity is oral squamous cell carcinoma (OSCC). Patients with OSCC indicated that a specific marker of oxidative stress, malondialdehyde (MDA) in saliva was a better diagnostic tool as MDA in blood (Rasool et al. 2014). Salivary IL-8 levels seem to be higher in patients who had experienced tumour diseases (Rathnayake et al. 2013a,b). To detect head and neck squamous cell carcinoma (HNSCC) microRNAs (miRNAs) of saliva was used, and the results showed that miR-9, miR-134 and miR-191 were differentially expressed between saliva from HNSCC patients and healthy controls. Additionally, the authors suggested that these saliva-derived miRNAs may serve as novel biomarkers to reliably detect HNSCC (Salazar et al. 2014).

There are number of cytokines and chemokins involved in the cancer progression, such as interferon-gamma (IFN-γ), TNF-α, IL-1β, transforming growth factor-beta-1 (TGF-β1), epidermal growth factor (EGF), IL-6 and -8, vascular endothelial growth factor (VEGF), interleukins-4 and -10, tumour necrosis factor (TNF) and endothelin. Saliva based testing of these biomarkers is promising depending on the methods of analysis (Prasad & McCullough 2013). About 5 % of all cancers of the head and neck are salivary gland carcinomas (SGCs). Thus there is a need to develop new molecular biomarkers for early diagnosis and to improve the diagnosis of SGCs. Further research in this is required.

To identify disease specific molecular biomarkers in whole saliva is challenging. There are certain biomarkers found in saliva of high sensitivity and specificity, particularly in oral diseases, such as periodontal disease and oral cancer. There are factors that have an influence for the expression and release of biomarkers, such as their intracellular location, the size of the proteins, and the characteristics of the local biological fluid flow. The type of saliva used for diagnostic purpose to detect systemic conditions has an impact. In this regard unstimulated saliva reveals more information than stimulated saliva since unstimulated saliva contains higher concentrations of diagnostic biomarkers. High sensitivity and sophisticated methods and techniques are required for valuable outcome of the analyses of saliva samples.

5. Conclusion remarks

Inflammatory saliva and GCF biomarkers can be used as an aid in periodontal diagnostics, but there is a need to define the range of physiological levels and cutoff for pathological bursts of periodontitis progression. However, using just one definite cutoff point or merely one biomarker is not rational for adults or adolescents. Adolescence might have certain character‐istics with different cutoff points compared to adults. The clinical use of salivary biomarkers to identify systemic conditions is another interesting area for developing non-invasive screening and diagnostic procedure. This might be the main goal for saliva research but in this regard it is important to consider the influence of oral health conditions which may confound the utility of the biomarkers. Modifying factors, such as smoking and pregnancy also should be taken into account when interpreting the results of the oral fluid inflammatory biomarkers.

Acknowledgements

This work was supported by grant from the National Fund for Scientific and Technological Development, Chilean Government (1120138), the Finnish Dental Society Apollonia and the

Research Foundation of Helsinki University Central Hospital. The authors declare that they have no competing interests. Timo Sorsa is an inventor of US-patents 5652227, 5736341, 5866432 and 6143476.

Author details

Anna Maria Heikkinen[1], Päivi Mäntylä[1], Jussi Leppilahti[1], Nilminie Rathnayake[3], Jukka Meurman[1,2] and Timo Sorsa[1,2,3]

1 Institute of Dentistry, Helsinki University, Central Hospital Helsinki, Finland

2 Departments of Oral and Maxillofacial Diseases and Periodontology, Helsinki University, Central Hospital Helsinki, Finland

3 Division of Periodontology, Department of Dental Medicine, Karolinska Institutet, Huddinge, Sweden

References

[1]   Alavi, A.L., R.M Palmer, E.W. Odell, P.Y. Coward, and R.F. Wilson. Elastase in gingival crevicular fluid from smokers and non-smokers with chronic inflammatory periodontal disease. Oral Dis 1995; 1: 110-4.

[2]   Albandar, J.M., and T.E. Rams. Global epidemiology of periodontal diseases: an overview. J Periodontology 2000 2002; 29:7-10.

[3]   Allam, J.P., Y. Duan, F. Heinemann, J. Winter, W. Gotz W, J. Deschner, M. Wenghoefer, T. Bieber, S. Jepsen, and N. Novak. IL-23-producing CD68(+) macrophage-like likecells predominate within an IL-17-polarized infiltrate in chronic periodontitislesions. J. Clin. Periodontol. 2011; 38, 879–886.

[4]   Anil, S., R.S. Preethanath, M. Alasqah, S.A. Mokeem, and P.S. AnandS. Increased levels of serum and gingival crevicular fluid monocyte chemoattractant protein-1 in smokers with periodontitis. J Periodontol 2013; 84: e23-8.

[5]   Bostanci, N., T. Ilgenli, G.Emingil, B. Afacan, B. Han, H. Töz H., G. Atilla, F.J. Hughes, and G.N. Belibasakis. Gingival crevicular fluid levels of RANKL and OPG in periodontal diseases: implications of their relative ratio. J Clin Periodontol 2007; 34: 370-6.

[6]   Boström, L., L.E. Linder, and J. Bergström. Clinical expression of TNF-alpha in smoking-associated periodontal disease. J Clin Periodontol 1998; 25: 767-73.

[7]   Boström, L., LE. Linder, and J. Bergström. Smoking and cervicular fluid levels of IL-6 and TNF-alpha in periodontal disease.J Clin Periodontol 1999; 26: 352-7.

[8]   Boström, L., L.E. Linder, and J. Bergström. Smoking and GCF levels of IL-1beta and IL-1ra in periodontal disease. J Clin Periodontol 2000; 27: 250-5.

[9]   Boström, L., L.E. Linder, and J. Bergström. Influence of smoking on the outcome of periodontal surgery. A 5-year follow-up. J Clin Periodontol 1998; 25: 194-201.

[10]   Boyle, J.O., L. Mao, J.A Brennan, W.M. Koch, D.W. Eisele, J.R. Saunders, and D. Sidransky. Gene mutations in saliva as molecular markers for head and neck squamous cell carcinomas. Am J Surg 1994;168: 429–432.

[11]   Fox, P.C. Salivary monitoring in oral diseases. Ann N Y Acad Sci 1993; 694: 234–237.

[12]   Chang, Y.C., F.M Huang, K.W Tai, L.C. Yang, and M.Y Chou. Mechanisms of cytotoxicity of nicotine in human periodontal ligament fibroblast cultures in vitro. J Periodontal Res 2002; 37: 279-85.

[13]   Chapple, I.L.C., and J.B. Matthews. The role of reactive oxygen and antioxidant species in periodontal tissue destruction. Periodontology 2000 2007;2:160-232.

[14]   Cutler, C.W., and R. Jotwani. Antigen-presentation and the role of dendritic cells in periodontitis. Periodontology 2000 2004; 35, 135–157.

[15]   Genco, R.J., and W.S. Borgnakke. Risk factors for periodontal disease. Periodontology 2000 2013; 62, 59–94.

[16]   Goodson, J.M., A.C. Tanner, A.D. Haffajee, G.C. Sornberger, and S.S. Socransky. Patterns of progression and regression of advanced destructive periodontal disease. J Clin Periodontol 1982; 9,472-481.

[17]   Goodson, J.M., A. Kantarci, M.L. Hartman, G.V. Denis, D. Stephens, H. Hasturk, T. Yaskell, J. Vargas, X. Wang, M. Cugini, R. Barake, O. Alsmadi, S. Al-Mutawa, J. Ariga, P. Soparkar, J. Behbehani, K. Behbehani, and F. Welty. Metabolic disease risk in children by salivary biomarker analysis. PLoS One 2014; 10: 9: e98799.

[18]   Floriano, P.N., N. Christodoulides, C.S Miller, J.L. Ebersole, J. Spertus, B.G. Rose,D.F. Kinane, M.J Novak, S. Steinhubl, S. Acosta, S. Mohanty, P. Dharshan, C.K. Yeh, S. Redding, W. Furmaga W, and J.T. McDevitt. Use of saliva-based nano-biochip tests for acute myocardial infarction at the point of care: a feasibility study. Clin Chem 2009; 55: 1530–1538.

[19]   Fraser, H.S., R.M. Palmer, R.F. Wilson, P.Y. Coward, and D.A. Scott. Elevated systemic concentrations of soluble ICAM-1 (sICAM) are not reflected in the gingival crevicular fluid of smokers with periodontitis. J Dent Res 2001; 80: 1643-7.

[20]   Giannopoulou, C., N. Roehrich, and A. Mombelli. Effect of nicotine-treated epithelial cells on the proliferation and collagen production of gingival fibroblasts. J Clin Periodontol 2001; 28: 769-75.

[21] Goutoudi, P., E. Diza, and M. Arvanitidou. Effect of periodontal therapy on crevicular fluid interleukin-1beta and interleukin-10 levels in chronic periodontitis. J Dent 2004; 32: 511-20.

[22] Graves, D. Cytokines that promote periodontal tissue destruction. J Periodontol 2008; 79, 1585–1591.

[23] Gursoy, M., E. Kononen, T. Tervahartiala, U.K. Gursoy, R. Pajukanta, and T. Sorsa. Longitudinal study of salivary proteinases during pregnancy and postpartum. J Periodontal Res 2010; 45,496-503.

[24] Gursoy, M., R. Pajukanta, T. Sorsa, and E. Kononen E. Clinical changes in periodontium during pregnancy and post-partum. J Clin Periodontol 2008; 35, 576-583.

[25] Gursoy, U.K., E. Könönen, P. Pradhan-Palikhe, T. Tervahartiala, P.J. Pussinen, L. Suominen-Taipale, and T. Sorsa. Salivary MMP-8, TIMP-1, and ICTP as markers of advanced periodontitis. J Clin Periodontol 2010; 37: 487-93.

[26] Gürsoy U.K., E. Könönen, P.J. Pussinen, T. Tervahartiala, K. Hyvärinen, A.L. Suominen, V.J. Uitto, and S. Paju. Use of host- and bacteria-derived salivary markers in detection of periodontitis: A cumulative approach. Dis Markers 2011; 30, 299-305.

[27] Haytural, O., D.,Yaman, E.C. Ural, A. Kantarci, and K. Demirel. Impact of periodontitis on chemokines in smokers. Clin Oral Investig 2014; Sep 6.

[28] Heikkinen, A.M., R. Pajukanta, J. Pitkäniemi, U. Broms, T. Sorsa, M. Koskenvuo, and J.H.

[29] Meurman. The effect of smoking on periodontal health of 15- to 16-year-old adolescents J Periodontol 2008; 79: 2042-2047.

[30] Heikkinen, A.M., T. Sorsa, J. Pitkäniemi, T. Tervahartiala, K. Kari, U. Broms,

[31] M. Koskenvuo, and J.H. Meurman. Smoking affects diagnostic salivary periodontal disease biomarker levels in adolescents. J Periodontol 2010; 81: 1299-1307.

[32] Heikkinen, A.M. (2011). Oral health, smoking and adolescence. University of Helsinki, Faculty of Medicine, Institute of Dentistry. http://urn.fi/URN:ISBN: 978-952-10-7250-5.

[33] Hernandez, M., J. Gamonal, T. Tervahartiala, P. Mantyla, O. Rivera, A. Dezereg,

[34] N. Dutzan, and T. Sorsa. Associations between matrix metalloproteinase-8 and-14 and myeloperoxidase in gingival crevicular fluid from subjects with progressive chronic periodontitis: A longitudinal study. J Periodontol 2010; 81, 1644-1652.

[35] Hind, C.R., H. Joyce, G.A. Tennent, M.B. Pepys,and N.M.Pride. Plasma leukocyte elastase concentrations in smokers. JClin Pathol 1991; 44: 232-235.

[36] Hu, S. and M. Arellano, P. Boontheung, J. Wang, H. Zhou, J. Jiang, D. Elashoff, R. Wei,

[37] J.A. Loo, and D.T. Wong. Salivary proteomics for oral cancer biomarker discovery. Clin Cancer Res 2008; 14: 6246–6252.

[38] Irfan, U.M., D.V. Dawson, and N.F. Bissada. Epidemiology of periodontal disease: a review and clinical perspectives. J Int Acad Periodontol 2001; 3: 14-21.

[39] Johannsen, A., C. Susin, and A. Gustafsson A. Smoking and inflammation: evidence for a synergistic role in chronic disease. Periodontol 2000 2014; 64: 111-126.

[40] Julkunen, I., O. Silvennoinen and M. Hurme. Sytokiinit, niiden toiminta ja kliininen merkitys. In book: Huovinen, P., S. Meri, H. Peltola, M. Vaara, A. Vaheri and V. Valtonen (eds.). Mikrobiologia ja infektiosairaudet, book I. Kustannut Oy Duodecim. Gummerus Kirjapaino Oy. Jyväskylä 2003; 734-747.

[41] Kaufman, E., and I.B. Lamster. Analysis of saliva for periodontal diagnosis–a review. J Clin Periodontol 2000; 27: 453–465.

[42] Kaufman, E.,and I.B. Lamster. The diagnostic applications of saliva-a review. Crit Rev Oral Biol Med 2002; 13: 197–212.

[43] Kumar, A., S.S. Masamatti, and M.S. Virdi. Periodontal diseases in children and adolescents: a clinician's perspective part 2. Dent Update 2012; 39:639-642, 645-646, 649-652.

[44] Kraft-Neumärker, M., K. Lorenz, R. Koch, T. Hoffmann, P. Mäntylä, T. Sorsa, and L. Netuschil. Full-mouth profile of active MMP-8 in periodontitis patients. J Periodontal Res 2012; 47: 121-8.

[45] Koundouros, E., E. Odell, P. Coward, R. Wilson, and R.M. Palmer. Soluble adhesion molecules in serum of smokers and non-smokers, with and without periodontitis. J Periodontal Res 1996; 31: 596-599.

[46] Lee, Y.H., and D.T. Wong. Saliva: an emerging biofluid for early detection of diseases. Am J Dent 2009; 22, 241–248.

[47] Leppilahti, J.M., M. Ahonen, M. Hernández, S. Munjal, L. NetuschilL, V. Uitto, T. Sorsa, and P. Mäntylä. Oral rinse MMP-8 point-of-care immuno test identifies patients with strong periodontal inflammatory burden. Oral Diseases 2011; 17, 115-122.

[48] Leppilahti, J.M., M.A. Kallio, T. Tervahartiala, T. Sorsa, and P. Mäntylä. Gingival crevicular fluid matrix metalloproteinase-8 levels predict treatment outcome among smokers with chronic periodontitis. J Periodontol 2014a; 85: 250-260.

[49] Leppilahti, J.M., P.A. Hernández-Ríos, J.A. Gamonal, T. Tervahartiala, R. Brignardello-Petersen, P. Mantyla, T. Sorsa and M. Hernández. Matrix metalloproteinases and myeloperoxidase in gingival crevicular fluid provide site-specific diagnostic value for chronic periodontitis. J Clin Periodontol 2014b; 41: 348-356.

[50] Liede, K.E., J.K. Haukka, J.H. Hietanen, M.H. Mattila, H. Rönkä H, and T. Sorsa. The association between smoking cessation and periodontal status and salivary proteinase levels. J Periodontol 1999; 70: 1361-8.

[51] Malamud, D. Saliva as a diagnostic fluid. BMJ 1992; 305: 207–208.

[52] Matthews, J.B., F.M. Chen, M.R. Milward, M.R Ling, and I.L.C.Chapple. Neutrophil superoxide production in the presence of cigarette smoke extract, nicotine and cotinine. J Periodontol 2012; 39; 626-634.

[53] Miller,C.S., C.P. King, M.C. Langub, R.J. Kryscio, and M.V. Thomas. Salivary biomarkers of existing periodontal disease: a cross-sectional study. J Am Dent Assoc 2006; 137: 322–329.

[54] Mirrielees, J., L.I. Crofford, Y. Lin Y., R.J. Kryscio, D.R. 3 rd. Dawson, J.L. and Ebersole, and C.S. Miller. Rheumatoid arthritis and salivary biomarkers of periodontal disease. J Clin Periodontol 2010; 37: 1068-1074.

[55] Mirzaii-Dizgah, I., and E. Riahi. Salivary troponin I as an indicator of myocardial infarction. Indian J Med Res 2013; 138: 861–865.

[56] Mirzaii–Dizgah, I., S.F. Hejazi, E. Riahi, and M.M. Salehi MM. Saliva-based creatine kinase MB measurement as a potential point-of-care testing for detection of myocardial infarction. Clin Oral Invest 2012; 16: 775–779.

[57] Mueller,M., M. Vafaie, M. Biener, E. Giannitsis, and H.A. Katus. Cardiac troponin T: from diagnosis of myocardial infarction to cardiovascular risk prediction. Circ J 2013; 77: 1653-1661.

[58] Mäntyla, P., M. Stenman, D.F., Kinane, S. Tikanoja, H. Luoto, T. Salo, and T. Sorsa. Gingival crevicular fluid collagenase-2 (MMP-8) test stick for chair-side monitoring of periodontitis. J Periodontal Res 2003;38, 436-439.

[59] Mäntylä, P., M. Stenman, D.F. Kinane, T. Salo, K. Suomalainen, S. Tikanoja, and T. Sorsa. Monitoring periodontal disease status in smokers and nonsmokers using a gingival crevicular fluid matrix metalloproteinase-8-specific chair-side test. J Periodontal Res 2006; 41: 503-512.

[60] Nwhator, S.O., P.O. Ayanbadejo, K.A. Umeizudike, O.I. Opeodu, G.A. Agbelusi, J.A. Olamijulo, M.O. Arowojolu, T. Sorsa, B.S. Babajide, and D.O. Opedun. Clinical correlates of a lateral-flow immunoassay oral risk indicator. J Periodontol 2014; 85: 188-94.

[61] Palm, F., L. Lahdentausta, T. Sorsa, T. Tervahartiala, P. Gokel, F. Buggle, A. Safer, H. Becher, A.J. Grau, and P. Pussinen. Biomarkers of periodontitis and inflammation in ischemic stroke: A case-control study. Innate Immun 2013; 17; 20: 511-518.

[62] Palmer, R.M., R.F. Wilson, A.S. Hasan, and D.A. Scott. Mechanisms of action of environmental factors--tobacco smoking. J Clin Periodontol 2005; 32: 180-95.

[63] Papantonopoulos, G., K. Takahashi, T. Bountis, and B.G. Loos. Mathematical model-ing suggests that periodontitis behaves as a non-linear chaotic dynamical process. J Periodontol 2013; 84,e29-39.

[64] Papantonopoulos, G., K. Takahashi, T. Bountis, and B.G. Loos Artificial neural net-works for the diagnosis of aggressive periodontitis trained by immunologic parame-ters. PloS One 2014;9, e89757.

[65] Persson, L., J. Bergström, and A. Gustafsson A. Effect of tobacco smoking on neutro-phil activity following periodontal surgery. J Periodontol 2003; 74: 1475-1482.

[66] Persson, L., J. Bergström, H. Ito, and A. Gustafsson. Tobacco smoking and neutrophil activity in patients with periodontal disease. J Periodontol 2001; 72: 90-95.

[67] Petropoulos, G., I.J. McKay, and F.J. Hughes. The association between neutrophil numbers and interleukin-1alpha concentrations in gingival crevicular fluid of smok-ers and non-smokers with periodontal disease. J Clin Periodontol 2004; 31: 390-395.

[68] Prasad, G., and M. McCullough. Chemokines and cytokines as salivary biomarkers for the early diagnosis of oral cancer. Int J Dent 2013; 2013: 813756.

[69] Prescher, N., K. Maier, S.K. Munjal, T. Sorsa, C.D. Bauermeister, F. Struck, and L. Ne-tuschil. Rapid quantitative chairside test for active MMP-8 in gingival crevicular flu-id: first clinical data. Ann N Y Acad Sci 2007; 1098: 493-495.

[70] Ouellet-Morin, I., A. Danese, B. Williams, and L. Arseneault. Validation of a high-sensitivity assay for C-reactive protein in human saliva. Brain Behav Immun 2011; 25: 640–646.

[71] Ramseier, C.A., J.S. Kinney, A.E. Herr, T. Braun, J.V. Sugai, C.A. Shelburne, L.A. Ray-burn, H.M. Tran, A.K. Singh, and W.V. Giannobile.Identification of pathogen and host-response markers correlated with periodontal disease. J Periodontol 2009; 80, 436-446.

[72] Rasool, M., S.R. Khan, A. Malik, K.M.4. Khan, S. Zahid, A. Manan, M.H. Qazi, and M.I. Naseer. Comparative Studies of Salivary and Blood Sialic Acid, Lipid Peroxida-tion and Antioxidative Status in Oral Squamous Cell Carcinoma (OSCC). Pak J Med Sci 2014; 30: 466-471.

[73] Rathnayake, N., S. Akerman, B. Klinge, N. Lundegren, H. Jansson H, Y. Tryselius, T. Sorsa, and A. Gustafsson. Salivary biomarkers of oral health: a cross-sectional study. J Clin Periodontol 2013a; 40: 140-147.

[74] Rathnayake, N., S. Akerman, B. Klinge, N. Lundegren, H. Jansson, Y. Tryselius, T. Sorsa, A. Gustafsson. Salivary biomarkers for detection of systemic diseases. PLoS One. 2013b; 24; 8: e61356.

[75] Salazar, M.G., N. Jehmlich, A. Murr, V.M. Dhople, B. Holtfreter, E. Hammer, U. Völker, and T. Kocher. Identification of periodontitis associated changes in the pro-

teome of whole human saliva by mass spectrometric analysis. J Clin Periodontol 2013 ; 40: 825-832.

[76]   Salazar, C., R. Nagadia, P. Pandit, J. Cooper-White, N. Banerjee, N. Dimitrova, W.B Coman, and C. Punyadeera. A novel saliva-based microRNA biomarker panel to detect head and neck cancers. Cell Oncol 2014; 37: 331-338.

[77]   Seymour, G.J.,and E. Gemmell. Cytokines in periodontal disease: where to from here? Acta Odontol Scand 2001; 59: 167–173.

[78]   Seymour, G.J.,and J.J Taylor. Shouts and whispers: an introduction to immunoregulation in periodontal disease. Periodontology 2000 2004; 35, 9–13.

[79]   Sexton, W. M., Y. Lin, R.J. Kryscio, D.R.3rd. Dawson, J.L. Ebersole, and C.S. Miller. Salivary biomarkers of periodontal disease in response to treatment. J Clin Periodontol 2011; 38, 434-441.

[80]   Socransky, S.S., A.D. Haffajee, J.M. Goodson, and J. Lindhe. New concepts of destructive periodontal disease. J Clin Periodontol 1984; 11, 21-32.

[81]   Sorsa, T., P. Mäntylä, H. Rönkä, P. Kallio, G.B. Kallis, C. Lundqvist, D.F. Kinane, T. Salo, L.M. Golub, O. Teronen, and S. Tikanoja. Scientific basis of a matrix metalloproteinase-8 specific chair-side test for monitoring periodontal and peri-implant health and disease. Ann N Y Acad Sci 1999; 878: 130-40.

[82]   Sorsa, T., M. Hernández, J. Leppilahti, S. Munjal, L. Netuschil, and P. Mäntylä. Detection of gingival crevicular fluid MMP-8 levels with different laboratory and chairside methods. Oral Diseases 2010; 16, 39-45.

[83]   Souto, G.R., T.K. Segundo, F.O. Costa, M.C. Aguiar, and R.A. Mesquita. Effect of smoking on Langerhans and dendritic cells in patients with chronic gingivitis. J.Periodontol 2011; 82, 619–625.

[84]   Souto, G.R., C.M. Queiroz-Junior, F.O. Costa, and R.A. Mesquita. Smoking effect on chemokines of the human chronic periodontitis. Immunobiology 2014; 219, 633–636.

[85]   Srinivas, M., K.C. Chethana, R. Padma, G. Suragimath, M. Ani, B.S. Pai, and A. Walvekar. A study to assess and compare the peripheral blood neutrophil chemotaxisin smokers and non-smokers with healthy periodontium, gingivitis, and chronicperiodontitis. J. Ind. Soc. Periodontol 2012; 16, 54–58.

[86]   Stein, S.H., K.J. Wendell, M. Pabst, and M. Scarbecz. Profiling gingival crevicular fluid from smoking and non-smoking chronic periodontitis patients. J Tenn Dent Assoc 2006; 86: 20-4.

[87]   Söder, B. Neutrophil elastase activity, levels of prostaglandin E2, and matrix metalloproteinase-8 in refractory periodontitis sites in smokers and non-smokers. Acta Odontol Scand 1999; 57: 77-82.

[88] Söder, B., L.I. Jin, and S. Wickholm. Granulocyte elastase, matrix metalloproteinase-8 and prostaglandin E2 in gingival crevicular fluid in matched clinical sites in smokers and non-smokers with persistent periodontitis. J Clin Periodontol 2002; 29:384-91.

[89] Tanaka, H., N. Tanabe, M. Shoji, N. Suzuki, T. Katono, S. Sato, M. Motohashi, and M. Maeno M. Nicotine and lipopolysaccharide stimulate the formation of osteoclast-like cells by increasing macrophage colony-stimulating factor and prostaglandin E2 production by osteoblasts. Life Sci 2006; 78: 1733-1740.

[90] Tang, T.H., T.R. Fitzsimmons, and P.M. Bartold. Effect of smoking on concentrations of receptor activator of nuclear factor kappa B ligand and osteoprotegerin in human gingival crevicular fluid. J Clin Periodontol 2009; 36: 713-8.

[91] Tiwari, R.P., A. Jain, Z. Khan, V. Kohil, R.N. Bharmal, S. Kartikeyan, and P.S. Bisen. Cardiac Troponin I and T: Molecular markers for early diagnosis, prognosis, and accurate triaging of patients with acute myocardial infarction. Mol Diagn Ther 2012; 16: 371–381.

[92] Tymkiw, K.D., D.H. Thunell, G.K. Johnson, S. Joly, K.K. Burnell, J.E. Cavanaugh, K.A. Brogden, and J.M. Guthmiller. Influence of smoking on gingival crevicular fluid cytokines in severe chronic periodontitis. J Clin Periodontol 2011; 38: 219-28.

[93] Vernal, R., A. Chaparro, R. Graumann, J. Puente, M.A. Valenzuela, and J. Gamonal. Levels of cytokine receptor activator of nuclear factor kappaB ligand in gingival crevicular fluid in untreated chronic periodontitis patients. J Periodontol 2004; 75: 1586-1591.

[94] Yanagita, M., K. Mori, R. Kobayashi, Y. Kojima, M. Kubota, K. Miki, S. Yamada, M. Kitamura, and S. Murakami. Immunomodulation of dendritic cellsdifferentiated in the presence of nicotine with lipopolysaccharide from Porphy-romonas gingivalis. Eur. J. Oral. Sci. 2012b; 120, 408–414.

[95] Zalewska-Szajda, B., S. Dariusz Szajda, N. Waszkiewicz, S. Chojnowska, E. Gościk, U. Łebkowska, A. Kępka, A. Bossowski, A. Zalewska, J. Janica, K. Zwierz, J.R. Ładny, and D. Waszkiel D. Activity of N-acetyl-β-D-hexosaminidase in the saliva of children with type 1 diabetes. Postepy Hig Med Dosw 2013a; 67: 996-999.

[96] Zalewska, A., J. Szulimowska, N. Waszkiewicz, D. Waszkiel, K. Zwierz, and M. Knaś. Salivary exoglycosidases in the detection of early onset of salivary gland involvement in rheumatoid arthritis. Postepy Hig Med Dosw 2013b; 3; 1182-1188.

[97] Zhang, L., H. Xiao, S.K. Karlan, H. Zhou, and J. Gros. Salivary Transcriptomic and Proteomic Biomarkers for Breast Cancer Detection 2010; 5: 1–7.

Chapter 23

Oral Health From Dental Paleopathology

Hisashi Fujita

Additional information is available at the end of the chapter

http://dx.doi.org/10.5772/59263

1. Introduction

Since when have humans been afflicted with dental diseases? It is not easy to find an answer to this question. There are two main methods to examine what types of disease our ancestors suffered. One method involves the history of medicine or a study called "medical history," which mainly examines pathologies written in ancient documents and ancient writings and attempts to identify the diseases. Michinaga Fujiwara was a powerful individual in the Heian period of Japan (794-1192 AD) [1]. He was speculated to have died of complications of diabetes based on the records of his pathology in the literature. This type of finding is the result of research in the history of medicine (a study of medical history). The other method involves a field of study in physical anthropology called "paleopathology," in which the author of this paper specializes. In paleopathology, the research materials are hard tissues such as bones and teeth from humans of ancient times and obtained from archeological excavations (needless to say, the soft tissues have long decomposed and returned to soil). Thus, it is possible to learn about the frequency of certain diseases in the past in groups of people and about the true pathology at the time of death. In this paper, a few dental diseases were interpreted from the perspective of an anthropologist who handles ancient human skeletal remains. These diseases can be indicators of modern oral health.

2. Two major diseases in the oral cavity are caries and periodontal disease

This statement is believed to have been true since the ancient times. In a previous study, the author of this paper described that, before the introduction of modern dentistry, people were more affected by caries and periodontal disease, the main cause of tooth loss, because they were unable to receive scientific dental care. Modern humans can obtain nutrients parenterally and via gastrostomy with the advancement of modern medicine. For the majority of human

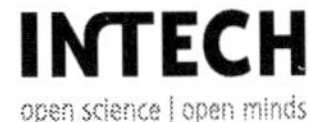

history, the mouth was the only means through which people have taken in nutrients. Therefore, tooth loss was speculated to have caused malnutrition and even death in many pre-modern individuals with numerous missing teeth. In the pre-modern times, longevity was likely dependent on the preservation of one's own teeth to obtain sufficient nutrients.

2.1. Tooth loss in human skeletal remains of Japan

Trinkaus reported on the problem of tooth loss in the La Chapelle-aux-Saints Neanderthal from approximately 60,000 years ago, the most ancient material that has been examined for this purpose [2]. He reported that 51.7% of the teeth were missing antemortem in this Neanderthal. In another study, Trinkaus also reported that 25% of the teeth were missing in the Shanidar Neanderthals [3]. It is difficult to obtain a large sample size of ancient human fossils, and consequently adequate statistical analysis cannot be performed due to small sample size. Therefore, the information from these ancient human fossils is merely for reference.

There are some case reports worldwide on tooth loss in Homo sapiens [4-8], but the number of studies on ancient human skeletal remains is not large. These researchers, except the author of this paper, used all examined individuals as materials. Thus, a bias likely occurred regarding the types of teeth, which were sometimes located in areas of defects in ancient human skeletal remains. The author of this paper examined remaining teeth in ancient human skeletal remains excavated from archeological sites of the pre-modern periods in Japan: the Kofun period (3rd–early7th century), Kamakura period (1192–1333 AD), Muromachi period (1335–1573 AD), and Edo period (1603–1868 AD). A total of 329 individuals were examined, of whom 145 individuals were selected as materials because their sex was determinable and their maxillary and mandibular alveolar bones were fully examinable (Table 1). This material selection method enabled data collection without bias for all tooth types. The estimation of age and determination of sex were performed by morphological observations of anthropological bones. Since the number of materials was not large, the individuals of different sexes were pooled together. The individuals were divided into three groups: early middle age group (approximately 20-39 years), late middle age group (approximately 40-49 years), and old age group (50 years or older).

In this study, the ancient human skeletal remains used as materials were grouped by time period and by age group. Table 1 shows the number of individuals and the number of examinable teeth. In all time periods as shown in Table 2, there was a tendency for the number of missing teeth to increase with age, progressing from early middle age to late middle age to old age. In the Kofun period, the mean number of missing teeth was 2.67 (SD: 1.63) in early middle age, 6.00 (SD: 2.00) in late middle age, and 16.00 in old age. In the Kamakura period, the mean number was 1.17 (SD: 1.47), 2.22 (SD: 2.10), and 4.50 (SD: 2.12), respectively. In the Muromachi period, the mean number was 1.80 (SD: 0.84), 5.80 (SD: 4.55), and 21.00, respectively. In the Edo period, the mean number was 2.31 (SD: 2.58), 5.18 (SD: 4.57), and 29.67 (SD: 4.04), respectively. Table 3 shows whether there is a difference in the number of missing teeth by age group after combining all the materials of different time periods. The results revealed that the number of missing teeth differed significantly (p<0.01) between the early middle age and late middle age groups and between the late middle age and old age groups, statistically indicating increasing tooth loss with age in pre-modern Japanese people. Table 4 shows the number of missing teeth in the maxilla and mandible. The number of missing teeth is shown by time period and by age group, but there were many time periods without a sufficient number of materials. Therefore, the lower portion of the table shows the number of maxillary missing teeth and the number of mandibular missing teeth of all time periods. A significance test was used to determine the difference in the number of missing teeth between the maxilla and mandible, and there was no significant difference between the jaws in any age group. Figures 1 and 2 show the percentages of missing teeth of all tooth types in the maxilla and mandible, respectively. In general, the percentage of missing teeth tended to be lower in the anterior teeth and the percentage tended to be higher in the posterior teeth.

Period	Group	Number of individuals	Number of Observed teeth[a]
Kofun	Early middle age	6	192
	Late middle age	7	224
	Old age	1	32
Kamakura	Early middle age	18	576
	Late middle age	18	576
	Old age	2	64
Muromchi	Early middle age	5	160
	Late middle age	5	160
	Old age	1	32
Edo	Early middle age	45	1440
	Larly middle age	34	1088
	Old age	3	96
Total		145	4640

[a]The number of observed teeth includes ante-mortem tooth loss and post-mortem tooth loss.

Table 1. The archaeological materials used from Kofun, Kamakura, Muromachi and Edo periods in Japan.

Period	Group	Lost teeth	Observed teeth	Average of number of ante-mortem teeth per person	SD
Kofun	Early middle age	16	192	2.67	1.63
	Late middle age	42	224	6.00	2.00
	Old age	16	32	16.00	-
Kamakura	Early middle age	21	576	1.17	1.47
	Late middle age	40	576	2.22	2.10
	Old age	9	64	4.50	2.12

Period	Group	Lost teeth	Observed teeth	Average of number of ante-mortem teeth per person	SD
Muromachi	Early middle age	9	160	1.80	0.84
	Late middle age	29	160	5.80	4.55
	Old age	21	32	21.00	-
Edo[a]	Early middle age	104	1440	2.31	2.58
	Late middle age	176	1088	5.18	4.57
	Old age	89	96	29.67	4.04

[a]Data were cited from Fujita[18].

Table 2. The number of ante-mortem tooth loss by age distribution.

	Significant
Early middle age-Late middle age	***
Late middleage-Old age	***

***: $P < 0.001$

Table 3. Comparison of number of missing teeth by age distribution.

	Tooth type						
	Upper			Lower			
Early middle age	URM1	ULM1	Total	LRM1	LLM1	Total	Grand total
Observed	36	34	70	31	31	61	131
Average	3.13	3.24	3.19	2.16	2.27	2.23	2.74
SD	0.99	1.05	1.01	0.9	0.87	0.86	1.06
Early middle age vs Late middle age	P=0.165 ns	P=0.104 ns	P<0.05 L>E	P<0.05 L>E	P=0.218 ns	P<0.01 L>E	P<0.05 L>E
Late middle age	URM1	ULM1	Total	LRM1	LLM1	Total	Grand total
Observed	11	9	20	8	7	15	35
Average	3.91	3.89	3.9	3.13	2.71	2.93	3.49
SD	1.64	1.05	1.37	1.25	0.76	1.03	1.31

ns: not significance

E: Early middle age; L: Late middle age

Table 4. Alveoler resession of Somali people in Early middle age and Late middle age.

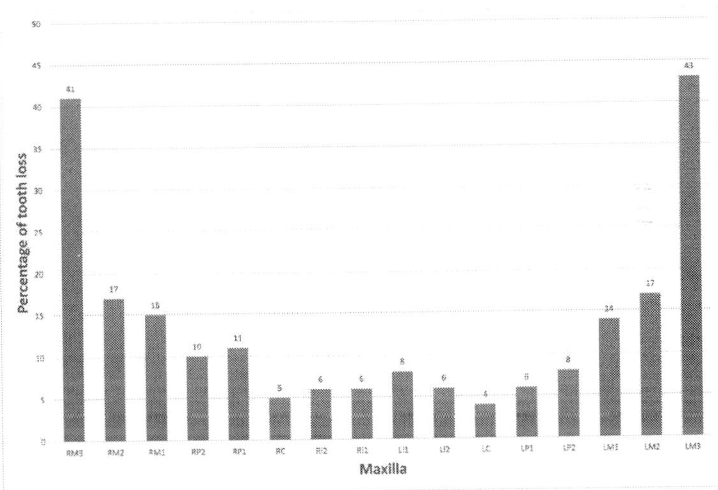

Figure 1. The rate of loss by tooth type in Maxilla in pre-modern periods in Japan.

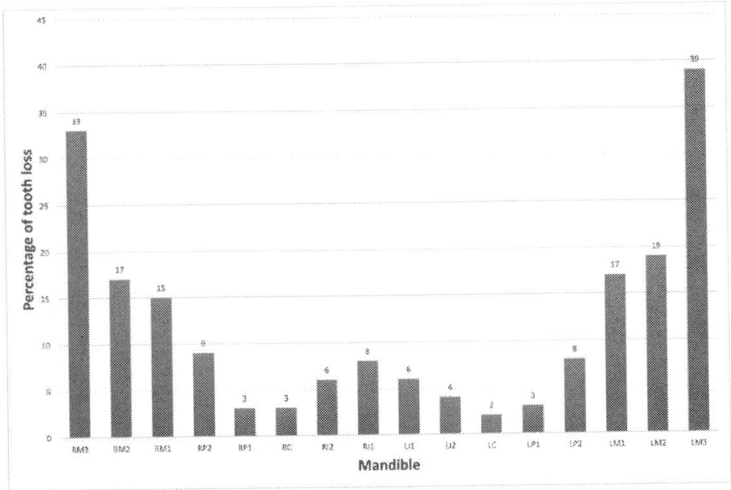

Figure 2. The rate of loss by tooth type in mandible in pre-modern periods in Japan.

In the early and late middle age individuals, the low number of missing teeth had been maintained at 1.11 to 6.00 teeth from the Kofun period to Edo period, spanning 1500 years. This result might be very surprising for health care providers as well as for the general public. The assumption is that people in olden times lost many teeth at an early age, but it is not consistent with the results of this study. At least to late middle age, the number of missing teeth was lower in pre-modern times than in modern time. Lopez *et al.* made a similar finding in a study comparing people of the Mediaeval Ages and modern people in Spain [5]. Sikanjic also made a similar finding in the number of missing teeth in human skeletal remains from the Iron Age in Croatia [6]. Diet and ingredients used in meals (i.e., nutrients) are expected to differ by country. Although it is difficult to generalize, modern people can receive scientific dental care, and tooth extraction can be performed easily and frequently. One cannot say that the dental treatment of tooth extraction was non-existent in the pre-modern times. However, it was likely not performed frequently, and the general public in those times were not as familiar with medical care as the general public of modern time [9].

The average lifespan of Japanese people is estimated to have been less than 15 years in the Jomon period and approximately 20 years in the Edo period [10]. The high mortality rates of infants and young children greatly decreased the average lifespan of the overall population. In these time periods, many adults also lost their lives due to various infections and parasitic diseases. Until the Edo period, Japanese people had a simple and plain diet, except for a small segment of the upper class. Such a diet did not contain much animal protein or fat. Diet in Japanese people began to change due to the introduction of more "American" foods, mainly with the post-war American occupation. Japanese people gradually began to consume more animal protein and fat. It is clearly consistent with the high correlation between increased average lifespan in Japanese people and increased consumption of animal protein and fat (Figures 3 and 4). Japan is currently a country with the longest lifespan in the world. This fact seems to suggest that there is a good balance of the two types of diet, a simple Japanese diet, mainly of vegetables and grains, and a Western-style diet.

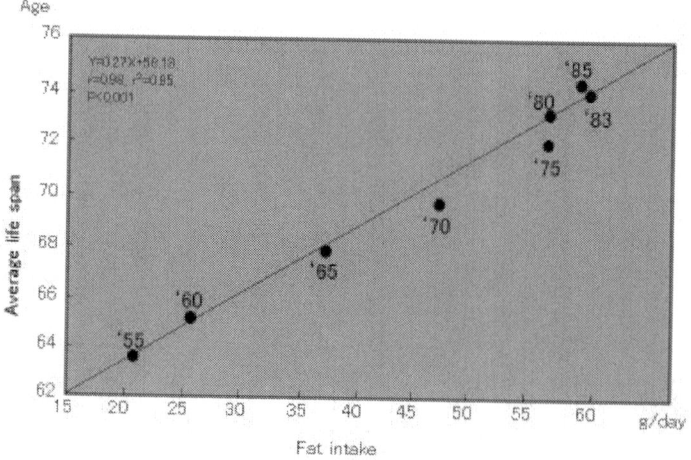

Figure 3. Relation between fat intake and Japanese life span

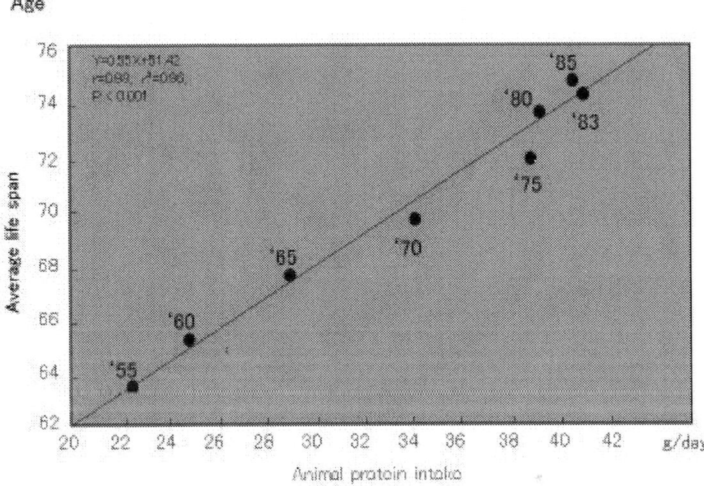

Figure 4. Relation between the animal protein intake and Japanese life span

Intravenous infusion was first introduced to Japan around 1960, and non-parenteral nutrition via gastrostomy was introduced much more recently. There are many restrictions and limitations when using these methods. In the time periods with only pre-modern medical care, the preservation of one's teeth was the only available way for people to get nutrients effectively. Thus, when people lost many of their teeth, they likely faced early death.

2.2. Tooth loss in ancient human skeletal remains from countries other than Japan

How was tooth loss in ancient human skeletal remains from other countries? The status of missing teeth was examined in human skeletal remains of the 3rd-7th centuries from the Yean-ri site in South Korea [11]. There were 2.7 missing teeth in the early middle age individuals and 8 missing teeth in the late middle age individuals, which are not large numbers. The status of missing teeth was also examined in modern Nigerian individuals who lived in the early 20th century and whose skeletal remains are stored at the University of Cambridge [12]. There were 1.3 missing teeth in the early middle age individuals and 3.3 missing teeth in the late middle age individuals, indicating very low numbers. No caries was observed in the examination of a total of 15 Nigerian individuals and 272 teeth. Similarly, when tooth loss was examined in Somali individuals living in the late 19th century to the early 20th century, AMTL was 2.60% in individuals in early middle age [13]. This percentage is a very low value, indicating the loss of at the most 1 tooth out of 32 teeth. In individuals in late middle age, AMTL was 17.02%, which is an approximate loss of 5.4 teeth. Thus, the number of missing teeth clearly increased with aging. There was a significant increase in alveolar bone loss with aging as shown in Table 4, while there was no change in caries rate with aging as shown in Table 5. It is speculated from these results that tooth loss in Somalis was due to periodontal disease and not caries. Although it is difficult to speculate on the details of their diet, they were believed to have had a low intake of simple sugars and carbohydrates. Thus, the diet of Somalis likely consisted of low cariogenic food. The Somali skeletal remains showed that they had periodontal disease from their early middle age. The disease progressed with age and caused alveolar bone loss, eventually leading to bone that could not support the teeth and consequently to tooth loss. The author observed an unexpectedly large number of remaining teeth in the late middle age individuals, much like in the Edo individuals in Japan. It indicated that Somali individuals also had low numbers of missing teeth.

	Tooth type										
	Upper					Lower					
Early middle age	I	C	P	M	Total	I	C	P	M	Total	Grand total
Observed	168	84	170	252	674	130	65	130	195	520	1194
Loss	9	3	1	8	21	0	0	3	7	10	31
SD	0.23	0.19	0.08	0.18	0.17	—	—	0.15	0.19	0.14	0.16
% AMTL	5.36	3.57	0.59	3.17	3.12	0	0	2.31	3.59	1.92	2.60
Early middle age vs Late middle age	P=0.135 ns	P=0.333 ns	P<0.01 L>E	P<0.001 L>E	P<0.001 L>E	P<0.001 L>E	P<0.05 L>E	P=0.051 ns	P<0.001 L>E	P<0.001 L>E	P<0.001 L>E
Late middle age	I	C	P	M	Total	I	C	P	M	Total	Grand total
Observed	52	26	52	78	208	44	22	43	65	174	382
Loss	7	3	5	18	33	6	3	5	18	32	65
SD	0.32	0.33	0.3	0.42	0.37	0.35	0.35	0.32	0.45	0.39	0.38
% AMTL	13.46	11.54	9.62	23.08	15.87	13.64	13.64	11.63	27.69	18.39	17.02

I: Incisors; C: Canines; P: Premolars; M: Molars in tooth type distribution.

ns: not significant

E: Early middle age; L: Late middle age

Table 5. Antemortem tooth loos (AMTL) of Somali people in Early middle age and Late middle age.

The lifespan remains short in developing countries of the 21st century. Similar types and proportions of disease are thought to have been maintained in modern populations (likely even in present-day populations) as in the populations of 1000-2000 years ago. It is speculated that missing teeth of populations of 1000-2000 years ago were maintained at very low numbers until late middle age despite the presence of periodontal disease, much like ancient human skeletal remains from Japan.

Early middle age				Late middle age				P-value
Tooth type	Observed	Caries	% Caries	Tooth type	Observed	Caries	% Caries	
UI	168	0	0	UI	52	0	0	-
UC	84	0	0	UC	26	0	0	-
UP	170	0	0	UP	52	1	1.92	P=0.537
UM	252	6	2.38	UM	78	0	0	P=0.384
U-total	674	6	0.89	U-total	208	1	0.48	P=0.896
LI	130	0	0	LI	44	0	0	-
LC	65	0	0	LC	22	0	0	-
LP	130	0	0	LP	43	0	0	-
LM	195	4	2.05	LM	65	2	3.08	P=0.991
L-total	520	4	0.77	L-total	174	2	1.15	P=0.994
Grand Total	1194	10	0.84	Grand Total	382	3	0.79	P=0.820

Table 6. Prevalence of dental caries of Somali people in Early middle age and Late middle age.

3. Stress markers and enamel hypoplasia

Stress in modern-day people signifies mainly "psychological stress" in the majority of cases. In ancient skeletal human remains, the focus is on the examination of signs of "physical stress" remaining in bones and teeth as a result of surviving in a very harsh environment. It is desirable to examine the level of such stress not in one or a few individuals but in a group, if possible in at least a few dozen to a few hundred individuals. Otherwise, the stress level in a certain group and differences in stress level among groups cannot be known.

Stress marker might not be a commonly used term. It is a lesion that is used to compare the level of health particularly among groups such as mentioned above. Stress markers on teeth are not very common. Enamel hypoplasia is one such marker and will be discussed below pertaining to ancient human skeletal remains.

Teeth are formed relatively early and enamel matrix is formed at approximately the sixth week of gestation for primary teeth. Enamel matrix formation begins early even for permanent teeth. For example, it begins to form at birth for permanent first molars. Enamel hypoplasia occurs when there is poor enamel formation at such stages. The cause is hypocalcemia due to conditions such as starvation and impaired food intake due to serious disease [14].

Enamel hypoplasia is a useful stress marker because: (1) it is a lesion which is found relatively frequently in ancient human skeletal remains, and (2) it is a lesion that occurs due to environmental factors such as those affecting the nutritional status. Briefly explained, the ancient human skeletal remains that we encounter represent one individual in a few thousands or a few tens of thousands of individuals who lived in the past from a certain time period. They represent a very fortunate discovery and are very important representatives. Therefore, if a disease occurred only in one in a few tens or hundreds of thousands, finding this disease in the excavated remains is greatly affected by chance. Therefore, such disease is not suitable for examining the stress level in a group or comparing the stress level with other groups.

As shown in Figure 5, enamel hypoplasia often appears linearly on the enamel surface. The crowns of healthy teeth should be smooth, but aplasia occurs in depressions of the crowns of teeth with enamel hypoplasia.

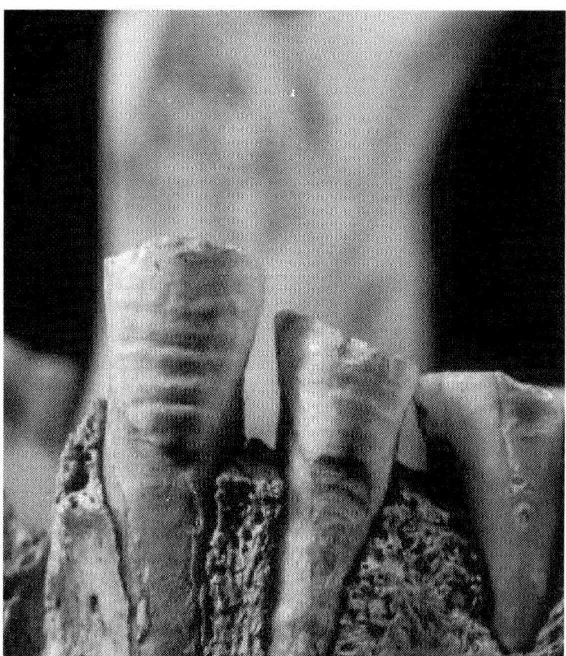

Figure 5. Linear enamel hypoplasia found in Jomon people of Japan

Although there are individual differences, the timing of crown formation by tooth type is roughly the same among individuals. Therefore, when enamel hypoplasia is seen in a certain site of a certain tooth, one can estimate the age at which the enamel hypoplasia occurred. If several lines can be seen in an individual (Figure 5), it can be speculated that this individual experienced multiple bouts of starvation or malnutrition due to serious disease. Some individuals have linear enamel hypoplasia of the entire dentition as in Figure 6. It shows that the individual was exposed to stress causing enamel hypoplasia during crown formation of different tooth types [14]. Therefore, this case is very important as such evidence.

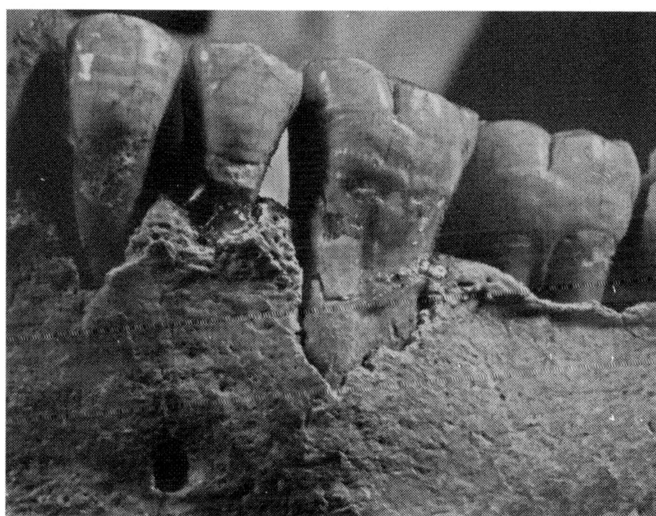

Figure 6. Linear enamel hypoplasia found some tooth type in Jomon people of Japan

When does enamel hypoplasia occur? There have been several studies on this topic, including one by Yamamoto, who examined ancient human skeletal remains of Japanese individuals [15]. According to the study of Yamamoto, enamel hypoplasia occurs repeatedly between 3.5-5.5 years of age in the majority of the cases and very rarely occurs at ages younger than 3 years. Yamamoto gave as reasons for the onset: such stress was likely fatal in individuals at ages younger than 3 years in a pre-modern environment, and even if individuals survived the stress, they could not have tolerated subsequent stress and would have died before the eruption of permanent teeth. In contrast, enamel hypoplasia in modern-day individuals occurs repeatedly at 0-12 months after birth but rarely beyond 34 months [15]. That is, it occurs repeatedly early after birth but rapidly decreases thereafter. Thus, the ancient skeletal remains indicate that timing of hypoplasia differed between ancient people and modern-day people. It is speculated that improved health status, including due to medical advancement, helps modern-day individuals face conditions recorded in crowns as enamel hypoplasia without causing death.

The above findings show that it was very difficult for very young children, particularly infants, to survive in pre-modern times during which bouts of starvation were common and medical care was not advanced. This tendency was likely stronger in more ancient times, and countless young lives must have been lost before these individuals were able to leave any signs of enamel hypoplasia.

Stress markers develop on bones and teeth when individuals continue to survive under a poor environment. If individuals die in a short period of time due to disease or malnutrition, then there will be no stress marker on bones or teeth. For example, when individuals die of acute infections, including dysentery and influenza, it is very difficult to find signs of such infections in excavated bones and teeth. If individuals had chronic diseases such as advanced tuberculosis, leprosy, and syphilis of the bone for a few years to decades, then signs of such diseases will remain in their bones.

The frequency of enamel hypoplasia was 48.1% in the Jomon population, 36.4% in the Kofun population, approximately 60% in the Edo population, and 39.5% in the present-day population of Japan [15]. These numbers seem to indicate that the environment in the Jomon period was better than that in the Edo period. However, these numbers can be explained in another way. When Jomon people suffered various diseases or malnutrition, they likely did not recover and died a short time later. Therefore, they probably did not live long enough to develop enamel hypoplasia, resulting in a lower frequency of enamel hypoplasia in the Jomon period. Edo people also likely lived in a much harsher environment than present-day people. However, medical care and nutritional conditions were improved in the Edo period compared with those in the Jomon period. Therefore, Edo people with various diseases and malnutrition likely had higher chances of survival than Jomon people with such conditions. As a result, signs of enamel hypoplasia remain in individuals from the Edo period. Present-day people can have high-quality medical care and nutrition readily and sufficiently, and the infant mortality rate has consequently decreased. Thus, only a modest frequency of enamel hypoplasia is seen. Therefore, in this type of a situation, one should conclude that a group with a low frequency of stress markers had a worse environment and that a group with a high frequency had a better environment. This phenomenon is called a "paleopathological paradox." One needs to be mindful of this paradox when examining nutritional conditions, health status, and the difference in frequency of disease among groups or time periods.

What are the frequencies of enamel hypoplasia in various countries? When the frequency of enamel hypoplasia was examined in former inhabitants of what is now the State of Illinois in the U.S., it was 45% in the excavated individuals from the hunting and gathering period, 60% in the excavated individuals from the transition to the agricultural period, and a high frequency of 80% in the excavated individuals from the agricultural period [16]. Similarly, when the frequency was examined in former inhabitants of what is now Ohio, it was higher in the excavated individuals from the agricultural period than those from the hunting and gathering period [17, 18]. These findings indicate that poor harvests more greatly affected people in an agricultural society than frequent food shortages affected people in a hunting and gathering society. In addition, the agricultural people who lived in these areas had a diet which depended heavily on corn. Such a diet resulted in increased caloric intake and nutritional quantity but decreased animal protein intake and nutritional quality. Weaning diets were deficient in protein, and nutritional stress occurred such as diarrhea due to bacterial infection. Some researchers interpret the high frequency of enamel hypoplasia as a result of increased population density in the agricultural period, leading to a higher risk for infection and increased environmental stress such as outbreaks of endemic diseases [19, 20].

The author of this paper is not in agreement with the above explanations. There is no evidence that a hunter-gatherer economy enabled people to maintain necessary and sufficient proteins. There is also no evidence that people in an agricultural economy had repeated poor harvests and had lower animal protein intake than people in a hunter-gatherer economy. The term "hunters and gatherers" gives the image of hunting. However, it is speculated that people in a hunter-gatherer economy did not necessary have sufficient animal-derived foods, and the majority of their diet consisted of plant-derived foods. Even natural-born hunters like lions have very low hunting success rates. Therefore, it is valid opinion that hunters and gatherers must have had great difficulties maintaining a constant intake of animal protein even with human intelligence and use of tools. The diet of an agricultural economy could not have consisted entirely of plant-derived foods. Instead, it is speculated that hunting must have continued, and its techniques must have evolved from previous time periods to the agricultural period. Therefore, people must have continued to consume animal-derived foods in the agricultural period.

Even when societies transitioned from a hunting-gathering type to an agricultural type, it is very unlikely that the consumption of animal protein decreased sharply. Instead, the afore-mentioned enamel hypoplasia frequencies should be interpreted in the following ways: the types of people who were unable to survive in a hunter-gatherer society were more likely to survive in an agricultural society, and the average lifespan, an index of cumulative stress, increased.

4. TMD in human skeletal remains from the Edo period in Japan

Prolonged retention of primary teeth rarely poses clinical problems in modern people if these teeth are extracted and the eruptive paths of permanent teeth are normalized. A report in a Japanese journal has shown that when primary teeth were retained beyond the normal period, their extraction resulted in gradual improvement of TMD and in normal occlusion. In the field of physical anthropology, very few report has been published that simultaneously discussed prolonged retention of primary teeth, temporomandibular joint (TMJ) arthritis, and TMD [21]. The material discussed in this section was skeletal human remains from the Edo period (17-19th centuries) in Japan. The mandible showed signs of TMJ arthritis and TMD likely due to bilateral primary second molars. The skeletal remains were excavated from the Suhgen temple site in Shinjuku-ku in Tokyo and were of a woman in the early part of early middle age. Retention of primary molars was observed in the left and right mandible (Figure 7). Since first premolars were present anterior to them, the over-retained primary teeth were both believed to be primary second molars. Radiographs showed no formation of left or right second premolars, confirming that they were missing congenitally (Figures 8a and 8b). It was speculated that bilateral primary second molars remained in adulthood because second premolars were missing congenitally. Other permanent mandibular teeth, including the third molars, were erupted bilaterally, and it is consistent with the individual being in the early part of early middle age. Bilateral primary molars had more severe occlusal attrition of the distal area than on the mesial area, and dentin was markedly exposed. The occlusal attrition of the mesial area was confined to near the proximal aspect adjacent to the first premolar.

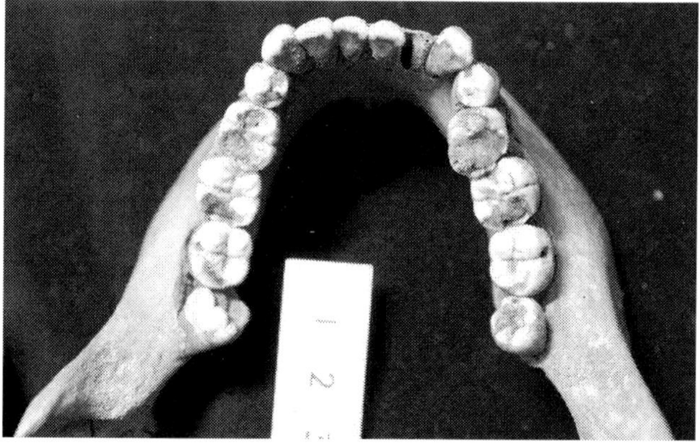

Figure 7. Persistence of both sides of second deciduous molars.

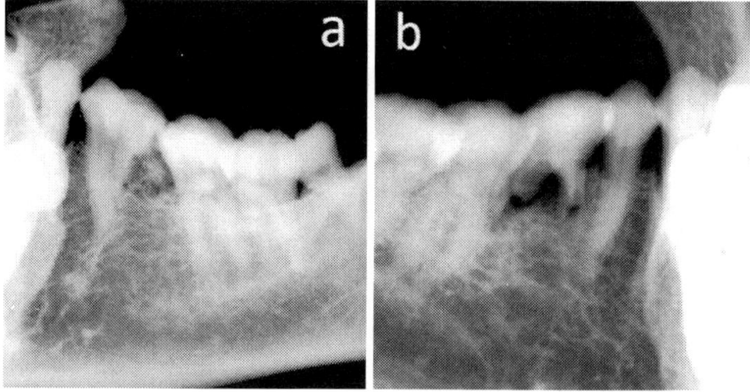

Figure 8. The lack of permanent second premolars are admitted in the roentgenograms. a: right side, b: left side, respectively. a: right mandibular condyle is normal. b: left mandibular condyle has caused the deformity by TMJ arthritis.

The right mandibular condyle was normal, but TMJ arthritis had developed in the left mandibular condyle with overall deformation (Figures 9a and 9b). It was of minimum expression under the Rando and Waldron classification [22]. The right mandibular fossa was normal. In the left mandibular fossa, a new articular facet had formed accompanying inflammation and deformation of the mandibular condyle, and it was evident that TMJ arthritis and accompanying TMD had developed (Figures 10a and 10b).

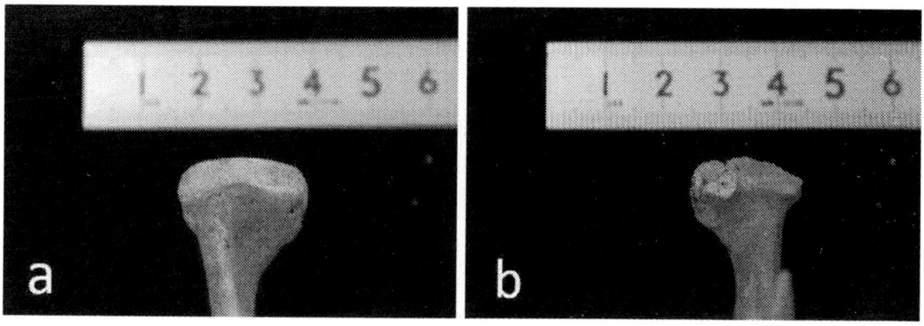

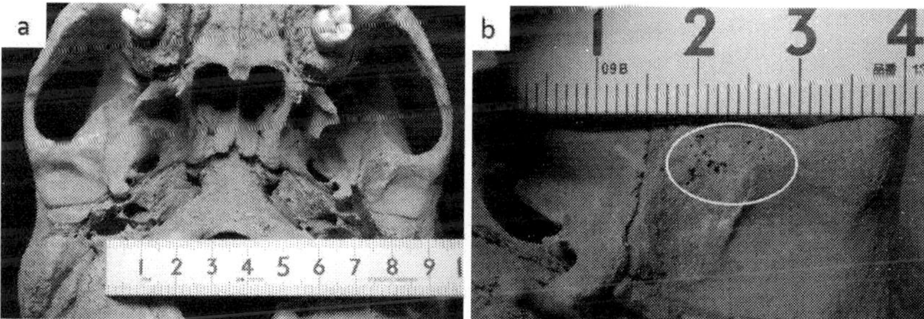

Figure 9. a: mandibular fossa of both sides. b: left mandibular fossa forms the false joint (arrow) and porosity is recognized in frame area.

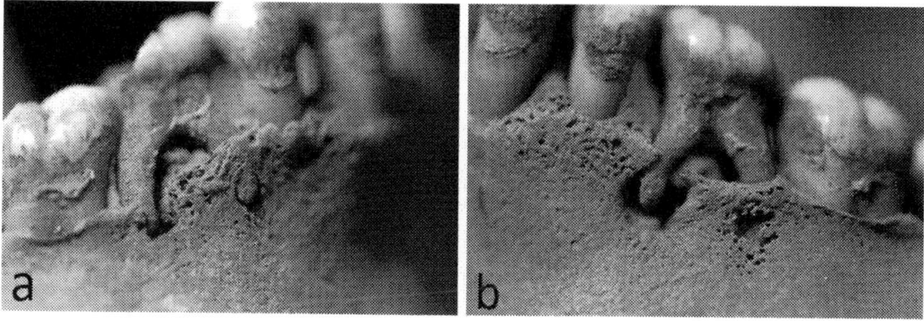

Figure 10. Periostitis found in the alveolar bone at right second deciduous molar (a) and left second deciduous molar (b).

There was bilateral periostitis of the alveolar bone supporting the primary teeth (Figures 11a and 11b). Periostitis was severe in the areas with over-retained primary second molars, and there was mild periostitis in all other areas, which was almost the entire maxilla and mandible.

Figure 11. Slight periostitis is admitted in the widespread area of the alveolar bone.

Sumiya reported that the prevalence of prolonged retention was 0.58% for primary second molars in both Japanese men and women aged 21-25 years [23]. Onizuka examined 151 teeth in 106 individuals with over-retained primary teeth who were aged 14-47 years and reported that 63% had one over-retained tooth and 32% had two over-retained teeth [24]. It should be noted that over-retained teeth occurred symmetrically in the left and right sides of the maxilla or mandible in 33 of 34 patients with two over-retained teeth, indicating a very high proportion of patients [24]. The most commonly over-retained tooth was the primary second molar at 52.3% [24]. In the individual from the Suhgen temple site, there was prolonged retention of two mandibular primary second molars with bilaterally symmetry. The occurrence rate was 0.19% based on simple calculation, suggesting that such prolonged retention occurred in approximately 2 in 1000 adults. When one takes into account that the excavated skeletal remains were of the Edo period, this individual can be said to represent a valuable case of over-retained primary teeth in ancient human skeletal remains.

Although some reports have discussed that over-retained primary teeth can frequently cause TMD, treatment such as extraction of such teeth has been reported to improve the symptoms. In the individual from the Suhgen temple site, occlusal attrition was observed in the distal area of the left and right first molars. In the right first molar, the occlusal surface gently sloped upward from the distal to the mesial direction until there was no attrition. One area of the left first molar showed severe attrition where its distal area contacted the left second molar. It is nearly impossible to reproduce an accurate antemortem occlusion using a mandible and maxilla without soft tissue. However, there was likely abnormal occlusal force on the areas with attrition. When the maxillary dentition was examined, the teeth had normal positions in the left and right molar regions and there was slight attrition confined to the enamel. Attrition was confined to the lingual aspect for the left and right maxillary first molars. In this individual, the findings were strongly suggestive of malocclusion such as cusp-to-cusp occlusion. It is not known whether TMD occurred at a transition period from primary teeth to permanent teeth or after eruption of all permanent teeth. In any case, prolonged retention of primary second molars was thought to have somehow contributed to the development of TMD.

There are limitations in discussing TMD based on archeological materials, but there can be reports of new valuable cases of archeological materials. Modern-day individuals can have prolonged retention of primary teeth causing TMD and can have concurrent periodontal disease. Therefore, it is desirable to appropriately treat individuals with such conditions in modern clinical dental medicine. The material from the Suhgen temple site was an excavated archeological sample, but the implication of its findings can be important in modern dental medicine.

5. Conclusions

This paper discussed three topics from the perspective of physical anthropology which handles ancient human skeletal remains: antemortem tooth loss and problems of periodontal disease and caries, enamel hypoplasia as a stress marker, and occurrence of TMD due to prolonged retention of primary teeth. There are many other oral diseases in ancient skeletal remains that the author of this paper would like to discuss but was unable to, due to limitation of space. The diseases discussed in this paper are all in the oral region and have afflicted people from a few thousand years ago until the present day, i.e., diseases which have also afflicted our ancestors. The author hopes that the readers were able to appreciate that many new findings can be obtained from examination of diseases in the past. It is important to focus on the present to save patients who suffer from modern-day diseases. However, when one examines only the present, one will likely be unable to properly envision dental health of the future. The author is of the opinion that "knowing the past" or "learning from the past" is a very important point. Modern humans have existed for a long time, the ancestors of whom emerged about 7 million years ago. Thus, humans have a long past and modern humans should be thought of as being on the leading edge of this long human history.

Cooperation of physical anthropologists will be important in the creation of guidelines in modern medicine and future oral health. Such an effort can organically link the past, present, and future for the first time and can contribute to a better future. Another hope of this author is that the information and findings of this paper will be useful to many readers.

Author details

Hisashi Fujita[*]

Address all correspondence to: rxh05535@nifty.com

Department of Bioanthropology, Niigata College of Nursing, Japan

References

[1] Sakai S. Japanese History from the diseases. Tokyo: Kodansha; 2014. (in Japanese)

[2] Trinkaus E.; Pathology and Posture of the La Chapelle-aux-Saints Neandertal. Am. J. Phys. Anthropol. 1985, 67, 19-41.

[3] Trinkaus E. The Shanidar Neandertals. Academic Press, New York, USA, 1983.

[4] Nelson GC, Lukacs JR, Yule P. Dates, Caries, and Early Tooth Loss During the Iron Age of Oman. Am J. Phys. Anthropol. 1999, 108, 333-343.

[5] Lopez B, Pardinas AF, Gacia-Vazquez E. Dopico E. Socio-cultural fractures in dental diseases in the Medieval and early Modern Age of northern Spain. Homo. 2012, 63, 21-42.

[6] Sikanjic PR. Bioarchaeology research in Croatia—a historical review. Coll Anthropol. 2005, 29(2): 763-768.

[7]   Fujita H. The number of missing teeth in people of the Edo period in Japan in the 17th to 19th centuries. Gerodontol. 2012, 29, e520-e524.

[8]   Oyamada J, Igawa K, Manabe Y, Kato K, Matsushita T, Rokutanda A, Kitagawa Y. Preliminary analysis of regional differences in dental pathology of early modern commoners in Japan. Anthropol. Sci. 2010, 118, 1-8.

[9]   Takehara T, Sakashita R, Fujita H, Matsushita T, Simoyama A. History of dental caries. : Tokyo; Sunashobo, 2001. (in Japanese)

[10]   Fujita H. Were the Jomon People healthy or not? Speculation of total health condition of ancient people. J. Lipid Nutrition, 2007 16(2), 205-210.

[11]   Fujita H., Suzuki, T., Shoda, S., Kawakubo, Y., Ohno, K., Giannakopoulou, P. and Harihara, S.: Contribution on antemortem tooth loss (AMTL) and dental attrition to oral palaeopathology in the human skeletal series from the Yean-ri site, South Korea. International Journal of Archaeology, 2013 1:1-5.

[12]   Fujita H. Dental Diseases and Stress Markers on Crania in the Early Modern People of Nigeria. Japanese Journal of Gerodontology, 2013 28(1): 10-19.

[13]   Fujita H. Health status in early modern Somali people from their skeletal remains. Int J Archaeol 2014, 2(3), 1-5.

[14]   Jalevik B, Noren JG. Enamel hypomineralization of permanent first molars: a morphological study and survey of possible aetiological factors. Int. J. Paediatr. Dent., 2000 10: 278-289.

[15]   Yamamoto M. Enamel Hypoplasia of the Permanent Teeth in Japanese from the Jomon to the Modern Periods. J. Anthrop. Soc. Nippon 1988 96(4) 417-433.

[16]   Goodman AH, Armelagos GJ, Rose JC. Enamel hypoplasia as as indicators of stress in three prehistoric populations from Illinois. Human Biol. 1980 52: 515-528.

[17]   Sciulli PW, Developmental abnormalities of the permanent dentition in prehistoric Ohio Valley Amerindians. Am. J. Phys. Anthropol., 1978 48: 193-198.

[18]   Cook DC. Subsistence and health in the Lower Illinois Valley: Osteological evidence. In: Cohen M and Aemelagos GJ (ed.) Paleopathology at the Origins of Agriculture. Academic Press, 1984 235-269.

[19]   Lallo JW, Rose JC. Patterns of stress, diseases and mortality in two prehistoric populations from North America. J. Human Evolution, 1979 8: 323-335.

[20]   Cassidy CM. Nutrition and health in agriculturalist and hunter-gatherers. In: Jerome NW, Kandel RF, Pelto GH (ed.) Nutritional Anthropology, Redgrave Press, 1980 117-145.

[21]   Fujita H, Suzuki T, Harihara S. Simultaneous Dental Anomalies (Polyanomalodontia) in Mediaeval Japanese Skeletal Remains. Jpn. J. Oral. Biol. 1997 39: 257-262.

[22] Rando C, Waldron T. TMJ Osteoarthritis: A New Approach to Diagnosis. Am. J. Phys. Anthropol. 2012 148: 45-53

[23] Sumiya Y. Statistic Study on Dental Anomalies in the Japanese. J. Anthropol. Soc. Nippon. 1959 64: 215-233. (in Japanese)

[24] Onizuka Y. Statistical Observation on the Multiple Cases (106 Cases) of the Retained Deciduous Teeth. Kyushu Shika Gakkai Zasshi 1979 33: 52-67. (in Japanese)

Chapter 24

Assorted Errands in Prevention of Children's Oral Diseases and Conditions

H.S. Mbawala, F.M. Machibya and F.K. Kahabuka

Additional information is available at the end of the chapter

http://dx.doi.org/10.5772/59768

1. Introduction

Children are young human beings; they are vulnerable to various ailments including oral diseases and conditions. In order to prevent the various oral diseases and conditions in children, all people responsible in looking after the children have a role to play so as to protect them from acquiring oral diseases or receive appropriate prompt management. This chapter presents responsibilities of various stakeholders in prevention of children's oral diseases and conditions. The impact of oral diseases in children's general health, growth and development is presented. The various oral diseases and conditions and the significance of their prevention is described. Finally, responsible stake holders and their various errands are elucidated.

2. Prevention of children's oral diseases and conditions

The word *prevent* comes from the Latin *"praeventus"*, which means anticipate or hinder. Prevention literally implies the act of putting a stop to something from happening. It refers to measures taken to make the occurrence of something from none existence or not progressing to a worse situation [1]. Subsequently, prevention of diseases is actions aimed at eradicating, eliminating or minimizing the impact of disease and disability, or if none of these are feasible, retarding the progress of the disease and disability. Prevention of oral diseases and conditions, therefore means to put a stop or to avoid the oral diseases and or conditions from occurring, control the already existing condition or disease not to progress further or take charge such that the impact of the condition or diseases is handled to improve quality of life of the affected individual. Disease preventive strategies are acting on the chain of disease causation where individuals who are at risk or have higher possibilities of contracting the disease or having the

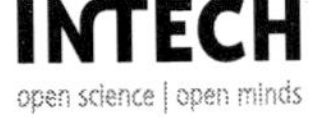

stated condition are made less likely to contract the disease by decreasing their susceptibility, for example action of fluoridated dentifrices on strengthening the teeth to prevent dental caries.

3. Essence of prevention of children's oral diseases and conditions

The rationale behind prevention of oral diseases in children lays back to the sense of widespread of the common oral diseases (dental caries and periodontal conditions) among them, where about 60-90% of children worldwide are affected [2].

Unfortunately, these oral diseases and conditions tend to create socio-demographic gradients [3]; where regardless of knowledge and scientific based evidence advances and achievement for the control and treatment, globally oral diseases have tended to accumulate in the most disadvantaged populations. In these populations the affected child usually have severe and multiple conditions or diseases. It is reported that about 50 million school hours are lost annually in USA due to dental pain as a result of dental caries and that dental pain is the second common condition at medical emergencies, hence oral diseases in children are a public health problem as they impact children's socio and psychological well being as well as restrict school activity [4]. Table 1 summarizes a range of research findings showing the socio-psychological impact of oral diseases to children. In most developing countries, the cost of treating dental caries among children alone will require their total health care budget [5]. Furthermore the clinical approach to dental treatment has proved to be an economic burden in industrialized countries where expenditure on oral health is about 3%-12% of total health expenditures.

Country	Age (yrs)	Dental pain prevalence (%)	Socio-psychological impact
South Australia [6]	5-15	31.8	Disturbed sleep and schoolwork
England [7]	8	47.5	Crying disturbed sleep, play, schoolwork, eating
Tanzania [8]	10-19	36.4	Disturbed eating, smiling, study and socializing
Thailand [10]	11-12	25.1	Disturbed eating, smiling, study and socializing
Uganda [11]	10-14.	42.1	Caries, subjective oral health indicators, dental attendance
Kerala, India [12]	12	68.0	Dissatisfaction with oral status and dental appearance

Table 1. Socio-psychological impacts of dental caries

4. Benefits of prevention of children's oral diseases and conditions

Children are young human beings who are dependent on adults to take care of their health issues both socially and economically. They are more vulnerable to diseases, and once sick it is their parents or guardians who decide and act for their health care. On the other hand, prevention of oral diseases through instituting most oral health related-behaviours like tooth brushing and use of fluoridated toothpaste are determined by the family. Likewise, associated expenses are to be incurred by a family earner.

Oral health is an integral part of overall well-being and essential for eating, growth, speech, social development, learning capacity and quality of life and tooth decay has been reported to have negative impact on childhood nutrition, growth and weight gain [13]. Additionally; World Federation of Public Health Associations [14] admits that oral health problems in children can impact on many aspects of their general health and development, causing substantial pain and disruption to their lives and often altering their behaviour.

Prevention of oral diseases is relatively less costly compared to curative dental services, therefore it is considered beneficial. For example, water fluoridation may appear expensive, but because of its wider coverage and its easy application versus dental treatment for a decayed tooth in an individual, it remains a better choice. Prevention of oral diseases is cost effective particularly in middle and low income countries where resources necessary for conventional dental treatment are scarce and a substantial proportion of their financial resources for health is directed to address infectious diseases.

Another benefit of preventing oral diseases in children is to minimize pain, discomfort and suffering; enable them to eat and socialize well, avoid loss of school hours ultimately contribute into their growth and development.

5. Levels of disease prevention

The concept of prevention is conveniently defined at four levels, namely primordial, primary, secondary and tertiary prevention though in reality the stages blur one into the next.

5.1. Primordial prevention

This is a relatively recent classification of disease prevention. It seeks to prevent at a very early stage, often before the risk factor is present in the particular context, the activities which encourage the emergence of lifestyles, behaviours and exposure patterns that contribute to increased risk of disease. Or it is actions and measures that inhibit the emergence of risk factors in the form of environmental, economic, social, and behavioral conditions and cultural patterns of living. In primordial prevention, efforts are directed towards discouraging children from adopting harmful lifestyles, the main intervention being through individual and mass education. According to Porta [15], primordial prevention consists of conditions, actions, and measures that minimize hazards to health and hence inhibit the emergence and establishment of processes and factors (environmental, economic, social, behavioral, cultural) known to increase the risk of diseases. Furthermore, Porta [15] states that primordial prevention is accomplished through many public and private healthy public policies and intersectoral action and that it may be seen as a form of primary prevention. Primordial prevention addresses broad health determinants rather than preventing personal exposure to risk factors, which is the goal of primary prevention. For instance, outlawing alcohol would represent primordial prevention, whereas a campaign against drinking would be an example of primary prevention. In dentistry primordial prevention will include enforcing a law on fluoride levels in various products and education on causes and prevention of oral diseases and conditions to individuals and to the community.

5.2. Primary prevention

Primary prevention can be defined in several ways. One of these definitions states that primary prevention is the action taken prior to the onset of disease, which removes the possibility that the disease will occur. It also can be defined as the first level of health care, designed to prevent the occurrence of disease and promote health, or as prevention of disease through the control of exposure to risk factors. Approaches for primary prevention include population-wide strategies and high-risk strategies focusing on population sub-groups. It may be accomplished by measures of "Health promotion" and "specific protection" that is; measures designed to promote general health and well-being, and quality of life of people or by specific protective measures. Examples of primary prevention in dentistry include fluoridation of public water, oral evaluation, dental prophylaxis, Fluoride use as preventive agent, fissure sealants, use of Xylitol, mouth guards, regular dental examinations and self-care such as tooth brushing, flossing, use of dental rinses and medicinal mouthwashes.

5.3. Secondary prevention

Is defined as the application of available measures to detect early departures from health and to introduce appropriate treatment and interventions. Others define secondary prevention as the second level of health care, based on the earliest possible identification of disease so that it can be more readily treated or managed and adverse sequelae can be prevented. This level of prevention is also defined as action which halts the progress of a disease at its incipient stage and prevents complications. Screening is a major component of secondary prevention. Examples of secondary prevention in dentistry are Fluoride use on incipient caries, dental restorations, periodontal debridement, root canal treatments, serial extraction, fixed and removable appliances, installation of caps and crowns. Removal of broken or impacted teeth, especially the third molars is also a type of secondary preventive dentistry.

5.4. Tertiary prevention

Is the application of measures to reduce or eliminate long-term impairments and disabilities, minimising suffering caused by existing departures from good health and to promote the patient's adjustments to his/her condition. In other words, it is the third phase or level of health care, concerned with promotion of independent function and prevention of further disease-related deterioration. It also can be defined as all the measures available to reduce or limit impairments and disabilities, and to promote the patients' adjustment to irremediable conditions. Examples of tertiary prevention in dentistry include; denture fabrication, bridges, implants, oro-maxillofacial surgery, periodontal surgery, fixed prosthodontics and space maintainers. Most dental procedures aiming at children fall under the first three levels of prevention.

6. Rationale of oral disease prevention in children

Although dental diseases are not among the feared killer diseases like ebola and malaria, their high prevalence inflict heavy pain in the community in terms of treatment cost, physical and physiological incapacitation and rarely death. Oral health is part and parcel of the general health in such a way that severe illness on orofacial region can lead to systemic problems like malnutrition, immunosupresion, septicaemia etc.

The rationale for preventing oral diseases and especially in children can be viewed under three areas; the disease burden inflicted by oral diseases to the community, the common risk factors shared by oral diseases and other chronic diseases and the lifelong effects to be gained if efforts for prevention are directed to children.

6.1. Disease burden

Despite great improvements in the oral health of populations in several countries, globally, oral health problems still persist [16]. Traditional treatment of oral diseases is extremely costly; it is the fourth most expensive disease to treat in most industrialized countries where 5–10% of public health expenditure relates to oral health [17, 18]. In most developing countries resources are primarily allocated to emergency oral care and pain relief; it is estimated that, if treatment were available in these countries, the costs of dental caries in children alone would exceed the total health care budget for children [5].

6.2. Relation to general health

There is a group of risk factors common to many chronic diseases and oral diseases. They include tobacco and alcohol use, frequent consumption of sugars and inadequate physical activity, especially when coupled with consumption of excess calories, [19-23]. Hence, addressing these factors will ultimately prevent other systemic diseases. The four most prominent non-communicable diseases sharing risk factors with oral diseases are cardiovascular diseases, diabetes, cancer and chronic obstructive pulmonary diseases; the factors are preventable and relate to lifestyles.

6.3. Lifelong effect in children

Children are young, easy to learn and usually what they learn at early age is retained for life. Therefore, efforts for directing disease prevention to children who are likely to practice preventive measures and maintain good oral health throughout adulthood are justified.

7. Oral diseases and conditions that affect children

There are many oral diseases affecting children. They may be congenitally transmitted or acquired through environmental interaction. The chapter describes some of the common oral diseases and conditions in children

7.1. Dental caries

Dental caries or tooth decay is the disease which causes destruction of tooth material, which includes: enamel, dentin, root and pulp. It is one of the most prevalent chronic diseases worldwide [16]. Dental caries forms over time through interaction between cariogenic bacteria and fermentable carbohydrates or cariogenic food particles left on the surface of the tooth. When bacteria feed on the sugars in the food they produce acids responsible for tooth demineralization. All people carry bacteria in their mouth which make them susceptible to tooth decay. In particular, risks for caries development include physical, biological, environmental, behavioural, and lifestyle-related factors such as poor oral hygiene, inappropriate methods of feeding infants, diet high in sugars, high numbers of bacteria, and frequent use of medications containing sugar or causing dry mouth, insufficient fluoride, malnutrition including vitamin and mineral deficiencies and some medical conditions, such as Sjogren's syndrome, that decreases the flow of saliva in the mouth. The teeth are susceptible to caries throughout lifetime, though host factors including tooth structure and saliva modify the progression of the disease. Children are susceptible to aggressive tooth decay of primary teeth known as early childhood caries.

Treatment of dental caries: Some initial dental caries process may stop if prevention actions (like oral hygiene improvement) are put in place. Nevertheless, treatment options for more severe caries include dental fillings. When decay reaches the dentin but not yet in the pulp, it can be treated by removing the decay using rotary or hand instruments; the cavity is then cleaned and filled with dental materials of choice. When the lesion extends into the pulp and/or root canal of the tooth, it is treated by root canal treatment procedure. The procedure involves preparation of an access cavity followed by removal of dead tissue, blood vessels and nerves from the canal and finally cleaning of the root canal(s). Biocompatible materials are filled in the cavity and the canals. When indicated, a crown is placed on the tooth to strengthen the restored tooth crown.

Tooth Extraction: Removal of the tooth is opted if the extent of tooth decay and/or tooth infection is beyond repair with filling or root canal treatment. When the tooth is extracted, it can be replaced with dental implant, partial bridge or denture.

7.2. Periodontal diseases

Periodontal disease refers to gingivitis (an inflammatory condition of the soft tissues surrounding a tooth or the gingiva) and periodontitis (involving the destruction of tooth supporting structures such as the periodontal ligament, bone, cementum and soft tissues). Periodontal disease is initiated by a complex of bacterial species, mainly composed of Gram-negative, anaerobic bacteria growing in subgingival areas. The persistent inflammation due to host response to pathogens causes the destruction of periodontal tissues, leading to clinical manifestations of the disease [24]. In general, most children and adolescents worldwide have signs of gingivitis. An aggressive periodontitis affects about 2% of young individuals during puberty and may lead to premature tooth loss.

Causes of periodontal diseases: Periodontal diseases are caused by bacteria in dental plaque-a sticky substance that forms on tooth surface, but other factors influence the disease progression. In reaction to bacterial invasion, the body immune system releases substances that inflame and damage the connective tissues of the gingiva, periodontal ligament or even the alveolar bone. This leads to swollen, bleeding gums which are signs of gingivitis. Further damage involving cementum, alveolar bone with periodontal pockets indicates severe form of periodontal disease. Some genetic and environmental factors put the host susceptible to periodontal diseases. Rare syndromes affecting phagocytes, the structure of the epithelia, connective tissue, or teeth, could have severe periodontal manifestations. For some disorders, the responsible gene or tissue defect has been identified.

Haim-Munk and Papillon-Lefèvre syndromes are rare autosomal recessive disorders associated with periodontitis onset at childhood and early loss of both deciduous and permanent teeth [25, 26].

Tobacco and alcohol use: Tobacco use is clearly a risk factor for periodontal disease. In contrast, a small but significant association exists between alcohol consumption and loss of periodontal support [27].

Infection like HIV and AIDS: An infection process impairs the immune response thereby lowering the gingival protection from local infection.

Nutrition: Historically, specific, overt nutritional deficiencies have been associated with periodontal disease. Vitamin C deficiency leads to scurvy with decreased formation and maintenance of collagen, increased periodontal inflammation, haemorrhage, and tooth loss.

Diabetes: The relation between periodontal health and diabetes has been described as bidirectional; although periodontitis is a potential complication of diabetes, evidence suggests that treatment of periodontal infections in diabetics could improve glycaemic control [28].

Stress: Emotional and psychosocial stresses clearly are factors in periodontal disease, but their precise role in the pathogenesis of this disease is unknown [29].

Impaired immune response: Severe periodontal disease and loss of tooth-supporting tissues often occurs if the individual's host response or immune function is impaired. Various systemic diseases such as leukaemia and thrombocytopenia could be associated with increased severity of periodontal disease.

Treatment for periodontal diseases: The foundation of periodontal therapy is anti-infective non-surgical treatment aimed at controlling the bacterial plaque and other prominent risk factors. Proper tooth brushing can prevent and treat initial stages of bacterial induced gingivitis. However, scaling and root planning is indicated for treating advanced periodontal disease.

Dental plaque and calculus can be removed from tooth-crown and root surfaces (scaling and root planing) by use of various manual or powered instruments. Special attention is devoted to biofilm debridement in periodontal pockets combined with improved personal oral hygiene. Additional use of local antibiotics, local antiseptic drugs, and systemic antibiotics provides some extra benefit compared with debridement alone.

7.3. Dental trauma

Dental trauma is any injury to the mouth, including teeth, lips, gums, tongue, and jawbones. About one third of 5 years old children have sustained traumatic dental injuries involving primary teeth mostly tooth luxation: boys have slightly higher frequency than girls. A prevalence of 5–12% has been found in children aged 6–12 years in the Middle East. A significant proportion of dental trauma relates to falls, sports, unsafe playgrounds or schools, road accidents and violence [30].

An important predisposing factor for dental trauma is large maxillary overjet and incomplete lip closure. Other risk factors associated with incisors injury in elementary school children are playing without mouthguard and/or faceguard and sociobehavour factors including gender (Male>Female) and increased participation in sport activities [31, 32].

Treatment of dental trauma varies according to the type or extent of injury like fracture, avulsion and luxation (tooth displacement). Tetanus booster and antibiotics should be administered whenever a dental injury is at risk for infection. Arrangements should be made for prompt follow-up with a dentist or an oral and maxillofacial surgeon [33, 34]. Specific procedural details of each type of fracture is beyond the scope of this chapter

7.4. Dental malocclusion

Malocclusion is not a disease but rather a set of dental deviations which in some cases can influence quality of life and interfere with oral functions. The prevalence of different traits of malocclusions varies with age, ethnicity and geographical location. The reported incidence ranges from 32 to 93 percent [35].

The causes of malocclusion include hereditary transmission, oral habits such as thumb sucking, tongue thrusting, pacifier use, prolonged use of a bottle early loss of teeth, impacted teeth, or abnormally shaped teeth, misalignment of jaws due to fractures after a severe injury, tumours of the mouth and jaw, congenital and acquired jaw deformities and abnormal orofacial muscle function.

Treatment: Every dentist who treats children practices orthodontics, whether knowingly or not. It is not enough to think of orthodontics as being solely concerned with appliances.

Orthodontics is the longitudinal care of the developing occlusion and any problems associated with it. All qualified dental practitioners should be encouraged to consider the orthodontic requirements of their patients. Orthodontic treatments include the uses of fixed and removable appliances, tooth extraction for space gain and surgery to correct dental and jaws relation [36].

7.5. Oral mucosal lesions

There are many mucosa lesions occurring in the mouth. Some are local due to local derangement, while others occur in the mouth manifesting systemic diseases like HIV/AIDS. Of the oral mucosa lesions, Leukoplakia is the most frequent form of oral precancer and appears in the oral cavity as a white patch that cannot be rubbed off [37]. Oral lesions may be in form of a swelling, blisters, cyst, ulcers and mucosa coulour change or mucosa plaque.

Oral manifestations of systemic diseases: Many systemic disease manifests with oral signs and symptoms, hence, the mouth is considered as the mirror of the general body health. Some oral lesions (e.g. Koplik's sport) are very specific thus are used in confirming diagnosis of some diseases. Some lesions appear at the initial stage of systemic diseases that should alert clinician to speculate and work for early diagnosis of particular systemic conditions. Before the introduction of Highly Active Antiretroviral Therapy (HAART), approximately 40–50% of people who were HIV-positive had oral disease caused by fungal, bacterial or viral infections that often occur early in the course of the disease [38]. The common systemic diseases with oral lesions include; HIV, Sickle cell anaemia, Hodgkin's lymphoma, Sjögren's syndrome, drugs side effects, Herpes simplex, Varicella-zoster, measles, oral hairy leukoplakia and syphilis.

Congenital anomalies: There are many orofacial conditions occurring congenitally. Of the developmental disorders, congenital diseases of the enamel or dentine, problems related to the number, size and shape of teeth, and craniofacial birth defects such as cleft lip and/or palate are most important [39].

8. Basic principles of prevention of oral diseases in children

WHO Global Oral Health Programme for public health has set down basic principle approaches underlying effective oral disease prevention namely; acting on socio-determinants of health, working as one through the common risk factor approach and implementation of multiple strategies of prevention in different settings.

Socio-determinants of health: It is now apparent that individual behaviours such as oral hygiene practices, dietary patterns and attendance for dental care, which are the bases for prevention of oral diseases and conditions are largely influenced by family, social and community factors, as well as political and economical measures [40]. Therefore, WHO recommends that oral disease prevention strategies (public health strategies) need to be directed at underlying socio-determinants of health. They include; socioeconomic and political context, social position and health care system [41].

Thecommon risk factors approach as one of the underlying strategies for public health approach recognizes that chronic non-communicable diseases such as obesity, cancers, diabetes and oral diseases share a set of common risk conditions and factors. Hence providing a rationale for partnership in disease prevention which is particularly applicable in countries with limited numbers of oral health personnel.

The multiple strategies of prevention: The other underlying principle is the multiple strategies to be implemented in different settings. There should be a mix of complementary public health approaches that focus both on assisting individuals and communities to avoid disease and on the other hand to create supportive environments that are conducive to sustain good health. In the prevention of oral diseases, the high-risk approach has been largely dominant. Finally, the WHO now increasingly acknowledges that the best preventive strategy for public health approach is a combination of the high-risk and directed population approaches, [42].

9. Available prevention approaches for specific oral diseases and their effectiveness

Evidence base of oral health interventions from systematic reviews and effectiveness studies conducted between 1994 to 2005 reveal that there are several approaches for diseases prevention [43]. Water fluoridation and use of topical flourides as toothpaste, mouthrinses and varnishes were effective in reducing caries prevalence of 14 to 46% respectively. Whereas fissure sealants are reported to have caries reduction of up to 86% in 12 months and 57% in 48 months time. Dental health education provided a short term improvement in oral health knoweledge and had limited effects on oral health behaviours. While the effectivenes of dieatary control on reducing caries was not revealed. Table 2 below, summarizes the prevention approaches for specific oral diseases and their effectiveness.

Oral Diseases/Conditions prevention approach	Effectiveness in oral disease prevention
Dental health education	• Short term improvement in oral health knowledge
	• Limited effect on oral health related behaviour
	• Not effective for caries reduction
	• Short-term effect on plaque control and gingival bleeding
Topical fluorides	Caries reduction when fluoridated:
	• Toothpaste 24%
	• Mouthwashes 26%
	• Gels 28%
	• Varnishes 46%
Fissure sealants	Caries reduction ranging from 86-57% in a year or two.
Water fluoridation	Caries reduction by 14%
Dietary approach	Not effective in reducing caries.

Table 2. Available prevention approaches for specific oral diseases and their effectiveness, modified from Watt, R. G. [40]

10. Different stakeholders responsible for children's oral health

There are diverse stakeholders for children's oral health who vary in accordance to the child's age or place where the child is located on a specified period of time. Another category is the overall universal stakeholder.

The stakeholders in accordance to the child's age are presented for three age groups namely; birth to three years, four to seven years and eight to twelve years.

10.1. From birth to three years

At birth children do not have teeth. Usually the mothers are the fundamental persons in charge of the children's oral health. Under special circumstances, for example a very sick mother or a mother who pass away after delivery, caretakers may become principally accountable. Whether the mother is available or not, more carers come in as the child grows to one year and further to three years. They include, fathers, siblings, helpers and other family members. Other important responsible groups for prevention of oral diseases in young children are the professionals that is; Medical personnel (Medical doctors and nurses) and Dental personnel (Dentists, Dental Hygienists, Dental Nurses).

10.2. Four to seven years

As children grow they also assume responsibility on their health issues. Thus the stakeholders for children aged four to seven years are the mothers, fathers, children themselves, siblings, helpers, other family members and nursery/school teachers. The Medical personnel (Medical doctors and nurses) and Dental personnel (Dentists, Dental Hygienists, Dental Nurses) are accountable in prevention of oral diseases in this age group.

10.3. Eight to twelve years

The primary responsible persons for the oral health of eight to twelve years old children are the children themselves. These are supported by mothers, fathers, siblings, helpers, other family members and school teachers. The Medical personnel (Medical doctors and nurses) and Dental personnel (Dentists, Dental Laboratory Technologists, Dental Hygienists, Dental Nurses) have a big role to play in prevention of oral diseases in this age group.

The stakeholders can also be looked at in terms of location. The various locations of interest are the homes, school, health facilities and institutions for children with special health care needs.

10.4. Responsible stakeholders for children's oral health at homes

At homes the stakeholders responsible for children's oral health are Parents and guardians, children themselves and other children carers (siblings, relatives or helpers).

10.5. Responsible stakeholders for children's oral health at school

The stakeholders responsible for children's oral health at schools are teachers, children themselves and other children carers depending on the school system.

10.6. Responsible stakeholders for children's oral health at health facilities

At Health facilities responsible stakeholders for children's oral health include Medical personnel (Medical doctors and nurses), Dental personnel (Dentists, Dental Laboratory Technologists, Dental Hygienists and Dental Nurses).

10.7. Responsible stakeholders for children's oral health at Institutions for children with special health care needs

The oral health of children living at institutions is a responsibility of children carers, parents/guardians and children themselves depending on their level of dependency.

10.8. Universal stakeholders

In this chapter, governments, professional associations, Dental products manufacturers, the media and NGOs are considered universal stakeholders because their responsibilities cut across ages and locations. The governments are responsible for policies and governance of all issues pertaining to health. Whereas, professional associations' responsibilities are to safeguard the health of the people they serve. The dental products manufacturers are responsible to supply products required at all levels of prevention regardless of age or place. The NGOs can at any age and location play any role that falls within the organisation's governing regulations.

11. Assorted errands

The different tasks of various stakeholders in the prevention of oral diseases among children are presented with the centre of attention being the four levels of prevention.

11.1. Tasks of various stakeholders in executing primordial prevention of oral diseases among children

Under primordial prevention the task is to give education before the risk factor for oral diseases has occurred. The target group is the community without the risk factors.

The responsible individuals and their responsibilities are presented below;

11.2. Oral health personnel

Dentists, Dental Therapists, Dental Hygienists, Dental Nurses and Community Dental Workers or any other oral health workers are primarily responsible to give oral health education (OHE). That is; to inform the community on the common oral diseases and conditions that affect children, their causes and measures to prevent them. Important messages for the community comprise proper and timely tooth brushing of children's teeth, sensible use of sugary containing food staffs including avoiding leaving a nipple in the child's mouth at night. Other messages include maintenance of playgrounds, blunting sharp edges, securing windows and stairs as well as shunning slippery floors to protect young children against injuries, regular visit to a dentist for check-up and discouraging misconceptions, beliefs and practices harmful to children's oral health. As Narksawat et al. [44] put it that parents must be motivated to consistently spend the time required to take care of the primary dentition of their children by regular cleaning and controlling the snacking behavior of their children. Emphasis should be directed to parents of children with special health care needs, motivating and empowering them to realize these preventive strategies. In order to execute primordial prevention, the oral health personnel ought to target the community because this stage is done to a community who do not have the risk factors.

11.3. Community

The obligation of the community that is; parents, school teachers, children and other family members is to receive OHE and make use of the received information in order to avoid the risk factors. Parents of children with special health care needs, require endurance in looking after their children's oral health.

11.4. School teachers

School teachers are responsible to supervise children's playing activities, maintenance of playgrounds and controlling availability of sugary foods within school premises.

11.5. Universal stakeholders

In order for the primordial prevention to succeed, support is required from universal stakeholders, that is; Governments, Professional Associations, the Media and NGOs. The support expected is through formulation and enforcement of policies on OHE, provision of funds and personnel to take part in OHE activities as well as support to the profession to air Oral Health Education messages/campaigns through various media.

11.6. Tasks of various stakeholders in executing primary prevention of oral diseases among children

Primary prevention targets the community and the children in particular. The goal is to prevent personal exposure to risk factors.

11.6.1. Governments

Governments are in charge of policy formulation and implementation. The governm520ents therefore are liable to have in place policies supporting primary prevention of oral diseases in children such as those governing school oral health programmes including those directed to children with special health care needs, where required fluoridation of public water and fostering availability of fluoride tablets. They should provide conducive working environment, avail funds and give any other support to preventive programmes.

11.6.2. Oral health personnel

Primary prevention requires oral health personnel (Dentists, Dental Therapists, Dental Hygienists, Dental Nurses, Community Dental Workers or any other oral health workers) collectively or individually to do oral evaluation, regular dental examinations, dental prophylaxis, fissure sealants and health education with emphasis on plaque control and use of fluoridated tooth paste twice per day in the morning and evening before retiring to bed. They are also responsible to correct oral habits, and monitor occlusal development so as to prevent malocclusions. These procedures can be done at the chair side but also in communities such as primary schools or reproductive and child health clinics. Moreover, oral health care workers need to devise special primary preventive programmes for children with special health care needs bearing in mind the challenges encountered during dental treatment to these children. It may require outreach programmes to visit children at their schools where tailor-made information and instructions are given to the children.

11.6.3. Medical personnel (Medical doctors and nurses)

The medical personnel who see children for various ailments should join oral health personnel by mentioning prevention of oral diseases when they talk about prevention of other diseases particularly those sharing common risk factors such as diabetes, heart diseases, hypertension and cancers. The medical personnel attending children with special health care needs are liable to emphasise prevention of oral diseases.

11.6.4. Parents and community at large

The responsibility of parents and other community members is to advocate the use of Fluoride as a caries preventive agent and plaque control for prevention of gum diseases. Fluoride tooth paste used during tooth brushing twice a day in the morning and before retiring to be bed is universally accepted to prevent dental caries. Therefore, parents are responsible to brush their children's teeth from the eruption of the first tooth to six years of age. From age seven to 10 years, parents should supervise children's tooth brushing. In older children, parents should supervise flossing, use of dental rinses and medicinal mouthwashes. Furthermore, parents are responsible to facilitate the use of Xylitol and mouth guards if indicated. Parents should take their children for regular dental visits so that children's oral health can be monitored. Supervision and facilitation of using dental rinses and medicinal mouthwashes is another parents' task. Parents of children with special health care needs should pay special attention to prevent oral diseases for their children. This is particularly important given the hassles encountered in the dental settings by parents and oral health workers during dental treatment of children with special health care needs.

11.6.5. School and sports teachers

School children spend most of their day time at schools and therefore in contact with school teachers. The teachers are obliged to facilitate preventive actions against oral and other diseases. They can supervise tooth brushing or mouth rinse activities. They can support other programmes like Fluoride application or fissure sealing.

11.6.6. NGOs

Various national and international NGOs have funds and volunteers to support preventive programmes. They can arrange and participate in community services such as oral health screening, Fluoride application or fissure sealing programmes by giving funds and organising for personnel to take part in various programmes.

11.6.7. Dental products manufacturers

The dental product manufactures supply a wide range of products that are used to realize primary prevention of oral diseases among children. They are responsible to avail good quality products at affordable prices the dental products for prevention of diseases; tooth brushes, tooth paste, mouthwashes, fissure sealants, fluorides, dental floss, mouth mirrors as well as dental supplies including gloves, antiseptics etc.

11.7. Tasks of various stakeholders in executing secondary prevention of oral diseases among children

Secondary prevention involves actions which halt the progress of a disease at its incipient stage and prevents complications.

11.7.1. Governments

In order to facilitate provision of services to children at early stages of oral diseases so as to halt their progress and prevent complications, governments are required to provide conducive dental clinic working environments, avail funds, have in place and enforce policies on dental supplies. Governments are also responsible to oversee activities related to prevention of oral diseases in children in public sectors, private sectors and insurance companies.

11.7.2. Oral health personnel (Dentists, dental therapists, dental hygienists, dental nurses, community dental workers or any other oral health workers)

The Oral health personnel working in public or private sectors are responsible to provide or take part in treatment of various oral diseases and conditions. They should use Fluoride [45] on incipient caries, restore decayed teeth or perform root canal treatments where necessary, professional tooth cleaning and if indicated periodontal debridement. They should keep abreast with new knowledge, procedures, techniques and materials to facilitate them offer quality treatment of oral diseases at their early stages. Oral health care workers providing dental treatment to children with special health care needs should equip themselves with techniques to address the challenges encountered during dental treatment to these children.

11.7.3. Medical personnel (Medical doctors and nurses)

The medical personnel who see children for various ailments are liable to do early diagnosis of oral diseases and make prompt referral. Whereas Rozier et al. [46] demonstrated that non-dental professionals can integrate preventive dental services into their practices, the American Academy of Pediatrics recommends physician interventions in addressing dental caries to include oral health screening and referral when indicated, provision of oral hygiene instructions, dietary information, and anticipatory guidance to parents, as well as prescription of fluoride supplements. In so doing they will facilitate early identification of oral diseases, promote their readily treatment and prevention of adverse sequelae.

11.7.4. Parents

Parents have a significant role to play to aid the oral health personnel in executing secondary prevention of oral diseases among children. They have to take their children for dental consultation at early stages of the disease. For the parents to achieve this task they have to develop a practice of looking into their children's mouths and consult dentists for any abnormal development principally so for children with special health care needs. After consulting the dentists they need to comply with appointments and instructions given by professionals.

11.7.5. Dental products manufacturers

A diverse list of materials and supplies is needed to support oral health personnel in delivering secondary prevention of oral diseases among children. The dental products manufacturers are responsible to avail required materials and supplies at affordable prices and of good quality. The requirements range from instruments, dental materials and dental supplies to dental equipment.

11.7.6. School teachers

Since school teachers spend most of their working time with children, their role in secondary prevention of oral diseases among children is to remind and motivate parents as well as children to consult dentists as per professional recommendations.

11.7.7. NGOs

The NGOs can support treatment programmes through volunteer services and provision of funds to buy required instruments, dental materials, dental supplies or dental equipment depending on the NGO's capacity.

11.8. Tasks of various stakeholders in executing tertiary prevention of oral diseases among children

There are a few actions at the level of tertiary prevention of oral diseases among children:

11.8.1. Governments

As for other levels of prevention, governments are responsible to provide conducive working environment, avail dental supplies and funds to allow provision of tertiary level prevention to those children who need such services. The governments should have policies to govern provision of tertiary level oral health care.

11.8.2. Oral health personnel (Dentists, dental therapists, dental hygienists, dental nurses, dental laboratory technologists or any other oral health workers)

It is the responsibility of oral health personnel to provide or take part in provision of tertiary level oral health care. This level is provided at health facilities. The oral health personnel should bear in mind that tertiary prevention in children at times implies primary prevention of oral problems in adult life.

11.8.3. Parents

The tertiary level care in children is important for future oral health of adults. Parents are therefore required to consult dentists for this care as will be advised by dentists and to comply with appointments and instructions given by professionals.

11.8.4. Dental products manufacturers

The dental products manufacturers should avail required materials and supplies for the preparation of children's tertiary level care because they are important for future oral health of adults. Tertiary prevention in children should not to considered as cosmetic therefore the required instruments, materials and other supplies should be availed at a reasonable cost.

11.8.5. NGOs

The NGOs should support treatment programmes as per individual organisation policy and capability.

Basically, oral disease prevention is difficult to attain but it is a responsibility that has to be fulfilled. It is worth to direct efforts of disease prevention to children because they are young, easy to learn and usually what they learn at early age is retained for life thus children are likely to adopt preventive measures and maintain good oral health throughout adulthood.

12. Conclusion

Diverse groups of people are responsible to execute prevention of oral diseases in children. If they work as a team and accountable on each individual errand, oral diseases in children can be minimized or controlled thus enable children to eat well and ultimately grow well which contribute to improved children's social development, learning capacity and thus good quality of life.

13. Recommendations

The different errands should be publicized and motivate all responsible groups or individuals to be accountable with their roles in order to realize prevention of oral diseases in children.

Author details

H.S. Mbawala, F.M. Machibya and F.K. Kahabuka[*]

*Address all correspondence to: kokukahabuka@yahoo.com

Department of Orthodontics, Paedodontics and Preventive Dentistry, School of Dentistry, Muhimbili University of Health and Allied Sciences, Dar es Salaam

References

[1] Leavell, Hugh R. Clark, E.G. (1958). Preventive Medicine for the doctor in his community: epidemilogic approach. New York: McGraw-Hill.

[2] World Health Organization (WHO 2002). Global Oral Health Data Base. Geneva: World Health Organization.

[3] Petersen, P. E. (2003). The World Oral Health Report 2003: continuous improvement of oral health in the 21st century–the approach of the WHO Global Oral Health Programme. *Community Dentistry and Oral Epidemiology*, 3-24.

[4] United States Department of Health and Human Services (USDHHS). (2000) Oral Health in America: A Report of the Surgeon General. National Institute of Health. http://www.nidcr.nih.gov/datastatistics/surgeongeneral/report/executivesummary.htm

[5] Yee R, Sheiham A. (2002). The burden of restorative dental treatment for children in third world countries. *International Dental Journal* 52:1-9.

[6] Slade, G. D., Spencer, A. J., Davies, M. J., & Burrow, D. (1996). Intra-oral distribution and impact of caries experience among South Australian school children. *Australian dental journal*, 41(5), 343-350.

[7] Shepherd, M. A., Nadanovsky, P., & Sheiham, A. (1999). Dental public health: the prevalence and impact of dental pain in 8-year-old school children in Harrow, England. *British dental journal, 187*(1), 38-41.

[8] Mashoto, K. O., Astrom, A. N., David, J., & Masalu, J. R. (2009). Dental pain, oral impacts and perceived need for dental treatment in Tanzanian school students: a cross-sectional study. *Health Qual Life Outcomes, 7,* 73.

[9] Nomura, L. H., Bastos, J. L. D., & Peres, M. A. (2004). Dental pain prevalence and association with dental caries and socioeconomic status in schoolchildren, Southern Brazil, 2002. *Brazilian oral research, 18*(2), 134-140.

[10] Kiwanuka, S. N., & Åstrøm, A. N. (2005). Self-reported dental pain and associated factors in Ugandan schoolchildren. *Norsk epidemiologi, 15*(2)

[11] Gherunpong, S., Tsakos, G., & Sheiham, A. (2004). The prevalence and severity of oral impacts on daily performances in Thai primary school children. *Health Qual Life Outcomes, 2*(1), 57.

[12] David, J., Åstrøm, A. N., & Wang, N. J. (2006). Prevalence and correlates of self-reported state of teeth among schoolchildren in Kerala, India. *BMC Oral Health, 6*(1), 10.

[13] Sheiham A. Dental caries affects body weight, growth and quality of life in preschool children British Dental Journal 2006; 201: 625-626

[14] World Federation of Public Health Associations (WFPHA) (2013). Oral Health for Children www.wfpha.org/tl_files/doc/about/.../OHWG_Child%20Declaration.pdf

[15] Porta M. A Dictionary of Epidemiology (2008). Fifth Edition, *Oxforn University Press Amazon.com*

[16] Petersen PE, Bourgeois D, Ogawa H, Estupinan-Day S, Ndiaye C. (2005). The global burden of oral diseases and risks to oral health. *Bulletin of the World Health Organization* 83:661-669.

[17] Griffin SO, Jones K, Tomar SL. (2001). An economic evaluation of community water fluoridation. *Journal of Public Health Dentistry* 61:78-86.

[18] Wang NJ, Källestaal C, Petersen PE, Arnadottir IB. (1998). Caries preventive services for children and adolescents in Denmark, Iceland, Norway and Sweden: strategies and resource allocation. *Community Dentistry and Oral Epidemiology* 26:263-71.

[19] Franceschi S, Talamini R, Barra S, Baron AE, Negri E, et al. (1990). Smoking and drinking in relation to cancers of the oral cavity, pharynx, larynx, and esophagus in northern Italy. *Cancer research 50*(20):6502-6507.

[20] Giovannucci E, Colditz GA, Stampfer MJ, Willett WC (1996). Physical activity, obesity, and risk of colorectal adenoma in women (United States). *Cancer Causes & Control* 7(2):253-263.

[21] Sanders TA (2004). Diet and general health: dietary counselling. *Caries Res* 38:3-8.

[22] Saito T, Shimazaki Y, Kiyohara Y, Kato I, Kubo M, et al. (2005). Relationship between obesity, glucose tolerance, and periodontal disease in Japanese women: the Hisayama study. *Journal of Periodontal Research* 40(4):346-353.

[23] Liang J, Matheson BE, Kaye WH, Boutelle KN (2013). Neurocognitive correlates of obesity and obesity-related behaviors in children and adolescents. *Int J Obes* doi: 10.1038/ijo.2013.142. [Epub ahead of print]

[24] Kornman KS, Page RC, Tonetti MS. (1997). The host response to the microbial challenge in periodontitis: assembling the players. *Periodontol.* 14:33–53.

[25] Hart TC, Hart PS, Bowden DW, et al. (1999). Mutations gene of the cathepsin C are responsible for Papillon-Lefevre syndrome. *J Med Genet* 36: 881–87.

[26] Toomes, C., James, J., Wood, A. J., Wu, C. L., McCormick, D., Lench, N.,... & Thakker, N. S. (1999). Loss-of-function mutations in the cathepsin C gene result in periodontal disease and palmoplantar keratosis. *Nature genetics,* 23(4), 421-424.

[27] Tezal M, Grossi SG, Ho AW, Genco R.J. (2004). Alcohol consumption and periodontal disease. The Third National Health and Nutrition Examination Survey. *J Clin Periodontol* 31: 484–88.

[28] Taylor GW. (2001). Bidirectional interrelationships between diabetes and periodontal diseases: an epidemiologic perspective. *Ann Periodontol* 6: 99–112.

[29] LeResche L, Dworkin SF. (2000). The role of stress in inflammatory disease, including periodontal disease: review of concepts and current findings. *Periodontol.* 30:2002; 91–103.)

[30] Glendor U. (2008). Epidemiology of traumatic dental injuries –a 12 year review of the literature. *Dental Traumatol* 24: 603–611

[31] Kania MJ, Keeling SD, McGorray SP, Wheeler TT, King GJK. (1996). Risk factors associated with incisor injury in elementary school children. *Angle Orthod* 66:423-432.

[32] Baldava P. and Anup N. Risk factors for traumatic dental injuries in an adolescent male population in India.*J Contemp Dent Pract* 2007; 8.6: 35-42.

[33] Harrison L. (2014). Dental trauma: guidelines for pediatricians updated. Medscape Medical News. January 27, 2014. Available at http://www.medscape.com/viewarticle/819755.

[34] Keels MA. (2014). Management of dental trauma in a primary care setting. *Pediatrics.* 133(2):e466-76.

[35] Carvalho JC, Vinker F, Declerck D. (1998). Malocclusion, dental injuries and dental anomalies in the primary dentition of Belgian children. *Int J Paediatr Dent.* 8(2): 137-41.

[36] McNair A and Morris D. (2008). Managing the Developing Occlusion: A guide for dental practitioners. 3rd Ed. British Orthodontic Society.

[37] Bokor-brati M. (2000). The prevalence of precancerous oral lesions. Oral leukoplakia. *Archive of Oncology* 8(4):169-70.

[38] Arendorf TM, Bredekamp B, Cloete CA, Sauer G. (1998). Oral manifestations of HIV infection in 600 South African patients. *Journal of oral pathology & medicine*. 27:176-9.

[39] Lidral AC, Murray JC, Buetow KH, Basart AM, Schearer H, Schiang R, Naval A, Layda E, Magee K, Magee W. (1997). Studies of the candidate genes *TGFB2,MSX1, TGFA*, and *TGFB3* in the etiology of cleft lip and palate in the Philippines. *Cleft Palate Craniofac J* 34(1):1-6.

[40] Newton J.T, Bower E.J. (2005). The social determinants of oral health: new approaches to conceptualising and researching complex causal networks. *Community Dentistry and Oral Epidemiology*. 33:25-34

[41] Watt, R. G. (2005). Strategies and approaches in oral disease prevention and health promotion. *Bulletin of the World Health Organization, 83*(9), 711-718

[42] World Health Organization (WHO 2000). Global strategy for the prevention and control of non-communicable diseases. Geneva

[43] Marinho, V. C., Higgins, J. P., Sheiham, A., & Logan, S. (2004). Combinations of topical fluoride (toothpastes, mouthrinses, gels, varnishes) versus single topical fluoride for preventing dental caries in children and adolescents. *Cochrane Database Syst Rev, 1.*

[44] Narksawat K, Boonthum A, Tonmukayakul U. (2011). Roles of parents in preventing dental caries in the primary dentition among preschool children in Thailand. *Asia Pac J Public Health*. 23(2):209-16. doi: 10.1177/1010539509340045. Epub 2009 Jul 2.

[45] American Academy of Pediatrics. Practice guideline endorsement. Recommendations for Using Fluoride to Prevent and Control Dental Caries in the United States. Available at: http://www.aap.org/policy/fluoride.html. (Accessed September 2014)

[46] Rozier R. G., Bawden, J. W., Slade, G. D. (2003) Prevention of Early Childhood Caries in North Carolina Medical Practices: Implications for Research and Practice. *Journal of Dental Education* 67:876-885

[47] Donovan D., McDowell I., Hunter D. (2008). AFMC Primer on Population Health A virtual textbook on Public Health concepts for clinicians. Association of Faculties of Medicine of Canada - AFMC http://phprimer.afmc.ca/inner/primer_contents

[48] Fendrychová J. Preventive Dentistry In Dostálová T, Seydlová. (2010). Dentistry and Oral Diseases for medical students. Chapter 12 Pg 191- 198. *Grada Publishing*

[49] Pine C. M., Harris R. (2007) Community Oral Health. 2nd edition Quintessence Pub.

[50] Vivekanand. (2004). Manual of Community Dentistry Chapter 9, pg 167 – 186 Jaypee Brothers Publishers.

Chapter 25

Drug-Induced Oral Reactions

Ana Pejcic

Additional information is available at the end of the chapter

http://dx.doi.org/10.5772/59261

1. Introduction

Oral Medicine is a specialty that deals with the diagnosis and medical management of the complex medical disorders involving the oral mucosa. The success of any treatment depends on a proper and correct diagnosis. A successful diagnostician has to have qualities like knowledge, interest, intuition, curiosity, and patience. 99.9% of systemic diseases have one or more oral manifestations which are diagnosed by oral physician even before the general physician. Early recognition and diagnosis are important for early treatment, improving survival and for limiting the complications of therapy.

In present day the number of elderly people is on the rise. This is a rapidly growing population who has chronic medical conditions, take multiple medications and require routine, safe and appropriate oral and general healthcare, which may be challenging for the dental physician. The oral medicine specialists require careful assessment of each elderly person to help in the formulation of a strategy for their care, maintenance of comfort, self-respect and, effective and sympathetic dental care for them [1].

Several systemic factors are known to contribute to oral diseases or conditions, and among those are the intakes of drugs. The pathogenesis of oral adverse reactions related to intake of medications is not well-understood, and the prevalence is not known. They are, however, believed to be a relatively common phenomenon, although medication-induced oral reactions are often regarded by the health profession as trivial complaints [2].

Drug-induced side effects are a frequent occurrence. Many commonly available drugs can produce untoward consequences, even when used according to standard or recommended methods of administration. Such adverse drug reactions can involve every organ and system of the body and may be seen in all age group, and present in many different forms [3]. Regarding different parts of the oral system, these reactions can be categorized to oral mucosa and tongue, periodontal tissues, dental structures, salivary glands, cleft lip and palate,

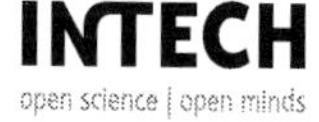

muscular and neurological disorders, taste disturbances, drug-induced oral infection, and facial edema. The oral drug reactions are often nonspecific, but they may mimic specific disease states such as Pemphigus vulgaris, Erythema multiforme, or Lichen planus [4,5]. The knowledge about drug-induced oral adverse effects helps health professionals to better diagnose oral disease, administer drugs, improve patient compliance during drug therapy, and may influence a more rational use of drugs [6].

Oral drug-reaction patterns with associated drugs and drug classes include:

2. Aphthous stomatitis

Aphthous stomatitis (also termed recurrent aphthous stomatitis, recurring oral aphthae or recurrent aphthous ulceration) is a common condition characterized by the repeated formation of benign and non-contagious mouth ulcers (aphthae), in otherwise healthy individuals. Aphthous–like ulcerations may occur from a variety of medications, including capropril and nonsteroidal anti-inflammatory drugs (NSAIDs), Asathiopurine, Losartan, and Gold compounds. It is unclear as to the mechanism leading to this reaction pattern [7,8].

The lesions may be single or multiple. Three clinical variations have been recognized: minor, major and herpetiforme ulcers. Minor form and herpetiforme ulcers heal without scarring in 7-12 days and major form persist for 3-6 weeks [9].

For treatment used topical steroids or, in severe cases, intralesional steroid injection or systemic steroids in low dose.

3. Burning mouth syndrome

Burning mouth syndrome (BMS) is a painful, frustrating condition often described as a scalding sensation in the tongue, lips, palate, or throughout the mouth. Signs and symptoms are: burning, scalding or tingling feeling on the tongue, lips, throat or palate, no specific lesion evident, with or without any sing of inflammation and discomfort usually worse at the end of the day. This syndrome may occur due to psychogenic factors, hormonal withdrawal, folate, iron, pyridoxine deficiency, or hypersensitivity reactions to the materials utilized in dental prostheses [10,11]. The most common medications that produce this side effect are: ACE inhibitors, antibiotics, hormone replacement therapy antidepressants and cephalosporin [12,13,14]. Possible treatments may include: replacing medication, treating existing disorder or treatment is aimed at the symptoms to try to reduce the pain associated with burning mouth syndrome.

- **Glossitis-**Glossitis is inflammation of the tongue. Signs and symptoms are: swollen intensely painful tongue, red and smooth tongue. Pain may be referred to the ears and salivation, fever and enlarged lymph nodes may develop if infection is present. Various drugs which can cause glossitis are: antibiotics, corticosteroids, methotrezole, and tricyclic antidepressants [15,16].

The goal of treatment is to reduce inflammation. Good oral hygiene is necessary, including thorough tooth brushing at least twice a day.

- **Oral ulcerations (nonspecific ulceration and mucositis)**

Oral ulcerations may occur in a different setting, including local irritation, chemotherapy, opportunistic infections and fixed drug reactions. Epithelial necrosis and ulceration may result from direct application of over-the-counter medications such as aspirin, hydrogen peroxide, potassium tablets, and phenol-containing compounds to the mucosa. [17]. Aspirin is often used by patients seeking relief from dental pain. The affected mucosa appears whitish and corrugated, with erosion and ulceration of the more severely damaged areas. The associated discomfort can be severe enough to require treatment. Oral drug reaction may be as small round /oval lesions/ with yellow or grey floor and may lead to difficulties in speck. Drugs including anti-neoplastics (methotrexate, 5-fluorouracil), barbiturates, dapsone, tetracyclines, nonsteroidal anti-inflammatory drugs (NSAIDs) (eg, indomethacin, salicylates, gold salts, naproxen), meprobamate, methyldopa, penicillamine, propranolol, spironolactone, thiazides, tolbutamide, alendronate, captopril, phenytoin, and (by direct contact) compounds containing aspirin can cause oral ulcerations. [18,19].

They are clinically diverse, but usually appear as a single, painful ulcer with a smooth red or whitish-yellow surface and a thin erythematous haloo. For treatment used removal of factors and topical steroids for a short time.

4. Vesico-bullous lesions

Oral drug reactions that bear striking clinical, histopathologic, and even immunopathologic resemblance to idiopathic Lichen planus, Erythema multiforme (EM), Pemphigoid, Pemphigus vulgaris, and Lupus erythematosus (LE) are well recognized, and the list of reactions in each category is constantly expanding. Clinically, any oral site can be affected; however, the posterior buccal mucosa (cheeks), the lateral borders of the tongue, and the alveolar mucosa are most commonly involved. Lesions may be isolated, although bilaterally symmetric involvement is not uncommon [20,21].

- Lichen planus – Lichen planus is a relatively common papulosquamous disorder involving the skin and mucous membranes. Often these lesions are asymptomatic. Lichen planus–like or lichenoid drug reactions are a heterogeneous group of lesions of the oral mucosa that show clinical and histopathological similarities to lichen planus. Lichenoid reactions have subsequently been reported in association with many agents (amalgam, composite resins, and dental restorative materials). A number of drugs have been implicated in lichen planus-like eruptions. The most common agents are nonsteroidal anti-inflammatory drugs and angiotensin converting enzyme inhibitors.

Although drug-induced lichenoid reactions tend to be erosive and unilateral compared with the typical bilateral presentation in idiopathic lichen planus, these associations are not consistently observed. Middle aged individuals are more commonly affected. The predilection sites are the buccal mucosa, tongue, and gingiva. The pathogenic mechanism by which drugs cause LP-like drug eruptions is not clear, T cell-mediated autoimmune phenomena are involved in the pathogenesis of Lichen planus [22,23,24,25].

Clinical characteristic oral lesions of the disease are white papules that usually coalesce, forming a net-work of lines (Wickham's striae). Six forms of the disease are recognized in the oral mucosa. The common forms are reticular and erosive, the less common are atrophic and hypertrophic, and the rare ere bullous and pigmented.

The disease can usually be diagnosed on clinical grounds alone. Histopathological examination is very helpful.

In treatment, topical steroids may be helpful, and intralesional injection. Systemic steroids in low doses can be used in severe and extensive cases.

- Erythema multiforme (EM) – like – Erythema multiforme is a syndrome consisting of symmetrical mucocutaneus lesions that have a predilection for the oral mucosa, hand, and feet. Initial bullae may rupture, giving rise to widespread superficial ulceration [26]. A spectrum of disease can be seen ranging from a benign cutaneus eruption to a severe mucocutaneous eruption. Steven-Johnson syndrome represents a severe manifestation of EM. Syndrome characterized by various clinical types of lesions. The lips are swollen, crusted, and bleeding. Drugs with potential to cause Erythema multiforme are: antibiotics (antimalarial, penicillin, sulfonamide, and tetracycline), allopurinol, barbiturates, protease inhibitors, and NSAIDs. Drug-induced EM represents approximately 25% of all reported cases. Drug-induced EM is frequently linked to agents such as sulfonamides, sulfonylureas, and barbiturates, among others [27,28,29].

- Pemphigoid – like – Drug-induced Pemphigoid can occur in the setting of a number of drugs. Antirheumatics (penicillamine, ibuprofen, phenacetin), cardiovascular drugs (furosemide, captopril, clonidine), antibiotics (penicillin's, sulfonamides), antimicrobials, thiol-containing drugs, and sulfonamide derivatives. Pemphigoid-like reactions can be limited to the oral mucosa, or they can affect other mucosal or cutaneous sites. Clinically, lesions appear as relatively sturdy vesicles or bullae that break down into shallow ulcerations. Generalized or multifocal involvement of the gingival tissues may be observed, with marked erythema and erosion of the superficial gingiva, a pattern that has been called Desquamative gingivitis. Thiol-containing drugs and sulfonamide derivatives are among the most commonly involved medications, as are the therapeutic classes of NSAIDs, cardiovascular agents, antimicrobials, and antirheumatics. Drug-induced pemphigoid patients may be younger and have more frequent oral involvement [30]. For treatment used steroids and, rarely, immunosuppressive drugs.

- Pemphigus – like – drug reactions have been reported to have similar clinical, histologic, and immunofluorescent patterns as Pemphigus vulgaris. Alpha-mercaptopropionylglycine, ampicillin, captopril, cephalexin, ethambutol, glibenclamide, gold, heroin, ibuprofen, penicillamine, phenobarbital, phenylbutazone, piroxicam, practolol, propranolol, pyritinol chlorohydrate, rifampin, and theobromine. Pemphigus-like reactions can have features of either pemphigus vulgaris or pemphigus foliaceous, although pemphigus foliaceous is uncommon in the oral cavity. Thiol-containing drugs are the most common cause of pemphigus-like reactions. In drug-induced pemphigus vulgaris, the relatively fragile vesicles are rarely observed at clinical examination, and most cases are characterized by irregular ulcerations with ragged borders that may coalesce to involve large areas of the mucosa. Patients may have circulating autoantibodies to the desmosomal components [31]. Treatment is used systemic steroides, immunosuppressive drugs and dapsone.

- Lupus erythematosus (LE) – like-Drug-induced LE is a well-recognized adverse reaction that is most commonly associated with procainamide and hydralazine, although more than 70 medications are implicated (Carbamazepine, chlorpromazine, ethosuximide, gold, griseofulvin, hydantoins, hydralazine, isoniazid, lithium, methyldopa, penicillamine, primidone, procainamide, quinidine, reserpine, streptomycin, thiouracils, and trimetha-dione.). Clinically, the oral lesions of drug-induced LE may simulate those of erosive lichen planus, with irregular areas of erythema or ulceration bordered by radiating keratotic striae. These lesions may affect the palate, buccal mucosa, and gingival or alveolar tissues. The rarity of lichen planus on the hard palate may be helpful in differentiating it from drug-induced LE [32]. In treatment used steroids and antimalarial drugs.

5. Color changes of oral mucosa and teeth (Pigmentation)

Pigmentation may by normal pigmentation which are a physiological finding, particularly in dark-skinned individuals because increased melanin production and deposition in the oral mucosa. No treatment is required. Abnormal oral pigmentation can result from a number of causes, including local and systemic medications (amiodarone, antimalarials, bisulfan, clofazimine, cyclophosphamide, estrogen). Discoloration can occur after direct contact with or following systemic absorption of a drug. Discoloration of the oral mucosa after drug use may be due to direct melanocytic stimulation, the deposition of pigmented drug metabolites, and erythrocyte degradation products. Local agents such as heavy metals (bismuth, lead) or dental amalgam (amalgam tattoo) may cause discoloration by traumatic implantation. Systemic medications may leave the patient with a bluish gray to yellowish-brown discoloration of the buccal mucosa, tongue, or hard palate. Typically, such pigmentation is most notable on the posterior regions of the hard palate, appears bluish-black to brown, and may be bilateral. Smoker's melanosis, or smoking-associated melanosis, is an abnormal melanin pigmentation of the oral mucosa [33].

Clinically, it appears as multiple brown pigmented areas, usually located on the anterior labial gingiva of the mandible. Teeth discoloration may be intrinsic or extrinsic. Intrinsic stains are caused by drugs (tetracycline) taken during development of tooth [34]. Extrinsic stains are taken up by tooth after development of tooth (tea, coffee, chlorhexidine) [35,36,37].

6. Black hairy tongue (Lingua villosa, Lingua nigra)

Hairy changes are on the upper side of the tongue (never on under side).Hairy tongue is a relatively common disorder that is due to marked accumulation of keratin on the filiforme papillae of the tongue. Lingua is black but may also be brown, white, green or pink. Normally asymptomatic and may develop secondary fungal infection (Candidosis). Hairy tongue may appear as a result of the growth of pigment-producing bacteria that colonize the elongate filiforme papillae. The black tongue may also be due to staining from food and tobacco. Black hairy tongue can be seen with the administration of oral antibiotics, corticosteroides, aldomet, sulfonamides and excessive smoking in adult's [38]. Treatment is elimination of predisposing factors, brushing of the tongue and local use of keratolytic agents.

7. Drug induced gingival enlargement

Gingival enlargement is seen in periodontitis, system disorders, and drug-induced states. The enlargement is usually generalized throughout the mouth but is more severe in maxillary and mandibular anterior regions. Drug-induced gingival overgrowth is a relatively common disorder of the gingiva due to several drugs. The drugs most commonly implicated are: Calcium channel blockers (amlodipine, diltiazem, felodipine, isradipine, nicardipine, nifedipine, nimodipine, nisoldipine, nitrendipine, oxidipine, and verapamil), other dihydropyridines (bleomycin), cyclosporine, phenytoin, and sodium valproate. Diffuse, non-neoplastic enlargement or overgrowth of the gingival tissues was initially recognized in patients who were using phenytoin. More recently, calcium channel blockers (members of the dihydropyridine class of medications), cyclosporine, and the antiepileptic drug sodium valproate have been associated with this reaction. Within the calcium channel blocker family, nifedipine, diltiazem, verapamil, and amlodipine are among the most commonly reported causative agents [39,40,41]. The gingival overgrowth is usually related to the dose of the drugs, the duration of therapy, the serum concentration, and the presence of dental plaque [42,43]. Clinically, both marginal gingiva and interdental papilla appear enlarged and firm, with a surface that may be smooth, stippled, or lobulated.

Treatment is discontinuation of the offending drug, improvement of oral hygiene and gingivectomy.

8. Xerostomia

Xerostomia, or dry mouth, is the most common adverse drug-related effect in the oral cavity. There are many causes of xerostomia. Pharmacologic therapy is a common cause. Xerostomia has been associated with more than 500 medications (antidepressants and antipsychotics, antihypertensives, antihistamines, anticholinergics, and decongestants). The synergistic effects of medications have been recognized and are increasingly common in elderly patients taking multiple medications (polypharmacy). In addition, habits such as smoking, alcohol consumption, and even long-term use of caffeinated drinks may contribute to oral dryness or the perception of dryness. Clinical signs and symptoms are: difficulty eating and swallowing, difficulty speaking and little saliva present in the mouth or may be thick stringy saliva [44,45].

9. Swelling

Several drugs can induce type I hypersensitivity reactions, or disease mediated by immuno-globulin E mast cells, that can range from isolated swelling of the oral tissues to full-blown anaphylaxis. Around the mouth, the lips are the most frequently involved site, followed by the tongue. The swelling is acute and is often transient. Lesions typically last for only several hours, but may last for days. Among the most common offending agents are ACE inhibitors, penicillin and penicillin derivatives, cephalosporins, barbiturates, and aspirin and other NSAIDs. Affected mucosa typically appears edematous and crythematous within minutes or hours after exposure to the offending drug. Similar contact reactions to latex had become increasingly problematic in oral health care settings until the recent shift towards non-latex replacement materials such as vinyl or nitrile rubber [46,47].

10. Oral thrush — Oral candidosis

The yeast, *Candida albicans* is the most common cause of infection of the oral cavity. Drug-induced oral candidosis is usually asymptomatic, but it may have an associated erythematous, ulcerated base. It is usually by *Candida albicans*, and less frequently by other fungal species. Predisposing factors may be local (xerostomia, dentures, antibiotic, poor oral hygiene) and systemic (steroids, HIV infections, immunosuppressive drugs). Clinical sing and symptoms are: Presents of creamy-white lesions on tongue, pain, slight bleeding if the lesions are rubbed or scraped, "cottony" feeling in the mouth, loss of taste (ageusia) and difficulty swallowing (if infection spreads to throat). This often follows the use of broad-spectrum antibiotics or the use of corticosteroid inhalers, and immunosuppressive agents such as cyclosporine, and cytotoxic therapies [48]. In treatment used topical antifungal agents and systemic.

11. Taste disturbance (Ageusia, Dysgeusia)

Numerous causes exist that can lead to a decreased ability to perceive taste or causing an unpleasant taste. The alteration in taste may be simply a blunting or decreased sensitivity in taste perception (hypogeusia), a total loss of the ability to taste (ageusia), or a distortion in perception of the correct taste of a substance, for example, sour for sweet (dysgeusia) [49].

The most common cause is due to an upper respiratory infection that affects olfaction, in turn, decreasing one's sense of taste. Drugs can also distort taste. Clinical signs and symptoms are:

total loss of ability to taste, complaints of metallic taste, impaired salty taste, reduced appetite and weight loss. Drugs causing taste disturbance are: antibiotics, ACE inhibitors, aspirin, diclofenac, diltiazem, metronidazole, propranolol, and sulphonamides [50].

12. Stomatitis — Contact allergy

Stomatitis or oral inflammation of the mouth is a nonspecific term that describes many oral drug reactions. This is a relatively common oral mucosal reaction to continuous contact of substances. Restorative materials, mouthwashes, dentifrices, food and other substances may be responsible. The clinical symptoms may include: nonspecific generalized inflamed gums, palate, lips, tongue and buccal mucosa, bleeding, oral lesions as ulcerations and erosions, and breathing difficulties if severe allergic reaction involving tongue. Lesions occur within 24 hours of ingesting the medication. The causative medication is withdrawn. Drugs are: antibiotics, food additives, mouthwashes, toothpastes, cosmetics, dental materials and topical steroids [51]. Stomatitis refers to an inflammatory process involving the mucous membrane of the mouth that may manifest itself through a variety of signs and symptoms including erythema, vesiculation, bulla formation, desquamation, sloughing, ulceration, pseudomembranous formation, and associated discomfort.

Stomatitis may arise due to factors that may be of either local, isolated conditions or of systemic origin. For example, a solitary oral ulcer with a history of a recurrent pattern may be classified as recurrent aphthous stomatitis, a purely local phenomenon. Another clinically-similar-appearing lesion, on the other hand, may represent an oral mucosal manifestation of a more generalized disease process such as Crohn's disease. Stomatitis may involve any site in the oral cavity, including the vermillion of the lips, labial/buccal mucosa, and dorsal/ventral tongue, floor of mouth and hard/soft palate, and gingivae [52].

The diagnosis is based on the history and clinical features.

Treatment is discontinuation of any the causative medication. In severe and extended lesions, low doses of steroids for one week help the lesions to heal.

13. Angular cheilitis

Angular cheilitis (AC), or perleche, is a common disorder of the angles of the mouth. This is soreness and cracks at the corners of the mouth. Several drugs may cause AC as a side effect, by various mechanisms, such as creating drug-induced xerostomia. Medication also contributes to the onset of cheilitis. There are certain medicines that have a side effect of dry lips which is potential for cheilitis. Less commonly, angular cheilitis is associated with primary hypervitaminosis A which can occur when as a result from an excess intake of vitamin A in the form of vitamin supplements. Drugs are: Aldomet, Zocor (statins), tetracycline and vitamin A [53,54].

The condition is characterized by erythema, maceration, fissuring, erosion, and crusting at commissures. Remissions and exacerbations are common. Diagnosis is based on the clinical findings.

Treatment is discontinuation of any the causative medication, and topical steroids.

14. Osteonecrosis

Osteonecrosis is a disease resulting from the temporary or permanent loss of blood supply to the bones. This is a serious oral complication of treatment with Bisphosphonates. Bone under teeth is exposed, usually triggered by a dental extraction. Most commonly associated with i.n. zoledronic acid. Clinical symptoms are: swelling and loosening of teeth, altered local sensation, facial pain, toothache, lose teeth, exposed bone, recurrent infection and marked oral odour [55,56].

15. Salivary glands

Salivary gland function can be affected by a variety of drugs that can by a variety of drugs that can produce xerostomia or ptyalismus. It is suggested this is due to both the reduced salivary flow rate and to a decrease in salivary calcium and phosphate concentration. Systemic drug therapy can also produce pain and swelling of the salivary glands. [57].

Salivary gland enlargement may be painless or associated with tenderness. The causes of salivary gland swelling are numerous, but they can be viewed as local causes or drug related (thiouracil, sulfonamides, NSAIDs, phenothiazines) [58].

16. Sialorrhoea

Sialorrhoea, or excessive salivation is commonly associated with many systemic conditions. Clinical signs and symptoms are: increased salivary floe, drooling or dribbling and increased swallowing. Drugs causing sialorrhorea are: pilocarpine, rivastigmin, nifedipine, lithium and dimercaptol [59,60]. The treatments currently available for sialorrhoea are unsatisfactory. Systemic anticholinergic drugs are often ineffective and produce unacceptable side effects.

17. Halitosis

Halitosis is the offensive breath resulting from poor oral hygiene, dental or oral infections, ingestion of certain foods, use of tobacco, and some systemic diseases. Halitosis, or bad breath, may have many different etiologies (alcohol, drugs, and foods, smoking). It may be association with an abnormal taste in the mouth. This association is commonly seen with smoking, various foods, alcohol, periodontal disease or other oral infection. Concern about halitosis is estimated to be the third most frequent reason for people to seek dental care, following tooth decay and gum disease) [61]. A number of systemic diseases can cause halitosis, especially cirrhosis and renal failure. In diabetic ketoacidosis, patient's breath may smell of acetone. Drugs are not frequently implicated, but disulfiram dimethylsulfoxide has been associated with halitosis. Effective treatment is not always easy to find. Gently cleaning the tongue surface twice daily is the most effective way to keep bad breath in control, than, eating a healthy breakfast with rough food and chewing gum [62].

18. Hemorrhage — Bleeding

Bleeding can occur internally, where blood leaks from blood vessels inside the body, or externally, either through a natural opening such as the mouth, nose, ear, urethra, vagina or anus, or through a break in the skin. Bleeding arises due to traumatic injury, underlying medical condition, or some drugs. Drugs such as aspirin, NSAIDS, anticoagulants which thin in the blood and drug induced thrombocytopenia as caused by chloramphenicol, penicillins, streptomycin and sulfonamides may lead to oral bleeding. Broad spectrum antibiotics such as cephalosporin's decrease Vitamin K level by altering gastrointestinal flora and may lead to bleeding disorder [63].

19. Taking care of your oral health during drug use

Some easy to prevent or reduce the adverse effects of various drug therapies are as follow:

- Use of soft bristle tooth brush

- Brush or rinse after every meal

- Use mild tooth paste

- Regular use of floss without injury in gums

- Eat dry nuts alters food that stimulate salivary flow.

- Have regular dental checkup

- Use of ice chips to decrease pain and dryness of mouth

When being prescribed a new medication, ask your doctor or pharmacist about all the possible side effects [64].

Whenever a patient comes with oral lesions ask about history of medications and if significant then either reduce to the minimum dose required or switch to alternative regimen depending upon the severity of symptoms. Sometimes active treatment of the concerned effect may also be required.

Author details

Ana Pejcic[*]

Address all correspondence to: dranapejcic@hotmail.com

Department of Periodontology and Oral medicine, Medical faculty, University of Nis, Serbia

References

[1] Cianco SG. Medication's impact on oral health. J Am Dent Assoc 2004; 135(10): 1440-1448.

[2] Porter SR, Scully C. Adverse drug reactions in the mouth. Clin Dermatol 2000; 18(5): 525-532.

[3] Scully C, Bagan JV. Adverse drug reactions in the orofacial region. Crit Rev Oral Biol Med 2004; 15(4): 221-239.

[4] Abdollahi M. Current opinion on drug-induced oral reactions: A comprehensive review. J Contemp Dent Pract 2008; (9)3: 001-015.

[5] Abdollahi M, Radfar M. A review of drug-induced oral reactions. J Contemp Dent Pract 2003; 4: 10-31.

[6] Abdollahi M, Radfar M. A Review of Drug-Induced Oral Reactions. J Contemp Dent Pract 2003; (4)1: 10-31.

[7] Vucicevic Boras V, Savage N, Mohamad Zaini Z. Oral aphthous-like ulceration due to tiotropiumbromide. Med Oral Patol Oral Cir Bucal 2007; 12(3): E209-210.

[8] Kharazmi M, Sjöqvist K, Warfvinge G. Oral ulcers, a little known adverse effect of alendronate: review of the literature. J Oral Maxillofacial Surg 2012; 70 (4): 830–836.

[9] Boulinguez S, Reix S, Bedane C, Debrock C, Bouyssou-GauthierML, Sparsa A, et al.). Role of drug exposure in aphthousulcers: a case-control study. Br J Dermatol 2000; 143: 1261-1265.

[10] Symour RA. Oral and dental disorders. In: Davies DM, Ferner RE, DeGlanville H. eds.,Davies'stextbook of adverse drugreactions, 5th ed., London, Chapman & Hall Medical, 1998: 234-250.

[11] Lorca SC, Minguez Serra PM, Silvestre FJ. Drug-induced burning mouth syndrome: a new etiological diagnosis.Med Oral Patol Oral Cir Bucal 2008; 13(3): E167-170.

[12] Fedele S, Fricchione G, Porter SR, Miggna MD. Burning mouth syndrome (stomatodynia). QJM 2007; 100(8): 527-530.

[13] Sardella A. An up-to-date view on burning mouth syndrome. Minerva Stomatol 2007; 56(6): 327-340.

[14] Culhane NS, Hodle AD. Burning mouth syndrome after taking clonazepam. Ann Pharmacother. 2001; 35(7-8): 874-876.

[15] Reamy BV, Derby R, Bunt CW. Common tongue conditions in primary care. Am Fam Physician 2010; 81(5): 627-634.

[16] Litt JZ. Drug eruption reference manual. London. The Parthenon Publishing Group, 2001: 274-421.

[17] Nordt SP. Tetracycline-induced oral mucosal ulcerations. Ann Pharmacother. 1996 May;30(5):547-8.

[18] Jones TA, Parmar SC: Oral mucosal ulceration due to ferrous sulphate tablets: report of a case. Dent Update 2006; 33(10): 632-633.

[19] Naranjo J, Poniachik J, Cisco D, et al.: Oral ulcers produced by mycophenolate mofetil in two liver transplant patients. Transplant Proc 2007, 39(3): 612-614.

[20] Criado PR, Brandt HR, Moure ER, Pereira GL, Sanches Júnior JA. Adverse mucocutaneous reactions related to chemotherapeutic agents: part II. An Bras Dermatol 2010; 85(5): 591-608.

[21] Scully C, Bagan JV. Adverse drug reactions in the orofacial region. Crit Rev Oral Biol Med 2004; 15: 221-239.

[22] Serrano-Sanchez P, Bagan JV, Soriano J, Sarrion G. Drug-induced oral lichenoid reactions. A literature review. J Clin Exp Dent 2010; 2(2): e71-75.

[23] Cobos-Fuentes MJ, Martínez-Sahuquillo-Márquez A, Gallardo-Castillo I, et al. Oral lichenoid lesions related to contact with dental materials: a literature review. Med Oral Patol Oral Cir Bucal 2009; 14: e514-520.

[24] Woo V, Bonks J, Borukhova L, Zegarelli D. Oral Lichenoid Drug Eruption: A Report of a Pediatric Case and Review of the Literature. Pediatric Dermatology 2009; 26: 458-464.

[25] Lage D, Juliano PB, Metze K, et al. Lichen planus and lichenoid drug-induced eruption: a histological and immunohistpchemical study. Int J Dermatol 2012; 51: 1199.

[26] Ayangco L, Rogers RS III. Oral manifestations of erythema multiforme. Dermatol Clin 2000; 321: 195-205.

[27] Joseph IT, Vergheese G, Gorge D, Sathyan P. Drug induced oral erythema multiforme: A rare and less recognized variant of erythema multiforme. J Oral Maxillofac Pathol 2012; 16: 145-148.

[28] Hazin R, Ibrahini OA, Hazin MI, et al: Stevens-Johnson syndrome: pathogenesis, diagnosis, and management. Ann Med. 2008; 40(2): 129-138.

[29] Iks R, Karakaya G, Erkin G, Kalyoncu AF. Multidrug-induced erythema multiforme. J Investig Allergol Clin Immunol 2007, 17(3):196-198.

[30] Vassileva S. Drug-induced pemphigoid: bullous and cicatricial. Clin Dermatol 1998; 16(3): 379-387.

[31] Civatte J. Drug-induced pemphigus diseases. Dermatol Monatsschr 1989; 175(1): 1-7.

[32] Rubin RL. Drug-induced lupus. Toxicology. 2005; 209(2):135-147.

[33] Eisen D. Disorders of pigmentation in the oral cavity. Clin Dermatol. 2000; 18(5): 579-587.

[34] Aschheim KW, Dale BG. Esthetic dentistry, a clinical approach to techniques and materials. 2nd ed., Phiadephia, Mosby, 2001:247-249.

[35] Eisen D. Disorders of pigmentation in the oral cavity. Clin Dermatol 2000; 18: 579-587.

[36] Sapone A, Basaglia R, Biagi GL. Drug-induced changes in the teeth and mouth. IJ Clin Ter. 1992; 140(6): 575-583.

[37] Meyerson MA, Cohen PR, Hymes SR. Lingual hyper pigmentation associated with minocycline therapy. Oral Surg Oral Med Oral Pathol Oral Radiol Endod 1995; 79: 180-184.

[38] Korber A, Dissemond J. Images in clinical medicine. Black hairy tongue. N Engl J Med 2006, 5; 354(1): 67.

[39] Shimizu Y, Kataoka M, Seto H, et. al. Nifedipine induces gingival epithelial hyperplasia in rats through inhibition of apoptosis. J Periodontol. 2002; 73(8): 861-867.

[40] Kataoka M, Kido J, Shinohara Y, Nagata T. Drug-induced gingival overgrowth–a review. Biol Pharm Bull 2005; 28(10):1817-1821.

[41] Nitin MN, Sandeep B, Arjun D, Surinder KS, Harsh M. Salivary gland tumor – our experience. Ind J Otolaryngol Head Neck Surg 2004; 56(1): 31-34.

[42] Pejcic A, Djordjevic V, Kojovic D, Zivkovic V, Minic I, Mirkovic D, Stojanovic M. Effectiveness of Periodontal Treatment in Renal Transplant Recipients. Medical Principles and Practice 2014; 23(2): 149-153.

[43] A Pejčić, Lj. Kesić, V. Živković, R. Obradović, M. Petrović, D. Mirković. Gingival overgrowth induced by nifedipine. Acta Stom Naissi 2011; 27: 1104-1109.

[44] Porter SR, Scully C, Hegarty AM. An update of the etiology and management of xerostomia. Oral Surg Oral Med Oral Radiol Endod 2004; 97(1): 28-46.

[45] Bardow A, Nyvad B, Nauntofte B. Relationships between medication intake, complaints of dry mouth, salivary flow rate and composition, and the rate of tooth demineralization in situ. Arch Oral Biol 2001; 46(5): 413-423.

[46] Kaplan AP, Greaves MW. Angioedema. J Am Acad Dermatol 2005; 53(3): 373-388.

[47]   Bas M, Adams V, Suvorava T, Niehues T, Hoffmann TK, Kojda G. Nonallergic angioedema: role of bradykinin. Allergy 2007; 62(8):842-5.

[48]   Muzyka BC. Oral fungal infections. Dent Clin North Am 2005; 49(1): 49-65.

[49]   Porter SR, Scully C. Adverse drug reactions in the mouth. Clin Dermatol. 2000 SepOct;18(5):525-32.

[50]   Drew H, Harasty L. Dysgeusia follow in a course of Zithromax: a case report. J N J Dent Assoc 2007; 78(2): 24-27.

[51]   Tack DA, Rogers ES. Oral drug reactions. Dermatol therap 2002; 15: 236-250.

[52]   P Lokesh, T Rooban Joshua Elisabeth, K Umadevi, K Ranganathan. Allergic Contact Stomatitis: A Case Report and Review of Literature. Indian J Clin Pract 2012; 22(9): 458-462.

[53]   Park KK, Brodell TR, Helm ES. Angular cheilitis, Part 2: Nutritional, systemic, and drug –related causes and treatment. Cutis 2011; 88 (1): 27-32.

[54]   Levin L, Laviv A, Schwartz-Arad D. Denture-related osteonecrosis of the maxilla associated with oral bisphosphonate treatment. J Am Dent Assoc 2007, 138(9): 1218-1220.

[55]   Woo SB, Kalmar JR. Osteonecrosis of the jaws and bisphosphonates. Alpha Omegan 2007; 100 (4): 194-202.

[56]   Knulst AC, Stengs CJ, Baart de la Faille H, et. al. Salivary gland swellingfollowingnaproxen therapy. Br J Dermatol. 1995; 133(4): 647-649.

[57]   Scully C. Drug effects on salivary glands; dry mouth. Oral Dis 2003; 9: 165-176.

[58]   Freudenreich O. Drug-induced sialorrhea. Drugs Today (Barc) 2005, 41(6):411-418.

[59]   Comeley C, Galletly C, Ash D. Use of atropeine eye drops for clozapine induced hypersalivation. Aust NZ J psychiatry 2000; 34: 1003-1034.

[60]   Yaegaki, K; Coil, JM. Examination, classification, and treatment of halitsis; clinical perspectives. Journal Canadian Dental Association 2000; 66 (5): 257–261.

[61]   Zalewska, A; Zatoński, M; Jabłonka-Strom, A; Paradowska, A; Kawala, B; Litwin, A. "Halitosis--a common medical and social problem. A review on pathology, diagnosis and treatment. Acta gastro-enterologica Belgica 2012; 75 (3): 300–309.

[62]   American Dental Association."How medications can affect your oral health."J Am Dent Assoc 2005; 136(6):831.

[63]   Alan Tack D, Rogers S R.Oral drug reactions. Dermatologic Therapy 2002; 15: 236-250.

[64]   P. Serrano-Sánchez, JV Bagán, Jiménez-Soriano, G Sarrión. Drug-induced oral lichenoid reactions. A literature review. J Clin Exp Dent. 2010; 2(2): e71-75.

Chapter 26

Epithelial-Mesenchymal Transition — A Possible Pathogenic Pathway of Fibrotic Gingival Overgrowth

Ileana Monica Baniţă, Cristina Munteanu,
Anca Berbecaru-Iovan, Camelia Elena Stănciulescu,
Ana Marina Andrei and Cătălina Gabriela Pisoschi

Additional information is available at the end of the chapter

http://dx.doi.org/10.5772/59267

1. Introduction

Gingival overgrowth (GO) or gingival enlargement refers to important changes of gums aspect and function. Even it seems an issue of little significance, health of gums is a prerequisite condition for a psychological and physical comfort because severe GO affects speech, mastication, and nutrition, causes aesthetic concerns and increases susceptibility for periodontal and systemic diseases. The treatment of severe cases needs gingivectomy that may be repeated if is necessary.

At clinical endo-oral examination, GO is characterized by increased gums volume, swollen and deepening of gingival sulcus. Thickening of soft tissues covering alveolar ridges is more than 1 mm comprising both the mobile and attached gums. The degree of overgrowth can be variable from the interdentally papilla to cover the entire tooth crown. Enlargement is painless, slowly progressive and depends to a great extend on the oral hygiene [1-6].

Usually, GO is classified according the clinical appearance and the etiological factor. Histological and cell molecular studies have uncovered some of the pathogenic pathways and cellular alterations associated with GO but still remain unknown aspects.

In this chapter we describe recent insights into the pathogenic mechanisms of GO overgrowth discussing in detail the role of epithelial-mesenchymal transition (EMT) in gingival fibrotic diseases.

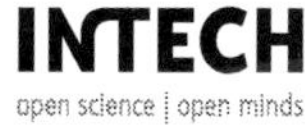

2. Terms definition, classification and risk factors for gingival overgrowth

Gingival overgrowth (GO), often named gingival hyperplasia or hypertrophy, is classified according the clinical appearance and the etiological factors, if these are known. If clinical examination displays rather an inflammatory aspect (gingivitis and periodontitis) the gums are red, soft, shiny, and bleed easily. Inflammatory gingivitis is induced frequently by poor dental hygiene resulting in bacterial plaque and causes reactive GO, named also focal reactive GO, inflammatory hyperplasia or epulis. Generally, the epulides are pedunculated or sessile lesions of gums; because this term, considered unsuitable, is clinico-topographical, without a histological description of the lesion, nowadays the preferred term is gums reactive lesion [7, 8]. Smoking, systemic diseases (diabetes mellitus, HIV infection) determine also inflammatory gums lesions.

Non inflamed gingival enlargement tends to have a darker red or purple color, is either firm or soft, when bleeds easily. Determinative causes are extremely polymorphous: (i) subjects with poor dental hygiene; (ii) specific hormonal states-puberty, pregnancy; (iii) nutritional deficiency, such as scurvy; (iv) blood conditions, such as acute leukemia, lymphoma or aplastic anemia; (v) genetic conditions – epulis or Neumann tumor; (vi) drug-induced GO (named also fibrotic gingival hyperplasia) appeared after administration of some anticonvulsivants (phenytoin), immunosupressants (cyclosporin A, CsA) and antihypertensive calcium channel blockers (verapamil, diltiazem, nifedipine); (vii) systemic diseases such as sarcoidosis, Crohn disease, acromegaly, primary amyloidosis or type I neurofibromatosis [6,9,10].

Gingival fibromatosis (GF) is the term frequently used for any GO when suspect a hereditary pattern (hereditary gingival fibromatosis, HGF), as part of a more extensive syndrome (Table 1) or the etiologic factor remains unknown-idiopathic gingival fibromatosis (IGF). Specialty literature is sometimes confuse or redundant regarding the relation between definition and the etiological factors. For the beginning, we tried to present a brief synthesis of these definitions.

Hereditary gingival fibromatosis (HGF), previously known as gingival elephantiasis, idiopathic gingival fibromatosis, hereditary gingival hyperplasia, non-bacterial plaque gingival lesion, gingival gigantism or just hypertrophic gums [11,12] can be classified as follows:

i.   Hereditary or isolated GF named also non-syndromic or type I GF seems to be determined by the mutation of SOS1 (*Sun of sevenless-1)* gene on chromosome 2. For the first time, this mutation was described in a large Brazilian family [13]. SOS1 is an oncogene involved in cell growth. This mutation was designated GINGF1 (Mendelian Inheritance in Man classification MIM135300) [10].

Recently a type 2 HGF, GINGF2 (MIM605544), was described in association to a mutation mapped on chromosome 5 but the specific gene involved has not yet been identified [10,14-16]. The presence of teeth in alveoli seems to be a condition for hereditary GO development as it disappears or reduces after tooth extraction. Some authors consider HGF an atypical pathology of childhood because it is present mainly during the mixed dentition stage [11]. Another type of HGF with family aggregation, GINGF3 (MIM 609955), a mutation mapped on chromosome

2 but not to the SOS 1 gene in which clinical signs appear earlier during the primary dentition stage was described by [17].

ii. Syndromic GF is associated with several clinical signs in some syndromes (Table 1). In syndromic GF, gingival events are caused by chromosomal abnormalities (duplications, deletions) of chromosomes 2p12-16 [18,19], 4q (MIM252500), 8 (MIM266270), 14q [20], 19p (MIM266200), 19q (MIM248500) and Xq [8,9,13,21-26].

Syndrome	Clinical signs
Zimmerman-Laband Syndrome	GF and facial deformability, changes of nose and ears, nail dystrophy, hypoplasia, epilepsy, hepato-splenomegaly, deafness, mental retardation
Rutherford Syndrome	GF and corneal dystrophy, aggressive behavior, mental retardation
Jones Syndrome	GF and progressive deafness, maxillary odontogenic cysts
Cross Syndrome	Gingival hypertrophy and microphthalmia, mental retardation, hypopigmentation
Murray-Puretic-Drescher Syndrome	GF and bone, cartilage, skin and muscle diseases
Ramon Syndrome	GF and cherubism, hypertrichosis, mental retardation, convulsions, growth retardation, juvenile rheumatoid arthritis
Cowden Syndrome	Localized GF with multiple hamartomas

Table 1. Syndromic gingival fibromatosis [adapted after 6,15,16,27]

Recently, in [28] is described a new syndrome that includes generalized thin *hypoplastic amelogenesis imperfecta* found in a family with multiple consanguineous marriages, this type having clinical and histological similarities with GINGF1 and GINGF3.

Genetic and syndromic fibromatosis are sometimes termed IGF [12,27,29-32].

Lacking specific immunohistochemical markers, the diagnosis of HGF is based exclusively on clinical examination, patient medical history and family pedigree.

It was recommended to use the term „idiopathic fibromatosis" only for GF that doesn't incriminate genetic and hereditary causes mentioned above, in order to avoid these confusions of classification [6,9].

GO incidence varies according the socioeconomic status and the risk factors involved being reported a rate of 1/9000 adults; the most numerous GO are inflammatory or induced by drugs-phenytoin increases gingival volume in 57% of cases, CsA in 30-46% and calcium channel blockers in 10% [3,33,34]. HGF is the most rare type of GO and estimated to affect 1/750,000 people with the same incidence in both sexes [2,6,10,35,36].

Under the influence of such risk factors, clinical increase of gums volume is due to the enlargement of both epithelial and connective tissue. Microscopically examination displays the coexistence of tissue hypertrophy and cellular hyperplasia which imposed the generic term of GO [2]. Irrespective the risk factor, presence of bacterial plaque and hereditary predisposition are constantly incriminated as etiological cofactors mainly for drug-induced GO [2]. To sustain this association, it was revealed that patients with inflammatory GO before the onset of treatment with CsA developed more severe forms of GO [37] and suggested that patients carriers of a genetic polymorphism related to IL-1A expression often develop GO after CsA treatment [38]; specialty literature reports cases of IGF or HGF associated with chronic or aggressive periodontitis [39-41].

3. Histological aspects of gingival fibromatosis

Histological studies that we performed on samples of fibrotic gingival tissues revealed common, non-specific aspects despite the numerous risk factors, generally characterized by an increase of gums volume to which contribute both the epithelium (cellular hyperplasia) and lamina propria (accumulation of extracellular matrix, ECM, and cells) (Figure 1). Various types of GF are characterized by different incidence of pro-inflammatory cells.

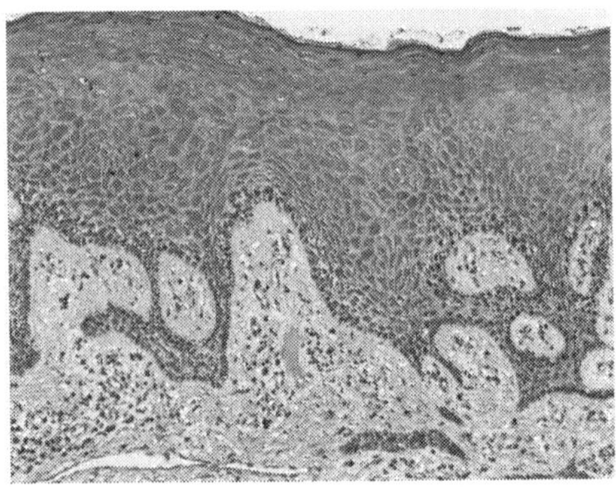

Figure 1. General view of a sample with gingival overgrowth (trichrome staining, x100)

In drug-induced GO, connective tissue is more rich in pro-inflammatory cells than in HGF or IGF. An exception is phenytoin-induced GO characterized mainly by fibrotic lesions unlike CsA or nifedipine-induced GO which determine important inflammatory reactions [23,42-45]. Due to its clinical and histological features, phenytoin-induced GO is often included in the category of fibromatous GO [11,15,23] which yield some confusions.

Histological changes of syndromic GO, HGF and phenytoin-induced GO are similar: epithelial hyperplasia with hyperkeratosis and elongated papillae, thickening of collagen bundles, increase of tissue differentiation and fluctuating number of fibroblasts (Figure 2a).

Enlargement and acanthosis of gingival epithelium with deep epithelial ridges was reported [46, 47]. Epithelial hyperplasia results from acanthosis but appears only in the areas of chronic inflammation [46-48]. In many areas epithelial hyperkeratosis was observed [17,26,47,49]. Regarding the sulcular epithelium we noted many signs of considerable degeneration, subpepithelial edema and extensive inflammatory cell infiltration (Figure 2b). Thick, densely wrapped collagen bundles with scattered resident cells of connective tissue were observed in lamina propria.

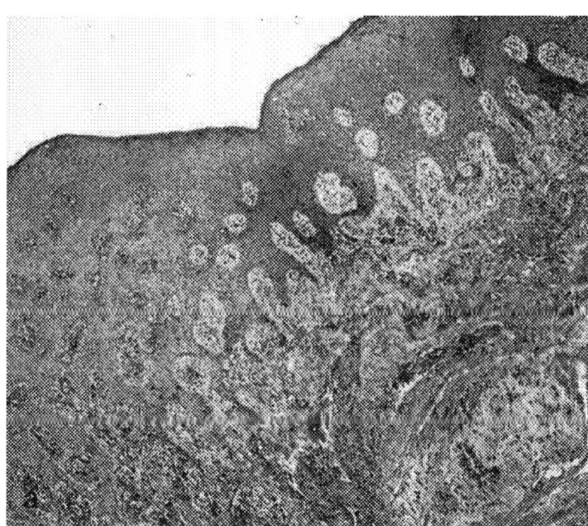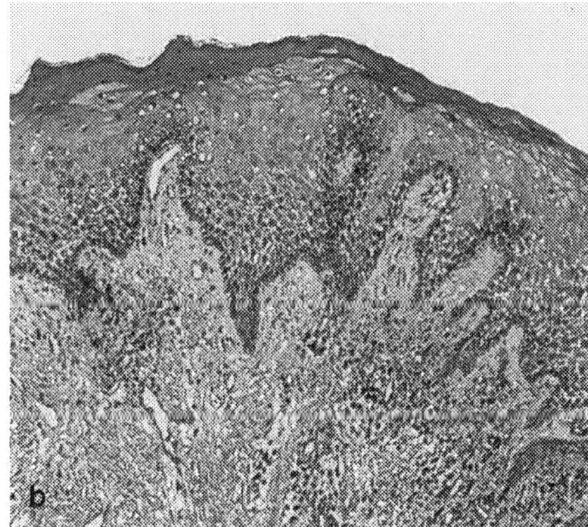

Figure 2. General view of syndromic GO: a) masticatory gingival mucosa; b) sulcular gingival mucosa (trichrome staining, x100)

The incidence of fibroblast is disputed; some authors reported numerous fibroblasts [16,31,45,50,51] while others claimed on the contrary a decreased number [17,41,43,52]. This variable number of fibroblasts even within HGF pointed attention to the different molecular mechanism underlying gingival fibrotic processes.

4. Pathogenic pathways of gingival overgrowth

Histological and cell molecular studies have uncovered some of the pathogenic pathways and cellular alterations associated with GO but still remain unknown aspects.

Studies revealed that the same molecules and biological events are involved in inflammation, wound repair and fibrosis. Theories and previous investigations on the morphology and molecular mechanisms by which the fibrotic deposition occurs have been widely published. Integrating these findings, Bartold and Narayanan state in [53] that fibrosis can evolve as a response to the action of a single factor or of a combination of various factors such as: (i) abnormal release of inflammatory mediators; synthesis of some molecules frees others and their crosstalk could have synergic, cumulative or antagonist effects; (ii) persistence of abnormal changes in the action of growth factors and cytokines; even the intensity of cell response to this stimulation is not so great the long lasting effect is cumulative and increased;

(iii) establishment of a pro-fibrotic cell phenotype; aberrant interaction of normal cell phenotypes with peptide mediators could induce the recruitment of abnormal cells.

These cell interactions determine the accumulation of gingival tissue through two main pathogenic pathways: (i) excessive synthesis of ECM and (ii) decrease of its breakdown [15,23,43,53-55]. Each of these pathways is initiated and sustained by growth factors, cytokines, molecules involved in ECM breakdown, matrix metalloproteinases – MMP, and their tissue inhibitors (TIMP) released by cellular elements that belongs both to the epithelium and gingival chorion. Recently, epithelial to mesenchymal transition (EMT) has been proposed as another pathogenic pathway promoting gingival fibrosis.

5. Role of epithelium in extracellular matrix accumulation — The epithelial-mesenchymal transition

Development of fibrotic lesions is indirectly related to the presence and histophysiology of epithelial cells. The interference of oral epithelial cells in ECM storage is sustained by the results of many studies reporting epithelial morphological changes besides the accumulation of connective tissue. In the same time, epithelial keratinocytes or inflammatory cells infiltrating the epithelium synthesize several biomolecules (growth factors, cytokines, MMPs and TIMPs) which alter collagen metabolism and ECM synthesis in the lamina propria. In a recent study, Menga and coworkers in [56] showed an intense expression of type 1 collagen and TIMP-1 in fibroblasts from mixed cultures of keratinocytes and fibroblasts obtained from patients with GF, in parallel to an increased rough endoplasmic reticulum. The authors suggested that keratinocytes play an important role in the pathogenesis of GF through increase of ECM storage. The epithelium suffers acanthosis and hyperkeratosis, increases the number of epithelial cells, and of many inflammatory cells infiltrating its deep layers. The increase of keratinocytes number determines not only the epithelial enlargement mainly in the spindle layer but also the appearance of many epithelial ridges ascending deep in the lamina propria. These epithelial ridges often branch and adhere one to another (Figure 1, and 2a, b).

These findings are constantly accompanied by the increase of keratinocyte mitotic activity proved by Ki-67 or PCNA immunostaining in [45,57-60]. In a recent study, using immunohistochemistry, [61] reported that Mcm-2 and Mcm-5 (members of minichromosome maintenance protein family), considered a novel class of proliferation markers, and geminin, also a proliferation marker according to [62], showed various expression in samples from three different families with GF. No differences between the expression of apoptotic markers Bcl-2 and Bax were observed among the group. Thus the authors concluded that an important heterogeneity of gingival fibrosis occurs. Epithelial cells proliferation is stimulated by pro-inflammatory cytokines and growth factors, such as KGF (Keratinocyte Growth Factor) or EGF (Epidermal Growth Factor). EGF and its receptors (EGfr) are positively correlated with the proliferative potential of the cells from rete pegs [63,64]. In a previous study, we observed that epithelial cells have an increased mitotic index in cases of GF highly infiltrated with inflammatory cells (Figure 3) (*unpublished data*).

Epithelial proliferation seems to have at least two functions in GO. First it ensure a continuous regeneration of keratinocytes, the regenerative capacity of the epithelium being compulsory when continuous desquamation of the superficial cells prevents bacterial colonization of the mucosa; second, epithelial proliferation could contribute to fibrosis by maintaining a cell pool to replace those cells involved in EMT and transformed in fibroblasts.

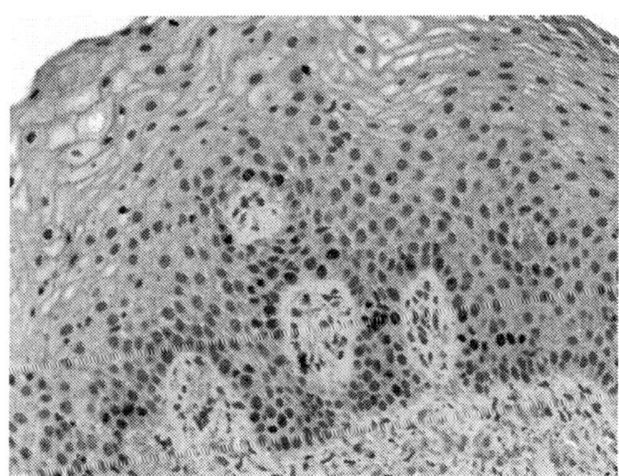

Figure 3. Gingival fibrosis. Increased number of Ki-67 positive cells in the basal epithelial layer (IHC, x200)

5.1. Concept of epithelial-mesenchymal transition

Epithelial-mesenchymal transition (EMT) is a concept first defined "epithelial–mesenchymal transformation" by G. Greenburg and E. Hay to characterize the conversion of epithelial cells to mesenchyme (EMT) and vice versa (mesenchymal-epithelial transition, MET) during chick embryonic development. This well-defined concept refers to a form of inherent plasticity of the epithelial phenotype that occurs normally in the developmental process. During EMT cells undergo a switch from a uniform, polarized epithelial phenotype to a motile mesenchymal phenotype. Current interest in this process stems from its importance in embryonic development and involvement in several pathologies (wound healing, fibrosis, cancer progression and metastasis) and has been extensively reviewed over the last 10 years in [65-78]. The conversion of an epithelial cell to a mesenchymal cell is critical to metazoan embryogenesis and a defining structural feature of organ development, and follows a common and conserved program with hallmarks [69,77]. As Lamouille and coworkers suggest in [77] it also has some variation which depend on the cell type, tissue environment and signals that activate the EMT program. During EMT, epithelial cell–cell and cell–ECM interactions are weakened and epithelial cells become able to trans-differentiate into fibrogenic fibroblast-like cells [68]. Turning an epithelial cell into a mesenchymal cell requires alterations in morphology, cellular architecture, adhesion, and migration capacity [69]. Loss of epithelial apical-basal polarity, acquisition of a front-rear polarity and motility result from the disappearance of cell adhesion molecules, reorganization of cytoskeleton and changes in cell shape [70]. In many cases cells gain an increased ability to break ECM proteins, acquire resistance to senescence and apoptosis [73].

Research in this field revealed that cellular events of EMT occurs in three distinct biological settings with different functional consequences: (i) type 1 EMT acts during implantation, embryogenesis and organ development when can generate mesenchymal cells (primary mesenchyme) and then secondary epithelia after the mesenchyme undergoes a reverse MET; (ii) type 2 EMT as a source of fibroblasts and other related cells involved in tissue regeneration and organ fibrosis in response to persistent inflammation; (iii) type 3 EMT occurs in neoplastic cells that have undergone genetic and epigenetic changes, notably of oncogenes and tumor suppressor genes, and contributes to cancer progression and metastasis [72,76,79]. A main distinction between the first two types of EMT is that type 1 EMT produces mesenchymal cells, whereas type 2 EMT results in fibroblasts in mature tissues. But other than the fact that mesenchymal cells have a shape similar to fibroblasts and, like fibroblasts, express fibronectin and fibrilar collagens, there is no evidence that fibroblasts originate in primitive mesenchymal cells [78].

EMT induction. Successful EMT depends upon a combination of growth factors and cytokines associated with the proteolytic digestion of the epithelial basement membranes (BM) under the action of MMPs. Local expression of TGF-β, EGF, IGF-II or FGF-2 facilitates EMT by binding membrane receptors with kinase activity [65]. The effect of TGF-β on EMT induction depends on β1-integrin transduction, Smad-dependent transcription, Smad-independent p38MAP kinase activation and Rho-like GTPase-mediated signaling [80,81]. IGF-II also facilitates the intracellular degradation of E-cadherin [82], while FGF-2 and TGF-β are required for the expression of MMP-2 and MMP-9 to assist in BM breakdown [83]. Indeed, decrease of type IV collagen from the BM was associated with increased expression of MMP-2 and MMP-9 during human pathologies involving EMT [54,84]. Loss of BM integrity is essential for the increased interactions between epithelial and connective tissue layers that contribute to fibrosis. Several lines of evidence indicate that TGF-β signaling is causally linked with EMT, plays an important role in regulating epithelial plasticity and is one of the most significant lines of communication between stroma and epithelium in different organ fibrosis (renal, cardiac, pulmonary, and hepatic) [81].

Consequent cell and molecular events are engaged to initiate EMT and enable it to complete: i) activation of transcription factors; ii) expression of cell surface specific proteins; iii) reorganization and expression of cytoskeletal proteins; iv) synthesis of ECM-degrading enzymes. In many cases, these factors are used as biomarkers to prove cell passage from one phenotype to the other and EMT involvement in tissue remodeling (Figure 4).

Transcriptional regulation of EMT. EMT involves changes in gene expression that induce the loss of proteins associated with the epithelial phenotype and increased expression of proteins associated with a mesenchymal and migratory cell phenotype with concomitant alterations in cytoskeletal organization, cell adhesion and production of ECM [72]. Cellular plasticity that is the switch of epithelial to mesenchymal features is achieved through a well orchestrated program that involves the action of three families of transcription factors: Snail, ZEB (zinc-finger E-box-binding) and bHLH (basic helix-loop-helix). Expression of these factors is induced in response to TGF-β through different mechanisms and their function is finely regulated at transcriptional, translational and post-translational levels [77].

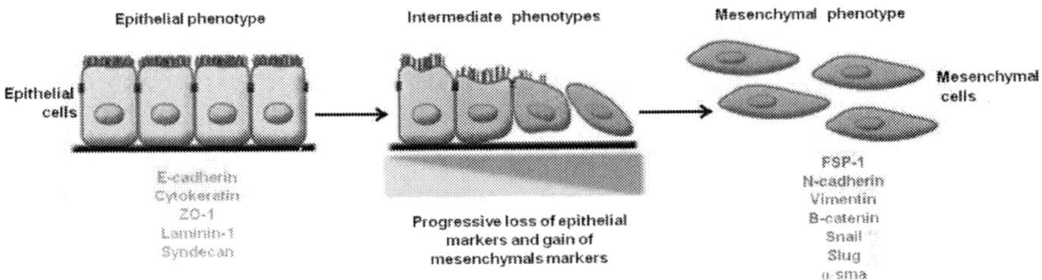

Figure 4. EMT is a functional transition from polarized epithelial cells into mobile cells able to secrete extracellular compounds (adapted after [72])

Snail family. Three Snail proteins have been identified in vertebrates: Snail 1 (Snail), Snail 2 (Slug) and Snail 3. They function as transcription repressors and their activity depend on the C-terminal zinc finger domain and the N-terminal SNAG domain [77]. Snail expression is induced in response to various growth factors. In cells that undergo TGF-β induced EMT Snail expression is mediated by Smad2/3 that form complexes with Smad4 and activates transcription by binding to Snail promoter [85]. Expression of Snails suppresses a spectrum of genes involved in maintaining the epithelial structure and function (Table 2) and enhances the expression of genes encoding vimentin and fibronectin leading to a full phenotype.

ZEB family. Two ZEB proteins have been identified in vertebrates, ZEB1 and ZEB2, which have two zinc-finger clusters at each end who mediates the interaction with DNA regulatory sequences. TGF-β induces the expression of ZEB proteins through an indirect mechanism mediated in part by Ets-1 and then ZEBs interact with Smad3 and repress the expression of epithelial marker genes (E-cadherin, claudins, ZO-3, plakophilin-2) and induce the expression of mesenchymal proteins (vimentin, N-cadherin, MMP-2) [86-88].

Helix-loop-helix family. HLH is a large family of transcription factors divided into seven classes based on their tissue distribution, dimerization ability and DNA-binding specificity [89]. The structure of HLH includes two parallel α-helices linked by a loop required for dimerization. E12, E47, Twist and Ids are involved in EMT. E12, E47 and Twist are able of DNA binding while Ids proteins are unable and act as dominant negative inhibitors [90]. Ectopic expression of E12 and E47 represses E-cadherin, plakoglobin or desmoplakin expression and induces mesenchymal markers, such as vimentin, fibronectin, N-cadherin or α5-integrin, and promotes migration and invasion [90]. Expression of Twist decreases E-cadherin, claudin-7 and occludin expression, increases that of N-cadherin and vimentin, and enhances migration and invasion [91]. Ids expression is repressed in response to TGF-β [92,93].

EMT proteome. Commonly used molecular markers of EMT could be grouped as follows: (i) decrease the amount of proteins associated with the epithelial phenotype; ii) abundance of some proteins; (iii) increased activity of selected proteins (Rho, GSK-3β); (iv) accumulation of proteins within the nucleus [69]. Table 2 listed common members of EMT proteome.

Delaminating of epithelia to facilitate movement is dependent on cell context and growth factor signaling and is accompanied by a decrease of apoptosis and mitosis [65].

In fibrotic diseases, TGF-β/Smad/Snail is a key signaling pathway [72,81]. Subsequently E-cadherin, cytokeratin, claudin and occludin are repressed, while FSP1 (fibroblast-specific protein-1), vimentin, fibronectin, Rho and MMP are increased [78].

According to [96] EMT represents the main source of fibroblasts in fibrotic pathology of connective tissues.

Generally, researches focused on few EMT markers and for this reason are not comprehensive. We specify that most information about the presence of EMT markers is indicated by the presence of proteins in epithelia and not only in fibroblasts, and as an example we'll discuss later the expression of FSP1.

	Name	EMT Type
Proteins that decrease in abundance	E-cadherin	1,2,3
	Cytokeratins	1,2,3
	Occludin	1,2,3
	Claudins	1,2,3
	ZO-1	1,2,3
	Collagen IV	1,2,3
	Laminin 1	1,2,3
Proteins that increase in abundance	N-cadherin	1,2
	Vimentin	1,2
	α-SMA	2,3
	Fibronectin	1,2
	FSP-1	1,2,3
	Snail, Slug	1,2,3
	ZEB	1,2,3
	Twist, E12/E47	1,2,3
	Ets-1	1,2,3
	MMP-2, MMP-9	2,3
	$\alpha v \beta 6$ Integrin	1,3
Proteins that accumulate in the nucleus	β-catenin	1,2,3
	Smad2/3	1,2,3
	NF-$\kappa\beta$	2,3
	Snail, Slug	1,2,3
	Twist	1,2,3
	LEF-1	1,2,3
	Ets-1	1,2,3
	ZEB	1,2,3

Table 2. Epithelial-mesenchymal transition proteome (modified after [69,78])

FSP1, also known as S100A4 is one of the most interesting proteins identified in the EMT proteome [94]. This is a fibroblast-specific protein member of the S100 superfamily of cytoplasmic, calcium-binding proteins. S100 members have been implicated in calcium signal transduction, cytoskeletal membrane interactions, microtubule dynamics, p53-mediated cell cycle regulation, cellular growth and differentiation. Because the precise function of FSP1 is not entirely clear, its interaction with cytoskeletal moieties suggest that FSP1 protein may be associated with mesenchymal cell shape to enable motility and its expression indicates the presence of a molecular program determining the fibroblast phenotype in many organ fibrosis (kidney, liver, heart, brain, lungs) [72,94,95]. FSP1 is a specific marker not only for fibroblasts but also for endothelial cells undergoing endothelial-mesenchymal transition (EndMT) [78,96].

5.2. Epithelial-mesenchymal transition in gingival overgrowth

The process of EMT is involved in the normal development and several pathologies of oral cavity. In oral tissues, type 1 EMT is associated to palate and root development, type 2 EMT could play a contributory role in GF and oral submucous fibrosis and type 3 EMT is responsible for progression, invasion and poor prognosis of oral squamous cell carcinoma [76,97].

Fibrosis which occurs in many epithelial organs (kidney, liver, lung, heart, intestine) begins as a part of a repair event, that normally generate fibroblasts by EMT mechanism in order to reconstruct tissues following inflammatory injury. It seems that in gingival fibrosis as in other organs, the main trigger for type 2 EMT is the cytokine bath released in response to persistent inflammation [78,98]. Inflammatory injury results in the recruitment of a diverse array of cells (mainly resident fibroblasts and macrophages) that release growth factors (TGF-β, PDGF, EGF, FGF-2) and MMPs, especially MMP2, MMP3 and MMP 9 [72]. Under the influence of these factors and others chemoatractants [83] the delaminated epithelial cells migrate towards the disruptions of the BM. In EMT a discontinuous BM accompanied by a decreased expression of collagen IV and laminin was reported [54]. First the epithelial cells loss the polarity, cell adhesion molecules are disrupted and cell-cell junctions disappears. The intermediate filament profile change from cytokeratins to vimentin, the F-actin rearranges to a mesenchymal shape and some cells begin to express α-smooth muscle actin (α-sma) [83]. Epithelial cells undergoing EMT are specifically labeled *in vitro* and also *in vivo* [65,99,100] by FSP1, collagen type 1 and α-sma [78,94].

Recently, was provided data about EMT origin of gingival fibroblasts in drug-induced GO. The authors reported that mesenchymal cells from the lamina propria raised after phenotypic changes of some cells from the basal and parabasal epithelial layers [54,60, 101]. These cells had a diminished expression of E-cadherin compared to others; meanwhile the majority of keratinocytes expressed FSP1. Besides phenytoin-induced GO, we reported similarly results in a case of syndromic GO (Figure 5.) [47].

As we mentioned before, the main growth factor involved in EMT is TGF-β1 that triggers activation of the transcription factors able to repress the expression of epithelial markers, for example E-cadherin.

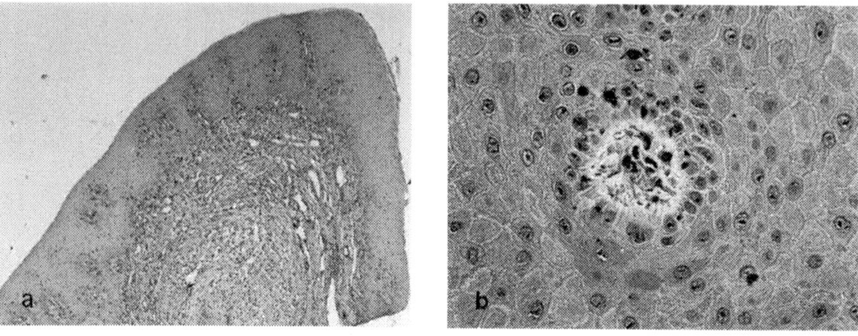

Figure 5. Syndromic GO. FSP1-positive reaction not only in fibroblasts but also in many keratinocytes, probably those that undergone EMT (IHC, a.x 100; b. x 400).

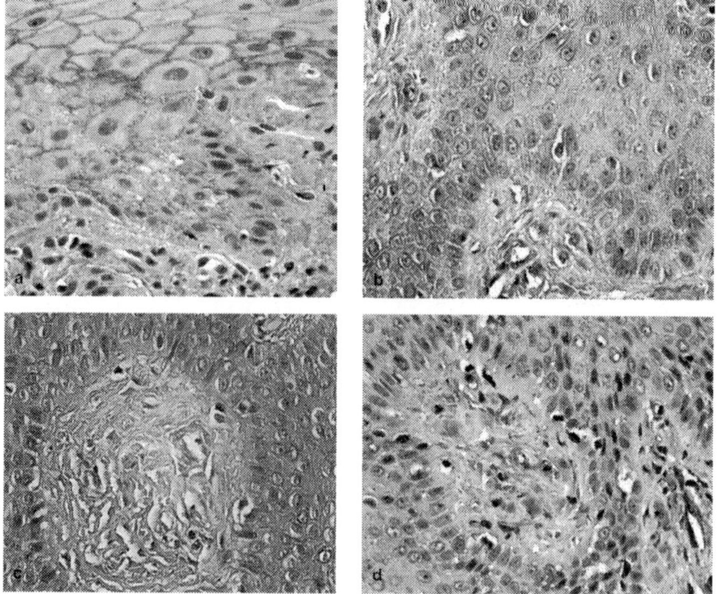

Figure 6. Idiopathic GO: a. Immunostaining for E-cadherin, x400; b. Immunostaining for TGF-β1, x200. c. Independent epithelial cells very close to the basal lamina, x400; d. FSP1 positive cells in the basal epithelium and the superficial connective tissue of the chorionic papilla, x 400.

Immunohistochemical studies that we performed on fibrotic GO samples revealed a diminished expression of E-cadherin in the basal epithelial layer in proximity of the BM suggesting that these cells undergo EMT while the immune reaction for TGF-β1 revealed many positive cells deep in the epithelium, mainly in the epithelial rete ridges [46,101]. A careful examination of these areas revealed independent epithelial cells detached from their neighbors, some of them extremely close to the basal lamina. In the lamina propria, adjacent to the BM we observed numerous intense FSP1 positive cells (Figure 6) (*unpublished data*).

The same results we reported in cases of phenytoin induced GO. Regarding the expression of FSP1 we observed an increased number of S100A4 positive cells both in the epithelium and lamina propria. At higher magnification we detected these FSP1 positive cells mainly in the basal epithelial layer nearby the disrupting BM and in the connective tissue close to the epithelium [101]. Tissues with phenytoin-induced GO showed significant reduction of E-cadherin expression in the epithelium compared with tissues from subjects without overgrowth where E-cadherin had a constant presence in the adherent junctions between keratinocytes. For the same samples we performed the assessment of the transcription factors Smad3 and Snail. We found an up-regulation in cells from profound epithelial layers. Often these positive cells were round or elongated, surrounded by a clear halo and we presumed that as a prove for lost of adhesion and the possibility to cross the disrupting BM to the connective tissue (Figure 7). Endothelial cells were also positive for these factors, especially for Smad3.

Overexpression of Snail, able to represses E-cadherin expression, and of MMP2 and MMP9 able to digest proteins from BM in the epithelium are downstream events of TGF-β1 biological effects [60, 102]. Experimental data proved that supplementation of epithelial cell cultures with TGF-β1 leads to loss of cell-cell adhesion through inhibition of E-cadherin gene expression and decrease of adherent junctions, tight junctions and desmosomes [72,102,103].

5.3. Connective tissue growth factor and the epithelial-mesechymal transition

As we mentioned before, besides TGF-β1 other growth factors could be involved in EMT such as IGF-II, EGF, FGF-2 and recently CTGF [104].

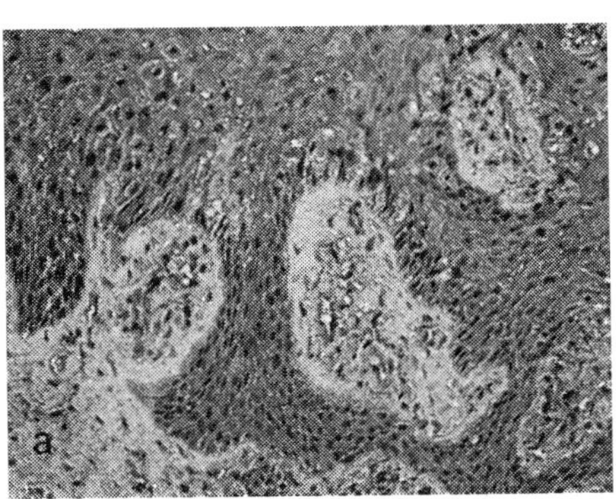
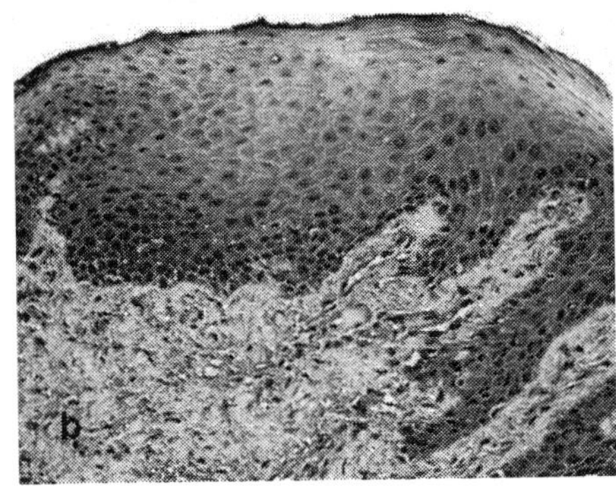

Figure 7. Phenytoin-induced GO. Expression of the transcription factors Smad 3 (a, x100) and Snail1 (b, x100).

TGF-β1 acts as a strong pro-fibrilogenetic factor through several mechanisms: (i) direct stimulation of collagen synthesis after the increase of number of highly collagen synthesizing fibroblasts through EMT; (ii) initiation of CTGF control on collagen synthesis [105]. Kantarci and coworkers in [104] showed a direct relation between the incidence of FSP1 positive cells and CTGF expression in drug-induced GO.

CTGF/CCN2 is a member of the CCN family whose members contain conserved cysteine-rich domains and have various biological activities, being important to stimulate proliferation of diverse cell types and to promote fibrosis [105]. CTGF/CCN2 is highly expressed in a wide variety of fibrotic lesions and was already demonstrated that CTGF levels are highest in gingival tissues from phenytoin induced lesions, intermediate in nifedipine-induced lesions, and nearly absent in CsA-induced overgrowth [44,106]. CTGF/CCN2 expression in connective tissue fibroblasts was positively related with the degree of fibrosis because CTGF is able to stimulate fibroblast proliferation and ECM synthesis.

We performed immunohistochemical studies to reveal the pattern of CTGF expression in various types of GO and we noted a constant intense CTGF positive reaction in all cases. We observed strong positivity in the epithelium and lamina propria not only in fibroblasts but also in endothelial and pro-inflammatory cells (Figure 8).

In phenytoin-induced GO and IGF, the most fibrotic types of GO, CTGF/CCN2 content was significantly higher compared to GO induced by other drugs (nifedipine, amlodipine) and controls. Similar results were reported by Kantarci and coworkers in [44] who revealed that CTGF/CCN levels were elevated in phenytoin-induced fibrotic lesions and HGF, the highest CTGF positive reaction being observed in the basal epithelial layer and the superficial connective tissue. Because the presence of CTGF in the epithelium is intriguing, they performed *in situ* hybridization to identify cells that express CTGF mRNA and confirmed the presence of a high amount of CTGF in the basal epithelial layer [44]. In the connective tissue, CTGF promotes local fibrosis but its presence in the epithelium could have a distinct significance as was mentioned for the uterine tissue where CTGF stimulates cell proliferation. The authors suggest that CTGF could also stimulate gingival cells proliferation, mesenchymal cells and also keratinocytes from the basal layer revealing an increased mitotic index in GO [44].

6. Role of mesenchymal cells in gingival overgrowth

The main cells of gingival connective tissue incriminated for increased collagen synthesis are logically the fibroblasts. Gingival fibroblasts are involved in ECM homeostasis through a dual effect. On the one hand, they are responsible for collagen synthesis and, on the other hand, by a process of phagocytosis, it performs ECM breakdown.

Under normal circumstances, but especially in organ fibrosis, fibroblasts show different origins. For example, in kidney fibrosis, the trans-differentiation of epithelial cells through EMT is responsible for 36% of fibroblasts, 14-15% originated in bone marrow stem cells-namely fibrocytes [99] and the rest from local fibroblast proliferation. [65]

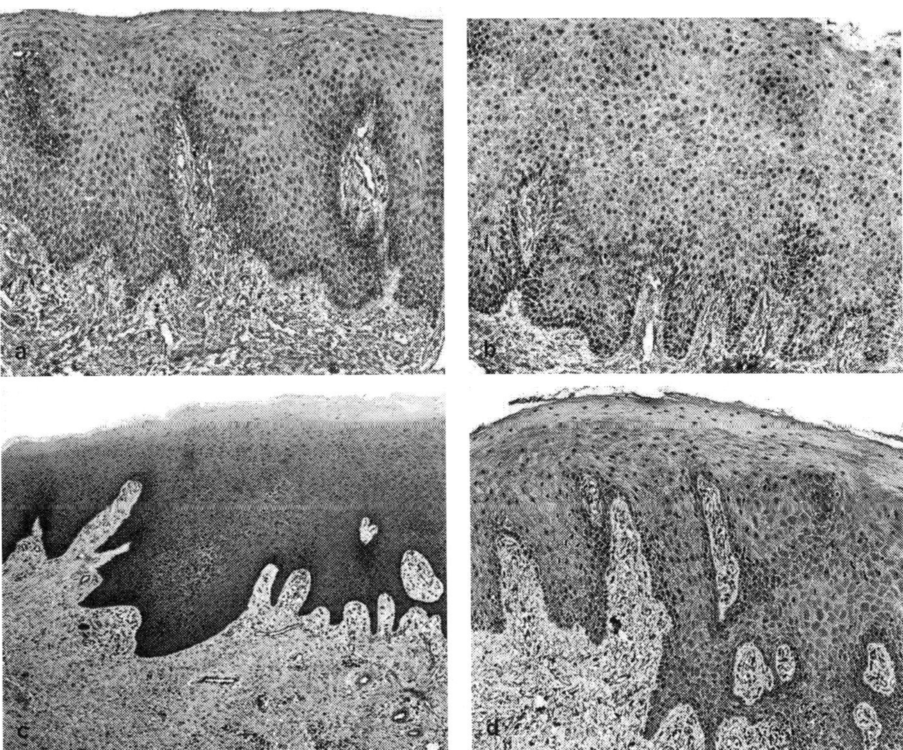

Figure 8. Immunostaining for CTGF in various samples of gingival fibromatosis: a, b. Idiopathic GF, x200, c. Phenytoin-induced GF, x100; d. Reactive GF, x200.

Kisseleva and Brenner showed in [99] that there are differences between the expression of several markers in fibrocytes and fibroblasts. The fibrocytes are cells involved in skin, kidney, liver and lung fibrosis. They have dual phenotypic features between fibroblasts and lymphocytes, and are defined as CD45+cells able to synthesize collagen with bone marrow origin, where they represents ≤1% of the cell population. Tissue injuries increase their number and after proliferation spread through blood into the damaged tissue where their proportion varies in relation to the tissue (5%-25%). [107,108]

In vitro the fibrocytes can differentiate into α-sma-positive myofibroblasts following stimulation by TGF-β1. The authors suggest that the role of these cells is not limited to tissue fibrilogenesis but to fulfill a role of intermediary in the biosignaling between the immune and fibrogenetic cells. This observation is based on the fact that fibrocytes express lymphoid markers (CD45, MHC II, MHC I), myeloid markers and adhesion molecules (CD54, ICAM-1) but also fibroblast markers (Thy-1, α-1 collagen). In addition, fibrocytes secrete growth factors and cytokines, for example TGF-β1, that stimulate the local deposition of ECM constituents. [109]

The second type of fibroblast-like cells derived still from bone marrow is represented by fibroblasts which in contrast to fibrocytes do not express myelo-monocytic markers and hyperexpress α-sma *in vitro* [110]. These are the main cells responsible for lung fibrosis.

Morphologically in fibrotic GO were described two populations of fibroblasts: one with little cytoplasm, considered inactive, and the other, well represented, with abundant cytoplasm, endoplasmic reticulum and Golgi apparatus-the active form. [29,111]

Kantarci and coworkers reported a reduction of fibroblasts apoptosis and at the same time an increased fibroblasts proliferation regardless of the inflammatory infiltration in phenytoin-induced GO and HGF which may explain the increased fibrosis. [45]

Through an autocrine signaling TGF-β1 seems to be the stimulus for increased collagen synthesis in fibroblasts. Hakkinen and Csiszar in [112] advanced the hypothesis that in GF the onset of overgrowth along with dental eruption can be placed either on account of the differentiation of abnormal phenotype fibroblasts or following their activation by pro-inflammatory cells or by mechanical trauma of eruption.

Recently there have been proposed two ways of stimulating fibroblasts proliferation either the pathway induced by increased FAS (fatty acid synthase) expression [112,113] or by increased expression of c-myc (a nuclear proto-oncogene) which hyperexpression is associated with disturbances of cell proliferation. [114] Conflicting results regarding the proliferative activity of fibroblasts in GF can be explained either by the genetic heterogeneity of the pathology itself or by the small number of cases studied. [112]

Cells that undergo EMT reorganize their actin cytoskeleton in order to facilitate formation of membrane projections that include sheet-like membrane protrusions or lamellipodia and spike-like extensions or filopodia that enable cells to directional motility. [115] Finally, the result of both EMT and EndMT is the myofibroblast, a mobile cell rich in actin stress fibers that expresses α-sma. These processes have been named EMyt and EndMyt. [77,116,117]. The mesenchymal phenotype resulting after EndMT is characterized by the acquisition of mesenchymal markers, such as α-sma and N-cadherin and the complementary loss of endothelial markers, such as CD31/Pecam-1 and VE-cadherin. [117] The mechanism of EndMT was discovered in the process of heart-development but actually it had been implicated in a wide variety of pathological conditions like several organs fibrosis and as well as in cancer. [98] There is not a consensus regarding the fact that myofibroblasts of fibrotic tissue occur exclusively as a result of EMT, these cells having a very heterogeneous origin. In tissue injury the local fibroblasts become activated by local cytokines released from inflammatory and resident cells or by the change of the mechanical microenvironment. These cells become first proto-myofibroblasts – cells acquiring contractile stress fibers composed of cytoplasmic actin. [118,119] *In vivo* such a protomyofibroblast became a differentiated myofibroblast by *de novo* expression of α-sma, used for this reason as a molecular marker. [119]

Since only certain subpopulations of myofibroblasts, previously called activated fibroblasts, express α-sma [120,121] it has advanced the hypothesis that actin of smooth muscle could actually label the cells detached from the blood vessel walls as a response to local injury. [122,123] At least three local events are needed to generate α-sma–positive differentiated myofibroblasts: (i). The accumulation of biologically active TGF-β1, the main promoter of fibroblasts differentiation into myofibroblasts and trigger of EMT; (ii) The presence of specialized ECM proteins, like the ED-A splice variant of fibronectin. Some authors argue that in the presence of the granulation tissue fibroblasts gain progressively features of myofibroblasts including α-sma expression [118,124] and (iii) High extracellular stress raised from the mechanical properties of ECM and cell remodeling activity. In addition, in [119] have been suggested that bone marrow derived circulating cells known as fibrocytes represent an alternative source of myofibroblasts in skin wound healing or organ fibrosis. There are few reports in the literature referring to the evidence of myofibroblasts in reactive focal GO, HGF and drug induced gingival hyperplasia. [25,47,126,127] Schor and coworkers reported in [128] that the only tissues that do not develop post lesion scars are embryonic and gingival tissues. This special reactivity was due to the fact that gingival fibroblasts and skin activates TGFβ1 by different signaling pathways. [129] Following the experiments authors suggested that the lack of scars in gingival mucosa is due to the fact that mechanical stress, a normal condition for functional periodontal tissues and remodeling processes is translated into fibroblast proliferation, production of TGF-β1 and CTGF, but not in activating genes responsible for α-sma synthesis.

7. Conclusions and perspectives

EMT is a dynamic physio-pathological event that depends upon a fine crosstalk between signaling pathways. Understanding the molecular mechanisms involved in EMT may reveal new biological targets for an effective therapeutic control of fibrosis in syndromic and IGF.

Further studies are needed regarding the expression of genes that control the synthesis of ECM under the particularities of structure and function of oral mucosa which normally is constantly remodeled and, on the other hand, is in a continuous state of inflammation due to the contact with different external agents. In this respect, special attention should be paid to factors that govern the relationship between innate immunity and EMT.

List of abbreviations

GO-Gingival Overgrowth

EMT – Epithelial-Mesenchymal Transition

GF-Gingival Fibromatosis

HGF-Hereditary Gingival Fibromatosis

IGF-Idiopathic Gingival Fibromatosis

IL1A – Interleukin 1A

ECM-Extracellular matrix

CsA-cyclosporin

MMP – Matrix Metalloproteinases

TIMP – Tissue Inhibitors of Matrix Metalloproteinases

KGF-Keratinocyte Growth Factor

EGF-Epidermal Growth Factor

EGFr – Epidermal Growth Factor receptor

MET – Mesenchymal Epithelial Transition

BM – Basement Membrane

TGF – Transforming Growth Factor

IGF – Insulin-like Growth Factor

FGF – Fibroblast Growth Factor

ZEB – Zinc finger E-box binding

bHLH – basic Helix-Loop-Helix

FSP1 – Fibroblast Specific Protein-1

EndMT – Endothelial Mesenchymal Transition

PDGF – Platelet Derived Growth Factor

α-sma-α-smooth muscle actin

CTGF – Connective Tissue Growth Factor

EMyt – Epithelial Myofibroblast Transition

EndMyt-Endothelial Myofibroblast Transition

Author details

Ileana Monica Baniţă[1], Cristina Munteanu[1], Anca Berbecaru-Iovan[2],
Camelia Elena Stănciulescu[2], Ana Marina Andrei[2] and Cătălina Gabriela Pisoschi[2*]

*Address all correspondence to: c_pisoschi@yahoo.com

1 Department of Dentistry, University of Medicine and Pharmacy, Craiova, Romania

2 Department of Pharmacy, University of Medicine and Pharmacy, Craiova, Romania

References

[1] Desai P & Silver JG. Drug-induced gingival enlargements. Journal of Canadian Dental Association 1998;64(4):263-268

[2] American Academy of Periodontology. Informational paper: drug associated gingival enlargement. Journal of Periodontology 2004;75:1424-1431

[3] Kataoka M, Kido J, Shinohara Y & Nagata T. Drug-Induced Gingival Overgrowth-a Review. Biological and Pharmaceutical Bulletin 2005;28(10):1817-1821

[4] Lin K, Guihoto LMFF & Yacubian EMT. Drug-Induced Gingival Enlargement – Part II. Antiepileptic Drugs Not Only Phenitoin is Involved. Journal of Epilepsy and Clinical Neurophysiology 2007;13(2):83-88

[5] Carey JC, Cohen MM Jr, Curry CJ, Devriendt K, Holmes LB & Verloes A. Elements of morphology: standard terminology for the lips, mouth, and oral region. American Journal of Medical Genetic part A. 2009;149A(1):77-92.

[6] www.maxillofacialcenter.com

[7] Kfir Y, Buchner A & Hansen LS. Reactive lesions of the gingiva. A clinicopathological study of 741 cases. Journal of Periodontology 1980;51(11):655-661

[8] Savage NW & Daly CG. Gingival enlargements and localized gingival overgrowths. Australian Dental Journal 2010;55(Suppl 1):55-60

[9] Clocheret K, Dekeyser C, Carels C &, Willems G. Idiopathic gingival hyperplasia and orthodontic treatment case report. Journal of Orthodontics 2003;30(1):13-19

[10] http://dermnetnz.org.

[11] Bittencourt LP, Campos V, Moliterno LFM, Ribeiro DPB & Sampaio RK. Hereditary Gingival Fibromatosis Review of the Literature and a case report. Quintessence International 2000;31:415-418

[12] Coletta RD & Graner E. Hereditary gingival fibromatosis: a systematic review. Journal of Periodontology 2006;77(5):753-764

[13] Hart TC, Zhang Y, Gorry MC, Hart PS, Cooper M, Marazita ML, Marks JM, Cortelli JR & Pallos D. A mutation in the SOS1 gene causes hereditary gingival fibromatosis type1. The American Journal of Human Genetics 2002;70(4):943-954

[14] Zhu Y, Zhang W, Huo Z, Zhang Y, Xia Y, Li B, Kong X & Hu L. A novel locus for maternally inherited human gingival fibromatosis at chromosome 11p15. Human Genetics 2007;121(1):113-123

[15] Douzgou S & Dallapicolla B. The gingival Fibromatoses, In: Underlying mechanisms of epilepsy, Kaneez FS (Editor), Intech, 2011, ISBN 978-953-307-765-9

[16] Ibrahim M, Abouzaid M, Mehrez M, Gamal El Din H. & El Kamah G. Genetic Disorders Associated with Gingival Enlargement, In: Gingival diseases – their aethiology,prevention and treatment. Panagos FD & Davies RB (Editors), Intech, 2011, ISBN 978-953-306-367-7

[17] Pampel M, Maier S, Kreczy A, Weirich-Schwaiger H, Utermann G & Janecke AR. Refinement of the GINGF3 locus for hereditary gingival fibromatosis. European Journal Pediatrics 2010;169(3):327-332

[18] Fryns JP. Gingival fibromatosis and partial duplication of the short arm of chromosome 2 (dup(2)(p13-p21). Annales de Genetique 1996;39(1):54-55

[19] Shashi V, Pallos D, Pettenati MJ, Cortelli JR, Fryns JP, von Kap-Herr C & Hart TC. Genetic heterogeneity of gingival fibromatosis on chromosome 2p. Journal of Medical Genetics 1999;36(9):683-686

[20] Rivera HM, Rramirez-Duenas L, Figuera LE, Gonzales-Montes RM & Vasquez AI. Opposite Inbalaces of distal 14q in two unrelated patients. Annales de Genetique 1992;35:97-100

[21] Marcias Flores MA, Garcia-Cruz D, Rovera H, Escobar-Lujan M, MelendezVeg A, Rivas-Campos D, Rodriguez-Colazzo F, Morello-Arellano I & Cantu JM. A new Form of Hipertrichosis inherited as an X-linked dominant trait. Human Genetics 1984:66(1):66-70

[22] Seymour RA, Ellis JS & Thomason JM. Risk factor for drug induced gingival overgrowth. Journal of Clinical Periodontology 2000;27:217-223

[23] Trackman PC & Kantarci A. Connective tissue metabolism and gingival overgrowth. Critical Review in Oral Biology and Medicine 2004; 15(3):165-175

[24] Taylor GW & Borgnakke WS. Periodontal disease: associations with diabetes, glycemic control and complications. Oral Disease 2008;14(3);191-203

[25] Damasceno LS., Gonçalves F da S, Costa e Silva E, Zenóbio EG, Souza PE & Horta MC. Stromal myofibroblasts in focal reactive overgrowths of the gingival. Brazilian Oral Research 2012;26(4):373-377

[26] Livada R & Shiloah J. Gummy smile: could it be genetic? Hereditary gingival fibromatosis. Journal of the Michigan Dental Association 2012;94(12):40-43

[27] Khan U, Mustafa S, Saleem Z & Azam A. Hereditary Gingival Fibromatosis, Diagnosis and treatment. Pakistan Oral & Dental Journal 2012;32(2):226-231

[28] Martelli-Júnior H, Bonan PR, Dos Santos LA, Santos SM, Cavalcanti MG & Coletta RD. Case reports of a new syndrome associating gingival fibromatosis and dental abnormalities in a consanguineous family. Journal of Periodontology 2008;79(7): 1287-1296

[29] DeAngelo S, Murphy J, Claman L, Kalmar J & Leblebicioglu B. Hereditary gingival fibromatosis: a review. Compendium of Continuing Education in Dentistry 2007;28(3):138-143

[30] Cekmez F, Pirgon O & Tanju IA. Idiopathic gingival hyperplasia. International Journal of Biomedical Sciences 2009;5(2):198-200

[31] Jaju PP, Desai A, Desai RS & Jaju SP. Idiopathic Gingival Fibromatosis: Case Report and Its Management. International Journal of Dentistry 2009, Vol.2009, Article ID 153603, 6 pages, doi:10.1155/2009/153603, ISSN 1687-8736

[32] Yadav VS, Chakraborty S, Tewari S & Sharma RK. An unusual case of idiopathic gingival fibromatosis. Contemporary Clinical Dentistry 2013;4(1):102-104

[33] Brunet L, Miranda J, Roset P, Berini L, Farre M & Mendieta C. Prevalence and risk of gingival enlargement in patients treated with anticonvulsant drugs. European Journal of Clinical Investigation 2001;31:781-788

[34] Seymour RA. Effects of medications on the periodontal tissues in health and disease. Periodontology 2000 2006;40:120-129

[35] Fletcher JP. Gingival Abnormalities of genetic origin: a preliminary communication with special reference to hereditary generalized gingival fibromatosis. Journal of Dental Research 1996;45:597-612

[36] Kather J, Salgado MA, Salgado UF, Cortelli JR & Pallos D. Clinical and histomorphometric characteristics of three different families with hereditary gingival fibromatosis. Oral Surgery Oral Medicine Oral Pathology Oral Radiology and Endodontology 2008;105(3):348-352

[37] Varga E, Lennon MA & Mair LH. Pre-transplant gingival hyperplasia predicts severe cyclosporin-induced gingival overgrowth in renal transplant patients. Journal of Clinical Periodontology 1998;25(3):225-230

[38] Bostanci N, Ilgenli T, Pirhan DC, Clarke FM, Marcenes W, Atilla G, Hughes FJ & McKay IJ. Relationship between IL-1A polymorphisms and gingival overgrowth in renal transplant recipients receiving cyclosporin A. Journal of Clinical Periodontology 2006;33(11):771-778

[39] Casavecchia P, Uzel MI, Kantarci A, Hasturk H, Dibart S, Hart TC, Trackman PC & Van Dyke T. Hereditary gingival fibromatosis associated with generalized aggressive periodontitis: a case report. Journal of Periodontology 2004;7(5):770-778

[40] Chaturvedi R. Idiopathic gingival fibromatosis associated with generalized aggressive periodontitis: a case report, Journal Canadian Dental Associattion 2009;75(4): 291-295

[41] Rizwan S. Gingival Fibromatosis with Chronic Periodontitis-A rare Case report. Inteernational e-Journal of Science, Medicine and Education 2009;3(2):24-27

[42] Uzel MI, Kantarci A, Hong HH, Uigur C, Sheff MC & Firatli E. Connective tissue growth factor in phenytoin induced gingival overgrowth. Journal of Periodontology 2001;72:921-931

[43] Uzel MI, Casavecchia P, Kantarci A, Gallagher G, Trackman PC & Van Dyke TE. 3000 Fibrosis Levels in Hereditary Gingival Fibromatosis, http//iadr.confex.com/iadr/2002 SanDiego

[44] Kantarci A, Black SA, Xydas CE, Murawel P, Uchida Y, Yucecal-Tuncer B, Atilla G, Emingil G, Uzel MI, Lee A, Firatli E, Sheff M, Hasturk H, Van Dyke TE, Trackman PC, Epithelial and Connective Tissue Cell CTGF/CCN Expression in Gingival Fibrosis, Journal of Pathology 2006; 210(1):59-66

[45] Kantarci A, Augustin P, Firatli E, Sheff MC, Hasturk H, Graves DT, Trackman PC., Apoptosis in gingival overgrowth tissues., Dental Research 2007;86(9):888-892

[46] Baniţă M, Pisoschi C, Stănciulescu C, Mercuţ V, Scrieciu M, Hâncu M & Crăiţoiu M. Phenytoin induced gingival overgrowth – an immunohistochemical study of TGF-β1 mediated pathogenic pathways. Farmacia 2011;59(1):24-34

[47] Pascu I, Pisoschi CG, Andrei AM, Munteanu C, Rauten AM, Scrieciu M, Taisescu O, Surpăţeanu M & Baniţă M. Heterogeneity of Collagen Secreting Cells in Gingival Fibrosis – an Immunohistochemical Assessment and a Review of the Literature. Romanian Journal of Morphology and Embryology (in press)

[48] Baniţă M, Pisoschi C, Stănciulescu C, Scrieciu M & Căruntu ID. Idiopathic gingival overgrowth – a morphological study an review of the literature. Revista Medico-Chirurgicală a Societăţii de Medici şi Naturalişti Iasi 2008;112(4):1076-1083

[49] Ramer M, Marrone J, Stahl B & Burakoff R. Hereditary gingival fibromatosis: identification, treatment, control. Journal of the American Dental Association 1996;127(4): 493-495

[50] Doufexi A, Mina M & Ioannidou E. Gingival overgrowth in children: epidemiology, pathogenesis, and complications. A literature review. Journal of Periodontology 2005;76(1):3-10

[51] Vishnoi SL. Hereditary Gingival Fibromatosis: Report of Four generations pedigree. International Journal of Case Reports and Images 2012;2(6):1-5.

[52] Tipton DA & Dabbous MK. Autocrine transforming growth factor beta stimulation of extracellular matrix production by fibroblasts from fibrotic human gingiva. Journal of Periodontology 1998; 69(6):609-619

[53] Bartold PM & Narayanan AS. Molecular and cell biology of healthy and diseased periodontal tissues. Periodontology 2000, 2006;40(1):29-49.

[54] Kantarci A, Nseir Z, Kim YS, Sume SS & Trackman PC. Loss of basement membrane integrity in human gingival overgrowth. Journal of Dental Research 2011;90(7): 887-893

[55] Aghili H & Goldani Moghadam M. Hereditary gingival fibromatosis: a review and a report of a rare case. Case Reports in Dentistry, Vol. 2013; Article ID:930972. doi: 10.1155/2013/930972

[56] Menga L, Yea X, Fan M, Xiong X, Von den Hoffb JW & Biana Z. Keratinocytes modify fibroblast metabolism in hereditary gingival fibromatosis. Archives of Oral Biology 2008;53(11):1050-1057

[57] Saito K, Mori S, Iwakura M & Sakamoto S. Immunohistochemical localization of transforming growth factor beta, basic fibroblast growth factor and heparan sulfate glycosaminoglycan in gingival hyperplasia induced by nifedipine and phenytoin. Journal of Periodontal Research 1996;31:545-555

[58] Ayanoglou CM & Lesty C. Cyclosporin A-induced gingival overgrowth in the rat: a histological, ultrastructural and histomorphometric evaluation Journal of Periodontal Research 1999;34(1):7-15

[59] Martelli-Júnior H, Lemos DP, Silva CO, Graner E & Coletta RD. Hereditary gingival fibromatosis: report of a five-generation family using cellular proliferation analysis. Periodontology 2005;76(12):2299-2305

[60] Sume SS, Kantarci A, Lee A, Hasturk H & Trackman PC. Epithelial to mesenchymal transition in gingival overgrowth. The American Journal of Pathology 2010;177(1): 208-218

[61] Martelli-Júnior H, Santos C de O, Bonan PR, Moura P de F, Bitu CC, León JE & Coletta RD. Minichromosome maintenance 2 and 5 expressions are increased in the epithelium of hereditary gingival fibromatosis associated with dental abnormalities. Clinics (Sao Paulo) 2011;66(5):753-757

[62] Gonzales MA, Tachibana KE, Chin SF Callagy G, Madine MA, Vowler SL, Pinder SE, Laskey RA & Coleman N. Geminin predicts adverse clinical outcome in breast cancer by reflecting cell-cycle progression. Journal of Pathology 2004;204(2):121-130

[63] Araujo CS, Graner E, Almeida OP, Sauk JJ & Coletta RD. Histomorphometric characteristics and expression of epidermal growth factor and its receptor by epithelial cells of normal gingival and hereditary gingival fibromatosis. Journal of Periodontal Research 2003;38(3):237-241

[64] Bulut S, Uslu H, Ozdemir BH, Bulut OE, Analysis of proliferative activity in oral gingival epithelium in immunosuppressive medication induced gingival overgrowth, Head Face Medicine 2006; 2:13

[65] Kalluri R & Neilson E.G. Epithelial-mesenchymal transition and its implications for fibrosis. Journal of Clinical Investigation 2003;112(12):1776–1784

[66] Thiery JP. Epithelial mesenchimal transition in development and pathologies. Current Opinion in Cell Biology 2003;15(6):740–746

[67] Liu Y. Epithelial to mesenchymal transition in renal fibrogenesis: pathologic significance, molecular mechanism, and therapeutic intervention. Journal of the American Society of Nephrology 2004;15(1):1-12

[68] Radisky DC. Epithelial-mesenchymal transition. Journal of Cell Science 2005;118(19): 4325–4326

[69] Lee JM, Dedhar S, Kalluri R & Thompson EW. The epithelial-mesenchymal transition: new insights in signaling, development, and disease. Journal of Cell Biology 2006;172(7):973-981.

[70] Thiery JP & Sleeman JP. Complex networks orchestrate epithelial–mesenchymal transitions. Nature Reviews. Mollecular Cell Biology 2006;7(2):131–142

[71] Hugo H, Ackland ML, Blick T, Lawrence MG, Clements JA, Williams ED & Thompson EW. Epithelial--mesenchymal and mesenchymal--epithelial transitions in carcinoma progression. Journal of Cell Physiology 2007;213(2):374-383

[72] Kalluri R & Weinberg RA. The basics of epithelial-mesenchymal transition. Journal of Clinical Investigation 2009;119:1420–1428

[73] Thiery JP, Acloque H & Nieto MA. Epithelial-Mesenchymal Transitions in Development and Disease. Cell 2009;139: 871-890

[74] Cannito S, Novo E, Valfrè di Bonzo L, Busletta C, Colombatto S & Parola M. Epithelial–Mesenchymal Transition: From Molecular Mechanisms, Redox Regulation to Implications in Human Health and Disease. Antioxidant Redox Signaling 2010;12:1383-1430

[75] Carew RM, Wang B & Kantharidis P. The role of EMT in renal fibrosis. Cell Tissue Research 2012;347:103–116

[76] Ghanta SB, Nayan N, Raj Kumar NG & Pasupuleti S. Epithelial–mesenchymal transition: Understanding the basic concept. Journal of Orofacial Sciences 2012;4(2): 82-86

[77] Lamouille S, Xu J & Derynck R. Molecular mechanisms of epithelial-mesenchymal transition. Nature Reviews. Molecular Cell Biology 2014;15(3):178-196

[78] Zeisberg M & Neilson EG. Biomarkers for epithelial-mesenchymal transitions. The Journal of Clinical Investigation 2009;119(6):1429–1437

[79] Kalluri R. EMT:when epithelial cells decide to become mesenchymal-like cells. The Journal of Clinical Investigation 2009;119(6):1417-1419

[80] Bhowmick NA, Zent R, Ghiassi M, McDonnell M & Moses HL. Integrin beta 1 signaling is necessary for transforming growth factor-beta activation of p38MAPK and epithelial plasticity. The Journal of Biological Chemistry 2001;276(50):46707-46713

[81] Xu J, Lamouille S & Derynck R. TGF-β-induced epithelial to mesenchymal transition. Cell Research 2009;19:156-172

[82] Morali OG, Delmas V, Moore R, Jeanney C, Thiery JP & Larue L. IGF-II induces rapid beta-catenin relocation to the nucleus during epithelium to mesenchyme transition. Oncogene 2001;20(36):4942-4950

[83] Strutz F, Zeisberg M, Ziyadeh FN, Yang CQ, Kalluri R, Müller GA & Neilson EG. Role of basic fibroblast growth factor-2 in epithelial-mesenchymal transformation. Kidney International 2002;61(5):1714-1728

[84] Zeng ZS, Cohen AM & Guillem JG. Loss of basement membrane type IV collagen is associated with increased expression of metalloproteinases 2 and 9 (MMP-2 and MMP-9) during human colorectal tumorigenesis. Carcinogenesis 1999;20(5):749-755.

[85] Cho HJ, Baek KE, Saika S, Jeong MJ & Yoo J. Snail is required for transforming growth factor-beta-induced epithelial-mesenchymal transition by activating PI3 kinase/Akt signal pathway. Biochemical and Biophysical Research Communication 2007;353(2):337-343

[86] Postigo AA. Opposing functions of ZEB proteins in the regulation of the TGFb/BMP signaling pathway. EMBO Journal 2003;22 (10):2443-2452

[87] Vandewalle C, Comijn J, De Craene B, Vermassen P, Bruynee E., Andersen H, Tulchinsky E, van Roy F & Berx G. SIP1/ZEB2 induces EMT by repressing genes of different epithelial cell-cell junctions. Nucleic Acids Research 2005; 33(20):6566-6578

[88] Bindels S, Mestdagt M, Vandewalle C, Jacobs, N, Volders L, Noel A, van Roy F, Berx G, Foidart JM & Gilles C. Regulation of vimentin by SIP1 in human epithelial breast tumor cells. Oncogene 2006; 25(36):4975-4985

[89] Massari ME & Murre C. Helix-loop-helix proteins: regulators of transcription in eucaryotic organisms. Molecular Cell Biology 2000;20:429-440

[90] Perez-Moreno MA, Locascio A, Rodrigo I, Dhondt G, Portillo F, Nieto MA & Cano A. A new role for E12/E47 in the repression of E-cadherin expression and epithelial-mesenchymal transitions. The Journal of Biological Chemistry 2001;276(29): 27424-27431

[91] Ansieau S, Bastid J, Doreau A, Morel AP, Bouchet BP, Thomas C, Fauvet F, Puisieux I, Doglioni C, Piccinin S, Maestro R, Voeltzel T, Selmi A, Valsesia-Wittmann S, Caron de Fromentel C & Puisieux A. Induction of EMT by twist proteins as a collateral effect of tumor-promoting inactivation of premature senescence. Cancer Cell 2008;14(1):79-89

[92] Kang Y, Chen CR & Massagué J. A self-enabling TGFb response coupled to stress signaling: Smad engages stress response factor ATF3 for Id1 repression in epithelial cells. Molecular Cell 2003;11(4):915-926

[93] Kowanetz M, Valcourt U, Bergstrom R, Heldin CH & Moustakas A. Id2 and Id3 define the potency of cell proliferation and differentiation responses to transforming growth factor beta and bone morphogenetic protein. Molecular Cell Biology 2004;24(10):4241-4254

[94] Strutz F, Okada H, Lo CW, Danoff T, Carone RL, Tomaszewski JE & Neilson EG. Identification and characterization of a fibroblast marker: FSP1. The Journal of Cell Biology 1995;130(2):393-405

[95] Schneider RK, Neuss S, Stainforth R, Laddach N, Bovi M, Knuechel R & Perez-Bouza A. Three-dimensional epidermis-like growth of human mesenchymal stem cells on dermal equivalents: contribution to tissue organization by adaptation of myofibroblastic phenotype and function. Differentiation 2008;76(2):156-167

[96] Iwano M, Plieth D, Danoff TM, Xue C, Okada H & Neilson EG. Evidence that fibroblasts derive from epithelium during tissue fibrosis. The Journal of Clinical Investigation 2002;110(3):341-350

[97] Yu W, Ruest LB & Svoboda KK. Regulation of epithelial-mesenchymal transition in palatal fusion. Experimental Biology and Medicine (Maywood) 2009;234(5):483-491

[98] Potenta S, Zeisberg E & Kalluri R. The role of endothelial-to-mesenchymal transition in cancer progression. British Journal of Cancer 2008;99(9):1375-1379

[99] Kisseleva T & Brenner DA. Mechanisms of fibrogenesis. Experimental Biology and Medicine (Maywood) 2008;233(2):109-122

[100] Guarino M, Tosoni A & Nebuloni M. Direct contribution of epithelium to organ fibrosis: epithelial-mesenchymal transition. Human Pathology 2009;40(10):1365-1376

[101] Pisoschi C, Stănciulescu C, Munteanu C, Fusaru AM & Baniţă M. Evidence for epithelial mesenchymal transition as a pathogenic mechanism of phenytoin induced gingival overgrowth. Farmacia 2012;60(2):168-176

[102] Zavadil J & Böttinger EP. TGF-beta and epithelial-to-mesenchymal transitions. Oncogene 2005;24(37):5764-5774

[103] Bolos V, Jorda M, Fabra A, Portillo F, Palacio J & Cano A. Genetic profiling of epitelial cells expressing E-cadherin repressors reveals a distinct role for Snail, Slug and E47 factors in epithelial-mesenchymal transition. Cancer Research 2006;66:9543-9556

[104] Kantarci A, Sume SS, Black SA, Lee A, Xydas C, Hasturk H & Trackman P. Epithelial and Connective Tissue cell CTGF/CCN2 Expression in Gingival Fibrosis: Role of Epithelial-Mesenchimal Transition) in CCN proteins in health and disease: An overview of the Fifth International Workshop of the CCN family of genes, Perbal A, Takigawa M & Perbal BV, Springer, 2010

[105] Holbourn KP, Acharya KR & Perbal B. The CCN family of proteins: structure-function relationships. Trends in Biochemical Sciences 2008;33(10):461-473

[106] Pisoschi CG, Stănciulescu CE, Munteanu C, Andrei AM, Popescu F & Baniţă IM. Role of Transforming Growth Factor β – Connective Tissue Growth Factor Pathway in Dihydropyridine Calcium Channel Blockers-Induced Gingival Overgrowth. Romanian Journal of Morphology and Embyology 2014;56(2):285-290

[107] Kisseleva T, Uchinami H, Feirt N, Quintana-Bustamante O, Segovia JC, Schwabe RF & Brenner DA. Bone marrow-derived fibrocytes participate in pathogenesis of liver fibrosis. Journal of Hepatology 2006;45(3):429-438

[108] Moore BB, Kolodsick JE, Thannickal VJ, Cooke K, Moore TA, Hogaboam C, Wilke CA & Toews GB. CCR2-mediated recruitment of fibrocytes to the alveolar space after fibrotic injury. The American Journal of Pathology 2005;166(3):675-684

[109] Quan TE, Cowper SE & Bucala R.The role of circulating fibrocytes in fibrosis. Current Rheumatology Reports 2006;8(2):145-150

[110] Hashimoto N, Jin H, Liu T, Chensue SW & Phan SH. Bone marrow-derived progenitor cells in pulmonary fibrosis. The Journal of Clinical Investigation 2004;113(2): 243-252

[111] Sakamoto R, Nitta T, Kamikawa Y, Kono S, Kamikawa Y, Sugihara K, Tsuyama S & Murata F. Histochemical, immunohistochemical, and ultrastructural studies of gingival fibromatosis: a case report. Medical Electron Microscopy 2002;35(4):248-254

[112] Häkkinen L & Csiszar A. Hereditary gingival fibromatosis: characteristics and novel putative pathogenic mechanisms. Journal of Dental Research 2007;86(1):25-34

[113] Almeida JP, Coletta RD, Silva SD, Agostini M, Vargas PA, Bozzo L &, Graner E. Proliferation of fibroblasts cultured from normal gingiva and hereditary gingival fibromatosis is dependent on fatty acid synthase activity. Journal of Periodontology 2005;76(2):272-278

[114] Secombe J, Pierce SB & Eisenman RN. Myc: a weapon of mass destruction. Cell 2004;117(2):153-156

[115] Ridley AJ. Life at the Leading Edge. Cell 2011;145(7):1012-1022

[116] Quaggin SE & Kapus A. Scar wars: mapping the fate of epithelial-mesenchymal-myofibroblast transition. Kidney International 2011;80(1):41-50

[117] van Meeteren LA & ten Dijke P. Regulation of endothelial cell plasticity by TGF-β. Cell Tissue Research 2012;347(1):177-186

[118] Tomasek JJ, Gabbiani G, Hinz B, Chaponnier C & Brown RA. Myofibroblasts and mechano-regulation of connective tissue remodelling. Nature Reviews Molecular Cell Biology 2002;3(5):349-363

[119] Hinz B, Phan SH, Thannickal VJ, Galli A, Bochaton-Piallat ML & Gabbiani G. The myofibroblast. One function, multiple origins. The Americal Journal of Pathology 2007;170(6):1807-1816

[120] Tang WW, Van GY & Qi M. Myofibroblast and alpha 1 (III) collagen expression in experimental tubulointerstitial nephritis. Kidney International 1997;51(3):926-931

[121] Serini G & Gabbiani G. Mechanisms of myofibroblast activity and phenotypic modulation. Experimental Cell Research 1999;250(2):273-283

[122] Okada H, Danoff TM, Kalluri R & Neilson EG. Early role of Fsp1 in epithelial-mesenchymal transformation. The American Journal of Physiology 1997;273(4 Pt 2):F563-574

[123] Eyden B. The myofibroblast: an assessment of controversial issues and a definition useful in diagnosis and research. Ultrastructural Pathology 2001;25(1):39-50

[124] Desmoulière A, Chaponnier C & Gabbiani G. Tissue repair, contraction, and the myofibroblast. Review. Wound Repair Regeneration 2005;13(1):7-12

[125] Castella LF, Buscemi L, Godbout C, Meister JJ & Hinz B. A new lock-step mechanism of matrix remodelling based on subcellular contractile events. Journal of Cell Science 2010;123(Pt 10):1751-1760

[126] Lombardi T & Morgan PR. Immunohistochemical characterisation of odontogenic cysts with mesenchymal and myofilament markers. Journal of Oral Pathology & Medicine 1995;24(4):170-176

[127] Miguel MC, Andrade ES, Rocha DA, Freitas R de A & Souza LB. Immunohistochemical expression of vimentin and HHF-35 in giant cell fibroma, fibrous hyperplasia and fibroma of the oral mucosa. Journal of Applied Oral Sciences 2003;11(1):77-82

[128] Schor SL, Ellis I, Irwin CR, Banyard J, Seneviratne K, Dolman C, Gilbert AD & Chisholm DM. Subpopulations of fetal-like gingival fibroblasts: characterisation and potential significance for wound healing and the progression of periodontal disease. Oral Disease 1996;2(2):155-166

[129] Guo F, Carter DE & Leask A. Mechanical tension increases CCN2/CTGF expression and proliferation in gingival fibroblasts via a TGFβ-dependent mechanism. PLoS One 2011;6(5):e19756. doi: 10.1371/journal.pone.0019756

Chapter 27

Ultrasonic Instrumentation

Ana Isabel García-Kass,
Juan Antonio García-Núñez and
Victoriano Serrano-Cuenca

Additional information is available at the end of the chapter

http://dx.doi.org/10.5772/59259

1. Introduction

Although ultrasounds (US) were discovered in the 18th Century due to their use in animal kingdom, they were not manufactured until the 19th Century, when certain devices facilitating the reproduction of these non audible for human sounds were developed. They constitute rare frequencies with several properties. First of all they were developed for their use in navy and in medicine. In the 20th Century it was noticed that they could have uses in dentistry, so the first applications for calculus removal were initiated, taking advantage of their mechanical energy and cavitation effect. The different possibilities achieved by conventional US together with those of sonicators, of lower frequency but with similar effects, resulted in a fast development of these technologies.

Since Michigan longitudinal studies demonstrated that the open flap radicular instrumentation techniques were in a long term as effective as the closed ones, the latter were developed, so treatment of periodontitis suffered a change of paradigm. From that moment on, periodontal treatment involved less open flaps and more mechanical treatments, limiting surgeries to very concrete cases, in order to enable access to the deepest pockets and furcations. The result was a reduction in discomfort for patients and a better long term prognosis. Prevention gained more importance and supportive periodontal therapies were regularly done adjusting them to the individual necessities of each patient, depending on the type of periodontitis and the severity of the case. To reduce the number of surgeries, it was crucial to develop instruments able to reach deep pockets. Small curettes and microcurettes were developed, and later on special ultrasonic tips which allowed the instrumentation of pockets of difficult access for Gracey and Universal curettes. Even when effectuating periodontal surgery, clinicians preferred US rather than curettes for the narrow furcations' instrumentation. The fewer fatigue

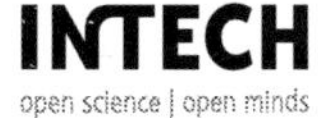

of the professional and the efficacy of the results have favoured the great development of these instruments during the last years.

A new progress occurred in dentistry with the introduction of piezoelectric US. These US produced less discomfort in patients, and with the development of special tips imitating microcurettes, deep and narrow pockets instrumentation was possible without doing surgery. With the important development of implant rehabilitations during the last twenty years and the subsequent peri-implantitis, the necessity of new instruments has arisen, as traditional and teflon curettes are not suitable for this purpose. To solve this problem, tips of teflon and other materials have emerged to facilitate the elimination of deposits settled over the irregular implants' surface, with controversial results.

The use of US in endodontics was introduced later to clean and disinfect root canals. It is quite useful basically to make easier the access to the root canals in certain conditions, in endodontic retreatments and to clean before the sealing of the root canal. One of the latest US applications in dentistry is in surgery, as they avoid discomfort of rotary instruments while preserving the soft tissues. The cut precision allows their use in implants' surgery, ostectomies and especially in those techniques where tearing of soft tissues could be produced due to their proximity, i.e., sinus lift procedures. These techniques are in continuous progress; they are linked to piezo-electric US and to those new materials allowing their use in favourable conditions.

The aim of this chapter is to revise the physical principles of US, the materials used and the historical evolution, their basic uses in perio and endodontics, as well as their efficacy when comparing with other techniques and finally the possibilities in maxilar surgery. Other less frequent applications are also mentioned.

2. History and physics of ultrasounds

Before 1700 man was unaware of ultrasounds because their frequency is below human's audible frequency. In 1700, Spallanzani described their use by bats when flying and capturing their preys. Later on, it was demonstrated that other animal species had the same faculties, and in the 19th Century, with the discovery of Doppler effect about deformation of light waves in movement, it was observed that this property could also be applied to ultrasounds. In fact, they are sound waves that are not audible for men due to their high frequency (Figure 1).

At the end of the 19th Century, the Curie brothers [1] described the piezoelectric effect (from greek *piezein*, mechanic pressure) of several crystals, property used later for the fabrication of ultrasonic devices with new characteristics. At this time, in 1883, Galton develops a high frequency whistle to find out the human hearing limit, and from that moment on ultrasounds (US) for different applications are developed. Although the first ultrasonic apparatus date from 1950, the first commercial application for dentistry was in periodontics in 1957 with Cavitron®, developed by Dentsply for doing prophylaxis and calculus removal. Its name comes from the cavitation effect produced by ultrasounds when working with water. When a liquid flows through a region where pressure is lower than its steam pressure, the liquid boils and produces

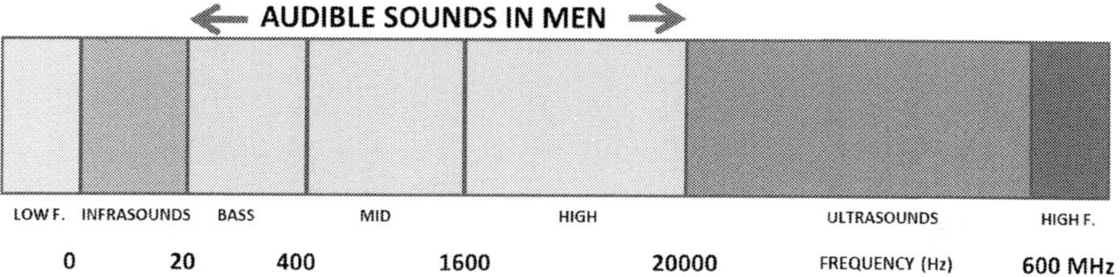

Figure 1. Human audition and ultrasound frequencies in Hz

vapour bubbles. The bubbles will be carried to a higher pressure area, where the steam returns immediately to the liquid phase, imploding the bubbles suddenly. Thus, a change from liquid to gaseous phase takes place, and again to liquid phase with water dissociation and formation of H^+ and OH^- (Figure 2).

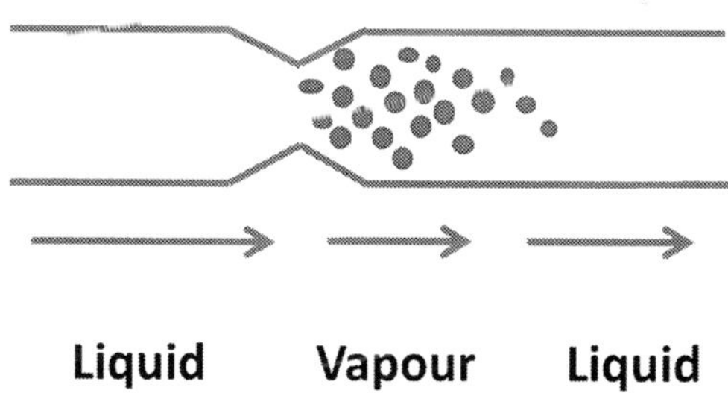

Figure 2. Representation of cavitation effect

Cavitation is defined as the formation of submicroscopic cavities or vacuums as a result of the vibration of a fluid due to the high frequency alternating movement of the tip of an instrument. When these vacuums implode, shock waves which spread through the medium are generated and produce energy (heat) release [2].

The basis of the ultrasonic action consists of an electric generator transmitting vibrations to the tip of the device with frequencies of 25,000 to 30,000 Hz, whose shock waves generate pressures and depressions which detach the calculus and break water molecules by the cavitation phenomenon. To the effect of cavitation it adds an acoustic streaming, with a great cleaning and bactericidal action, which potentiates the bactericidal effect of cavitation, effect that can increase adding an antiseptic product to the irrigation fluid.

There are two types of ultrasonic devices: the classical ones, laminated or magnetostrictive, with elliptical oscillation of the tip, and the piezoelectric ones, of quartz with lineal oscillation. Laminated US are based on the Joule magnetostriction phenomenon. According to this phenomenon, several ferromagnetic materials get deformed when they go through a magnetic field. The deformation degree depends on the material employed, the magnetization strength, the previous treatment of the material and the temperature. The metallic sheets are situated in the handle, i.e. in the handpiece where the insert is placed (Figure 3).

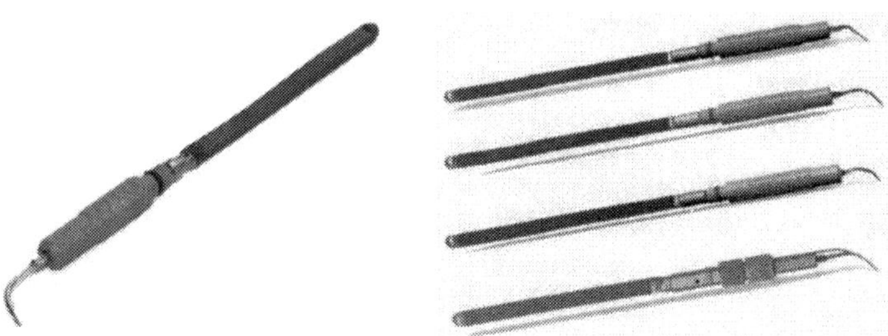

Figure 3. Laminated US device and several ultrasonic inserts for Cavitron

Piezoelectric US (Figure 4) are based on quartz clock principles. When applying an alternating current to the ceramic/quartz discs, changes in polarity produce expansion and contraction trasmitting the oscillation to the tip, applicator or insert. The sound thus generated, presents the same intensity, frequency and wavelength than the material employed in its fabrication (quartz, zinc blende, sodium borate...). Nowadays, the most used crystals are ceramic zirconate discs, which are less sensitive to temperature and blows.

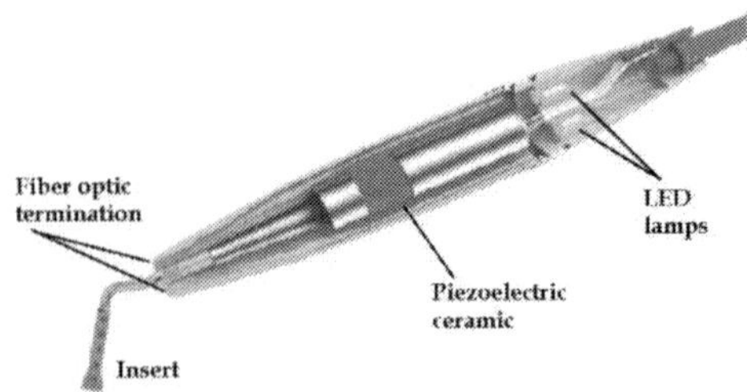

Figure 4. Piezoelectric US for surgery. Modified from Variosurg (NSK) catalogue

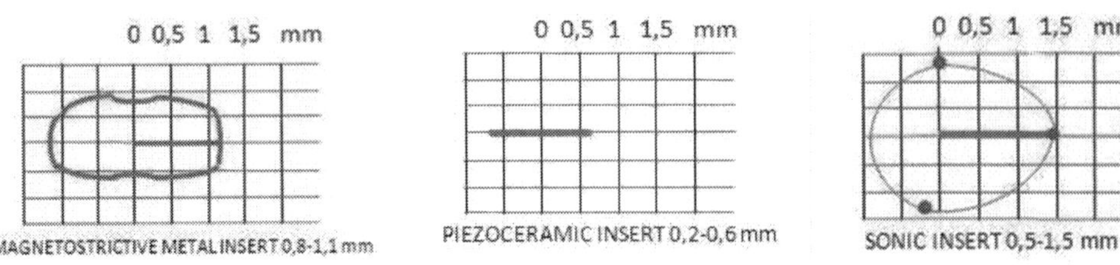

Figure 5. Oscillation of magnetostrictive US, piezoceramic US and sonicators

3. Biologic actions

US present several effects over the tissues which vary depending on the time, type of US and way of application. These effects are mechanical, thermal, biological, chemical, massage and placebo.

1. Mechanical effects. The most important, as vibration favours the removal of calculus, biofilm and of the cementum surface, damaged by bacterial toxins and sometimes contaminated by bacteria (Figure 6). Inside the root canals, US clean the pulpal detritus.

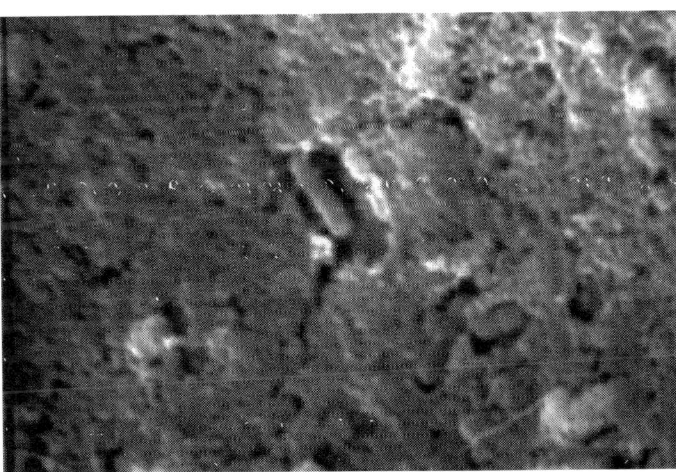

Figure 6. Bacterial presence inside cementum in periodontitis. Original magnification SEM x3000. Bacteria can be identified supragingivally, in the epithelial junction and in apical areas of cementum

2. Thermal effects. US are a way of energy and thus, during their application, heat is generated. This heat can be useful, as it favours the cleaning of the treated area and the elimination of detritus, blood debris, biofilm and calculus; but if it is excessive it could burn the tissues, especially gingiva and periostium. This is the reason why it is crucial to control the irrigation system, checking for possible obstructions of applicator/insert.

3. Biological effects. US produce an increase in permeability of the cellular membrane, known as phonophoresis, which facilitates the cellular function, and thus the recuperation of the inflamed soft tissues.

4. Chemical effects. Ultrasonic vibration favours the chemical processes in the area in which they are applied. Biological exchanges among the treated tissues improve; in addition, an increase of the blood supply takes place, helping to reduce inflammation and to facilitate the arrival of blood cells and anti-inflammatory mediators, favouring tissue normality. It

also produces oxidation and macromolecule depolymerization phenomena, due to the ions release.

5.   The massage and placebo effects, also associated to US, are of less interest in our field, but they should not be forgotten.

Due to the cavitation effect and the acoustic micro-streaming produced by oscillatory movements of ultrasonic inserts, US are used in humans in different ways for diagnosis and treatment. In the oral cavity they are mainly used for root instrumentation in periodontics, and less in endodontics, ostectomy, and sinus lift procedures. There are also other less frequent applications that we shall describe.

4. US in periodontics and implants

It is well known that periodontal disease is based on the presence of a mature biofilm with more than 700 bacterial species, being only a fraction of them related to periodontitis. The progression of the disease depends on the periodontopathogens, but also on the patient's immune system and its response to bacterial aggression. The elimination of bacteria, their toxins and calculus produced by saliva, is essential to keep under control the disease. Once local factors are removed, a strict hygiene is required, as well as a supportive periodontal treatment program, in order to eliminate calculus and subgingival biofilm, which is the main responsible of the bone and attachment loss and is formed shortly after its elimination.

Treatment was traditionally based on the mechanical elimination of plaque and calculus, which facilitate biofilm's survival, mainly using hand instruments and US, directly or by an open flap procedure. Longitudinal studies of the decades of 70's and 80's, showed that even most periodontally advanced cases, well treated and maintained, remained stable through the years [3], versus those patients who did not receive any treatment, who suffered a considerable tooth loss and worsening of periodontal parameters [4].

Since Michigan longitudinal studies [5-7] demonstrated that the open flap radicular instrumentation techniques were in a long term as effective as the closed ones [7], the latter were developed, so treatment of periodontitis suffered a change of paradigm. From that moment on, periodontal treatment involved less open flaps and more mechanical treatments, limiting surgeries to very concrete cases, in order to enable access to the most deep pockets and furcations [8]. The result was a reduction in discomfort for patients and a better long term prognosis. Prevention gained more importance and supportive periodontal therapies were regularly done adjusting them to the individual necessities of each patient, depending on the type of periodontitis and the severity of the case.

To reduce the number of surgeries, it was crucial to develop instruments able to reach deep pockets. Small curettes and microcurettes were developed, and later on special ultrasonic tips which allowed the instrumentation of pockets of difficult access for Gracey and Universal curettes.

The first device used in periodontal prophylaxis was Cavitron®, introduced in 1957 by Dentsply (USA). With the important development of implant rehabilitations during the last twenty years and the subsequent peri-implantitis, the necessity of new instruments has arisen, as traditional and teflon curettes are not suitable for this purpose. Ultrasonic instruments are very comfortable to use, they produce less fatigue in the operator than curettes and allow the combination of different tips and products in order to improve the treatment efficacy. Several authors [9] even demonstrate better results when instrumentation is done with US instead of curettes.

During the 80's, we demonstrated in several publications that prophylaxis done *in vitro* with US resulted at least equal or even more effective than with curettes [10, 11] (Figure 7).

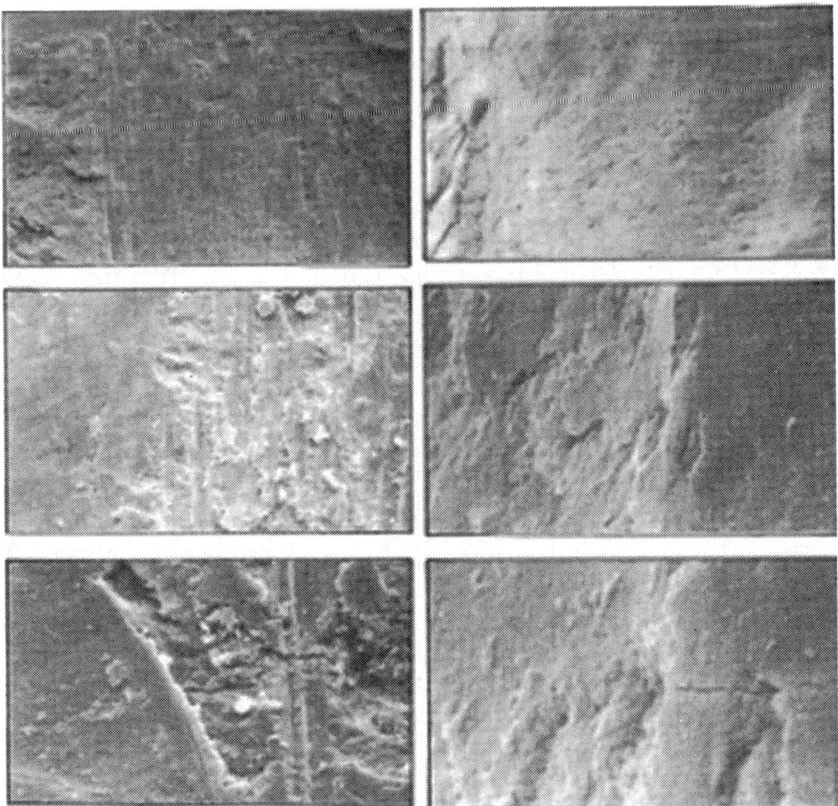

Figure 7. Cementum of the same tooth treated with curettes (left) and US (right). Original magnification SEM x352, x1136 and x3000

In Drisko's 1993 review, it is suggested that a thorough radicular debridement can be achieved without overinstrumentation, using certain sonic and ultrasonic scalers. The evaluation of residual plaque and calculus after hand and mechanical instrumentation with sonic and ultrasonic scalers, shows that sonic and US instruments obtain similar, and in some cases, better results than those obtained with manual instrumentation. When comparing modified ultrasonic inserts with unmodified ultrasonic inserts and manual scalers, it is observed that the modified ones generate smoother surfaces, better plaque and calculus removal, less damage and better access to the bottom of the pocket, which together with a less operating time lead to a lower fatigue [12].

Several years later, another review of the same author shows that US, through their cavitation effect, are able to eliminate toxins from the cementum surface without damaging it. This, together with the irrigation action, improves healing, as it is not necessary an excessive instrumentation of cementum to achieve satisfactory results. The additional benefits of the chemical irrigation during ultrasonic instrumentation are the weakly attached subgingival plaque removal and a better access to difficult areas such as narrow and deep pockets, root grooves and furcations. Thus, microultrasonic tips, of smaller diameter, allow the penetration 1 mm farther than manual instruments [13].

In a position paper of 2000, US and sonicators were compared, reaching similar results than hand instruments in terms of plaque, calculus and endotoxins removal. Ultrasonic scalers used at medium power produced less damage in root surfaces than manual instruments or sonicators. Furcations seemed to be more accesible when using sonic or ultrasonic scalers than when using manual instruments. It was still not clear if root roughness was more or less pronounced when using US or curettes, and if the roughness produced in radicular cement affected long term wound healing. Although the aim of root instrumentation is the highest as possible elimination of calculus and toxins, it is necessary to preserve cementum. According to the reviewed papers, toxins remain in the root surface, thus being easily removed with US. One of the main problems of the intervention with US and sonicators is the aerosols production, which involves the risk of transmitting infectious diseases, therefore it is essential the use of barriers against aerosols. Concerning the use of chemical agents there is no evidence of their additional clinical benefit [14].

To avoid the potential damage of the cementum surface done by sonic and US instruments and curettes, and looking after an effective treatment of the root surface, a sonic instrument covered by teflon was introduced in order to compare it with the standard instrumentation and with Per-io-Tor in extracted teeth. Per-io-Tor and the mentioned sonic instrument seemed to be adequate for soft deposits' elimination in the root surface, but not for calculus removal [15].

Another study compared *in vivo* the effect of two piezoelectric US, Vector scaler and Enac scaler, with a hand scaler. Instrumentation was completed until the obtaining of a hard surface. Roughness, amount of remaining calculus and loss of dental substance were examined by SEM. Vectorial US provided a smooth root surface with minimal dental substance loss [16].

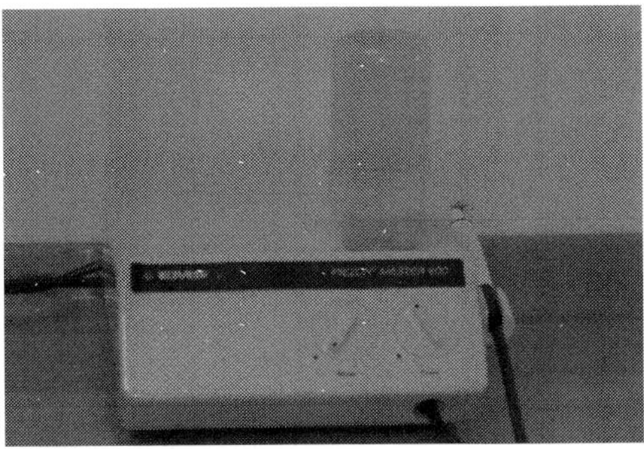

Figure 8. EMS piezoelectric US Piezon Master

The effects of US were described in 1969 by Clark [17]: they depend on the vibratory movement amplitude, the pressure applied, the instrument's tip sharpness, and the tip's application angle and time by surface unit. Their effects condition the way of use: they should be used at 40-50% of their power to avoid the metal fatigue and to favour the long-term duration of device and tip, they should be applied tangentially (parallel to the root surface) to avoid damage in the cementum surface (Figure 9), they should never be applied with the tip perpendicular to the cementum and the tip should be in a continuous movement (Figure 10) in order to avoid the production of holes in enamel and cementum. To avoid an excessive increase of temperature, the irrigation should be abundant (Figure 11), and to achieve an optimal efficacy the most suitable tip should be selected for each indication. It should be taken into account that it is different to work over a thick layer of supragingival calculus than over a thin subgingival layer, which is more adhered. This is the reason why large tips are used for superficial calculus, small tips for subgingival calculus, curette-like for scaling and thin and long for narrow and deep pockets (Figure 11).

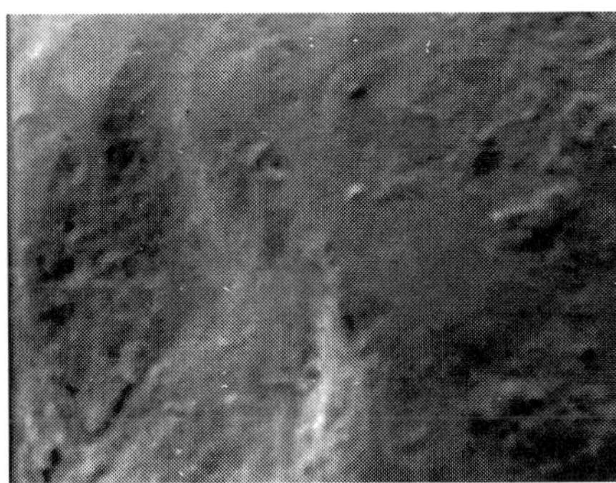

Figure 9. Hole in cementum due to a wrong ultrasonic instrumentation. Original magnification x600

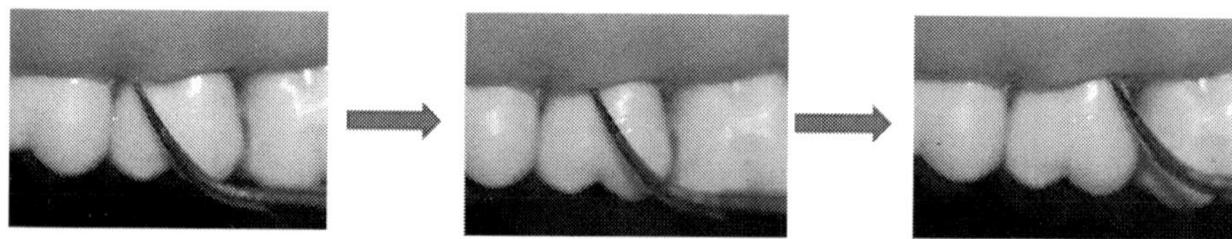

Figure 10. Insert application and displacement for calculus removal

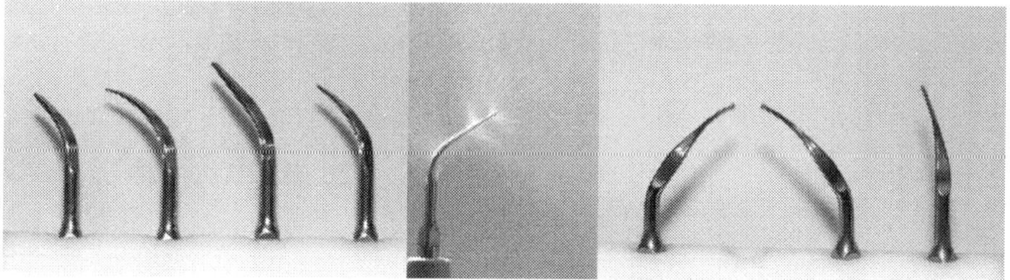

Figure 11. Supra (left) and thin subgingival (right) ultrasonic tips should always work with abundant irrigation

When US are used with complementary water tank and an antiseptic liquid, it is convenient to wash the whole circuit with demineralized water after its use, so the obstruction of tubes with the substances used is avoided. In case of using only water, it is recommended to fill in the deposit with low mineralized water, in order to facilitate the cleaning and prevent obstructions in tubes and inserts.

Due to their lineal oscillation over the dental surface, the actual rounded-tip piezoelectric US, reduce abrasion and obtain a uniform and smooth surface. With 32.000 oscillations per second, they are autoregulated and their cavitation effect and acoustic streaming reduce discomfort and have limited effects over gingival epithelium (Figure 12).

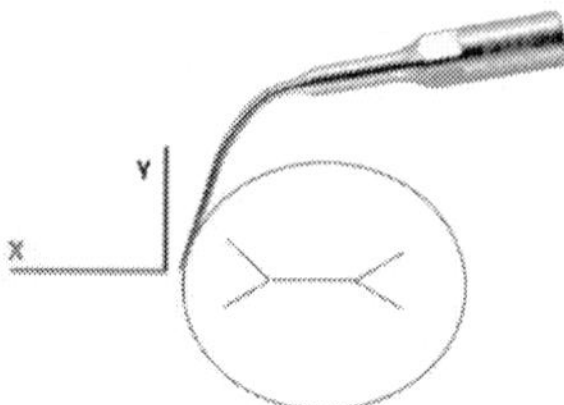

Figure 12. Vector decomposition of ultrasonic oscillation

Some of these US may incorporate two bottles, one for the bactericidal agent and the other for water for clearing or cleaning. They are also equipped with perio and endodontic tips.

Ultrasounds present few contraindications. They are not recommended in children except in very concrete cases. They should be avoided in the proximity of composite resins, as they could produce roughness or even detachment of the filling. They should not be used directly over ceramic partial fixed prosthesis or veneers, as ceramic could detach or break. In patients with certain types of pacemakers, interferences could be produced with inhibition and increase of the stimulation frequency. It is recommended the intermittent use of ultrasounds, avoiding the support of instruments over the generator as well as deprogramming the frequency modulation during the sessions. With a magnet, the pacemaker, which usually works at demand mode, converts into fixed-rate, not being sensitive to electromagnetic fields. In case of non sensible to electromagnetic interferences pacemakers, US could be used in the same way as in patients without pacemakers. Another option in these patients is the use of sonicators (Figure 13) because they use an air flow so they don't generate electromagnetic fields.

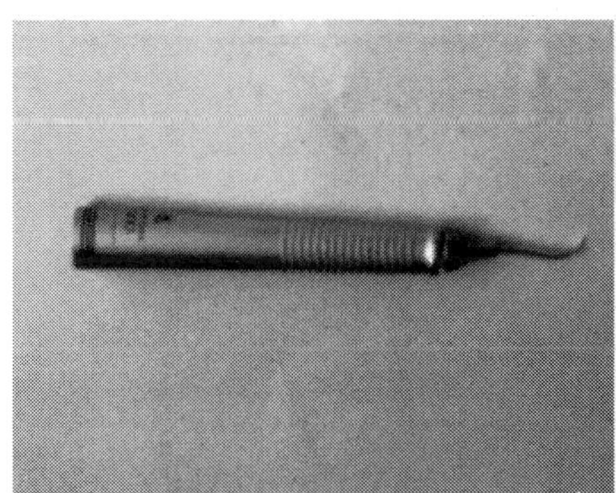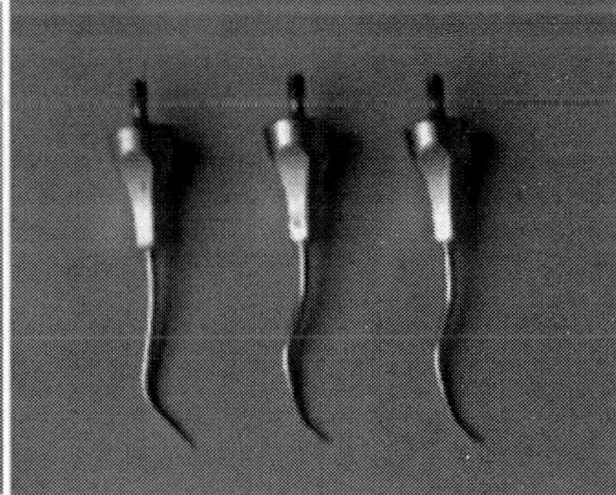

Figure 13. Sonicator and varied tips

These instruments present certain advantages and disadvantages in relation to ultrasounds. Their oscillation frequency is much lower, of 2,000 Hz, because the oscillation is produced by the air that arrives directly from the equipment and generates an orbital oscillation in the application tip. Their efficacy is similar to that of ultrasounds, but they can only use water instead of antiseptic liquids and the set of tips is much more reduced than the ultrasounds.

Ultrasounds are used as preventive and complementary to surgery treatment in implants. In this case the tip should not be metallic but of teflon, in order to avoid the damage of the implants ' surface (Figure 14).

Fox *et al.* compared plastic and metal curettes in titanium implants in an *in vitro* study. Plastic instruments produced an insignificant alteration of the implants' surface after instrumentation, in contrast with metal instruments, which significantly altered this surface [18].

Something similar occurs when using Piezoelectric Ultrasonic Scalers with carbon, plastic and metallic tips on titanium implants. Remaining plaque and calculus index seemed to be similar with the three treatments. When using a laser profilometer and a laser scanning electron

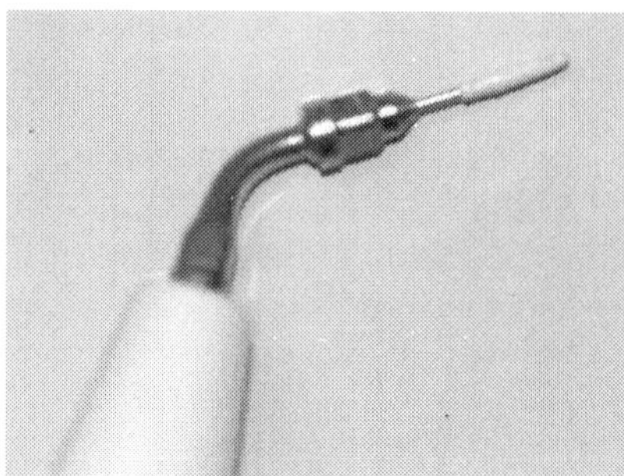

Figure 14. EMS Teflon insert for implants' instrumentation

microscope to evaluate the treated abutment surface characteristics, implants treated with carbon and plastic tips presented smoother surfaces than those treated with metallic tips, which were more damaged [19].

5. US in endodontics

US were incorporated into this field in 1957 when Richman used them for root canal cleaning and instrumentation [20]. In 1976, Martin improved endodontic treatment adding simultaneous irrigation, but its commercialization and use only were extended from 1980 by Martin *et al.* [21]. There are sonic apparatus in which special files are used, and several ultrasonic devices which work with standard files, with the usual colours and diameters (Figure 15).

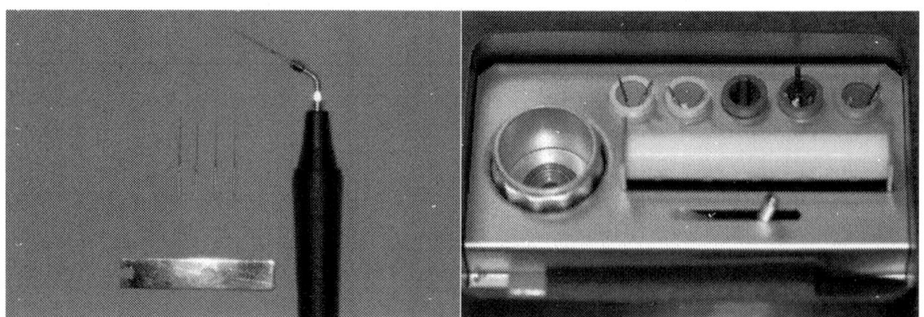

Figure 15. EMS ultrasonic handle and several endodontic K-files.

In endodontics US work by a transversal vibration, with a characteristic pattern of nodes and antinodes along the file's length (Figure 16) [22, 23], and may work in two different ways: with simultaneous ultrasonic instrumentation and irrigation (UI) or with passive ultrasonic irrigation (PUI), which works in an alternating way.

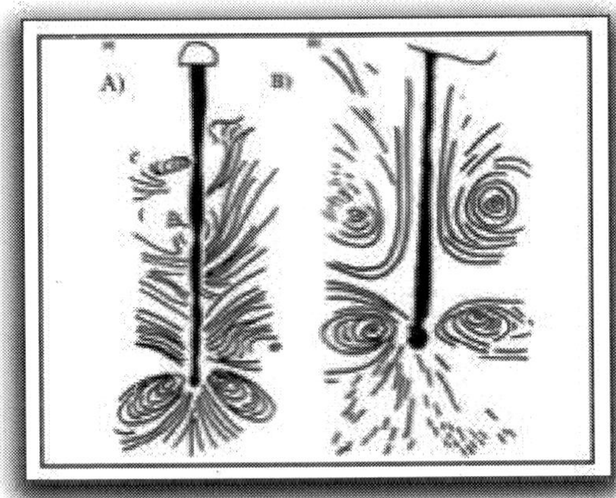

Figure 16. Diagrammatic representation of the current observed in ultrasonic (A) and sonic (B) activated files [24].

As for ultrasonic instrumentation UI, it is discussed if the root canals thus instrumented are significantly cleaner than those prepared with files in the usual way. Some authors support UI cleaning is better [25-29], while other studies affirm the cleaning is similar [30-36]. For Ruddle, these differences could be due to the limited space available in the root canal to let the ultrasonic vibration [37]. Also the lack of space could be responsible of the lesions produced during ultrasonic instrumentation, such as perforations and deficient root canal preparations [38]. This is the reason why this technique is only recommended after the complete root canal preparation [39], by what is known as PUI.

Passive ultrasonic irrigation was described by Weller [40] as a technique in which the effect of the ultrasonic tip reduces the risk of contact with the root canal surface, thus reducing the risk of perforation, while the cavitation and cleaning effects are preserved. As the root canal has already been prepared, the file moves freely and the irrigant penetrates easily in the apical area of the root canal system [41]. In this technique two ways of irrigation may be used: continuous or discontinuous, in which irrigation works intermittently after each ultrasonic cycle. Both of them allow control of irrigation, so they seem to be equally efficient [42].

Sonic instruments may also be used for root canal therapy with similar results. Jensen *et al.* compare the sonic and ultrasonic cleaning efficacy after manual instrumentation in molars with curved roots. Results are analysed with photomicrographs with a grid in order to quantify the debris and evaluate the root canal cleaning level in the three groups. Sonic and ultrasonic treated molars after manual instrumentation seemed to be cleaner than those only manually treated, while the level of cleaning among sonic and ultrasonically treated molars was similar [43].

Another recent *in vitro* study compares the ability of different ultrasound irrigation procedures to eliminate debris and to open the dentine tubules. Previously instrumented with mechanical rotatory technique single-rooted extracted teeth are treated with US. The amount of debris and the number of open dentinal tubules were established by SEM. In the apical third, ultrasonic activation of the irrigation with Irrisafe tips seemed to be the most effective method to eliminate debris and open dentinal tubules [44].

According to Martí-Bowen *et al.*, the use of US in periapical surgery with retrograde filling, it is feasible to reach difficult access root canals with sacrifice of few root tissue. Nowadays, good results are obtained in teeth with periapical pathology which previously were condemned to failure [45].

Van der Sluis *et al.* summarize the potential uses of US in endodontics with the following options: to improve the endodontic access (for example elimination of calcifications), irrigation of root canals, to remove broken posts and other obstructions inside the root canals, humectation with sealer of the root canal walls, guttapercha condensation of the obturations of root canals, mineral trioxide aggregate (MTA) application, endodontic surgery, and increase of the dentinal permeability in dental bleaching [46]; also to break fillings due to their shock effect, to remove old fillings and make easier the access to root canals, and in endodontic retreatments. There are available different applicators with the most adequate form for each use (Figures 17, 18).

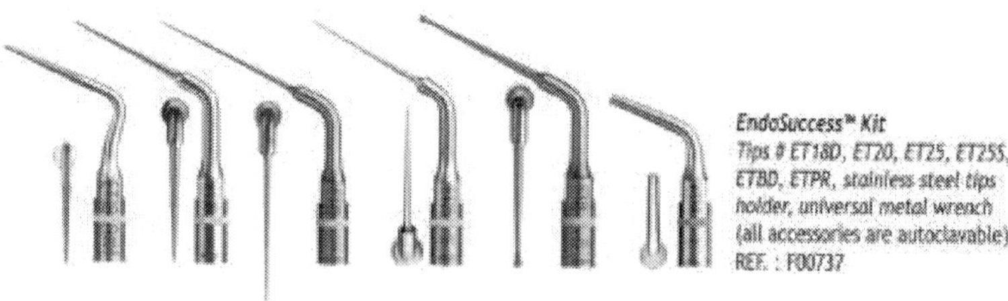

Figure 17. Satelec EndoSuccess Retreatment Kit. From left to right, tips for dentinal overhangs, calcificatons or filling materials elimination; for treatments in the coronal third; for treatments in the medium and apical thirds; for retreatment in coronal third and isthmus; for canal probing; and for loosening of posts and crowns. (Courtesy of Satelec, Merignac Cedex, France)

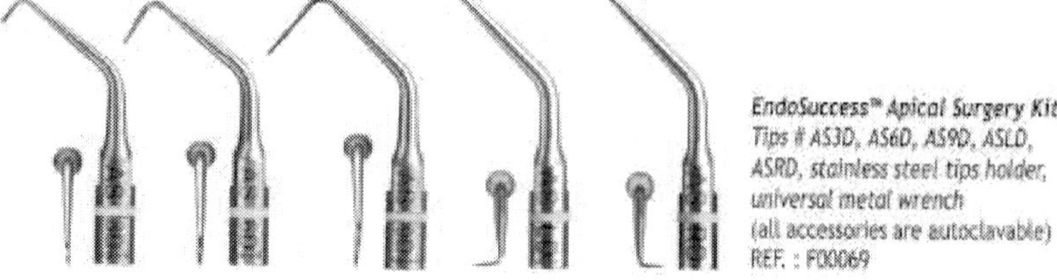

Figure 18. Satelec EndoSuccess Apical Surgery Kit. From left to right, universal apical surgery tip; second instrument; complicated cases (up to the coronal third), premolar left-orientated tip; premolar right orientated tip. (Courtesy of Satelec, Merignac Cedex, France)

6. US in surgery

Another application of US in dentistry is in oral and maxillofacial surgery to cut hard tissues. Experimental studies show that their application present better histological results than the rotary techniques. The precision of the cut with the different available inserts allows their use in our specialization in different fields such as general oral surgery, osseous grafts and implantology.

Although initially their use was reduced to sinus lift procedures, because they preserve the sinus membrane, their use has been extended to obtain bone grafts, osseous distraction and cortical split procedures, inferior dental nerve surgery, implant surgeries, extractions, etc. These biophotonic equipments allow changes in vibration's frequency from standard mode, with constant vibrations and frequency (used over soft tissues), to surgery mode (for hard tissues), where the modulation of amplitude and continuous vibration improves the efficacy over bone. Several applicators are designed for each osseous intervention (Figure 19).

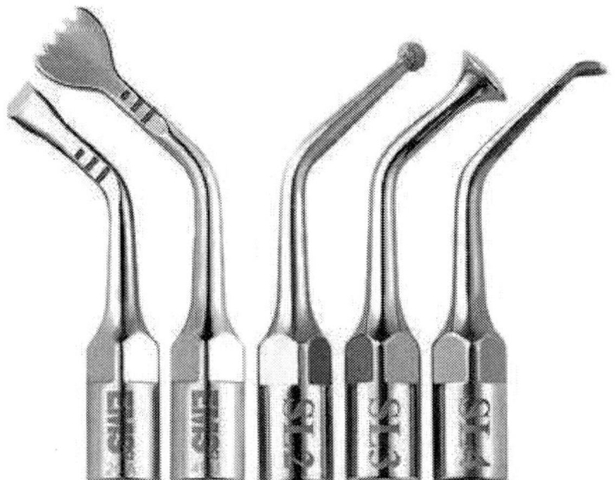

Figure 19. EMS Piezon Master Surgery US presents tips (from left to right) for vertical non-traumatic osseous incision, horizontal non-traumatic osseous incision, non-traumatic osteotomy, detachment of Schneider's membrane during sinus lift procedures and obtaining of bone fragments for bone augmentation.

The tips are different depending on the application: they present multiple lateral impact for surgery; curved, thin and scalpel-like for osteotomy; thin for non-traumatic extractions; cone-shaped diamond covered and calibrated for guiding during preparation; rounded or flat, diamond covered or scaler-shaped for sinus lift procedures. There are multiple surgical possibilities, as it is possible to do thin incisions for grafts, cysts elimination, sinus lift procedures with alveolar or lateral access, extractions, osteoplasties, osteotomies and other.

The advantages justifying their use are less bleeding and thus better visibility during the intervention, higher cut precision than with traditional instruments and less increase of temperature, less discomfort for patients as ultrasonic vibration is less noisy than drilling, and especially that the action over the soft tissues is minimal when they are accidentally applied over them, without tearing them up.

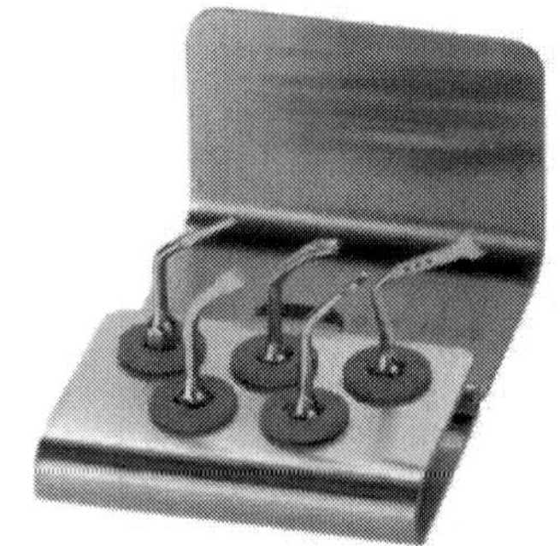

Basic Kit Piezosurgery

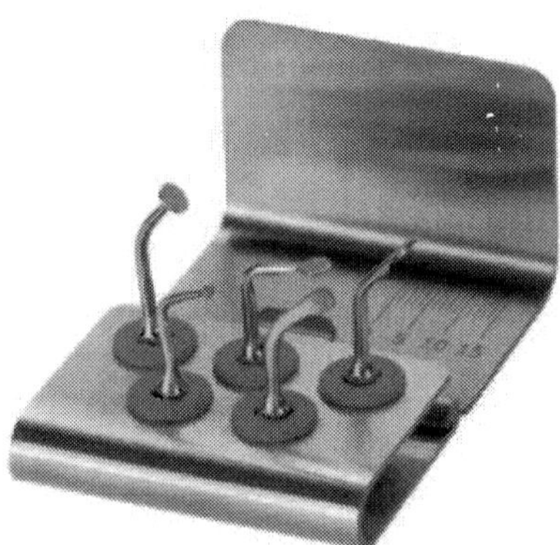

Figure 20. Mectron Piezosurgery´s basic surgery and sinus lift procedure kits.

The action of the tip is effectuated by two mechanical effects: direct and indirect. In the direct mechanical effect, the tissues in contact with the tip are under a very high frequency. It is the effect of a hammer working only over the hard tissues. In the indirect one, positive and negative pressures are generated over the fluids; they are known as cavitation, and they displace the osseous tissue and potentiate the mechanical effects. This produces localized osseous destruction in a continuous or discontinuous way, being the surgeon who decides one or another possibility depending on the osseous density and the required refrigeration. This makes the cut selective without neither microscopic osseous nor soft tissue alterations. Refrigeration should be abundant with saline solution, in order to avoid heating and wash up the field to obtain a better vision.

Kits are usually available for each type of indication. The insert size and angulation allow the use depending on the necessities of the case. There are basic kits, kits for surgery, osseous distraction, implants, endodontic surgery, alveolar and lateral sinus lift procedures, osteoplasy and ostectomy, etc (Figure 20).

7. US trays

US trays deserve to be mentioned. Their utilization is essential in the dental office as intermediate step between the washing with soap and the sterilization of instrumental. They allow the elimination of organic debris that remain adhered in the instrument gaps facilitating the sterilization (Figure 21).

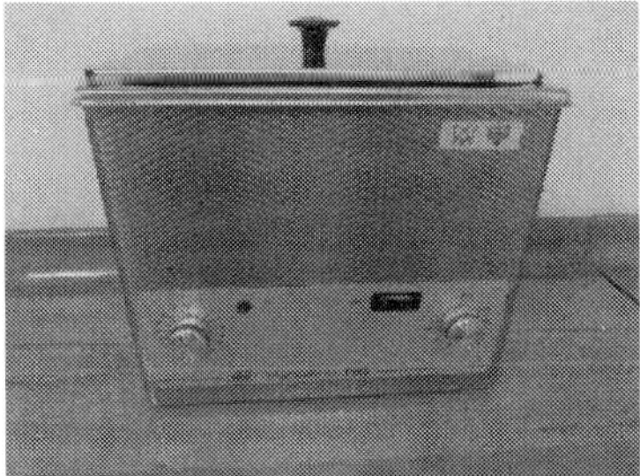

Figure 21. US tray.

Other applications of ultrasounds in Dentistry are removal of broken screws in implants, posts and crowns removal, etc. (Figure 22), but these applications are less frequent, they are not standardized and each professional acts according to his guidelines.

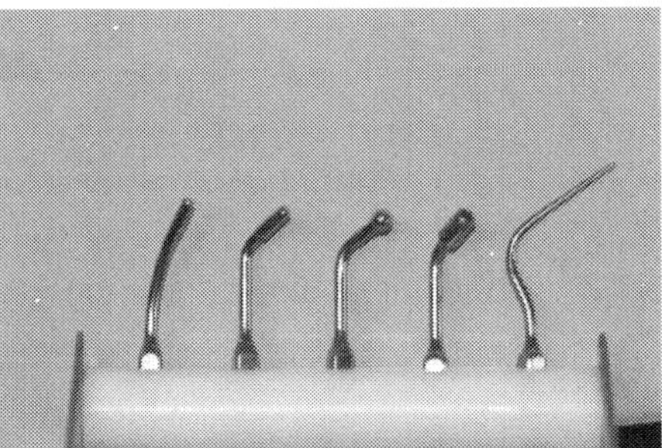

Figure 22. Set of diverse US tips

8. Conclusion

The evolution of US in dentistry during the last 65 years has been revised. The first laminated devices, only used for supragingival and slightly subgingival tartrectomies, have lead to sonicators and newer piezoelectric US with multiple inserts which allow the performance of tartrectomies reducing patient's discomfort and subgingival instrumentation. The variety of available tips lets us choose those which better adapt to our necessities and to the clinical situation, even in cases of periimplantitis. In endodontics, tips to facilitate the access, to clean the root canal and to carry out retreatments are available.

The industry offers the clinician optimal possibilities to achieve retrograde fillings more difficult or even impossible to carry out with other techniques. Among the latest applications, new possibilities emerge to effectuate certain surgical treatments, sinus lift procedures, implants placement, removal of fillings and crowns and other clinical situations.

Taking into account the great advance in US technology during the last years, it is reasonable to anticipate a great future for these devices. We are commited to regularly revisit the literature in order to know new opportunities provided by technology so the most suitable device is used in each clinical situation.

Author details

Ana Isabel García-Kass, Juan Antonio García-Núñez* and Victoriano Serrano-Cuenca

*Address all correspondence to: garcinu@odon.ucm.es

Department of Stomatology III, School of Dentistry, Complutense University of Madrid, Madrid, Spain

References

[1] Curie J, Curie P. Dévélopements par presión de l'électricité polaire dans les cristaux hémièdres à faces inclinées. In: Editeurs G-V, ed. Compte rendu hebdomadaire des séances de l'Académie des Sciences. Paris, 1880.

[2] American Association of endodontist Glossary, 6° Ed Chicago, 1998.

[3] Lindhe J, Nyman S. Long-term maintenance of patients treated for advanced periodontal disease. J Clin Periodontol 1984: 11: 504-514.

[4] Becker W, Berg L, Becker B. Untreated periodontal disease: a longitudinal study. J Periodontol 1979: 50: 234-244.

[5] Ramfjord S, Knowles J, Nissle R, Shick R, Burgett F. Longitudinal study of periodontal therapy. J Periodontol 1973: 44: 66-77.

[6] Knowles J, Burgett F, Nissle R, Shick R, Morrison E, Ramfjord S. Results of periodontal treatment related to pocket depth and attachment level. Eight years. J Periodontol 1979: 50:225-33.

[7] Ramfjord S, Caffesse R, Morrison E, et al. 4 modalities of periodontal treatment compared over 5 years. J Clin Periodontol 1987: 14: 445-452.

[8] Rateitschak-Pluss E, Schwarz J, Guggenheim R, Duggelin M, Rateitschak K. Non-surgical periodontal treatment: where are the limits? An SEM study. J Clin Periodontol 1992: 19: 240-244.

[9] Matia J, Bissada N, Maybury J, Ricchetti P. Efficiency of scaling of the molar furcation area with and without surgical access. Int J Periodontics Restorative Dent 1986: 6: 24-35.

[10] Bascones-Martínez A, García-Núñez J, Herrera I, et al. MEB en superficies dentarias tratadas con diferentes aparatos de limpieza. Prot Dental 1983: 11: 5-12.

[11] García-Núñez J, Ramos-Navarro J, Cerero-Lapiedra R, Esparza-Gómez G. Resultado de las técnicas de profilaxis a la luz de la MEB. Av Odontoestomatol 1986: 7: 83-86.

[12] Drisko C. Scaling and root planing without overinstrumentation: hand versus power-driven scalers. Curr Opin Periodontol 1993: 78-88.

[13] Drisko C. Root instrumentation. Power-driven versus manual scalers, which one? Dent Clin North Am 1998: 42: 229-244.

[14] Drisko C, Cochran D, Blieden T, et al. Position paper: sonic and ultrasonic scalers in periodontics. Research, Science and Therapy Committee of the American Academy of Periodontology. J Periodontol 2000: 71: 1792-1801.

[15] Kocher T, Langenbeck M, Rühling A, Plagmann H. Subgingival polishing with a teflon-coated sonic scaler insert in comparison to conventional instruments as assessed on extracted teeth. (I) Residual deposits. J Clin Periodontol 2000: 27: 243-249.

[16] Kawashima H, Sato S, Kishida M, Ito K. A comparison of root surface instrumentation using two piezoelectric ultrasonic scalers and a hand scaler in vivo. J Periodontal Res 2007: 42: 90-95.

[17] Clark S. The ultrasonic dental unit: a guide for the clinical application of ultrasonics in dentistry and in dental hygiene. J Periodontol 1969: 40: 621-629.

[18] Fox S, Moriarty J, Kusy R. The effects of scaling a titanium implant surface with metal and plastic instruments: an in vitro study. J Periodontol 1990: 61: 485-490.

[19] Kawashima H, Sato S, Kishida M, Yagi H, Matsumoto K, Ito K. Treatment of titanium dental implants with three piezoelectric ultrasonic scalers: an in vivo study. J Periodontol 2007: 78: 1689-1694.

[20] Richman R. The use of ultrasonics in root canal therapy and root resection. Med Dent J 1957: 12: 12-18.

[21] Martin H, Cunningham W, Norris J, Cotton W. Ultrasonic versus hand filing of dentin: a quantitative study. Oral Surg Oral Med Oral Pathol 1980: 49: 79-81.

[22] Walmsley A. Ultrasound and root canal treatment: the need for scientific evaluation. Int Endod J 1987: 20: 105-111.

[23] Walmsley A, Williams A. Effects of constraint on the oscillatory pattern of endosonic files. J Endod 1989: 15: 189-194.

[24] Lumley P, Walmsley A, Laird W. Streaming patterns produced around endosonic files. Int Endod J 1991: 24: 290-297.

[25] Cunningham W, Martin H. A scanning electron microscope evaluation of root canal debridement with the endosonic ultrasonic synergistic system. Oral Surg 1982: 53: 527-531.

[26] Cunningham W, Martin H. Endosonics-the ultrasonic synergistic system of endodontics. Endod Dent Traumatol 1985: 1: 201-206.

[27] Stamos D, Sadeghi E, Haasch G, Gerstein H. An in vitro comparison study to quantitate the debridement ability of hand, sonic, and ultrasonic instrumentation. J Endod 1987: 13: 434-440.

[28] Lev R, Reader A, Beck M, Meyers W. An in vitro comparison of the step-back technique versus a step-back/ultrasonic technique for 1 and 3 minutes. J Endod 1987: 13: 523-530.

[29] Archer R, Reader A, Nist R, Beck M, Meyers W. An in vivo evaluation of the efficacy of ultrasound after step-back preparation in mandibular molars. J Endod 1992: 18: 549-552.

[30] Reynolds W, Madison S, Walton R, Krell K, Rittman B. An in vitro histological comparison of the step-back, sonic, and ultrasonic instrumentation techniques in small, curved root canals. J Endod 1987: 13: 307-314.

[31] Goldman M, White R, Moser C, Tanca J. A comparison of three methods of cleaning and shaping the root canal in vitro. J Endod 1988: 14: 7-12.

[32] Baker M, Ashrafi S, Van Cura J, Remeikis N. Ultrasonic compared with hand instrumentation: a scanning electron microscope study. J Endod 1988: 14: 435-440.

[33] Pugh R, Goerig A, Glaser C, Luciano W. A comparison of four endodontic vibratory systems. Gen Dent 1989: 37: 296-301.

[34] Walker T, del Río C. Histological evaluation of ultrasonic and sonic instrumentation of curved root canals. J Endod 1989: 15: 49-59.

[35] Ahmad M, Pitt Ford T, Crum L. Ultrasonic debridement of root canals: acoustic streaming and its possible role. J Endod 1987: 13: 490-499.

[36] Goodman A, Reader A, Beck M, Melfi R, Meyers W. An in vitro comparison of the efficacy of the step-back technique versus a step-back/ultrasonic technique in human mandibular molars. J Endod 1985: 11: 249-256.

[37] Ruddle C. Endodontic disinfection: tsunami irrigation. Endo Prac 2008: 2008: 7-16.

[38] Lumley P, Walmsley A, Walton R, Rippin J. Effect of precurving endosonic files on the amount of debris and smear layer remaining in curved root canals. J Endod 1992: 18: 616-619.

[39] Zehnder M. Root canal irrigants. J Endod 2006: 32: 389-398.

[40] Weller R, Brady J, Bernier W. Efficacy of ultrasonic cleaning. J Endod 1980: 6: 740-743.

[41] Krell K, Johnson R, Madison S. Irrigation patterns during ultrasonic canal instrumentation. Part I. K-type files. J Endod 1988: 14: 65-68.

[42] van der Sluis L, Gambarini G, Wu M, Wesselink P. The influence of volume, type of irrigant and flushing method on removing artificially placed dentine debris from the apical root canal during passive ultrasonic irrigation. Int Endod J 2006: 39: 472-476.

[43] Jensen S, Walker T, Hutter J, Nicoll B. Comparison of the cleaning efficacy of passive sonic activation and passive ultrasonic activation after hand instrumentation in molar root canals J Endod 1999: 25: 735-738.

[44] Mozo S, Llena C, Chieffi N, Forner L, Ferrari M. Effectiveness of passive ultrasonic irrigation in improving elimination of smear layer and opening dentinal tubules. J Clin Exp Dent 2014: 6: 47-52.

[45] Martí-Bowen E, Peñarrocha-Diago M, García-Mira B. Periapical surgery using the ultrasound technique and silver amalgam retrograde filling. A study of 71 teeth with 100 canals. Med Oral Patol Oral Cir Bucal 2005: 10: 67-73.

[46] van der Sluis L, Cristescu R. Ultraschall in der Endodontie. Die Quintessenz 2009: 60: 1281-1292.

Chapter 28

Oral Health and Adverse Pregnancy Outcomes

Sukumaran Anil, Raed M. Alrowis,
Elna P. Chalisserry, Vemina P. Chalissery,
Hani S. AlMoharib and Asala F. Al-Sulaimani

Additional information is available at the end of the chapter

http://dx.doi.org/10.5772/59517

1. Introduction

Maternal health has long been recognized as an important determinant in reducing the risk for pregnancy-related complications such as preterm birth and preeclampsia. Preterm (PTB) delivery and low birth weight (LBW) are considered to be the most relevant biological determinants of newborn infant survival in both developed and developing countries. The oral changes that can occur in pregnancy have been a focus of interest for many years. Physiological changes that occur in pregnant women can adversely affect oral health. Elevations in estrogen and progesterone enhance the inflammatory response and consequently alter the gingival tissue (Mascarenhas et al., 2003). During pregnancy, the incidences of gingivitis and periodontitis are increased, and many pregnant women suffer from bleeding and spongy gums.

Periodontal disease, a persistent bacterial infection, leads to a chronic and systemic challenge with bacterial substances and host-derived inflammatory mediators that are capable of initiating and promoting systemic diseases (Williams et al., 2000; Gibbs, 2001). The mechanisms underlying this destructive process involve both direct tissue damage resulting from bacterial products and indirect damage through bacterial induction of the host inflammatory and immune responses. Even though controversy exists regarding the role of oral health as an independent contributor to abnormal pregnancy outcomes, the recognition and understanding of the importance of oral health has led to significant research into the role of maternal oral health in pregnancy outcomes (Sanz et al., 2013). Adequate oral hygiene habits are mandatory to control the development of periopathogenic oral biofilms, which have been reported to be associated with poor obstetric outcomes (Lieff et al., 2004; Han, 2011).

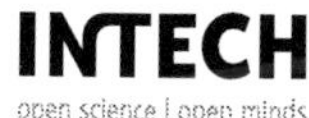

The chapter will cover the following aspects on oral health and adverse pregnancy outcomes including a systematic analysis of the studies linking preterm delivery, low birth weight, preeclampsia and periodontal disease.

- Association between periodontitis and pregnancy.

- Pre term birth, low birth weight and periodontal disease.

- Preeclampsia and periodontal disease.

- Biological mechanism linking periodontal disease to adverse pregnancy outcome.

- Evidence based literature analysis.

- Observational and systematic studies.

- Intervention studies on the impact of periodontal therapy

- Other expected oral outcomes due to pregnancy

- Early childhood caries.

- Gingival enlargement.

2. Association between periodontitis and pregnancy

Several studies have revealed the role and influence of periodontitis on adverse pregnancy outcomes. During pregnancy, the changes in hormone levels promote an inflammatory response that increases the risk of developing gingivitis and periodontitis. Even with good plaque control, 50%-70% of all women will develop gingivitis during their pregnancy, commonly referred to as pregnancy gingivitis, due to the variations in hormone levels. Pregnancy gingivitis generally manifests during the second and eighth months of pregnancy and is considered a consequence of the observed increased levels of the hormones progesterone and estrogen, which can effect small blood vessels of the gingiva, making it more permeable (Jensen et al., 1981; Barak et al., 2003).

Research suggests that the presence of maternal periodontitis has been associated with adverse pregnancy outcomes such as preterm birth (Offenbacher et al., 1996; Jeffcoat et al., 2001; Offenbacher et al., 2001), preeclampsia (Boggess et al., 2003), gestational diabetes (Xiong et al., 2006), delivery of a small-for-gestational-age infant, and fetal loss (Moore et al., 2004; Boggess et al., 2006). These increased risks suggest that periodontitis may be an independent risk factor for adverse pregnancy outcomes.

3. Preterm, Low Birth Weight (LBW) and periodontal disease

Preterm (PTB) delivery is defined as delivery before 37 weeks of gestation. The international definition of low birth weight (LBW), adopted by the 29th World Health assembly in 1976, is a birth weight of less than 2,500 grams (WHO, 1984). The primary cause of LBW is PTB delivery or premature rupture of membranes. Preterm infants who are born with a low birth weight are termed preterm low birth weight (PLBW). PTB and LBW are considered to be the most relevant biological determinants of newborn infants survival, both in developed and in developing countries. Preterm birth is a major cause of infant mortality and morbidity and poses considerable medical and economic burdens on society (Alves and Ribeiro, 2006). The rate of preterm birth appears to be increasing worldwide, and efforts to prevent or reduce its prevalence have been largely unsuccessful. The importance of PTB and LBW deliveries comes from their capacity to predict the increased risk of mortality among infants born with this condition. Preterm births account for 75% of perinatal mortality and more than half of long-term morbidity (Goldenberg et al., 2008). Moreover, one of the targets of the World Health Organization is to reduce the number of births in which the child weighs less than 2,500 g because this is a known predictor of childhood morbidity and mortality (Cruz et al., 2005).

The primary factors causing LBW infant deliveries are high or low maternal age (>34 yrs or <17 yrs.), smoking, alcohol or drug use during pregnancy, inadequate prenatal care, race, maternal demographic characteristics, hypertension, psychological characteristics, adverse behaviors, multiple pregnancies, nutritional status, diabetes, genitourinary tract infections, uterine contractions and cervical length, and biological and genetic markers (Verkerk et al., 1993; Copper et al., 1996; Nordstrom and Cnattingius, 1996; Romero et al., 2002; Marakoglu et al., 2008).

Microbiological studies suggest that intrauterine infection might account for 25–40% of preterm births. Microorganisms can gain access to the amniotic cavity by (1) ascending from the vagina and the cervix; (2) hematogenous dissemination through the placenta; (3) accidental introduction during invasive procedures; and (4) retrograde spreading through the fallopian tubes (Goldenberg et al., 2000). It has been suggested that spontaneous preterm labor is commonly associated with bacterial vaginosis, a vaginal condition characterized by the prevalence of anaerobes (Gibbs, 2001). This has been shown to elicit an inflammatory burden that results in placental damage and distress and, hence, fetal growth restriction. In addition, the cascade of disordered cytokine response can lead to the stimulation of prostaglandin synthesis and the release of matrix metalloproteinases (MMPs), which account for the uterine contractions and membrane rupture, respectively, and lead to the induction of labor (Romero et al., 1992; Winkler et al., 1998). This suggests that distant sites of infection (oral cavity) or sepsis may target the placental membranes. The maternal susceptibility to oral infections during pregnancy increases the sensitivity of the gingiva to the pathogenic bacteria found in dental biofilms (Barak et al., 2003). Studies have reported the presence of higher levels of *Porphyromonas gingivalis, Bacteroides forsythus, Actinobacillus actinomycetemcomitans* and *Treponema denticola*, organisms normally associated with periodontal disease, in mothers of PTB and LBW babies as compared to normal controls (Offenbacher et al., 1996). Approximately 25% of PLBW deliveries occur without any of the risk factors discussed in this section, which emphasizes the limited understanding of the causes and pathophysiology of the problem (McGaw, 2002).

In 1996, researchers first reported a relationship between maternal periodontal disease and the delivery of a preterm infant. The 1996 study by Offenbacher and colleagues suggested that maternal periodontal disease could lead to a seven-fold increased risk of delivering a PLBW infant. Since then, researchers have investigated these possible associations for over a decade. It is important to understand the underlying biologic mechanisms for the relationship between periodontal disease and adverse pregnancy outcomes such as preterm birth to provide a rationale for therapeutic interventions and exploration of other methods that may be used as adjuncts to the standard treatment. These authors concluded that approximately 18% of PLBW cases might be attributable to periodontal disease (Offenbacher et al., 1996).

4. Preeclampsia and periodontal disease

Preeclampsia is a complication recognized by gestational hypertension and proteinuria. It is one of the most significant health problems during pregnancy and affects 8% to 10% of all pregnancies (Roberts et al., 2003). Intravascular inflammation and endothelial cell dysfunction with altered placental vascular development is believed to be central to the pathogenesis of preeclampsia. To prevent fetal morbidity due to preeclampsia, preterm delivery is induced (Boggess et al., 2006). Maternal clinical periodontal disease at delivery has been associated with an increased risk for the development of preeclampsia (Canakci et al., 2007).

Boggess et al. (2003) were the first investigators to report an association between maternal clinical periodontal infection and the development of preeclampsia. In this longitudinal study, they found a two-fold increased risk for preeclampsia among women with periodontal disease during pregnancy compared with controls. A few other studies also reported an association between preeclampsia and periodontal disease (Table). Canakci et al. (2007) reported that women with preeclampsia were three times more likely to have periodontal infections than healthy women and that periodontal disease also affects the severity of preeclampsia. Barak and colleagues (2007) also found that women with preeclampsia experienced more severe periodontitis than healthy controls. They found a significant elevation in the gingival crevicular fluid levels of PGE-2, interleukin (IL)-1 P, and tumor necrosis factor alpha (TNF-a). In their study, Contreras et al. (2006) found more severe periodontal infections in pregnant women with preeclampsia with the presence of *P. gingivalis, T. forsythensis,* and *E. corrodens* than in controls.

5. Biological mechanism linking periodontal disease to adverse pregnancy outcomes

Two potential mechanisms have been put forward to explain the underlying link between oral health and adverse pregnancy outcomes (Han, 2011). First, periodontal disease causes systemic abnormal immunological changes, leading to pregnancy complications. The elevated systemic inflammation leads to elevated C-reactive protein (CRP) levels, which increase the risk for preeclampsia. Translocation of oral bacteria into the placenta has been demonstrated in animal models of both chronic and acute infections (Lin et al., 2003b; Han et al., 2004).

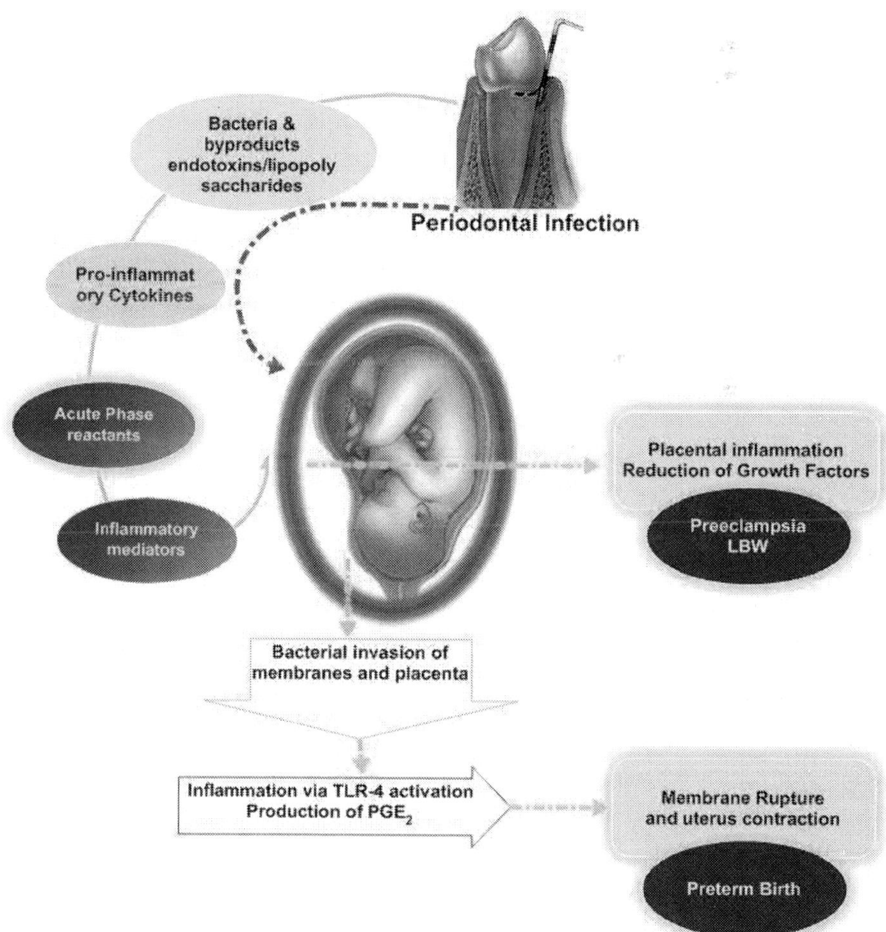

Figure 1. Possible biological mechanism linking periodontal disease and pregnancy complications.

The biological mechanisms proposed to explain the link between maternal periodontitis and PLBW involve the translocation of either inflammatory mediators such as IL-1 β, TNFα and PGE$_2$ or periodontal bacteria and their products from the periodontal tissues to the fetal-placental unit via the systemic circulation, thereby triggering preterm labor (Hillier et al., 1988). Increased levels of interleukin-1 beta (IL-1β), IL-6, tumor necrosis factor alpha (TNF-α, beta-glucuronidase (β–glucuronidase), prostaglandin E2 (PGE2), aspartate aminotransferase (AST), and metalloproteinase-8 (MMPT-8) and decreased levels of osteoprotegerin (OPG) have been detected not only in the gingival tissues, gingival crevicular fluid (GCF), and saliva but also in the serum/plasma of patients affected by periodontal disease (Lin et al., 2003a; Offenbacher et al., 2006; Furugen et al., 2008; Trindade et al., 2008; Wright et al., 2008; Duarte et al., 2010; Buduneli and Kinane, 2011).

Cytokines such as IL-1, IL-6, and TNF-α are all potent inducers of both prostaglandin synthesis and labor, and the levels of these cytokines have been found to be elevated in the amniotic fluid of patients with amniotic fluid infections in preterm labor (Romero et al., 2006). The intra-amniotic levels of PGE_2 and TNF-α rise steadily throughout pregnancy until a critical threshold is reached to induce labor, cervical dilation, and delivery (Offenbacher et al., 1996). Lipo poly sacchrides (LPS), one of the microbial components, can activate macrophages and other cells to synthesize and secrete a wide array of molecules, including the cytokines IL-16, TNF-α, and IL-6, PGE2 and matrix metalloproteinases (Darveau et al., 1997).

The second hypothesis suggests that oral bacteria directly colonize the placenta, causing a localized inflammatory response that results in prematurity and other adverse outcomes. The ratio of anaerobic gram-negative bacterial species to aerobic species increases in dental plaques during the second trimester of pregnancy (Kornman and Loesche, 1980), which may lead to increased cytokine production. If these bacteria escape into the general circulation and cross the placental barrier, they could augment the physiologic levels of PGE_2 and TNF-α in the amniotic fluid and induce premature labor. Animal studies have shown that chronic maternal exposure to the periodontal pathogen *P. gingivalis* results in systemic dissemination, transplacental passage, and fetal exposure (Lin et al., 2003b; Boggess et al., 2005). Studies in murine models have shown that *P. gingivalis* infection compromises normal fetal development by systemic dissemination and direct targeting of the fetal-placental unit.

6. Observational studies

The increasing number of case control studies investigating a link between periodontal disease and various adverse pregnancy outcomes in humans has produced conflicting findings (Table 1, 2, 3). Several studies suggest a significant association between maternal periodontal disease and pregnancy complications, including premature delivery, low birth weight and preeclampsia. Periodontal disease and progression during pregnancy appear to confer risk for preterm delivery, and the strength of the association increases at earlier gestational deliveries. However, not all studies supported this contention. Differences in the ethnicity and levels of periodontal disease in patients have been proposed as possible reasons for the conflicting findings reported in these studies. Periodontal disease is twice as prevalent among African-Americans, and this might possibly explain the observed increased risk in preterm delivery and fetal growth restriction among African-Americans (Madianos et al., 2001).Adverse pregnancy outcome and periodontal disease share a number of common risk factors, including age, ethnicity, socioeconomic status and smoking. The majority of studies investigating this association have used a dichotomous definition based on the number of teeth or sites with predefined levels of probing depth and attachment loss. Other studies have employed a range of continuous variables to reflect periodontal status, including probing depth, attachment loss and bleeding on probing. Several studies focused on the clinical measures of periodontal disease, which may not adequately reflect the infectious/ inflammatory burden present in pregnant women. The effect of periodontal disease on adverse pregnancy outcome suggests that periodontal infection as a risk factor but the evidence is insufficient to establish a cause and effect relationship.

7. Interventional studies

Several studies have examined the effects of periodontal treatment on preterm birth and low birth weight outcomes with conflicting findings (Table.4). Studies showed that periodontal therapy provided to women with periodontitis or gingivitis during pregnancy reduced the incidence of preterm low birth weight compared to those whose treatment was delayed until after birth (Lopez et al., 2002; Jeffcoat et al., 2003; Lopez et al., 2005).

Another study reported that significantly reduced rates of preterm births and low birth weight infants were observed for pregnant women who received plaque control instructions and scaling and root planing (Tarannum and Faizuddin, 2007). A three-year retrospective examination of a large insurance company database suggested that receiving preventive dental treatment is associated with a lower incidence of adverse birth outcomes compared with instances in which no dental services are delivered (Albert et al., 2011). However, a large multi-center study that included over 800 patients reported that periodontal treatment had no effect on pregnancy outcomes, recording the occurrence of preterm birth as 12% in the treatment group and 12.8% in the control group (Michalowicz et al., 2006).

Notably, the incidence of adverse birth outcomes from the various studies was lower among women who received some dental care and more so among those who received post-delivery periodontal care or those who received prophylactic treatment compared with those who received no dental care. The beneficial effect of dental care during the gestation period among these health-conscious and care-seeking women might also represent a coincidence. Good oral hygiene practices, however, can minimize gingival disease during pregnancy (Gibbs, 2001). Therefore, it has been recommended that all women should have a dental examination and appropriate dental hygiene care at least once during their pregnancy (Lieff et al., 2004). The American Academy of Periodontology recommends that women considering pregnancy or who are pregnant undergo a periodontal examination and receive the appropriate preventive and/or therapeutic services, if indicated.

8. Conclusions from the meta-analysis

The association between maternal periodontitis with adverse pregnancy outcomes such as low birthweight, pre-term birth and pre-eclampsia has been investigated for the past 20 years.

Several systematic reviews and meta-analysis has been conducted on various aspect of the association (Table 5). However, the strength of the observed associations based on clinical parameters is modest and seems to vary according to the population studied, the method used to assess periodontal diseases (Ide and Papapanou, 2013)

Khader and Ta'ani (2005) conducted a meta-analysis of periodontal disease in relation to the risk of preterm birth/low birth weight (PTB/LBW) based on two case-control studies and three prospective cohort studies. The sample sizes in the studies ranged from 80 to 1,313 women, with an age range between 12 and 40 years old. The odds ratio in these studies ranged from 3.5 to 7.5. Pregnant women with periodontal disease had an overall adjusted odds ratio of preterm birth that was 4.28 times higher than the odds ratio for healthy subjects (95% CI: 2.62 to 6.99; $P < 0.005$). They concluded that periodontal disease in pregnant mothers significantly increases the risk of subsequent preterm births or low birth weights.

Based on the meta-analysis, Xiong et al. (2006) concluded that periodontal disease might be associated with an increased risk of adverse pregnancy outcomes. They analyzed 44 studies (26 case-control studies, 13 cohort studies, and five controlled trials). The authors observed that the findings from observational studies yielded inconsistent conclusions on the relationship between periodontal disease and various pregnancy outcomes. Of the 39 observational studies, 25 studies (16 case-control and nine cohort) suggested that periodontal disease was associated with an increased risk of adverse pregnancy outcomes. Several studies demonstrated a direct relationship between the intensity of the periodontal disease and the risk of adverse pregnancy outcomes.

Vergnes and Sixou (2007) too echoed the same association when they reviewed 17 observational studies (11 case/controls, four cohorts, and two cross-sectionals) resulting in preterm low birth weight with an OR = 2.83 (95% CI: 1.95-4.10, $P < 0.0001$) and low birth weight with OR = 4.03 (95% CI: 2.05-7.93, $P < 0.0001$)

Though most of the studies have focused on the pregnancy outcome and periodontitis, very few studies have addressed the effect of periodontal treatment on adverse pregnancy outcome. One such review (Michalowicz et al., 2013) analyzed the same and resulted in a lone study on 303 Brazilian women 18 to 35 years of age with a gestational age ≤20 weeks. Randomization was stratified on smoking. All women, regardless of their periodontal status, received comprehensive non-surgical treatment (test group: oral hygiene instruction, scaling and root planing, and at least monthly follow-up visits) or supragingival scaling and oral hygiene instruction (control group).Despite statistically significant and substantial improvements in clinical periodontal measures with treatment (e.g. bleeding on probing (BOP) was reduced from 50% to 11%), there were no significant differences between test and control groups in preterm birth rates at <37 weeks (11.7 versus 9.1%, respectively, p = 0.57) or at <35 weeks (5.5% versus 5.8%, p = 0.99), or in fractions of infants weighing <2500 g (5.6% versus 4.1%,p = 0.59).

In a meta-analysis of the seven randomized trials, Polyzos and colleagues (2009) summarized that overall treatment of periodontal problems substantially reduced the rate of preterm delivery. They evaluated seven randomized controlled trials (n=2,663). There was a statistically significant reduction in incidence of preterm birth (OR 0.55, 95% CI 0.35 to 0.86, p<0.05) and low birth weight (OR 0.48, 95% CI 0.23 to 1.00, p<0.05) in women who received periodontal treatment compared to those who did not. The review findings suggested that treatment of periodontal disease during pregnancy reduced the rate of preterm birth and may reduce the incidence of low birth weight in infants.

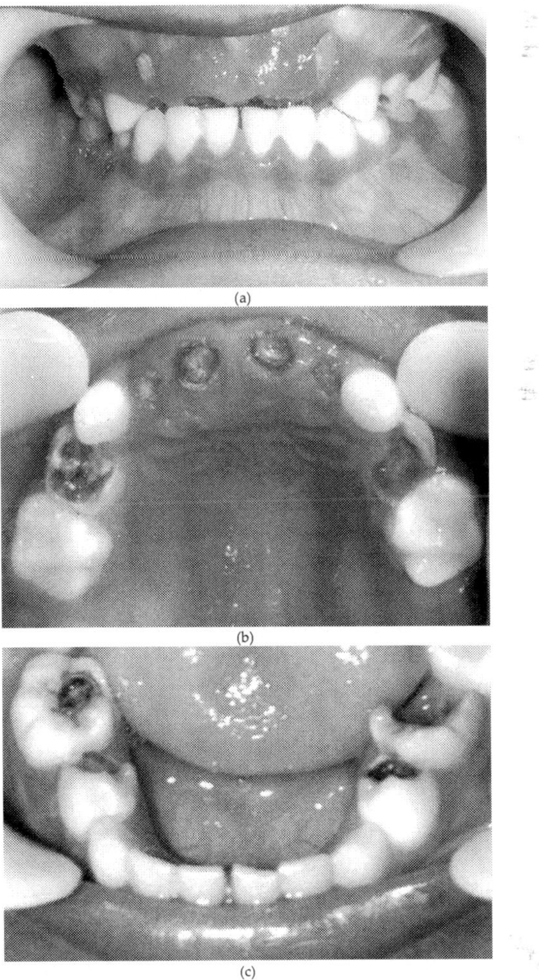

Figure 2. Early childhood caries

Polyzos et al (2010) examined whether treatment of periodontal disease with scaling and root planing during pregnancy is associated with a reduction in the preterm birth rate in randomized controlled trials. Of the 11 trials (with 6558 women), five trials were considered to be of high methodological quality (low risk of bias), whereas the rest were low quality (high or unclear risk of bias). It is noteworthy to see that the results among low and high quality trials were consistently diverse; low quality trials supported a beneficial effect of treatment, and high quality trials provided clear evidence that no such effect exists (odds ratio 1.15, 95% confidence interval 0.95 to 1.40; P=0.15).

9. Maternal oral health and early childhood caries

Early childhood caries (ECC) is an infectious disease that can present as soon as an infant's teeth erupt. ECC can progress rapidly and may have a lasting detrimental impact on the health and well-being of the child. Mothers with poor oral health and high levels of cariogenic oral bacteria are at greater risk for infecting their children with bacteria and increasing the risk of their children developing caries at an early age (Ramos-Gomez et al., 2002). *Streptococcus mutans* (MS) colonization of an infant may occur from the time of birth (Berkowitz, 2006), and significant colonization occurs after dental eruption, as the teeth provide non-shedding and other surfaces for adherence. (Wan et al., 2001; Tanner et al., 2002).

Cariogenic bacteria can be transmitted from mother to child by behaviors that directly pass saliva such as sharing a spoon when tasting baby food, cleaning a dropped pacifier by mouth or wiping the baby's mouth with saliva (Berkowitz, 2003). Reducing the transmission of cariogenic bacteria can be accomplished by reducing the maternal reservoir, avoiding vectors, and increasing the child's resistance to colonization (Li et al., 2003). Studies have demonstrated the effectiveness of a primary prevention program initiated during pregnancy to significantly improve the oral health of mothers and their children (Gunay et al., 1998; Soderling et al., 2001). Hence, comprehensive dental care for pregnant women is imperative to safeguard their oral and general health, as well as to reduce their children's caries risk (Brambilla et al., 1998; Boggess and Edelstein, 2006).

10. Gingival overgrowth related to pregnancy

Hormonal changes during pregnancy have been associated with varying types of gingival enlargement. These changes can potentiate the effects of local irritants on gingival connective tissue. Localized gingival overgrowth (pregnancy gingival tumor) is found in 0.2-0.5% of pregnant females. It occurs as a benign, rapidly growing lesion, usually in the 1st trimester of pregnancy and extending up to 3rd trimester. A pregnancy gingival tumor is a smooth or lobulated exophytic lesion with a pedunculated or sessile base (Srivastava et al., 2013) (Figure 3.). Several theories and speculations have been suggested to explain its occurrence during pregnancy, and meticulous maintenance of oral hygiene during pregnancy is important in reducing its incidence and the severity of gingival inflammation. Hormonal factors might play a role in aggravating gingivitis and gingival overgrowth (Oettinger-Barak et al., 2006; Andrikopoulou et al., 2013)

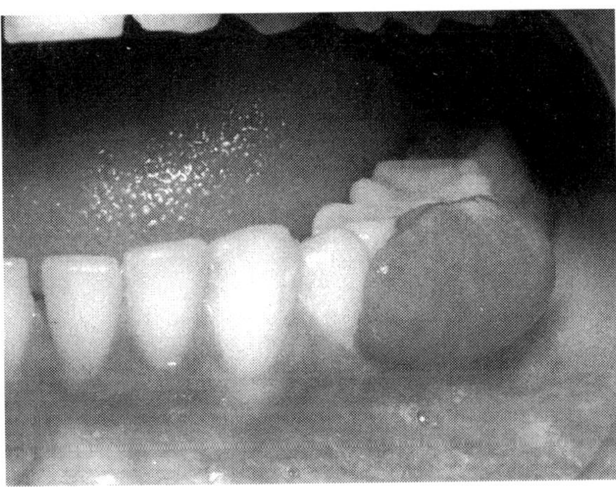

Figure 3. Pregnancy gingival overgrowth

11. Conclusion

Birth weight is considered to be an important determinant of the chances that an infant survives, grows, and matures. Maternal risk factors include age, height, weight, socio-economic status, ethnicity, smoking, alcohol use, nutritional status, and stress (Copper et al., 1996; Davenport et al., 2002). A review of the available literature has shown an association between periodontal disease and early pregnancy loss, preterm birth, low birth weight and preeclampsia (Jeffcoat et al., 2001; Gomes-Filho et al., 2007; Vergnes and Sixou, 2007; Xiong et al., 2007). However, the results regarding the treatment of oral disease during pregnancy are conflicting; some studies suggest a reduction in the rate of preterm births and dental caries (Brambilla et al., 1998; Jeffcoat et al., 2003; Lopez et al., 2005), whereas others show no impact (Michalowicz et al., 2006; Offenbacher et al., 2009; Macones et al., 2010).

The hypothesis that infection elsewhere in the body may influence PLBW has led to an increased awareness of the potential role of chronic bacterial infections. Periodontal disease is associated with a chronic Gram-negative infection of the periodontal tissues that results in a long-term local elevation of pro-inflammatory prostaglandins and cytokines and an increase in systemic levels of some of these inflammatory mediators (Page and Kornman, 1997). The evidence suggests that periodontitis can have a significant effect on systemic health. Periodontal disease is associated with many adverse pregnancy outcomes such as preterm delivery (Xiong et al., 2006), preeclampsia (Canakci et al., 2004), abortion and stillbirth (Moore et al., 2004), low birth weight (LBW) infants (Jarjoura et al., 2005) and preterm LBW infants (Xiong et al., 2006).

The strength of the association between periodontal disease and PTLB ranges from a two-fold to a seven-fold increase in risk. Although there are several data suggesting a relationship between maternal periodontal infection and preterm birth, several studies have failed to demonstrate such an association (Davenport et al., 2002; Holbrook et al., 2004; Moore et al., 2004; Buduneli et al., 2005; Rajapakse et al., 2005). Some of the factors that might have affected these observations are the lack of a consistent clinical definition and the failure to control for potential confounders (Holbrook et al., 2004; Moore et al., 2004; Buduneli et al., 2005). Another potential reason for the disparate findings among studies is the differences in the populations studied.

Several common risk factors are responsible for PLBW, such as age, socioeconomic status, and smoking, along with periodontal diseases. Because the inflammatory mediators that occur in periodontal diseases also play an important part in the initiation of labor, it is possible that a biological mechanism links the two conditions. Furthermore, intervention studies, animal studies, and more detailed mechanistic examinations are needed to directly correlate periodontal diseases to PLBW babies and eliminate the confounding effects of various other risk factors.

Author, year	Subjects, cases/ controls	Adverse pregnancy outcome	Periodontitis evaluation	Findings	Association
Jacob and Nath (2014), India	170/170	LBW	BOP,PD, CAL	Periodontitis represents a strong, independent, and clinically significant risk factor for LBW	Significant
Bulut et al. (2014), Turkey	50/50	PTB	PPD, CAL	The findings indicated that maternal periodontitis was not a possible risk factor for pre-term delivery	Significant
Santa Cruz et al. (2013), Spain	54/116	PTB	Microbiological tests	Clinical periodontal condition was not associated with adverse pregnancy outcomes in a Spanish Caucasian population with medium-high educational level	Non-significant
Kumar et al. (2013), India	61/132	LBW	Periodontal examination	Maternal periodontitis is associated with an increased preterm delivery and low birthweight infants.	Significant
Cruz et al (2009) Brazil	164/388	LBW	PI,BOP, PD, CAL	The findings suggest an association between periodontal disease and low birth weight among mothers with low education levels	Significant
Vettore et al. (2008)	150/66	PTB / LBW	PI, CI, BOP, PD, CAL	PD was significantly higher in non-preterm low birth weight controls than in subjects in the preterm low birthweight.	Non- significant

Author, year	Subjects, cases/ controls	Adverse pregnancy outcome	Periodontitis evaluation	Findings	Association
Brazil					
Santo-Pereira (2007) Brazil	124	PTB	Periodontitis was classified based on CAL	Periodontal disease more prevalent in women with preterm vs. term labor	Significant
Bassani et al. (2007), Brazil	304/611	LBW	PD, CAL	Similar rate of periodontal disease among cases and controls	Non-significant
Gomes-Filho et al. (2006), Brazil	44/177	PLBW	PI, PD, BOP, CAL	No statistically significant difference in the periodontal clinical parameters between the groups	Non-significant
Wood et al. (2006), Canada	50/101	PTB	Oral hygiene index simplified, PD, CAL, BOP	There was no difference in the proportion of sites with significant attachment loss.	Non-significant
Skuldbol et al. (2006), Denmark	21/33	PTB	PI, PD, BOP, Bitewing radiographs	No association between periodontal disease and preterm birth was found	Non-significant
Radnai et al. (2006), Hungary	77/84	PTB	PI, CI, BOP, PD	A significant association was found between PB and initial chronic localized periodontitis	Significant
Bosnjak et al. (2006) , Croatia	17/64	PTB	CAL, PD, Papillary bleeding index	Periodontal disease was a significant independent risk factor for PTB.	Significant
Alves and Ribeiro (2006), Brazil	19/40	PLBW	The periodontal screening and recording	There was a higher rate of periodontal disease in cases (84.21%-16/19) as compared with controls (37.5% -15/40).	Significant
Moore et al. (2005) UK	61/93 (154)	PTB	PI, PD, CAL, BOP	No association between periodontal disease and pregnancy outcome	Non-significant
Noack et al. (2005), Germany	59/42	PLBW	PI, BOP, PD, CAL	Periodontitis was not a detectable risk factor for preterm low birth weight.	Non-significant
Buduneli et al. (2005) Turkey	53/128 (181)	PTB/LBW	BOP, PD, PI	No difference in periodontal disease between cases and controls	Non-significant
Jarjoura et al. (2005) USA	83/120 (203)	PTB/LBW	PI, BOP, PD, CAL	Periodontal disease associated with PTB/LBW	Significant

Author, year	Subjects, cases/ controls	Adverse pregnancy outcome	Periodontitis evaluation	Findings	Association
Moliterno et al. (2005), Brazil	76/75	PLBW	PD, CAL	Significant associations with low birth weight babies was periodontitis	Significant
Moore et al. (2004), UK	48/82	PTB	PI, PD, CAL, BOP	No statistically significant difference in the carriage of the IL-1P + ^{3953} allelic variant between cases and controls	Non-significant
Goepfert et al. (2004) USA	95/44	PTB	CAL	Multivariable analyses supported the association between severe periodontal disease and spontaneous preterm birth.	Significant
Mokeem et al. (2004) Saudi Arabia	30/60	PLBW	PD, BOP, CI, CPITN,	There is a correlation between periodontal disease and PLBW	Significant
Radnai et al. (2004)Hungary	41/44	PTB /LBW	PD,BOP ,CI	Periodontitis can be regarded as an important risk factor for PTB	Significant
Davenport et al. (2002) UK	236/507(743)	PLBW	PD, BOP, CPITN	No evidence for an association between periodontal disease and PLBW.	Non-significant
Louro et al. (2001)Brazil	13/13	LBW	Extension and severity index	Periodontal disease may be a risk factor for LBW	Significant
Dasanayake et al. (2001) USA	17/63	LBW	*Porphyromonas gingivalis (P.g),* Serum IgG levels	Women with higher levels of P.g. IgG had higher odds of giving birth to LBW infants	Significant
Sembene et al (2000). Senegal	26/87	LBW	CPITN score: <1 1- 1.99 2- 2.99 "/>3	Periodontal disease is a potential risk factor for LBW	Significant
Dasanayake et al(1998) Thailand	50/ 50	LBW	DMFT and CPITN	Periodontal disease associated with LBW	Significant
Offenbacher et al. (1996) USA	93/31	PTB/LBW	CAL	Periodontal disease associated with PTB/LBW	Significant

PTB- Preterm Birth; PLBW- Preterm Low Birthweight; LBW- Low Birth Weight; PI-Plaque Index; GI- Gingival Index ; PD- Probing Depth; CAL- Clinical Attachment Level; CI calculus index; BOP- Bleeding On Probing; CAL - Clinical Attachment Level; CPITN- Community Periodontal Index for Treatment Needs ; DMFT - Decayed, Missing, and Filled Teeth

Table 1. Case-control studies on the relationship between adverse pregnancy outcome and periodontal disease

Study/Country	Sample size	Periodontal disease - Parameters	Conclusions	Association
Muwazi et al (2014)	400	PPD, BOP,CD GR, CPI	Significant association only between gingival recession and low birth weight	Significant
Kothiwale et al (2014)	770	PPD , CPI	The severity of periodontal disease was associated with an increased rate of pre-term infants. Severe anemia and periodontal infection may have an adverse effect on pregnancy and fetal development.	Significant
Ammanagi (2014) India	290	Not Known	Periodontal disease is a risk factor for PLBW	Significant
Abati et al (2013) Italy	750	Comprehensive oral and dental examination	Data failed to demonstrate the association between periodontitis and preterm birth and low birth weight.	Non - significant
Srinivas et al. (2009) India	786	CAL	No association between Periodontal disease and Pre term birth	Non - significant
Agueda et al. (2008) Spain	1200	PD,CAL,BOP	No significant association between periodontitis and low birth weight	Non - significant
Mobeen et al. (2008) Pakistan	1152	PD, CAL,PI, GI	Preterm birth and low birthweight were not related to measures of periodontal disease.	Non - significant
Pitiphat et al. (2008) USA	1635	Self-reported periodontitis Radiographs	The results suggest that periodontitis is an independent risk factor for poor pregnancy outcome among middle-class women.	Significant
Sharma et al. (2007) Fiji Islands	670	CPITN	There is a highly significant association between pre-term birth and moderate to severe periodontal disease	Significant
Toygar et al., (2007) Turkey	3576	CPITN	Maternal periodontal disease may be a risk factor for PTB and LBW	Significant
Rajapakse et al (2005) Sri Lanka	227	PI,CAL,BOP	Suggestive association between pre term low birth weight and periodontitis	Significant
Dortbudak et al. (2005) Austria	36	PD	Periodontitis can induce a primary host response in chorioamnnion leading to PTB	Significant
Moore et al (2004) UK	3738	PI,CAL,BOP,PD	No association between either PTB or LBW and periodontal disease.	Not Significant
Holbrook et al. (2004)	96	PD, gingival culture	No link between low grade periodontal disease and PTB	Not Significant

Study/Country	Sample size	Periodontal disease - Parameters	Conclusions	Association
Iceland				
Romero et al (2002) Venezuela	69	PI- Russell's Index	Periodontal disease is a risk factor for PTB &LBW	Significant
Lopez et al (2002) Chile	639	PD,CAL	Periodontal disease is an independent risk factor for PTB and LBW	Significant
Offenbacher et al (2001) USA	767	PD, CAL	Periodontal disease is a risk factor for PTB and LBW	Significant
Jeffcoat et al. (2001) USA	1313	CAL, PD	Periodontal disease is an independent risk for PTB	Significant

PTB- Preterm Birth; PLBW- Preterm Low Birthweight; LBW- Low Birth Weight; PI-Plaque Index; GI- Gingival Index ; PD- Probing Depth; CAL- Clinical Attachment Level; CI calculus index; BOP- Bleeding On Probing; PI - Periodontal Index ; CAL - Clinical Attachment Level; PPD-Probing Pocket Depth; CD - Calculus Deposit; CPI- Community Periodontal Index

Table 2. Adverse outcomes of pregnancy, pregnancy : Pre term birth weight/ low birth weight and Pre term weight- Cohort Studies

Author, year, country	Subjects, cases/controls	Periodontitis evaluation	Observations	Association
Kumar et al. (2013) India	61/132	PI,CAL,BOP	Maternal periodontitis is associated with an increased risk of pre-eclampsia.	Significant
Chaparro et al (2013) Chile	43/11	PI,CAL,BOP	Increased IL-6 levels in GCF in early pregnancy were associated with increased preeclampsia risk.	Significant
Taghzouti et al (2012) Canada	92/245	CAL,PD	No association between periodontal disease and preeclampsia	Significant
Hirano et al. (2012) Japan	18/109	PI,CAL,BOP	No statistically significant association between preeclampsia and periodontitis.	Not Significant
Wang et al. (2012) Japan	13/106	CAL	Polymorphism and subgingival DNA level of A. actinomycetemcomitans were significantly associated with preeclampsia.	Significant
Ha et al. (2011) Korea	16/48	CAL	Periodontal disease could be associated with preeclampsia	Significant
Politano et al (2011) Brazil	58/58	CAL,BOP,PD	There was an association between preeclampsia and periodontitis	Significant

Author, year, country	Subjects, cases/controls	Periodontitis evaluation	Observations	Association
Shetty et al. (2010) India	30/100	PD,CAL,GI	Periodontitis both at enrolment (OR = 5.78, 95% CI 2.41-13.89) as well as within 48 hours of delivery (OR = 20.15, 95% CI 4.55-89.29), may be associated with an increased risk of preeclampsia.	Significant
Nabet et al. (2010) France	1108/1094	CAL.PD,BOP	Maternal periodontitis is associated with an increased risk of induced preterm birth due to pre-eclampsia.	Significant
Lohsoonthorn et al. (2009) Thailand	150/150	PD,CAL	No association between periodontal disease and preeclampsia	Not Significant
Srinivas et al (2009) India	786	CAL	No association between periodontitis and pre-eclampsia	Not Significant
Siqueira et al.(2008) Brazil	164/1042	PD,CAL,BOP	Maternal periodontitis is a risk factor associated with preeclampsia.	Significant
Canakci et al (Canakci et al., 2007) Turkey	38/21	PD, CAL, BOP	Mild to severe periodontal disease is associated with an increased risk for development of preeclampsia	Significant
Kunnen et al (2007) Netherlands	17/35	PI, CI, BOP, R, PD	Severe periodontal disease was associated with increase of early onset preeclampsia	Significant
Barak et al (2007) Israel	16/14		Women with preeclampsia had higher prevalence of periopathogenic in bacterial placental tissue than controls	Significant
Contreas et al (2006) Columbia	130/243	PD, CAL	Periodontal disease is associated with an increased risk for development of preeclampsia	Significant
Cota et al (2006) Brazil	109/479	PI, CI, BOP, R, PD	Periodontal disease is associated with an increased risk for development of preeclampsia	Significant
Khader et al (2006) Jordan	115/230	PD, CAL,PI,CI	No association between periodontal disease and preeclampsia	Significant
Oettinger et al. (2005) Israel	15/15	PD, CAL,PI,CI	Periodontal disease is associated with an increased risk for development of preeclampsia	Significant

Author, year, country	Subjects, cases/controls	Periodontitis evaluation	Observations	Association
Canakci et al. (2004) Turkey	41/41	PD, CAL, BOP	Periodontal disease is associated with an increased risk for development of preeclampsia	Significant
Castaldi et al (2006) Argentina	1562	CAL, PD	No association between periodontal disease and preeclampsia	Not significant
Boggess et al (2003) USA	763	PI,CAL,BOP, PD	Association between periodontal disease and preeclampsia	Significant

CAL- Clinical Attachment Level; PTB- Preterm Birth; PLBW- Preterm Low Birthweight; LBW- Low Birth Weight; PD- Probing Depth; BOP- Bleeding On Probing; CAL - Clinical Attachment Level; PPD-Probing Pocket Depth; CD - Calculus Deposit; CPI- Community Periodontal Index

Table 3. The relationship between periodontal disease and Preeclampsia : Observational studies

Author, year	Subjects cases/controls	Adverse pregnancy outcome	Type of Periodontal Therapy/intervention	Results
Albert (2011)	464/12321	LBW,PTB	Periodontal treatment	Significant
Tarannum and Faizuddin (2007)	53/68	PTB, LBW	Scaling and root planning (SRP) and Plaque control instructions	Significant
Michalowicz et al.(2006)	413/410	PTB, LBW	Scaling and oral hygiene instructions	Non-significant
Offenbacher et al.(2006)	40/34	PTB	SRP and advised to use of a sonic toothbrush	Significant
Sadatmansouri et al. (2006)	30/30	PLBW	Oral hygiene instructions, 0.2% Chlorhexidine mouth	Significant
Lopez et al.(2005)	580/290	PLBW	Scaling, Plaque control, 0.12% chlorhexidine	Significant
Jeffcoat et al. (2003)	366/723	PTB	Scaling and root planning	Significant
Lopez et al.(2002)	163/188	PLBW	scaling and root planing (SRP) and Oral Hygiene instructions	Significant
Mitchell-Lewis et al (2001)	74/ 90	PLBW	Oral prophylaxis	Significant

PTB- Preterm Birth; PLBW- Preterm Low Birthweight; LBW- Low Birth Weight

Table 4. Studies showing the relationship of periodontal therapy on preventing adverse pregnancy outcomes

Authors	Studies included	Outcomes	Conclusions
Ide and Papapanou (2013)	Cross-sectional, case-control or prospective cohort epidemiological studies on the association between periodontal status and preterm birth, low birthweight (LBW) or preeclampsia.Preterm birth (<37 weeks gestation), LBW (<2500 g), gestational age, small for gestational age, birthweight, pregnancy loss or miscarriage, or pre-eclampsia.	Although significant associations emerge from case-control and cross-sectional studies using periodontitis "case definitions," these were substantially attenuated in studies assessing periodontitis as a continuous variable.	Maternal periodontitis is modestly but significantly associated with LBW and preterm birth, but the definition of periodontitis appears to impact the findings. Data from prospective studies followed a similar pattern, but associations were generally weaker. Maternal periodontitis was significantly associated with pre-eclampsia. It is suggested that future studies employ both continuous and categorical assessments of periodontal status. Further use of the composite outcome preterm LBW is not encouraged.
Michalowicz et al. (2013)	To identify randomized controlled trials (RCTs) published between January 2011 and July 2012 and discuss all published RCTs testing whether periodontal therapy reduces rates of preterm birth and low birthweight.	The single RCT identified showed no significant effect of periodontal treatment on birth outcomes.	Non-surgical periodontal therapy, scaling and root planing, does not improve birth outcomes in pregnant women with periodontitis.
Polyzos et al. (2010)	11 Case control studies trials (with 6558 women)	Periodontal treatment had no significant effect on the overall rate of preterm birth (odds ratio 1.15, 95% confidence interval 0.95 to 1.40; P=0.15).Furthermore, treatment did not reduce the rate of low birthweight infants (odds ratio 1.07, 0.85 to 1.36;P=0.55).	Treatment of periodontal disease with scaling and root planing during pregnancy does not reduce the risk of preterm birth and should not be routinely recommended as a measure to prevent preterm birth
Polyzos et al (2009)	Seven randomized trials were included based on the criteria.There were 2663 patients: 1491 had been randomized to receive periodontal treatment and 1172 to no treatment.	Treatment resulted in significantly lower PTB (odds ratio [OR], 0.55; 95% confidence interval [CI], 0.350.86; P = .008) and borderline significantly lower LBW (OR, 0.48; 95% CI, 0.23-1.00;P = .049), whereas no difference was found for spontaneous abortion/stillbirth (OR, 0.73; 95% CI, 0.41-1.31; P = .292).	The analysis showed that treatment with scaling and/or root planing during pregnancy significantly reduces the rate of PTB and may reduce the rate of LBW infants.
Vergnes and Sixou (2007)	17 observational studies (11 case/controls, four cohorts, and two cross-sectionals)	Preterm low birth weight:OR = 2.83 (95% CI: 1.95-4.10, P < 0.0001)LBW:	These findings indicate a likely association, but it needs to be

Authors	Studies included	Outcomes	Conclusions
		OR = 4.03 (95% CI: 2.05-7.93, P < 0.0001)	confirmed by large, well- designed, multicenter trials
Xiong et al. (2006)	44 studies (26 case-control studies, 13 cohort studies, and five controlled trials)	Twenty nine suggested an association between periodontal disease and increased risk of adverse pregnancy outcome (ORs ranging from 1.10 to 20.0) and 15 found no evidence of an association (ORs ranging from 0.78 to 2.54) Preterm Low birth weight:RR = 0.53, 95% CI: 0.30-0.95, P < 0.05Preterm birth: RR = 0.79, 95% CI: 0.55-1.11, P "/> 0.05 Low birth weight: RR = 0.86, 95% CI: 0.58%1.29, P "/> 0.05	The published literature is not vigorous to clinically link periodontal disease and/or its treatment to specific adverse pregnancy outcomes
Khader and Ta'ani (2005)	5 studies (two case-control and three prospective cohorts)	PTB: OR = 4.28 (95% CI: 2.62-6.99; P < 0.005)PTLBW: OR = 5.28 (95% CI: 2.21-12.62; P < 0.005)Either PTB or LBW: OR = 2.30 (95% CI: 1.21-4.38; P < 0.005)	Periodontal diseases in the pregnant mother significantly increase the risk of subsequent preterm birth or low birth weight

PTB- Preterm Birth; PLBW- Preterm Low Birthweight; LBW- Low Birth Weight; PI-Plaque Index; GI- Gingival Index ; PD- Probing Depth; CAL- Clinical Attachment Level; CI calculus index; BOP- Bleeding On Probing; PI - Periodontal Index ; CAL - Clinical Attachment Level; PPD-Probing Pocket Depth; CD - Calculus Deposit; CPI- Community Periodontal Index ;

Table 5. Meta-analysis on periodontal disease and adverse pregnancy outcomes

Author details

Sukumaran Anil[1*], Raed M. Alrowis[1], Elna P. Chalisserry[2], Vemina P. Chalissery[3], Hani S. AlMoharib[1] and Asala F. Al-Sulaimani[4]

*Address all correspondence to: drsanil@gmail.com

1 Department of Periodontics and Community Dentistry, College of Dentistry, King Saud University, Riyadh, Saudi Arabia

2 College of Dentistry, King Saud University, Riyadh, Saudi Arabia

3 Mahatma Gandhi Dental College and Hospital, Jaipur, Rajasthan, India

4 King Saud University, Riyadh, Saudi Arabia

References

[1] Abati S, Villa A, Cetin I, Dessole S, Luglie PF, Strohmenger L, Ottolenghi L, Campus GG. 2013. Lack of association between maternal periodontal status and adverse pregnancy outcomes: a multicentric epidemiologic study. The journal of maternal-fetal & neonatal medicine : the official journal of the European Association of Perinatal Medicine, the Federation of Asia and Oceania Perinatal Societies, the International Society of Perinatal Obstet 26:369-372.

[2] Agueda A, Ramon JM, Manau C, Guerrero A, Echeverria JJ. 2008. Periodontal disease as a risk factor for adverse pregnancy outcomes: a prospective cohort study. Journal of clinical periodontology 35:16-22.

[3] Albert DA, Begg MD, Andrews HF, Williams SZ, Ward A, Conicella ML, Rauh V, Thomson JL, Papapanou PN. 2011. An examination of periodontal treatment, dental care, and pregnancy outcomes in an insured population in the United States. American journal of public health 101:151-156.

[4] Alves RT, Ribeiro RA. 2006. Relationship between maternal periodontal disease and birth of preterm low weight babies. Brazilian oral research 20:318-323.

[5] Ammanagi R. 2014. Low birth weight among newborns and maternal poor periodontal status. Indian journal of public health 58:69.

[6] Andrikopoulou M, Chatzistamou I, Gkilas H, Vilaras G, Sklavounou A. 2013. Assessment of angiogenic markers and female sex hormone receptors in pregnancy tumor of the gingiva. Journal of oral and maxillofacial surgery : official journal of the American Association of Oral and Maxillofacial Surgeons 71:1376-1381.

[7] Barak S, Oettinger-Barak O, Machtei EE, Sprecher H, Ohel G. 2007. Evidence of periopathogenic microorganisms in placentas of women with preeclampsia. Journal of periodontology 78:670-676.

[8] Barak S, Oettinger-Barak O, Oettinger M, Machtei EE, Peled M, Ohel G. 2003. Common oral manifestations during pregnancy: a review. Obstetrical & gynecological survey 58:624-628.

[9] Bassani DG, Olinto MT, Kreiger N. 2007. Periodontal disease and perinatal outcomes: a case-control study. Journal of clinical periodontology 34:31-39.

[10] Berkowitz RJ. 2003. Causes, treatment and prevention of early childhood caries: a microbiologic perspective. Journal 69:304-307.

[11] Berkowitz RJ. 2006. Mutans streptococci: acquisition and transmission. Pediatric dentistry 28:106-109; discussion 192-108.

[12] Boggess KA, Beck JD, Murtha AP, Moss K, Offenbacher S. 2006. Maternal periodontal disease in early pregnancy and risk for a small-for-gestational-age infant. American journal of obstetrics and gynecology 194:1316-1322.

[13] Boggess KA, Edelstein BL. 2006. Oral health in women during preconception and pregnancy: implications for birth outcomes and infant oral health. Maternal and child health journal 10:S169-174.

[14] Boggess KA, Lieff S, Murtha AP, Moss K, Beck J, Offenbacher S. 2003. Maternal periodontal disease is associated with an increased risk for preeclampsia. Obstetrics and gynecology 101:227-231.

[15] Boggess KA, Madianos PN, Preisser JS, Moise KJ, Jr., Offenbacher S. 2005. Chronic maternal and fetal Porphyromonas gingivalis exposure during pregnancy in rabbits. American journal of obstetrics and gynecology 192:554-557.

[16] Bosnjak A, Relja T, Vucicevic-Boras V, Plasaj H, Plancak D. 2006. Pre-term delivery and periodontal disease: a case-control study from Croatia. Journal of clinical periodontology 33:710-716.

[17] Brambilla E, Felloni A, Gagliani M, Malerba A, Garcia-Godoy F, Strohmenger L. 1998. Caries prevention during pregnancy: results of a 30-month study. Journal of the American Dental Association 129:871-877.

[18] Buduneli N, Baylas H, Buduneli E, Turkoglu O, Kose T, Dahlen G. 2005. Periodontal infections and pre-term low birth weight: a case-control study. Journal of clinical periodontology 32:174-181.

[19] Buduneli N, Kinane DF. 2011. Host-derived diagnostic markers related to soft tissue destruction and bone degradation in periodontitis. Journal of clinical periodontology 38 Suppl 11:85-105.

[20] Bulut G, Olukman O, Calkavur S. 2014. Is there a relationship between maternal periodontitis and pre-term birth? A prospective hospital-based case-control study. Acta odontologica Scandinavica:1-8.

[21] Canakci V, Canakci CF, Canakci H, Canakci E, Cicek Y, Ingec M, Ozgoz M, Demir T, Dilsiz A, Yagiz H. 2004. Periodontal disease as a risk factor for pre-eclampsia: a case control study. The Australian & New Zealand journal of obstetrics & gynaecology 44:568-573.

[22] Canakci V, Canakci CF, Yildirim A, Ingec M, Eltas A, Erturk A. 2007. Periodontal disease increases the risk of severe pre-eclampsia among pregnant women. Journal of clinical periodontology 34:639-645.

[23] Castaldi JL, Bertin MS, Gimenez F, Lede R. 2006. [Periodontal disease: Is it a risk factor for premature labor, low birth weight or preeclampsia?]. Rev Panam Salud Publica 19:253-258.

[24] Chaparro A, Sanz A, Quintero A, Inostroza C, Ramirez V, Carrion F, Figueroa F, Serra R, Illanes SE. 2013. Increased inflammatory biomarkers in early pregnancy is associated with the development of pre-eclampsia in patients with periodontitis: a case control study. Journal of periodontal research 48:302-307.

[25] Contreras A, Herrera JA, Soto JE, Arce RM, Jaramillo A, Botero JE. 2006. Periodontitis is associated with preeclampsia in pregnant women. Journal of periodontology 77:182-188.

[26] Copper RL, Goldenberg RL, Das A, Elder N, Swain M, Norman G, Ramsey R, Cotroneo P, Collins BA, Johnson F, Jones P, Meier AM. 1996. The preterm prediction study: maternal stress is associated with spontaneous preterm birth at less than thirty-five weeks' gestation. National Institute of Child Health and Human Development Maternal-Fetal Medicine Units Network. American journal of obstetrics and gynecology 175:1286-1292.

[27] Cota LO, Guimaraes AN, Costa JE, Lorentz TC, Costa FO. 2006. Association between maternal periodontitis and an increased risk of preeclampsia. Journal of periodontology 77:2063-2069.

[28] Cruz SS, Costa Mda C, Gomes-Filho IS, Rezende EJ, Barreto ML, Dos Santos CA, Vianna MI, Passos JS, Cerqueira EM. 2009. Contribution of periodontal disease in pregnant women as a risk factor for low birth weight. Community dentistry and oral epidemiology 37:527-533.

[29] Cruz SS, Costa Mda C, Gomes Filho IS, Vianna MI, Santos CT. 2005. [Maternal periodontal disease as a factor associated with low birth weight]. Revista de saude publica 39:782-787.

[30] Darveau RP, Tanner A, Page RC. 1997. The microbial challenge in periodontitis. Periodontology 2000 14:12-32.

[31] Dasanayake AP. 1998. Poor periodontal health of the pregnant woman as a risk factor for low birth weight. Annals of periodontology / the American Academy of Periodontology 3:206-212.

[32] Dasanayake AP, Boyd D, Madianos PN, Offenbacher S, Hills E. 2001. The association between Porphyromonas gingivalis-specific maternal serum IgG and low birth weight. Journal of periodontology 72:1491-1497.

[33] Davenport ES, Williams CE, Sterne JA, Murad S, Sivapathasundram V, Curtis MA. 2002. Maternal periodontal disease and preterm low birthweight: case-control study. Journal of dental research 81:313-318.

[34] Dortbudak O, Eberhardt R, Ulm M, Persson GR. 2005. Periodontitis, a marker of risk in pregnancy for preterm birth. Journal of clinical periodontology 32:45-52.

[35] Duarte PM, da Rocha M, Sampaio E, Mestnik MJ, Feres M, Figueiredo LC, Bastos MF, Faveri M. 2010. Serum levels of cytokines in subjects with generalized chronic

and aggressive periodontitis before and after non-surgical periodontal therapy: a pilot study. Journal of periodontology 81:1056-1063.

[36] Furugen R, Hayashida H, Yamaguchi N, Yoshihara A, Ogawa H, Miyazaki H, Saito T. 2008. The relationship between periodontal condition and serum levels of resistin and adiponectin in elderly Japanese. Journal of periodontal research 43:556-562.

[37] Gibbs RS. 2001. The relationship between infections and adverse pregnancy outcomes: an overview. Annals of periodontology / the American Academy of Periodontology 6:153-163.

[38] Goepfert AR, Jeffcoat MK, Andrews WW, Faye-Petersen O, Cliver SP, Goldenberg RL, Hauth JC. 2004. Periodontal disease and upper genital tract inflammation in early spontaneous preterm birth. Obstetrics and gynecology 104:777-783.

[39] Goldenberg RL, Culhane JF, Iams JD, Romero R. 2008. Epidemiology and causes of preterm birth. Lancet 371:75-84.

[40] Goldenberg RL, Hauth JC, Andrews WW. 2000. Intrauterine infection and preterm delivery. The New England journal of medicine 342:1500-1507.

[41] Gomes-Filho IS, Cruz SS, Rezende EJ, Dos Santos CA, Soledade KR, Magalhaes MA, de Azevedo AC, Trindade SC, Vianna MI, Passos Jde S, Cerqueira EM. 2007. Exposure measurement in the association between periodontal disease and prematurity/low birth weight. Journal of clinical periodontology 34:957-963.

[42] Gomes-Filho IS, da Cruz SS, Rezende EJ, da Silveira BB, Trindade SC, Passos JS, de Freitas CO, Cerqueira EM, de Souza Teles Santos CA. 2006. Periodontal status as predictor of prematurity and low birth weight. J Public Health Dent 66:295-298.

[43] Gunay H, Dmoch-Bockhorn K, Gunay Y, Geurtsen W. 1998. Effect on caries experience of a long-term preventive program for mothers and children starting during pregnancy. Clinical oral investigations 2:137-142.

[44] Ha JE, Oh KJ, Yang HJ, Jun JK, Jin BH, Paik DI, Bae KH. 2011. Oral health behaviors, periodontal disease, and pathogens in preeclampsia: a case-control study in Korea. Journal of periodontology 82:1685-1692.

[45] Han YW. 2011. Oral health and adverse pregnancy outcomes - what's next? Journal of dental research 90:289-293.

[46] Han YW, Redline RW, Li M, Yin L, Hill GB, McCormick TS. 2004. Fusobacterium nucleatum induces premature and term stillbirths in pregnant mice: implication of oral bacteria in preterm birth. Infection and immunity 72:2272-2279.

[47] Hillier SL, Martius J, Krohn M, Kiviat N, Holmes KK, Eschenbach DA. 1988. A case-control study of chorioamnionic infection and histologic chorioamnionitis in prematurity. The New England journal of medicine 319:972-978.

[48] Hirano E, Sugita N, Kikuchi A, Shimada Y, Sasahara J, Iwanaga R, Tanaka K, Yoshie H. 2012. The association of Aggregatibacter actinomycetemcomitans with preeclamp-

sia in a subset of Japanese pregnant women. Journal of clinical periodontology 39:229-238.

[49] Holbrook WP, Oskarsdottir A, Fridjonsson T, Einarsson H, Hauksson A, Geirsson RT. 2004. No link between low-grade periodontal disease and preterm birth: a pilot study in a healthy Caucasian population. Acta odontologica Scandinavica 62:177-179.

[50] Ide M, Papapanou PN. 2013. Epidemiology of association between maternal periodontal disease and adverse pregnancy outcomes--systematic review. Journal of clinical periodontology 40 Suppl 14:S181-194.

[51] Jacob PS, Nath S. 2014. Periodontitis among poor rural Indian mothers increases the risk of low birth weight babies: a hospital-based case control study. Journal of periodontal & implant science 44:85-93.

[52] Jarjoura K, Devine PC, Perez-Delboy A, Herrera-Abreu M, D'Alton M, Papapanou PN. 2005. Markers of periodontal infection and preterm birth. American journal of obstetrics and gynecology 192:513-519.

[53] Jeffcoat MK, Geurs NC, Reddy MS, Cliver SP, Goldenberg RL, Hauth JC. 2001. Periodontal infection and preterm birth: results of a prospective study. Journal of the American Dental Association 132:875-880.

[54] Jeffcoat MK, Hauth JC, Geurs NC, Reddy MS, Cliver SP, Hodgkins PM, Goldenberg RL. 2003. Periodontal disease and preterm birth: results of a pilot intervention study. Journal of periodontology 74:1214-1218.

[55] Jensen J, Liljemark W, Bloomquist C. 1981. The effect of female sex hormones on subgingival plaque. Journal of periodontology 52:599-602.

[56] Khader YS, Jibreal M, Al-Omiri M, Amarin Z. 2006. Lack of association between periodontal parameters and preeclampsia. Journal of periodontology 77:1681-1687.

[57] Khader YS, Ta'ani Q. 2005. Periodontal diseases and the risk of preterm birth and low birth weight: a meta-analysis. Journal of periodontology 76:161-165.

[58] Kornman KS, Loesche WJ. 1980. The subgingival microbial flora during pregnancy. Journal of periodontal research 15:111-122.

[59] Kothiwale SV, Desai BR, Kothiwale VA, Gandhid M, Konin S. 2014. Periodontal disease as a potential risk factor for low birth weight and reduced maternal haemomglobin levels. Oral health & preventive dentistry 12:83-90.

[60] Kumar A, Basra M, Begum N, Rani V, Prasad S, Lamba AK, Verma M, Agarwal S, Sharma S. 2013. Association of maternal periodontal health with adverse pregnancy outcome. The journal of obstetrics and gynaecology research 39:40-45.

[61] Kunnen A, Blaauw J, van Doormaal JJ, van Pampus MG, van der Schans CP, Aarnoudse JG, van Winkelhoff AJ, Abbas F. 2007. Women with a recent history of early-

onset pre-eclampsia have a worse periodontal condition. Journal of clinical periodontology 34:202-207.

[62] Li Y, Dasanayake AP, Caufield PW, Elliott RR, Butts JT, 3rd. 2003. Characterization of maternal mutans streptococci transmission in an African American population. Dental clinics of North America 47:87-101.

[63] Lieff S, Boggess KA, Murtha AP, Jared H, Madianos PN, Moss K, Beck J, Offenbacher S. 2004. The oral conditions and pregnancy study: periodontal status of a cohort of pregnant women. Journal of periodontology 75:116-126.

[64] Lin D, Smith MA, Champagne C, Elter J, Beck J, Offenbacher S. 2003a. Porphyromonas gingivalis infection during pregnancy increases maternal tumor necrosis factor alpha, suppresses maternal interleukin-10, and enhances fetal growth restriction and resorption in mice. Infection and immunity 71:5156-5162.

[65] Lin D, Smith MA, Elter J, Champagne C, Downey CL, Beck J, Offenbacher S. 2003b. Porphyromonas gingivalis infection in pregnant mice is associated with placental dissemination, an increase in the placental Th1/Th2 cytokine ratio, and fetal growth restriction. Infection and immunity 71:5163-5168.

[66] Lohsoonthorn V, Kungsadalpipob K, Chanchareonsook P, Limpongsanurak S, Vanichjakvong O, Sutdhibhisal S, Sookprome C, Wongkittikraiwan N, Kamolpornwijit W, Jantarasaengaram S, Manotaya S, Siwawej V, Barlow WE, Fitzpatrick AL, Williams MA. 2009. Maternal periodontal disease and risk of preeclampsia: a case-control study. Am J Hypertens 22:457-463.

[67] Lopez NJ, Da Silva I, Ipinza J, Gutierrez J. 2005. Periodontal therapy reduces the rate of preterm low birth weight in women with pregnancy-associated gingivitis. Journal of periodontology 76:2144-2153.

[68] Lopez NJ, Smith PC, Gutierrez J. 2002. Periodontal therapy may reduce the risk of preterm low birth weight in women with periodontal disease: a randomized controlled trial. Journal of periodontology 73:911-924.

[69] Louro PM, Fiori HH, Filho PL, Steibel J, Fiori RM. 2001. [Periodontal disease in pregnancy and low birth weight]. J Pediatr (Rio J) 77:23-28.

[70] Macones GA, Parry S, Nelson DB, Strauss JF, Ludmir J, Cohen AW, Stamilio DM, Appleby D, Clothier B, Sammel MD, Jeffcoat M. 2010. Treatment of localized periodontal disease in pregnancy does not reduce the occurrence of preterm birth: results from the Periodontal Infections and Prematurity Study (PIPS). American journal of obstetrics and gynecology 202:147 e141-148.

[71] Madianos PN, Lieff S, Murtha AP, Boggess KA, Auten RL, Jr., Beck JD, Offenbacher S. 2001. Maternal periodontitis and prematurity. Part II: Maternal infection and fetal exposure. Annals of periodontology / the American Academy of Periodontology 6:175-182.

[72] Marakoglu I, Gursoy UK, Marakoglu K, Cakmak H, Ataoglu T. 2008. Periodontitis as a risk factor for preterm low birth weight. Yonsei medical journal 49:200-203.

[73] Mascarenhas P, Gapski R, Al-Shammari K, Wang HL. 2003. Influence of sex hormones on the periodontium. Journal of clinical periodontology 30:671-681.

[74] McGaw T. 2002. Periodontal disease and preterm delivery of low-birth-weight infants. Journal 68:165-169.

[75] Michalowicz BS, Gustafsson A, Thumbigere-Math V, Buhlin K. 2013. The effects of periodontal treatment on pregnancy outcomes. Journal of clinical periodontology 40 Suppl 14:S195-208.

[76] Michalowicz BS, Hodges JS, DiAngelis AJ, Lupo VR, Novak MJ, Ferguson JE, Buchanan W, Bofill J, Papapanou PN, Mitchell DA, Matseoane S, Tschida PA, Study OPT. 2006. Treatment of periodontal disease and the risk of preterm birth. The New England journal of medicine 355:1885-1894.

[77] Mitchell-Lewis D, Engebretson SP, Chen J, Lamster IB, Papapanou PN. 2001. Periodontal infections and pre-term birth: early findings from a cohort of young minority women in New York. Eur J Oral Sci 109:34-39.

[78] Mobeen N, Jehan I, Banday N, Moore J, McClure EM, Pasha O, Wright LL, Goldenberg RL. 2008. Periodontal disease and adverse birth outcomes: a study from Pakistan. American journal of obstetrics and gynecology 198:514 e511-518.

[79] Mokeem SA, Molla GN, Al-Jewair TS. 2004. The prevalence and relationship between periodontal disease and pre-term low birth weight infants at King Khalid University Hospital in Riyadh, Saudi Arabia. J Contemp Dent Pract 5:40-56.

[80] Moliterno LF, Monteiro B, Figueredo CM, Fischer RG. 2005. Association between periodontitis and low birth weight: a case-control study. Journal of clinical periodontology 32:886-890.

[81] Moore S, Ide M, Coward PY, Randhawa M, Borkowska E, Baylis R, Wilson RF. 2004. A prospective study to investigate the relationship between periodontal disease and adverse pregnancy outcome. British dental journal 197:251-258; discussion 247.

[82] Moore S, Randhawa M, Ide M. 2005. A case-control study to investigate an association between adverse pregnancy outcome and periodontal disease. Journal of clinical periodontology 32:1-5.

[83] Muwazi L, Rwenyonyi CM, Nkamba M, Kutesa A, Kagawa M, Mugyenyi G, Kwizera G, Okullo I. 2014. Periodontal conditions, low birth weight and preterm birth among postpartum mothers in two tertiary health facilities in Uganda. BMC oral health 14:42.

[84] Nabet C, Lelong N, Colombier ML, Sixou M, Musset AM, Goffinet F, Kaminski M, Epipap G. 2010. Maternal periodontitis and the causes of preterm birth: the case-control Epipap study. Journal of clinical periodontology 37:37-45.

[85] Noack B, Klingenberg J, Weigelt J, Hoffmann T. 2005. Periodontal status and preterm low birth weight: a case control study. Journal of periodontal research 40:339-345.

[86] Nordstrom ML, Cnattingius S. 1996. Effects on birthweights of maternal education, socio-economic status, and work-related characteristics. Scandinavian journal of social medicine 24:55-61.

[87] Oettinger-Barak O, Barak S, Ohel G, Oettinger M, Kreutzer H, Peled M, Machtei EE. 2005. Severe pregnancy complication (preeclampsia) is associated with greater periodontal destruction. Journal of periodontology 76:134-137.

[88] Oettinger-Barak O, Machtei EE, Ofer BI, Barak S, Peled M. 2006. Pregnancy tumor occurring twice in the same individual: report of a case and hormone receptors study. Quintessence international (Berlin, Germany : 1985) 37:213-218.

[89] Offenbacher S, Beck JD, Jared HL, Mauriello SM, Mendoza LC, Couper DJ, Stewart DD, Murtha AP, Cochran DL, Dudley DJ, Reddy MS, Geurs NC, Hauth JC, Maternal Oral Therapy to Reduce Obstetric Risk I. 2009. Effects of periodontal therapy on rate of preterm delivery: a randomized controlled trial. Obstetrics and gynecology 114:551-559.

[90] Offenbacher S, Katz V, Fertik G, Collins J, Boyd D, Maynor G, McKaig R, Beck J. 1996. Periodontal infection as a possible risk factor for preterm low birth weight. Journal of periodontology 67:1103-1113.

[91] Offenbacher S, Lieff S, Boggess KA, Murtha AP, Madianos PN, Champagne CM, McKaig RG, Jared HL, Mauriello SM, Auten RL, Jr., Herbert WN, Beck JD. 2001. Maternal periodontitis and prematurity. Part I: Obstetric outcome of prematurity and growth restriction. Annals of periodontology / the American Academy of Periodontology 6:164-174.

[92] Offenbacher S, Lin D, Strauss R, McKaig R, Irving J, Barros SP, Moss K, Barrow DA, Hefti A, Beck JD. 2006. Effects of periodontal therapy during pregnancy on periodontal status, biologic parameters, and pregnancy outcomes: a pilot study. Journal of periodontology 77:2011-2024.

[93] Page RC, Kornman KS. 1997. The pathogenesis of human periodontitis: an introduction. Periodontology 2000 14:9-11.

[94] Pitiphat W, Joshipura KJ, Gillman MW, Williams PL, Douglass CW, Rich-Edwards JW. 2008. Maternal periodontitis and adverse pregnancy outcomes. Community dentistry and oral epidemiology 36:3-11.

[95] Politano GT, Passini R, Nomura ML, Velloso L, Morari J, Couto E. 2011. Correlation between periodontal disease, inflammatory alterations and pre-eclampsia. Journal of periodontal research 46:505-511.

[96] Polyzos NP, Polyzos IP, Mauri D, Tzioras S, Tsappi M, Cortinovis I, Casazza G. 2009. Effect of periodontal disease treatment during pregnancy on preterm birth incidence: a metaanalysis of randomized trials. American journal of obstetrics and gynecology 200:225-232.

[97] Polyzos NP, Polyzos IP, Zavos A, Valachis A, Mauri D, Papanikolaou EG, Tzioras S, Weber D, Messinis IE. 2010. Obstetric outcomes after treatment of periodontal disease during pregnancy: systematic review and meta-analysis. Bmj 341:c7017.

[98] Radnai M, Gorzo I, Nagy E, Urban E, Novak T, Pal A. 2004. A possible association between preterm birth and early periodontitis. A pilot study. Journal of clinical periodontology 31:736-741.

[99] Radnai M, Gorzo I, Urban E, Eller J, Novak T, Pal A. 2006. Possible association between mother's periodontal status and preterm delivery. Journal of clinical periodontology 33:791-796.

[100] Rajapakse PS, Nagarathne M, Chandrasekra KB, Dasanayake AP. 2005. Periodontal disease and prematurity among non-smoking Sri Lankan women. Journal of dental research 84:274-277.

[101] Ramos-Gomez FJ, Weintraub JA, Gansky SA, Hoover CI, Featherstone JD. 2002. Bacterial, behavioral and environmental factors associated with early childhood caries. The Journal of clinical pediatric dentistry 26:165-173.

[102] Roberts JM, Pearson G, Cutler J, Lindheimer M, Pregnancy NWGoRoHD. 2003. Summary of the NHLBI Working Group on Research on Hypertension During Pregnancy. Hypertension 41:437-445.

[103] Romero BC, Chiquito CS, Elejalde LE, Bernardoni CB. 2002. Relationship between periodontal disease in pregnant women and the nutritional condition of their newborns. Journal of periodontology 73:1177-1183.

[104] Romero R, Espinoza J, Goncalves LF, Kusanovic JP, Friel LA, Nien JK. 2006. Inflammation in preterm and term labour and delivery. Seminars in fetal & neonatal medicine 11:317-326.

[105] Romero R, Mazor M, Sepulveda W, Avila C, Copeland D, Williams J. 1992. Tumor necrosis factor in preterm and term labor. American journal of obstetrics and gynecology 166:1576-1587.

[106] Sadatmansouri S, Sedighpoor N, Aghaloo M. 2006. Effects of periodontal treatment phase I on birth term and birth weight. Journal of the Indian Society of Pedodontics and Preventive Dentistry 24:23-26.

[107] Santa Cruz I, Herrera D, Martin C, Herrero A, Sanz M. 2013. Association between periodontal status and pre-term and/or low-birth weight in Spain: clinical and microbiological parameters. Journal of periodontal research 48:443-451.

[108] Santos-Pereira SA, Giraldo PC, Saba-Chujfi E, Amaral RL, Morais SS, Fachini AM, Goncalves AK. 2007. Chronic periodontitis and pre-term labour in Brazilian pregnant women: an association to be analysed. Journal of clinical periodontology 34:208-213.

[109] Sanz M, Kornman K, Working group 3 of joint EFPAAPw. 2013. Periodontitis and adverse pregnancy outcomes: consensus report of the Joint EFP/AAP Workshop on Periodontitis and Systemic Diseases. Journal of clinical periodontology 40 Suppl 14:S164-169.

[110] Sembene M, Moreau JC, Mbaye MM, Diallo A, Diallo PD, Ngom M, Benoist HM. 2000. [Periodontal infection in pregnant women and low birth weight babies]. Odontostomatol Trop 23:19-22.

[111] Sharma R, Maimanuku LR, Morse Z, Pack AR. 2007. Preterm low birth weights associated with periodontal disease in the Fiji Islands. International dental journal 57:257-260.

[112] Shetty M, Shetty PK, Ramesh A, Thomas B, Prabhu S, Rao A. 2010. Periodontal disease in pregnancy is a risk factor for preeclampsia. Acta obstetricia et gynecologica Scandinavica 89:718-721.

[113] Siqueira FM, Cota LO, Costa JE, Haddad JP, Lana AM, Costa FO. 2008. Maternal periodontitis as a potential risk variable for preeclampsia: a case-control study. Journal of periodontology 79:207-215.

[114] Skuldbol T, Johansen KH, Dahlen G, Stoltze K, Holmstrup P. 2006. Is pre-term labour associated with periodontitis in a Danish maternity ward? Journal of clinical periodontology 33:177-183.

[115] Soderling E, Isokangas P, Pienihakkinen K, Tenovuo J, Alanen P. 2001. Influence of maternal xylitol consumption on mother-child transmission of mutans streptococci: 6-year follow-up. Caries research 35:173-177.

[116] Srinivas SK, Sammel MD, Stamilio DM, Clothier B, Jeffcoat MK, Parry S, Macones GA, Elovitz MA, Metlay J. 2009. Periodontal disease and adverse pregnancy outcomes: is there an association? American journal of obstetrics and gynecology 200:497 e491-498.

[117] Srivastava A, Gupta KK, Srivastava S, Garg J. 2013. Massive pregnancy gingival enlargement: A rare case. Journal of Indian Society of Periodontology 17:503-506.

[118] Taghzouti N, Xiong X, Gornitsky M, Chandad F, Voyer R, Gagnon G, Leduc L, Xu H, Tulandi T, Wei B, Senecal J, Velly AM, Salah MH, Fraser WD. 2012. Periodontal disease is not associated with preeclampsia in Canadian pregnant women. Journal of periodontology 83:871-877.

[119] Tanner AC, Milgrom PM, Kent R, Jr., Mokeem SA, Page RC, Riedy CA, Weinstein P, Bruss J. 2002. The microbiota of young children from tooth and tongue samples. Journal of dental research 81:53-57.

[120] Tarannum F, Faizuddin M. 2007. Effect of periodontal therapy on pregnancy outcome in women affected by periodontitis. Journal of periodontology 78:2095-2103.

[121] Toygar HU, Seydaoglu G, Kurklu S, Guzeldemir E, Arpak N. 2007. Periodontal health and adverse pregnancy outcome in 3,576 Turkish women. Journal of periodontology 78:2081-2094.

[122] Trindade SC, Gomes-Filho IS, Meyer RJ, Vale VC, Pugliese L, Freire SM. 2008. Serum antibody levels against Porphyromonas gingivalis extract and its chromatographic fraction in chronic and aggressive periodontitis. Journal of the International Academy of Periodontology 10:50-58.

[123] Vergnes JN, Sixou M. 2007. Preterm low birth weight and maternal periodontal status: a meta-analysis. American journal of obstetrics and gynecology 196:135 e131-137.

[124] Verkerk PH, van Noord-Zaadstra BM, Florey CD, de Jonge GA, Verloove-Vanhorick SP. 1993. The effect of moderate maternal alcohol consumption on birth weight and gestational age in a low risk population. Early human development 32:121-129.

[125] Vettore MV, Leal M, Leao AT, da Silva AM, Lamarca GA, Sheiham A. 2008. The relationship between periodontitis and preterm low birthweight. Journal of dental research 87:73-78.

[126] http://en.wikipedia.org/wiki/Vaccine

[127] Wang Y, Sugita N, Kikuchi A, Iwanaga R, Hirano E, Shimada Y, Sasahara J, Tanaka K, Yoshie H. 2012. FcgammaRIIB-nt645+25A/G gene polymorphism and periodontitis in Japanese women with preeclampsia. International journal of immunogenetics 39:492-500.

[128] WHO. 1984. The incidence of low birth weight: an update. World Health Organisation Wkly Epidemiol Rec 59:205-211.

[129] Williams CE, Davenport ES, Sterne JA, Sivapathasundaram V, Fearne JM, Curtis MA. 2000. Mechanisms of risk in preterm low-birthweight infants. Periodontology 2000 23:142-150.

[130] Winkler M, Fischer DC, Hlubek M, van de Leur E, Haubeck HD, Rath W. 1998. Interleukin-1beta and interleukin-8 concentrations in the lower uterine segment during parturition at term. Obstetrics and gynecology 91:945-949.

[131] Wood S, Frydman A, Cox S, Brant R, Needoba S, Eley B, Sauve R. 2006. Periodontal disease and spontaneous preterm birth: a case control study. BMC pregnancy and childbirth 6:24.

[132] Wright HJ, Matthews JB, Chapple IL, Ling-Mountford N, Cooper PR. 2008. Periodontitis associates with a type 1 IFN signature in peripheral blood neutrophils. Journal of immunology 181:5775-5784.

[133] Xiong X, Buekens P, Fraser WD, Beck J, Offenbacher S. 2006. Periodontal disease and adverse pregnancy outcomes: a systematic review. BJOG : an international journal of obstetrics and gynaecology 113:135-143.

[134] Xiong X, Buekens P, Vastardis S, Yu SM. 2007. Periodontal disease and pregnancy outcomes: state-of-the-science. Obstetrical & gynecological survey 62:605-615.

Chapter 29

Periodontal Disease — A Physician's Viewpoint

Myers J.B.

Additional information is available at the end of the chapter

http://dx.doi.org/10.5772/59264

1. Introduction

From the physician's viewpoint teeth and the periodontal framework are relatively ignored. How many physicians actually inspect the teeth of their patients let alone their patients' gums? Increasingly though, awareness of integration and holistic appreciation of organ function has penetrated the formal divides that separate clinical practice according to body parts and organ function.

2. A deeper look in a clinical context

Metabolic function that is general and common to all body parts, and the inflammatory basis of disease highlight the commonality that underlies these processes. It is therefore not surprising to find that, in theory, changes in nail capillaries reflect capillary integrity in other body parts and signs of inflammatory disease that is present elsewhere may be seen in peripheral nail capillaries.

It has been proposed that periodontal disease is a factor resulting in inflammatory changes, raised C-reactive protein levels and loss of capillaries through inflammatory thrombotic events that results in increased cardiovascular risk and cognitive loss [1], as all body parts including brain become affected [2]. Thus if an association exists between capillary loss and rarefaction with cognitive decline and silent or ischaemic cardiomyopathy and ischaemic heart disease periodontal disease is a risk factor that needs to be considered. Similarly stroke occurs more commonly after an infection such as upper respiratory infection or urinary tract infection [3]. Thus inflammation resulting in stroke may also arise as a result of periodontal disease [1].

Microcirculatory changes involving capillary may be attributable to periodontal disease on the basis of inflammatory products being generated on a persistent basis [1,2]. There is also the

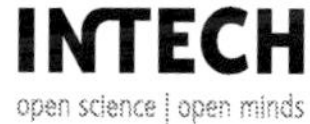

theoretical proposition that large vessels too are or become affected. Atheroma formation may be an inflammatory process [4]. It could result from the interaction of inflammatory proteins or monocytes acting on a dysfunctional endothelial surface such as may affect the lining of major blood vessels in the presence of underlying atheromatous change. These inflammatory cytokines [interleukin [IL]-1, IL-6] may be generated by periodontal disease and be linked to atheroma formation [5].

The effect on both micro-circulation i.e. capillaries and on the large vessels could result in increasing blood pressure and aggravate hypertension or even cause it if damage sufficient to impair capillary reserve capacity occurs, on challenge with a higher sodium intake, leads to the development of hypertension [6,7]. Similarly, renal effects would lead to renal impairment and even failure, as occurs in autoimmune [8] or hypertensive disease [9,10] or result in stroke and cerebral infarction or white matter degenerative change that manifest as vascular dementia [11] and even states of confusion depending on the severity and acuteness of the microcirculatory rarefaction and /or dysfunction.

Thus periodontal disease affects microcirculation integrity as well as larger vessels predisposing to cardiovascular risk through microvascular rarefaction and atheroma formation. Microvascular changes are themselves the cause of large vessel changes. Dysfunction or loss of perivascular capillaries affect large vessel compliance [12] in much the same way that periodontal vessels have an effect on dental health and function.

3. Treatment — Preventive, prophylactic and after the fact

Treatment of risk factors and complications such as stroke or cognitive loss must address the question is periodontal disease present. Diabetic disease is also related to this.

4. Periodontal health and general health and wellbeing

Periodontal disease causes halitosis and dentition. The presentation of a person relies on the ability to smile and is enhanced by having a set of healthy teeth and healthy breath. In Jewish law, bad breadth is a sufficient reason for divorce. A smile is everything. It secures a job, makes friends, is high profile as well as high society and it ensures the willingness of others to help when behaviour is amicable and is accompanied by a smile, that, I contend, is as important a factor as incontinence or continence in either resulting in institutionalised care or willing helpers to assist in home based care if that is their preferred choice rather than institutionalisation.

Mouth breathing: upper respiratory complaints are the source. Chronic upper respiratory blockage leads to snoring and poor sleep. It causes those who cannot breathe through their nose to gulp, not chew their food and to put on weight. The answer is to clear the nose with steam inhalation and to practice "how to breathe when you eat", Breathe in then out then insert a small amount of food into your mouth and chew, then swallow before you breathe in again, through your nose. Eat with your mouth closed and practice breathing in through your nose using the abdominal transverse muscles and diaphragm to aerate the lungs through your nose. It is not uncommon for these people to present with what appears to be an asthma attack on a cold night. The dentist, too, as well as the physician, has to be aware of this [13].

What does dental form tell you? By this I mean the effect of thumb sucking, which is a transient phase, but could persist or recur, indicates a psychological effect or emotional disturbance that could influence adult behaviour, which is notional on my part, not researched. Yet, when the individual takes steps to overcome this, to have the cosmetic treatments that correct this, they are at the same time overcoming the insecurity that led to the "buck-teeth" and building confidence to deal with situations from within. This is healthy and surely indicates the place of cosmetic dentistry in the recovery motivated by inner strength to change, i.e. the place of dental treatments in psychological and emotional wellbeing. For the same reason, treatments that overcome or help to contain periodontal disease that cause bad breath through simple oral hygiene, especially in those patients predisposed to this, whether through mouth breathing or on anti-epileptic agents that produce gum hypertrophy, such as phenytoin, is important.

Smoking habit and oral health. I believe that is not uncommon that people who mouth breathe smoke. In this situation smoking warms the air and damages the cilia on the bronchial cell lining. The reflex that responds to cold air with a cough is therefore overcome and mucus production in the bronchi remains there as the cilia of ciliated bronchial cells that are paralysed cannot move it up. Smoking also discolours the teeth, pipe smoking breaks them. When the sinuses are blocked the air cannot be warmed nor humidified. Treatment may be given for asthmatic attack or long term for asthma, that may be an incorrect assessment of events. Steroid inhalator therapy may result in fungal overgrowth in the oral mucosa without therapeutic benefit either long term or during an acute attack [13].

Too many sweets. But its not the fruit. Its the sticky stuff and sticky stuff combined with acids that corrode or vehicles such as flour that stick to one's teeth.

Geriatric dentistry: care of the elderly includes attention to oral health and diet. Access to clinic and to the dental chair have to be user friendly. Assistance may be needed. Lowering the dental chair to a convenient level to get onto and off, safely. Head up tilt and back support may be required. Rheumatoid arthritis does affect the neck, so neck extension is to be prevented.

Visits to nursing homes and now routine; medications and poly-pharmacy remain sources of notable concern. All medications cannot be listed here. The newer oral anticoagulants [NOAC's] used as prophylaxis against stroke in patients with non-valvular atrial fibrillation, e.g. Dabigatran, a direct thrombin inhibitor [DTI] and Apixaban, Rivaroxaban [Factor Xa inhibitors] are increasingly being used to replace Warfarin/Vitamin K depleting anticoagulants [14]. Since new information is becoming available at a rapid pace, an "EHRA" web site with the latest updated information accompanies the guide able to be accessed on its website [www.NOACforAF.eu]. It also contains links to the ESC AF Guidelines, a key message pocket booklet, print-ready files for a proposed universal NOAC anticoagulation card, and feedback possibilities. Side-effect hazards include anti-fungal agents and calcium channel blockers, Verapamil and Diltiazem, which increases the level and effects of NOAC's manifold as do "ketokonazole" and like anti-fungal medications that render unacceptable NOAC's risk of haemorrhage. Quinine also increases the level of drug and risk. Partial thromboplastin time may be used to check Dabigatran effects. Renal function also affects the dose and needs to be regularly checked [up to six monthly]. Refer to www.NOACforAF.eu]. Ceasing treatment for dental treatments for at least twelve hours is advised, see paragraph 10 of the guide.

It is important to hand to the elderly patient written instructions for the patient if they are able and/or to a carer or accompanying person who may also be able to supervise, assist if necessary and give to you information regarding what other medications the person is taking, to bring in the dosette box, which is pre-packed by the pharmacy or by the carer or by the patient who is able and willing – it's a good mental exercise, as well as non-medications or unprescribed treatments.

Nutritional intake and health; role of carer; dental replacements – inserts, implants for nutrition and comfort; the importance of nutrition and type of foods available as well as types of diet, vitamised, soft can maintain health and prevent ill-health.

Aging is the inexorable loss of functional reserve capacity. There is a functional metabolic reserve, that could apply to anaesthetic agents, number of teeth, ability to chew, ability to swallow and ability to transfer to a chair, which maintains independence as the person is able to get onto and off a toilet and to mobilise. Exercise and nutrition are central to maintaining independence.

Cosmetic dentistry in the elderly is now available but not the only reason to undertake having new implants. At ninety three years, my mother chose to have implants as her dentures bothered her so much. Painful dentures can ruin any person's life, spoil one's appreciation of food, cause ulcers as everyone knows but also determine what one can eat or not eat. Loss of weight through poor dentition or ill fitting dentures can have devastating results, leading to a fall by having a mat in the wrong place and not lifting up one's feet, just once. Fracture, having to recuperate and being placed is the greatest risk of being admitted to a hospital, at least in Australia, where the maxim, we have a duty of care – to maintain safety" overtakes the right of privilege and free choice. Here, the word of an expert, whom the patient only trusts, is shunned by those with agenda's of their own, including seeking power and feeling of self importance. With less knowledge and greater inferiority everyone has their say. The Office of the Public Advocate, the bureaucrats on Tribunals and Medical Boards, who know less and are lesser individuals because they wish to control those who have made it, live it and enjoy it. What has this got to do with oral health? The answer is nutrition, trust, and confidence and an ability to communicate positively to one's environment, which is more likely to happen when one has a smile and a good set of teeth and friends in support. It will determine who will be prepared to care for you and who will not. It will ensure that where you live is where you wish to live and with whom.

Inflammation and infection is not as obvious in the elderly as immune mechanisms are not as intense, or able to marshalled, but tissue turgor is also not as dense and therefore pain is less. On the other hand recovery takes time. Even after extractions one needs to be cared for. One ought to take in higher protein drinks before and to continue to do so afterwards. The advent of bisphosphonates, which inhibit osteoclast recruitment and reduces bone loss in the treatment of osteoporosis and secondary prevention in cases with fracture of the femur or vertebrae has resulted in fear of osteonecrosis of the jaw [15], which is more likely to occur in patients who are receiving chemotherapy. Pretreatment dental surgery is suggested as well as use of antibiotics and an oral antiseptic solution when the condition occurs to treat and control pain [15].

5. Social dentistry

I have likened the loss of a tooth to the social situation of an elderly person. When one loses a friend one also loses support and one's own position becomes more vulnerable. This leads to lack of confidence, to isolation from society and to becoming depressed. Living in a residential home is akin to having a set of dentures. They are not yours, but they are there and do provide some comfort, but not always.

Tooth extraction is a metaphor for diminution of social interaction; support and social functioning in the elderly; isolation and depression, effect of loss and deprivation, while restoration is akin to the effect of nutrition on wellbeing, psychological, physical and spiritual.

Behaviour and institutionalisation: The effect of oral health, hygiene and behaviour can ensure that you will stay longer in your own home and even die there in familiar memory clad surroundings. Nothing insures this better than behaviour characterised by appreciation, thanks and a smile.

In old age, in adults and teens; the effect is the same. Confidence, radiating happiness and achievement are related to dental pride and appearance.

6. Oral function as a driver in social evolution

Stomal drive in evolution. Food and water intake determines survival.

Setting down roots led to stomatal development; to vegetative and sessile development.

Stomal development led to cortical development and permitted mobility.

Senses in animals included two eyes and two ears. Dentition permitted there to be one mouth for fluids and solids and determined strength development on the basis of what could be eaten when caught, the consistency of foods. Eyes and ears were used as warning signs to prevent being eaten and to survey what could be eaten or caught.

Amphibian and reptilian evolutionary dichotomy occurred as amphibians developed a buccal respiration pattern, using the floor of the mouth to create air movement into and out of the lungs, whereas reptiles developed ribs and birds developed air sacks in those ribs to lighten the weight and developed beaks as the driver rather than alligator teeth, though the Cretaceous creatures, Pterosaurs, that flew such as Pterodactylus had a small number of teeth, while Pteranodon was completely toothless. This fact, combined with Pteranodon's vaguely albatross-like build, has led paleontologists to conclude that this pterosaur flew along the seashores of late Cretaceous North America and fed mostly on fish [16].

Snakes developed the tooth to the utmost by having a venom ejaculation mechanism in them used in forward fanged snakes such as Viperidae [vipers] to blind or poison their prey before they ate them. Ear ossicles later incorporated into the middle ear in higher vertebrates, that are part of the mandibular system in snakes enabled the snake to dislocate his mandible to swallow large prey whole, and their fangs to catch prey, as least in the forward fanged snakes, whose body lengths are shorter than constrictors, rather than masticate. The extra ossicles also permitted vibration detection in preparedness to catch their prey as well as to swallow it, indicating the economy of form in relation to function that appears to be a formula for successful evolution; the combining of survival mechanisms: energy acquisition, through ingestion and metabolism, which also requires excretion, to live, grow and mate and energy expenditure to escape or, alternatively to develop further and adapt.

In the invertebrate world helminths developed suckers and they became tapeworm parasites, while special insertion of sperm techniques used by spiders ended by self sacrifice, with the male being eaten to provide ready nourishment for the newly fertilised eggs, taking the survival pitch of stomal drive to its ultimate.

Years ago, the rabbis recognised that food which is visually tempting increases appetite [17]. Plants use colour to attract insects to feast on the nectar as the lure to pollinate inadvertently and by the design of the plant while the insects eat. The latter example has a message – when you help others eat by providing nectar and food, they share in the benefits that you reproduce, which ensures that their progeny have energy in the form of nectar to eat.

Primal instinct and stomal drive – in the 21st century. A primal instinct demands our focus. In today's world while success can be founded on dental presentation, it can also be one's undoing, when stomal drive is for one's own sake, rather than for survival.

Obsession with desire that may attend one who has achieved success, in detracting from the focus of what one eats and gratitude for every morsel that appreciation of survival demands, results in a change in priorities, such that desire overtakes survival. Dependency results, as does pleasure drive and desire, to hedonism, loss of survival focus and breakdown.

It is true that eating can be fashioned to ensure body health and looks. It can also induce anorexia or bulimia. We need to be in tune with our primal instincts. They are a survival mechanism. Stomal health, includes oral hygiene and cortical awareness.

The stomal society. Society has cultural values that are tied to eating patterns. Nations are distinguished by their cultural or national cuisine. Japanese food is unique to Japan. Middle

Eastern food is particular to the middle east. African food to Africa. It ties us to the land. Chinese food is unique to Chinese. Is it fair to ask whether Italian culture would be what it is today if Marco Polo (1254-1324) had not brought back noodles from the Far East?

Cultures with traditions that incorporate food as symbols of significance and ethical values, as is the case with traditional Jewish customs, ensures that there is focus on survival as they are enjoyed and partaken to ensure history and moral values and ethics of daily life are transmitted to future generations. Therefore they do survive and can impart ethical values and morality to the world, for generations.

Stomal drive remains the focus during development as well as into old age. The application of implant techniques to old age in order to be able to masticate and enjoy a wholesome meal will ensure longer life and a more pleasing one. On the other hand cosmetic dentistry which forsakes nutritional and masticatory functions may shorten lifespan by changing focus and permitting distraction from survival to creep in.

7. Lips and buccal function

Although the lips have not been addressed in this chapter, lip function and the cheeks, ensures swallowing without spillage, as occurs in lower motor neurone facial palsy or paralysis. Lips have a prehensile function working with the tongue in almost mitten like clasp that enables giraffe to selectively eat the leaves they desire from the top of trees. Lips also reveal features of human emotion and desire. They also permit breath-holding and labial sounds.

8. General systems theory and stomal drive

The concept of the "constancy of the milieu extérieur"[7] i.e. maintaining one's environment in terms of Eco-social© harmony [18] even in response to change, this means ensuring diversity of activity, and diversity of flora and fauna. External milieu is also the lymph and plasma bathing cells [7]. What ensures this? Oral hygiene, oral health and what passes through it, liquids, solids, sounds and words.

9. Conclusion

Oral health and development determine both quality of life and quantity, as a survival mechanism essential for life the importance of stomal function for physical and emotional wellbeing as well as social functioning has been understated in the past. In addition stomal drive as a evolutionary mechanism has not been appreciated or previously understood in terms of both plant (stomata) and of invertebrate and vertebrate, animal, evolution and development, on land, in fresh water and the sea.

Author details

Myers J.B.*

Address all correspondence to: rebdoc1@bigpond.net.au

Department of Medical Science, Wellspring's Universal Environment P/L, Australia

References

[1] Myers JB. Infection, periodontal disease, inflammation, vascular (capillary) injury and cognitive decline with ageing: an hypothesis. J Neurological Sciences. 2005, 236 (Suppl.1) p518, P1650.

[2] Myers JB. "Capillary Band Width", "the Nail Sign: A clinical Marker of inflammation, vascular integrity, cognition and age. Personal Viewpoint and Hypothesis. Journal of the Neurological Sciences, Official Bulletin of the World Federation of Neurology, Suppl. 2009, 283(1-2) pp.86-90 Elsevier Publications, NY.

[3] Smeeth L, Thomas SL, Hall AJ, Hubbard R, Farrington P, Vallance P. Risk of Myocardial Infarction and Stroke after Acute Infection or Vaccination. N Engl J Med 2004;351:2611-8.

[4] Hansson GK. Immune Mechanisms in Atherosclerosis. Arteriosclerosis, thrombosis and Vascular Biology. 2001; 21: 1876-1890 doi: 10.1161/hq1201.100220

[5] Beck J, Garcia R, Heiss G, Vokonas PS, Offenbacher S. Periodontal Disease and Cardiovascular Disease. Journal of Periodontology 1996; 67(10s):1123-1137. doi:10.1902/jop.1996.67.10s.1123

[6] Myers, JB. "Sodium Sensitivity" in Man. Medical Hypotheses. 1987; 23: 265-276.

[7] Myers, JB. Biochemical response to change in the environment and the nature of "essential" hypertension. Medical Hypotheses. 1982; 9: 241-257.

[8] Kronbichler A, Mayer G. Renal involvement in autoimmune connective tissue diseases. BMC Medicine. http://www.biomedcentral.com/1741-7015/11/95

[9] Ebringer A, Doyle AE. Raised Serum IgG Levels in Hypertension. Brit Med J. 1970;2:146-148.

[10] Daniel W. Trott and David G. Harrison The immune system in hypertension. doi: 10.1152/advan.00063.2013 Adv Physiol Educ March 1, 2014 vol. 38 no. 1 20-24.

[11] Myers JB. Sodium intake, cognitive decline and Ageing. Sixth international Congress on Vascular Dementia, Barcelona Spain. 2009; November 19-22. Abstract p83. www.Kenes.com/vascular.

[12] Stefanidis C, Vlachopoulos C, Karayannacos P, Boudoulas H, Stratos C, Filippides T, Agapitos M, Toutouzas P. Effect of Vasa Vasorum Flow on structure and Function of the Aorta in Experimental Animals. Circulation 1995; 91; 2669-2678.

[13] Myers JB. COPD exacerbations. What else is wrong with the patient? An internist's viewpoint for the benefit of patients. Internal Medicine Society of Australia and New Zealand (IMSANZ) 2011 Annual Scientific Meeting. Lorne, Vic, Australia. November 11-13, 2011.

[14] Heidbuchel H, Verhamme P, Alings M, Antz M, Hacke W, Oldgren J, Sinnaeve P, Camm AJ, Kirchhof P. EHRA Practical Guide on the use of new oral anticoagulants in patients with non-valvular atrial fibrillation: executive summary. European Heart Journal doi:10.1093/eurheartj/eht134

[15] Marx RE, Sawatari Y, Fortin M, Broumand V. Bisphosphonate-Induced Exposed Bone [Osteonecrosis/Osteopetrosis] of the Jaws: Risk Factors, Recognition, Prevention, and Treatment. J Oral Maxillofac Surg 2005; 63:1567–1575.

[16] Strauss B. 10 Facts About Pterodactyls. Everything You Need to Know About Pterodactylus and Pteranodon. http://dinosaurs.about.com/od/dinosaurbasics/a/pterodactyl-facts.htm (accessed 16 September 2014)

[17] Yoma, 74-5. In: Ayin Yaacov.

[18] Myers JB. The Eco-society or Eco-social© environment and heart disease. A General Systems Approach. PM358. World Heart Federation's World Congress of Cardiology 2014. May 4-7, Melbourne, Australia.

Chapter 30

Salivary Diagnostics, Current Reality and Future Prospects

Andréa Cristina Barbosa da Silva, Diego Romário da Silva,
Sabrina Avelar de Macedo Ferreira, Andeliana David de Sousa Rodrigues,
Allan de Jesus Reis Albuquerque and Sandra Aparecida Marinho

Additional information is available at the end of the chapter

http://dx.doi.org/10.5772/59417

1. Introduction

1.1. Saliva: Composition and functions

Saliva is a aqueous, transparent and odorless liquid produced and secreted by the major and minor salivary glands, which combined with the gingival crevicular fluid, cellular debris, upper airway secretions and microorganisms of the oral cavity, makes up the total human saliva [1, 2].

The saliva is responsible for maintaining the homeostasis of the oral cavity and its pH normally lies around 6-7, which makes it slightly acidic. Initially, it shows up isotonic, becoming hypotonic as it passes through the network of ducts [3].

The daily average flow of total saliva in healthy people varies between 500 and 1500 mL, and the mean volume of saliva in the oral cavity is approximately 1 mL; however, there is always a great variability in individual rates of salivary flow [3]. This flow provides important information about the health quality not only oral but also systemic [4, 5].

The main constituent of saliva is water, which accounts for 99% of its composition. Solid components, which are characterized by organic and inorganic molecules, are dissolved in the aqueous medium. The salivary composition has significant changes from one individual to another and in the same individual under different circumstances; however, the rate of salivary flow is considered the main factor affecting its composition [6].

Saliva is composed of a number of inorganic ions, including sodium, potassium, chloride, calcium, magnesium, bicarbonate, phosphate, sulfate, thiocyanate and fluoride, which are

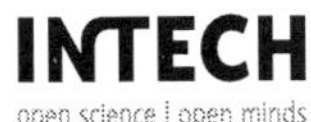

responsible for osmotic balance, buffering capacity and dental remineralization [7]. Humphrey and Williamson (2001), [3] consider that bicarbonate, phosphate and urea act as pH modulators being responsible for salivary buffering capacity.

The salivary organic components are represented by immunoglobulins, proteins, enzymes, mucins, and nitrogen products such as urea and ammonia. The salivary proteins (amylase, lipase, proteases, nucleases, mucins and gustin) act assisting in the digestive process, with antibacterial properties for hydrolysis of cellular membranes (lactoferrin, lysozyme and lactoperoxidase) besides inhibiting the adherence of microorganisms (immunoglobulins) [7].

The saliva keeps the oral health and creates a proper ecological balance. Among its functions (Figure 1) are the protection and lubrication of oral tissues, acting as a barrier against irritants, with buffering and cleaning action, maintaining the integrity of the teeth and antibacterial activity, besides acting improving the taste and starting the digestive process [8]. The saliva's lubricity capacity is provided mainly by mucins, they are secreted by the minor salivary glands, having low solubility, high viscosity, high elasticity and strong adhesiveness [6, 9, 10].

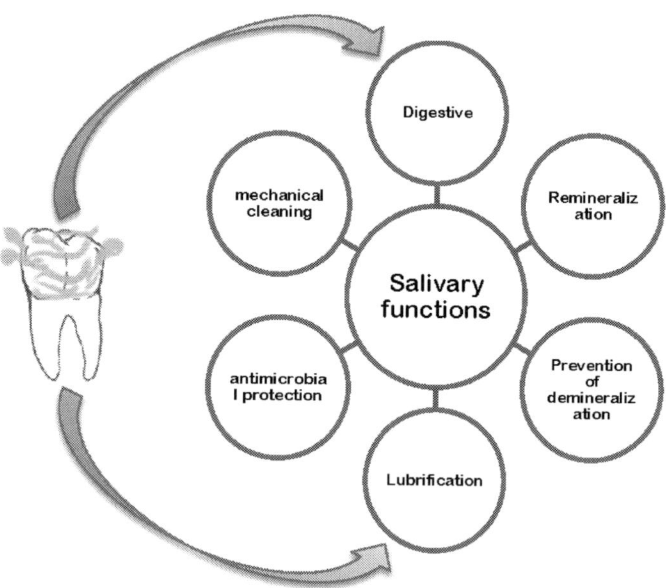

Figure 1. Saliva functions

Saliva was used for a long time as a method to monitor the caries risk, being used as biological environment extremely useful as buffering capacity and microbiological evaluation. Today, it is an object of detailed study for the diagnosis of systemic diseases that affect the function of the salivary glands and saliva composition, for example, Sjögren's syndrome, alcoholic cirrhosis, cystic fibrosis, sarcoidosis, diabetes mellitus and adrenal cortex diseases [11, 12]).

According to [13], saliva is a valuable source of clinically relevant information, since its many components, besides protecting the oral tissues integrity, act as biomarkers of diseases and systemic conditions of the individual. The qualitative changes in the composition of these biomarkers have been used to identify patients with increased susceptibility to some diseases, identification of sites with active disease, prediction of sites with greater disease activity in the future and / or serving as a tool for monitoring effectiveness of therapies.

2. The role of salivary biomarkers for diagnosis

There have been significant advances in techniques for detection of biomarkers in the oral cavity in recent years, especially by ELISA for proteins and PCR for RNA and DNA. With these advances in biotechnology, it has become possible to use saliva as a diagnostic mean for different conditions such as caries and periodontal disease, infectious and autoimmune diseases, genetic and psychological disorders, malignancies, legal issues, among others (Figure 2).

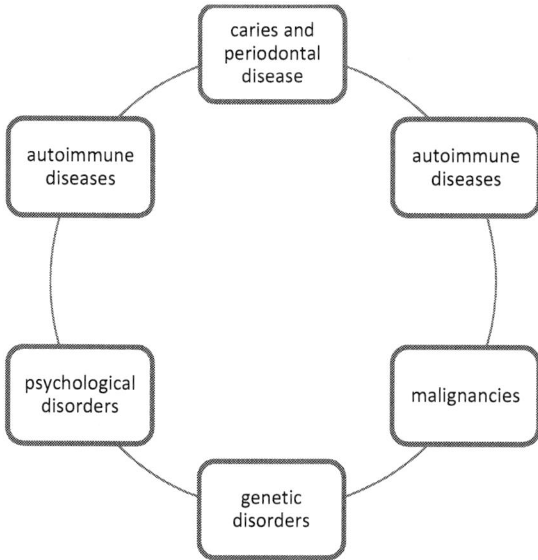

Figure 2. Major diseases with possibility of salivary diagnostics.

2.1. Caries and periodontal disease

Caries [14] and periodontal disease [15]) are the most occurring diseases in the oral cavity. Both considered infectious diseases and primarily responsible for tooth loss in adults. In recent years, remarkable achievements have been made in the field of oral microbiology, especially with regard to diagnosis. Techniques have been sought to predict the availability of patients to certain diseases; and this is not different with caries. The counts of bacteria present in saliva associated with other factors, such as diet and systemic conditions, may provide an estimate of the risk of caries in the individual. The increased number of lactobacilli and *Streptococcus mutans* in saliva have been associated with increased prevalence of caries and root caries [16]. Similarly, the methods of diagnosis in current clinical practice are able not only to detect the presence of inflammation, but also to identify patients at higher risk for progression of periodontal disease [17].

The human salivary buffer systems consist of an important natural defense against tooth decay [18]. The saliva's buffer capacity varies with glandular activity. The bicarbonate raises the pH of saliva and its buffering capacity, especially during stimulation [19]). Thus, the levels of bicarbonate and other important ions showing abnormalities can also suggest a predisposition to dental caries.

There has been an association between periodontal disease and increased levels of aspartate aminotransferase (AST) and alkaline phosphatase (ALP). The salivary AST can be used as a marker for monitoring periodontal disease. In addition, lower uric acid levels and albumin in saliva were associated with periodontitis and diabetes [20]. The development of new devices for periodontal monitoring probably would require less training and fewer resources than current diagnostic tests and may lead to better use by properly trained professionals for simpler and less intensive treatment, and may result in the provision of health care at low cost [21]. For determination of periodontal disease, it would be necessary a large body of research previously focused on fluid gingival biomarkers that provide the local disease status, but represents a technically difficult approach to implement in the clinical area [13, 17].

Currently, it is possible to use saliva tests for evaluating the microbiota associated with periodontal diseases, regardless of the degree of periodontal impairment of the patient. PCR tests can detect DNA of periodontal bacteria in oral fluids, such as *ggregatibacter actinomyce-temcomitans, Porphyromonas gingivalis, Campylobacter rectus, Eikenella corrodens* and *Fusobacterium nucleatum.* The analysis of the salivary microbial content reflects periodontal conditions and various socio-economic, cultural and behavioral aspects of patients [22].

2.2. Infectious diseases

In addition to exercising extremely important functions for the organism's homeostasis, saliva is currently an important tool for the diagnosis of infectious diseases. Besides the usual microorganisms in oral cavity, saliva may contain viruses and/or bacteria responsible for systemic diseases that can be identified by PCR. Another way to diagnose infectious disease by the salivary examination is through monitoring the presence of antibodies to the organisms [23].

Today, it is possible to identify, for example, the herpes virus associated with Kaposi's sarcoma and the presence of bacteria such as *Helicobacter pylori,* which is associated with gastritis, peptic ulcers and possible stomach cancer [11, 12]. Studies conducted in order to detect immunoglobulin M (IgM) against rubella showed 96% specificity when compared to standard considered as ideal test blood serum, which means that the use of saliva for epidemiological surveillance and control of this virus can be valid [24, 25]. It is also possible to detect the presence of Epstein-Barr virus (EBV) associated with infectious mononucleosis, highly communicable disease by contacting saliva and hairy leukoplakia [26].

The disease that generates more discussion regarding the use of saliva for diagnostic procedures is undoubtedly the Acquired Immunodeficiency Syndrome (AIDS). Until recently, oral HIV transmission through saliva of infected individuals during dental treatment or as a result of biting or contact stemmed by cough or kiss droplets has been considered less likely than vaginal or rectal transmission [27]. However, concerns about the way of transmission have increased. Studies have shown that these tests based on specific salivary antibodies are equivalent in reliability as compared to those in the serum, therefore being useful in the clinical use and epidemiological studies [28]. In recent years, researchers have shown that salivary tests for detection of antibodies to HIV [29] represents a non-invasive alternative for quantification of antibodies in blood to monitor the effectiveness of antiretroviral therapy and progression of Acquired Immunodeficiency Syndrome [30].

2.3. Autoimmune diseases

For this class of diseases, the most studied in parameters of salivary diagnostics is the Sjogren's syndrome. It is an autoimmune disease characterized by decreased secretion of the salivary and lacrimal glands, associated with endocrine disorders. The sialochemistry (analysis of saliva's chemical components) offers great value for the diagnosis of this syndrome. Increased immunoglobulin levels, inflammatory mediators, albumin, sodium and chloride and, decreased phosphate level are indicative of Sjögren's syndrome. Analysis of proteins in saliva showed increased level of lactoferrin, beta 2 microglobulin, lysozyme C, and cystatin C. However, levels of salivary amylase and carbonic anhydrase showed reduced [31, 32]. Thus, these references of protein chemical analysis associated with detailed history may show effectiveness for an accurate diagnosis.

Salivary changes that may reveal the presence of multiple sclerosis, an inflammatory disease characterized by loss of myelin and scarring caused due to failure in producing cells by the immune system have also sought. However, no significant changes were found except for a reduction in the production of IgA, which is inconclusive to suggest the diagnosis [33].

Sarcoidosis is an autoimmune and inflammatory disease, which affects the lymph nodes, lungs, liver, eyes, skin, or other tissues. Salivary diagnostics has demonstrated a decreased amount of saliva secretion associated with reduced activity of the enzyme alpha-amylase and kallikrein in most patients carrying the disease. However, there was no correlation between the decrease in enzyme activity and the volume of secretion, which complicates the understanding of salivary changes and possible diagnosis [34].

2.4. Psychological and genetic disorders

The total salivary flow and its characteristics had already been correlated with xerostomia, symptoms of anxiety, depression, Burning Mouth Syndrome and aphthous stomatitis [35, 36, 37]. The salivary cortisol levels may represent an important biological marker of stress. The salivary cortisol concentration increases after 20 the beginning of a stressful situation, besides increased pH and protein levels. However, there are no indications of changes in concentrations of fluoride under conditions of acute mental stress [38, 39].

The sialochemistry evaluation reveals significant elevation in the levels of phosphate, chloride and potassium in subjects with BSA symptoms, and also differences in expression pattern of salivary proteins of low molecular weight compared to healthy individuals. Levels of phosphate, potassium and chloride are increased in individuals with intense activity of the sympathetic nervous system, something common in situations of emotional stress [40].

The salivary alpha-amylase has its release regulated by the sympathetic autonomic nervous system, and has importance in the psychobiology of stress. The levels of salivary alpha-amylase in humans increase under various conditions of physical and psychological stress before any other clinical signs can be perceived [37, 41, 42]. Therefore, the salivary alpha-amylase may act as effective biomarker which can be used alternatively non-invasive way to evaluate psychological and metabolic stress, or including diseases whose etiology just seems to be related to stress.

Results are controversial and not always enlightening. For aphthous stomatitis significant changes in the levels of TCD4+ and TCD8+ lymphocytes have been associated and abnormal cytokine cascade arising from the oral mucosa. It is known that for aphthous stomatitis there are 41 genes expressed differently and increased activity of lymphocytes T-helper 1 (Th1), responsible for the production of interferon-gamma, interleukin 2 (IL-2) and alpha tumor necrosis factor (TNF-α). The levels of IL-2 are higher in patients with aphthous stomatitis compared with control subjects and may serve as markers in immunodiagnoses [43, 44, 45, 46, 47].

The secretory immunoglobulin A (IgA-s) can be used as the oral mucosa immune status parameter. It acts as a barrier to infectious agents, environmental allergens and carcinogens, as well as it participates in innate protection mechanisms. IgA deficiency is the most common humoral immune defect in humans and causes, in a large proportion, gastrointestinal and respiratory infections [48, 49, 50, 51].

The identification of exogenous genetic material in saliva may have forensic significance, or in cases of sexual assaults. The genetic material shared after a kiss is present and can be detected up to an hour after the kiss [52].

Cystic fribose, an autosomal recessive genetic disease caused by a disturbance in salivary glands secretions. Cystic fibrosis affects the chromosome 7, which is responsible for the production of a protein which will regulate the passage of sodium and chloride throuh cell membranes. The effects of this regulation can be analyzed through saliva. The Sodium and Potassium elements showed higher levels, while the trace elements vanadium, chromium, selenium and arsenic have lower levels in individuals with cystic fibrosis [53].

2.5. Malignancy

There is a growing interest worldwide for the saliva analysis through genomics, transcriptomics and proteomics, since this is a non-invasive source of rich genetic information. In the case of saliva, two main aspects of cancer diagnosis must be distinguished - one being the diagnosis of oral cancer (which has direct contact with saliva) and other the cancer diagnoses in other locations. Mouth cancer in advanced stages can usually be detected by inspection of the oral cavity. On the other hand, initial oral carcinomas are not visible and cannot be diagnosed and treated on time. The salivary proteomecan also be used for tumor detection [54].

The study of Streckfus et al. (2000) [55], demonstrated the role of saliva in the diagnosis of breast cancer, in which salivary tests for markers of disease were studied combined with mammography. From the analysis in saliva, the soluble fragment of the oncogene c-erbB-2, a prognostic marker for breast cancer, as well as the antigen for cancer were significantly higher in the saliva and serum of women diagnosed with cancer than that observed in a control group of healthy women and patients with benign tumors group, indicating that the saliva test for this oncogene is sensitive and reliable, and it is potentially useful in the early detection and monitoring of screening for breast cancer [56].

Additionally, the use of saliva test may be important in monitoring the levels of c-erbB-2 in patients undergoing chemotherapy and/or surgery, so that serves as an assessment of therapy effectiveness in question, and may be useful in preservation [57].

Franzmann et al. (2005) [58], evaluated the soluble CD44 in saliva as a potential molecular marker for head and neck cancer and concluded that the test can be effective to detect this cancer at all stages.

In the past, biomarkers were used primarily as prognostic indicators for patients with tumors of the head and neck. More recently, the role of biomarkers has been greatly expanded to cover all aspects of patient care, from early cancer detection to the more accurate tumor staging and even the selection of those patients most likely to benefit from specific therapies to post-treatment tumor surveillance. One of the most promising avenues regarding the early diagnosis of cancer has been the ability to use saliva as a substrate for the evaluation of biomarkers [59].

Recently, Jiang et al. (2005)[60], reported increased content of mitochondrial DNA in saliva of patients with head and neck cancer. Multivariate analysis revealed a significant and independent association of SCC diagnosis of head and neck, age and smoking with increased content of mitochondrial or nuclear DNA. Salivary proteins such as CEA, defensin-1, TNF-alpha, IL-1, 6 and 8 and CD44 showed increase in their detection in patients with oral cancer.

Most of these studies relied on immunological assays of individual gene products 2,137. It is expected that proteomic biomarkers, when combined, increase the sensitivity and specificity of detection of human cancer [61, 62].

Increased levels of salivary defensin-1, CA15-3 cancer antigen, tumor marker proteins, such as c-erbB-2 or CA-125 and antibodies against tumor suppressor protein p53 are promising markers of oral malignant neoplasms and other cancers. In the future, a global proteomic profile of saliva with methods newly developed for proteome analysis is likely to result in other peptide sequences candidates for detection with high sensitivity [62, 54].

When compared to blood, saliva can express more sensitive and specific markers for certain local oral diseases. For example, saliva contains expressed proteins locally different from serum that can be best indicators of the oral disease. There are compelling reasons to use saliva as a diagnostic fluid to monitor the onset and progression of oral cancer. Saliva is the fluid that drains the lesions and there is increased RNA and proteins of oral cancer on it [63].

2.6. Forensic evidence

The forensic dentistry method is efficient for human identification, but is endowed with certain limitations: it suffers distortion from the moment of the bite until the act of expertise, especially when the mark is left on the skin. The salivary DNA emerges as a complement or even to replace the first, since it is a test of excellence [64]. However, the use of saliva in the identification was only feasible after the development of molecular biology techniques applied to forensic dentistry. In forensic uses, the PCR technique is the most used as it drastically increases the chances of DNA analysis, allowing determining the individual's molecular profile. It was from then that saliva became a great focus on looking for traces, as they provide enough genetic material and excellent qualities for the exam in most cases [65].

The DNA can be degraded depending on the conditions of their preservation. Moisture, excessive heat, pH, enzymes and other are variables for its ideal preservation under the various surfaces that can be found [66].This being the object of several recent studies. In the study by [67], the authors concluded that saliva is able to provide genetic material, even when stored under conditions below those considered optimal.

The human salivary proteome (HSP), using 2D gel electrophoresis coupled to mass spectrometry, is able to identify approximately 100 different salivary proteins [68]. A significant number of spots on a typical 2-DE gel can capture fragments of abundant salivary proteins such as amylases, cystatins and immunoglobulins [69]. For the identification of less abundant salivary proteins, analysis by advanced techniques of mass spectrometry ensures a significant increase in resolution when compared to two-dimensional gel electrophoresis [70]. Generally, a pre fractionation of intact salivary proteins employing high resolution separation techniques is required to achieve a wide coverage of the human salivary proteome [71].

Human saliva stains can be found at crime scenes, alone or mixed with other biological fluids. The most common sites of occurrence are: the surface of objects such as envelopes [72], tissues cigarette butts, cups, sites near bites and often victims of rape [73].

3. Clinical application of salivary diagnosis in the era of "omics"

For the salivary diagnosis become routine in clinical practice, it is necessary to know specific salivary biomarkers of disease states or health, besides technology necessary for their detection [74]. The genomics, epigenomics, transcriptomics, proteomics and metabolomics (Figure 3) approaches are currently being used to characterize these diagnostic biomarkers in saliva [75].

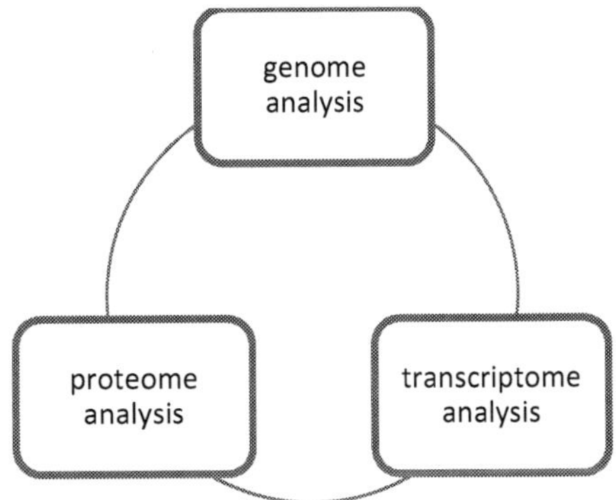

Figure 3. Study of omics to identify salivary biomarkers.

Biomarkers of DNA, mRNA, or protein biomarkers can provide useful diagnostic information that can identify the effect of disease or medication on salivary constituents. However, there is still not a complete characterization of the salivary proteome for disease biomarkers. Five hundred salivary proteins have been described, but this number is very small when compared to the more than 4,000 proteins listed for plasma [76].

The analysis of salivary genome and epigenoma allows identification of the presence of invading pathogens, as well as profiles transcription of anomalous genes that reflect genetic pathological processes such as cancer. The salivary genome consists of DNAs representing the individual's genome and the oral microbiota. The quality and yield of DNA that can be obtained from saliva is relatively good compared to blood and urine, which can be used for genotyping, amplification or sequencing [54], and can be stored for a long time without significant degradation [77].Thus, the salivary DNA is an analyte suitable for diagnosis but limited to reflect the presence or absence of specific genes or alterations in the sequences (mutations) and also cannot provide information about upregulation and downregulation of gene expression.

Regarding the salivary transcriptome, mRNAs and miRNAs are secreted by cells into the extracellular medium and can be found in biofluids remote cellular sources [78, 79, 80]. In the disease state, the transcription of specific miRNAs and mRNAs has changed. Despite suffering some criticism initially, the use of salivary RNAs as diagnostic biomarkers, is now widely accepted [81]. However, the precise sources of salivary RNAs and other molecules remain unclear.

The standard procedures for the isolation and analysis of salivary mRNA require low temperatures, besides being expensive and time consuming, precluding its clinical application. Currently, simple methods of stabilization of mRNA in saliva samples have been developed, allowing for storage at room temperature without the use of stabilizers, and are so-called 'direct-saliva-transcriptomic-analysis' [82]. However, this approach also involves centrifugation. An alternative method has been described [83], but it was based on the use of an expensive stabilizing agent (expensive). Thus, neither method is completely suitable for all applications. The mRNAs of saliva and plasma can be remarkably stable. The microarray technology is considered the gold standard for the identification of salivary transcripts. In this technique, the salivary transcriptome is determined using microarrays and is validated by means of qPCR. However, low concentrations of certain biomarkers, as well as small sample volumes require innovations in technology [84].

For proteins detection, the use surface - enhanced laser desorption/ionization time - of - flight (SELDI - TOF) mass spectrometry (MS), has been reported for several diseases. Recently, analysis of saliva for protein biomarker discovery has mainly been performed using two - dimensional difference gel electrophoresis (2D - DIGE) coupled with MS (which can identify around 300 proteins in a sample, and liquid chromatograpy - MS (LC - MS) based techniques (which can identify more than 1,050 proteins in a sample; reviewed in [85]. Thus, liquid chromatographic separation appears to resolve protein species more precisely than gel electrophoresis methods. A multiplex protein array was also employed, providing high - throughput analysis [86]; however, this method requires some prior knowledge of likely analytes. Despite these advances, the discovery and validation of protein salivary biomarkers still has some challenges. Proteins have short half-lives, making them unstable. Both the nature of peptides, as the oral environment makes them vulnerable to degradation. Thus, the diagnosis based on salivary protein requires immediate processing of samples, or the use of freezers and expensive protease inhibitors. In the clinical environment, these requirements are not easily circumvented.

The metabolome is the set of small metabolites and changes continuously, reflecting the gene and protein expression. Metabolomics investigations can generate quantitative data to elucidate metabolic dynamics related to disease and exposure to drugs [87]. However, a metabolomics limitation comparative to genomics, transcriptomics and proteomics is the inability to identify differentially the metabolites expressed [88, 89, 90].

4. Future prospects

In recent years, many important biological questions have been answered by the study of the "omics" (genomics, transcriptomics, proteomics, metabolomics, etc.), allowing the discovery of various salivary biomarkers. However, few of these markers have exceeded the identifica-tion phase. The transfer of scientific knowledge of salivary biomarkers for clinical applications is a challenging process that rarely has resulted in clinical implementation. Its successful application in clinical practice will depend on collaborative studies including physicians, epidemiologists, molecular biologists and bioinformaticians with a relevant clinical question and with well-defined parameters of recruitment and characterization of patients and samples. Thus, the use of saliva as a diagnostic fluid will be increasingly accepted, allowing for enhanced systemic and oral health.

Author details

Andréa Cristina Barbosa da Silva[1*], Diego Romário da Silva[1],
Sabrina Avelar de Macedo Ferreira[1], Andeliana David de Sousa Rodrigues[2],
Allan de Jesus Reis Albuquerque[3] and Sandra Aparecida Marinho[1]

*Address all correspondence to: andreacbsilva@gmail.com

1 Graduate Program in Dentistry, Center of Sciences, Technology and Health, State University
of Paraiba, UEPB, Araruna, Paraíba, Brazil

2 Graduate Program in Dentistry, Integrated College of Patos, FIP, Patos, Paraíba, Brazil

3 Brazilian Northeast Network on Biotechnology, RENORBIO, Federal University of Paraiba,
UFPB, João Pessoa, Paraíba, Brazil

References

[1] Nagler RM, Hershkovich O, Lischinsky S, Diamond, E, Reznick, AZ. Saliva analysis
in the clinical setting: revisiting an underused diagnostic tool. J. Investig. Med
2002;50(3) 214–225.

[2] Aps JKM, Martens, LC. Review: the physiology of saliva and transfer of drugs into
saliva. Forensic Sci. Int 2005;150(2-3) 119–131.

[3] Humphrey SP, Williamson RT. A review of saliva: normal composition, flow, and
function. J. Prosthet. Dent 2001;85(2) 162-169.

[4] Leite GJ, Mamede RCM, Leite, MGJ. Medida do Fluxo Salivar: Refinamentos ao Mé-
todo do Cuspe e Uso do Papel de Filtro. Rev. Brasil. Otorrinolaringol 2002;68(6)
826-832.

[5] Jenkins GN. The Physiology of the Mouth. 3rd ed. London: The Alden Press, 1970.

[6] Edgar WM. Saliva and dental health. Clinical implications of saliva: report of a consensus meeting. Br. Dent. J 1990;169(3-4) 96-98.

[7] Arnold AMD, Marek CA. The impact of saliva on patient care: A literature review. J.
Prosthet. Dent 2002;88(3) 337-343.

[8] Mandel, ID. The function of saliva. J. Dent. Res 1987;66, 623-627.

[9] Slomiany BL, Murty VL, Poitrowski J, Slomiany A. Salivary mucins in oral mucosal
defense. Gen Pharmacol 1996;27(5) 761-771.

[10] Tabak LA. Stucture and function of human salivary mucins. Crit. Rev. Oral Biol. Med
1990;1(4) 229-234.

[11] Koelle DM, Huang ML, Chandran B, Vieira J, Piepcorn M, Corey L. Frequent detection of Kaposi's sarcoma-associated herpesvirus (human herpesvirus 8) DNA in saliva of human immunodeficiency virus-infected man: clinical and immunologic correlates. J Infect Dis 1997;176, (1) 94-102.

[12] Reilly TG, Poxon V, Sanders DS, Elliott TS, Walt RP. Comparison of serum, salivary, and rapid whole blood diagnostic tests for *Helicobacter pylori* and their validation against endoscopy based tests. Gut, London 1997;40(4).

[13] Giannobile WV, Beikler T, Kinney JS, Ramseier CA, Morelli T, Wong DT. Saliva as a diagnostic tool for periodontal disease: current state and future directions. Periodontology 2000;50, 52-64. DOI: 10.1111/j.1600-0757.2008.00288.x.

[14] Keyes, PH. The infectious and transmissible nature of experimental dental caries. Arch. Oral Biol 1960;1, 304-320. Doi: 10.1016/0003-9969(60)90091-1.

[15] Pihlstrom BL, Michalowicz BS, Johnson NW. Periodontal diseases 2005; Lancet 366(9499) 1809-1820.

[16] Mittal S, Bansal V, Garg S, Atreja G, Bansal S. The diagnostic role of Saliva—a review 2011; Journal of Clinical and Experimental Dentistry 2011;3(4) 314–320.

[17] Zhang L, Henson BS, Camargo PM, Wong DT. The clinical value of salivary biomarkers for periodontal disease 2009; Periodontol 2000;51, 25-37. Doi: 10.1111/j. 1600-0757.2009.00315.x.

[18] Bretas LP, Rocha ME, Vieira MS, Rodrigues ACP. Fluxo Salivar e Capacidade Tamponante da Saliva como Indicadores de Susceptibilidade à Doença Cárie. Pesq Bras Odontoped Clin Integr 2008;8(3) 289-293. Doi: 10.4034/1519.0501.2008.0083.0006.

[19] Bardow A, Moe D, Nyvad B, Nauntofte B. The buffer capacity and buffer systems of human whole saliva measured without loss of CO2. Arch Oral Biol 2000;45(1) 1-12.

[20] Totan A, Greabu M, Totan C, Spinu T. Salivary aspartate aminotransferase, alanine aminotransferase and alkaline phosphatase: possible markers in periodontal diseases? Clinical Chemistry and Laboratory Medicine 2006;44(5) 612–615.

[21] Ramseier CA, Morelli T, Kinney JS, Dubois M, Rayburn LA, Giannobile WV (2008). Periodontal disease: salivary diagnostics. In: Salivary diagnostics. Wong DT, editor. Ames, IA: Wiley Blackwell, pp.156-168.

[22] Shimada M.H, Angelis L, Ciesielsky FIN, Gaetti-Jardim EC, Gaetti-Jardim JR E. Emprego de saliva na determinação do risco às doenças periodontais: aspectos microbiológicos e clínicos. Revista de Odontologia da UNESP 2008;37(2) 183-189.

[23] Lawrence HP. Salivary Markers of Systemic Disease: Noninvasive Diagnosis of Disease and Monitoring of General Health. Journal of the Canadian Dental Association 2002;68(3) 170-174.

[24] Vyse AJ, Brown DWG, Cohen BJ, Samuel R, Nokes DJ. Detection of rubella virus-specific immunoglobulin G in saliva by an amplification-based enzyme-linked immuno-

sorbent assay using monoclonal antibody to fluorescein isothiocyanate. J Clin Microbiol 1999;37(2) 391-395.

[25] Oliveira SA, Siqueira MM, Brown DWG, LITTON P, CAMACHO LAB, Castro ST, Cohen BJ. Diagnosis of rubella infection by detecting specific immunoglobulin M antibodies in saliva samples: a clinicbased study in Niterói, RJ, Brazil. Rev Soc Bras Med Trop 2000;33(4) 335-339.

[26] Mbulaiteye SM, Walters M, Engels EA, Bakaki PM, Ndugwa CM, Owor AM et al. High levels of Epstein-Barr virus DNA in saliva and peripheral blood from Ugandan mother-child pairs. J Infect Dis 2006;193(3) 422-426.

[27] Baron S. Oral transmission of HIV, a rarity: emerging hypotheses. J Dent Res 2001;80(7) 1602-1604.

[28] Malamud, D. Saliva as a diagnostic fluid. BMJ, London 1992;305(6847) 207-208.

[29] Malamud D. Oral diagnostic testing for detecting human immunodeficiency virus-1 antibodies: a technology whose time has come. Am J Med 1997;102(4A) 9-14.

[30] Shugars DC, Slade GD, Patton LL, Fiscus SA. Oral and systemic factors associated with increased levels of human immunodeficiency virus type 1 RNA in saliva. Oral Surg Oral Med Oral Pathol Oral Radiol Endod 2000;89(4) 432-40.

[31] Greabu M, Battino M, Mohora M et al., Saliva—a diagnostic window to the body, both in health and in disease. Journal of Medicine and Life 2009;2(2), 124–132.

[32] Malamud D. Saliva as a diagnostic fluid. Dental Clinics of North America 2011;55(1) 159–178.

[33] Ahmadi Motamayel F, Davoodi P, Dalband, M, Hendi SS. Saliva as a mirror of the body health. DJH Journal 2010;1(2), 1–15.

[34] Bhoola KD, McNicol MW, Oliver S, Foran J. Changes in salivary enzymes in patients with sarcoidosis. The New England Journal of Medicine 1969;281(16) 877–879.

[35] Bradley K, Formaker BK, Frank ME. Taste function in patients with oral burning. Chem Senses 2000;25(5), 575-81.

[36] Hershkovich O, Nagler RM. Biochemical analysis of saliva and taste acuity evaluation in patients with burning mouth syndrome, xerostomia and/or gustatory disturbances. Arch Oral Biol 2004;49(7) 515-22.

[37] Nater UM. et al. Human salivary alpha-amilase reactivity in a psychosocial stress paradigm. Int J Psychophysiol 2005;55(3) 333-342.

[38] Kristenson M, Garvin P, Lundberg U, editors. The role of saliva cortisol measurement in health and disease. EAE: Bentham Science Publishers; 2012.

[39] Naumova, E.A., Sandulescu, T., Bochnig, C., Al Khatib, Lee WK, Zimmer S, Arnold WH. Dynamic changes in saliva after acute mental stress. Scientific Reports 2014;4, 1-9. Doi: 10.1038/srep04884.

[40] Rhoades, R. A.; Tanner, G. A. Fisiologia médica. 2. Ed. Rio de Janeiro: Guanabara-Koogan, 741p, 2005.

[41] Nierop, A. et al. Prolonged salivary cortisol recovery in second-trimester pregnant women and attenuated salivary α-amylase responses to psychosocial stress in human pregnancy. J Clin Endocrinol Metab 2006;91(4), 1329-35.

[42] Kang, Y. Psychological stress-induced chances in salivary alpha-amylase and adrenergic activity. Nurs Health Sci 2010;12(4), 477-484.

[43] Savage NW, Seymour, GJ, Kruger, B.J. T-lymphocyte subset changes in recurrent aphthous stomatitis. Oral Surg Oral Med Oral Pathol 1985;60(2) 175-181.

[44] Buño, IJ. et al. Elevated levels of interferon gamma, tumor necrosis factor α, interleukins 2, 4 and 5, but not interleukin 10, are present in recurrent aphthous stomatitis. Arch Dermatol 1999;134(7) 827-831.

[45] Volkov, I. et al. Case Report: Recurrent aphthous stomatitis responds to vitamin B12 treatment. Can Fam Physician 2005;51(6) 844-845.

[46] Jurge S. et al. Recurrent aphthous stomatitis. Oral Dis 2006;12(1) 1-21.

[47] Chavan M. et al. Recurrent aphthous stomatitis: a review. J Oral Pathol Med 2012;41(8) 577-583.

[48] Lamm ME, Nedrud JG, Kaetzel CS, Mazanec MB. IgA and mucosal defense. APMIS - Acta Pathol Microbiol Immunol Scand 1995;103(4) 241-6.

[49] Truedsson L, Baskin B, Pan Q, Rabbani H, Vorechovsky I, Smith CI. Genetics of IgA deficiency. Acta Pathol Microbiol Immunol Scand 1995;103(12) 833-72.

[50] Kilian M, Reinholdt J, Lomholt T, Poulsen K, Frandsen EV. Biological significance of IgA1 proteases in bacterial colonization and pathogenesis: critical evaluation of experimental evidence. APMIS - Acta Pathol Microbiol Immunol Scand 1996;104(5) 321-38.

[51] Hucklebridge F, Lambert S, Clow A, Warburton DM, Evans PD, Sherwood N. Modulation of secretory immunoglobulin A in saliva; response to manipulation of mood. Biol Psychol 2000;53(1) 25-35.

[52] Kamodyová N, Durdiaková J, Celec P, Sedláčková T, Repiská G, Sviežená B, Minárik G. Prevalence and persistence of male DNA identified in mixed saliva samples after intense kissing. Forensic Sci Int Genet 2013;7(1) 124-8.

[53] Vieira LAC, Feijó GCS, Zara LF, Castro, CFS, Bezerra ACB. Atomic Spectroscopy Identifies Differences in Trace Element Parameters in theSaliva of Patients with Cystic Fibrosis. Pesq Bras Odontoped Clin Integr 2011;11(2) 211-216.

[54] Fabian TK, Fejerdy P, Csermely, P. Salivary Genomics, Transcriptomics and Proteomics: The Emerging Concept of the Oral Ecosystem and their Use in the Early Diagnosis of Cancer and other Diseases. Curr Genomics 2008;9(1) 11-21.

[55] Streckfus C et al., The presence of soluble cerbB-2 concentrations in the saliva and serum among women with breast carcinoma: a preliminary study. Clin Cancer Res 2000;6(6) 2363-2370.

[56] Streckfus C et al., Reliability assessment of soluble c-erbB-2 concentrations in the saliva of healthy women and men. Oral Surg Oral Med Oral Pathol Oral Radiol Endod 2001;91(2) 174-179.

[57] Bigler LR. et al. The potential use of saliva to detect recurrence of disease in women with breast carcinoma. J Oral Pathol Med 2002;31(7) 421-431.

[58] Franzmann EJ et al. Salivary soluble CD44: a potential molecular marker for head and neck cancer. Cancer Epidemiol Biomarkers Prev 2005;14(3) 735-739.

[59] Pai SI, Westra WH. Molecular pathology of head and neck cancer: implications for diagnosis, prognosis, and treatment. Annu Rev Pathol 2009;4(49) 70.

[60] Jiang WW et al., Increased mitochondrial DNA content in saliva associated with head and neck cancer. Clin Cancer Res 2005;11(7) 2486-2491. 2005.

[61] Arellano-Garcia ME et al., Multiplexed immunobead-based assay for detection of oral cancer protein biomarkers in saliva. Oral Dis 2008;14(8) 705-712.

[62] HU S, LOO JA, WONG DT. Human body fluid proteome analysis. Proteomics 2006;6(23) 6326-6353.

[63] Hu S, Loo JA, Wong DT. Human saliva proteome analysis and disease biomarker discovery. Expert Rev Proteomics 2007;4(4) 531-538.

[64] Silva RHA et al., Human bite identification and DNA technology in forensic dentistry. Brazilian Journal Oral Science 2006;19(5) 1193-1197.

[65] FARAH, S.B. DNA: segredos & mistérios. São Paulo: Sarvier; 1997.

[66] Burger J et al,. DNA preservation: a microsatellite-DNA study on ancient skeletal remains. Eletrophoresis 1999;20(8) 1722-1728.

[67] Nq, DP, Koh D, Choo SG, Ng V, Fu Q. Effect of storage conditions on the straction of PCR-quality genomic DNA from saliva. Clinica Chimica Acta 2004;343(1-2) 191-194, 2004

[68] Ghafouri B. et al. Mapping of proteins in human saliva using two-dimensional gel electrophoresis and peptide mass fingerprinting. Proteomics 2003;3(6) 1003 -1015.

[69] TZ, C., F. et al. Complexity of the human whole saliva proteome. Physiol. Biochem 2005; 61(3) 469–480.

[70] Hirtz C et al. MS characterization of multiple forms of alpha-amylase in human saliva. Proteomics 2005;5(17) 4597-607.

[71] Messana I, Cabras T, Inzitari R, et al. Characterization of the human salivary basic proline-rich protein complex by a proteomic approach. J Proteome Res 2004;3(4) 792-800.

[72] Xie H et al., A Catalogue of Human Saliva Proteins Identified by Free Flow Electrophoresis-based Peptide Separation and Tandem Mass Spectrometry. Proteomics 2005;4(11) 1826–1830.

[73] Fridez F, Coquoz R. PCR DNA typing of stamps: evaluation of the DNA extraction. Forensic Sci Int 1996;78(2) 103–110.

[74] Barni F, Berti A, Rapone CB, Lago G. a-Amylase Kinetic Test in Bodily Single and Mixed Stains. Journal of Forensic Science 2006;51(6) 1389-1396.

[75] Wong DT. Salivary diagnostics powered by nanotechnologies, proteomics and genomics. JADA 2006;137(3) 313-321.

[76] Bonne NJ, Wong DTW. Salivary biomarker development using genomic, proteomic and metabolomic approaches. Genome Medicine 2012;4(82) 1-12.

[77] Ramachandran P, Boontheung P, Xie Y, Sondej M, Wong DT, Loo JA. Identification of Nlinked glycoproteins in human saliva by glycoprotein capture and mass spectrometry. JProteome Res 2006;5(6) 1493-1503.

[78] Nunes AP, Oliveira IO, Santos BR, Millech C, Silva LP, Gonzalez DA, Hallal PC, Menezes AM, Araujo CL, Barros FC. Quality of DNA extracted from saliva samples collected with the Oragene DNA self-collection kit. BMC Med Res Methodol 2012.

[79] Park NJ, Zhou H, Elashoff D, Henson BS, Kastratovic DA, Abemayor E, Wong DT. Salivary microRNA: discovery, characterization, and clinical utility for oral cancer detection. Clin Cancer Res 2009;15(17) 5473-5477.

[80] Garcia JM, Garcia V, Pena C, Dominguez G, Silva J, Diaz R, Espinosa P, Citores MJ, Collado M, Bonilla F. Extracellular plasma RNA from colon cancer patients is confined in a vesicle-like structure and is mRNA-enriched. RNA 2008;14(7) 1424-1432.

[81] Tinzl M, Marberger M, Horvath S, Chypre C. DD3 RNA analysis in urine? A new perspective for detecting prostate cancer. Eur Urol 2004;46(2) 182-187.

[82] Kumar SV, Hurteau GJ, Spivack SD. Validity of messenger RNA expression analyses of human saliva. Clin Cancer Res 2006;12(17) 5033-5039.

[83] Lee YH, Zhou H, Reiss JK, Yan X, Zhang L, Chia D, Wong DT. Direct saliva transcriptome analysis. Clin Chem 2011;57(9) 1295-1302.

[84] Park NJ, Yu T, Nabili V, Brinkman BM, Henry S, Wang J, Wong DT. RNA protect saliva. An optimal room-temperature stabilization reagent for the salivary transcriptome. Clin Chem 2006;52(12) 2303-2304.

[85] Hu Z, Zimmermann BG, Zhou H, Wang J, Henson BS, Yu W, Elashoff D, Krupp G, Wong DT. Exon-level expression profiling: a comprehensive transcriptome analysis of oral fluids. Clin Chem 2008;54(5) 824-832.

[86] Liu J, Duan Y. Saliva: A potential media for disease diagnostics and monitoring. Oral Oncol 2012;48(7) 569-577.

[87] Lee A, Ghaname CB, Braun TM, Sugai JV, Teles RP, Loesche WJ, Kornman KS, Giannobile WV, Kinney JS. Bacterial and salivary biomarkers predict the gingival inflammatory profile. J Periodontol 2012;83(1) 79-89.

[88] Spielmann N, Wong DT. Saliva: diagnostics and therapeutic perspectives. Oral Dis 2011;17(4) 345-354.

[89] Sugimoto M, Wong DT, Hirayama A, Soga T, Tomita M. Capillary electrophoresis mass spectrometry-based saliva metabolomics identified oral, breast and pancreatic cancer-specific profiles. Metabolomics 2010;6(1) 78-95.

[90] Wei J, Xie G, Zhou Z, Shi P, Qiu Y, Zheng X, Chen T, Su M, Zhao A, Jia W. Salivary metabolite signatures of oral cancer and leukoplakia. Int J Cancer 2011;129(9) 2207-2217.

[91] Li X, Yang T, Lin J. Spectral analysis of human saliva for detection of lung cancer using surface-enhanced Raman spectroscopy. J Biomed Opt 2012;17(037003).

Chapter 31

Oral Health Related Quality of Life

Javier de la Fuente Hernández,
Fátima del Carmen Aguilar Díaz and
María del Carmen Villanueva Vilchis

Additional information is available at the end of the chapter

http://dx.doi.org/10.5772/59262

1. Introduction

Data about the impacts on people's life caused by oral condition has been gathered recently in the last decades. Functional consequences of oral disease have been documented and also the emotional and social ones. It is accepted and recognized by dental community that oral health status can cause considerable pain and suffering, if oral symptoms remain untreated would be a major source of diminished quality of life; disturbing people's food choices or their speech, or may lead to sleep deprivation, depression, and multiple adverse psychosocial outcomes. Influencing how people grow, enjoy life, chew, taste food and socialize, as well as their feelings of social well-being. There are so many oral affections that impact negatively on quality of life like caries, periodontal disease, tooth loss, cancer, dental injuries, dental fluorosis, and dental anomalies, craniofacial disorders among others. In fact not only dental disease but also treatment experience can negatively affect the oral health related quality of life. The relationship among these anomalies or conditions with quality of life are recently findings in literature in different populations. To evaluate these impacts different instruments have been developed for pediatric and adult population.

2. Oral health concept

2.1. Health

If there are complexities in defining disease, there are even more in defining health. Definitions have evolved over time. In the biomedical perspective, early definitions of health focused on the theme of the body's ability to function; health was seen as a state of normal function that could be disrupted from time to time by disease. An example of such a definition of health is: "a state characterized by anatomic, physiologic, and psychological integrity; ability to perform personally, in family, work, and in community roles; ability to deal with physical, biologic, psychological, and social stress". Then, in 1948, the World Health Organization (WHO) proposed a definition that aimed higher, linking health to well-being, in terms of "physical, mental, and social well-being, and not merely the absence of disease and infirmity". Although this definition is most accepted one it is also criticized as being vague, excessively broad, and unmeasurable.

This brought in a new conception of health, not as a state, but in dynamic terms, in other words, as "a resource for living". [1] The WHO in 1984 revised the concept of health and defined it as "the extent to which an individual or group is able to realize aspirations and satisfy needs, and to change or cope with the environment. Health is a resource for everyday life, not the objective of living; it is a positive concept, emphasizing social and personal resources, as well as physical capacities". [2] Thus, health referred to the ability to maintain homeostasis and recover from illness. Mental, intellectual, emotional, and social health referred to a person's ability to handle stress, to acquire skills, to maintain relationships, which are important for resources for resiliency and independent living. As seen the concept of health is wide and the way we define health also depends on individual perception, religious beliefs, cultural values, norms, and social class.

2.2. Oral health

As in 1948 WHO expanded the definition of health to mean "a complete state of physical, mental, and social well-being, and not just the absence of infirmity", oral health concept followed this change aiming not minimized oral health as having or not caries. So the concept of oral health (OH) has changed over time, going from a biologist approach, in which the oral cavity contributes to protect the body from infections by chewing and swallowing, to a social and psychological approaches, that take into account other roles of the oral cavity as the contribution that it has in self-esteem, communication and interaction and facial aesthetics. There is a concept of oral health defined by Dolan, who mention that OH means "a comfortable and functional dentition which allows individuals to continue in their desired social role." [3]. This definition already includes the role of OH in the performance of daily activities of the individual. With this we see that oral health is not just a medical condition, but an aggregate of aspects such as the impact that pain may have in daily or the degree of disability or dysfunction. Nowadays the importance of the oral cavity is recognized, as vital part of the human body. It is conceptualized as not only the teeth but others structures as gums, supporting tissues, ligaments, bone, hard and soft palate, soft mucosal tissue tongue, lips, salivary glands, chewing muscles, jaws, and the temporomandibular joints.

Similarly, the Canadian Dental Association defines oral health as "a state of the oral and related tissues and structures that contributes positively to physical, mental and social well-being and enjoyment of life's possibilities, by allowing the individual to speak, eat and socialize unhindered by pain, discomfort or embarrassment". Oral Health and oral cavity should be viewed as a part of a complete body, we must see human beings and their activities and not teeth and tooth decay, thus to recognized the play that oral health has on daily life activities. Clearly, there is an interaction between how we experience quality of life and how we perceive our oral health.

3. Health Related Quality of Life (HRQoL)

The term "quality of life" (QoL) was first used by the British economist Arthur Cecil Pigou in 1920. Later, after World War II, this term was expanded into other areas such as sociology, politics [4] and health, among others. Within the area of health the concept of quality of life was introduced and initially applied in patients with neoplastic disease [5], having a peak in the 90s and essentially incorporating the patient's perception. 4

The World Health Organization (WHO) in 1952 defined the concept of QoL, as "the proper and correct perception that a person has of itself in the cultural context and values on which it is embedded, in relation to its objectives, standards, hopes and concerns. [6]

This perception may be influenced by their physical, psychological, level of independence and social relationships. [7] Later it was considered good health and quality of life to "the absence of disease or defect and the sense of physical, mental and social well-being" or "personal sense of well-being and life satisfaction." Another proposal definition in 2003 by Ventegodt is "to have a nice life and live a life of high quality." [8] Later on it was postulated that "the quality of life has to do with the degree to which an individual can enjoy the possibilities of life". This concept was proposed by the Centre for Health Promotion, University of Toronto. [9]

The variety of definitions and the lack of consensus lead us to think that the term quality of life is only understood on a personal level or as Campbell mentioned: "The QoL is a vague and ethereal concept, something that many people talk about but anybody knows clearly what it really means. [10]

On the other hand, all the above definitions are general definitions of quality of life and not quality of life related to health (HRQoL). Furthermore, it becomes evident that these terms within the medical field have been used interchangeably. Strictly research in the field of health should address processes or limit the scope of the study quality of life related to health, which refers to the effects that the sufferings directly or these treatments can occur in people. [11, 12] HRQoL is the quality of life that relates directly to the state of health of the individual. It is clear and recognized that HRQoL refers to something much broader than health.

The HRQoL assessment in a patient represents the impact that a disease and its subsequent treatment has on the patient's perception of their well-being. One of the existing definitions consider HRQoL as "the subjective assessment of the influence of health status, health care and health promotion on an individual's ability to maintain a level of functioning that allows him to perform activities that are important, and affect overall welfare." [8]

Or, as Patrick and Erickson proposed, HRQoL is the "extent to which the value assigned to duration of life in terms of the perception of physical, psychological, social and diminishing opportunities limitations because of illness value is changed, its sequelae, treatment and / or health policy ". It has also been conceptualized as "the subjective perception, influenced by the current health status, ability to perform those activities important for the individual".4

For this assessment it has been proposed that the most important dimensions of HRQoL are: social, physical and cognitive functioning, mobility and personal care and emotional wellbeing.

HRQoL is an important subjective component so it will depend on the relationship that each individual has with his life. This concept will vary and depend largely on the perception that people has about their physical, mental, social and spiritual state, largely depending on their own values, convictions and beliefs, as well as their personal cultural context and history. [13]

Given the above, to assess HRQoL should be considered the values in which each person lives, that is, the cultural context in which he is immersed, and in the individual expectations and achievements. Similarly, the perception of HRQoL is not equal over time because people change their expectations and aspirations adjusting them to different circumstances.

Clinicians interested in knowing the effects of interventions or treatments also find useful information on HRQoL, as it evaluates the final result of medical interventions at one point, not assessing only according to biological or physiological standards but at emotional and social functional level, it means to evaluate everything that a person represents.

Similarly, this information is also relevant to patients and family members making them aware of areas where their performance is affected by their health, identifying where they may need further help or therapy or supporting them to choose between various options of treatments. Moreover, it has been identified that the assessment of HRQoL in children can be used as a predictor of costs of health care and can help to identify risk groups or to evaluate health services. [14, 15].

4. Oral Health Related Quality of Life (OHRQoL)

Although oral health problems are rarely a matter of life and death they remain a major public health problem because of its prevalence and there are significant indications that oral health problems have social, economic and psychological consequences, this means that they have impact of quality of life.

Nowadays there is a growing interest in recognizing oral health as a component of quality of life, currently the dental research efforts are not only focus on rehabilitating oral-dental diseases, but in exploring the relationship between oral health status and quality of life, in order to evaluate it, improve it and maintain it. In fact, OHRQoL is an integral part of general health and well-being and is recognized by the WHO as an important segment of the Global Oral Health Program. [16]

Oral health-related quality of life was defined as a "self-report specifically pertaining to oral health–capturing both the functional, social and psychological impacts of oral disease" [17]

There is another definition that conceptualizes OHRQoL mentioning that it "reflects people's comfort when eating, sleeping and engaging in social interaction; their self-esteem; and their satisfaction with respect to their oral health". Locker suggested that it is the result of an interaction between and among oral health conditions, social and contextual factors [18] and the rest of the body as Atchison mentioned. [19]

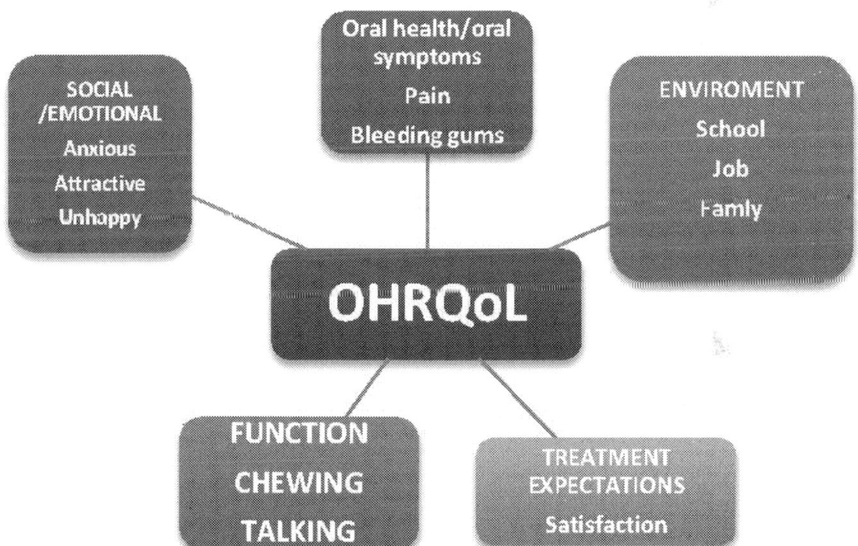

We must keep in mind that OHRQoL deals with conditions that vary in intensity and importance, some of them are life-threatening (e.g. oral cancers) some chronic (caries, periodontitis, etc.) some other dealing with aesthetics (fluorosis, dental anomalies, etc) and other are related to oral pain (pulpitis, dental treatments etc.).

As HRQoL oral health related quality of life is highly subjective and has to be assessed within the framework of patients' conditions, sociocultural environments and own experiences and states of mind: because OHRQoL is related to daily life and is unique to each individual, even patients with severe conditions can report having good quality of life. Furthermore, Quality of Life is by itself multi-faceted, showing variation over time for each individual. [20]

A long the time several oral conditions have been reported in literature as conditions having impact on OHRQoL. An example is **edentulism**, condition that can affect masticatory function, dietary choice, and nutritional level. It has been reported that wearing dentures may interfere with the ability to eat satisfactorily, talk clearly, and laugh freely.

Tooth loss is one of the worst types of damage to oral health, causing esthetic and functional problems. In addition to the biological causes of tooth loss, socioeconomic factors contribute to oral health associated with tooth loss. Socioeconomic status is related to inequalities in health, and socioeconomically disadvantaged people have higher risks of disease and suffer more from health conditions. [21] Several studies have reported an association between tooth loss and OHRQoL.

Some other common oral conditions, such as caries, periodontal disease, which are almost universal in prevalence, and which are chronic but with acute recurring episodes, also impact on QoL. In the same way other condition that might not be as common as the ones mentioned before but which prevalence cannot be considered low as dental fluorosis, craniofacial disorders and oral cancer which can be life treating.

There are several reports showing that **dental caries** has negative impacts on OHRQoL in populations of various ages across the globe, in children [22] and adults. Specially, children with caries whose scores can be about 50% greater than scores for children without caries [23]. Among toddlers and preschool-age early childhood caries (ECC) is one of the most common health problems among children with periodontal disease have lower OHRQoL compared with the general population

Another alteration that affects quality of life is **malocclusio**n. Authors as Onyeaso and Aderinokun in 2003, who conducted a study involving 614 Nigerian children aged 12-18 years, found a correlation between the malocclusion severity and the perception that children have about their dental appearance.

There is an association between the presence of malocclusion with worse OHRoQL. Particularly the one related to lack of space, facial pain has adversely effects of body image, social interaction and daily behavior of the individual. Given the fact that face and mouth appearance influence judgments of facial attractiveness, playing an important role in the development of social and occupational goals. Not only malocclusion but also its treatment has an effect on OHRQoL may also affect QoL through their effect on function and esthetics.

For instance, reports have been made demonstrating striking changes in self-concept and emotional health after **orthodontic and/or surgical treatment** of malocclusions and orofacial defects.

Another alteration that has an impacto n OHRQoL is severe **hypodontia**. It was associated with worse quality of life. Wong and cols. observed that 100% of children reported having impact in the area of oral symptoms, functional limitations in 88%, 55% to 100% emotional and social welfare. The number of missing teeth was associated moderately with the level of impact. One of the main impacts of OHQRL noted in literature was the difficulty chewing, especially among the elderly.

In Uganda, a study aiming to describe the OHRQoL in 12 years of age rural children showed that more than half of them reported oral impact "often" or "every day". Authors concluded that the presence of caries experience or treatment were associated with higher impacts on quality of life. The socially significant fluorosis was associated with greater number of impacts, but not with higher total scores. Despite low levels of oral problems these children experienced impacts on quality of life due to oral problems. Finding that most responsible for these impacts is the presence of caries and fluorosis a lower level. Also **severe fluorosis** can have a negative effect on smile aesthetics and produce functional problems, affecting self-confidence, causing discomfort, and probably disturbing social roles from a young age. [24]

Also **craniofacial disorders** cause impact on OHRQoL including limitations in verbal and nonverbal communication, social interaction, and intimacy. Individuals with facial disfigurements due to craniofacial diseases and conditions and their treatments may experience loss of self-image and self-esteem, anxiety, depression, and social stigma; these in turn may limit educational, career, and marital opportunities and affect other social relations. Diet, nutrition, sleep, psychological status, social interaction, school, and work are affected by impaired oral and craniofacial health.

Documented data, reported in Thailand, suggest that in ninety per cent of pre-adolescents have an impact related to oral health, 74% of 35–44-year olds had daily performances affected by their oral state; 46% reported their emotional stability was affected. Earlier, end points such as recurrence rates and survival were used to evaluate the efficacy of various therapeutic measures in head and neck cancer while patient's quality of life was usually ignored. Presently, the multitudinal impact of maxillofacial tumors on a patient's life has been recognized, which led various researchers to investigate the quality of life of those patients. However, studies evaluating the quality of life of patients with maxillectomy defects and the effect of prosthodontic therapy with obturator prostheses on their quality of life remain rare. A obturator prosthesis is a highly positive and non-invasive approach to improve the quality of life of patients with maxillectomy defects. [25]

Andiappan and cols. performed a meta-analysis and revealed that those receiving treatment for malocclusion and in individuals without malocclusion have significantly better OHRQoL compared to those with such condition [26]

Recent studies of the impact on OHRQoL on children's under general anesthesia treatment have shown significant improvement in oral health and psychological, social and overall wellbeing as well as a positive impact on the family.

Besides clinical conditions, there are other factors that contributed in the impact on OHRQoL as lower family income and sex. In general, women reported a greater impact on OHRQoL than men, although no differences are observed between clinical conditions present in each gender. Differences in the perception of OHRQoL between the genders may be caused by individual and subjective concepts related to beauty and personal esthetic standards, imposed by the social demands and personal needs [27].

5. Instruments to assess OHRQoL

As aforementioned, in the literature has been identified OHRQoL as a multidimensional construct containing physical, social and psychological domains. [28] The clinical indexes do not evaluate these aspects, they only measure the presence and severity of illness, and give scarce consideration to the functionality of the oral cavity as a whole, or to the impact of the symptoms on the patients' quality of life. So the clinical indexes that are commonly used to establish the presence and severity of pathological conditions should be complemented with indicators of social and emotional aspects related to the individual experience and subjective perception of changes in the patients' physical, mental, and social health. [29]

Over the years several socio-dental indicators have been developed, since Cohen and Jago first advocated the development of sociodental indicators. These indicators range from single item to composite inventories or scoring systems, covering the aforementioned OHRQoL domains. So since the 70's, several authors have been given the task to develop and test instruments that may assess the functional, emotional and social effects of oral abnormalities.

All these questionnaires around the world have been developed to measure the impact of oral disease on quality of life which comprising different domains including: pain and inability to perform normal functions of the mouth, sleep disturbances, loss of school days, degree of emotional and social wellbeing. These questionnaires could also potentially be a valuable outcome for evaluating oral health promotion programs and/or service initiatives. 30

5.1. OHRQoL instruments for adults

5.1.1. The Social Impacts of Dental Disease (SIDD) [31]

The SIDD developed in the early 1980s, was one of first socio-dental indicators. Created under a model that defines dental health status in socio-dental terms; the clinical indicators are largely determined by vulnerability whilst the social elements are more directly linked with the degree of social and psychological impact arising from dental diseases. The indicator was tested on large randomly selected samples of industrial workers in Warrington, in the North of England and skilled manual workers and their wives in the South of England.

It was developed as a component of a much broader socio-dental model of dental disease and health behavior so that both the clinical and socio-psychological aspects could be considered within an integrated framework. The model assumes that an individual's present oral health status and treatment needs are influenced by an interplay of three 'dimensions' of background and behavioural factors, namely vulnerability, motivational and preventive dimensions. The score for each individual was constructed from responses to questions relating to those five categories. A total impact score is derived by adding the number of categories. A score of 1 is given to the impact category if a positive response has been given to any of the questions in the category. Two total impact scores were used, one including (total score 0-5) and one excluding discomfort (totaL score 0-4) to see the difference if this relatively common problem was excluded.

5.1.2. Geriatric (General) Oral Health Assessment Index (GOHAI) [32]

The GOHAI is one of the most commonly used scales in assessment of OHRQoL it was developed by Kathryn Atchison and Dolan in 1990 in the USA for use with elderly populations. It is compounded by 12-items developed with three months' time reference, with five (six in the original) Likert scale options, scoring as 'often', always', 'seldom 'or 'sometimes' and 'never' reflecting the aspects that are considered to have an impact upon the quality of life of the older population. Nonetheless it was created for geriatric populations some author have used it with younger adult populations, which is reflected in the interchangeable us of the names Geriatric or General Oral Health Assessment Index. It was developed to evaluate three dimensions of OHRQoL including physical functions like eating, chewing, speech, swallowing; psychosocial functions like worry, limitations and discomfort with social contacts, dissatisfaction with appearance; and self-consciousness about oral health, pain or discomfort including the use of medication or discomfort from the mouth. The GOHAI score is determined by summing the final score of each of the12 items.

The GOHAI gives a greater weight to functional limitations or pain and discomfort. According to the research of Hassel et al., the GOHAI seems to be more appropriate when focusing on subjective oral health with minor clinical changes and immediate clinical aspects. [33]

This questionnarie has been tested on a variety of sample of subjects, of different ages, races and the reliability testes show that this instrument is acceptable in all samples tested thus far. It has also been translated and validated to a wide range of languages.

5.1.3 The Dental Impact Profile (DIP) [34]

This instrument was developed by Ronald Strauss. It consist in twenty-five items that have been placed in non-apparent order and respondents are offered three ordinal response choices (good effect, bad effect, no effect) about whether teeth or dentures have had an effect on various aspects of life. A response of "good effect" was seen as likely to be most socially acceptable and the potential for response bias in the positive direction exists. While "good effect" and "bad effect" response categories have meaning independently, they may be combined in the estimation of dental impact. Dental impact is noted for an item if teeth are seen to have an effect on that aspect of life, whether that effect is positive or negative. Responses of "no effect" are seen as indication of no dental impact. The four subscales and component items were:

1. Eating Subscale: Eating, Chewing and Biting, Enjoyment of eating, Food choice, Tasting

2. Health/Well-Being Subscale: Feeling comfortable, Enjoyment of life, General happiness, General health, Appetite, Weight, Living a long life

3. Social Relations Subscale: Facial appearance to other people, Facial appearance (to self), Smiling and laughing, Moods, Speech, Breath, Confidence around others, Attendance at activities, Success at work

4. Romance Subscale: Social Life, Romantic relationships, Having sex appeal, Kissing,

5.1.4. Dental impact on daily living (DIDL) [35]

Developed by Leao & Sheiham in 1996. The Dental Impact on Daily Living (DIDL) is a socio-dental measure which assesses five dimensions of quality of life comfort, appearance, pain, daily activities, eating. Comfort, related to complaints such as bleeding gums and food packing; Appearance, consisting of self-image; Pain; Performance, the ability to carry out daily activities and to interact with people; and Eating restriction, relating to difficulties in biting and chewing. The measure consists of a questionnaire of 36 items, which assesses the oral impacts on daily living, and a scale, which is a graphical representation of a method developed by Leao to assess the importance respondents attribute to the different dimensions involved. Items are summed into a score for each dimension. To compute the score, coded responses within each dimension were summed and divided by the number of items, resulting in a dimension score (For example, Appearance has four questions. The score for this dimension would be the sum of coded responses for all four questions divided by four). Impacts were coded as '+1' for positive impacts, 0 for impacts not totally negatives and '-1' for negative impacts. To construct a final score, questions within each category are summed and divided by the number of items, giving a score for each dimension. Before adding the different dimensions, they receive the respective weight attributed on the scale, otherwise it would be assumed that they were equally important. Then the five dimensions are finally added to give a final score.

One aspect to be highlighted in DIDL is the degree of flexibility offered in terms of aggregating and disaggregating data (either individual items, dimension scores or total score). Although criticized, a total score reproduces the total impact subjects are experiencing, and since dimensions sometimes may not impact separately, it appears important to have this view of the individual as a whole. Another point to be stressed is that in the total score generated by DIDL, weights attributed to dimensions (by each respondent) are personal. That is, the importance attributed to a dimension by a given individual is directly associated with his or her own impacts on that dimension. [36]

5.1.5. Oral health quality of life inventory

Developed by Cornell et al. in 1997, they included 56 questions divided 4 domains: oral health, nutrition, self-rated oral health, overall quality of life. It is part of a larger home-based interview, the Oral Health Quality of Life Interview (OHQOLI)*. In addition to the OH-QoL, OHQOLI includes self-report assessments of oral health and functional status (SROH), a Nutrition Quality of Life Index (NutQoL), and an interview version of the Quality of Life Inventory (QOLI). [37] The final OHQOLI interview has 40 SROH items, 15 OH-QoL items, and 9 NutQoL items. The OH-QoL items are distributed among the related SROH items. Thus, the subjective well-being items appear immediately following the related objective functional status items in the questionnaire. The overall format of the OHQOLI is designed for interviewer administration.

5.1.6. Oral Health Impact Profile (OHIP) [38]

The OHIP, developed by Slade & Spencer is the most widely used OHRQoL questionnaire. It is based on Locker's adaptation of the World Health Organisation's classification of impairments, disabilities and handicaps (Locker, 1988). The OHIP contains 49 assessing seven dimensions of impacts of oral conditions on people's OHRQoL including functional limitation, physical pain, psychological discomfort, physical disability, psychological disability, social disability and handicap.

A short version, OHIP-14, was later developed based on a subset of 2 questions for each of the 7 dimensions. [39] It is patient-centered, gives a greater weight to psychological and behavioral outcomes, is better at detecting psychosocial impacts among individuals and groups, and better meets the main criteria for the measurement of OHRQoL.[33] The OHIP 14 responses, "never", "hardly ever", "occasionally", "fairly often", and "very often", were codified from 0 to 4, respectively. Each of the 14 questions was assigned a score of 0 if the response was "never," and a score of 1 if the response was "hardly ever", "occasionally", "fairly often," or "very often," dichotomizing responses into no impact versus some impact. The scores assigned to the responses to the 14 questions are added to obtain values between 0 and 14. [40]

There also exist the OHIP-aesthetic which is a modified short form of the OHIP derived (OHIP-conceptual) that is most favorable in discriminating dental aesthetics, showing to be reliable and most sensitive to the dental aesthetics intervention-tooth whitening. [41]

5.1.7. Oral Impacts on Daily Performance (OIDP)

The OIDP aims to provide an alternative sociodental indicator which focuses on measuring the serious oral impacts on the person's ability to perform daily activities. It is one of many self-reported inventories to assess OHRQoL in terms of adverse impacts that oral conditions can have on everyday life experiences.

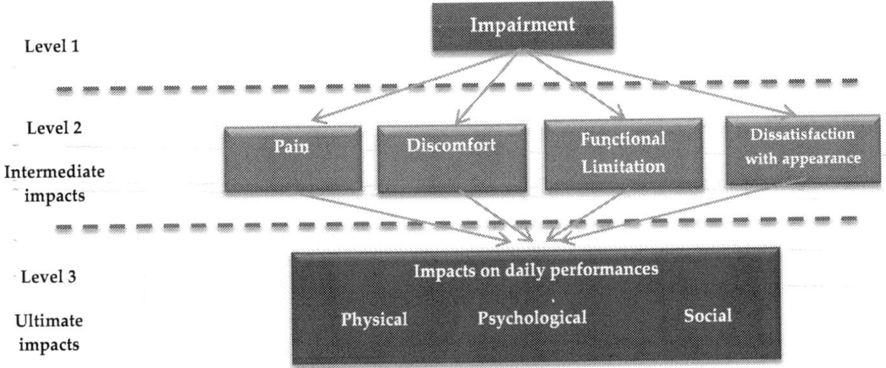

Figure 1. Theoretical framework of consequences of oral impacts

The theoretical framework of OIDP is presented in Figure 1. This is a modified model from the WHO International Classification of Impairments, Disabilities and Handicaps amended for dentistry by Locker. [42] In this modification different levels of consequence variables were established. The first level refers to the oral status, including oral impairments, which most clinical indices attempt to measure. The second level, "the intermediate impacts", includes the possible earliest negative impacts caused by oral health status: pain, discomfort or functional limitation. Dissatisfaction with appearance was added in this level since studies indicated that it was a major dimension of oral health outcomes. In addition, functional limitation may cause pain, discomfort or dissatisfaction with appearance and vice versa. The third level, or the "ultimate impacts" represents impacts on ability to perform daily activities which consists of physical, psychological and social performances. Any of the dimensions in the second level may impact on performance ability. This third level is equivalent to disability and handicap dimensions in the WHO model. The OIDP concentrates only on the measurement of "ultimate" oral impacts, thus covering the fields of disability and handicap.

The OIDP has been demonstrated to have appropriate psychometric properties when applied in population based cross-sectional surveys of elderly in Norway 43, Sweden 44, Greece and UK, Tanzania, Bosnia 45, Brazil, Thailand, among others. Studies have shown that OIDP is associated in the expected direction with self-reported oral health and clinical indicators and that personal-, socio-demographic-, and health care service related factors modify those relationships.

There are other questionnaires adapted to specific conditions/domains as the Orthognathic QOL Questionnaire, SOOQ for orthodontic surgery, OHRQOL for Dental Hygiene, The prosthetic quality of life (PQL), Quality of Life with Implant-Prostheses' (QoLIP-10)

5.1.8. The prosthetic quality of life (PQL) [46]

The PQL, created by Javier Montero and collaborators, is compounded by 11 items and can be applied in epidemiological studies or clinical trials with no special cost as regards the time required for exploration. It has a bipolar design of the responses of the items of the PQL that allows both negative and positive impacts to be recorded, such that the assessment of the physical, psychological and social well-being deriving from the use of dental prostheses, condition that makes it more complete than questionnaires limited to evaluating the presence of negative impact. Responses: Yes, a lot (1),Yes, slightly (2), It's more or less the same (3), I think it's worse (4), It's much worse (5).

5.1.9. Quality of Life with Implant-Prostheses' (QoLIP-10) [47]

Preciado and colaborators designed this instrumet of the 10-item scale that gather information on global oral satisfaction, socio-demographic, health-behavioural, clinical and prosthetic-related data. This questionnaire has shown to be reliable and valid. The factor analysis confirmed the existence of three dimensions and meaningful inter-correlations among the 10 items. The QoLIP-10 index confirmed its psychometric capacity for assessing the OHRQoL of implant overdenture and hybrid prosthesis wearers. Authors suggest that this instrument may be recommended for determining the influence of implant-retained overdentures and hybrid prostheses on the well-being of future patients.

5.2. OHRQoL instruments for children

During the past decade, several instruments have been developed to detect the impact of oral health on children's quality of life.

Questionnaire	Abbreviation	Original Language	Year	Validated in other languages as
Social Impacts of Dental Disease	SIDD	English	1980	
Sickness Impact Profile	SIP	English	1985	
The General (Geriatric) Oral Health Assessment	GOHAI	English	1990	French [48], German [49], Mandarin Chinese [50], Arabic [51], Swedish [52], Malay [53], Arabic [54], Turkey [55], Hindi [56] Spanish [57], Portuguese [58]
Dental Impact Profile	DIP	English	1993	
Oral Health Impact Profile	OHIP	English	1994	Korean, Chinese. Swedish, Portuguese, Japanese, Hungarian, Dutch, German, Hebrew, Croatian, Slovenian, Sinhalese, Persian, Italian
Dental Impact on Daily Living	DDIDL	English	1996	
Oral Impact Daily Performance	OIDP	English	2011	Portugues, Greece, Thai, Kannada [59], Swedish, Bosnian, Norwegian
	OIDP abreviado		2012	India [60], Albanian
Prosthetic quality of life questionnaire	PQL	English	2007	
Quality of Life with Implant-Prostheses'	QoLIP-10	English	2013	

Table 1. Questionnaires to asses OHRQoL in adults

5.2.1. Child Perception Questionnaire (CPQ11–14) [61]

In 2002, Jokovic et al. developed the Child Perceptions Questionnaire (CPQ), which is one of the first instruments used to evaluate OHRQoL in children. In addition to the CPQ, there is a Parent's Perceptions Questionnaire (P-CPQ) [62] and a Family Impact Scale (FIS) [63], which is compound a battery of instruments that provide information at different levels and perspectives for OHRQoL in children.

The CPQ has two versions, one is the CPQ_{11-14} for children from 11 to 14 years of age; the other, which is the CPQ_{8-10}, is for children aged 8 to 10 years. Both aim to evaluate the impact of oral and orofacial conditions in children at a functional, emotional, and social level.

The CPQ_{11-14} was constructed using a systematic multistage process based on the theory of measurement and scale development. It is one of the most used instruments which is composed of 37 items divided into four domains or subscales: oral symptoms (n=6), functional limitations (n=9), emotional well-being (n=9) and social well-being (n=13). The questions ask about the frequency of events in the previous three months in relation to the child's oral/oro-facial condition. The response options are: 'Never'=0; 'Once/twice'=1; 'Sometimes'=2; 'Often'=3;

'Everyday/almost every day'=4. The questionnaire also contains global ratings of the child's oral health and the extent to which the oral/oro-facial condition affected his/her overall well-being. They are worded as follows: "Would you say that the health of your teeth, lips, jaws and mouth is..." and "How much does the condition of your teeth, lips, jaws or mouth affect your life overall?" A 5-point response format ranging from 'Excellent'=0 to 'Poor'=4 and from 'Not at all'=0 to 'Very much'=4, respectively, is offered for these ratings.

The CPQ_{11-14} performs well as a discriminative measure, being able to distinguish between the three groups. Jokovic and co-workers developed short-forms versions of the CPQ_{11-14} using two different approaches. This resulted in developed two short versions to facilitate the administration of the questionnaire in clinical settings (16-item short-form) and in epidemiological surveys involving general populations (8-item short-form). Important to mention is that if an 8-item version could be used as an overall scale scores but not analysis is possible at the level of the individual domains. The number of items per domain is insufficient for this purpose. [64]

5.2.2. Child Perceptions Questionnaire 8-10 (CPQ 8-10) [65]

The CPQ_{8-10} contains 29 questions. The first two relate to demographic information; the next two pertain to global items; and the remaining twenty-five are divided into four domains: oral symptoms (OS), functional limitation (FL), emotional well-being (EW), and social well-being (SW). The questionnaire registers problems occurring during a prior four-week period. The responses are recorded in a Likert scale from 0 to 4, where 0=never; 1=once or twice; 2=sometimes; 3=often; and 4=every day or almost every day. The maximum score is 100, and the minimum is 0. For the global question concerning the general perception of oral health, the possible responses are 0=very good, 1=good, 2=OK, 3=poor. Regarding the second global question: How much does oral health affect daily living? With a scale as follows: 0=not at all, 1=a little bit, 2=some, 3=a lot.

Recently Foster and cols. suggested that these two questionnaires to be acceptable to be used in younger age group, since 5 years of age. They proposed to use a single questionnaire, CPQ_{8-10} or the short CPQ_{11-14}, to evaluated OHRQoL in children from 5 to 14 years of age [66], thus facilitating the use in prospective studies following children through different life stages.

5.2.3. Parental-Caregiver Perceptions Questionnaire — P-CPQ lxii and Family Impact Scale — FIS

The P-CPQ has 31 items distributed into 4 subscales: 6 oral symptoms (OS), 8 functional limitations (FL), 7 emotional wellbeing (EWB) and 10 social wellbeing (SWB). The questions refer only to the frequency of events in the previous 3 months. The items have 5 Likert response options: 'never=0', 'once or twice=1', 'sometimes=2', 'often=3', 'every day or almost every day=4'. A 'don't know' response also was permitted and scored as 0. Global ratings of the child's oral health and impact of the oral condition on his or her overall wellbeing were obtained from the parents/caregivers. The global ratings had a 5-point response format from 'excellent=0' to 'poor=4' for oral health and 'not at all=0' to 'very much=4' for wellbeing. The P-CPQ score is calculated by summing the response codes to all 31 items and dividing this sum by the number of items for which a valid response is obtained. The P-CPQ was developed for use with younger children and provides a measure of a child's OHRQoL. Where both parental and child reports are used, the P-CPQ can be regarded as complementing the latter, thus providing a comprehensive profile of a child's health and well-being.

The FIS is included in the P-CPQ and consists of 14 items that attempted to capture the effect of a child's oral or oro-facial condition on four domains: related to parental and family activities with 5 questions, parental emotions (4questions), family conflict (4 questions) and family finances (1 question). The questions ask about the frequency of events in the previous 3 months. Response options for the four domains and the respective scores were: 'Never' (scoring 0); 'Once or twice' (1); 'Sometimes' (2); 'Often' (3); and 'Everyday' or 'Almost every day' (4). A 'Don't know' (DK) response was also allowed. The FIS scores are computed by summing all of the item scores. Scores for each of the four domains can also be computed. The final score could vary from 0 to 56, for which a higher score denoted a greater degree of the impact of child's oral conditions on the functioning of parents-caregivers and the family as a whole.

In 2013 Thomson and cols developed the short form of the P CPQ [67] obtaining a 16 and 8 item short-form versions of the P-CPQ and FIS-8 short forms that were developed using data from two New Zealand pre/post-test interventional studies. The internal reliability, validity and responsiveness of the short-form versions were acceptable. [68]

5.2.4. Child Oral Impacts on Daily Performances [69]

The C-OIDP index is specifically designed to show the final impact of a number of oral health related conditions which can affect child's daily life. it is a short and enjoyable questionnaire, and relatively quick to administer. The modification of the OIDP included adjusting the language, changing the sequence of questions, simplifying index scales and shortening the recall period. When the index had been validated, pictures of performances were developed and tested in order to make the interview more practical. It was developed and tested among 11–12 year old Thai children. Eight activities are considered: eating, speaking, cleaning teeth, relaxing, emotion, and smiling, studying, and social contact.

The 0–5 scale was changed into 0–3 scale on the computer, by grouping together scores of 1 and 2, and scores of 4 and 5.

The index score is based on the score for each of these eight daily activities. The score for each activity is obtained by multiplying the frequency value by the severity value; the maximum score is therefore 3x3=9. Thus, the score scale for each activity is between 0 and 9. The total score is calculated by adding the scores for all activities, divided by the maximum score possible (8x9=72) and multiplying by 100. The index score ranges therefore between 0 100.

The C-OIDP has two modes of the same questionnaire: bone is interviewer-administered and the other is self-administered, and the latter is used in this validation for adolescents. Both modes have been shown to produce similar results.

5.2.5. *The Child Oral Health Impact Profile [70]*

The COHIP consists of 34 questions grouped into five domains measuring: oral health, functional well-being, socio-emotional well-being, school performance and self-image. This instrument was designed to measure self-reported OHRQoL in children 8-15 years of age, using both positive and negative questions. It was created by an international study and was simultaneously validated in the U.S.A., Great Britain, Spain, Portugal, China, France and Holland in 2007. Data reported suggest that this instrument has an acceptable validity and reliability (Cronbach's alpha 0.91, 0.84 CCI) to be applied in population of 8 to 15 years.

	Questionnaire	Original Language	Abbreviation	year	Validated in other languages
Child Oral Health Quality of Life Questionnaire COHQOL	Child Perception Questionnaire 11-14	English	CPQ_{11-14}	2005	Árabic, [73] Portugués [74], Chinese, [75] German [76], Italian, Cambodian [77], Danish [78]
	CPQ11-14 Short form	English		2006	Portuges, Arabic 79
	Child Perception Questionnaire 8-10	English	CPQ_{8-10}	2004	Spanish [80] Portugués, Danés, Bosnian
	Family Impact Scale	English	FIS	2007	Chinese, Portugués [81]
	Parental-Caregiver Perceptions Questionnaire	English	P-CPQ	2003	Chinese, Peruvian Spanish [82]
Child Oral Impacts of Daily Performance		English	Child-OIDP	2008	Spanish [83] Canarain Portugues, Swahilli, Malayan, French, Hebrew [84]
OIDP abreviated		English		2012	Indial [9] Albanian
Child Oral Health Impact Profile		English	COHIP[29]	2008	Spanish Persian [85] Corean [86]
Early Childhood Oral Health Impact Scale		English	ECOHIS[27]		Turkey [87], Persian [88] Chinese [89]. French [90] Lituan [91], Portugues [92]
Scale of Oral Health Outcomes		English	SOHO-5	2013	Portugues

Table 2. Questionnaires to asses OHRQoL in children

5.2.6. The Early Childhood Oral Health Impact Scale (ECOHIS) [71]

It was designed to evaluate OHRQoL of children of preschool age and younger. The ECOHIS consists of 13 questions relevant to preschool-age children. The survey questionnaire relies on parental ratings of the 13 items grouped in two main parts: the child impact section and the family impact section. The child impact section covers four domains: child symptoms (1 item), child functions (4 items), child psychology (2 items), and child self-image and social interaction (2 items). The family impact section covers two domains: parental distress (2 items) and family function (2 items). Each question asks about the frequency of an oral health-related problem and is scored on a scale from 0–5, as follows: never (score 0), hardly ever (score 1), occasionally (score 2), often (score 3), very often (score 4), don't know (score 5).

5.2.7. Scale of Oral Health Outcomes (SOHO) [72]

As dental caries is a chronic disease that can affect children from a very young age and it is important to measure its impacts on quality of life, as they may affect the psychological, social and educational development of the first self-reported OHRQoL measure among 5 year-old children. All inter-item correlations were positive and none was very high, and all item total correlation coefficients were above the recommended level of 0.2

Cronbach's alpha was 0.74. Despite the positive initial results, the assessment of this questionnaire should be an on-going process, by extending psychometric testing to properties not evaluated so far, and assessing its applicability and performance in other populations.

6. Conclusions

Multiple definitions have been postulated to conceptualize HRQoL and OHRQoL and in spite of there are different concepts we can see in every single one that quality of life refers to something much broader than health than physical status, it promotes to see a human being and his environment.

Important to mention that the assessments in the area of health are usually performed by the "professional" and although this is deemed appropriate, they often do not reflect the complex set of feelings that patient has about having or not having good health and quality of life. Therefore, relevant information about the quality of life is of practical importance for various actors in the health sector such as the health policy makers, health services researchers, epidemiologists, health program evaluators, who should underpin and complement their decisions based on this information. The evaluation of these concepts should not substitute clinical ones; rather those should complement them so to take into account the patient's own perception of their health, expectations, desires and needs. In this sense it is accepted and recognized by dental community that oral health status can cause considerable pain and suffering, dentists should not be only focus on physical status but in subjective evaluations about how people feel and how much they are satisfied or affected with their own oral condition.

The evaluation of OHRQoL promotes a shift from traditional dental criteria assessment and care that focus on a person's social and emotional experience and physical functioning in defining appropriate treatment goals and outcomes.

Author details

Javier de la Fuente Hernández, Fátima del Carmen Aguilar Díaz* and María del Carmen Villanueva Vilchis

*Address all correspondence to: fatimaguilar@gmail.com

Escuela Nacional de Estudios Superiores Unidad León – UNAM, León, Gto, México

References

[1] World Health Organization. Ottawa charter for health promotion. 1986.

[2] World Health Organization. Health promotion: a discussion document; 1984. 1984.

[3] Dolan T. Identification of appropriate outcomes for an aging population. SpecCareDent 1993;13(1):35–9.

[4] Schawartzmann L. Calidad de vida relacionada a la salud: aspectos conceptuales. Ciencia y Enfermería IX (2):9.21, 2003.

[5] Leplege A, Hunt S. The problem of quality of Life in Medicine. JAMA. 1997;278(1): 47-50.

[6] The World Health Organization Quality of Life assessment (WHOQOL): position paper from the World Health Organization. SocSci Med 1995;41:1403-9.

[7] World Health Organization, Concepts and methods of community-based initiatives. Community-Based Initiatives Series, Geneva: World Health Organization; 2003.

[8] Monés J. ¿Se puede medir la calidad de vida? ¿Cuál es su importancia?. CirEsp 2004; 76(2):71-1.

[9] Slade Gary D. Measuring Oral Health and Quality of Life, Department of Dental Ecology, School of Dentistry, University of North Carolina, September, 1997.

[10] Palomino B, López PG. (Programa de la Socialdemocracia Alemania 1974:58), Nota crítica: Reflexiones sobre la Calidad de Vida y el Desarrollo, Región y Sociedad, Ene-Jun, vol XI, número 17, El colegio de Sonora, pp.171-185.

[11] Testa MA, Simonson DC. Assessment of quality of life outcomes. N Enl J Med 1996;334:835-840.

[12] Gill T, Feinstein A. A critical appraisal of the quality of life measurements. JAMA 1994;272:619-625.

[13] Locker, D. Measuring Oral Health And Quality Of Life: Concepts Of Oral Health, Disease And Quality Of Life; University of North Carolina, Canada; 1997; 11-24.

[14] Williams J, Wake M, Hesketh. Health–Related Quality of Life of Overweight and Obese Children. JAMA. 2005;293(1):70-6

[15] Seid M, Varna JW, Segall D, Kurtin PS. Health-related quality of life as a predictor of pediatric healthcare costs: a two year prospective cohort analysis. Health and Quality of Life Outcomes. 2004, 2:48.

[16] WHO (2003). The World Oral Health Report 2003: continuous improvement of oral health in the 21st century—the approach of the WHO Global Oral Health Programme. Geneva, Switzerland: World Health Organization

[17] Gift HC, Atchison KA. Oral health, health, and health-related quality of life. Medical Care 1995; 33:NS57-NS77.

[18] Locker D, Jokovic A, Tompson B (2005). Health-related quality of life of children aged 11 to 14 years with orofacial conditions. Cleft Palate Craniofac J 42:260-266

[19] Atchison KA, Shetty V, Belin TR, Der-Martirosian C, Leathers R, Black E, et al. (2006). Using patient self-report data to evaluate orofacial surgical outcomes. Community Dent Oral Epidemiol34:93-102.

[20] Jean-Louis SixoubHow to make a link between Oral Health-Related Quality of Life and dentin hypersensitivity in the dental office?Clin Oral Investig. 2013 March; 17(Suppl 1): 41–44. Published online 2012 December 23. doi: 10.1007/s00784-012-0915-x

[21] Sheiham A, Alexander D, Cohen L, Marinho V, Moysés S, Petersen PE, et al. Global Oral Health Inequalities: Task Group-Implementation and delivery of oral health strategies. Adv Dent Res. 2011May;23(2):259-67.

[22] Lee, G. H., McGrath, C., Yiu, C. K., & King, N. M. (2010). A comparison of a generic and oral health-specific measure in assessing the impact of early childhood caries on quality of life. Community Dentistry and Oral Epidemiology, 38, 333–339.

[23] Huntington, N. L., Spetter, D., Jones, J. A., Rich, S. E., Garcia, R. I., & Spiro, A, 3rd. (2011). Development and validation of a measure of pediatric oral health-related quality of life: the POQL. Journal of Public Health Dentistry, 71, 185–193.

[24] Robinson, P.G., Nalweyiso, N., Busingye, J., Whitworth, J. (2005). Subjective impacts of dental caries and fluorosis in rural Uganda children. Community Dental Health, 22(4), 231-236.

[25] Pradeep Kumar, Habib Ahmad Alvi, JitendraRao, BalendraPratap Singh, Sunit Kumar Jurel, Lakshya Kumar, Himanshi Aggarwal. Assessment of the quality of life in maxillectomy patients: A longitudinal study. J AdvProsthodont 2013;5:29-35

[26] Andiappan M, Gao W, Bernabé E, Kandala NB, Donaldson AN, Malocclusion, orthodontic treatment, and the Oral health Impact Profile (OHIP-14) Systematic review and meta-analysis.Angle Orthod. 2014 Aug 26. [Epub ahead of print]

[27] BATISTA, MariliaJesus, PERIANES, Lílian Berta Rihs, HILGERT, Juliana Balbinot, HUGO, Fernando Neves, & SOUSA, Maria da Luz Rosário de. (2014). The impacts of oral health on quality of life in working adults. Brazilian Oral Research, 28(1), 1-6. Epub August 26, 2014. Retrieved September 15, 2014, from http://www.scielo.br/scielo.php?script=sci_arttext&pid=S1806-83242014000100249&lng=en&tlng=en. 10.1590/1807-3107BOR-2014.vol28.0040

[28] Slade GD, Assessing oral health outcomes: Measuring oral health and quality of life : proceedings of a conference held June 13-14, at the University of North Carolina-Chapel Hill, North Carolina. Chapel Hill, N.C., Department of Dental Ecology, School of Dentistry, University of North Carolina; 1997:IX, 160 s.

[29] Gherunpong S, Tsakos G, Sheiham A. A sociodental approach to assessing dental needs of children: Concept and models. Int J PaediatrDent. 2006;16:81-8.

[30] Sischo L, Broder HL.Oral health-related quality of life: what, why, how, and future implications.J Dent Res. 2011 Nov;90(11):1264-70. doi: 10.1177/0022034511399918. Epub 2011 Mar 21.

[31] Aubrey Sheiham, Annie M. Cushing, Joan Maizels M.A.,THE SOCIAL IMPACTS OF DENTAL DISEASE. MEASURING ORAL HEALTH AND QUALITY OF LIFE, 1996

[32] Atchison KA, Dolan TA: Development of the Geriatric Oral Health Assessment Index. J Dent Educ 1990, 54:680-687. /

[33] Locker D, Matear D, Stephens M, Lawrence H, Payne B: Comparison of the GOHAI and OHIP-14 as measures of the oral health-related quality of life of the elderly. Community Dent Oral Epidemiol 2001, 29:373-381

[34] Strauss RP, Hunt RJ. Understanding the value of teeth to older adults: Influences on quality of life. Journal of Am. Dent. Assoc. 1993; 124: 105-110.

[35] Leao AT, Sheilam A. The development of a socio-dental measure of dental impacts on daily living. Community Dent. Health 1996; 13: 22-26.

[36] Aubrey Sheiham, Anna T. Leao. THE DENTAL IMPACT ON DAILY LIVING..Measuring Oral Health and Quality of Life, 1996;98:1351–87.

[37] Frisch MB, Cornell J, Villanueva M, Retzlaff PJ. Clinical Validation of the quality of life inventory: A measure of life satisfaction for use in treatment planning and outcome assessment. Psychological Assessment

[38] Slade G D, Spencer A S: Development and evaluation of the oral health impact pro‐ file. Community Dent Health 11: 3–11 (1994)

[39] Slade, G.D.Derivation and validation of a short-form oral health impact profile. Com‐ munity Dentistry Oral Epidemiology 1997 25: 284-290

[40] Locker D, Allen PF. Developing short-form measures of oral health-related quality of life. J Public Health Dent. 2002 Winter; 62(1):13-20

[41] Wong AH, Cheung CS, McGrath C. Developing a short form of Oral Health Impact Profile (OHIP) for dental aesthetics: OHIP-aesthetic.Community Dent Oral Epide‐ miol. 2007 Feb;35(1):64-72.

[42] Locker D. Measuring oral health: A conceptual framework. Community Dent Health 1988; 5:3-18.

[43] Astrom AN, Haugejorden O, Skaret E, Trovik TA, Klock KS: Oral Impacts on Daily Performance in Norwegian adults: the influence of age, number of missing teeth, and socio-demographic factors.Eur J Oral Sci 2006, 114(?):115-121.

[44] Ostberg AL, Andersson P, Hakeberg M: Cross-cultural adaptation and validation of the oral Iimpacts on daily performances (OIDP) in Swedish. Swed Dent J 2008, 32(4): 187-195

[45] Eric J, Stancic I, Sojic LT, JelenkovicPopovac A, Tsakos G: Validity and reliability of the Oral Impacts on Daily Performance (OIDP) scale in the elderly population of Bos‐ nia and Herzegovina.Gerodontology 2012, 29(2):e902-e908

[46] Montero J, Bravo M, Lo´pez-Valverde A. Development of a specific indicator of the well-being of wearers of removable dentures. Community Dent Oral Epidemiol 2011; 39: 515–524

[47] Preciado A1, Del Río J, Lynch CD, Castillo-Oyagüe R. A new, short, specific ques‐ tionnaire (QoLIP-10) for evaluating the oral health-related quality of life of implant-retained overdenture and hybrid prosthesis wearers J Dent. 2013 Sep;41(9):753-63. doi: 10.1016/j.jdent.2013.06.014. Epub 2013 Jul 2.

[48] Tubert-Jeannin S, Riordan PJ, Morel-Papernot A, Porcheray S, Saby-Collet S: Valida‐ tion of an oral health quality of life index (GOHAI) in France. Community Dent Oral Epidemiol 2003, 31:275-284.

[49] Hassel AJ, Rolko C, Koke U, Leisen J, RammelsbergP.Community Dent Oral Epide‐ miol. 2008 Feb;36(1):34-42. doi: 10.1111/j.1600-0528.2007.00351.

[50] A-Dan W, Jun-Qi L. Factors associated with the oral health-related quality of life in elderly persons in dental clinic: validation of a Mandarin Chinese version of GOHAI. Gerodontology. 2011 Sep;28(3):184–91.

[51] AtiehMA.Gerodontology. 2008 Mar;25(1):34-41. doi: 10.1111/j.1741-2358.2007.00195.x. Epub 2008 Jan 13.

[52] Hägglin C, Berggren U, Lundgren J. A Swedish version of the GOHAI index. Psychometric properties and validation. Swed Dent J. 2005;29(3):113–24.

[53] Othman WN, Muttalib KA, Bakri R, Doss JG, Jaafar N, Salleh NC, et al. Validation of the Geriatric Oral Health Assessment Index (GOHAI) in the Malay language. J Public Health Dent. 2006 Ago 18;66(3):199-204.

[54] Daradkeh S, Khader YS. Translation and validation of the Arabic version of the Geriatric Oral Health Assessment Index (GOHAI). J Oral Sci. 2008 Dec;50(4):453–9.

[55] Ergül S, Akar GC. Reliability and validity of the Geriatric Oral Health Assessment Index in Turkey. J GerontolNurs. 2008 Sep;34(9):33–9.

[56] Deshmukh SP, Radke UM. Translation and validation of the Hindi version of the Geriatric Oral Health Assessment Index. Gerodontology. 2012 Jun;29(2):e1052–8.

[57] Sánchez-García S, Heredia-Ponce E, Juárez-Cedillo T, Gallegos-Carrillo K, Espinel-Bermúdez C, de la Fuente-Hernández J et al. Psychometric properties of the General Oral Health Assessment Index (GOHAI) and dental status of an elderly Mexican population. J PublicHealthDent. 2010;70(4):300–7.

[58] CAMPOS, Juliana Alvares Duarte Bonini, CARRASCOSA, AndréaCorrêa, ZUCOLOTO, MirianeLucindo, & MAROCO, João. (2014). Validation of a measuring instrument for the perception of oral health in women. Brazilian Oral Research, 28(1), 1-7. Epub August 18, 2014. Retrieved September 12, 2014, from http://www.scielo.br/scielo.php?script=sci_arttext&pid=S1806-83242014000100244&lng=en&tlng=en. 10.1590/1807-3107BOR-2014.vol28.0033.

[59] Agrawal N, Pushpanjali K, GargAK.The cross cultural adaptation and validity of the child-OIDP scale among school children in Karnataka, South India. Community Dent Health. 2013 Jun;30(2):124-6

[60] Usha GV, Thippeswamy HM, Nagesh L. Validity and reliability of Oral Impacts on Daily Performances Frequency Scale: a cross-sectional survey among adolescents. J ClinPediatr Dent. 2012 Spring;36(3):251-6.

[61] Jokovic A, Locker D, Stephens M, Kenny D, Tompson B, Guyatt G. Validity and reliability of a questionnaire for measuring child oral-health-related quality of life. J Dent Res. 2002 Jul; 81(7):459-63.

[62] Jokovic A, Locker D, Stephens M, Kenny D,Tompson B, Guyatt G. Measuring parental perceptions of child oral health-related quality of life.J Public Health Dent. 2003;63:67-72.

[63] Locker D, Jokovic A, Stephens M, Kenny D, Tompson B, Guyatt G. Family impact of child oral and oro-facial conditions. Community Dent Oral Epidemiol. 2002;30:438-48

[64] Jokovic A, Locker D, Guyatt G. Short forms of the Child Perceptions Questionnaire for 11–14-year-old children (CPQ11–14): Development and initial evaluation. Health

Qual Life Outcomes. 2006; 4: 4.Published online Jan 19, 2006. doi: 10.1186/1477-7525-4-4

[65] Jokovic A, Locker D, Tompson B, Guyatt G. Questionnaire for measuring oral health-related quality of life in eight-to ten-year-old children. Pediatr Dent. 2004;26:512-8.

[66] Foster Page et al. Do we need more than one Child Perceptions Questionnaire for children and adolescents? BMC Oral Health 2013, 13:26

[67] Thomson WM, Foster Page LA, Gaynor WN, Malden PE. Short-form versions of the Parental-Caregivers Perceptions Questionnaire and the Family Impact Scale. Community Dent Oral Epidemiol 2013; 41: 441–450.

[68] Thomson WM, Foster Page LA, Gaynor WN, Malden PE. Short-form versions of the Parental-Caregivers Perceptions Questionnaire and the Family Impact Scale. Community Dent Oral Epidemiol 2013; 41: 441–450.

[69] Gherunpong S, Tsakos G, Sheiham A: Developing and evaluating an oral health-related quality of life index for children; the CHILD-OIDP. Community Dent Health 2004, 21(2):161-169.

[70] Broder HL, McGrath C, Cisneros GJ, Questionnaire development: face validity and item impact testing of the Child Oral Health Impact Profile. Community Dent Oral Epidemiol 2007; 35 (Suppl.1): 8-19.

[71] Pahel BT, Rozier RG, Slade GD: Parental perceptions of children's oral health: the Early Childhood Oral Health Impact Scale (ECOHIS). Health Qual Life Outcomes 2007, 5:6.

[72] Tsakos et al.: Developing a new self-reported scale of oral health outcomes for 5-year-old children (SOHO-5). Health and Quality of Life Outcomes 2012 10:62

[73] Brown A, Al-Khayal Z: Validity and reliability of the Arabic translation of the child oral health related quality of life questionnaire (CPQ11-14) in Saudi Arabia.Int J Paediatr Dent 2006, 16:405-411

[74] Goursand D, Paiva SM, Zarzar PM, Ramos-Jorge ML, Cornacchia GM, Pordeus IA, Allison PJ: Cross-cultural adaptation of the Child Perceptions Questionnaire 11–14 (CPQ11-14) for the Brazilian Portuguese language.HealthQual Life Outcomes 2008, 14:2

[75] McGrath C, Pang HN, Lo EC, King NM, Hägg U, Samman N: Translation and evaluation of a Chinese version of the Child Oral Health-related Quality of Life measure. Int J PaediatrDent 2008, 18:267-274.

[76] The German version of the Child Perceptions Questionnaire (CPQ-G11-14): translation process, reliability, and validity in the general population.Bekes K, John MT, Zyriax R, Schaller HG, Hirsch

[77] Turton BJ, Thomson WM, Foster Page LA, Saub RB, Razak IA Validation of an Oral Health-Related Quality of Life Measure for Cambodian Children.. Asia Pac J Public Health. 2013 Oct 4. [Epub ahead of print]

[78] Wogelius P, Gjørup H, Haubek D, Lopez R, Poulsen S. Development of Danish version of child oral-health-related quality of life questionnaires (CPQ8-10 and CPQ11-14).BMC Oral Health. 2009 Apr 22;9:11. doi: 10.1186/1472-6831-9-11

[79] Bhayat A, Ali MA Validity and reliability of the Arabic short version of the child oral health-related quality of life questionnaire (CPQ 11-14) in Medina, Saudi Arabia..EastMediterr Health J. 2014 Aug 19;20(8):409-14

[80] del Carmen Aguilar-Díaz F, Irigoyen-Camacho ME. Validation of the CPQ8-10ESP in Mexican school children in urban areas. Med Oral Patol Oral Cir Bucal. 2011 May 1;16(3):e430-5.

[81] Goursand D, Paiva SM, Zarzar PM, Pordeus IA, Allison PJ..Family Impact Scale (FIS): psychometric properties of the Brazilian Portuguese language version.Eur J Paediatr Dent. 2009 Sep;10(3):141-6.

[82] Albites U, Abanto J, Bönecker M, Paiva SM, Aguilar-Gálvez D, Castillo JL. Parental-caregiver perceptions of child oral health-related quality of life (P-CPQ): Psychometric properties for the peruvianspanish language.

[83] Bernabé E, Sheiham A, Tsakos G. A comprehensive evaluation of the validity of Child-OIDP: further evidence from Peru.Community Dent Oral Epidemiol. 2008 Aug;36(4):317-25.

[84] Kushnir D, Natapov L, Ram D, Shapira J, Gabai A, Zusman SP. Validation of a Hebrew Version of the Child-OIDP Index, an Oral Health-related Quality of Life Measure for Children. Oral Health Prev Dent. 2013 Jul 18. doi: 10.3290/j.ohpd.a30173. [Epub ahead of print]

[85] Asgari I, Ahmady AE, Broder H, Eslamipour F, Wilson-Genderson M. Assessing the oral health-related quality of life in Iranian adolescents: validity of the Persian version of the Child Oral Health Impact Profile (COHIP). Oral Health Prev Dent. 2013;11(2):147-54. doi: 10.3290/j.ohpd.a29367.

[86] Ahn YS, Kim HY, Hong SM, Patton LL, Kim JH, Noh HJ. Validation of a Korean version of the Child Oral Health Impact Profile (COHIP) among 8-to 15-year-old school children. Int J Paediatr Dent. 2012 Jul;22(4):292-301. doi: 10.1111/j.1365-263X. 2011.01197.x. Epub 2011 Nov 17.

[87] Peker K, Uysal Ö, BermekG.HealthQual Life Outcomes. 2011 Dec 22;9:118. doi: 10.1186/1477-7525-9-118. Cross-cultural adaptation and preliminary validation of the Turkish version of the early childhood oral health impact scale among 5-6-year-old children.

[88] Jabarifar SE, Golkari A, Ijadi MH, Jafarzadeh M, Khadem P. Validation of a Farsi version of the early childhood oral health impact scale (F-ECOHIS).

[89] Lee GH, McGrath C, Yiu CK, King NM. Translation and validation of a Chinese language version of the Early Childhood Oral Health Impact Scale (ECOHIS).

[90] Li S, Veronneau J, Allison PJ. Validation of a French language version of the Early Childhood Oral Health Impact Scale (ECOHIS). Health Qual Life Outcomes. 2008 Jan 22;6:9. doi: 10.1186/1477-7525-6-9

[91] Jankauskienė B, Narbutaitė J, Kubilius R, Gleiznys A. Adaptation and validation of the early childhood oral health impact scale in Lithuania. Stomatologija. 2012;14(4): 108-13.

[92] Martins-Júnior PA, Ramos-Jorge J, Paiva SM, Marques LS, Ramos-Jorge ML. Validations of the Brazilian version of the Early Childhood Oral Health Impact Scale (ECOHIS). Cad SaudePublica. 2012 Feb;28(2):367-74

Chapter 32

Periodontal Health and Orthodontics

Mourad Sebbar, Zouhair Abidine,
Narjisse Laslami and Zakaria Bentahar

Additional information is available at the end of the chapter

http://dx.doi.org/10.5772/59249

1. Introduction

The most common objectives of an orthodontic treatment are facial and dental aesthetics and the improvement in the masticatory function. There is a continuously increasing number of adult patients who actively seek orthodontic treatment, and it is also an undeniable fact that the incidence of periodontal disease increases with age. Therefore, the number of patients with periodontal problems that attend orthodontic practices is significantly greater than in the past [1].

There are many links between periodontology and orthodontics. After all, every orthodontic intervention has a periodontal dimension: orthodontic biomechanics and treatment planning are basically determined by periodontal factors such as the length and shape of the roots, the width and height of the alveolar bone, and the structure of the gingiva [2].

The main objective of periodontal therapy is to restore and maintain the health and integrity of the attachment apparatus of teeth. Additionally, orthodontic therapy can facilitate management of several restorative and aesthetic problems relating to fractured teeth, tipped abutment teeth, excess spacing, inadequate pontic space, malformed teeth, and diastema.

Generally, the main reasons routinely cited to justify the provision of orthodontic treatment are improvement of facial and dental aesthetics and of dental health and function. However, association between malocclusions and periodontal condition is still controversial [3].

Ngom [4] found significant correlations between malocclusions and periodontal condition and suggested that malocclusions are risk markers for periodontal diseases. However, a real inference about a cause/effect relationship between malocclusions and periodontal condition in this study was not possible.

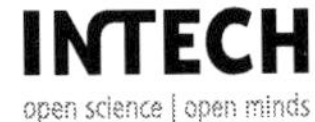

A review of the literature conducted by Van Gastel [5] showed contradictory findings on the impact of malocclusion and orthodontic appliances on periodontal health, since only a few studies reported attachment loss during orthodontic treatment. It has been suggested that this contradiction may be partly due to the selection of materials and differences in the research methods employed [6].

All evidence-based literature concerning the orthodontic-periodontic relationships show that a good orthodontic treatment of patients, who have excellent oral hygiene and do not suffer any periodontal breakdown, is a non-harmful treatment for the periodontium, it has been also demonstrated that a diminished oral hygiene in corporation with periodontal disorder would make the orthodontic treatment a real high risk for the periodontium [7.8].

In the modern and serious dental practice, such synergy is fundamental. Besides systemic variables, genetic heritance, age, collaboration, correct and complete diagnosis and good execution, the factor that isexplicitly mentioned in the literature as a must for success of the orthodontic therapy and of the periodontal therapy is the patient adequate oral hygiene [9].

A multidisciplinary approach is often necessary to treat and prevent dental problems in patients. This chapter will address basic considerations for orthodontists as well as periodontists for successful outcome of various treatments. Several clinical cases will be presented to illustrate the orthodontic-periodontic relationships.

2. Orthodontic treatment and oral hygiene

A high standard of oral hygiene is essential for patients undergoing orthodontic treatment. Without good oral hygiene, plaque accumulates around the orthodontic appliance, causing gingivitis and, in some cases, periodontal breakdown. To avoid such problems, the orthodontist has a double obligation: to advise the patient about methods of plaque control and, at routine visits, to monitor the effectiveness of the oral-hygiene regime. However, despite receiving appropriate advice, many patients undergoing orthodontic treatment fail to maintain an adequate standard of plaque control. It is important that the orthodontist is able to communicate the importance of oral hygiene to motivate patients to maintain a satisfactory standard of oral hygiene during orthodontic treatment [10].

Before any orthodontic treatment an initial diagnosis and referral for treatment to control active periodontal disease is to be considered. Moreover, all general, dental and periodontal treatment should be completed before the orthodontic treatment. Once the orthodontic appliances are placed, the patients need to be instructed in how to manage the new oral environment and how to maintain the health of the dental and periodontal structures. The orthodontist has to provide the patient with initial brushing instructions with either a conventional toothbrush or a powered one when the appliances are first placed. However, if the orthodontists correctly advice their patients to follow proper oral hygiene instructions during the orthodontic treatment is still an opened question.

Manual tooth brushing, one of the oldest methods of plaque removal, remains the basis of oral hygiene and plaque control. It is often used as the standard or control against which other methods of plaque removal are assessed [10,11]. Instruction should emphasize the need to use sufficient pressure to remove plaque; a pressure sensitive toothbrush would be a valuable aid to patients undergoing orthodontic treatment.

Chlorhexidine mouthwashes, as an adjunct to tooth brushing, have been found effective in the control of gingival inflammation [12], although prolonged use may cause problems with staining as Chlorhexidine rinses can potentially stain the margins of composite restorations that cannot be easily removed. More recently, pre-brushing rinses have been introduced, though these show no differences in effect on plaque accumulation or gingival health [13]. Chlorhexidine is also useful for patients after orthognathic surgery, especially when inter-maxillary fixation is to be used.

On the other hand, Fluoride mouth rinses significantly reduce the extent of enamel decalcification and gingival inflammation during orthodontic treatment [13.14]. A number of studies evaluated the effect of mechanical aids, as compared with manual tooth brushing, on oral hygiene in orthodontic patients [11.12] and it has been shown that the use of electric toothbrushes brought a significant improvement in oral hygiene. The orthodontist can follow some suggestions in order to improve plaque removal by the patient. Bonding of molars results in better periodontal health than banding. Whenever possible the use of single arch wires is recommended. The removal of excess composite around brackets, especially at the gingival margin, and avoiding the use of lingual appliances whenever possible are also important ideas in order to keep healthy periodontal tissue during any orthodontic treatment.

3. Periodontal tissue and orthodontics

3.1. Periodontal tissue and orthodontic forces

Tooth movement during orthodontic therapy is the result of placing controlled forces on teeth. Removable appliances place intermittent tipping forces on teeth while fixed appliances can create continuous multidirectional forces to create torquing, intrusive, extrusive, rotational and bodily movement [15.16]. Bone surrounding a tooth subjected to a force responds in the following manner: resorption occurs where there is pressure and new bone forms where there is tension. When pressure is applied to a tooth, there is an initial period of movement for six to eight days as the periodontal ligament (PDL) is compressed. Compression of the PDL results in blood supply being cut off to an area of the PDL and this produces an avascular cell-free zone by a process termed "hyalinization". When hyalinization occurs, the tooth stops moving. Once the hyalinized is removed, tooth movement can occur again [16.17].

3.2. Mechanisms of tissue damage

Unfestooned orthodontic bands are particularly suspects as possibly complicating factors jeopardizing interproximal periodontal support, and at the present time "special periodontally friendly bands" are being designed in research and design laboratories. These challenging effects of band impingement may directly compromise local resistance related to subgingival pathogens in susceptible patients and result in damage to both interproximal gingival tissues and alveolar crestal bone in a manner similar to that produced by faulty crown margins. Periodontal support might also be damaged during tooth intrusion where patients have active periodontitis or gingival infection significant enough to convert to periodontal disease.

The etiology of periodontal problems may not simply rely on exaggerated host immunologic reactions. Mattingly and coworkers [18] and others [19.20.21] reflect the view that long-term fixed appliances can contribute to unfortunate but predictable qualitative alterations in the subgingival bacterial biofilms that become progressively periodontopathic with time.

On a practical level it seems that an absence of bleeding on probing is a better forecasting parameter of health than bleeding on probing is a predictor of progressive disease. In other words, an absence of bleeding on probing, despite the pocket depth can justifiably be used as a test of "healthy gums." On the other hand, while bleeding on probing is certainly an indication of infection of the gingivae, it is one of many risk factors associated with progressive bone loss due to periodontitis. However, the test is not spontaneous bleeding or even bleeding on brushing and flossing. That elicits only superficial disease, one that contributes significantly to caries and marginal decalcification. The best test is "bleeding on probing" elicited by stroking the sulci with a flexible plastic periodontal probe at a comfortable range of force between 10 and 20 g. Those orthodontic patients who present with persistent bleeding on such probing should be notified that they are "at risk" and that prudence dictates a more intensive regimen of periodontal therapy than those who present with little or no bleeding on probing. Since bleeding swollen gingiva is ubiquitous in the orthodontic population, universal caution should be employed and supportive periodontal care recommended routinely as an integral part of orthodontic therapy. Studies have pointed out the importance of a full-mouth examination, six sites per tooth, for a comprehensive description of periodontal status in orthodontic patients [22.23].

3.3. Orthodontic treatment in periodontally susceptible or compromised patients

Under severe control against formation of dental biofilm and elimination or surveillance of periodontal pockets, patients who present susceptible or compromised periodontal status can be submitted to orthodontic treatment [24.25.26]. Moreover, the orthodontic treatment allows that the stable periodontal status is maintained [27.28.29.30]

Although there is no clear correlation between malocclusion and periodontal disease or between the effects of orthodontic treatments on periodontal improvement the literature describes clear interaction between Orthodontics and Periodontics [9].

Probable contributions of orthodontics in the periodontics field are:

1. It allows better oral hygiene by the patient, since it provides well shaped dental arches. Without dental crowding, malocclusion as a periodontal disease facilitator is eliminated;

2. It allows vertical occlusal impact parallels to the long axes of the teeth. Therefore, the applied muscle force is uniformly distributed all over the dental arch;

3. It contributes, along with prosthetic rehabilitations, for a normal vertical dimension;

4. In selected cases, it allows that the adequate dental crown-root relationship is achieved with induced orthodontic extrusion, with no bone loss;

5. It facilitates that bone vertical defects are corrected or improved with dental uprighting;

6. It improves the positioning of prosthetic pillars for fixed prostheses and of the next teeth of osteointegrated implants;

7. It decreases or eliminates effects of bruxism, as pain or muscle spasms, during the orthodontic therapy;

8. With the current available orthodontic technology and with correct planning and execution, it allows precise, light and efficient orthodontic movements.

Summarizing, when the periodontal inflammatory/infectious process is controlled and the periodontal health is stabilized, the orthodontic treatment is indicated. However, orthodontic movements in periodontal susceptible or compromised patients in active status of inflammation /infection increase significantly the risk of loss of attachment and of bone loss. In extreme cases, they can provoke periodontal collapse and condemnation of the teeth to extraction [9].

4. Combined periodontal/orthodontic treatment

4.1. Periodontal treatment schedule

When planning orthodontic treatment in adults with a history of periodontal disease, it is suggested to allow 2– 6 months from the end of periodontal therapy until bracket placement, for periodontal tissue remodelling, restoration of health and evaluation of patient's compliance. The patient should practise sound oral hygiene and fully understand the potential risks in case of non-compliance [8]. It should be kept in mind that the critical pocket depth for maintaining periodontal health with ordinary oral hygiene is 5–6 mm [31].

During orthodontic treatment, professional cleaning and examination of periodontal tissues should be performed routinely [8]. The specific interval varies for each patient (few weeks to 6 months), and it should be determined considering the analysis of risk factors for periodontal disease and the planned tooth movements. Thorough tooth cleaning and scaling is suggested at short intervals when intrusion and new attachment is attempted 32]. If the patient fails to maintain high level of oral hygiene, orthodontic treatment should be interrupted.

Elective periodontal treatment should be implemented during the final stages of orthodontic treatment or even later, when the final position of hard and soft tissues can be safely determined. The decision is individualized depending on the clinical characteristics of the case and the comprehensive treatment plan [33.34.35].

After the end of active orthodontic treatment and appliance removal, the patient should receive renewed oral hygiene instructions for reducing the risk of recession, because plaque removal and tooth cleaning will be more easily performed. Also, patients should be introduced to a programme of regular follow-up visits to the periodontist and the orthodontist. The timing between follow-up visits is prescribed by the team according to the severity of the patient's pre-treatment condition and the prognosis of the post-treatment condition.

4.2. Treatment phases

4.2.1. Preorthodontic phase

Preorthodontically, the emphasis is on reducing marginal inflammation, augmenting the soft tissue volume in patients with critical mucogingival findings, and improving hygiene conditions through caries therapy and temporary restorations.

The control of periodontal infection by oral hygiene instruction, professional plaque removal and root planing is a fundamental prerequisite for subsequent orthodontic therapy. Many studies have shown that teeth with a reduced but healthy periodontium can be moved without further attachment loss. On the other hand inflammatory periodontal destruction is accelerated by plaque-infected teeth with destroyed connective tissue attachment.

If periodontal regeneration is indicated, a surgical approach is inevitable. Resective bone surgery during flap surgery is contraindicated because orthodontically induced remodeling processes may have a positive influence on osseous topography. Orthodontic treatment can be started 4–6 weeks after the regenerative periodontal therapy; the interaction of progressing regenerative wound healing and orthodontic tissue remodeling may result in additional attachment gain [2].

4.2.2. Orthodontic phase

The orthodontic therapy is determined by two key factors:

- Findings-oriented biomechanics, calculation of active and reactive forces as well as moments as far as possible

- Continuous monitoring of periodontal health. Thorough planning of biomechanics reduces the risk of root resorptions as well as of bone and gingival dehiscences.

A further loss of bone sup-port or attachment induced by uncontrolled force systems should be avoided in all events – especially in patients with periodontally affected teeth.

Maintenance of periodontal health requires meticulous plaque removal in all hygiene-critical areas: bracket periphery, and interproximal and gingival tooth surfaces. If uncontrollable aggravation of the periodontal destruction occurs or if the patient's oral hygiene deteriorates, orthodontic therapy has to be stopped to ensure a reasonable risk/benefit ratio [2].

4.2.3. Postorthodontic phase

The postorthodontic retention phase should last at least six months to permit complete mineralization of osteoid tissues. Only then can the periodontal status be re-evaluated and a decision made on definitive prosthetic measures and the individual retention strategy. For many reasons postorthodontic stability requires semi-permanent or permanent retention:

- to prevent the risk of relapse

- to offset any imbalance of soft tissue/reduced bone support • to eliminate secondary occlusal trauma • to improve masticatory comfort in the presence of increased tooth mobility.

Fixed lingual retainers, passive plates or acrylic foils serve for semi-permanent stabilization, while intracoronal titanium pins are suitable for permanent retention [2].

5. Aspects in periodontic-orthodontic interrelationships

Generally, the main reasons routinely cited to justify the provision of orthodontic treatment are improvement of facial and dental aesthetics and of dental health and function. However, association between malocclusions and periodontal condition is still controversial.

Ngom and co-workers [4] found significant correlations between malocclusions and periodontal condition and suggested that malocclusions are risk markers for periodontal diseases. However, a real inference about a cause/effect relationship between malocclusions and periodontal condition in this study was not possible.

A review of the literature conducted by Van Gastel [5] showed contradictory findings on the impact of malocclusion and orthodontic appliances on periodontal health, since only a few studies reported attachment loss during orthodontic treatment. It has been suggested that this contradiction may be partly due to the selection of materials and differences in the research methods employed. However, our previous studies showed that orthodontic treatment in general does not have any negative effects on the periodontal tissues when a high level of oral hygiene is maintained [6.36].

Actually, between the year 1964 and 2007, sufficient studies had been conducted in terms of orthodontic treatment and possible related periodontal changes. Thus, it sounds plausible to extract evidence-based conclusions from those studies by means of systematic reviews.

In 2008, Bollen [36] conducted two systematic reviews to address the following questions: does a malocclusion affect periodontal health, and does orthodontic treatment affect periodontal health? The first review found a correlation between the presence of a malocclusion and periodontal disease. Subjects with greater malocclusion have more severe periodontal disease. The second review identified an absence of reliable evidence on the effects of orthodontic treatment on periodontal health. The existing low-quality evidence suggests that orthodontic therapy results in small detrimental effects to the periodontium. It has been suggested that the results of both reviews do not warrant recommendation for orthodontic treatment to prevent future periodontal problems, except for specific unusual malocclusions.

In 2010, Van Gastel and co-workers showed in his study [37] that placement of fixed ortho-dontic appliances has an influence both on microbial and clinical periodontal parameters, which were only partly normalized, 3 months following the removal of the appliances.

On the other side, it seems that there still are studies that give the orthodontic treatment positive points regarding periodontal health. Gray and McIntyre [38] conducted a systematic literature review to determine the effectiveness of orthodontic oral health promotion (OHP) upon gingival health, and it has been found that an OHP program for patients undergoing fixed appliance orthodontic treatment produces a short-term reduction (up to 5 months) in plaque and improvement in gingival health.

The results of Gomes and co-workers [39] indicate that use of orthodontics appliances is not necessarily related to a worsening of periodontal conditions. The results of this study reinforce the importance of susceptibility to periodontal disease independent of a well-known retentive plaque factor, i.e. orthodontic appliances and/or bands.

The existing evidence, in general, does not seem to support the claim that orthodontic therapy results in overall improvement in periodontal health.

6. Contribution of orthodontics to periodontal therapy

Orthodontics can serve as an adjunct to periodontal treatment procedures to improve oral health in a number of situations. Pathological tooth migration is one of the few evident signs of periodontitis that affects dentofacial esthetics. This phenomenon is more commonly seen in the anterior dentition due to lack of stable occlusal and sagittal contacts with the opposing teeth [39.40].

Achieving an esthetically acceptable result in such cases may require various orthodontic tooth movements like intrusion, rotation, and uprighting. This can also help control periodontal breakdown and restore good oral function [41].

Tulloch [42] is of the opinion that fixed appliance therapy is more preferable if orthodontic tooth movement is desired in a patient suffering from periodontitis. Fixed appliance allows easy splinting of teeth to achieve stable anchorage. He also highlights the importance of reducing the force magnitude and applying counteracting moments to reduce the stress on periodontal ligament fibres.

Lijian [24] has enlisted the various precautions to be taken when attempting tooth movement in height-reduced periodontium, which includes achieving stable anchorage and long-term periodontal maintenance care.

Deepa [43] reported the use of orthodontic soft aligners in repositioning a periodontally involved tooth. Light and intermittent forces generated by the soft aligner allow regeneration of tissue during tooth movement. Along with periodontal procedures, orthodontically assisted occlusal improvement may be required in treatment of patients with severely attrited lower anterior teeth.

Patient's compliance, motivation, and oral hygiene maintenance will help determine the best time to start adjunctive orthodontic treatment. It is suggested that tooth movement can be undertaken 6 months after completion of active periodontal treatment if there is sufficient evidence of complete resolution of inflammation [44].

Sanders [45] has recommended a three-step comprehensive protocol to be followed before, during, and after adjunctive orthodontic therapy. In patients diagnosed with vertical bony defects, adjunctive orthodontic procedures can help improve the condition. The authors reported improvement in alveolar bone defects, gingival esthetics, and the crown-root ratio in patients with one-or two-wall isolated vertical infrabony defects with a combination of tooth extrusion and periodontal treatment. Orthodontic intrusion has also been shown to improve periodontal condition [46]. However, elimination of pockets was undertaken prior to intrusion in order to prevent apical displacement of plaque [47].

Orthodontic treatment could improve adjacent tooth position before implant placement or tooth replacement. This is especially true for the patient who has been missing teeth for several years and had drifting and tipping of the adjacent dentition

7. Contribution of periodontics to orthodontic therapy

On many occasions, a stable and esthetically acceptable outcome cannot be achieved with orthodontics without adjunctive periodontal procedures. For instance, a high labial frenum attachment is considered to be a causative factor of midline diastema. Frenectomy is recommended in such cases as the fibres are thought to prevent the mesial migration of the central incisors. However, the timing of periodontal intervention has been a topic of much debate [37].

According to Vanarsdall, [49] surgical removal of a maxillary labial frenum should be delayed until after orthodontic treatment unless the tissue prevents space closure or becomes painful and traumatized.

Forced eruption of a labially or palatally impacted tooth is now a common orthodontic treatment procedure. Careful exposure of the impacted tooth while preserving keratinized tissue requires the expertise of a periodontist. Preservation of keratinized tissue is important to prevent loss of attachment. The preferred surgical procedure is primarily an apically or laterally positioned pedicle graft [50].

Retention of orthodontically achieved tooth rotation is a problem that has always plagued the orthodontist. Circumferential supracrestal fiberotomy (CSF) is a procedure that is frequently used to enhance post-treatment stability [50]. Edwards [51] concluded from his long-term prospective study that CSF is more successful in preventing relapse in the maxillary arch. According to him, CSF does not affect the periodontium adversely.

Mucogingival surgeries may be needed during the course of orthodontic treatment to maintain sufficient width of attached gingival [52]. Also, crown lengthening procedures can facilitate easy placement of orthodontic attachments on teeth with short clinical crowns. This procedure can also be used for smile designing [53]. Alveolar ridge augmentation and placements of dental implants [54] are the other adjunctive periodontal treatment procedures undertaken to facilitate achievement of orthodontic treatment goals.

Panwar *et al.* [55] in 2010 presented a case report on combined periodontal and orthodontic treatment of pathologic migration of anterior teeth. Comprehensive orthodontics was initiated with pre-adjusted edgewise appliances using very light force, which resulted in optimal biological response. Since there was trauma from lower anterior teeth, anterior bite plane allowed posterior eruption of teeth, which resulted in the opening of the bite. The periodontal health improved the moment trauma was relieved. Periodontal treatment and the patient's co-operation in oral hygiene were also continued as supportive therapy.

Michael *et al.* in 2009 provided the treatment options for the significant dental midline diastema. After the required prosthetic intervention, periodontal tissues were altered by gingivoplasty and crown lengthening and provided optimal result with favorable esthetic, functional, and biologic consequences [56].

8. Case report

8.1. Case n°1

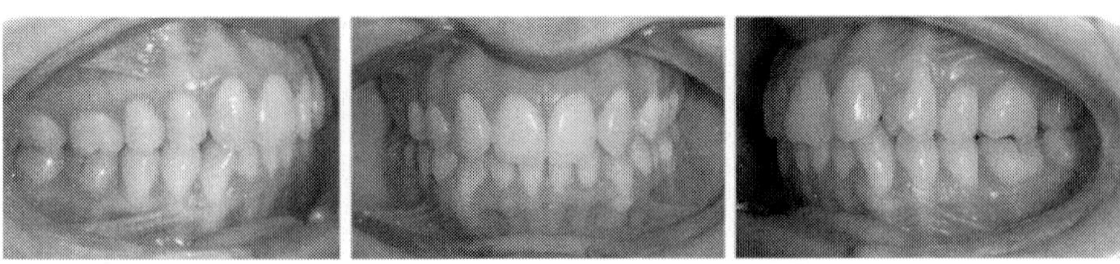

Figure 1. A patient who consults for gingival recession at the 24

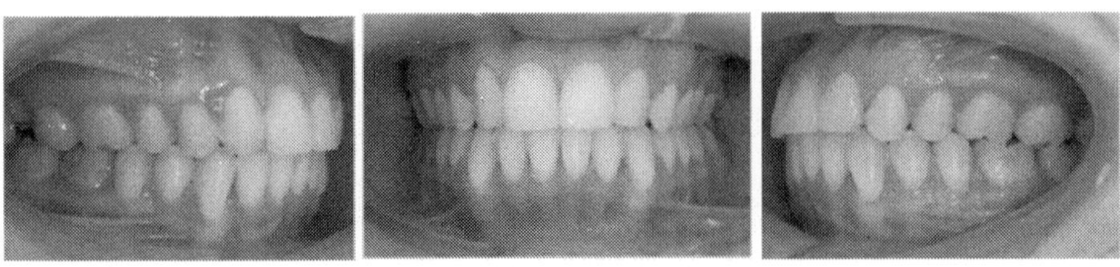

Figure 2. Orthodontic treatment has been used to correct the malocculsion and to correct the rotation of the 24. A gingival grafting was performed to cover the recession

8.2. Case n°2

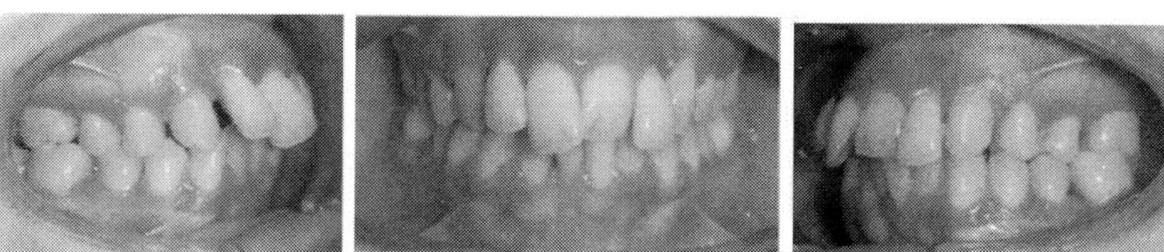

Figure 3. A patient who consults for malpositions and dental extrusions

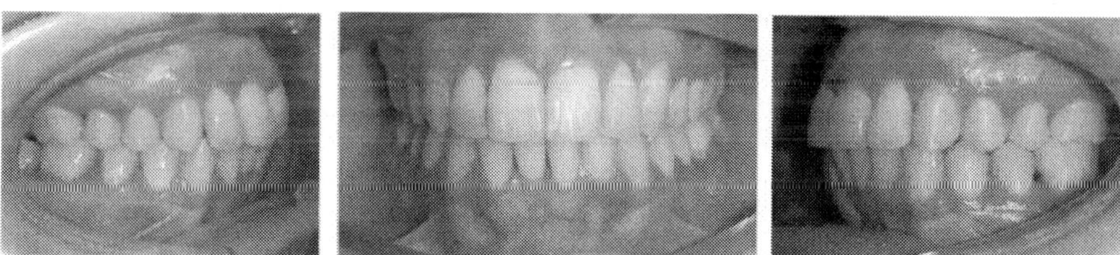

Figure 4. Orthodontic treatment was aimed at correcting dental malposition and regain proper alignment will facilitate the oral hygiene.

8.3. Case n°3

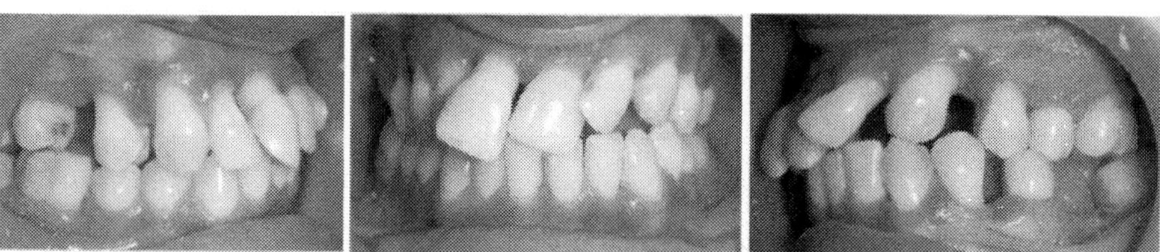

Figure 5. A patient with dental malposition and higher gingival recession secondary to periodontal disease

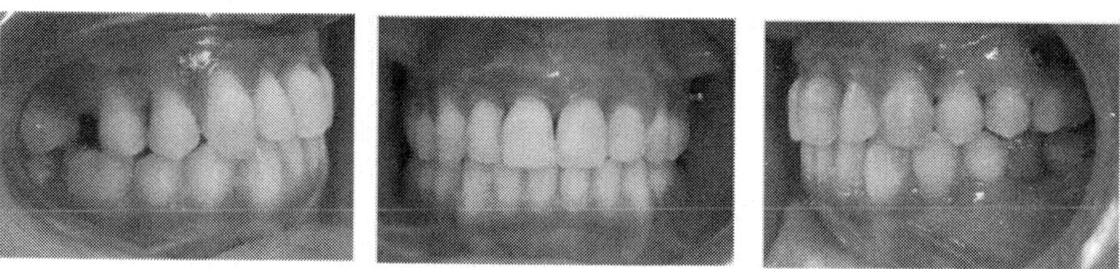

Figure 6. Orthodontic treatment was able to obtain dental and periodontal balance while maintaining good oral hygiene.

8.4. Case n°4

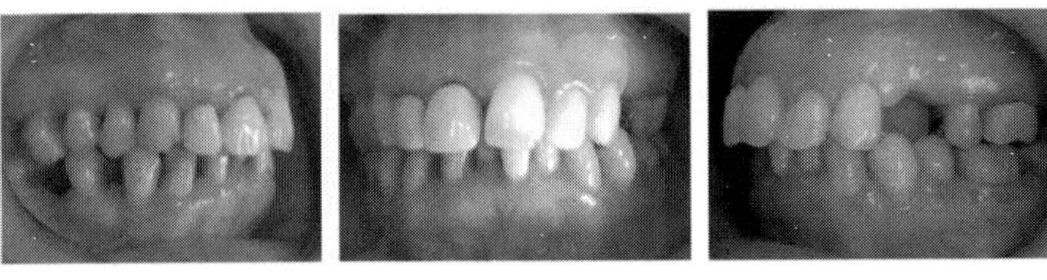

Figure 7. Clinical examination in this patient showed defective prostheses with poor periodontal status.

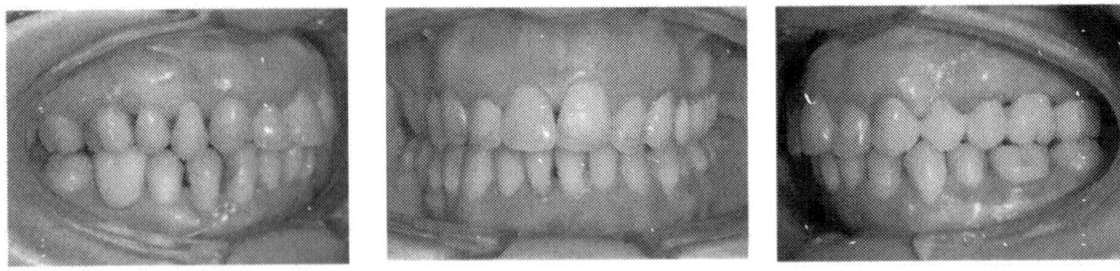

Figure 8. Orthodontic treatment was performed to correct the malocclusion. The patient also received a prosthetic rehabilitation.

9. Conclusion

Harmonious cooperation of the general dentist, the periodontist and the orthodontist offers great possibilities for the treatment of combined orthodontic–periodontal problems. Undoubtedly, application of oral hygiene measures is difficult during orthodontic treatment. Orthodontic treatment along with patient's compliance and absence of periodontal inflammation can provide satisfactory results without causing irreversible damage to periodontal tissues. Furthermore, orthodontic treatment can expand the possibilities of periodontal therapy in certain patients, contributing to better control of microbiota, reducing the potentially hazardous forces applied to teeth and finally improving the overall prognosis. Participation of the periodontist is also essential, either in management of orthodontic–periodontal problems or in specific interventions aiming to prevent orthodontic treatment's relapse.

Author details

Mourad Sebbar[1*], Zouhair Abidine[1], Narjisse Laslami[2] and Zakaria Bentahar[2]

*Address all correspondence to: mouradsebbar@hotmail.com

1 Hospital Moulay Abdellah, Mohammedia, Morocco

2 Department of orthodontics, Faculty of dentistry, Casablanca, Morocco

References

[1] Gkantidis N, Christou P, Topouzelis N. The orthodontic–periodontic interrelationship in integrated treatment challenges: a systematic review. J Oral Rehabilitation 2010;37:377-390.

[2] Diedrich P, Fritz U, Kinzinger G. Interrelationship between Periodontics and Adult Orthodontics Perio 2004,1(3): 143-149.

[3] Dannan A. An update on periodontic-orthodontic interrelationships. J Indian Soc Periodontol 2010,14: 66-71.

[4] Ngom PI, Benoist HM, Thiam F, Diagne F, Diallo PD. Influence of orthodontic anomalies on periodontal condition. Odontostomatol Trop 2007;301:9-16.

[5] Van Gastel J, Quirynen M, Teughels W, Carels C. The relationships between malocclusion, fixed orthodontic appliances and periodontal disease: A review of the literature. Aust Orthod J 2007;23:121-9.

[6] Dannan A, Darwish MA, Sawan MN. Effect of orthodontic tooth movements on the periodontal tissues. Damascus Univ Journal for Health Sciences [Master Thesis] 2005;21:306-7.

[7] Dannan A, Darwish MA, Sawan MN. How do the periodontal tissues react during the orthodontic alignment and leveling phase? Virtual J Orthod 2008;8:1-7.

[8] Sanders NL. Evidence-based care in orthodontics and periodontics: a review of the literature. J Am Dent Assoc. 1999;130(4):521-7.

[9] Del Santo M. Periodontium and Orthodontic Implications: Clinical Applications. Int J Stomatol Res 2012, 1(3): 17-23.

[10] Jackson CL. Comparison between electric toothbrushing and manual toothbrushing, with and without oral irrigation, for oral hygiene of orthodontic patients. Am J Orthod Dentofacial Orthop. 1991;99(1):15-20.

[11] Wilcoxon DB, Ackerman RJ, Jr., Killoy WJ, Love JW, Sakumura JS, Tira DE. The effectiveness of a counterrotational-action power toothbrush on plaque control in orthodontic patients. Am J Orthod Dentofacial Orthop. 1991;99(1):7-14.

[12] Brightman LJ, Terezhalmy GT, Greenwell H, Jacobs M, Enlow DH. The effects of a 0.12% chlorhexidine gluconate mouthrinse on orthodontic patients aged 11 through 17 with established gingivitis. Am J Orthod Dentofacial Orthop. 1991;100(4):324-9.

[13] Pontier JP, Pine C, Jackson DL, DiDonato AK, Close J, Moore PA. Efficacy of a pre-brushing rinse for orthodontic patients. Clin Prev Dent. 1990;12(3):12-7.

[14] Denes J, Gabris K. Results of a 3-year oral hygiene programme, including amine fluoride products, in patients treated with fixed orthodontic appliances. Eur J Orthod. 1991;13(2):129-33.

[15] Lindhe J. Textbook of clinical periodontology. 2nd ed. Copenhagen: Munksgaard; 1989.

[16] Proffit WR, Fields HW. Contemporary orthodontics. 2nd ed. St Louis: CV Mosby; 1993.

[17] Reitan K. Biomechanical principles and reactions. In: Graber X, Swain BF, editors. Current orthodontic concepts and techniques. St Louis: CV Mosby; 1985. p. 101-92.

[18] Mattingly JA, Sauer GJ, Yancey JM, Arnold RR. Enhancement of 27. streptococcus mutans colonization by direct bonded orthodontic appliances. J Dent Res 1983;62:1209-11.

[19] Paolantonio M, Festa F, di Placido G, D'Attilio M, Catamo28. G, Piccolomini R. Site-specific subgingival colonization by actinobacillus actinomycetemcomitans in orthodontic patients. Am J Orthod Dentofacial Orthop 1999;115:423-8.

[20] Sallum A, et al. Clinical and microbiologic changes after removal of orthodontic appliances. Am J Orthod Dentofacial Orthop 2004;126:363-6.

[21] Perinetti G, Paolantonio M, Serra E, D'Archivio D, D'Ercole S, Festa F, et al. Longitudinal monitoring of subgingival colonization by actinobacillus actinomycetemcomitans, and crevicular alkaline phosphatise and aspartate aminotransferase activities around orthodontically treated teeth. J Clin Periodontol 2004;31:60-7.

[22] Lijian L. Periodontic-orthodontic interactions—rationale, sequence and clinical implications. Hong Kong Dent J 2007;4:60-4.

[23] Lang NP, Loe H. The relationship between the width of keratinized gingiva and gingival health. J Periodontol 1972;43:623-7.

[24] Elliasson LA, Hugoson A, Kurol J, Siwe H. The effects of orthodontic treatment on periodontal tissues in patients with reduced periodontal support. Eur J Orthod 1982;4:1-9.

[25] Boyd RL, Leggot PJ, Quinn RS, Eakle WS, Chambers DW. Periodontal implications of orthodontic treatment in adults with reduced or normal periodontal tissues versus those of adolescents. Am J Orthod Dentofac Orthop 1989;96:191-8.

[26] Ong M A Wang HL. Periodontic and orthodontic treatment in adults. Am J Orthod Dentofac Orthop 2002;122:420-8.

[27] Brown S The effect of orthodontic therapy on certain types of periodontal defects (I). Clinical findings. J Periodontol 1973;44:742-56.

[28] Ingber JS. Forced eruption. Part I. A method of treating isolated one and two wall infrabony osseous defects – rationale and case report. J Periodontol 1974;45:199-206.

[29] Ingber JS. Forced eruption. Part II. A method of treating nonrestorable teeth – periodontal and restorative considerations. J Periodontol 1976;47:203-16.

[30] Kraal JH, Digiancinto JJ, Dail RA. Lemmerman K, Peden JW. Periodontal conditions in patients after molar uprighting. J Prosth Dent 1980;43:156-62.

[31] Socransky SS, Haffajee AD. The nature of periodontal diseases. Ann Periodontol. 1997;2:3–10.

[32] Melsen B, Agerbaek N, Markenstam G. Intrusion of incisors in adult patients with marginal bone loss. Am J Orthod Dentofacial Orthop. 1989;96:232–241.

[33] Spear FM, Kokich VG, Mathews DP. Interdisciplinary man-agement of anterior dental esthetics. J Am Dent Assoc 2006;137:160–169.

[34] Konikoff BM, Johnson DC, Schenkein HA, Kwatra N, Waldrop TC. Clinical crown length of the maxillary anterior teeth preorthodontics and postorthodontics. J Periodontol. 2007;78:645–653.

[35] Theytaz GA, Kiliaridis S. Gingival and dentofacial changes in adolescents and adults 2 to 10 years after orthodontic treatment. J Clin Periodontol. 2008;35:825–830.

[36] Bollen AM. Effects of malocclusions and orthodontics on periodontal health: Evidence from a systematic review. J Dent Educ 2008;72:912-8.

[37] Van Gastel J, Quirynen M, Teughels W, Coucke W, Carels C. Longitudinal changes in microbiology and clinical periodontal parameters after removal of fixed orthodontic appliances. Eur J Orthod 2011;33:15-21.

[38] Gray D, McIntyre G. Does oral health promotion influence the oral hygiene and gingival health of patients undergoing fixed appliance orthodontic treatment? A systematic literature review. J Orthod 2008;35:262-9.

[39] Gomes SC, Varela CC, da Veiga SL, Rösing CK, Oppermann RV. Periodontal conditions in subjects following orthodontic therapy. A preliminary study. Eur J Orthod. 2007;29(5):477-81.

[40] Vinod K, Reddy YG, Reddy VP, Nandan H, Sharma M. Orthodontic-periodontics interdisciplinary approach. J Indian Soc Periodontol. 2012;16(1):11-5.

[41] Zachrisson BU. Orthodontics and periodontics. In: Lindhe J, Karring T, Lang NP, editors. Clinical periodontology and implant dentistry. 4th ed. Oxford: Blackwell Munksgaard; 2003:744-80.

[42] Tulloch JF. Adjunctive treatment for adults. In: Proffit WR, Fields J r HW, editors. Contemporary orthodontics. 3rd ed. St. Louis: Mosby; 2000:616-43.

[43] Deepa D, Mehta DS, Puri VK, Shetty S. Combined periodontic-orthodontic-endodontic interdisciplinary approach in the treatment of periodontally compromised tooth. J Indian Soc Periodontol 2010;14:139-43.

[44] Padmanabhan S, Reddy VL. Inter-disciplinary management of a patient with severely attrited teeth. J Indian Soc Periodontol 2010;14:190-4.

[45] Sanders NL. Evidence-based care in orthodontics and periodontics: A review of the literature. J Am Dent Assoc 1999;130:521-7.

[46] Lino S, Taira K, Machigashira M, Miyawaki S. Isolated vertical infrabony defects treated by orthodontic tooth extrusion. Angle Orthod 2008;78:728-36.

[47] Sam K, Rabie AB, King NM. Orthodontic intrusion of periodontally involved teeth. J Clin Orthod 2001;35:325-30.

[48] Melsen B. Tissue reaction following application of extrusive and intrusive forces to teeth in adult monkeys. Am J Orthod 1986;89:469-75.

[49] Vanarsdall RE. Periodontal/orthodontic interrelationships. In: Graber TM, Vanarsdall RE, editors. Orthodontics-current principles and technique. 3rd ed. St. Louis: Mosby; 2000:801-38.

[50] Vanarsdall RL, Corn H. Soft-tissue management of labially positioned unerupted teeth. Am J Orthod 1977;72:53-64.

[51] Edwards JG. A surgical procedure to eliminate rotational relapse. Am J Orthod 1970;57:35-46.

[52] Edwards JG. A long-term prospective evaluation of the circumferential supracrestal-fiberotomy in alleviating orthodontic relapse. Am J Orthod Dentofacial Orthop 1988;93:380-7.

[53] Kokich VG. Esthetics: The orthodontic-periodontic restorative connection. Semin Orthod 1996;2:21-30.

[54] Huang LH, Shotwell JL, Wang HL. Dental implants for orthodonticanchorage. Am J Orthod Dentofacial Orthop 2005;127:713-22.

[55] Panwar M, Jayan B. Combined periodontal and orthodontic treatment of pathologic migration of anterior teeth. MJAFI 2010;66:67-9.

[56] Michael R. Treatment options for the significant dental midline diastema inside dentistry 2009. http:/www.dentalaegis.com/id/2009/05/clinical-treatment-options-treatment-optionsfor-the-significant-dental-midline-diastema.

Chapter 33

Panoramic Radiography — Diagnosis of Relevant Structures That Might Compromise Oral and General Health of the Patient

Ticiana Sidorenko de Oliveira Capote,
Marcela de Almeida Gonçalves,
Andrea Gonçalves and Marcelo Gonçalves

Additional information is available at the end of the chapter

http://dx.doi.org/10.5772/59260

1. Introduction

The chapter provides information about panoramic radiography, showing the principal indications, advantages and disadvantages of this examination. Moreover, focus is given to some anatomical variations that can be detected on panoramic radiographs such as bifid mandibular canal, retromolar canal, and alterations such as calcified stylohyoid complex, arterial calcifications, phleboliths, sialolithiasis and tonsilloliths. Such structures/alterations are not reasons for indication of panoramic radiography, but they are radiographic findings, being important their identification, indication of more accurate examinations, and even referring to other professionals. Therefore, a literature review was conducted, citing relevant anatomy textbooks and scientific papers, and it was illustrated with panoramic radiographs showing these described structures/alterations.

2. Indications and contraindications of panoramic radiographs

Panoramic radiography is a radiologic technique that provides an overview of the jaws and surrounding structures. It is frequently indicated when professionals want to evaluate some structures such as unerupted third molars, orthodontic treatment, tooth development, developmental abnormalities, trauma, large lesions, and others [1, 2]. The panoramic radio-

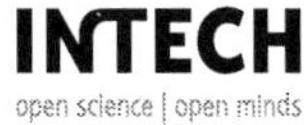

graph allows the dental professional to view a large area of the maxilla and mandible on a single film [2].

The panoramic radiography is frequently used as initial diagnostic image of some alterations and based on it, the professional will verify the need of other more detailed and more accurate examinations [1].

If you have a full-mouth series, the panoramic radiography shows no more or little useful information for a patient receiving general dental care [1].

Some contraindications of panoramic radiographs are clinical situations that require detail and definition, such as carious lesions, visualization of alveolar crests, level of root canal filling [3], periodontal disease or periapical lesions [2].

In dental clinical practice, panoramic radiography is one of the most indicated radiographic examinations by dentists because it provides a general overview of dentomaxilomandibular structures and it is not so costly for patients.

3. Advantages and disadvantages of panoramic radiography

Panoramic radiography has many advantages including short time for the procedure, greater patient acceptance and cooperation, overall coverage of the dental arches and associated structures (more anatomic structures can be viewed on a panoramic film than on a complete intraoral radiograph series), simplicity, low patient radiation dose [2, 4]. The dose to the patient is approximately ten times less than full-mouth survey using the long cone and E+ film and it is four times less than four bitewings using the long round cone and E+ film [4].

The panoramic radiograph is less confusing to the patient than a series of small separate intraoral radiographs, making it easier for the dentist to explain the diagnosis and treatment plan to the patient [5].

The panoramic radiograph is an excellent imaging modality in patients with trismus or trauma, because such patients cannot open their mouths and this is not needed to take a panoramic film [4]. It is an excellent projection of diverse structures on a single film, which no other imaging system can achieve. Individual structures may be imaged by other methods, once pathologic conditions have been detected using the panoramic radiography [3, 4].

Nevertheless, this radiographic examination presents a lack of details and resolution of some structures due to overlapping of anatomical structures in the image, mild distortion and magnification [1, 3]. Objects of interest that are located outside the focal trough (it is the area of the dental anatomy that is reproduced distinctly on the panoramic radiograph) [5] are not seen [2], and artifacts are commom and may easily be misinterpreted [5].

These features limit the indications of panoramic radiographs in cases where details and accurate measurements are needed [1, 3].

4. Anatomical variations observed on panoramic radiographs

The term "normal" in Anatomy refers to the shape and position most frequently found in individuals, that is, the typical shape. Anatomical variation is the deviation from the normal that does not bring any noticeable functional disorder [6].

Not very unusual, the bifid mandibular canals are observed on panoramic radiographs (Figure 1).

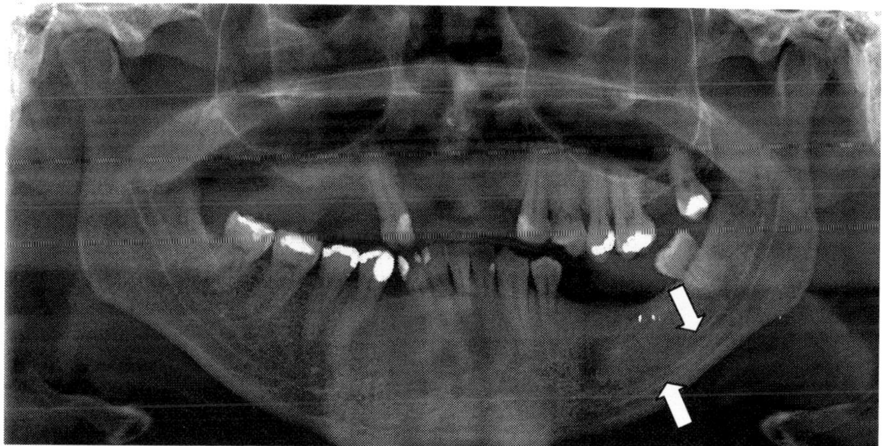

Figure 1. Digital panoramic radiography with a bifid mandibular canal image on the left side.

There are different frequencies and shapes in the literature.

Only 4 panoramic radiographs (0.08%) from 5,000 were highly suggestive of bifurcation [7]. Seven cases (0.35%) from 2,012 radiographs presented a suggestive image of a double man-dibular canal [8]. From 700 panoramic radiographs evaluation, 3 cases (0.43%) showed bifid mandibular canal [9]. Duplication or division of the mandibular canal was found in 33 individuals (0.9%) from the 3,612 evaluated panoramic radiographs [10]. It is important to observe the presence of bifid mandibular canals to prevent potential complications during surgical dental procedures. A total of 6,000 panoramic radiographs were studied, and there were 57 bifid mandibular canals (0.95%) [11].

Three main patterns of duplication were found radiographically [10]. The first variety (Type 1) consisted of two canals originating from one foramen. The second variety of duplication or division (Type 2) was produced by a short upper canal extending to the second molar or third molar teeth. Type 3 was seen as two mandibular canals of equal dimensions apparently arising from separate foramina in the mandibular ramus and joining together to form one canal in the molar region of the body of the mandible. Other variations (Type 4) included duplication or division of the canal, apparent partial or complete absence of the canal or lack of symmetry.

The most common supplemental mandibular canals are duplicate canals commencing from a single mandibular foramen and the least common arising from two distinctly separate foramina [10]. A different classification was used by reference [9], which verified that type III (the canal is located close to the lower border of the mandible) is the most common, followed by the type II (the canal is noted between the apices of the first and second molars and the lower border of the mandible) and the type I (the canal is in close contact with the apices of the first and the second molars).

No great difference in frequency between males and females was found by reference [10] and there was no statistical significance between sex and types of the mandibular canal in the study of reference [9]. Women presented more bifid mandibular canals than men (63.5% vs. 36.5%) [8].

When bifid mandibular canals were evaluated by cone beam computed tomography (CBCT), a higher frequency was found. An incidence of 15.6% from 301 mandible sides was observed by [12] and, in a recent study an incidence of 10.2% was found in CBCT of 1933 patients [13]. However, different results were found by reference [8]. In their study, computed axial tomography was used in 3 of the 7 cases with apparent double inferior alveolar nerve images on panoramic radiographs. The existence of a bifid canal could only be confirmed in 2 of these patients. The authors suggested that the true incidence of bifid mandibular canals might be lower than reported by other studies. The possible causes underlying a false double-canal radiograph may include the imprint of the mylohyoid nerve on the internal mandibular surface where it separates from the inferior alveolar nerve and travels to the floor of the mouth [8, 14, 15]. Another explanation could be the radiologic osteocondensation image produced by the insertion of the mylohyoid muscle into the internal mandibular surface, with a distribution parallel to the dental canal [8, 16].

Bifurcation of the mandibular nerve may be a cause of inadequate anesthesia in a small percentage of cases [7, 8]. One of the seven patients who presented bifid mandibular canals on panoramic radiographs commented that her dentist had experienced problems in performing inferior alveolar nerve block in the past. Another patient had no such problems, and the remaining five patients had either never undergone anesthesia or remembered no associated problems [8]. This problem is usually resolved by performing inferior alveolar nerve anesthesia at a somewhat higher level (the so-called "Gow-Gates" technique) [8, 17]. Other possible complications can occur during surgery of the lower third molar, in orthognathic or reconstructive mandibular surgery, and in the placement of dental implants [8, 18], because of possible damage to an unidentified second mandibular canal [8].

Another anatomical variation that can be observed on panoramic radiographs is the retromolar canal, and it can be considered a type of mandibular canal division.

Retromolar canal has been observed in dry mandibles, cadaveric dissections, panoramic radiographs and cone beam computed tomography. Variability in the prevalence of the retromolar canal is also verified in different studies, 1.7% [19], 12.19% [20], 12.9% [21], 14.08% [22], 17% [23], 18% [24], 21.9% [25], 25% [26], 26.58% [27] (studies with dry mandibles); 5.8% [28], 16.8% [29] (studies with panoramic radiography); 16% [30], 75.4% in individuals assessed by tomography exams, 72% in cadavers [31], 52.5% [13], 75.4% [32] (studies with computed tomography).

In the retromolar canals there were found striated muscle fibers, myelinated nerve fibers and blood vessels [26]. In the retromolar canal an artery was found, being the branch of the inferior alveolar artery, and the existing nerve derived from the inferior alveolar nerve and went to the third-molar region, the retromolar triangle mucosa, the buccal mucosa, the vestibular gingiva of the premolar region and inferior molars [33]. Accessory canals in the retromolar region are functionally important in providing the neural and/or vascular components of the mandible [34]. Figure 2 shows one retromolar canal bilaterally.

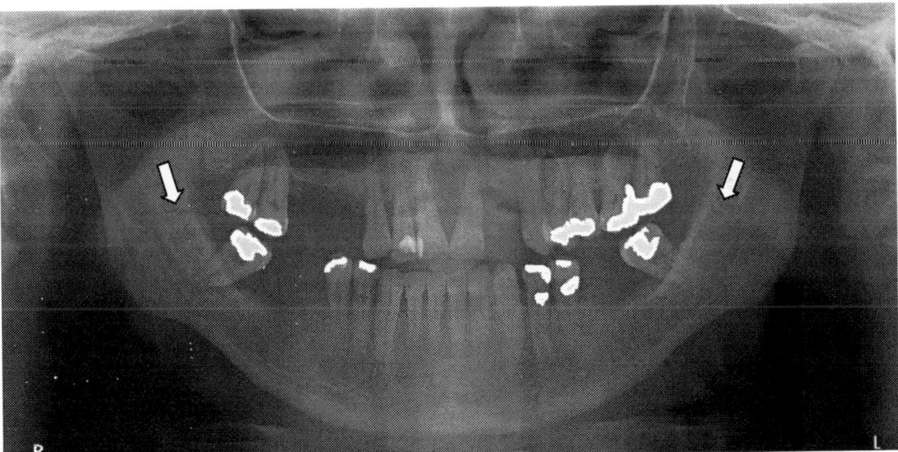

Figure 2. Digital panoramic radiography presenting a retromolar canal image on both sides.

Therefore, the content of the mandibular retromolar canal, usually of nerve fibers and/or blood vessels, is very important for surgical and anesthetic procedures involving the retromolar area. The confirmation of retromolar foramen and canal locations prior to surgical procedures, such as extraction of an impacted molar and bone harvesting as a donor site for bone graft surgery [35]. Complications such as traumatic neuroma, paraesthesia, and bleeding could arise because of failure to recognize the presence of mandibular canal variation [36, 37].

Studies have demonstrated the advantage of computed tomography over panoramic radiography in identification of anatomical variations [30, 36, 38].

It is clinically significant to accurately localize a bifid mandibular canal before dentoalveolar surgery especially when their presence is suspected by panoramic radiography [39]. Therefore, when professionals have suspicious of accessory mandibular canals on panoramic radiography, computed tomography should be done to confirm them and avoid complications.

5. Alterations observed on panoramic radiographs that might compromise oral and general health

Due to the broad coverage of panoramic radiographs, sometimes we can visualize some structures that affect more than the patient's oral health, but also general health. Many changes are asymptomatic and can be identified casually, as when the panoramic radiography is required for dental evaluation.

Among them, there are the calcified stylohyoid complex, arterial calcifications and other soft tissue calcifications.

5.1. Calcified stylohyoid complex

The styloid process is a cylindrical bone originated on the temporal bone [40-44] in front of the stylomastoid foramen [41-43], being located between the internal and external carotid arteries and laterally to the tonsillar fossa [43, 45, 46].

According to reference [47], elongated styloid process defines a styloid process that is longer than normal and thus associated with calcification of the process and its ligament, but some authors preferred the term calcified stylohyoid complex to describe the elongated process with advanced calcification [47].

The stylohyoid ligament is attached to the lesser horn of the hyoid bone [43, 48] and the calcification of the stylohyoid complex includes the stylohyoid ligament which connects the styloid process to the lesser horn of the hyoid bone [43].

The etiology of elongated styloid process is unknown [40, 43-45, 49, 50]. It was suggested that calcified styloihyoid complex could be resulted from local chronic irritations, history of trauma, endocrine disorders in female at menopause, persistence of mesenchymal elements, bone tissue growth and mechanical stress or trauma during stylohyoid ligament development [40, 43, 45, 46, 49], although no significant difference between females at menopause or not were showed [43]. A case report of twins suggested a possibility that calcified stylohyoid complex might be originated from genetic factors [44].

Only one report commented about the positive correlation that was found between the length of the styloid process and serum calcium concentration, heel bone density and body height and weight [47]. Previous studies reported difference in age for calcified stylohyoid ligament [51], i.e., the length increased with the age [41-43, 52], and its occurrence is rare in children [46]. Thus, dentists should pay attention not only for pathosis of the teeth and jaws, but also for information on general health conditions [47].

The measurements of the calcified stylohyoid complex on the panoramic radiography consist on the distance from the point where the styloid process left the tympanic plate to the tip of the process, involving mineralized parts of the ligament [42, 47, 50].

The literature reports that calcified styloid process is considered normal when it does not extend below the mandibular foramen. It is considered elongated when it extends below the mandibular foramen [51]. Finally, calcification of the stylohyoid ligament occurs when the calcification extends below the mandibular foramen and does not appear to be continuous with the base of the skull [51]. Figure 3 presents a panoramic radiography showing a calcified stylohyoid complex on both sides.

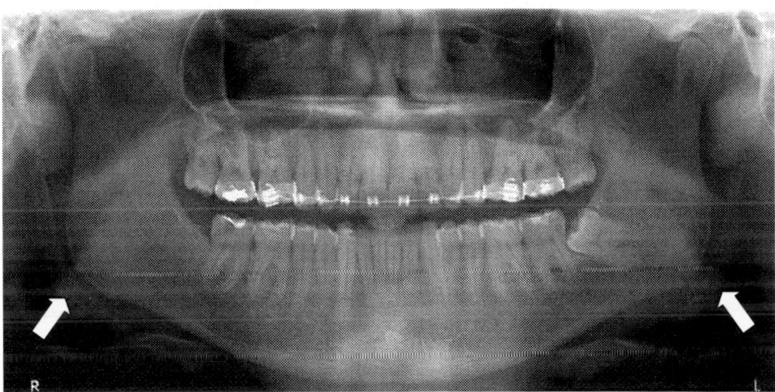

Figure 3. Digital panoramic radiography with a calcified stylohyoid complex on both sides. On the right side we can observe the stylohyoid ligament calcification near the hyoid bone. On the left side a fragmented stylohyoid ligament calcification can be seen.

Cervicalpharyngeal pain is classified into 3 entities: Eagle syndrome, stylohyoid syndrome and pseudostylohyoid syndrome [46]. Eagle's syndrome comprises elongated styloid process when it causes clinical symptoms, including dysphagia, foreign body sensation [45, 46, 48, 50, 53, 54], odynophagia, hypersalivation, and more rarely, temporary voice changes [53]. Eagle syndrome needs a history of trauma or neck surgery and painful symptoms on clinical palpation of the elongation or ossification of the stylohyoid process complex [46]. It may also cause stroke when compresses carotid arteries [40].

Stylohyoid syndrome does not comprise a history of trauma or surgery [46], and it occurs due to the compression of the internal and external carotid arteries and vascular structures [43, 53], resulting in a persistent pain to the carotid region, as headache, chronic neck pain, pain upon head movement and pain radiating to the eye [53]. It also shows radiographic elongation or ossification of the stylohyoid process complex [46] and it affects patients older than 40 years [46, 48]. This condition is more prevalent than Eagle syndrome [48].

In pseudostylohyoid syndrome there is no evidence of any elongation or ossification, but the patient describes the symptoms [46].

In Eagle syndrome, the styloid process is longer than 25mm [46]; from 25mm to 30mm it is considered elongated [42], although it varies in length in different people and even on the two sides of the same person [41, 42]. There is a significant prevalence for men concerning the styloid process length [42, 47]. However, there was no difference between sexes on the pattern distribution of calcified stylohyoid complex [43, 47, 51, 52]. The calcified stylohyoid complex bilaterally is prevalent [1, 41-43, 49, 52].

Radiographic imaging may include panoramic radiography, lateral cephalometry, Towne projection film, or computed tomogragphy (CT) scan [42, 43, 45, 46, 48, 53].

Calcified stylohyoid complex is usually visualized on panoramic radiography [1, 40, 51] as an incidental finding [49], as a long, thin, radiopaque process that is thicker at its base, posteriorly to the external acoustic meatus, with a trajectory downward and forward [1, 46]. A thicker calcified stylohyoid complex is uncommon. Figure 4 presents a very thick calcified stylohyoid complex.

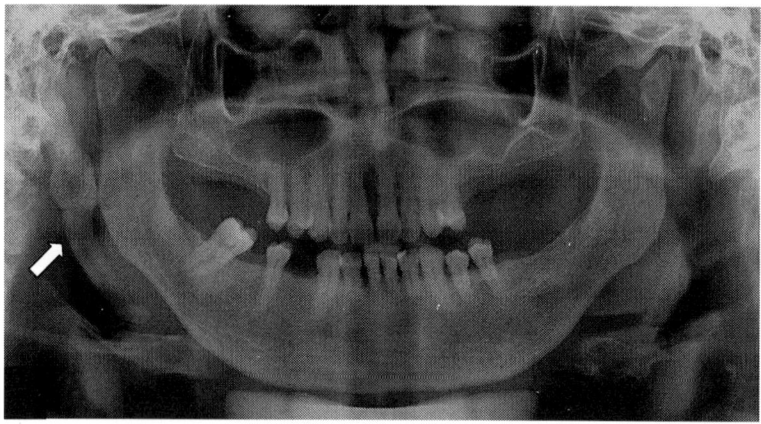

Figure 4. Digital panoramic radiography shows a thick calcified stylohyoid complex on the right side.

Panoramic radiography is the best imaging modality to visualize the styloid process bilaterally [42, 45] in patients with or without symptoms, and helps avoid misinterpretation of symptoms as tonsillar pain or dental pain, pharyngeal or muscular origin [42]. Panoramic radiography may be the first choice as imaging modality, because of its availability, low cost, diagnostic performance, and less patient dose compared to other imaging methods [43]. Nevertheless, panoramic radiography is not appropriate for measuring the length, and to show direction and anatomical variation of calcified stylohyoid complex compared to the multislice computed tomography [40, 46, 48, 54] and cone beam computed tomography do [43].

Data from clinical history, physical and radiographic examination must be considered when diagnosing Eagle's syndrome [46, 47, 54]. In the physical examination the calcified stylohyoid complex can be palpated on the tonsillar fossa as a hard and pointed structure [45, 49, 54].

The differentiation diagnosis of styloid ligament calcification may include calcified carotid artery atheromas, pheboliths and lymph node calcification [47] and for symptomatic elongated styloid process may comprise temporomandibular joint disorder, glossopharyngeal and trigeminal neuralgias, temporal arteritis, migraine, myofacial pain, atypical odontalgia, sialadenitis, sialolithiasis, cervical arthritis and tumors [46, 49], pain secondary to unerupted or impacted third molars, histaminic headache [46].

Most patients with calcified stylohyoid complex are asymptomatic [1, 44, 52] and no treatment is required [1]. The first choice of treatment is the use of analgesics and anti-inflammatory medications [46, 49]. However, for severe symptomatic patients with Eagle's syndrome the surgical excision of the stylohyoid complex is recommended [1, 44, 46, 54]. Regardless the cervicalpharyngeal pain it is important for the dentist who is involved in the diagnosis and treatment of these syndromes to identify on the panoramic radiography the calcified stylo-hyoid complex and to refer the patient to a specialized team.

5.2. Arterial calcifications

The common carotid artery originates from the aorta artery and in the height of the upper edge of the thyroid cartilage branches into two terminal branches: internal and external carotid artery. The identification of the point of bifurcation is often located 3 cm below the lower edge of the mandible [55].

It is considered a dystrophic calcification where there are deposited calcium salts in chronically inflamed or necrotic tissues. The presence of an atheromatous plaque in the extracranial carotid vascular path is the main cause for vasculocerebral embolism and obstructive diseases [1].

Carotid artery atherosclerotic plaques develop when fatty substances, cholesterol, platelets, cellular waste products, and calcium are deposited in the lining of the artery [56]. Some risk factors for atherosclerosis are: diabetes mellitus, obesity, hypertension, smoking, inadequate diet, chronic kidney disease and menopause among others [57].

Panoramic radiographs, obtained during professional dental examinations, are a potential method for early detection of Calcified Carotid Artery Atheroma (CCAA) [58]. Patients found to have carotid calcification on panoramic radiographs should be referred for cerebrovascular and cardiovascular evaluation and aggressive management of vascular risk factors [59]. Patients who have risk factors and CCAA on panoramic radiographs have a higher chance of suffering a vascular event compared with patients without image CCAA on panoramic radiographs, indicating that the incidental finding of calcifications on a panoramic dental radiograph is a powerful marker for future adverse, nonfatal, vascular events, with cardio-vascular events being more common than cerebrovascular events [56].

The prevalence of CCAA in HIV+patients was assessed by reference [60] through review of medical records and on panoramic radiography and the authors concluded that infection and the treatment used to treat HIV infection can influence the identification of CCAA. Thus, a careful examination of panoramic radiographs in these patients is recommended and the need for further studies related to the subject is reinforced.

Authors [61] observed hypertension as the major risk factor associated with carotid artery calcification followed by diabetes mellitus and hyperlipidemia in the Thai population. A standard panoramic dental radiography detected the presence of calcified cervical carotid artery disease in approximately 31% of postmenopausal women with no history of transient ischemic attack or stroke. It was demonstrated that hypertension was a significant risk factor for the development of atheromas [62]. Other authors [63] observed that patients who had evidence of calcified carotid plaque on panoramic radiographs had lower incidence of diabetes mellitus and hyperlipidemia but were more likely to have stroke, compared with patients with negative panoramic radiography for calcification.

The utility of observing calcification will obviously depend on the prevalence and amount of calcium within these lesions, which varies according to each patient [64].

A high interobserver agreement (92.4%) on the detection of carotid artery calcification (CAC) on panoramic radiographs of male patients above 50 years old was observed by reference [65]. No significant difference in the prevalence CCA in HIV+patients using conventional and digital panoramic radiograph was found [60]. Authors [66] emphasized that digital panoramic radiograph allow low intensity calcifications to be visualized due to the possibility of changing the contrast, density and expansion.

Radiographically, calcified carotid atheroma is initially developed at the bifurcation of arteries, soft tissues of the neck, and adjacent to the greater horn of the hyoid bone and the cervical vertebrae C3 and C4 or the intervertebral space between them. They are radiopaque, usually multiple and irregularly shaped, with a vertical distribution and they have an internally heterogeneous radiopacity [1]. The shape varies from circular to mostly linear with irregular margins and appears punctate containing areas of radiolucencies [67]. Figures 5 and 6 present panoramic radiographs with images suggesting the presence of atheromas.

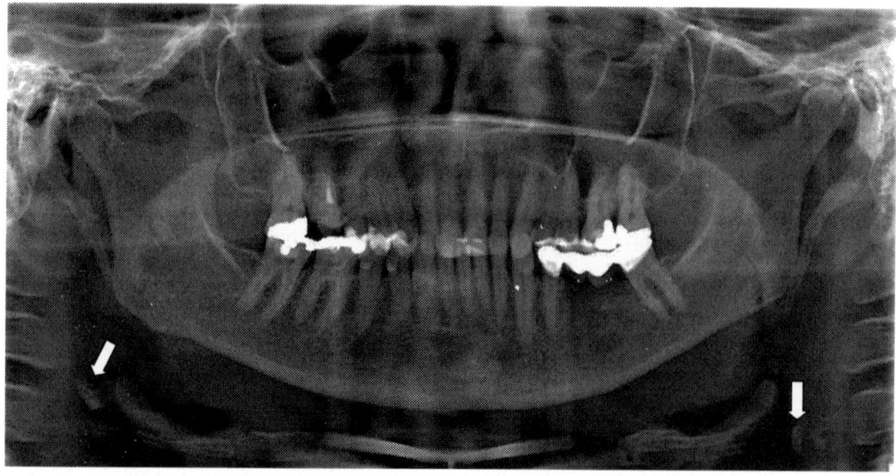

Figure 5. Digital panoramic radiography with images suggesting the presence of atheroma on both sides.

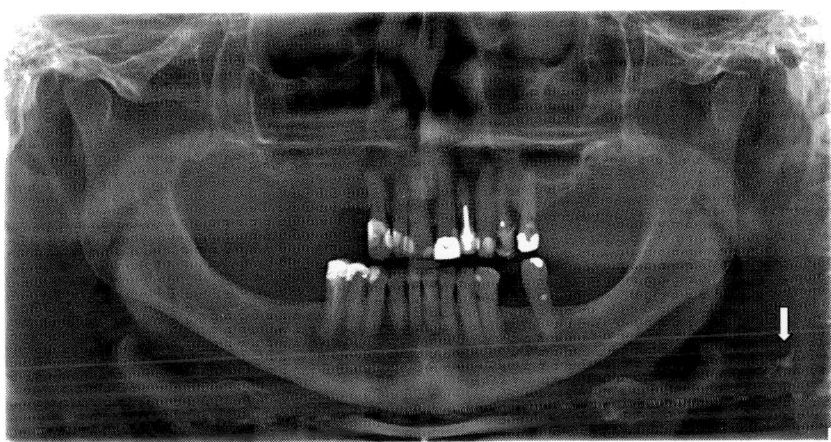

Figure 6. Digital panoramic radiography with image suggesting the presence of atheroma on left side.

Panoramic radiographs of a 67-year-old white woman were evaluated, and observed the presence of multiple, irregular, nonhomogenous radiopacities lying overboth the right and the left carotid bifurcations [64]. The calcifications were located inferior to the angle of the mandible and the tip of the hyoid bone, and to the top tip of the thyroid cartilage and the C3, C4 and C5 vertebrae [64]. Other authors [61] evaluated panoramic radiographs in 1370 patients and reported the presence of calcified carotid artery as irregular, heterogenous, vertcolinear or circular radiopaque lower to the neck at the level of the C3 and C4 intervertebral junction in the Thai population. The carotid artery calcifications were located within the soft tissues of the neck, approximately 2 centimeters inferior and posterior to the angle of the mandible, at about the level of the lower margin of the third cervical vertebra [62].

The differential diagnosis of CCAA image can be performed with several nearby anatomical structures such as the hyoid bone, styloid process, especially the thyroid cartilage and triticeous cartilage.

The triticeous cartilage often occurs in each lateral thyrohyoid ligament forming the edges of the thyrohyoid membrane [68].

The calcified triticeous cartilage can be confused with an atheromatous plaque but the shape, outline and location help in discriminating the triticeous cartilage from calcification in the carotid arteries [1, 67].

Triticeous cartilages and calcified carotid atheromas are located in a similar region on panoramic radiographs; the shape and outline help in differentiating these 2 calcifications in the neck. Triticeous cartilage is specifically located between the greater horn of the hyoid and superior horn of the thyroid cartilage, and the shape is mostly well-defined oval, with a smooth, well-defined corticated border [67]. Figure 7 shows a panoramic radiography with triticeous cartilages on both sides.

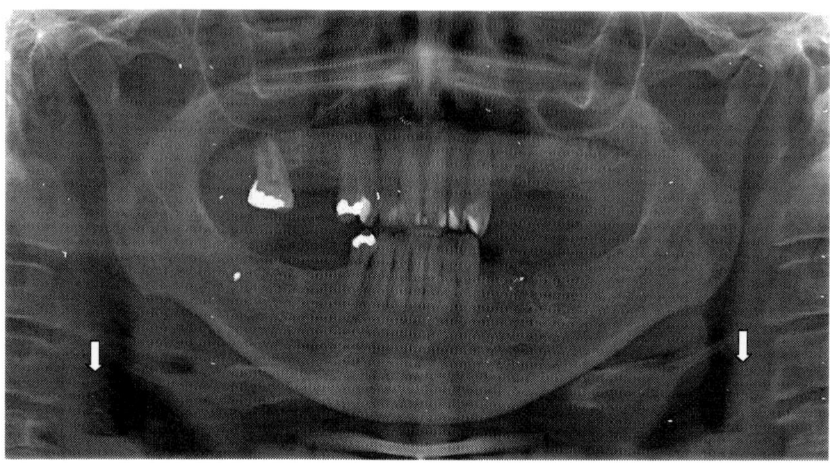

Figure 7. Digital panoramic radiography with image suggesting triticeous cartilage on both sides (between the greater horn of the hyoid and superior horn of the thyroid cartilage).

Authors [57] emphasized that although the panoramic radiography is not the test of choice, it is possible to identify atheroma in the carotid artery and therefore the dentist may instruct the patient to seek medical advice as soon as possible.

In order to confirm the presence of CACs, advanced imaging techniques such as duplex ultrasound, magnetic resonance imaging, and angiography should be performed [61].

The reliability of digital panoramic radiographs in detecting atheroma in the carotid artery was assessed [69] and the authors compared with ultrasound examinations. The results showed that digital panoramic radiography has a high level of agreement with ultrasonography with 76% of sensitivity and 98.66% of specificity. The authors concluded that the panoramic radiograph should not be routinely used in the detection of calcified carotid atheromatous plaques although when detected on a routine dental examination it is very useful.

The image of CCAA on panoramic radiograph was confirmed utilizing duplex ultra-sonography, which revealed carotid artery stenosis (CAS) [64]. The authors suggested that calcifications seen lying over the carotid bifurcation on panoramic radiographs should prompt further evaluation for CAS.

The dystrophic calcification of the tunica intima resulting in CCAA can be distinguished radiographically from another calcified form of arteriosclerosis, medial artery arteriosclerosis (MAA) or Mönckeberg's medial calcific sclerosis. The calcification in MAA is generalized because it affects the tunica media of medium and smaller muscular arteries. Calcifications are typically diffuse, multiple, and circumferential along the wall of the arterial vessel. MAA may be an indicator of peripheral artery disease, including diabetes mellitus or chronic kidney disease. MAA is generally observed in the limbs and rarely reported in the head and neck [70]. MAA can be identified on the panoramic radiography when the facial artery is affected.

According to reference [71], the panoramic radiography can be the first auxiliary in diagnosis for detecting facial artery calcification in patients in hemodialysis. The authors suggested that more studies should be performed, in order to determine the incidence of that alteration in those patients.

Radiographically, the calcium deposited in the arterial wall outlines the artery contour, being identified as a pair of parallel, thin radiopaque lines, or with circular aspect, depending on the evaluated view [1].

5.3. Sialolithiasis

Sialolithiasis is the most common disease of the salivary glands [72-74] characterized by obstruction of salivary secretion by a calculus, associated with swelling, pain [72, 75, 76] and infection of the affected gland [75]. More than 80% of the salivary gland calculi occurs in the submandibular gland [1, 72, 74-78] and 5%-20% in the parotid gland [72, 75-78] and rarely in the sublingual gland and the minor salivary glands (1% to 2%) [72, 75-77]. It is common in adults (1.2% of the population), with a male predominance [1, 72, 74, 76, 77], although previous investigators cited that sialolithisis occurs more frequently in white woman [73]. Children are rarely involved and sialolithiasis is more frequently in the third to the sixth decades of life [72, 74-77].

Patients with sialolithiasis may complain of moderate to intense pain when it involves the duct of a major salivary gland, particularly at mealtimes, when salivary flow is stimulated [1, 73], associated with enlargement of the gland [73].

Sialoliths are stones found within the ducts of salivary glands [1] and may be single or multiple [72, 76]. Single sialolith is more common seen [1, 79]. Figure 8 shows a panoramic radiography with a single sialolith on the right side in the submandibular gland. They measure from 1 mm to less than 1 cm [72, 74, 75]. Giant sialoliths are rare, bigger than 3.5 cm and also occur in male patients and are commonly located in the submandibular gland [74].

According to reference [74], several factors seem to be involved in the development of salivary calculi in the submandibular gland tissues such as: the submandibular excretory duct is wider in diameter and longer than the Stensen's duct; the secretion against gravity [74, 77]; the secretion is more alkaline compared with pH of the parotid saliva; the submandibular saliva contains a higher quantity of mucin proteins, while parotid saliva is entirely serous; then its saliva presents high calcium and phosphate content [73, 74, 77].

Initial events that contribute for the formation of a nidus that later will be the site for the precipitation of mineral salts contained in the salivary secretion include infection, inflammation, physical trauma, salivary stagnation, introduction of foreign bodies and the presence of desquamated ephitelial cells [73, 74].

The likely mechanism of sialolith formation in the sublingual gland is mechanical trauma with mucus extravasation, which serves as a nidus for stone formation [77]. In summary, the formation of a sialolith requires salivary stagnation, a nidus and a precipitation of salivary salts [75].

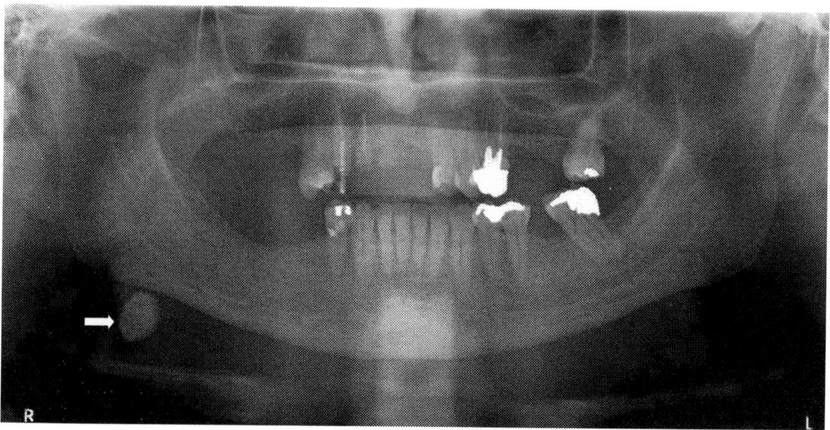

Figure 8. Digital panoramic radiography with image suggesting a single sialolith in the right submandibular gland.

Depending on the sialolith size and calcification degree, it can be visible in conventional radiographs. In panoramic radiography, the calcification image may appear superimposed on the mandible; therefore, it may be mistaken by an intrabone lesion [73]. Plain film radiography demonstrates dystrophic calcifications and the possible involvement of adjcent osseous structures [1].

Panoramic radiography usually shows sialoliths in the submandibular gland if they are located in the posterior duct [1]. If calculi can not be visualized in conventional radiographs, other imaging examinations may be necessary [73]. Sialography is used to evaluate obstructive and inflammatory conditions of the ductal system. If the patient is allergic to the iodine contrast agent used in sialography, the alternative imaging examination is ultrasonography or scintilography [1].

Computed tomography or magnetic resonance imaging are appropriate if the sialography suggests the presence of a space-occupying mass [1]. According to previous investigation, panoramic radiography and CT scan estimation appeared to be somewhat closer to the surgical specimen size [75].

Sialoliths in the sublingual gland are usually round or oval shaped. However, stones in Wharton's duct may be elongated. Parotid stones are usually smaller and more often multiple [77]. A single mass of calcification of the parotid gland with a calcification of part of its duct can be seen in the Figure 9.

Giant sublingual sialolith was previous described as a large single calcified mass in sublingual area on panoramic radiography. Giant sublingual sialolith has already been associated with dysphagia as well as eating and speaking difficulty [76]

Sialolith is usually homogeneously radiopaque, although it can show evidence of multiple layers of calcification if large [1, 79]. Salivary stones are usually shaped by the duct and then

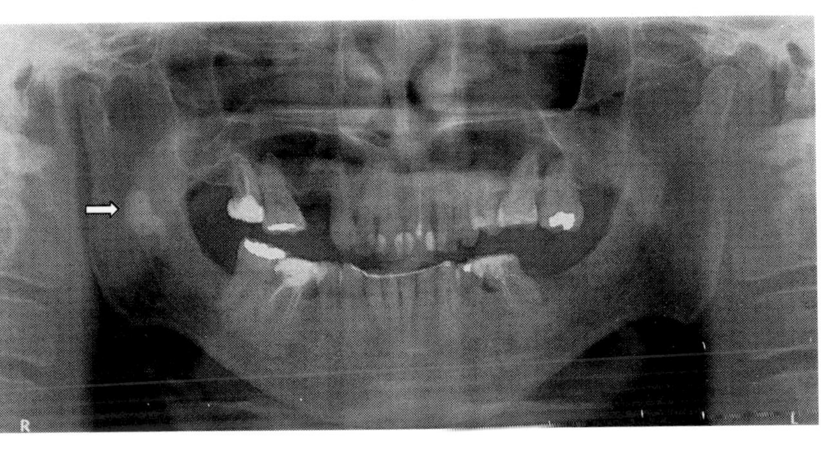

Figure 9. Digital panoramic radiography showing a image suggesting a calcification in the right parotid gland and in its duct.

they are elongated [77, 79]. Sialoliths are more likely localized in the Wharton's duct (submandibular gland) than in the Stensen's duct (parotid gland) [79]. Figure 10 shows calcifications in the submandibular and parotid glands.

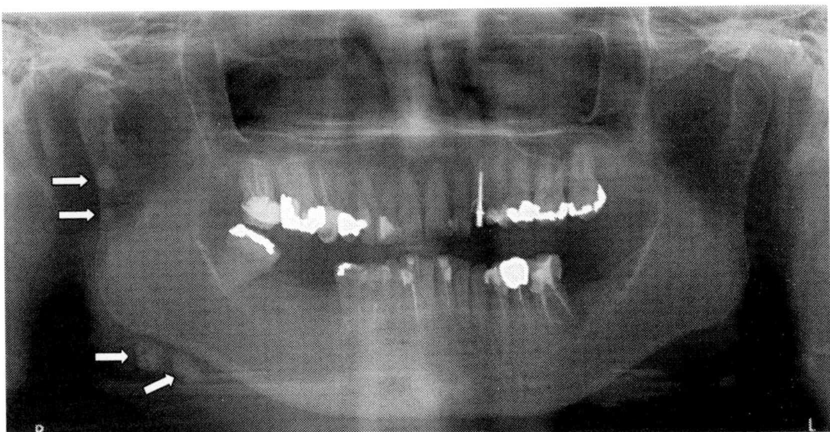

Figure 10. Digital panoramic radiography with image suggesting calcifications in the right submandibular and parotid glands.

A previous report descibed 3 cases with multiple microliths in their parotid parenchyma in Sjögren's syndrome showing panoramic radiography with many spots-like calcifications observed around the gonial angle and in the posterior part of the ramus [78]. According to previous publication, parotid calculi are frequently seen about halfway up on the ramus and may be multiple [80] as cited above. We can observe a panoramic radiography with multiple microliths in the parotid gland on both sides in the Figure 11.

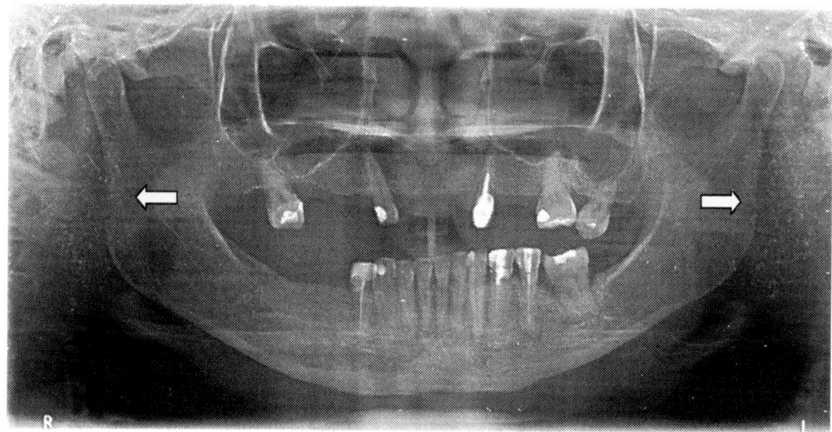

Figure 11. Digital panoramic radiography with image suggesting multiple microliths in the parotid gland on both sides.

Although this report is about panoramic radiography, previous investigations comment about cone beam computed tomography (CBCT) and reported that for visualization of the delicate structures of the parotid and submandibular salivary glands and for identification of sialoliths and single ductal strictures, CBCT sialography may be better than plain film sialography [81]. CBCT is the preferable imaging modality for salivary calculus diagnosis considering its high diagnostic-information-to-radiation-dose ratio [82] and to show the shapes of stones more clearly [75].

Vascular malformation with phleboliths must be included in the differential diagnosis of salivary gland obstruction and magnetic resonance imaging may be able to distinguish between them, but sialography is the most effective diagnostic modality to this differentiation [79].

According to [72], sialolithiasis treatment depends on the localization of the salivary calculus [72, 73]. The sialolith should be removed via a transoral sialolithotomy avoing sialadenectomy. Intraglandular sialoliths necessitate sialadenectomy [73, 75]. Solitary sialoliths usually do not recur [72].

5.4. Phleboliths

Phleboliths are idiopathic calcification (or calcinosis) that results from deposition of calcium in the normal tissue. This calcification results from deposition of calcium in the normal tissue, despite normal serum levels of calcium and phosphate [1]. Phleboliths are calcified thrombi found within vascular channels, often in the presence of hemangiomas or vascular malformations. They may originate from injury to a vessel wall or result from stagnation of the flow of blood [83, 84]. A case of intramuscular hemangioma was related by reference [85], where it was observed the large number of phleboliths of the tongue due to the long-term presence of hemangioma and stagnant blood flow. The authors [86], when reporting an intramuscular hemangioma also suggested that the cause of the large number of phleboliths is the long-term presence of hemangioma and stagnant blood.

The presence of vascular anomalies in the head and neck has a great importance for the professionals working in this area, since any procedure performed in this region without the due caution may trigger the onset of an emergency, as bleeding, which can lead to the patient's death. Therefore, there is a need to conduct a thorough diagnosis in order to help in the discovery of the existence of these defects, so that such situations are avoided [87]. Those authors reviewed the charts of 108 patients with vascular anomalies and observed in 31% of the cases that the changes were in the region of the mouth and tongue, being the period of childhood and adolescence the most affected (64%).

Clinically, the vascular changes may have a swollen soft tissue, which is throbbing and with its modified coloration and some noises when auscultating [1].

A case of a patient with multiple swellings on the surface and in the mouth with a purplish coloration in intraoral examination was reported by reference [88]. Radiographic examination showed small phleboliths in the left submandibular region, and ultrasound also showed calcifications. Histological examination showed that the characteristics are originated from venous malformation. Three cases of hemangioma of the head and neck varying like the clinical characteristics presented were presented by reference [89], however some commonalities between them could be noticed as swelling, absence of pulse or noise, and two cases showed discoloration.

Phleboliths calcification starts in the center of the thrombus and consists of apatite crystals of calcium phosphate and carbonate [1]. Initially, calcification of the thrombus occurs, forming the core of the phlebolith. The fibrinous component then undergoes secondary calcification and becomes attached. Repetition of this process causes enlargement of the phlebolith [86].

Radiographically, the phlebolith features radiopaque, rounded or oval image measuring more than 6mm in diameter and uniform periphery. Internally, it can present a homogeneous radiopacity, but it commonly presents a laminated appearance with a target aspect [1]. A patient with an oral mixed mucosal and submucosal venous malformation with multiple phleboliths, which the panoramic radiograph revealed multiple round-to-oval radiopaque bodies located in the soft tissues of the left retromolar trigone. Those structures had a laminated pattern and were interpreted as phleboliths [90].

A patient presented a small mass that contained calcification in the anterior part of the masseter muscle and the plain radiograph showed a round, uniformly radiopaque lesion [91]. The same was observed by other authors [92], who reported about a patient with a masseteric intramuscular hemangioma, which other than a mild facial asymmetry, was subjectively asymptomatic. This diagnosis could not be reached without computed tomography (CT) scan that identified the presence of the calcified body confirmed by the panoramic radiograph. The patient did not exhibit the lamellated feature of a phlebolith. MRI with contrast was ordered for further evaluation and diagnosis that clearly visualized an enhanced vascular lesion within the left masseter muscle, and confirmed the presence and location of the phlebolith. However, phleboliths are not easily recognized in magnetic resonance image (MRI) film because of their very low signal intensity. They are best identified on plain radiograph and CT scan. Authors [93] observed in occlusal radiograph of a patient with vascular malformation, two oval radiopaque images, diagnosed after microscopic examination as being phlebolith.

Studies about hemangiomas and venous malformations associating imaging methods have been reported in literature aiming to improve the diagnosis of these changes and the presence of phleboliths. CT was used in 3 cases that revealed phleboliths so no other imaging was considered to be necessary [89]. Phlebolith was observed on radiography and ultrasonography of paranasal sinus [88]. Plain x-rays may also help with the diagnosis because of the typical appearance of the calcified bodies and computed tomography, magnetic ressonance, and ultrasonography are more useful for making an accurate diagnosis [91]. A case of intramuscular hemangioma and another one of vascular malformation presenting phleboliths by the use of sialography and occlusal radiographs was presented by reference [84]. Occlusal radiography and Doppler ultrasonography also were used in a case of vascular malformation [93].

The radiographic image of phlebolith can be similar to a sialolith [1]. Phleboliths are usually multiple, with oval shape, randomly located and lamellated [92]. Figure 12 shows a panoramic radiography with multiple phleboliths on the right side.

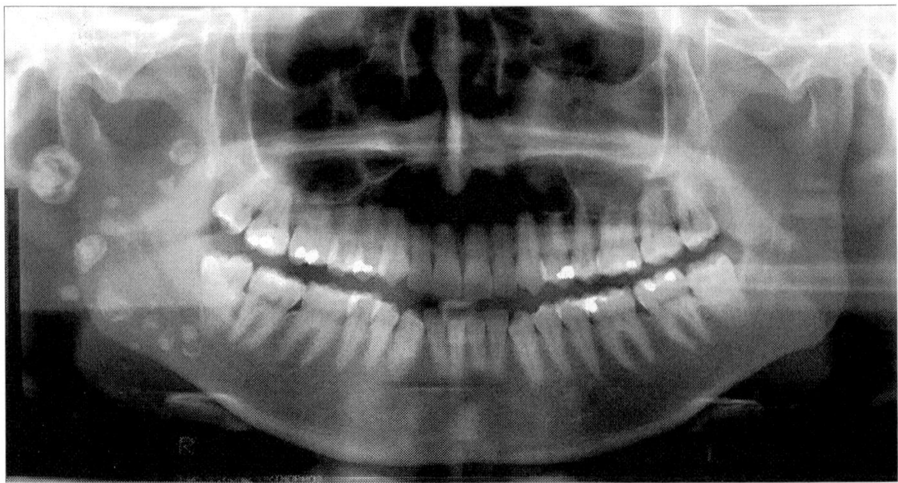

Figure 12. Panoramic radiography with image suggesting multiple phleboliths on the right side.

The sialoliths are frequently elliptically or elongated shaped due to the anatomic contour of the salivary duct [90, 92]. According to reference [90], sialography usually reveals a filling defect at the site of the salivary calculus, whereas phleboliths appear to be external to the duct system [90]. A case of recurrent episodes of pain and swelling in the right submandibular region was reported by reference [79]. Radiopaque images were identified in occlusal and panoramic radiographs, being diagnosed as sialoliths. The sialendoscopy was indicated and no intraductal stones were detected. A vascular network of capillaries was detected in all the ductal lumen altering the sialolithiasis diagnostic to a vascular malformation with phleboliths. The authors concluded that the vascular malformation obstructing the duct of the salivary gland is overlooked by physicians, and that phleboliths may be confounded with sialoliths.

5.5. Tonsilloliths

Tonsilloliths are calcifications within a tonsillar crypt, which involve primarily the palatine tonsil caused by dystrophic calcification as a result of chronic inflammation [94]. Small concretions are not uncommon findings especially in the aged population [95], however large tonsillar concretions occur with a much lower incidence [95-98].

The prevalence of tonsilloliths (measuring above 2 mm) in 1524 patients attending the oral and maxillofacial radiology clinic of The University of Iowa was observed to be 8.14% by reference [99]. The age range of subjects was 9.2–87 years (mean 52.6 years), the average size of tonsillolith was 4mm (range: 3–11 mm), with no sex predilection.

The large tonsilloliths occur in males and females equally [98, 100], and on the fifth decade of life [100]. Tonsilloliths in children are rare and they are more common in young adults with long stories of recurrent tonsillar inflammation [98, 100].

The exact etiology and pathogenesis is unknown. Repeated episodes of inflammation may produce fibrosis at the openings of the tonsillar crypts. Bacterial and epithelial debris then accumulates within these crypts and contributes to the formation of retention cysts. Calcification occurs subsequent to the deposition of inorganic salts and the enlargement of the formed concretion takes place gradually. The tonsilloliths derive their phosphate and carbonate of lime and magnesia from saliva secreted by salivary glands [94-98, 101]. The mineral content of tonsilloliths can be composed by phosphorus, calcium, carbonate or magnesium [95].

On the panoramic radiography, tonsilloliths commonly appear as multiple, small, and ill-defined radiopacities [99]. On the other hand, other authors [94] described tonsilloliths as usually being single and unilateral, but occasionally they may be multiple or bilateral. Tonsilloliths should be the first differential diagnosis when multiple opaque lesions with ill-defined borders, which are superimposed on the palatal uvula and the ramus are detected on the panoramic radiography [94]. The radiographic appearance of tonsilloliths was predominantly multiple and well defined (62.90%) and the single, well-defined tonsillolith in a similar location constituted 28.23% in the study of reference [99]. The authors verified that the majority of the cases were located in the lower one third of the mandibular ramus (93.55%). Figures 13 and 14 shows panoramic radiographs with multiple tonsilloliths in the lower one third of the mandibular ramus on both sides.

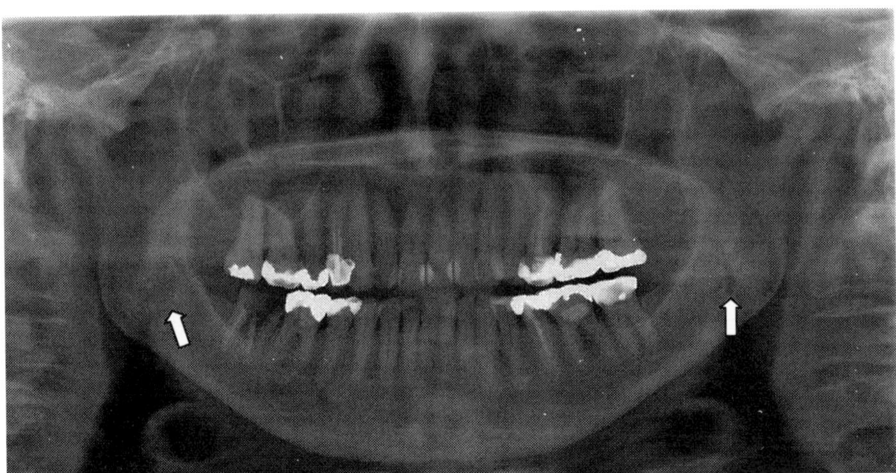

Figure 13. Digital panoramic radiography with image suggesting multiple tonsilloliths in the lower one third of the mandibular ramus on both sides.

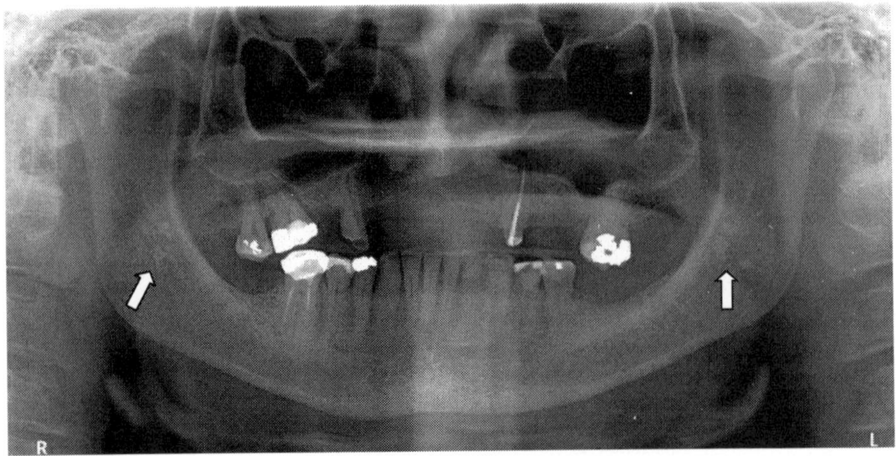

Figure 14. Digital panoramic radiography with image suggesting multiple tonsilloliths in the lower one third of the mandibular ramus on both sides.

Calcifications in the carotid arterial, lymph nodes, salivary gland and stylohyoid ligament are some of the differential diagnosis that might be considered [101].

On the clinical examination, it should be considered malignancy or calcified granulomatous disease such as tertiary syphilis, tuberculosis and deep fungal infection as differential diagnosis [98].

When no predisposing causes can be discovered (like chronic obstructive sialolithiasis of the salivary glands, past medical history of kidney stone), the medical history represents the most important element to recognise the tendency of some patients to develop calcifications, as in the case reported [96]. The observations in the study of [99] do not support any correlations between tonsilloliths and calcifications in other body organs, tissues, or ducts.

Patients with tonsilloliths may be asymptomatic probably when the calcifications have small size [101], and their lesions discovered incidentally on panoramic radiographs or they can present pain or soreness, dysphagia, halitosis, otalgia, infection, a foreign body-like sensation, irritable cough, difficulty in swallowing, bad/altered taste [94-96, 98-100].

Incidental findings of large tonsilloliths are reported using panoramic radiography [96, 98, 100]. The panoramic radiography helps to observe the location of opacities, but considering its two-dimensional limitations, a computed tomography or cone beam computed tomography scan is necessary to accurately position the calcifications [96, 100].

Treatment is usually removal of concretions by curettage and larger lesions may require local excision [96, 98, 99]. If there is evidence of chronic tonsillitis, tonsillectomy offers definitive therapy; however it is advisable to postpone tonsillectomy until all acute symptoms have subsided [98].

The diagnosis of tonsillar calculi, exploring their etiology, evaluating them for removal, and not dismissing them as clinically insignificant it is important because of the significant morbidity via chronic infection, pain, and/or swallowing abnormalities, with the potential of further pulmonary complications [95].

6. Conclusion

Panoramic radiograph is a radiological technique that provides an overview of the jaws and adjacent structures. Asymptomatic patients may show anatomical variations or alterations that may be randomly displayed on panoramic radiographs. These alterations may contribute to clinical complications and damage the patient's oral and general health. Therefore, it is of utmost importance that dentists be able to recognize the evidence of these variations and alterations on panoramic radiographs and request additional examinations that provide a more accurate diagnosis. Thus, we conclude that the panoramic radiograph, within its limitations, contributes effectively to the initial diagnosis of anatomic variations and alterations, and the dental professional can identify the risks and refer their patients to a specialist.

Author details

Ticiana Sidorenko de Oliveira Capote[1*], Marcela de Almeida Gonçalves[1],
Andrea Gonçalves[2] and Marcelo Gonçalves[2]

*Address all correspondence to: ticiana@foar.unesp.br

1 Dental School at Araraquara, Univ. Estadual Paulista, UNESP, Department of Morphology, Araraquara, São Paulo, Brazil

2 Dental School at Araraquara, Univ. Estadual Paulista, UNESP, Department of Diagnostic and Surgery, Araraquara, São Paulo, Brazil

References

[1] White SC, Pharoa MJ. Oral Radiology: Principles and Interpretation. 5th ed. Saint Louis: Mosby; 2007.

[2] Haring JI, Jansen L. Dental radiography: principles and techniques. 2nd ed. Philadelphia: Saunders; 2000. 569 p.

[3] Alvares LC, Tavano O. Curso de radiologia em odontologia. 4th ed. São Paulo, Brazil: Livraria Santos Editora Ltda; 2002. 248 p.

[4] Langland OE, Langlais RP, Preece JW. Principles of dental imaging. 2nd ed. Lippincott Williams & Wilkins; 2002. 459 p.

[5] De Lyre WR, Johnson ON. Essentials of dental radiography for dental assistants and hygienists. 4th ed. Norwalk, Conn.: Appleton & Lange; 1990. xvii, 446 p.

[6] Aumuller G. Anatomia. Rio de Janeiro: Guanabara Koogan; 2009.

[7] Grover PS, Lorton L. Bifid mandibular nerve as a possible cause of inadequate anesthesia in the mandible. Journal of oral and maxillofacial surgery : official journal of the American Association of Oral and Maxillofacial Surgeons 1983;41(3):177-179.

[8] Sanchis JM, Penarrocha M, Soler F. Bifid mandibular canal. Journal of oral and maxillofacial surgery : official journal of the American Association of Oral and Maxillofacial Surgeons 2003;61(4):422-424.

[9] Zografos J, Kolokoudias M, Papadakis E. [The types of the mandibular canal]. To Helleniko periodiko gia stomatike & gnathoprosopike cheirourgike / episemo organo tes Hetaireias Stomatognathoprosopikes Cheirourgikes. The Greek Journal of Oral & Maxillofacial Surgery 1990;5(1):17-20.

[10] Nortje CJ, Farman AG, Grotepass FW. Variations in the normal anatomy of the inferior dental (mandibular) canal: a retrospective study of panoramic radiographs from 3612 routine dental patients. The British Journal of Oral Surgery 1977;15(1):55-63.

[11] Langlais RP, Broadus R, Glass BJ. Bifid mandibular canals in panoramic radiographs. Journal of the American Dental Association 1985;110(6):923-926.

[12] Kuribayashi A, Watanabe H, Imaizumi A, Tantanapornkul W, Katakami K, Kurabayashi T. Bifid mandibular canals: cone beam computed tomography evaluation. Dentomaxillofacial Radiology 2010;39(4):235-239.

[13] Kang JH, Lee KS, Oh MG, Choi HY, Lee SR, Oh SH, et al. The incidence and configuration of the bifid mandibular canal in Koreans by using cone-beam computed tomography. Imaging Science in Dentistry 2014;44(1):53-60.

[14] Wilson S, Johns P, Fuller PM. The inferior alveolar and mylohyoid nerves: an anatomic study and relationship to local anesthesia of the anterior mandibular teeth. Journal of the American Dental Association 1984;108(3):350-352.

[15] Sillanpaa M, Vuori V, Lehtinen R. The mylohyoid nerve and mandibular anesthesia. International Journal of Oral and Maxillofacial Surgery 1988;17(3):206-207.

[16] Kiersch TA, Jordan JE. Duplication of the mandibular canal. Oral Surgery, Oral Medicine, and Oral Pathology 1973;35(1):133-134.

[17] Meechan JG. How to overcome failed local anaesthesia. British Dental Journal 1999;186(1):15-20.

[18] Quattrone G, Furlini E, Bianciotto M. [Bilateral bifid mandibular canal. Presentation of a case]. Minerva Stomatologica 1989;38(11):1183-1185.

[19] Ossenberg NS. Temporal crest canal: case report and statistics on a rare mandibular variant. Oral Surgery, Oral Medicine, and Oral Pathology 1986;62(1):10-12.

[20] Bilodi AKS, Singh S, Ebenezer DA, Suman P, Kumar K. A study on retromolar foramen and other accessory foramina in human mandibles of Tamil Nadu region. International Journal of Health Sciences and Research 2013;3(10):61-65.

[21] Galdámes IS, Matamala DZ, López MC. Retromolar Canal and Forame prevalence in dried mandibles and clinical implications. International Journal of Odontostomatology 2008;2(2):183-187.

[22] Athavale SA, Vijaywargia M, Deopujari R, Kobayashi K. Bony and cadaveric study of retromolar region. People's Journal of Scientific Research 2013;6(2):14-18.

[23] Motta-Junior J, Ferreira ML, Matheus RA, Stabile GAV. Forame retromolar: sua repercussão clínica e avaliação de 35 mandíbulas secas. Revista de Odontologia da UNESP 2012;41(3):164-168.

[24] Gupta S, Soni A, Singh P. Morphological study of accessory foramina in mandible and its clinical implication. Indian Journal of Oral Sciences 2013;4(1):12-16.

[25] Narayana K, Nayak UA, Ahmed WN, Bhat JB, Devaiah BA. The retromolar foramen and canal in south Indian dry mandibles. European Journal of Anatomy 2002;6(3): 141-146.

[26] Bilecenoglu B, Tuncer N. Clinical and anatomical study of retromolar foramen and canal. Journal of oral and maxillofacial surgery : official journal of the American Association of Oral and Maxillofacial Surgeons 2006;64(10):1493-1497.

[27] Rossi AC, Freire AR, Prado BG, Prado FB, Botacin PR, Caria PHF. Incidence of retromolar foramen in human mandibles: ethinic and clinical aspects. International Journal of Morphology 2012;30(3):1074-1078.

[28] von Arx T, Hanni A, Sendi P, Buser D, Bornstein MM. Radiographic study of the mandibular retromolar canal: an anatomic structure with clinical importance. Journal of Endodontics 2011;37(12):1630-1635.

[29] Muinelo-Lorenzo J, Suarez-Quintanilla JA, Fernandez-Alonso A, Marsillas-Rascado S, Suarez-Cunqueiro MM. Descriptive study of the bifid mandibular canals and retromolar foramina: cone beam CT vs panoramic radiography. Dentomaxillofacial Radiology 2014;43(5):20140090.

[30] Lizio G, Pelliccioni GA, Ghigi G, Fanelli A, Marchetti C. Radiographic assessment of the mandibular retromolar canal using cone-beam computed tomography. Acta Odontologica Scandinavica 2013;71(3-4):650-655.

[31] Schejtman R, Devoto FC, Arias NH. The origin and distribution of the elements of the human mandibular retromolar canal. Archives of Oral Biology 1967;12(11): 1261-1268.

[32] Patil S, Matsuda Y, Nakajima K, Araki K, Okano T. Retromolar canals as observed on cone-beam computed tomography: their incidence, course, and characteristics. Oral Surgery, Oral Medicine, Oral Pathology, and Oral Radiology 2013;115(5):692-699.

[33] Kodera H, Hashimoto I. [A case of mandibular retromolar canal: elements of nerves and arteries in this canal]. Kaibogaku Zasshi Journal of Anatomy 1995;70(1):23-30.

[34] Haveman CW, Tebo HG. Posterior accessory foramina of the human mandible. The Journal of Prosthetic Dentistry 1976;35(4):UNKNOWN.

[35] Kawai T, Asaumi R, Sato I, Kumazawa Y, Yosue T. Observation of the retromolar foramen and canal of the mandible: a CBCT and macroscopic study. Oral Radiology 2012;28(1):10-14.

[36] Kaufman E, Serman NJ, Wang PD. Bilateral mandibular accessory foramina and canals: a case report and review of the literature. Dentomaxillofacial Radiology 2000;29(3):170-175.

[37] Anderson LC, Kosinski TF, Mentag PJ. A review of the intraosseous course of the nerves of the mandible. The Journal of Oral Implantology 1991;17(4):394-403.

[38] Lee J, Yoon S, Kang B. Mandibular canal branches supplying the mandibular third molar observed on cone beam computed tomographic images: reports of four cases. Korean Journal of Oral and Maxillofacial Radiology 2009;39:209-212.

[39] Fukami K, Shiozaki K, Mishima A, Kuribayashi A, Hamada Y, Kobayashi K. Bifid mandibular canal: confirmation of limited cone beam CT findings by gross anatomical and histological investigations. Dentomaxillofacial Radiology 2012;41(6):460-465.

[40] Gokce C, Sisman Y, Sipahioglu M. Styloid Process Elongation or Eagle's Syndrome: Is There Any Role for Ectopic Calcification? European Journal of Dentistry 2008;2(3): 224-228.

[41] MK OC. Calcification in the stylohyoid ligament. Oral Surgery, Oral Medicine, and Oral Pathology 1984;58(5):617-621.

[42] More CB, Asrani MK. Evaluation of the styloid process on digital panoramic radiographs. The Indian Journal of Radiology & Imaging 2010;20(4):261-265.

[43] Alpoz E, Akar GC, Celik S, Govsa F, Lomcali G. Prevalence and pattern of stylohyoid chain complex patterns detected by panoramic radiographs among Turkish population. Surgical and Radiologic Anatomy : SRA 2014;36(1):39-46.

[44] Kim JE, Min JH, Park HR, Choi BR, Choi JW, Huh KH. Severe calcified stylohyoid complex in twins: a case report. Imaging Science in Dentistry 2012;42(2):95-97.

[45] Rizzatti-Barbosa CM, Ribeiro MC, Silva-Concilio LR, Di Hipolito O, Ambrosano GM. Is an elongated stylohyoid process prevalent in the elderly? A radiographic study in a Brazilian population. Gerodontology 2005;22(2):112-115.

[46] Valerio CS, Peyneau PD, de Sousa AC, Cardoso FO, de Oliveira DR, Taitson PF, et al. Stylohyoid syndrome: surgical approach. The Journal of Craniofacial Surgery 2012;23(2):e138-140.

[47] Okabe S, Morimoto Y, Ansai T, Yamada K, Tanaka T, Awano S, et al. Clinical significance and variation of the advanced calcified stylohyoid complex detected by panoramic radiographs among 80-year-old subjects. Dentomaxillofacial Radiology 2006;35(3):191-199.

[48] Kaushik A, Kaushik M, Panwar R, Tanwar R, Garg P, Garg S. Calcified stylohyoid ligaments: A diagnostic dilemma. SRM Journal of Research in Dental Sciences 2012;3(4):275.

[49] Koivumaki A, Marinescu-Gava M, Jarnstedt J, Sandor GK, Wolff J. Trauma induced eagle syndrome. International Journal of Oral and Maxillofacial Surgery 2012;41(3): 350-353.

[50] Sudhakara Reddy R, Sai Kiran C, Sai Madhavi N, Raghavendra MN, Satish A. Prevalence of elongation and calcification patterns of elongated styloid process in south India. Journal of Clinical and Experimental Dentistry 2013;5(1):e30-35.

[51] MacDonald-Jankowski DS. Calcification of the stylohyoid complex in Londoners and Hong Kong Chinese. Dentomaxillofacial Radiology 2001;30(1):35-39.

[52] Ferrario VF, Sigurta D, Daddona A, Dalloca L, Miani A, Tafuro F, et al. Calcification of the stylohyoid ligament: incidence and morphoquantitative evaluations. Oral Surgery, Oral Medicine, and Oral Pathology 1990;69(4):524-529.

[53] Jain S, Bansal A, Paul S, Prashar DV. Styloid-stylohyoid syndrome. Annals of Maxillofacial Surgery 2012;2(1):66-69.

[54] Moon CS, Lee BS, Kwon YD, Choi BJ, Lee JW, Lee HW, et al. Eagle's syndrome: a case report. Journal of the Korean Association of Oral and Maxillofacial Surgeons 2014;40(1):43-47.

[55] Figún ME, Garino RR. Anatomia odontológica funcional e aplicada. São Paulo: Panamericada; 1989. 658 p.

[56] Friedlander AH, Cohen SN. Panoramic radiographic atheromas portend adverse vascular events. Oral Surgery, Oral Medicine, Oral Pathology, Oral Radiology, and Endodontics 2007;103(6):830-835.

[57] Guimaraes Henriques JC, Kreich EM, Helena Baldani M, Luciano M, Cezar de Melo Castilho J, Cesar de Moraes L. Panoramic radiography in the diagnosis of carotid artery atheromas and the associated risk factors. The Open Dentistry Journal 2011;5:79-83.

[58] Bayram B, Uckan S, Acikgoz A, Muderrisoglu H, Aydinalp A. Digital panoramic radiography: a reliable method to diagnose carotid artery atheromas? Dentomaxillofacial Radiology 2006;35(4):266-270.

[59] Cohen SN, Friedlander AH, Jolly DA, Date L. Carotid calcification on panoramic radiographs: an important marker for vascular risk. Oral Surgery, Oral Medicine, Oral Pathology, Oral Radiology, and Endodontics 2002;94(4):510-514.

[60] da Silva NG, Pedreira EN, Tuji FM, Warmling LV, Ortega KL. Prevalence of calcified carotid artery atheromas in panoramic radiographs of HIV-positive patients undergoing antiretroviral treatment: a retrospective study. Oral Surgery, Oral Medicine, and Oral Pathology 2014;117(1):67-74.

[61] Pornprasertsuk-Damrongsri S, Thanakun S. Carotid artery calcification detected on panoramic radiographs in a group of Thai population. Oral Surgery, Oral Medicine, Oral Pathology, Oral Radiology, and Endodontics 2006;101(1):110-115.

[62] Friedlander AH, Altman L. Carotid artery atheromas in postmenopausal women. Their prevalence on panoramic radiographs and their relationship to atherogenic risk factors. Journal of the American Dental Association 2001;132(8):1130-1136.

[63] Griniatsos J, Damaskos S, Tsekouras N, Klonaris C, Georgopoulos S. Correlation of calcified carotid plaques detected by panoramic radiograph with risk factors for stroke development. Oral Surgery, Oral Medicine, Oral Pathology, Oral Radiology, and Endodontics 2009;108(4):600-603.

[64] Almog DM, Illig KA, Khin M, Green RM. Unrecognized carotid artery stenosis discovered by calcifications on a panoramic radiograph. Journal of the American Dental Association 2000;131(11):1593-1597.

[65] Yoon SJ, Shim SK, Lee JS, Kang BC, Lim HJ, Kim MS, et al. Interobserver agreement on the diagnosis of carotid artery calcifications on panoramic radiographs. Imaging Science in Dentistry 2014;44(2):137-141.

[66] Garay I, Netto HD, Olate S. Soft tissue calcified in mandibular angle area observed by means of panoramic radiography. International Journal of Clinical and Experimental Medicine 2014;7(1):51-56.

[67] Ahmad M, Madden R, Perez L. Triticeous cartilage: prevalence on panoramic radiographs and diagnostic criteria. Oral Surgery, Oral Medicine, Oral Pathology, Oral Radiology, and Endodontics 2005;99(2):225-230.

[68] William PL, Warwick R, Dyson M, Bannister LH. Gray Anatomia. 37 ed. Rio de Janeiro: Guanabara Koogan; 1995.

[69] Khambete N, Kumar R, Risbud M, Joshi A. Evaluation of carotid artery atheromatous plaques using digital panoramic radiographs with Doppler sonography as the ground truth. Journal of Oral Biology and Craniofacial Research 2012;2(3):149-153.

[70] MacDonald D, Chan A, Harris A, Vertinsky T, Farman AG, Scarfe WC. Diagnosis and management of calcified carotid artery atheroma: dental perspectives. Oral Surgery, Oral Medicine, Oral Pathology, and Oral Radiology 2012;114(4):533-547.

[71] Miles DA, Craig RM. The calcified facial artery. A report of the panoramic radiographic incidence and appearance. Oral Surgery, Oral Medicine, and Oral Pathology 1983;55(2):214-219.

[72] Eyigor H, Osma U, Yilmaz MD, Selcuk OT. Multiple sialolithiasis in sublingual gland causing dysphagia. The American Journal of Case Reports 2012;13:44-46.

[73] Jardim EC, Ponzoni D, de Carvalho PS, Demetrio MR, Aranega AM. Sialolithiasis of the submandibular gland. The Journal of Craniofacial Surgery 2011;22(3):1128-1131.

[74] Ledesma-Montes C, Garces-Ortiz M, Salcido-Garcia JF, Hernandez-Flores F, Hernandez-Guerrero JC. Giant sialolith: case report and review of the literature. Journal of Oral and Maxillofacial Surgery 2007;65(1):128-130.

[75] Bodner L. Giant salivary gland calculi: diagnostic imaging and surgical management. Oral Surgery, Oral Medicine, Oral Pathology, Oral Radiology, and Endodontics 2002;94(3):320-323.

[76] Gungormus M, Yavuz MS, Yolcu U. Giant sublingual sialolith leading to dysphagia. The Journal of Emergency Medicine 2010;39(3):e129-130.

[77] Hong KH, Yang YS. Sialolithiasis in the sublingual gland. The Journal of Laryngology and Otology 2003;117(11):905-907.

[78] Shimizu M, Yoshiura K, Nakayama E, Kanda S, Nakamura S, Ohyama Y, et al. Multiple sialolithiasis in the parotid gland with Sjogren's syndrome and its sonographic findings--report of 3 cases. Oral Surgery, Oral Medicine, Oral Pathology, Oral Radiology, and Endodontics 2005;99(1):85-92.

[79] Su YX, Liao GQ, Wang L, Liang YJ, Chu M, Zheng GS. Sialoliths or phleboliths? The Laryngoscope 2009;119(7):1344-1347.

[80] Langland OE, Langlais RP, Morris CR. Principles and practice of panoramic radiology : including intraoral radiographic interpretation. Philadelphia: Saunders; 1982. xiv, 458 p.

[81] Jadu FM, Lam EW. A comparative study of the diagnostic capabilities of 2D plain radiograph and 3D cone beam CT sialography. Dentomaxillofacial Radiology 2013;42(1):20110319.

[82] Dreiseidler T, Ritter L, Rothamel D, Neugebauer J, Scheer M, Mischkowski RA. Salivary calculus diagnosis with 3-dimensional cone-beam computed tomography. Oral Surgery, Oral Medicine, Oral Pathology, Oral Radiology, and Endodontics 2010;110(1):94-100.

[83] Shemilt P. The origin of phleboliths. The British Journal of Surgery 1972;59(9): 695-700.

[84] Mandel L, Perrino MA. Phleboliths and the vascular maxillofacial lesion. Journal of Oral and Maxillofacial Surgery 2010;68(8):1973-1976.

[85] Kamatani T, Saito T, Hamada Y, Kondo S, Shirota T, Shintani S. Intramuscular hemangioma with phleboliths of the tongue: A case report. Indian Journal of Dentistry 2014.

[86] Kanaya H, Saito Y, Gama N, Konno W, Hirabayashi H, Haruna S. Intramuscular hemangioma of masseter muscle with prominent formation of phleboliths: a case report. Auris, nasus, larynx 2008;35(4):587-591.

[87] Silva MI, Sassi LM, Rapoport A, Benedito VO, Machado R, Quebur MI. Aspectos clínicos e histológicos das anomalias vasculares da boca. Revista Brasileira de Cirurgia de Cabeça e Pescoço 2004;33(2):63-69.

[88] Chava VR, Shankar AN, Vemanna NS, Cholleti SK. Multiple venous malformations with phleboliths: radiological-pathological correlation. Journal of Clinical Imaging Science 2013;3(Suppl 1):13.

[89] Altug HA, Buyuksoy V, Okcu KM, Dogan N. Hemangiomas of the head and neck with phleboliths: clinical features, diagnostic imaging, and treatment of 3 cases. Oral Surgery, Oral Medicine, Oral Pathology, Oral Radiology, and Endodontics 2007;103(3):e60-64.

[90] Scolozzi P, Laurent F, Lombardi T, Richter M. Intraoral venous malformation presenting with multiple phleboliths. Oral Surgery, Oral Medicine, Oral Pathology, Oral Radiology, and Endodontics 2003;96(2):197-200.

[91] Kato H, Ota Y, Sasaki M, Arai T, Sekido Y, Tsukinoki K. A phlebolith in the anterior portion of the masseter muscle. The Tokai Journal of Experimental and Clinical Medicine 2012;37(1):25-29.

[92] Gordon JS, Mandel L. Masseteric Intramuscular Hemangioma: Case Report. Journal of Oral and Maxillofacial Surgery 2014.

[93] Mohan RP, Dhillon M, Gill N. Intraoral venous malformation with phleboliths. The Saudi Dental Journal 2011;23(3):161-163.

[94] Babu BB, Tejasvi MLA, Avinash CK, B C. Tonsillolith: a panoramic radiograph presentation. Journal of Clinical and Diagnostic Research 2013;7(10):2378-2379.

[95] Cooper MM, Steinberg JJ, Lastra M, Antopol S. Tonsillar calculi. Report of a case and review of the literature. Oral Surgery, Oral Medicine, and Oral Pathology 1983;55(3): 239-243.

[96] Giudice M, Cristofaro MG, Fava MG, Giudice A. An unusual tonsillolithiasis in a patient with chronic obstructive sialoadenitis. Dentomaxillofacial Radiology 2005;34(4): 247-250.

[97] Mesolella M, Cimmino M, Di Martino M, Criscuoli G, Albanese L, Galli V. Tonsillolith. Case report and review of the literature. Acta Otorhinolaryngologica Italica 2004;24(5):302-307.

[98] Sezer B, Tugsel Z, Bilgen C. An unusual tonsillolith. Oral Surgery, Oral Medicine, Oral Pathology, Oral Radiology, and Endodontics 2003;95(4):471-473.

[99] Bamgbose BO, Ruprecht A, Hellstein J, Timmons S, Qian F. The prevalence of tonsilloliths and other soft tissue calcifications in patients attending oral and maxillofacial radiology clinic of the University of Iowa. International Scholarly Research Notices Dentistry 2014;2014:839635.

[100] Guevara C, Mandel L. Panoramic radiographic demonstration of bilateral tonsilloliths. The New York State Dental Journal 2011;77(3):28-30.

[101] de Moura MD, Madureira DF, Noman-Ferreira LC, Abdo EN, de Aguiar EG, Freire AR. Tonsillolith: a report of three clinical cases. Medicina Oral, Patologia Oral y Cirugia Bucal 2007;12(2):E130-133.

Chapter 34

Advances in Radiographic Techniques Used in Dentistry

Zühre Zafersoy Akarslan and Ilkay Peker

Additional information is available at the end of the chapter

http://dx.doi.org/10.5772/59129

1. Introduction

Conventional radiographic techniques have been used in dental radiography since the discovery of the x-rays. With the revolution in electronic systems, equipment's have been produced to achieve a radiographic image in a digital format. Digital images are in numeric format and differ from conventional radiographs in terms of pixels, and the different shades of gray given to these pixels [1].

A digital image is produced by analog-to-digital conversion (ADC). First, the small ranges of voltage values in the signal are grouped together as a single value. Second, every sampled signal is assigned a value and stored in the computer. Last, the computer organizes the pixels in their proper locations and displays a shade of gray corresponding the number assigned and the image becomes visible on the computer screen [1].

Two dimensional and three dimensional digital imaging modalities have been developed for dentomaxillofacial diagnosis, treatment planning and several clinical applications. These modalities consist of digital intraoral imaging, digital panoramic and cephalometric imaging and cone-beam computed tomography.

The knowledge of advances regarding radiographic techniques and proper use of them gives the opportunity to the practitioner for improvement in diagnostic tasks and treatment planning. Therefore, the aim of this chapter is to focus on the requirements, applications, advantages and disadvantages and artifacts of the currently available digital imaging techniques according to the literature.

2. Two dimensional digital imaging in dentistry

Two dimensional imaging is an adjunct of clinical examination in dentistry. It has an important role in the diagnosis of dental pathologies and treatment planning.

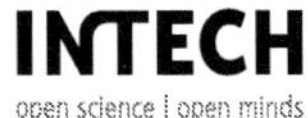

Two dimensional imaging could be broadly categorized as intraoral and extraoral imaging. Intraoral imaging includes periapical, bitewing and occlusal projections, while extraoral imaging includes panoramic and cephalometric projections. These both were acquired with conventional radiography; which is a technique using films, cassettes and wet film processing for long time, but nowadays with the introduction of digital systems they could be achieved with digital imaging.

Two dimensional digital imaging systems have been considerably improved since their initial introduction. This improvement in type, size, shape, radiation effective dose, and resolution of the sensors made them to be adopted in routine use in dental clinics [2,3]. The diagnostic performance of two dimensional digital imaging systems was found to be comparable with conventional radiography. Studies reported the usefulness of digital imaging in caries diagnosis [4-6], periodontal bone defects [7-9], endodontic applications and diagnosis of periapical lesions [10,11], root fractures [12] and root resorption [13,14].

2.1. Digital intraoral imaging

Digital intraoral imaging could be achieved by periapical, bitewing and occlusal projections. Periapical images show the crown and root of the investigated tooth/teeth and some of the surrounding structures. It is useful in dentistry as it shows the entire image of tooth/teeth, periapical region and some of the surrounding structures. Bitewing images show only the crown of the tooth/teeth and part of the root(s), but allow the visualization of both the maxillary and mandibular teeth crowns and alveolar crest in one image. Occlusal images show the palate and the floor of the oral cavity and a larger area of teeth and surrounding structures compared to periapical and bitewing projections. Assessment of bucco-lingual direction of interested regions is also possible with the cross-sectional occlusal technique. It is useful for the examination of the palate and floor of mouth and for the anterior teeth when patients are unable to open their mouth wide enough for the placement of receptors in periapical projections. Although two dimensional intraoral digital imaging is useful and has several advantages, the superimposition of unwanted structures is the main problem in capable of decision-making for correct diagnosis and treatment planning [15].

Intraoral digital imaging could be achieved with indirect, semi-direct and direct digital intraoral techniques. The dentists should have knowledge about the requirements, advantages and disadvantages of these systems in detail to maximize benefits and safe use of the systems.

Indirect Digital Intraoral Imaging: In this method, conventional radiographs (analog images) are transferred to digital medium with the aid of a flatbed scanner with a transparency adapter, a slide scanner and a digital camera. It is a simple way to obtain a digital image and it is less expensive compared to semi-direct and direct digital systems. This technique was used more commonly at the beginning of digital image acquisition. With the improvement and widespread of other digital techniques, it has lost its popularity nowadays [16].

Semi-Direct Digital Intraoral Imaging: Semi-direct digital intraoral imaging is possible with a system using photo-stimulable phosphor coated plates (PSP) (Figure 1). These plates are placed in the mouth of the patient and exposed to x-rays. After the exposure, they are scanned with a special laser scanner system and the latent image becomes visible on the computer monitor [17]. The latent image is erased by exposing the plates with bright light prior to a new x-ray exposure after the plates are scanned [18,19].

The plates should not be exposed to light because this will release some of the energy captured by the plate before it is scanned and degrade the quality of the radiographic image. Hence, the plates exposed to x-ray should be kept in subdued light environment prior to scanning. [18]

Different types of scanners are present. Some of the scanners scan only one plate in each step, and other are capable of scanning more than one at each scan. [19] Scanning time also differ among modalities from 4 seconds to several minutes and according to the spatial and contrast resolution of the image.

Similar to films used in conventional radiography there are different sizes of plates, including child size, adult size, adult bitewing size and occlusal size and they can be used with the film holders used in conventional radiography [20].

Semi-direct digital imaging is a more comfortable technique for patients' compared to direct digital intraoral imaging as the plates' are flexible to some extent and the size, shape and thickness are similar to films used in conventional radiography [21].

Direct Digital Intraoral Imaging: Direct digital intraoral images could be achieved with solid-state sensors. There are two types of solid state-sensors; charged-coupled device (CCD) and complementary metal oxide semiconductor (CMOS).

CCD sensors: A solid state silicon chip is used to record the image in this technology. Silicon crystals convert absorbed radiation to light and the electrons constitutes the latent image according to the light intensity. This signal is sent to the computer with a cable connecting the sensor and the computer, and the image becomes visible on the screen (Figure 2) [1,19].

CMOS sensors: This technology was adapted to intraoral digital imaging after the CCD sensors were invented. These sensors have a similar working principle with CCD, only the chip design differ in terms of integration of the control circuitry directly into the sensor [16]. CMOS sensors are less expensive than CCD's [1]. Initial CMOS systems had a cable connected to the sensor and computer, but nowadays cable-free type is also produced. In cable-free type, the radiographic data stored in the chip are transferred to the computer in radio-waves with the aid of a stationary radio-wave receiver connected to the computer. The manufactures instruction recommends the distance between the sensor and this receiver should not be more than 180cm, but in a study it was reported that this distance could be more than this, but should not exceed 350cm [22].

2.2. Digital extraoral imaging

The revolution in digital extraoral radiography includes digital panoramic imaging and digital cephalometric imaging. Digital extraoral and panoramic systems have not been widely adopted since their first introduction in the dental market (Figure 3). This was due to their very high costs. Sometime after their invention, relatively cost effective systems with improved computer settings (computer speed, data storage capacities) have been manufactured and they

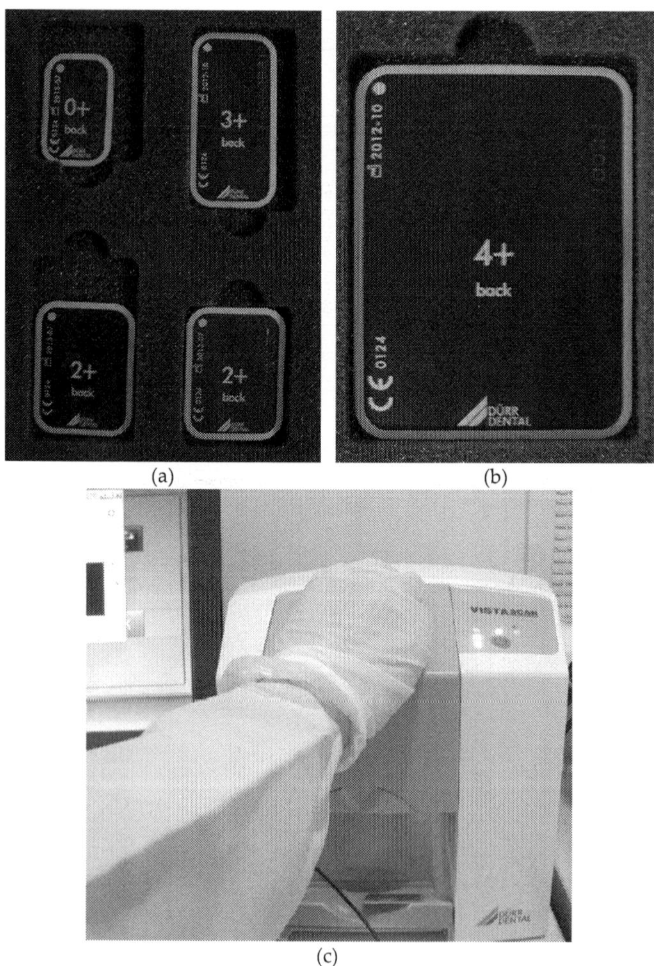

Figure 1. PSP plates (a,b) and plate scanning system (c)

have been started to be adopted in dental practice [23]. The image quality of direct digital panoramic images has been reported to be equal to conventional panoramic radiographs [24].

Panoramic radiography has been one of the most common imaging method among dentists. This technique provides facial structures that includes both maxillary and mandibular teeth and their supporting structures to be imaged on a single film with a single exposure. It is simple and could be applied in cases when mouth opening is not enough to place an intraoral receptor, and an extreme gag reflex (Figure 4) [25].

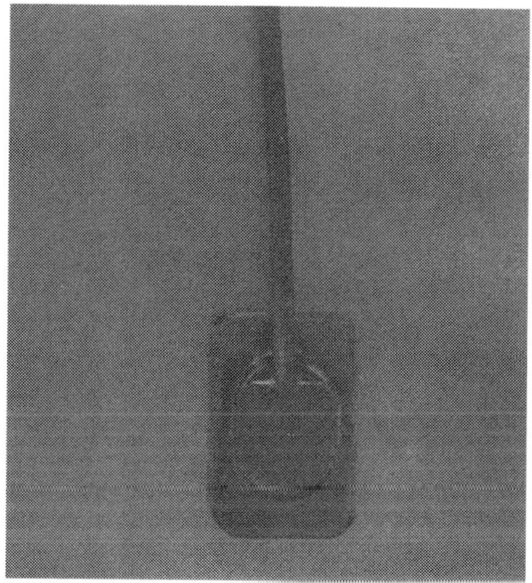

Figure 2. Cabled CCD sensor

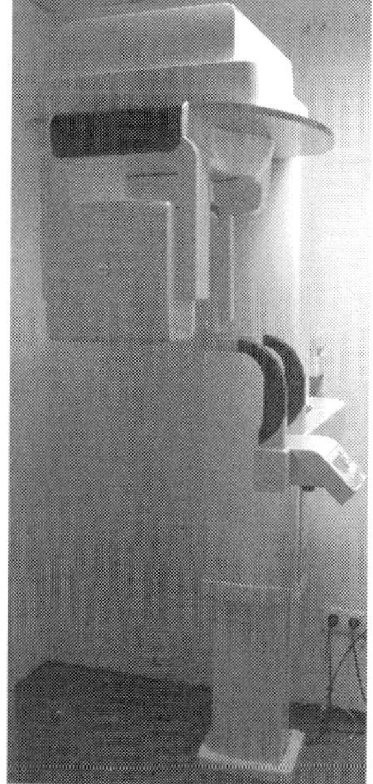

Figure 3. A digital panoramic unit

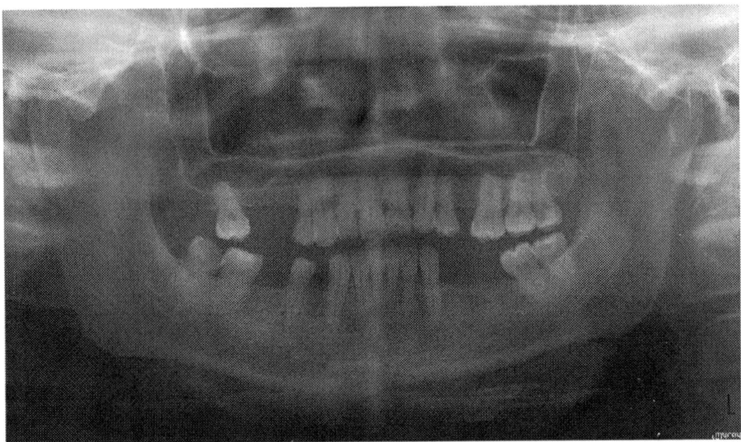

Figure 4. An example of digital panoramic image

Similar to panoramic imaging the same revolution took place in cephalometric radiography. Cephalometric radiography is a technique providing the image of the head in lateral and posterioanterior view (Figure 5). It is frequently used by orthodontists as a treatment planning tool. Some manufacturers made special digital units with a cephalometric attachment to allow exposure of standardized skull views. Digital cephalometric images make it possible to perform cephalometric analysis and superimposition on chair side computer, enhancement of the images for further aid in diagnosis, ease of storage and data transmission [26].

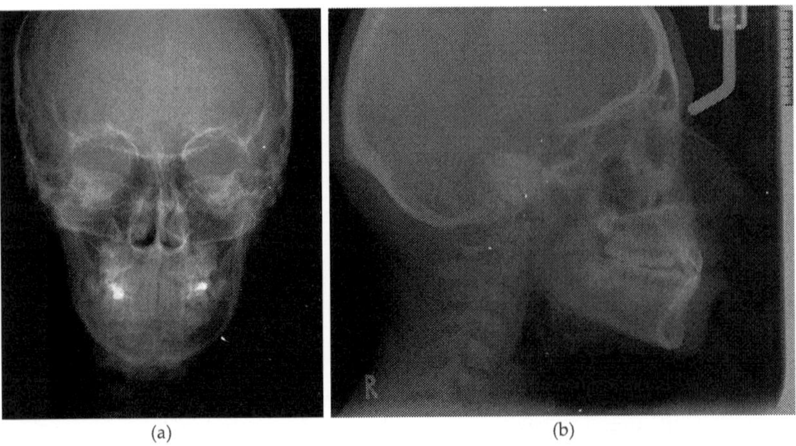

(a)   (b)

Figure 5. Digital posterioanterior (a) and lateral cephalometric image (b)

CCD sensor and PSP plate technology have been used in panoramic and cephalometric devices to capture the image. Compared with digital intraoral sensors, CCD's used in extraoral imaging contains more quantity of pixels to make the image wide and long compared with intraoral imaging. In panoramic units, the CCD is placed opposite to the x-ray source and the long axis of the array is oriented to the x-ray beam. The mechanics used for digital panoramic machine is similar to conventional technique however, it differs for cephalometric imaging. A CCD receptor in a size which could completely take the image of the skull simultaneously is very expensive; therefore to reduce the cost a different mechanic was constructed. In this system, a linear CCD array and a slit shaped x-ray beam with a scanning motion is present and this provides scanning of the skull in short time. The disadvantage of this mechanic is the increased possibility of patient movement artifacts during scanning [1].

2.3. Advantages and disadvantages of two dimensional digital imaging in comparison with conventional radiography

Digital intraoral and extraoral systems have some advantages and disadvantages compared with conventional radiographic techniques. Recently, with the routine use of these systems some aspects which were stated to be advantages initially have been started to be questioned also.

Image enhancement: Image enhancement is the improvement of the original image to make the image visually more appealing. This could be both applied to digital intraoral and extraoral images. Image enhancement could be made by adjusting the contrast and brightness, applying various filters to reduce unsharpness and noise and zooming the image [27].

Radiographic contrast describes the range of densities on a radiograph. It is defined as the differences in densities between light and dark regions [15]. First generation digital sensors performed suboptimal images in terms of contrast and spatial resolution. This has been improved with the new detector technology [2]. The resultant image of an underexposed or overexposed digital detector could be corrected in terms of density and contrast. This especially helps to prevent the retakes due to improper contrast and density [28]. It was reported that contrast enhancement was useful for the detection of low contrast objects both in solid-state and PSP systems [29] and contrast and brightness-enhanced digital images enabled better signal detection and showed a comparable performance with film for detection of artificially induced recurrent caries [30].

There are various filters in each system which could be applied to the digital images for image enhancement. In general, there are filters which sharpen, smooth and emboss the image [31] Filters that smooth the image remove high frequency noise. Filters that sharpen the images either remove low frequency noise or enhance boundaries between regions with different intensities. (edge enhancement) [1]. Filters that emboss the image make it appear as an image with depth. This is named as "3D" in some software's as the resultant image resembles a three dimensional image. It was reported that filtration of a digital panoramic image with the emboss filter may have a value in detecting approximal caries especially in the mandibular molar region [31] and the sharpen filter may be useful for detecting subtle approximal caries [32].

However, controversial results were reported also. Digitally enhanced images with sharpness, zoom and pseudocolour were found not to be effective for the detection of occlusal caries [33].

Image processing is task dependent. Filters should be applied in special cases and they should be used properly and carefully by the clinicians. An edge enhancement filter could be useful for marginal bone height measurements around implants [29] while, it may not improve the level of accuracy for cephalometric points detection [34].

A study demonstrated digital image magnification at X3, X6 and X12 had a significant influence on observer performance in the detection of approximal caries but magnification over these values reduced the diagnostic accuracy [35]. In another study, it was reported that three digital magnifications; 1 : 1, 2 : 1, and 1 : 2 did not affect the detection of root fractures [36].

The operator should be very careful during image enhancement, because inaccurate application of these functions may lead to inaccurate diagnosis of pathology! [1]

Image analysis: Image analysis functions help to obtain diagnostically relevant information from the image. Linear, curved and angle measurements, area calculation, densitometric analysis, complex tools and procedures are present in this extent. Simple linear, curved and angle measurements, area calculation and densitometric analysis functions are generally present in the software of digital imaging devices, but complex tools and procedures require special software [1].

Measurements can be performed with a special digital ruler and are expressed as pixels and in millimeters or inches in digital images. The operator could measure something with the aid of the electronic ruler by drawing lines or curves with the cursor. If the measurement is going to be expressed as pixels the detector should be exposed with an object with known dimensions for the conversation of the pixels into real length [19]. It was reported that radiographic measurements of bone height around implants in images obtained from a PSP system was accurate and precise as much as conventional radiographs [29].

Computer aided cephalometric analysis is faster in data acquisition and analysis than conventional radiographic techniques. Special programs have been developed to perform computer aided cephalometric analysis directly on the screen displayed images. This could reduce the potential errors occurring form digitizing of the radiographs and the need of hardcopies. [37, 38] The reliability of landmark identification and linear and angular measurements in conventional and digital lateral cephalometry was found to be comparable with each other, but all landmarks were not accurately identified in both techniques [39]. A software developed for quantitative analysis of cervical vertebrae maturation was found to be useful [40].

Decrease in radiographic working time: CCD and CMOS sensors provide an important decrease in radiographic working time, especially for radiographic evaluation during endodontic treatment or surgical procedures. Reduction in radiographic working time differs among sensors and plates. Images with sensors are obtained simultaneously after the exposure on the screen, but the PSP plates require an additional scanning procedure after exposure and this increases working time. Working time differ between cable-free and cabled sensors. Cable-free sensors require less time compared with cabled sensors [20,22,41].

Ease in archiving and electronically transmission of the images: Images can be easily archived in digital medium and can be electronically transferred to other clinics or for consultation without any impairment in the image quality by web or CD, flash disk etc. in a very short time and little effort. In addition, other operators have the chance to enhance the image when required [1, 26].

Elimination of film processing step and hazardous wastes: One of the important advantages of digital systems is the elimination of a dark room, film processing equipment's and hazardous wastes such as processing chemicals, lead foil present in the film package and rare earth products in extraoral film cassettes [1,26,27].

In direct digital panoramic and cephalometric imaging the step of inserting and removing a film in cassette in a dark room is eliminated. Besides, the elimination of film processing step puts away the artifacts due to improper processing which could be a reason for retakes of radiographs both in digital intraoral and extraoral radiology [1].

Radiation dose: It was suggested that direct digital intraoral systems [1,26,42,43,44] and direct digital cephalometric systems require less radiation dose to obtain an image compared with conventional film in the first presentation of the systems [45,46].

The radiation dose required for CCD and CMOS sensors for a single exposure is lower compared to that of films. PSP plates require less radiation exposure than conventional film while, they require higher radiation dose compared with CCD and CMOS sensors [1].

The active imaging area of CCD and CMOS sensors are smaller than films thus, they do not show the same number of teeth or area [20]. According to a study additional retakes of images due to placement errors compared with films were higher in these sensors as they have a smaller active imaging area [47]. Therefore the number of images required for the radiographic examination of the same region increases. Due to these factors the effect in radiation dose decrease in sensor systems may be speculated [20].

The dynamic range of the sensors is lower from the PSP plates. This means that, the quality of the image decrease in systems using sensors when overexposed, however, the quality remains unchanged even at overexposure of the PSP plates. This could be an advantage for decreasing the retakes, but a disadvantage which may result in unnecessary high patient radiation dose [48].

Disadvantages

Cost: The cost of shifting from film based systems to digital intraoral and extraoral systems is very expensive [1,26]. This leads to a decrease in the popularity of these systems especially in countries having low income rates.

Lack in cross infection control: Compared with films, the sensors and plates used in digital imaging are not disposable and could not be sterilized thus; special attention is required for infection control. The sensors and plates could be covered with a special film protecting cover, traditional plastic sheaths or latex finger cots. The traditional plastic sheath covering the sensor during exposure was found to leak in some cases [49] and although latex finger cot stretched over the sensor resulted in less contamination it did not fully eliminate the risk [50]. Therefore, authors suggested the use of both a plastic sheath and a latex finger cot especially during invasive procedures [20,49,50].

Wiping the plates covered with a special plastic cover with soap or alcohol before placing in the scanner was reported as a useful method in disinfection control [21,51].

Structures of sensors and plates: CCD and CMOS sensors are thicker and stiff than conventional films and the patients feel more uncomfortable during the radiographic process compared with film. Besides, the cable attached to the sensor makes sensor placement in the oral cavity difficult [1,22,52].

PSP plates are similar to films in terms of dimension and thickness. Reports indicated that PSP plates were more tolerable by both adult [21] and pediatric patients than sensors [53] Although PSP plates are similar to films some kinds of plastic envelopes used for covering the plates have sharp edges, and their corners could not be bent. This leads to difficulty during placement of the plates in the oral cavity and the patients may feel uncomfortable [20].

Physical damage could occur if the patient bites the cable of the CCD and CMOS sensors and PSP plates. In addition PSP plates are prone to damage if they are dropped to floor, bended, and scratched. Mechanical wear and trauma influences the life span of the plates and sensors. This affects the cost-effectiveness of these systems compared with conventional radiography [20].

It is not possible to distinguish images from plates that have been exposed backward in most PSP systems [1,26]. One manufacturer has developed a PSP system with a metal disk present on the hard cover which protects the plates. In the case of opposite insertion of the plate, this object becomes visible on the radiographic image.

Ability of manipulation of the images for fraudulent purposes: Digital technology also brings the capability of manipulation of the original image. This is an important issue for legal purposes. Manufacturers are developing systems which keep the original of the image obtained subsequently after x-ray exposure. With this security key if anyone alters the contrast, density and other characteristics of the image, it is possible to acquire the original data. Thus if one could show the source of the original data these images are considered to be reliable [19,54].

2.4. Artifacts in two dimensional digital imaging

The term artifact describes any distortion or error in the image that is unrelated to the subject being studied [55]. Image artifacts decrease the rate of accurate diagnosis and treatment planning. Additionally, radiographic retakes cause unnecessary radiation dose exposure to patients, clinicians, radiology staff and the environment, as well as the loss of time and money [56]. These are going to be presented as artifacts in intraoral digital imaging and digital panoramic imaging in this section.

2.4.1. Artifacts in digital intraoral imaging

Although image artifacts in film-based radiography are well-known, digital radiography, like any emerging technology, produces new and different challenges. Thus, knowing the reasons of image artifacts is very important for the clinicians [57]. The artifacts of digital imaging can be categorized in three parts: **I)** Operator artifacts during exposed image receptors **II)** Image processing artifacts: and **III)** Defective sensor artifacts

I) Operator artifacts during exposed image receptors

Cone-cut image: It is resulted from improper alignment of the position-indicating device; partial image occurs.

Distorted images: These artifacts occur because bending of phosphor plates during intraoral placement [1].

Double images: It appears due to incomplete erasure of previous image in PSP plates.

Underexposed images: This could be related with i) placement of the opposite side of the PSP plate facing the x-ray tube, ii) noisy images and iii) overlapped sensor plate images.

Opposite side of the sensor plate wrongly placed facing the x ray tube: This is a significant problem for most phosphor plate systems due to backward placement of the phosphor plate in the mouth cannot be distinguished from correct placement. The images have little x-ray attenuation from the polyester base when exposed backward [1]. On the other hand, very few manufacturers had placed a metal disc back of the sensor plates to distinguish by the clinician.

The sensor plate wrongly placed in protector envelope.

Noisy images: It appears as a result of excessive exposure to ambient light between image acquisition and scanning [1].

Overlapped sensor plate images: It appears when plates are overlapped before scanning.

II) Image processing artifacts: This type of artifacts can be corrected thorough rescanning by another scanner without the need to retakes [57].

a. Incorrect usage of image processing tools: This type of artifact occurs form incorrect use of filters [1].

b. The artifacts resulting from image scanning resolution: Scanning under the 300 dpi causes lack of detail [1].

c. Undefined image artifacts [57].

The image of a horizontal white line after scanning

Brightness of images although scanning with optimal conditions and procedures

Half images after scanning

Reduction of the image size

Overlapped images after scanning of two different intraoral sensor plates in two different slots.

III) Defective sensor artifacts [1].

The image artifact resulting from scratching or biting mark.

The image artifact resulting from partial peeling of the coating of the intraoral sensor plate.

The image artifact resulting from surface contamination by glove powder smudging.

Geometric image artifacts resulting from mishandling of CCD sensors.

Examples of intraoral image artifacts are presented in Figure 6-13.

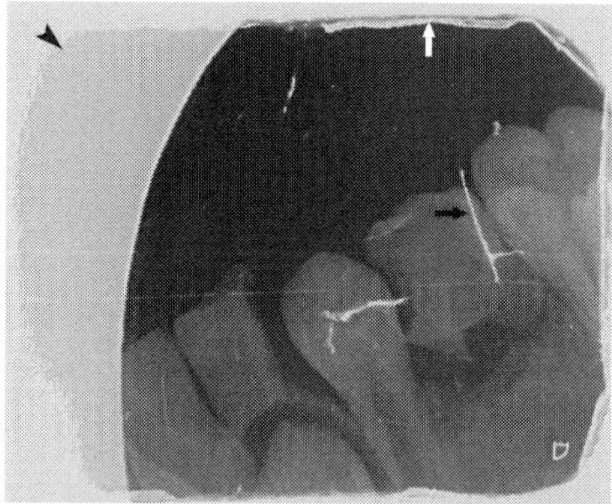

Figure 6. Cone-cut image (black arrowhead), the image artifact resulting from excessive bending of the plate within the mouth (black arrow) and image artifact resulting from partial peeling of the coating of the plate (white arrow).

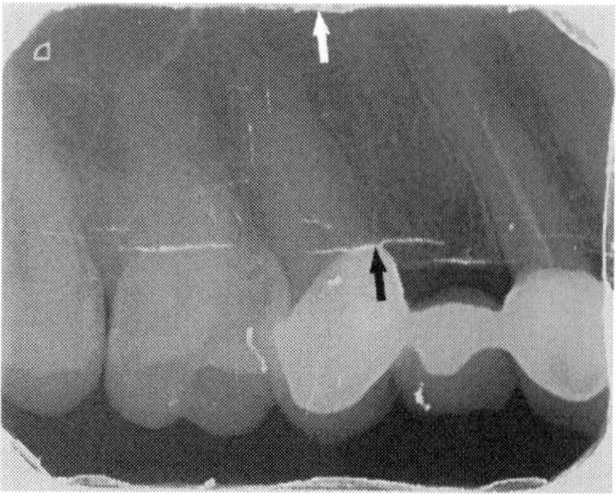

Figure 7. The image artifact resulting from excessive bending of the plate within the mouth (black arrow) and image artifact resulting from partial peeling of the coating of the plate (white arrow).

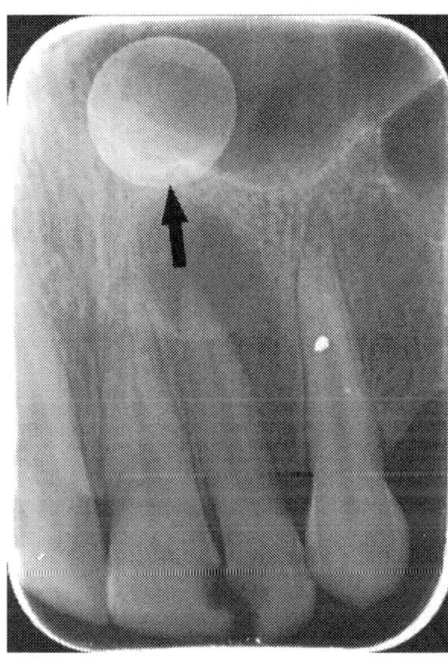

Figure 8. The image of metal disc resulting from opposite insertion of the plate facing the x ray tube (black arrow).

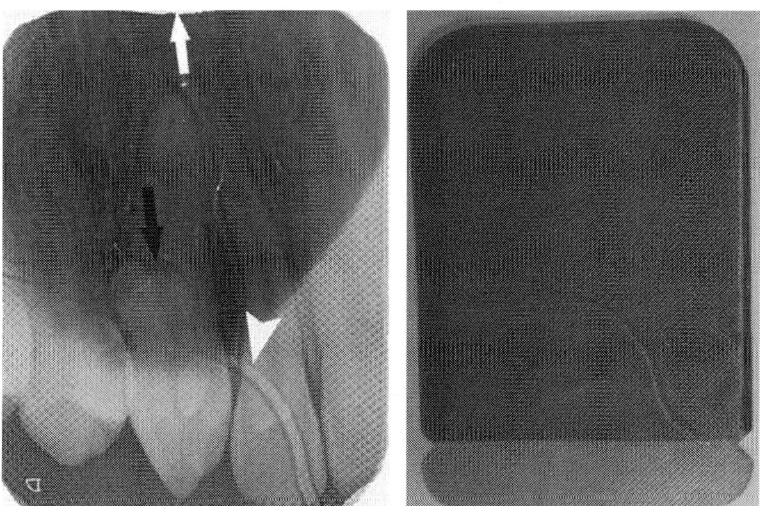

Figure 9. The image artifact resulting from opposite insertion of the plate in protector envelope (white arrowhead) and partial peeling of the coating of the plate (white arrow). Also overlapped sensor plate image is seen. Note the odontoma in the canine region (black arrow).

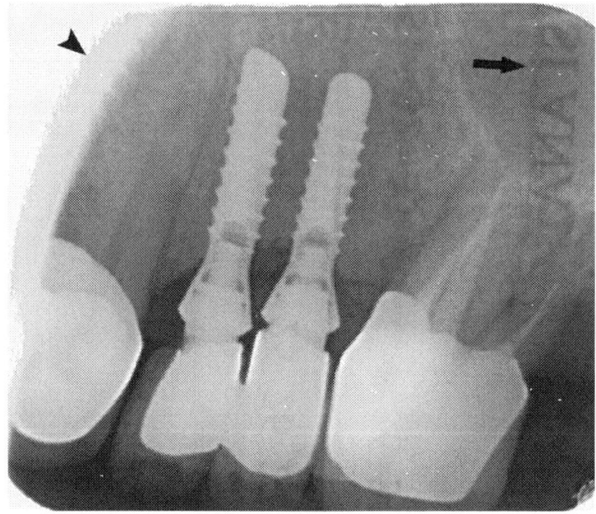

Figure 10. The image artifact resulting from cone-cut (black arrowhead) and image of letters due to contact of plate and letters before scanning (black arrow).

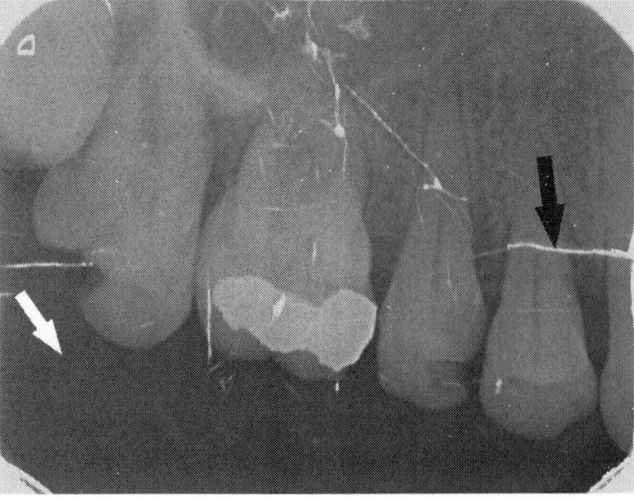

Figure 11. The bright image artifact resulting from non-uniform image density (white arrow), the image artifact resulting from excessive bending of the plate within the mouth (black arrow).

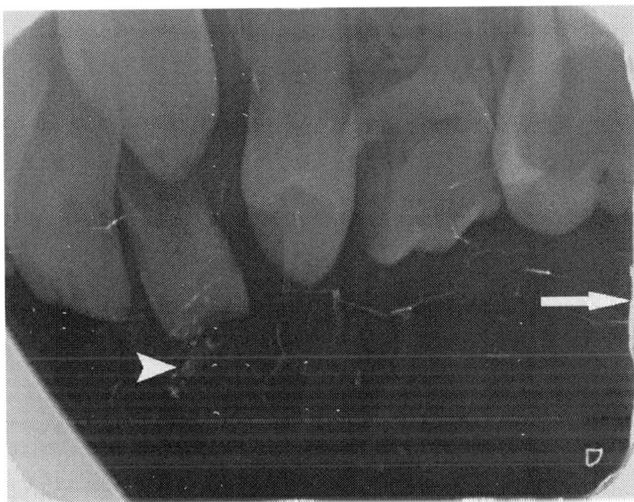

Figure 12. The image artifact resulting from scratching or biting mark the image artifact resulting from excessive bending of the plate within the mouth (white arrowhead) and generalized brightness of the image

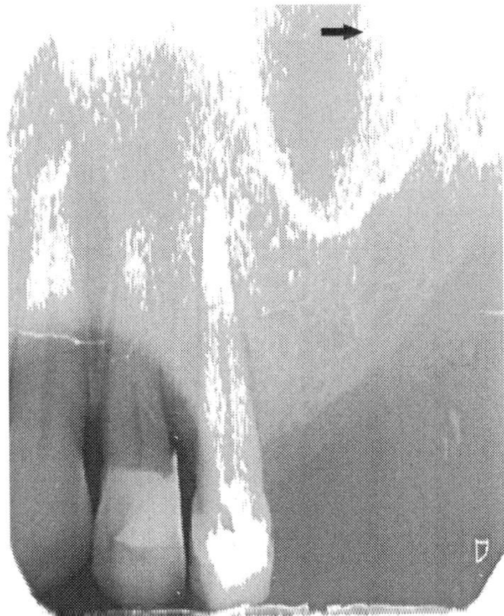

Figure 13. The image artifact resulting from surface contamination by glove powder smudging (black arrow) and image artifact resulting from partial peeling of the coating of the plate (white arrow).

2.4.2. Artifacts in digital panoramic imaging

Artifacts in digital panoramic imaging are similar to the errors occurring in conventional panoramic radiography. One of the advantages of digital panoramic imaging is that errors associated with film radiographs; such as static electricity and image processing are not present as in this technique.

Artifacts could occur due to I)technical errors, II)improper patient positioning and III)during x-ray exposure in digital panoramic imaging [58-60].

i.   **Artifacts due to technical errors**

  1. Radiopaque artifacts (earrings, necklace, prosthesis, lead apron, spectacles, apron/thyroid shield etc.)

ii.   **Artifacts due to improper patient positioning**

  1. Occlusal plane rotated downwards, the condyles approaching the upper edge of the image or are cut-off by its upper edge due to chin tipped too low.

  2. Occlusal plane rotated upwards, the condyles approach the lateral edges of the image or are projected off its edges symmetrically and bilaterally due to chin raised too high.

  3. Overlapped or unclear appearance of the anterior teeth because of patient not biting on the bite-block

  4. Narrowed or blurring anterior teeth, superimposition of the spine on the condyles or rami caused due to patients biting the bite-block too far forward.

  5. Widening of anterior teeth due to the patient biting the bite-block too far back.

  6. Asymmetrical placement of teeth, the condyle is enlarged and is above the contra lateral condyle, which is smaller and lower in the image due to the rotation of the head in sagittal plane.

  7. Radiolucency above the maxillary teeth roots due to the patient not raising the tongue against the palate.

  8. The patient's neck is stretched forward on a slant, vertebral column causing extreme lightness in the anterior region as a result of the superimposed shadow of the spine.

  9. Superimposition of the hyoid bone with the body of the mandible according to the patient's Frankfurt plane not being parallel to the floor

iii.   **Artifacts occurring during x-ray interpretation**

  1. Missing or doubled objects or abrupt shifting of image vertically due to the horizontal or vertical movement of the patient during exposure.

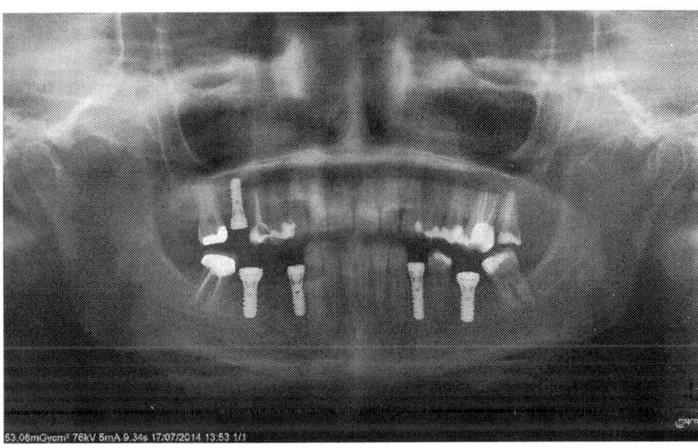

Figure 14. Digital panoramic image demonstrating occlusal plane rotated downwards, the condyles approach the upper edge of the image superimposition of the hyoid bone with the body of the mandible according to the patient's Frankfurt plane not being parallel to the floor.

It was reported that artifacts of digital panoramic images differed between patients with mixed dentition and permanent dentition and more artifacts were seen in permanent dentition. Positioning the patient too forward was seen more common in the mixed dentition. Slumped position and improper chin position were more commonly seen in the permanent dentition. Blurred or shortened upper incisors were more prevalent in the mixed dentition [61]. Training of dental personnel and a discussion of technical measures to be taken if errors occur are essential to maximize the quality of panoramic radiographs [59].

Examples of digital panoramic image artifacts are presented in Figure 14-17.

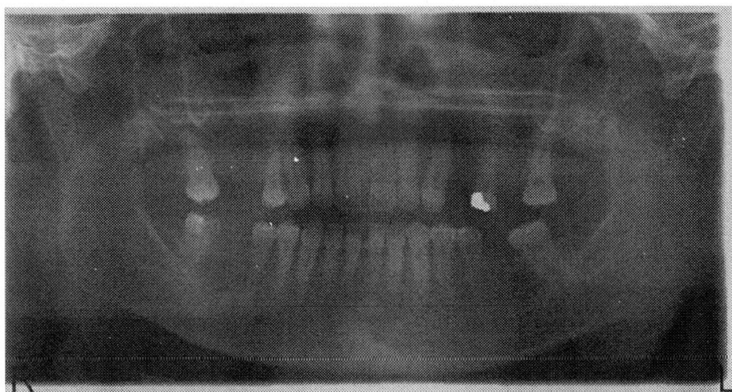

Figure 15. Digital panoramic image demonstrating radiolucency above the maxillary teeth roots due to the patient not raising the tongue against the palate.

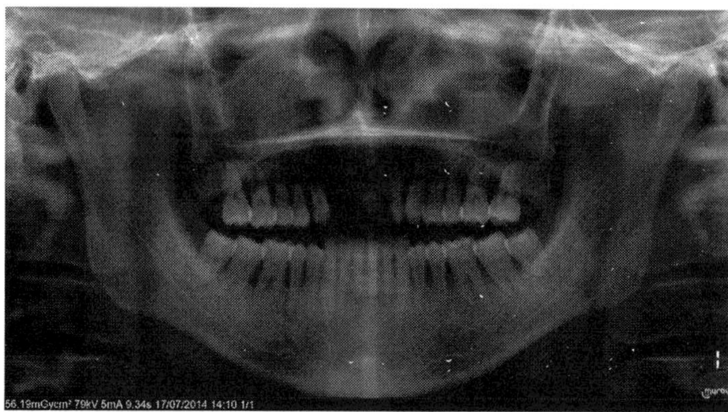

Figure 16. Digital panoramic image demonstrating narrowed anterior teeth, superimposition of the spine on the condyles or rami caused due to patients biting the bite-block too far forward and radiolucency above the maxillary teeth.

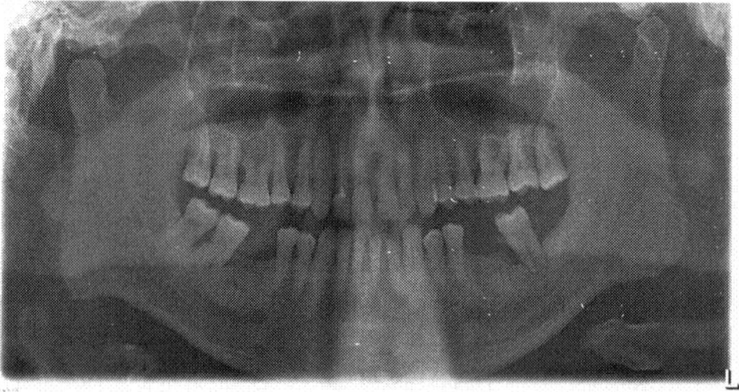

Figure 17. Digital panoramic image demonstrating vertebral column causing extreme lightness in the anterior region as a result of the superimposed shadow of the spine and noisy image.

3. Three dimensional digital imaging in dentistry

Three dimensional imaging gives the opportunity to the practitioner to examine the dento-maxillofacial region without superimposition and distortion of the image. Three dimensional imaging was acquired with conventional tomography [62] and tuned aperture computed tomography techniques in the past years [63] but, with the introduction of cone-beam computed tomography (CBCT) it left its place to this new imaging modality. Details about CBCT technique and its clinical applications are going to be discussed in this section.

3.1. Cone-beam computed tomography

CBCT is a relatively new digital imaging technology. Although, it has been given several names including dental volumetric tomography (DVT), cone beam volumetric tomography (CBVT), dental computed tomography (DCT) and cone beam imaging (CBI), the most preferred name is cone-beam computed tomography (CBCT) [55].

This technique was initially developed for angiography in 1982 and was applied to dental imaging some after. It has the advance of three dimensional imaging of the area of interest without superimposition of other structures. Multiplanar and 3D images could be achieved with this technique with lower radiation dose and higher spatial resolution relative to computed tomography (CT) providing better visualization of structures with mineralized tissue. Although CBCT images have high spatial resolution, the data from which images are created contains considerable noise caused by scattered radiation. Thus, soft tissue contrast in CBCT images is inferior to that in CT images [64]. Another problem which can affect the image quality and diagnostic accuracy of the images is the scatter and beam hardening caused by high density neighboring structures, such as enamel, metal posts and restorations [65].

The CBCT system works with a flat panel detector and special scanner using collimated x-ray source that produces a cone-or pyramid-shaped beam of x-radiation making a single full or partial circular rotation around the head of the patient. A sequence of discrete planar projection images using a digital detector is produced after exposure. Subsequently, these two-dimensional images are reconstructed into a three-dimensional volume [55,66].

Examples of multiplanar and three dimensional CBCT images are presented in Figure 19-22.

Patient positioning differs among CBCT devices (Figure 18). An image could be achieved with the patient seated, standing or supine position. CBCT is not a complex device to use and three dimensional image reconstruction can be made easily with appropriate software [55,67].

Compared with two dimensional imaging, the effective radiation dose can be higher in CBCT depending on the machine, field of view, and the resolution of the image [3,68]. The effective doses for various devices range from 52 to 1025 microsieverts [55]. This is an important issue because all imaging modalities using x-rays for the acquisition of radiographic images rely on a basic principle; *'As Low As Reasonably Possible (ALARA)'*. This principle maintains the protection of patients and staff during the acquisition of images. Therefore, the selection criteria of the CBCT examination should weigh potential patient benefits against the risks associated with the level of radiation dose. This could be achieved by appropriate clinical usage and optimizing technical factors such as; using the smallest field of view necessary for diagnostic purposes, and using appropriate personal and patient protective shielding [66,69].

Although dental exposure only contributes a few percent to the populations' total medical exposure, it is curial to adopt certain measures to avoid unnecessary repeated examinations, especially with the advent of CBCT in dentistry [70].

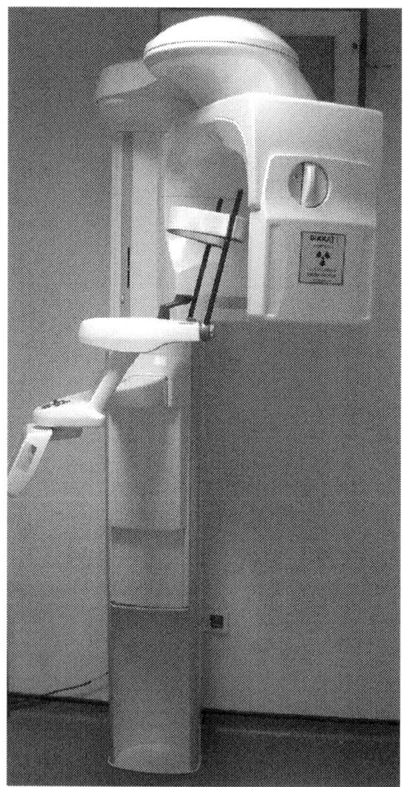

Figure 18. A CBCT unit

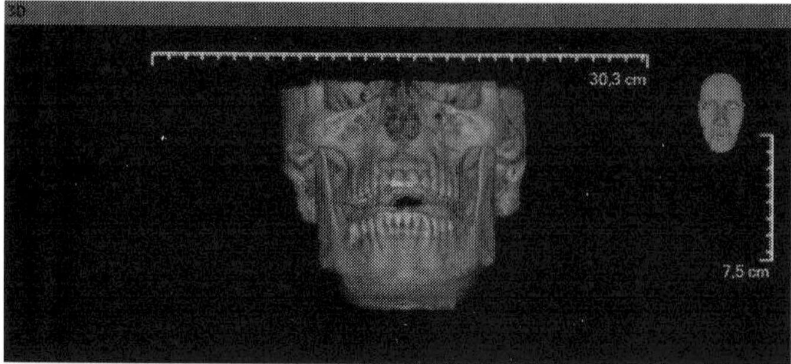

Figure 19. An example of a three dimensional CBCT image

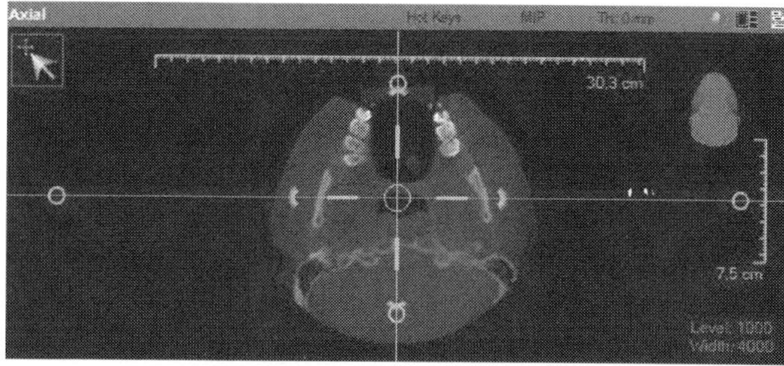

Figure 20. An example of an axial slice of CBCT image

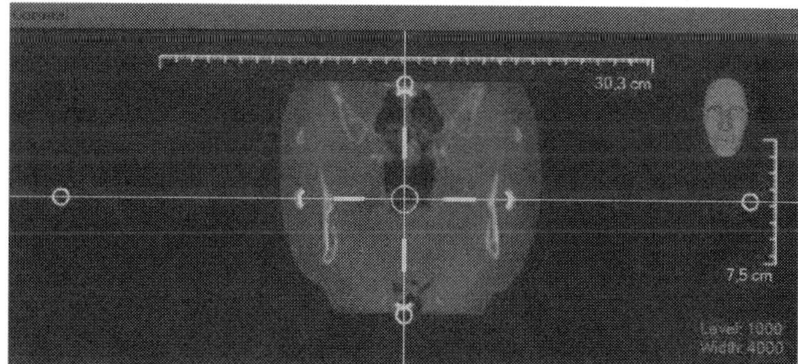

Figure 21. An example of a coronal slice of CBCT image

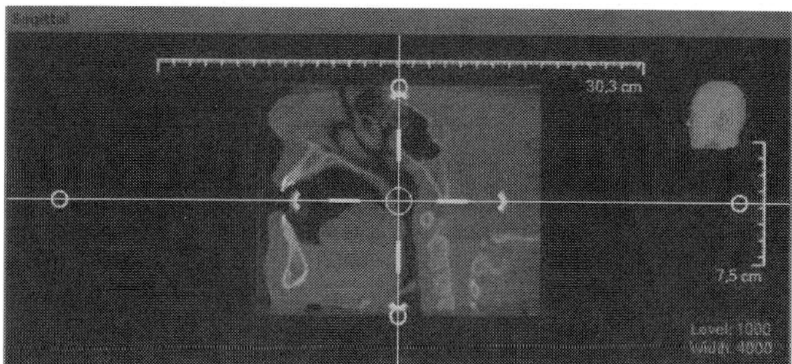

Figure 22. An example of a sagittal slice of CBCT image

3.2. Applications of CBCT in Dentistry

CBCT is used in all areas of dentistry including oral and maxillofacial surgery, orthodontics, pediatric dentistry, periodontology and endodontics. It has been recommended that the use of CBCT could benefit the diagnosis and treatment outcomes for specific cases [55,71].

3.2.1. Oral and maxillofacial surgery

Radiographic methods for the assessment of bone quantity and quality are traditionally used in preoperative planning of dental implant placement. The American Academy of Oral and Maxillofacial Radiology (AAOMR) recommended the evaluation of a potential implant site should include cross-sectional imaging, orthogonal to the site of interest [72]. CBCT is one of the techniques which could be used for cross sectional imaging orthogonal to the site of interest. It is a popular method of planning dental implant placement [73]. It provides the visualization of the alveolar bone height, width and buccolingual dimensions and spatial localization of the neighboring anatomic structures, such as inferior alveolar canal, incisive canal and maxillary sinus. Accurate measurements could be performed directly, as the images are free from distortion however; errors in patient positioning can lead to alterations in these distances. It was concluded that improper patient positioning led to imprecise measurements of bone height and width, which may cause damage to anatomical structures [74].

In addition to implant site assessment, CBCT is used in the pre-surgical evaluation of impacted teeth, supernumerary teeth, and relationship of the inferior alveolar canal to the roots of mandibular third molars, lesions localized on the jaws, osteomyelitis, and osteonecrosis etc. This will benefit to the maxillofacial surgeon to visualize the accurate location of the pathology and its relationship with adjacent structures and important anatomical landmarks [55,75].

Maxillofacial fractures could be also diagnosed with CBCT, but the limits and thus an indication for medical computed tomography exist where there is extensive fractures with suspicion of craniocerebral trauma [76].

Degenerative pathologies or abnormalities in the bony structures of temporomandibular joint, such as cortical erosion, condylar sclerosis and/or articular eminence, articular surface flattening, presence of osteophytes and ankylosis can also be visualized with CBCT [55].

Examples of CBCT images acquired for a radiolucent lesion (Figure 23), preoperative implant planning (Figure 24), TMJ (Figure 25) and a fracture in the mandible (Figure 26).

3.2.2. Orthodontics and pediatric dentistry

Radiographic assessment has always been an important aspect in orthodontics for diagnosis and treatment planning. Two dimensional radiographic techniques have been used for a long time but it has some well documented limitations such as magnification, geometric distortion, superimposition of structures, projective displacements (which may elongate or foreshorten an object's dimensions), rotational errors and linear projective transformation [77,78]. However, CBCT allows for evaluation and analysis of the area of interest without any distortion, magnification and superimposition of other structures.

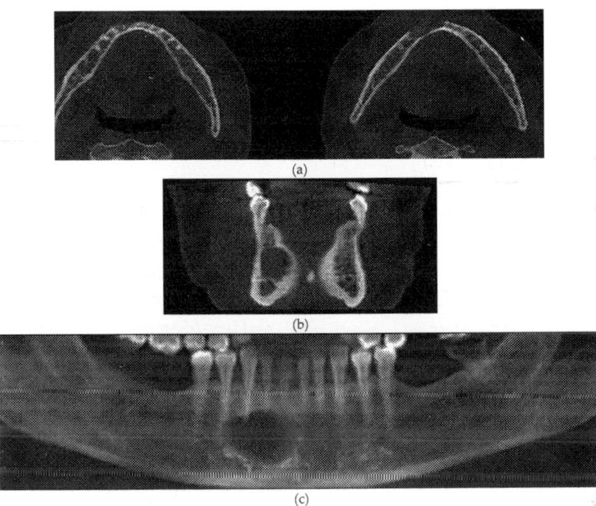

Figure 23. The axial (a), coronal (b) and panoramic (c) CBCT images of a radiolucent lesion seen in the anterior region of the mandible.

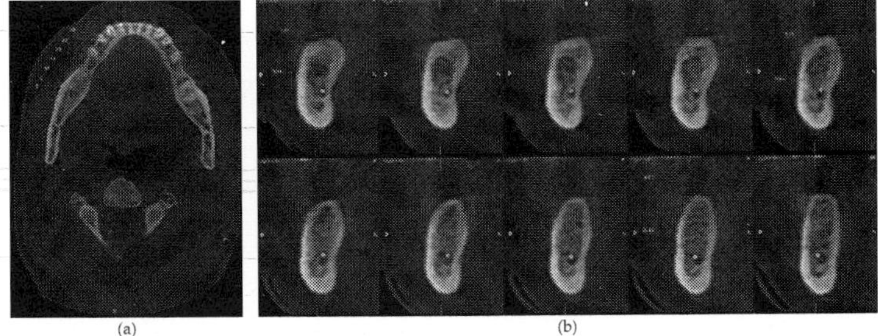

Figure 24. The axial (a) and cross sectional (b) images of a CBCT scan for preoperative implant planning.

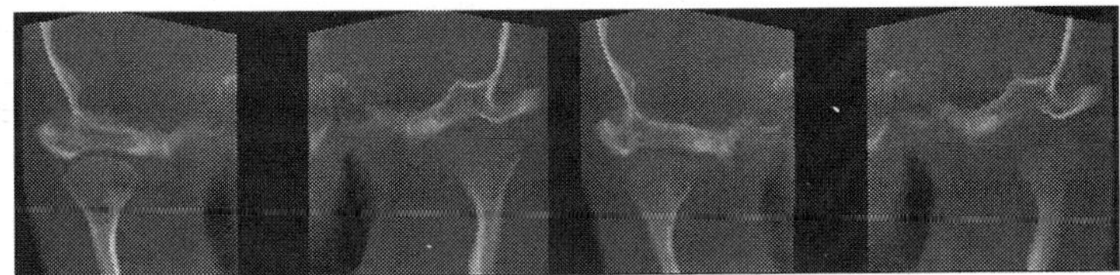

Figure 25. The coronal CBCT images of the TMJ.

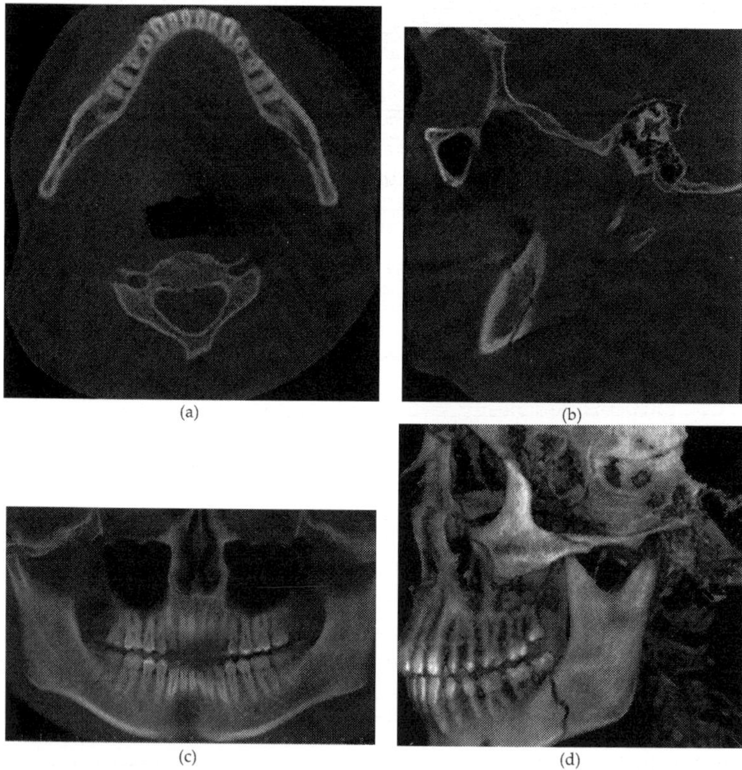

Figure 26. The axial (a), sagittal (b), panoramic (c) and 3D CBCT image (d) of a fracture in the left third molar region in mandible.

It has been suggested that information obtained from a CBCT scan has the potential to improve orthodontic diagnosis and treatment planning in airway analysis before and after orthognathic surgical planning, [79] cleft lip palate [80,81] root position and structure [82] and mini screw placement [83,84].

A study evaluated the impact of CBCT on orthodontic diagnosis and treatment planning and reported the most frequently diagnosis and treatment plan changes occurred in cases of unerupted teeth, severe root resorption, or severe skeletal discrepancies. Contrary, they found no benefit for abnormalities of the temporomandibular joint, airway, or crowding [85].

During the past decade, CBCT imaging has been a popular method in orthodontics, but the disability of showing 'minor external root resorption or not providing treatment at a microscopic level' still are disadvantages [86].

An example of CBCT image acquired for cleft palate is presented in Figure 27.

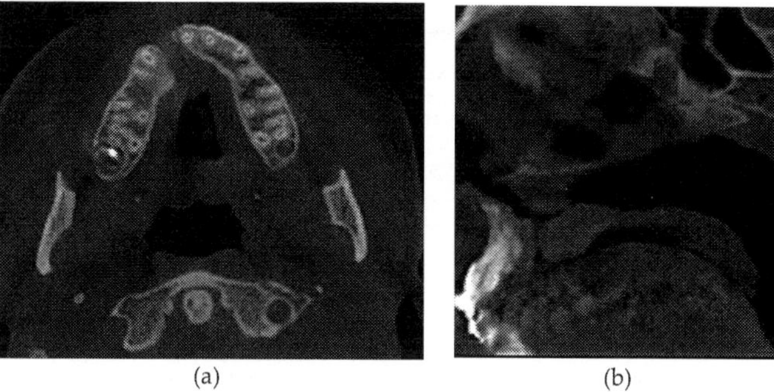

(a)   (b)

Figure 27. The axial (a) and sagittal (b) CBCT images of a cleft palate.

The use of CBCT in pediatric dentistry has been mentioned in the dental literature. A research from Korea demonstrated the most prevalent usage of CBCT among children and adolescents were for diagnosis and monitoring of the growth of cysts and other tumors, following by localization of impacted teeth, and supernumerary teeth [87].

Children are more suspicious to dental trauma on anterior teeth than adults. Thus, teeth fracture is a common sequel. From a database search it was concluded that CBCT was useful in cases in which conventional radiographic techniques yield inconclusive results or showed a fracture in the middle third of a root. CBCT may rule out or confirm an oblique course of fracture involving the cervical third in the labiolingual dimension. Although there are considerable advantages of CBCT in the diagnosis of fractures, more experimental and clinical studies are warranted to determine the exact impact on outcomes [88].

CBCT generates a higher effective radiation dose to the tissues than conventional radiographic techniques. The effective radiation dose should not be underestimated, especially in children, who are much more susceptible to stochastic biological effects [89].

Similar CBCT exposure settings are predicted to result in higher equivalent doses to the head and neck organs in children than in adults. Some CBCT scanners present in the dental market provide a pediatric option to the user. A study evaluated the equivalent radiation doses of two CBCT machines; one with a pediatric preset option and the other with an adult setting. They demonstrated significantly higher equivalent radiation dose when the child phantom was scanned with adult settings. When the pediatric preset was used for the scans, there was a decrease in the ratio of equivalent dose to the child mandible and thyroid. Thus, the practitioner must put pressure on the machine settings during scanning pediatric patients. If not, this will result in excessive radiation to children [90].

A CBCT scan must be only used in cases when the radiographic data is going to change the treatment modality and treatment outcome in orthodontics and pediatric dentistry!

An example of CBCT image acquired from a child having an impacted permanent canine and an odontoma is presented in Figure 28.

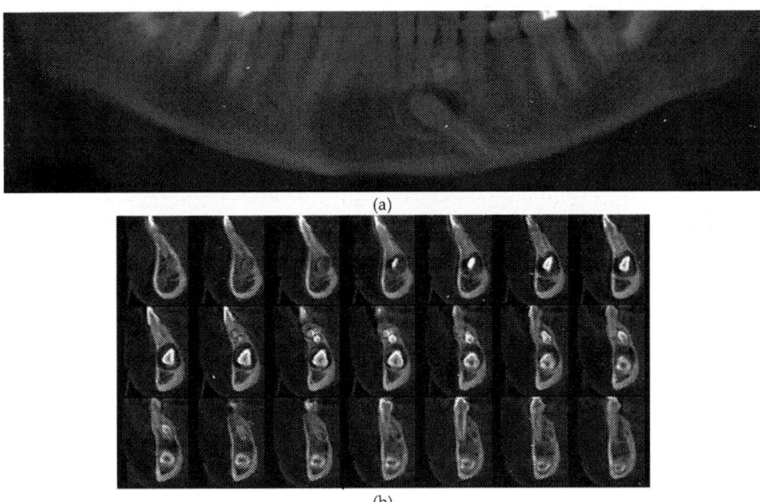

Figure 28. The panoramic (a) and cross sectional (b) CBCT image of a child having an impacted permanent canine and an odontoma.

3.2.3. Periodontology

Diagnosis of periodontal pathologies; such as, gingival hyperplasia, gingival recession and bleeding, depends on clinical signs and symptoms. However, radiographic imaging is essential in the diagnosis of pathologies related with alveolar bone. Two dimensional imaging techniques are routinely used for the assessment of alveolar bone defects in peridontology, but diagnosis of bone craters and alveolar bone support is limited by projection geometry and superimpositions of adjacent anatomical structures. CBCT has the capability of imaging these areas without the limitations of two dimensional imaging techniques [91,92].

Studies have evaluated the role of CBCT in periodontal diagnosis. In vitro studies reported the usefulness of CBCT in the imaging of periodontal defects [93-95]. A study explored the diagnostic values of digital intraoral radiography and CBCT in the determination of periodontal bone loss, infrabony craters and furcation involvements. The authors reported that the detection of crater and furcation involvements failed in 29% and 44% for the CCD, respectively. On the other hand all defects were visualized with CBCT. Besides, the panoramic reconstruction and cross sectional images of CBCT allowed comparable measurements of periodontal bone levels and defects as with intraoral radiography [96]. In a clinical study it was reported that CBCT may provide detailed radiographic information in furcation involvements present in patients with chronic periodontitis and so may have an effect on treatment planning decisions [97].

Although CBCT provide benefits in periodontal diagnosis, it should be used only in cases having the necessity of three dimensional imaging! [91]

An example of CBCT image acquired for periodontal pathology is presented in Figure 29.

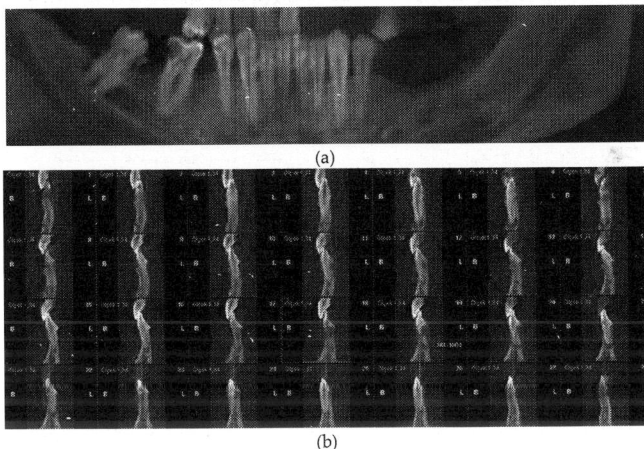

Figure 29. The panoramic (a) and cross sectional (b) CBCT image showing periodontal alveolar bone loss. Note the apical lesion and also external root resorption in the incisor.

3.2.4. Endodontics

Radiographic imaging has an important role in the diagnosis of periapical lesions and treatment procedure. Radiographic data not only helps the diagnosis of the pathology but also gives us the possibility to assess the anatomy of the tooth, such as the root number and curvature, pulp horns, coronal and radicular pulp tissue, root apex, lamina dura and periradicular alveolar bone. Until recently, the assessment of these structures relied on two dimensional radiographs. However, such images have inherent limitations in endodontics [98,99].

Endodontic applications of CBCT include the diagnosis of periapical lesions due to pulpal inflammation, identification and localization of internal and external resorption, detection of vertical root fractures, visualization of accessory canals, elucidation of causes of non-healing endodontically treated teeth, [99] and pre-surgical assessment of apical lesions for the planning of endodontic surgery [100,101].

A study evaluated the sensitivity and specificity of CBCT and digital periapical radiography in the detection of mesial root perforations of mandibular molars and demonstrated that CBCT could be used for detection of perforation *before* obturating root canals. Contrary, periapical radiography (with three different horizontal angulations) would be trustworthy in filled root canals [102].

A study compared the accuracy of CBCT scans and periapical radiographs in diagnosis of vertical root fractures and the influence of root canal filling on this issue. The results showed that the specificity of CBCT was reduced by the presence of root canal filling but its overall accuracy was not influenced. Both the sensitivity and overall accuracy of periapical radiographs were reduced by the presence of root canal filling but still CBCT showed a higher accuracy than periapical radiographs for detecting vertical root fracture [103].

CBCT is also useful for the diagnosis of the origin of pain in the maxillary posterior region. Maxillary premolar and molar teeth show a close relationship with sinus maxillaries. This may cause the periradicular infection to spread and erode the cortical border of sinus maxillaries and cause an infection in the sinus. Similarly, an infection occurring in the periradicular region of teeth having root apexes localized directly in the sinus lead to sinus infection also. In such cases the patient has both a tooth infection and sinus maxillaries infection and a correct diagnosis is essential for successful treatment. One other situation is that in some cases sinus infection leads to the posterior teeth give false positive signs and symptoms of periapical infection. It was reported that compared with periapical radiographs CBCT revealed a higher number of correct diagnosis of periapical pathology. This technique also allowed appreciate evaluation of expansion of the lesions into the maxillary sinuses, thickening of the sinus mucosa, missed canals and apicomarginal communications [104].

CBCT has become an important imaging modality for diagnosis and treatment planning in endodontics. However, the higher effective dose of ionizing radiation compared to two dimensional imaging modalities limits the routine usage of this technique. Concerning the utility of CBCT in treatment planning decisions, the gain of radiographic information with this technique has to be evaluated carefully on an individual basis. Moreover, radioopaque materials such as root canal filling and posts often create artifacts, which may compromise diagnosis [105].

An example of CBCT image acquired for periapical pathology is presented in Figure 30.

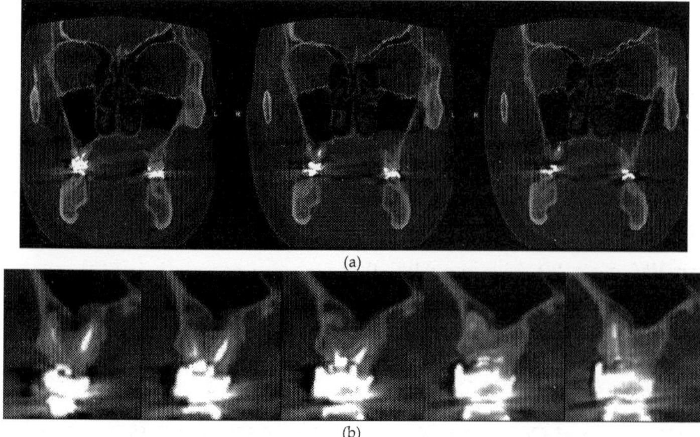

Figure 30. The coronal (a) and cross sectional (b) CBCT images of a periapical lesion present in the maxillary first molar.

4. Conclusion

Tremendous advances have been made for improvements of digital imaging systems since their initial introduction on the market and it seems that their adaption will be increasing in the future. Dentists should have knowledge of the working principles, requirements, clinical benefits and hazardous effects of these systems for proper usage.

Author details

Zühre Zafersoy Akarslan and Ilkay Peker

*Address all correspondence to: dtzuhre@yahoo.com

Gazi University Faculty of Dentistry, Department of Dentomaxillofacial Radiology Ankara, Turkey

References

[1] Ludlow JB, Mol A. Digital Imaging In: White SC, Pharoah MJ. 6th ed Oral Radiology. Principles and Interpretation. St. Louis Mosby/Elsevier; 2009. p78-99.

[2] Farman AG, Farman TT. A Comparison of 18 Different X-Ray Detectors Currently Used in Dentistry. Oral Surgery Oral Medicine Oral Pathology Oral Radiology Endodontics 2005;99(4):485-489.

[3] Eshraghi T, McAllister N, McAllister B. Clinical Applications of Digital 2-D and 3-D Radiography for the Periodontist. Journal of Evidence Based Dental Practice 2012;12(3):36-45.

[4] Erten H. Akarslan ZZ, Topuz Ö. The Efficiency of Three Different Films and Radiovisiography in Detecting Approximal Carious Lesion. Quintissence International 2005;36 (1):65-70.

[5] Castro VM, Katz JO, Hardman PK, Glaros AG, Spencer P. In Vitro Comparison of Conventional Film and Direct Digital Imaging in the Detection of Approximal Caries. Dentomaxillofacial Radiology 2007;36(3):138-42.

[6] Bottenberg P, Jacquet W, Stachniss V,Wellnitz J, Schulte AG. Detection of Cavitated or Non-Cavitated Approximal Enamel Caries Lesions Using CMOS and CCD Digital X-Ray Sensors and Conventional D and F-Speed Films at Different Exposure Conditions. American Journal of Dentistry 2011;24(2):74-78.

[7] Jorgenson T, Masood F, Beckerley JM, Burgin C, Parker DE. Comparison of Two Imaging Modalities: F-Speed Film and Digital Images for Detection of Osseous De-

fects in Patients with Interdental Vertical Bone Defects. Dentomaxillofacial Radiology 2007;36(8):500-505.

[8] de Molon RS, Morais-Camillo JA, Sakakura CE, Ferreira MG, Loffredo LC, Scaf G. Measurements of Simulated Periodontal Bone Defects in Inverted Digital Image and Film-Based Radiograph: An In Vitro Study. Imaging Sciences in Dentistry 2012;42(4): 243-247.

[9] Vandenberghe B, Corpas L, Bosmans H, Yang J, Jacobs R. A Comprehensive in Vitro Study of Image Accuracy and Quality for Periodontal Diagnosis. Part 1: The Influence of X-Ray Generator on Periodontal Measurements Using Conventional and Digital Receptors. Clinical Oral Investigation 2011;15(4):537-549.

[10] Paurazas SB, Geist JR, Pink FE, Hoen MM, Steiman HR. Comparison of Diagnostic Accuracy of Digital Imaging by Using CCD and CMOS-APS Sensors With E-Speed Film in The Detection of Periapical Bony Lesions. Oral Surgery Oral Medicine Oral Pathology Oral Radiology Endodontics 2000;89(3):356-362.

[11] Wallace JA, Nair MK, Colaco MF, Kapa SF. A Comparative Evaluation of the Diagnostic Efficacy of Film and Digital Sensors for Detection of Simulated Periapical Lesions. Oral Surgery Oral Medicine Oral Pathology Oral Radiology Endodontics 2001;92(1):93-97.

[12] Shintaku WH, Venturin JS, Noujeim M, Dove SB. Comparison between Intraoral Indirect and Conventional Film-Based Imaging for the Detection of Dental Root Fractures: An Ex Vivo Study. Dental Traumatology 2013;29(6):445-449.

[13] Kamburoğlu K, Tsesis I, Kfir A, Kaffe I. Diagnosis of Artificially Induced External Root Resorption Using Conventional Intraoral Film Radiography, CCD, and PSP: An Ex Vivo Study. Oral Surgery Oral Medicine Oral Pathology Oral Radiology Endodontics 2008;106(6):885-891.

[14] Kamburoğlu K, Barenboim SF, Kaffe I. Comparison of Conventional Film with Different Digital and Digitally Filtered Images in the Detection of Simulated Internal Resorption Cavities--An Ex Vivo Study in Human Cadaver Jaws. Oral Surgery Oral Medicine Oral Pathology Oral Radiology Endodontics 2008;105(6):790-797.

[15] White SC, Pharoah MJ. Oral Radiology. Principles and Interpretation. 6th Ed St. Louis Mosby/Elsevier; 2009.

[16] Wakoh M, Kuroyanagi K. Digital Imaging Modalities for Dental Practice. The Bulletin of Tokyo Dental College 2001;42(1):1-14.

[17] Pai SS, Zimmerman JL. Digital Radiographic Imaging in Dental Practice. Dentistry Today 2002;21(6):56-61.

[18] Molteni R. Effect of Visible Light on Photo-Stimulated-Phosphor Imaging Plates. International Congress Series 1256 (2003) 1199– 1205.

[19] Van Der Stelt PF. Filmless Imaging: The Uses of Digital Radiography in Dental Practice. Journal of American Dental Association 2005;136(10):1379-1387.

[20] Wenzel A, Møystad A.Work Flow with Digital Intraoral Radiography: A Systematic Review. Acta Odontologica Scandinavia 2010;68(2):106-114.

[21] Wenzel A, Frandsen E, Hintze H. Patient Discomfort and Cross-Infection Control in Bitewing Examination with a Storage Phosphor Plate and a CCD-Based Sensor. Journal of Dentistry 1999;27(3):243-246.

[22] Tsuchida R, Araki K, Endo A, Funahashi I, Okano T. Physical Properties and Ease of Operation of a Wireless Intraoral X-Ray Sensor. Oral Surgery Oral Medicine Oral Pathology Oral Radiology Endodontics. 2005;100(5):603-608.

[23] Farman AG, Farman TT. Extraoral and Panoramic Systems. Dental Clinics of North America 2000;44(2):257-272.

[24] Molander B, Gröndahl HG, Ekestubbe A. Quality of Film-Based and Digital Panoramic Radiography. Dentomaxillofacial Radiology 2004;33(1):32-36.

[25] Alan G L. Panoramic Imaging. In: White SC, Pharoah MJ. Oral Radiology. Principles and Interpretation. 6th Ed St. Louis Mosby/Elsevier; 2009.

[26] Brennan J. An Introduction to Digital Radiography in Dentistry. Journal of Orthodontics 2002;29(1)66-69.

[27] Wenzel A. Computer-Aided Image Manipulation of Intraoral Radiographs to Enhance Diagnosis in Dental Practice: A Review. International Dental Journal 1993;43(2):99-108.

[28] Van Der Stelt PF.Better İmaging: The Advantages of Digital Radiography. Journal of American Dental Association 2008;139 Suppl:7S-13S.

[29] Borg ESome Characteristics of Solid-State and Photo-Stimulable Phosphor Detectors for Intra-Oral Radiography. Swedish Dental Journal Suppl. 1999;139:i-viii, 1-67.

[30] Nair MK, Ludlow JB, May KN, Nair UP, Johnson MP, Close JM. Diagnostic Accuracy of Intraoral Film and Direct Digital Images for Detection of Simulated Recurrent Decay. Operative Dentistry 2001;26(3):223-230.

[31] Akarslan ZZ, Akdevelioğlu M, Güngör K, Erten H. A Comparison of the Diagnostic Accuracy of Bitewing, Periapical, Unfiltered and Filtered Digital Panoramic Images for Approximal Caries Detection in Posterior Teeth. Dentomaxillofacial Radiology 2008;37(8):458-463.

[32] Belém MD, Ambrosano GM, Tabchoury CP, Ferreira-Santos RI, Haiter-Neto F. Performance of Digital Radiography with Enhancement Filters for the Diagnosis of Proximal Caries. Brazilian Oral Research 2013;27(3):245-251.

[33] Kositbowornchai S, Basiw M, Promwang Y, Moragorn H, Sooksuntisakoonchai N. Accuracy of Diagnosing Occlusal Caries Using Enhanced Digital Images. Dentomaxillofacial Radiology 2004;33(4):236-240.

[34] Leonardi RM, Giordano D, Maiorana F, Greco M. Accuracy Of Cephalometric Landmarks on Monitor-Displayed Radiographs with and without Image Emboss Enhancement. European Journal Of Orthodontics 2010;32(3):242-247.

[35] Møystad A, Svanaes DB, Larheim TA, Gröndahl HG. Effect of Image Magnification of Digitized Bitewing Radiographs on Approximal Caries Detection: An In Vitro Study. Dentomaxillofacial Radiology 1995;24(4):255-259.

[36] Kositbowornchai S, Sikram S, Nuansakul R, Thinkhamrop B. Root Fracture Detection on Digital Images: Effect of the Zoom Function. Dental Traumatology 2003 19(3): 154-159.

[37] Gotfredsen E, Kragskov J, Wenzel A. Development of a System for Craniofacial Analysis from Monitor-Displayed Digital Images. Dentomaxillofacial Radiology 1999;28(2):123-126.

[38] Chen YJ, Chen SK, Chang HF, Chen KC. Comparison of Landmark Identification in Traditional Versus Computer-Aided Digital Cephalometry. Angle Orthodontics 2000;70(5):387-392.

[39] Akhare PJ, Dagab AM, Alle RS, Shenoyd U, Garla V. Comparison of Landmark Identification and Linear and Angular Measurements in Conventional and Digital Cephalometry. International Journal of Computerized Dentistry 2013;16(3):241-254.

[40] Santiago RC, Cunha AR, Júnior GC, Fernandes N, Campos MJ, Costa LF, Vitral RW, Bolognese AM. New Software for Cervical Vertebral Geometry Assessment and its Relationship to Skeletal Maturation--A Pilot Study. Dentomaxillofacial Radiology 2014;43(2):20130238.

[41] Wenzel A, Kirkevang LL. Students' Attitudes to Digital Radiography and Measurement Accuracy of Two Digital Systems in Connection with Root Canal Treatment. European Journal of Dental Education 2004;8:167–171.

[42] Horner K, Shearer AC, Walker A, Wilson NH. Radiovisiography: An Initial Evaluation. British Dental Journal 1990;168(6):244-248.

[43] Walker A, Horner K, Czajka J, Shearer AC, Wilson NH. Quantitative Assessment of a New Dental Imaging System. British Journal of Radiology 1991;64(762):529-536.

[44] Soh G, Loh FC, Chong YH. Radiation Dosage of a Dental Imaging System. Quintessence International 1993;24(3):189-191.

[45] Näslund EB, Møystad A, Larheim TA, Øgaard B, Kruger M. Cephalometric Analysis with Digital Storage Phosphor Images: Extreme Low-Exposure Images with and

without Postprocessing Noise Reduction. American Journal of Orthodontics and Dentofacial Orthopedics 2003;124(2):190-197.

[46] Näslund EB, Kruger M, Petersson A, Hansen K. Analysis of Low-Dose Digital Lateral Cephalometric Radiographs. Dentomaxillofacial Radiology 1998;27(3):136-139.

[47] Hellén-Halme K, Johansson PM, Håkansson J, Petersson A. Image Quality of Digital and Film Radiographs in Applications Sent to the Dental Insurance Office in Sweden for Treatment Approval. Swedish Dental Journal 2004;28(2):77-84.

[48] Berkhout WE, Beuger DA, Sanderink GC, Van Der Stelt PF. The Dynamic Range of Digital Radiographic Systems: Dose Reduction or Risk of Overexposure? Dentomaxillofacial Radiology 2004;33(1):1-5.

[49] Hokett SD, Honey JR, Ruiz F, Baisden MK, Hoen MM. Assessing the Effectiveness of Direct Digital Radiography Barrier Sheaths and Finger Cots. Journal of American Dental Association 2000;131:463–467.

[50] Hubar JS, Gardiner DM. Infection Control Procedures in Conjunction with Computed Dental Radiography. International Journal of Computerized Dentistry 2000;3(4): 259–267.

[51] Negron W, Mauriello SM, Peterson CA, Arnold R. Cross-Contamination of the PSP Sensor in a Preclinical Setting. Journal Of Dental Hygiene 2005;79(3):1–10.

[52] Al-Rawi W, Teich S. Evaluation of Physical Properties of Different Digital Intraoral Sensors. Compendium of Continuing Education in Dentistry 2013;34(8):E76-83.

[53] Russo JM, Russo JA, Guelmann M. Digital Radiography: A Survey of Pediatric Dentists. Journal of Dentistry for Children (Chic). 2006;73(3):132-135.

[54] Berg EC. Legal Ramifications of Digital Imaging in Law Enforcement. Forensic Science Communications 2000;2(4).

[55] Scarfe WC, Farman AG. Cone Beam Computed Tomography. In: White SC, Pharoah MJ. Oral Radiology. Principles and Interpretation. 6th Ed St. Louis Mosby Elsevier; 2009. P.225-243

[56] Peker I, Alkurt MT. Evaluation of Radiographic Errors Made by Undergraduate Dental Students in Periapical Radiography. The New York State Dental Journal 2009;75(5):45-48.

[57] Chiu HL, Lin SH, Chen CH, Wang WC, Chen JY, Chen YK, Lin LM. Analysis of Photostimulable Phosphor Plate Image Artifacts in an Oral and Maxillofacial Radiology Department. Oral Surgery Oral Medicine Oral Pathology Oral Radiology Endodontics 2008;106(5):749-756.

[58] Brezden NA, Brooks SL. Evaluation of Panoramic Dental Radiographs Taken in Private Practice. Oral Surgery Oral Medicine Oral Pathology 1987;63(5):617-621.

[59] Akarslan ZZ, Erten H, Güngör K, Celik I. Common Errors on Panoramic Radiographs Taken in a Dental School. Journal of Contemporary Dental Practice 2003;4(2): 24-34.

[60] Rondon RH, Pereira YC, Do Nascimento GC. Common Positioning Errors in Panoramic Radiography: A Review. Imaging Science in Dentistry 2014;44(1):1-6.

[61] Peretz B, Gotler M, Kaffe I. Common Errors in Digital Panoramic Radiographs of Patients with Mixed Dentition and Patients with Permanent Dentition. International Journal of Dentistry 2012;2012:584138. Doi: 10.1155/2012/584138.

[62] Frederiksen NL. Advanced Imaging. In: Oral Radiology Principles and Interprtation, 6th Ed, St. Louis, Mosby/Elsevier 2009,P. 207-224.

[63] Yamamoto K, Hayakawa Y, Kousuge Y, Wakoh M, Sekiguchi H, Yakushiji M, Farman AG. Diagnostic Value of Tuned-Aperture Computed Tomography versus Conventional Dentoalveolar Imaging in Assessment of Impacted Teeth. Oral Surgery Oral Medicine Oral Pathology Oral Radiology Endodontics 2003;95(1):109-118.

[64] Tyndall DA, Price JB, Tetradis S, Ganz SD, Hildebolt C, Scarfe WC; American Academy of Oral and Maxillofacial Radiology. Position Statement of the American Academy of Oral and Maxillofacial Radiology on Selection Criteria for the use of Radiology in Dental Implantology with Emphasis on Cone Beam Computed Tomography. Oral Surgery Oral Medicine Oral Pathology Oral Radiology 2012;113(6): 817-826.

[65] Soğur E, Baksi BG, Gröndahl HG. Imaging of Root Canal Fillings: A Comparison of Subjective image Quality Between Limited Cone-Beam CT, Storage Phosphor and Film Radiography. International Endodontic Journal 2007;40(3):179-185.

[66] American Dental Association Council On Scientific Affairs. The Use of Cone-Beam Computed Tomography in Dentistry. An Advisory Statement from the American Dental Association Council on Scientific Affairs. Journal of American Dental Association 2012;143(8):899-902.

[67] Hatcher DC, Dial C, Mayorga C. Cone Beam CT for Presurgical Assessment of Implant Sites. Journal of the California Dental Association 2003;31(11):825-833.

[68] Scarfe WC, Levin MD, Gane D, Farman AG. Use of Cone Beam Computed Tomography in Endodontics. International Journal of Dentistry 2009;2009:634567. Doi: 10.1155/2009/634567.

[69] Dawood A, Patel S, Brown J. Cone Beam CT in Dental Practice. British Dental Journal 2009;207(1):23-28.

[70] Farman AG. ALARA Still Applies. Oral Surgery Oral Medicine Oral Pathology Oral Radiology Endodontics 2005;100(4):395-397.

[71] Alamri HM, Sadrameli M, Alshalhoob MA, Sadrameli M, Alshehri MA. Applications of CBCT in Dental Practice: A Review of the Literature. General Dentistry 2012;60(5): 390-400.

[72] Tyndall DA, Brooks SL. Selection Criteria for Dental Implant Site Imaging: A Position Paper of the American Academy of Oral and Maxillofacial Radiology. Oral Surgery Oral Medicine Oral Pathology Oral Radiology Endodontics 2000;89(5):630-637.

[73] Horner K. Cone-Beam Computed Tomography: Time for an Evidence-Based Approach. Primary Dental Journal 2013;2(1):22-31.

[74] Visconti MA, Verner FS, Assis NM, Devito KL. Influence of Maxillomandibular Positioning in Cone Beam Computed Tomography for Implant Planning. International Journal of Oral And Maxillofacial Surgery 2013;42(7):880-886.

[75] Stoetzer M, Nickel F, Rana M, Lemound J, Wenzel D, Von See C, Gellrich NC. Advances in Assessing the Volume of Odontogenic Cysts and Tumors in the Mandible: A Retrospective Clinical Trial. Head And Face Medicine 2013; 20;9:14.

[76] Kaeppler G. Applications of Cone Beam Computed Tomography in Dental and Oral Medicine. International Journal of Computerized Dentistry 2010;13(3):203-219.

[77] Tsao DH, Kazanoglu A, Mccasland JP. Measurability of Radiographic Images. American Journal of Orthodontics 1983; 84(3): 212–216.

[78] Adams GL, Gansky SA, Miller AJ, Harrell WE Jr, Hatcher DC. Comparison between Traditional 2-Dimensional Cephalometry and a 3-Dimensional Approach on Human Dry Skulls. American Journal of Orthodontics and Dentofacial Orthopedics 2004;126(4):397-409.

[79] Burkhard JP, Dietrich AD, Jacobsen C, Roos M, Lübbers HT, Obwegeser JA. Cephalometric and Three Dimensional Assessment of the Posterior Airway Space and Imaging Software Reliability Analysis before and after Orthognathic Surgery. Journal of Craniomaxillofacial Surgery. 2014; Pii: S1010-5182(14)00128-0. Doi: 10.1016/J.Jcms. 2014.04.005. Article in Press

[80] Cheung T, Oberoi S. Three Dimensional Assessment of the Pharyngeal Airway in Individuals with Non-Syndromic Cleft Lip and Palate. 2012;7(8):E43405. Doi: 10.1371/Journal.Pone.0043405

[81] Garib DG, Yatabe MS, Ozawa TO, Da Silva Filho OG. Alveolar Bone Morphology in Patients with Bilateral Complete Cleft Lip and Palate in the Mixed Dentition: Cone Beam Computed Tomography Evaluation. The Cleft Palate Craniofacial Journal 2012;49(2):208-214.

[82] Baysal A, Ucar FI, Buyuk SK, Ozer T, Uysal T. Alveolar Bone Thickness and Lower Incisor Position in Skeletal Class I and Class II Malocclusions Assessed with Cone-Beam Computed Tomography. Korean Journal of Orthodontics 2013;43(3):134-140.

[83] Morea C, Hayek JE, Oleskovicz C, Dominguez GC, Chilvarquer I. Precise Insertion of Orthodontic Miniscrews with a Stereolithographic Surgical Guide Based on Cone Beam Computed Tomography Data: A Pilot Study. International Journal of Oral and Maxillofacial Implants 2011;26(4):860-865.

[84] Chang HP, Tseng YC. Miniscrew Implant Applications in Contemporary Orthodontics. The Kaohsiung Journal of Medical Sciences 2014;30(3):111-115.

[85] Hodges RJ, Atchison KA, White SC. Impact of Cone-Beam Computed Tomography on Orthodontic Diagnosis and Treatment Planning. American Journal of Orthodontics and Dentofacial Orthopedics 2013;143(5):665-674.

[86] Noar JH, Pabari S. Cone Beam Computed Tomography--Current Understanding and Evidence for its Orthodontic Applications? Journal of Orthodontics 2013;40(1):5-13.

[87] Shim YS, Kim AH, Choi JE, An SY. Use of Three-Dimensional Computed Tomography Images in Dental Care of Children and Adolescents in Korea. Technology Health Care 2014; 4. Epub Ahead of Print

[88] May JJ, Cohenca N, Peters OA. Contemporary Management of Horizontal Root Fractures to the Permanent Dentition: Diagnosis--Radiologic Assessment to Include Cone-Beam Computed Tomography. Pediatric Dentistry 2013;35(2):120-124.

[89] Aps JK. Cone Beam Computed Tomography in Paediatric Dentistry: Overview of Recent Literature. European Archievs of Paediatric Dentistry 2013;14(3):131-140.

[90] Al Najjar A, Colosi D, Dauer LT, Prins R, Patchell G, Branets I, Goren AD, Faber RD. Comparison of Adult and Child Radiation Equivalent Doses from 2 Dental Cone-Beam Computed Tomography Units. American Journal of Orthodontics and Dentofacial Orthopedics 2013;143(6):784-792.

[91] Acar B, Kamburoğlu K. Use of Cone Beam Computed Tomography in Periodontology. World Journal of Radiology 2014; 28;6(5):139-147.

[92] Corbet, EF Ho DK, Lai SM. Radiographs in Periodontal Disease Diagnosis and Management. Australian Dental Journal 2009;54(1): S27–S43.

[93] Mengel R, Candir M, Shiratori K, Flores-De-Jacoby L. Digital Volume Tomography in the Diagnosis of Periodontal Defects: An In Vitro Study on Native Pig and Human Mandibles. Journal of Periodontology 2005;76(5):665–673.

[94] Misch KA, Yi ES, Sarment DP. Accuracy of Cone Beam Computed Tomography for Periodontal Defect Measurements. Journal of Periodontology 2006;77(7):1261–1266.

[95] Mol A, Balasundaram A. In Vitro Cone Beam Computed Tomography Imaging of Periodontal Bone. Dentomaxillofacial Radiology 2008;37(6):319–324.

[96] Vandenberghe B, Jacobs R, Yang J. Detection of Periodontal Bone Loss Using Digital Intraoral and Cone Beam Computed Tomography Images: An In Vitro Assessment of Bony and/or Infrabony Defects. Dentomaxillofacial Radiology 2008;37(5):252-260.

[97] Walter C, Kaner D, Berndt DC, Weiger R, Zitzmann NU. Three-Dimensional Imaging as a Pre-Operative Tool in Decision Making for Furcation Surgery. Journal of Clinical Periodontology 2009;36(3):250–257.

[98] Patel S. New Dimensions in Endodontic Imaging: Part 2. Cone Beam Computed Tomography. International Endodontic Journal 2009;42(6): 463–475.

[99] Tyndall DA, Kohltfarber H. Application of Cone Beam Volumetric Tomography in Endodontics. Australian Dental Journal 2012;57(L):72-81.

[100] Rigolone M, Pasqualini D, Bianchi L, Berutti E, Bianchi SD. Vestibular Surgical Access to the Palatine Root of the Superior First Molar: "Low-Dose Cone-Beam" CT Analysis of the Pathway and its Anatomic Variations. Journal of Endodontics 2003;29(11):773-775.

[101] Tsurumachi T, Honda K. A New Cone Beam Computerized Tomography System for use in Endodontic Surgery. International Endodontics Journal 2007;40(3):224-232.

[102] Haghanifar S, Moudi E, Mesgarani A, Bijani A, Abbaszadeh N. A Comparative Study of Cone-Beam Computed Tomography and Digital Periapical Radiography in Detecting Mandibular Molars Root Perforations. Imaging Science in Dentistry 2014;44(2): 115-119.

[103] Hassan B, Metska ME, Ozok AR, Van Der Stelt P, Wesselink PR. Detection of Vertical Root Fractures in Endodontically Treated Teeth by a Cone Beam Computed Tomography Scan. Journal of Endodontics 2009;35(5):719-722.

[104] Low KM, Dula K, Burgin W, Von Arx T. Comparison of Periapical Radiography and Limited Cone-Beam Tomography in Posterior Maxillary Teeth Referred for Apical Surgery. Journal of Endodontics 2008;34(5):557–562.

[105] Jeger FB, Lussi A, Bornstein MM, Jacobs R, Janner SF. [Cone Beam Computed Tomography in Endodontics: A Review for Daily Clinical Practice][Article in German] Schweiz Monatsschr Zahnmed 2013;123(7-8):661-668.

Chapter 35

Evidence-Based Control of Oral Malodor

Nao Suzuki, Masahiro Yoneda and Takao Hirofuji

Additional information is available at the end of the chapter

http://dx.doi.org/10.5772/59229

1. Introduction

Concern regarding halitosis is estimated to be the third most frequent reason for people to seek dental care, following tooth decay and periodontal disease [1]. Compared with tooth decay and periodontal disease, there are a diverse number of causes of halitosis. Table 1 shows a commonly used classification of halitosis [2 – 4]. Obvious bad breath is termed genuine halitosis, which is classified as physiological and pathological halitosis. Pathological halitosis is further sub-classified into halitosis as a result of oral and extra-oral causes. Physiological and oral pathological halitosis occur in the oral cavity, and comprise 85% or more of genuine halitosis [5, 6]. Physiological halitosis generally occurs at the time of waking or starving, and likely results from increased microbial metabolic activity that is aggravated by a physiological reduction in salivary flow, oral cleaning, and inadequate mouth cleaning before sleep or after eating [4]. Clinical causes of oral pathological halitosis include poor oral hygiene, tongue debris, periodontitis, inadequately fitted restorations, deep caries, endodontic lesions, ulceration, and low salivary flow [7 – 11]. The most common malodorous compounds that cause oral-derived malodor are volatile sulfur compounds (VSCs) such as hydrogen sulfide (H_2S) and methyl mercaptan (CH_3SH), which are associated with microbial amino acid metabolism [12, 13]. Halitosis derived from extra-oral causes is less common, but causes include respiratory disorders, gastrointestinal diseases, metabolic disorders, and drugs [2 – 4]. The smell of gases that have accumulated in organs during respiratory disorders and gastrointestinal diseases can be emitted directly from the oral cavity and nose. Malodorous components caused by some metabolic disorders and drugs circulate in the bloodstream and are exhaled in the breath after alveolar gas exchange. Components of extra-oral malodor include those due to disease, such as acetone in uncontrolled diabetes and trimethylamine in trimethylaminuria ("fish odor syndrome" [14]). Dimethyl sulfide (CH_3SCH_3), a VSC, is the main contributor to extra-oral or blood-borne halitosis via an as-yet-unknown metabolic disorder [15]. Some patients that complain of halitosis do not have bad breath. Although

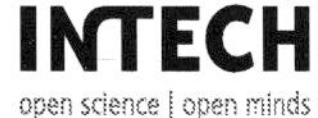

pseudo-halitosis is not diagnosed as a psychiatric disorder, some patients with this condition exhibit neurotic tendencies more frequently than do patients with genuine halitosis [6]. Halitophobia is characterized by a patient's persistent belief that he or she has halitosis, despite reassurance, treatment, and counseling. Many patients with halitophobia have slight bad breath at their first visit to a dental clinic. However, the presence of a mental condition together with bad breath has been suggested in these individuals.

Classification (treatment needs)	Description
Genuine halitosis	Obvious malodor, and of an intensity beyond the socially acceptable level is perceived.
Physiological halitosis (TN-1)	Malodor arises through putrefactive processes within the oral cavity. No specific diseases or pathological conditions that could cause halitosis are found.
Pathological halitosis	
Oral (TN-1 and TN-2)	Halitosis caused by a disease or a pathological condition that causes malfunction of the oral tissues.
Extra-oral (TN-1 and TN-3)	Malodor that originates from a respiratory system, gastrointestinal tract, metabolic disorders, or drugs.
Pseudo-halitosis (TN-1 and TN-4)	No objective evidence of malodor, although the patient thinks they have it.
Halitophobia (TN-1 and TN-5)	The patient persists in believing they have halitosis despite reassurance, treatment, and counseling.

Table 1. Classification of halitosis [2-4].

All patients that complain of halitosis should receive an explanation of halitosis and instructions for oral hygiene (TN-1; Table 2) [16]. Further professional instruction, education, and reassurance are necessary for patients with pseudo-halitosis (TN-4). Professional cleaning and treatment of oral diseases are performed in patients with oral pathological halitosis (TN-2), and treatment and control of the systemic causative disease by a physician or medical specialist is provided for patients with extra-oral pathological halitosis (TN-3). Medical treatment by a psychological specialist is required for the treatment of halitophobia, regardless of the presence of bad breath (TN-5).

Category	Treatment regimen
TN-1	Explanation of halitosis and instructions for oral hygiene.
TN-2	Oral prophylaxis, professional cleaning, and treatment for oral diseases, particularly periodontal diseases.
TN-3	Referral to a physician or medial specialist.
TN-4	Explanation of the examination data, further professional instructions, education, and reassurance.
TN-5	Referral to a clinical psychologist, psychiatrist, or other psychological specialist.

Table 2. Treatment needs (TN) for halitosis [2, 16] useful for clinical dentists.

Most genuine halitosis occurs in the oral cavity, and is known as oral-derived malodor. As mentioned above, VSCs are produced during the metabolism of the sulfur-containing amino acids cysteine and methionine by bacteria [12, 13]. Gram-negative anaerobes in the oral cavity are important producers of VSCs. Periodontopathic bacteria isolated from subgingival plaques, such as *Porphyromonas gingivalis*, *Prevotella intermedia*, *Tannerella forsythia*, and *Treponema denticola*, generate significant amounts of H_2S and CH_3SH [17]. The genera *Veillonella*, *Actinomyces* and *Prevotella* are H_2S-producing normal inhabitants of the tongue coating [18]. *Solobacterium moorei* is present in the tongue dorsa of subjects with halitosis, specifically [19]. A recent investigation of the bacterial composition of saliva reported that high proportions of the genera *Neisseria*, *Fusobacterium*, *Porphyromonas*, and SR1 were present in patients with high H_2S and low CH_3SH, whereas high proportions of the genera *Prevotella*, *Veillonella*, *Atopobium*, *Megasphaera*, and *Selenomonas* were detected in patients with high CH_3SH and low H_2S [20]. The human oral cavity contains more than 500 bacterial species that interact both with each other and host tissues, suggesting that various bacteria might play roles in malodor production. The treatment strategy for oral-derived malodor is the acquisition of a normal microbiota, as well as reducing the numbers of bacteria. The prevention and treatment of oral malodor involve primarily the removal of any causative clinical conditions, predominantly via oral hygiene instructions and the treatment of oral diseases. Persistent malodor usually originates from the posterior dorsum of the tongue and/or oral/dental diseases, including periodontal diseases. Tongue cleaning and the treatment of periodontal diseases are effective for improving oral malodor [21, 22]. In addition, many products such as mouthwash, dentifrice, gel, gum, oil, tablets, and lozenges can play supporting roles in controlling oral malodor. Such products improve oral malodor by reducing bacterial load and/or nutrient availability, exerting anti-inflammatory effects, and converting VSCs into non-volatile substances. The active ingredients used for controlling oral malodor can be separated into chemical agents and naturally derived compounds. Examples of chemical agents include chlorhexidine, cetylpyridinium chloride, zinc chloride, triclosan, stannous fluoride, hydrogen peroxide, chlorine dioxide, and sodium fluoride. Naturally derived compounds can be sub-classified into natural botanical extracts (e.g., actinidine, hinokitiol, eucalyptus-extract, green tea, magnolia bark extract, and pericarp extract of garcinia mangostana L), salivary components (lactoferrin and lactoperoxidase), and probiotic bacteria (*Lactobacillus salivarius*, *Lactobacillus reuteri*, *Weissella cibaria*, and *Streptococcus salivarius*). In this chapter, these various approaches to the prevention and treatment of oral malodor are summarized.

2. Chemical agents

Chlorhexidine (CHX), cetylpyridinium chloride (CPC), triclosan, zinc ions (Zn^{2+}), and chlorine dioxide (ClO_2) are all known to inhibit oral malodor [23, 24]. In many cases, these active ingredients have been used in mouthwashes and dentifrices, both individually and in combinations. CHX digluconate has been used most frequently to treat oral cavities as an active ingredient in mouthwash that is designed to reduce dental plaque and oral bacteria. CHX is used in mouthwashes at 0.12% or 0.2%, and a previous study revealed that these two concentrations of CHX had an identical effect on gingival inflammation [25]. Young et al. [26] evaluated the inhibitory effects of CHX, CPC, and Zn^{2+} on VSC production. Data revealed that 0.2% CHX and 1% Zn^{2+} exhibited excellent inhibitory effects, and had similar effects on VSC production; however, the two agents had different anti-VSC kinetics. Briefly, 0.2% CHX had a sustained inhibitory effect, whereas Zn^{2+} had an immediate effect. In contrast, 0.2% CPC had only a mild inhibitory effect on VSC production. These ingredients are found in commercial mouthwashes, often in combination. Roldán et al. [27] compared five commercial mouthwashes in a randomized, double-blind, crossover trial: 0.12% CHX alone, 0.12% CHX plus 5% alcohol, 0.12% CHX plus 0.05% CPC, 0.12% CHX plus sodium fluoride, and a combination of 0.05% CHX, 0.05% CPC, and 0.14% Zn^{2+}. In this study, the combination of 0.12% CHX plus 0.05% CPC resulted in the greatest reduction in oral bacterial numbers. In contrast, the combination of 0.05% CHX, 0.05% CPC and 0.14% Zn^{2+} provided the most immediate reduction in VSC levels. Zn^{2+} can be effective in reducing the activity of VSCs directly, in addition to its antimicrobial effect [28]. It has been reported that a combination of Zn^{2+} and CHX or CPC inhibited VSC formation synergistically [29]. ClO_2 and chlorite anion (ClO_2^-) also oxidize VSCs directly into non-malodorous products, which consumes the amino acids that act as precursors to VSCs [30, 31]. A randomized double-blind crossover placebo-controlled clinical trial found that mouth rinsing with ClO_2 effectively reduced morning malodor for 4 h in healthy volunteers [32]. Triclosan is a broad-spectrum antibacterial agent that blocks lipid synthesis in susceptible bacteria [33]. A double-blind, crossover, randomized study comparing the VSC-reducing effects of mouthwashes on morning bad breath in healthy subjects reported that VSC formation was inhibited by, in descending order, mouthwashes containing 0.12% CHX gluconate, 0.03% triclosan, essential oils, and 0.05% CPC [34].

However, there are concerns regarding the potential side effects of these chemical agents. The use of 0.2% CHX results in an unpleasant bitter taste, perturbs taste, causes desquamative lesions and soreness of the oral mucosa, and yellow/brown staining of the teeth and dorsum of the tongue [35]. Hypersensitivity to CHX is rare, but several immediate-type allergies such as contact urticarial, occupational asthma, and anaphylactic shock have been reported [36, 37]. In Japan, based on these reports, the concentration of CHX used near a wound is limited to 0.05%, which is lower than its effective concentration. Recently, the possibility that triclosan is hazardous to human health has been suggested. Several studies reported that triclosan might contribute to bacterial resistance to antibiotics, or interfere with endocrine functions in rats [38, 39]. The US Food and Drug Administration (FDA) named triclosan in the National Toxicology Program (NTP) for toxicological evaluation.

3. Naturally derived compounds (Table 3)

3.1. Natural botanical extracts

Due to the increase in health consciousness, many flavors and natural botanical extracts have been added to foods and medicine to reduce oral malodor. In addition, the effects of natural botanical extracts on oral malodor have been evaluated in randomized controlled trials.

Study	Conditions for the assessment (the period that avoided oral activities, mouth cleaning, etc.)	Study population (Age)	Study design	Follow-up time	Active ingredient	Study group	Sample size	Pretreatment	Vehicle	Frequency (washout period)	Malodor assessment	Results
Natural botanical extracts												
Tanaka et al [41].	4:30–6:30 pm (at least 4 h)	Volunteers with gingivitis or mild periodontitis (20–50 years)	Double-blind, randomized, placebo-controlled parallel trial	14 weeks	Eucalyptus extract	High-concentration (0.6%), low-concentration (0.4%), and placebo	32, 32, and 33, respectively	Full-mouth supragingival scaling	Chewing gum	Two tablets for 5 min, five times daily for 12 weeks	OLT score, VSCs by GC	The OLT score decreased significantly at 4, 8, 12 and 14 weeks in the 0.4%- and 0.6%-eucalyptus extract groups but not in the placebo group. The group–time interactions revealed significant reductions in the OLT score and VSCs in both experimental groups compared with the placebo group.
Rassameemasmaung et al [47].	7:00–8:30 am (at least 2 h)	Gingivitis patients (18–55 years)	Double-blind, placebo-controlled parallel trial	4 weeks	Green tea extract	Green tea and placebo	Both $n = 30$	None	Mouthwash	Twice daily for 4 weeks	VSCs by Halimeter	The VSC levels decreased significantly at 30 min, 3 h, and day 28 in the green tea group. On day 28 there was a significant difference between the green tea and placebo group.
Rassameemasmaung et al [49].	8:00 am (at least 2 h)	Gingivitis patients (17–37 years)	Double-blind, randomized, placebo-controlled parallel trial	8 weeks	The pericarp extract of *Garcinia mangostana* L.	Garcinia and placebo	Both $n = 30$	1) None 2) Scaling	Mouthwash	Twice daily for 2 weeks (4 weeks)	VSCs by Halimeter	1) The VSC levels decreased significantly in the Garcinia group compared with baseline and the placebo group. 2) The VSC levels in the Garcinia group was reduced significantly compared with the placebo group, but not with baseline.
Iha et al [52].	At the same time of day (at least 5 h)	Patients with oral malodor (33–71 years)	Randomized, open-label, parallel trial	4 weeks	Hinokitiol	Hinokitiol and 0.01% CPC	Both $n = 9$	None	Gel	Three times daily, for 4 weeks	OLT score, H_2S and CH_3SH levels using GC	The OLT score, and the levels of H_2S and CH_3SH were reduced significantly in the hinokitiol group, whereas the OLT score was improved significantly in the 0.01% CPC group.
Nohno et al [54].	Morning (at least 4 h)	Male volunteers (24–54 years)	Double-blind, randomized, placebo-controlled crossover trial	4 weeks	Actidinine	Actidinine and placebo	Both $n = 14$	None	Tablet	Three times daily, for a week (2 weeks)	VSCs by Oral Chroma	The VSC levels were reduced significantly in both the test and placebo groups after just taking a tablet. The VSC level was reduced significantly in the test group, but not in the placebo group, after use for 1 week.

Study	Conditions for the assessment (the period that avoided oral activities, mouth cleaning, etc.)	Study population (Age)	Study design	Follow-up time	Active ingredient	Study group	Sample size	Pretreatment	Vehicle	Frequency (washout period)	Malodor assessment	Results
Salivary components												
Shin et al [57].	Morning (from the midnight before)	Volunteers with oral malodor (26–54 years)	Double-blind, randomized, placebo-controlled crossover trial	1 week	Lactoferrin and Lactoperoxidase	Lactoferrin and Lactoperoxidase, and placebo	Both $n = 15$	None	Tablet	Twice at a 1-h interval in the morning (1 week)	H_2S, CH_3SH, and total VSCs by GC	The CH_3SH level was significantly lower in the test group compared with the placebo group 10 min after the first ingestion. The median concentration of CH_3SH in the test group was below the olfactory threshold from 10 min until 2 h, whereas the level in the placebo group remained above the threshold during the experimental period.
Probiotic bacteria												
Kang et al [58].	7:00–8:00 am (from the evening before)	Student volunteers (20–30 years)	Open label crossover trial	1 day	Weissella cibaria CMU	W. cibaria CMU, Lactobacillus casei, Weissella confuse, and distilled water	46, 10, 10, and 46, respectively	None	Solution	15 mL. for 2 min, twice daily	H_2S and CH_3SH using Oral Chroma	Rinsing of the mouth with solutions containing W. cibaria CMU twice a day significantly reduced H_2S and CH_3SH the next morning; L. casei, W. confuse, and distilled water had no effect.
Burton et al [63].	Morning (from awakening)	Subjects with oral malodor (18–69 years)	Open label parallel trial	1 week	Sterptococcus salivarius K12	S. salivarius K12 and placebo	13 and 10	Mechanical and chemical oral cleansing treatment	Lozenge	Day 1: at 2-h intervals over 8 h. Afterwards: twice daily for a week	VSCs by Halimeter	The VSC levels 1 week after treatment initiation was reduced significantly in the test group compared with the placebo group.
Keller et al [70].	Morning (from the evening before)	Young adult volunteers (19–25 years)	Double-blind, randomized, placebo-controlled crossover trial	7 weeks	Lactobacillus reuteri DSM 17938 and ATCC PTA 5289	L. reuteri and placebo	Both $n = 25$	None	Chewing gum	Twice daily for 2 weeks (3 weeks)	OLT, VSCs by Halimeter	The OLT score was significantly lower in the probiotic group compared with the placebo group. The VSC levels were not significantly different between groups.
Suzuki et al [76].	At the same time of day (at least 5 h)	Patients with oral malodor (22–67 years)	Double-blind, randomized crossover trial	6 weeks	Lactobacillus salivarius WB21	L. salivarius WB21 and placabo	Both $n = 23$	None	Tablet	Three daily for 2 weeks (2 weeks)	OLT, VSCs by GC	The OLT score was reduced significantly in both the probiotic and placebo periods. VSC levels were reduced significantly in the probiotic period but not in the placebo period.

OLT, organoleptic test; VSCs, volatile sulfur compounds; GC, gas chromatography; H_2S, hydrogen sulfide; CH_3SH, methyl mercaptan.

Table 3. Clinical trials to evaluate the effects of naturally derived compounds on reducing oral malodor.

Eucalyptus extract is one of the four active ingredients of Listerine® mouthwash (Pfizer Inc., Morris Plains, NJ, USA), which was created in 1879 and was formulated originally as a surgical antiseptic. It has antibacterial activity against several periodontopathic bacteria including *P. gingivalis* and *P. intermedia*, which produce VSCs [40]. The effect on oral malodor of chewing gum containing eucalyptus extract was evaluated in a double-blind randomized trial over a 12-week period [41]. Relative to baseline, organoleptic test (OLT) scores decreased significantly at 4, 8, 12, and 14 weeks in the 0.4%-and 0.6%-eucalyptus extract groups, but not in the placebo group. In addition, the group-time interactions revealed significant reductions in OLT scores, VSC levels, and tongue-coating scores in both eucalyptus concentration groups compared with the placebo group.

The catechins present in green tea have *in vitro* bactericidal activity against the odor-producing periodontal bacteria *P. gingivalis* and *Prevotella* spp. [42], inhibit the adherence of *P. gingivalis* to oral epithelial cells [43], and reduce periodontal breakdown by inhibiting the collagenase and cysteine proteinase activity of *P. gingivalis* [44, 45]. It was reported that green tea powder reduced VSC concentrations in mouth air immediately after administration [46]. A double-blind placebo-controlled clinical trial found that rinsing the mouth with green tea containing mouthwash twice per day significantly reduced VSC levels at 30 min, 3 h, and day 28, compared with baseline [47]. There was a significant difference between the green tea group and the placebo group at day 28 [47].

Pericarp extracts of *Garcinia mangostana*, which is commonly known as the mangosteen tree, exert antimicrobial activity against the oral bacteria *Streptococcus mutans* and *P. gingivalis*, and exhibit anti-inflammatory effects [48]. The use of mouthwash containing pericarp extracts of *G. mangostana* twice daily for 2 weeks reduced VSC levels significantly compared with baseline and the placebo group [49]. Furthermore, rinsing with mouthwash containing *G. mangostana* L for 2 weeks after scaling and polishing reduced VSC level significantly compared with placebo, whereas there was no significant difference between baseline and day 15 [49].

Hinokitiol (β-thujaplicin), a component of essential oils isolated from Cupressaceae, shows antibacterial activity against various bacteria, including periodontopathic bacteria and fungi [50, 51], and has been used as a therapeutic agent against periodontal disease and oral *Candida* infections. An open-label, randomized, controlled trial was performed in patients with genuine halitosis to evaluate the effects of mouth cleaning using hinokitiol-containing gels on oral malodor [52]. Mouth cleaning, including the teeth, gingiva, and tongue, was performed three times per day for 4 weeks. Organoleptic test (OLT) scores, levels of H_2S and CH_3SH, the frequency of bleeding on probing, mean probing pocket depths, and plaque indices were improved significantly in the group treated using the hinokitiol-containing gel. In contrast, only OLT scores improved significantly in the control group treated using 0.01% CPC-containing control gel.

Actidinine is a cysteine protease derived from the kiwi fruit. Tongue coating is understood to be an important factor in oral malodor and is composed of proteins [22, 53]. The effect of a tablet containing actidinine on oral malodor was evaluated in a double-blind, randomized crossover trial [54]. The subjects sucked the tablets three times per day for 1 week. VSC levels and tongue-coating ratios decreased significantly on the first day in both the test and placebo groups immediately after taking a tablet. VSC levels were significantly lower after 7 days only in the test group. There was no significant reduction in tongue-coating ratios in either group after 7 days of use.

3.2. Salivary components

Saliva contains a variety of antimicrobial proteins including lactoferrin, peroxidase, lysozyme, and secretory immunoglobulin A. Lactoferrin is an iron-binding glycoprotein that chelates two ferric ions per molecule, and decreases bacterial growth, biofilm development, iron overload, reaction oxygen formation, and inflammatory processes [55]. Salivary peroxidase, in the presence of H_2O_2 and SCN-, can reversibly inhibit bacterial enzyme and transport systems by oxidizing the sulfhydryl groups of proteins [56]. A reduction in salivary flow might inhibit antimicrobial defense systems in saliva. A relationship between low salivary flow and the generation of H_2S and CH_3SH in mouth air has been reported previously [8].

The effect of a tablet containing lactoferrin and lactoperoxidase purified from bovine milk on oral malodor was evaluated in a randomized, double-blind, crossover, placebo-controlled clinical trial [57]. According to that study, CH_3SH levels were significantly lower in the test group compared with the placebo group 10 min after taking a tablet. The median CH_3SH concentration in the test group was below the olfactory threshold between 10 min and 2 h, whereas the level in the placebo group was above the threshold throughout the experimental period.

3.3. Probiotic bacteria

The use of probiotics as preventative and therapeutic products for oral healthcare is a novel antimicrobial approach that has been proposed as an alternative to chemotherapeutics. Probiotics are defined as "live microorganisms that confer a health benefit on the host when administered in adequate amounts" by the World Health Organization and the Food and Agriculture Organization of the United States (http://www.who.int/foodsafety/fs_manage-ment/en/probiotic_guidelines.pdf). Probiotics have been used traditionally to treat diseases related to the gastrointestinal tract. Recently, the use of such probiotics to improve oral health has attracted increasing attention, although this field is still in its infancy. Nevertheless, there are several reports related to the use of probiotics to ameliorate oral malodor.

Kang et al. isolated three peroxide-generating lactobacilli, identified as *W. cibaria*, from the saliva of kindergarten children aged 4–7 years who had little supragingival plaque and no oral disease, including dental caries [58]. These isolates co-aggregated with *F. nucleatum*, inhibited VSC production by *F. nucleatum*, and prevented proliferation by *F. nucleatum in vitro*. Subsequently, the effect of *W. cibaria* CMU on morning odor was evaluated in a clinical trial of healthy volunteers. Rinsing the mouth using solutions containing *W. cibaria* CMU twice per day reduced production of H_2S and CH_3SH the next morning significantly. Conversely, use of solutions containing distilled water, *Lactobacillus casei,* and *Weissella confusa* had no effect.

Streptococcus salivarius K12 has been used to prevent the pharyngitis and tonsillitis induced by *Streptococcus pyogenes. S. salivarius* was selected as an oral probiotic because it is an early colonizer of oral surfaces and is the predominant member of tongue microbiota numerically in 'healthy' individuals [19, 59]. *S. salivarius* K12 produces two bacteriocins: salivaricin A and salivaricin B [60, 61]. It exerts inhibitory activities against oral malodor-related oral bacteria, such as *Atopobium parvulum*, *Eubacterium sulci*, and *S. moorei*, to varying extents [62]. According to an additional *in vitro* study, inhibitory effects were observed against *Streptococcus anginosus*, *Eubacterium saburreum*, and *Peptostreptococcus micros*, but not *P. gingivalis* and *P. intermedia* [63]. This report described the results of a preliminary clinical trial that administered lozenges containing either *S. salivarius* K12 or placebo. The subjects undertook a 3-day regimen of CHX mouth rinsing followed by the use of lozenges at specific intervals. The VSC levels 1 week after the initiation of treatment were reduced significantly in the *S. salivarius* K12 group compared with the placebo group. The salivary bacterial composition was examined using PCR-denaturing gradient gel electrophoresis, and data revealed that it changed in most subjects following K12 treatment, albeit to differing extents.

Lactobacillus reuteri is a member of the indigenous oral microbiota in humans, and it exerts antibacterial properties by converting glycerol into reuterin, a broad-spectrum antimicrobial substance [64]. Products that contain *L. reuteri* have been marketed for the prevention and treatment of gingivitis and periodontal disease [65-67]. However, data are conflicting regarding the potential of *L. reuteri* for caries management, as some studies reported useful effects whereas other did not [68, 69]. The effect of chewing gum containing two strains of probiotic lactobacilli (*L. reuteri* DSM 17938 and *L. reuteri* ATCC PTA 5289) on oral malodor was evaluated in a randomized double-blinded placebo-controlled crossover trial [70]. The study populations were healthy volunteers, and the study design included two intervention periods of 2 weeks with a 3-week washout period. The organoleptic scores were significantly lower in the probiotic group compared with the placebo group. However, there were no differences in VSC levels between the two groups, either before or after rinsing with L-cysteine. The researchers hypothesized that the probiotic gum might have affected bacteria that produce malodorous compounds other than VSCs.

Lactobacillus salivarius WB21 is an acid-tolerant lactobacillus derived from *L. salivarius* WB1004 [71], and is a potentially effective probiotic against *Helicobacter pylori*. Oral consumption of tablets containing *L. salivarius* WB21 was reported to improve periodontal conditions in healthy volunteer smokers and reduce the numbers of the periodontopathic bacterium *T. forsythia* in subgingival plaque [72, 73]. A double-blind, randomized, placebo-controlled clinical trial using oils containing *L. salivarius* WB21 in patients with periodontal disease reported reduced bleeding on probing compared with the placebo group after 2 weeks [74]. We performed an open-label pilot study previously to evaluate whether oral administration of a tablet containing *L. salivarius* WB21 altered oral malodor or clinical conditions in patients complaining of oral malodor [75]. The organoleptic scores and concentrations of H_2S and CH_3SH were reduced in patients without periodontitis after 2 weeks of treatment, and the organoleptic scores and bleeding on probing were decreased in patients with periodontitis after 4 weeks. Subsequently, we performed a 14-day, double-blind, randomized, placebo-controlled crossover trial using tablets containing *L. salivarius* WB21 or placebo taken orally by patients with oral malodor [76]. The organoleptic scores were decreased significantly in both the probiotic and placebo periods compared with the baseline scores, and there was no difference between periods. Compared with the values at baseline, the concentrations of total VSCs decreased significantly in the probiotic period but not in the placebo period, and significant differences were observed between the two periods. In addition, the mean probing pocket depth decreased significantly in the probiotic period compared with the placebo period. Quantitative analysis of the bacteria in saliva found significantly lower levels of ubiquitous bacteria and *F. nucleatum* during the probiotic period.

4. Conclusions

Chemical agents have been used widely to prevent and treat oral malodor. However, long-term use of some antiseptic agents such as CHX might result in complications such as staining of teeth and the development of microbial resistance. In addition, recent studies have raised concern regarding the potentially harmful effects of triclosan on the human body. These phenomena and consumers' increasing health consciousness have led to the development of alternative antimicrobial approaches, including herbs, natural botanical extracts, salivary components, and probiotics. Diverse natural products have been marketed as effective for preventing and treating oral malodor, and an increasingly diverse range of strategies for oral malodor is available. However, few studies have demonstrated effectiveness of new products against oral malodor clinically. Furthermore, most studies evaluated the short-term effects of products on oral malodor, either immediately or only a few weeks after taking the products. However, the products used for preventing and treating oral malodor, including mouthwash, toothpaste, tablets, and lozenges, are generally used for the long term. Therefore, the long-term effects of agents on oral malodor, as well as their safety and side effects, should be evaluated in randomized controlled trials.

Author details

Nao Suzuki*, Masahiro Yoneda and Takao Hirofuji

*Address all correspondence to: naojsz@college.fdcnet.ac.jp

Section of General Dentistry, Department of General Dentistry, Fukuoka Dental College, Japan

References

[1] Loesche WJ, Kazor C. Microbiology and treatment of halitosis. Periodontol 2000 2002;28:256–79.

[2] Yaegaki K, Coil JM. Examination, classification, and treatment of halitosis; clinical perspectives. J Can Dent Assoc 2000;66:257–61.

[3] Murata T, Yamaga T, Iida T, Miyazaki H, Yaegaki K. Classification and examination of halitosis. Int Dent J 2002;52:181–6.

[4] Scully C, Greenman J. Halitosis (breath odor). Periodontol 2000 2008;48:66–75.

[5] Delanghe G, Ghyselen J, van Steenberghe D, Feenstra L. Multidisciplinary breath-odour clinic. Lancet 1997;350:187.

[6] Suzuki N, Yoneda M, Naito T, Iwamoto T, Hirofuji T. Relationship between halitosis and psychologic status. Oral Surg Oral med Oral Pathol Oral Radiol Endod 2008;106:542–7.

[7] Morita M, Wang HL. Association between oral malodor and adult periodontitis: a review. J Clin Periodontol 2001;28:813–9.

[8] Koshimune S, Awano S, Gohara K, Kurihara E, Ansai T, Takehara T. Low salivary flow and volatile sulfur compounds in mouth air. Oral Surg Oral Med Oral Pathol Oral Radiol Endod 2003;96:38–41.

[9] Yoneda M, Naito T, Suzuki N, Yoshikane T, Hirofuji T. Oral malodor associated with internal resorption. J Oral Sci 2006;48:89–92.

[10] Garrett NR. Poor oral hygiene, wearing dentures at night, perceptions of mouth dryness and burning, and lower educational level may be related to oral malodor in denture wearers. J Evid Based Dent Pract 2010;10:67–9.

[11] Tangerman A, Winkel EG. Extra-oral halitosis: an overview. J Breath Res 2010;4:017003.

[12] Scully C, Porter S, Greenman J. What to do about halitosis. BMJ 1994;308:217–8.

[13] Tonzetich J. Production and origin of oral malodor: a review of mechanisms and methods of analysis. J Periodontol 1977;48:13–20.

[14] Whittle CL, Fakharzadeh S, Eades J, Preti G. Human breath odors and their use in diagnosis. Ann N Y Acad Sci 2007;1098:252–66.

[15] Tangerman A, Winkel EG. Intra-and extra-oral halitosis: finding of a new form of extra-oral blood-borne halitosis caused by dimethyl sulphide. J Clin Periodontol 2007;34:748–55.

[16] Coil J, Yaegaki K, Matsuo T, Miyazaki H. Treatment needs (TN) and practical remedies for halitosis. Int Dent J 2002;52:187–91.

[17] Persson S, Edlund MB, Claesson R, Carlsson J. The formation of hydrogen sulfide and methyl mercaptan by oral bacteria. Oral Microbiol Immunol 1990;5:195–201.

[18] Washio J, Sato T, Koseki T, Takahashi N. Hydrogen sulfide-producing bacteria in tongue biofilm and their relationship with oral malodour. J Med Microbiol 2005;54:889–95.

[19] Kazor CE, Mitchell PM, Lee AM, Stokes LN, Loesche WJ, Dewhirst FE, Paster BJ. Diversity of bacterial populations on the tongue dorsa of patients with halitosis and healthy patients. J Clin Microbiol 2003;41:558–63.

[20] Takeshita T, Suzuki N, Nakano Y, Yasui M, Yoneda M, Shimazaki Y, Hirofuji T, Yamashita Y. Discrimination of the oral microbiota associated with high hydrogen sulfide and methyl mercaptan production. Sci Rep 2012;2:215.

[21] Kuo YW, Yen M, Fetzer S, Lee JD. Toothbrushing versus toothbrushing plus tongue cleaning in reducing halitosis and tongue coating: a systematic review and meta-analysis. Nurs Res 2013;62:442–9.

[22] Pham TA, Ueno M, Zaitsu T, Takehara S, Shinada K, Lam PH, Kawaguchi Y. Clinical trial of oral malodor treatment in patients with periodontal diseases. J Periodontal Res 2011;46:722–9.

[23] Fedorowicz Z, Aljufairi H, Nasser M, Outhouse TL, Pedrazzi V. Mouthrinses for the treatment of halitosis. Cochrane Database Syst Rev 2008;8:CD006701.

[24] Riley P, Lamont T. Triclosan/copolymer containing toothpastes for oral health. Cochrane Database Syst Rev 2013;12:CD010514.

[25] Berchier CE, Slot DE, Van der Weijden GA. The efficacy of 0.12% chlorhexidine mouthrinse compared with 0.2% on plaque accumulation and periodontal parameters: a systematic review. J Clin Periodontol 2010;37:829–39.

[26] Young A, Jonski G, Rölla G. Inhibition of orally produced volatile sulfur compounds by zinc, chlorhexidine or cetylpyridinium chloride--effect of concentration. Eur J Oral Sci 2003;111:400–4.

[27] Roldán S, Herrera D, Santa-Cruz I, O'Connor A, González I, Sanz M. Comparative effects of different chlorhexidine mouth-rinse formulations on volatile sulphur compounds and salivary bacterial counts. J Clin Periodontol 2004;31:1128–34.

[28] Young A, Jonski G, Rölla G, Wåler SM. Effects of metal salts on the oral production of volatile sulfur-containing compounds (VSC). J Clin Periodontol 2001;28:776–81.

[29] Young A, Jonski G, Rölla G. Combined effect of zinc ions and cationinc anitibacterial agents on intraoral volatile sulphur compounds (VSC). Int Dent J 2003;53:237–42.

[30] Lynch E, Sheerin A, Claxson AW, Atherton MD, Rhodes CJ, Silwood CJ, Naughton DP, Grootveld M. Multicomponent spectroscopic investigations of salivary antioxidant consumption by an oral rinse preparation containing the stable free radical species chlorine dioxide (ClO$_2$). Free Radic Res 1997;26:209–34.

[31] Kim JS, Park JW, Kim DJ, Kim YK, Lee JY. Direct effect of chlorine dioxide, zinc chloride and chlorhexidine solution on the gaseous volatile sulfur compounds. Acta Odontol Scand 2014;72:645–50.

[32] Shinada K, Ueno M, Konishi C, Takehara S, Yokoyama S, Kawaguchi Y. A randomized double blind crossover placebo-controlled clinical trial to assess the effects of a mouthwash containing chlorine dioxide on oral malodor. Trials 2008;9:71.

[33] Levy CW, Roujeinikova A, Sedelnikova S, Baker PJ, Stuitje AR, Slabas AR, Rice DW, Rafferty JB. Molecular basis of triclosan activity. Nature 1999;398:383–4.

[34] Carvalho MD, Tabchoury CM, Cury JA, Toledo S, Nogueira-Filho GR. Impact of mouthrinses on morning bad breath in healthy subjects. J Clin Periodontol 2004;31:85–90.

[35] Gürgan CA, Zaim E, Bakirsoy I, Soykan E. Short-term side effects of 0.2% alcohol-free chlorhexidine mouthrinse used as an adjunct to non-surgical periodontal treatment: a double-blind clinical study. J Periodontol 2006;77:370–84.

[36] Nikaido S, Tanaka M, Yamato M, Minami T, Akatsuka M, Mori H. Anaphylactoid shock caused by chlorhexidine gluconate. Masui (Japanese) 1998;47:330–4.

[37] Krautheim AB, Jermann TH, Bircher AJ. Chlorhexidine anaphylaxis: case report and review of the literature. Contact Dermatitis 2004;50:113–6.

[38] Aiello AE, Larson EL, Levy SB. Consumer antibacterial soaps: effective of just risky? Clin Infect Dis 2007;45 Suppl 2:S137–47.

[39] Stoker TE, Gibson EK, Zorrilla LM. Triclosan exposure modulates estrogen-dependent responses in the female wistar rat. Toxicol Sci 2010;117:45–53.

[40] Nagata H, Inagaki Y, Yamamoto Y, Maeda K, Kataoka K, Osawa K, Shizukuishi S. Inhibitory effects of macrocarpals on the biological activity of *Porphyromonas gingivalis* and other periodontopathic bacteria. Oral Microbiol Immunol 2006;21:159–63.

[41] Tanaka M, Toe M, Nagata H, Ojima M, Kuboniwa M, Shimizu K, Osawa K, Shizukuishi S. Effect of eucalyptus-extract chewing gum on oral malodor: a double-masked, randomized trial. J Periodontol 2010;81:1564–71.

[42] Hirasawa M, Takada K, Makimura M, Otake S. Improvement of periodontal status by green tea catechin using a local delivery system: a clinical pilot study. J Periodontal Res 2002;37:433–8.

[43] Sakanaka S, Aizawa M, Kim M, Yamamoto T. Inhibitory effects of green tea polyphenols on growth and cellular adherence of an oral bacterium, *Porphyromonas gingivalis*. Biosci Biotechnol Biochem 1996;60:745–9.

[44] Makimura M, Hirasawa M, Kobayashi K, Indo J, Sakanaka S, Taguchi T, Otake S. Inhibitory effect of tea catechins on collagenase activity. J Periodontol 1993;64:630–6.

[45] Okamoto M, Sugimoto A, Leung KP, Nakayama K, Kamaguchi A, Maeda N. Inhibitory effect of green tea catechins on cysteine proteinases in *Porphyromonas gingivalis*. Oral Microbiol Immunol 2004;19:118–20.

[46] Lodhia P, Yaegaki K, Khakbaznejad A, Imai T, Sato T, Tanaka T, Murata T, Kamoda T. Effect of green tea on volatile sulfur compounds in mouth air. J Nutr Sci Vitaminol 2008;54:89–94.

[47] Rassameemasmaung S, Phusudsawang P, Sangalungkarn V. Effect of green tea mouthwash on oral malodor. ISRN Prev Med 2012;2013:975148.

[48] Nakatani K, Nakahata N, Arakawa T, Yasuda H, Ohizumi Y. Inhibition of cyclooxygenase and prostaglandin E2 synthesis by gamma-mangostin, a xanthone derivative in mangosteen, in C6 rat glioma cells. Biochem Pharmacol 2002;63:73–9.

[49] Rassameemasmaung S, Sirikulsathean A, Amornchat C, Hirunrat K, Rojanapanthu P, Gritsanapan W. Effects of herbal mouthwash containing the pericarp extract of *Garcinia mangostana* L on halitosis, plaque and papillary bleeding index. J Int Acad Periodontol 2007;9:19–25.

[50] Shih YH, Chang KW, Hsia SM, Yu CC, Fuh LJ, Chi TY, Shieh TM. In vitro antimicrobial and anticancer potential of hinokitiol against oral pathogens and oral cancer cell lines. Microbiol Res 2013;168:254–62.

[51] Komaki N, Watanabe T, Ogasawara A, Sato N, Mikami T, Matsumoto T. Antifungal mechanism of hinokitiol against *Candida albicans*. Biol Pharm Bull 2008;31:735–7.

[52] Iha K, Suzuki N, Yoneda M, Takeshita T, Hirofuji T. Effect of mouth cleaning with hinokitiol-containing gel on oral malodor: a randomized, open-label pilot study. Oral Surg Oral Med Oral Pathol Oral Radiol 2013;116:433–9.

[53] Yaegaki K, Sanada K. Biochemical and clinical factors influencing oral malodor in periodontal patients. J Periodontol 1992;63:783–9.

[54] Nohno K, Yamada T, Kaneko N, Miyazaki H. Tablets containing a cysteine protease, actinidine, reduce oral malodor: a crossover study. J Breath Res 2012;6:017107.

[55] Valenti P, Antonini G. Lactoferrin: an important host defence against microbial and viral attack. Cell Mol Life Sci 2005:62;2576–87.

[56] Thomas EL, Aune TM. Lactoperoxidase, peroxide, thiocyanate antimicrobial system: correlation of sulfhydryl oxidation with antimicrobial action. Infect Immun 1978;20:456–63.

[57] Shin K, Yaegaki K, Murata T, Ii H, Tanaka T, Aoyama I, Yamauchi K, Toida T, Iwatsuki K. Effects of a composition containing lactoferrin and lactoperoxidase on oral malodor and salivary bacteria: a randomized, double-blind, crossover, placebo-controlled clinical trial. Clin Oral Investig 2011;15:485–93.

[58] Kang MS, Kim BG, Chung J, Lee HC, Oh JS. Inhibitory effect of *Weissella cibaria* isolates on the production of volatile sulphur compounds. J Clin Periodontol 2006;33:226–32.

[59] Carlsson J, Grahnén H, Jonsson G, Wikner S. Early establishment of *Streptococcus salivarius* in the mouth of infants. J Dent Res 1970;49:415–8.

[60] Upton M, Tagg JR, Wescombe P, Jenkinson HF. Intra-and interspecies signaling between *Streptococcus salivarius* and *Streptococcus pyogenes* mediated by SalA and SalA1 lantibiotic peptides. J Bacteriol 2001;183:3931–8.

[61] Hyink O, Wescombe PA, Upton M, Ragland N, Burton JP, Tagg JR. Salivaricin A2 and the novel lantibiotic salivaricin B are encoded at adjacent loci on a 190-kilobase transmissible megaplasmid in the oral probiotic strain *Streptococcus salivarius* K12. Appl Environ Microbiol 2007;73:1107–13.

[62] Masdea L, Kulik EM, Hauser-Gerspach I, Ramseier AM, Filippi A, Waltimo T. Antimicrobial activity of *Streptococcus salivarius* K12 on bacteria involved in oral malodour. Arch Oral Biol 2012;57:1041–7.

[63] Burton JP, Chilcott CN, Moore CJ, Speiser G, Tagg JR. A preliminary study of the effect of probiotic *Streptococcus salivarius* K12 on oral malodour parameters. J Appl Microbiol 2006;100:754–64.

[64] Talarico TL, Casas IA, Chung TC, Dobrogosz WJ. Production and isolation of reuterin, a growth inhibitor produced by *Lactobacillus reuteri*. Antibicrob Agents Chemother 1988;32:1854–8.

[65] Teughels W, Durukan A, Ozcelik O, Pauwels M, Quirynen M, Haytac MC. Clinical and microbiological effects of *Lactobacillus reuteri* probiotics in the treatment of chronic periodontitis: a randomized placebo-controlled study. J Clin Periodontol 2013;40:1025–35.

[66] Twetman, S, Derawi B, Keller M, Ekstrand K, Yucel-Lindberg T, Stecksén-Blicks C. Short-term effect of chewing gums containing probiotic *Lactobacillus reuteri* on the levels of inflammatory mediators in gingival crevicular fluid. Acta Odontol Scand 2009;67:19–24.

[67] Vicario M, Santos A, Violant D, Nart J, Giner L. Clinical changes in periodontal subjects with the probiotc *Lactobacillus reuteri* Prodentis: a preliminary randomized clinical trial. Acta Odontol Scand 2013;71:813–9.

[68] Çaglar E, Cildir SK, Ergeneli S, Sandalli N, Twetman S. Salivary mutans streptococci and lactobacilli levels after ingestion of the probiotic bacterium *Lactobacillus reuteri* ATCC 55730 by straws or tablets. Acta Odontol Scand 2006;64:314–8.

[69] Keller MK, Hasslöf P, Dahlén G, Stecksén-Blicks C, Twetman S. Probiotic supplements (*Lactobacillus reuteri* DSM 17938 and ATCC PTA 5289) do not affect regrowth

of mutans streptococci after full-mouth disinfection with chlorhexidine: a randomized controlled multicenter trial. Caries Res 2012;46:140–6.

[70] Keller MK, Bardow A, Jensdottir T, Lykkeaa J, Twetman S. Effect of chewing gums containing the probiotic bacterium *Lactobacillus reuteri* on oral malodour. Acta Odontol Scand 2012;70:246–50.

[71] Aiba Y, Suzuki N, Kabir AM, Takagi A, Koga Y. Lactic acid-mediated suppression of *Helicobacter pylori* by the oral administration of *Lactobacillus salivarius* as a probiotic in a gnotobiotic murine model. Am J Gastroenterol 1998;93:2097–101.

[72] Shimauchi H, Mayanagi G, Nakaya S, Minamibuchi M, Ito Y, Yamaki K, Hirata H. Improvement of periodontal condition by probiotics with *Lactobacillus salivarius* WB21: a randomized, double-blind, placebo-controlled study. J Clin Periodontol 2008;35:897–905.

[73] Mayanagi G, Kimura M, Nakaya S, Hirata H, Sakamoto M, Benno Y, Shimauchi H. Probiotic effects of orally administered *Lactobacillus salivarius* WB21-containing tablets on periodontopathic bacteria: a double-blinded, placebo-controlled, randomized clinical trial. J Clin Periodontol 2009;36:506–13.

[74] Suzuki N, Tanabe K, Takeshita T, Yoneda M, Iwamoto T, Oshiro S, Yamashita Y, Hirofuji T. Effects of oil drops containing *Lactobacillus salivarius* WB21 on periodontal health and oral microbiota producing volatile sulfur compounds. J Breath Res 2012;6:017106. doi:10.1088/1752-7155/6/1/017106.

[75] Iwamoto T, Suzuki N, Tanabe K, Takeshita T, Hirofuji T. Effects of probiotic *Lactobacillus salivarius* WB21 on halitosis and oral health: an open-label pilot trial. Oral Surg Oral Med Oral Pathol Oral Radiol Endod 2010;110:201–8.

[76] Suzuki N, Yoneda M, Tanabe K, Fujimoto A, Iha K, Seno K, Yamada K, Iwamoto T, Masuo Y, Hirofuji T. *Lactobacillus salivarius* WB21-containing tablets for the treatment of oral malodor: a double-blind, randomized, placebo-controlled crossover trial. Oral Surg Oral Med Oral Pathol Oral Radiol 2014;117:462–70.

Chapter 36

Periodontal Changes and Oral Health

Petra Surlin, Anne Marie Rauten,
Mihai Raul Popescu, Constantin Daguci and
Maria Bogdan

Additional information is available at the end of the chapter

http://dx.doi.org/10.5772/59248

1. Introduction

Periodontal disease is represented by inflammatory processes that affect the tooth's support / anchoring system and lead to tooth loss and negative effects on the oral health. Tooth loss and decreasing number of contacts between antagonist teeth was placed in relation to the educational level, marital status and incomes. Changes in periodontal status have been associated with oral factors and different systemic diseases.

2. Oral factors and periodontal changes

2.1. Caries, edentation and occlusal trauma

Maxillary represents a morphofunctional very complex entity, consisting of various components whose smooth work ensures performance of specific key like mastication, phonation, physiognomy and self-preservation, contributing in the same time, cooperation with other organs and tissues, to swallowing and respiration.

All physiological interrelationships of the components of the ensemble: the jaws including teeth with periodontal tissues, buccal mucosa, tongue, salivary glands, temporomandibular joint, neuromuscular complex and the veins that irrigate the functional territory providing nutrition, are directed by the central nervous system [1,2]. This dependence is due to the permanently received information by cortex from the entire reception network of maxillary. It satisfies the balance and health of each organ this way, in which the occlusion coordinates integrates.

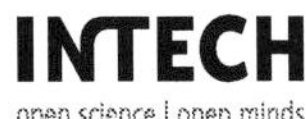

It is acknowledged that any pain occurred in the maxillary area generated by a traumatogenic occlusion occurs not only locally, but also away from the mouth. Any alteration occurred in one of the components of the maxillary (under the action of certain triggers cumulated with the favoring ones), happens on a common ground: occlusion. On the other hand, disorganisation at the dental arches level, with a disruption of movement, can affect one of the elements of the same assembly, occurring dysfunctional disorders.

As teeth are dependent on their supporting tissues which keep them in the pockets of the maxillary bones, the periodontal complex depends on the activity of dental arches, normal occlusal function leading to a morphofunctional mechanical stimulation that manages the responsible biological mechanisms for the proper integrity of the periodontium [3].

The analysis of functional occlusion should be used as the basis for all conservative dental treatment, periodontal, prosthetic and orthodontic surgery.

Due to the functional differentiation structure of periodontal tissues and topographical situation of the two components (shell and supportive) defenses and resistance against aggressive risk factors direct or indirect is special, being conditioned by their character. On periodontal coating will act primarily micro-irritation local agents and at the periodontal support component factors of functional order, resulting dysfunction appearance. Risk factors that contribute to the disturbance or alteration action of periodontal can be classified into three big categories:

i.   General favorable factors with dysmetabolic character that alters nutrition of the body, including the marginal periodontium.

ii.   Local disturbing or precipitating factors that can be very divers, responsible for local trophicity change of periodontium.

iii.   Aggravating regional factors that alter regional trophicity due to the presence of mandibular dysfunction caused by premature occlusal contacts and interference.

Studies performed on occlusal function and dysfunction shows that traumatic dental pain can be caused by traumatic injury to periodontal, cracks or fractures of teeth vital and a change of direction forces acting on periodontal dental units [1].

The occlusion was defined as the ratio of static contact between the two arches, regardless of the position occupied by the jaw to the cranium, unlike the interdental articulation, which requires dynamic contact of the dental arch.

Dynamic occlusal reports are made by the two arches during the performance of the stomatognathic system and during parafunctions. Occlusion is considered one of the three determinants of mandibular dynamics. In the same time, occlusion shows a anterior determinant (the front arches) and a posterior determinant (the arch side), between which there is a balance and interaction summarized in the context of mutual protection. Under this concept between the two determinants of occlusion there is a mutual protection, acting on static and dynamic phases of occlusion [4].

Dental occlusion is meant to stabilize the mandible position to the skull, participating in the development of systemic functions. Occlusal disorders occur as a result of dental anomalies of number, volume, position, dental crown injuries, dental migrations, edentulous, change of occlusion parameters, and secondary musculoskeletal joint dysfunction. Clinically it manifests as premature contacts (characterized by occlusion static phases), occlusal interference (in mandibular dynamic with dental contact), localized abrasion (at a tooth or dental group that takes over occlusal) or generalized to the whole arch.

Occlusal contacts can occur in the static and dynamic positions the jaw. Any occlusal contact that prevents uniform coaptation of support areas and occlusal contact points is called premature occlusal contact. Occlusal contact occurs early in the static occlusion (at the end of the terminal occlusion trajectory), or in the dynamic occlusion when the path of the jaw movement interferes with the dental contact.

Premature contact is always traumatizing for stomatognathic system elements. Traumatogenic capacity of a contact point depends on several factors such as the point of contact location, the size of the contact point, the state of the contact surfaces [5].

This way, if the point of contact is on a bigger surface, the friction force increases with it, and its pathogen potential. A reduced in size contact point, but between two rough surfaces can be as traumatic or even more than one big point on a polished surface, due to the high friction coefficient. Contacts may be multiple and symmetrical, while maintaining the mandible in a position close to or almost identical to the centric relation or intercuspation position without deviations above it, the rear or side. This rarely happens because the presence of small occlusal contacts creates what is called an occlusal instability. Clinical evaluation of static and dynamic occlusion cannot be made without registration cranio-mandibular relations. Within the tendency to establish maximum intercuspation contact (in patients with long-centric) and centric occlusion (in patients with point-centric), jaw moves from rest position, rising to the jaw with the action of high muscles [4].

Dynamic occlusion analysis is performed through a test movement printed to the jaw, and also during mastication, phonation and deglutition movements. The analysis of the test movements (retrusion, protrusion, left and right laterality) often reveals the presence of occlusion block-ages or of some traumatic sliding slopes. The retrusion movement performed between maximum intercuspation and centric relation can be blocked by some premature contacts, thus preventing the mandible excursion to centric relation during deglutition. The protrusion can register early contacts in the lateral area which would prevent the previous guidance of the occlusion on the retro incisive slope. The deeper is the occlusion, the larger is the trajectory of the protrusion. The premature contact points of the previous area in the protrusion movement prevent balanced contact of the whole frontal group in the guide movement, creating an overload of the teeth which keep the contact [6].

The test movements with left and right side orientation can reveal an inequality of the trajectories due to movement blocking through occlusal obstacles or due to their different orientation depending on the inclined planes which produce them. In the laterality movement there is recorded the most intense traumatogenic activity at the level of the interferences that may occur on the inactive or swing area, by turning the mandibular into lower grade leverage, therefore, more traumatic. In many cases, laterality or protrusion movement also causes a slight mobilization of the teeth which are in premature contact [4].

Occlusal force action on periodontal unit depends on the intensity, duration, direction of force, and the effects are also influenced by the state of tissue over which the force acts. The periodontal occlusal trauma is the degenerative injury that occurs when the occlusal forces exceed the adaptive capacity of the supporting tissue. Given that the dento-dental gearing is a cusp – fossa kind, the efforts leading is made in the long axis of the teeth. In normal circumstances, this condition is achieved by the way in which the teeth are implanted in the dental alveoli since their arcade eruption and through the manner in which are realized the dento-dental contacts in centric relation and maximum intercuspation, moments in which the masticatory pressures are maximum. In the teeth and periodontal tissue normal function, a particular importance has the correct position of dental organs, this being possible due to the presence of the balance between the multiple factors that are interrelated (presence of dental arcade integrity, the nature of the existing relations between adjacent teeth through contact areas and their character, dental morphology and cusps inclination, physiological mesial migration of teeth, physiological abrasion of teeth and their axial tilt, biological resistance of the healthy periodontium, lips, cheeks and tongue tone.

In the moment of integrity loss of dental arches, there occur multiple changes not only in the expense of odonto-periodontal units, but also for other components of the stomatognathic system, which demonstrates once again the present physiological interrelations between constituents of the complex.

Closely related to biomechanical homeostasis specific of the periodontium, the whole structural complex of the dento-maxillary system is conditioned by a series of morphological and functional elements that fit in the principle of inclined planes, among which the most important ones would be:

- Maximum and proximal vestibule-oral convexities of teeth ensure self-defense and self-stimulation of marginal periodontium through its protection against micro traumas that occur during mastication.

- The specific morphology of the frontal inferior teeth, vestibule-oral flattened in the third incisal and mesial-distal cervical narrowed to align them in a circle, defends the periodontium from pressures coming from the vestibule to the oral.

- Teeth roots' number and conical shape avoid the uneven application of the cementum-alveolar walls.

- Oral tilt of lower molars and vestibular tilt of the upper ones direct the masticatory pressures in the axial direction of these teeth while concentrating inwards massive facial.

When masticatory pressures are routed and transmitted in the long axis of the teeth, the ligaments that form the periodontal membrane are not crushed, but they act almost entirely, and are subject to forces with functional direction that determine their uniform extent, in functional limits with trophic effect on alveolar bone. After force's cessation, ligaments return to their spiral resting shape [7]. Taking into account that masticatory pressures are not permanent, periodontal ligaments are submitted to a real functional gymnastics, functional tasks interspersed with periods of rest, which stimulates periodontium, periodontal membrane and alveolar bone, and keeps it in normal parameters.

Local causes of traumatic occlusion with its negative consequences on the dento-maxillary are varied:

- Untreated caries, besides pulpal and periapical complications, they may also lead to occlusal disharmony and dysfunction by horizontal migration of proximal caries teeth or of their neighbors disturbing occlusal curves, vertical migration of antagonist teeth, of one tooth with occlusal caries or which considerably reduced the height of its crown, tipping of neighboring or antagonist caries teeth.

Through the loss of interdental contact point due to proximal caries, the fibrous foods can directly damage the marginal periodontium, which leads to periodontal damage and possible installation of a secondary occlusal trauma.

- The edentation without prosthesis acts by cancelling the dental arches continuity, due to loss of contact points, interrupting the continuity of the over alveoli ligaments system that normally form a connecting strap between teeth.

Also, the horizontal migration of teeth which border the edentulous breaches makes possible the spaces appearance between teeth and traumatic food impact of interdental gums papillae.

- Dental iatrogenic is often represented by inadequate fillings, inappropriate prosthetic marginal axial or transversal or which does not restore correctly proximal contact surfaces or natural convexities vestibule-oral and /or determine at the level of soft tissue rejection reactions, caused by prosthetic material.

The erroneous occlusal articular balancing compromised by grinding the occlusal stops and slopes guide altering vertical occlusal dimension and interdental space also produce occlusal dysfunction.

- Alteration of the morphology of dental crowns by pathological abrasion produces a broadening of the occlusal plane, constituting a cause of overload of odonto-periodontal units by masticatory forces.

- Primary malposition of some permanent teeth which erupt vicious in the three spatial planes. In this category, there are included anomalies of position: infra, over, predental, retrodental, vestibular or oral of some teeth, different combinations of malposition: mesio-vestibular position and distovestibular position.

- Isolated dental anomalies of form and volume can be generating occlusal interference by inconsistencies that appear in reports to other normally developed teeth. It produces a change in the position of teeth, bone implant base change, changing cuspid plans finally affecting occlusion reports.

- Occlusal vicious habits and tics are multiple and a source of risk factors for a dysfunctional maxillary. The most common harmful habits are: onychophagy (nail biting), biting objects (pipe, rubber, glasses frames), the practice of keeping and tighten between teeth, needle, nails, pencil, while working.

- Dentoalveolar fractures or maxillary bones may lead to dysfunctional occlusal interference. When the traumatic accident caused significant displacement of bone fragments of jaw, they rarely can be reduced in such a manner that there will be no significant occlusal changes after consolidation.

- Multiple parafunctions are the most common sources of occlusal dysfunction, bruxism holding priority. It is conditioned by the existence of occlusal disharmonies caused by premature dental contacts and occlusal interferences with an important role for multi-causal dysfunctional factors of the maxillary.

With a change of direction of force, normal pressure of normal muscle contractions become traumatic for periodontal membrane crushed between the tooth and alveolar wall it has no irrigation and normal metabolism anymore, and on the other hand, not all ligaments take functional tasks. Besides periodontal membrane suffering appears a harmful effect on alveolus: pressure causes bone lysis. Bone lysis always occurs in the way the force that causes pressure on the bone acts, which results in a stronger inclination of the tooth, like this appears traumatic periodontal conditions. By tilting the teeth it can escape the occlusal pressures making even dental contact to disappear; periodontal pain does not disappear with the disappearance of dental tooth contact as lack of stimuli periodontium undergoes hyaline degeneration of hypofunction [8]. Following these considerations to set the concept of primary occlusal trauma which means the harmful effect of occlusal forces on initial healthy periodontal when the direction, intensity or duration of occlusal force are beyond functional parameters: direction outside the long axis of the tooth, too long time, too much intensity. In this context, it should be emphasized that most studies are in agreement that the primary occlusal trauma (in the absence of superimposed etiologic factors, inflammatory, degenerative-dystrophic) does not causes periodontal disease but isolated periodontal lesions. Experience has shown that when the periodontium is weakened, initial periodontal suffering having other causes than occlusal, occlusal requests, even with optimal direction, the long axis of the teeth, even if they are intermittent, or even if the intensity normal, all lead to a periodontal trauma [9,10,11]. In this case, it is a secondary occlusal trauma in which the occlusal forces act on a previously weakened tooth periodontium. Obviously for already weaken teeth periodontium faulty forces within that direction, intensity or duration, have bad effects. Great difficulty occurs when, after periodontal is affected by an occlusal trauma, inflammatory component is superimposed, because at the moment it is hard to tell whether it is a primary or secondary occlusal trauma.

We can describe the three stages of occlusal trauma: stage of aggression, stage of repair and periodontal adaptation stage. During the stage of aggression collagen and osteogenic activity is inhibited, so that when the injury is not too strong to stimulate repair possibilities. If the trauma is not excessive, overcoming repair potential has serious periodontal consequences. If trauma is not excessive, it can reach the third stage, the periodontal adaptation. [12].

Disorders at the level of occlusive parameters characterized by shortening and cutting of occlusal areas, their artificial or mixed incorrectly realization, discontinuities, incorrect reconstructions of retroincisal slope, changes in the integrity and shape of support and guidance cusps, altered occlusion curves, uneven occlusal plane, are important factors of occlusal dysfunction, resulting in changes in jaw dynamic patterns, with muscle and joint response, taking into account the role of the dental determinant in achieving mandibular dynamics.

It is worth noting that the teeth in occlusal trauma, especially those with pathological abrasion, fractures may occur in low varnish areas, which can go up to an aspect of,, shelling " of dental crown [4].

True cuneiform lesions (mylolysis) are missing carious dentin being located strictly in the varnish. These are considered by many authors as pathognomonic lesions for teeth in occlusal trauma [13,14]. These lesions with lack of dental hard tissues are located on the vestibular side. The section looks like an obtuse angle open to the mouth vestibule. The lesion affects hard coronary tissues but extends to the root cementum, in the same time with marginal periodontal retraction [5,15,16]. The color of the cuneiform lesions walls is slightly modified and they have a hard consistency, heat sensitivity or chemical is inconsistent and injury has a slow progress. If you are creating a five grade cavity lesion evolves rapidly while getting the characteristics of dental cavity. Occlusal obstacles and / or occlusal parafunctions often cause appearance of pathological abrasion [13]. It should be clinically noted how the abrasion is dependent on other factors. It is demonstrates that the patient's age, degree of abrasion of tooth of specific subject, the presence of eccentric abrasion (which betrays occlusion function) are factors that cause pathological abrasion [4].

Studies show that reducing the masticatory field by edentation accelerates abrasion. Local hyperacidity (by diet or acid regurgitation) can lead to erosion (as opposed to abrasion) [17]. Presence of enamel dystrophy and dysplasia, in one word the quality of dental hard tissues is an important factor that causes tooth wear [18].Another extremely important factor that can cause tooth wear is the abrasive capacity of prosthetic restoration materials.Isolated clinical examination makes it virtually impossible to determine the rate of pathological abrasion. Therefore it is prudent that in such cases to make exploratory therapeutic methods (selective grinding, temporary dentures) before major restaurateurs interventions. In this way, the dentist is able to identify more precisely the primary determinant of pathological abrasion and abrasion evolution speed.General pathological abrasion-is the abrasion inconsistent with biological age. The generalized pathological abrasion is a major sign of dysfunctional occlusal [18,19].

Periodontal pockets do not occur in primary occlusal trauma, but usually in secondary, on a periodontium already affected in the presence of infectious and local irritative factors. As long as the inflammation is limited to the gum, it is not aggravated by traumatic occlusal forces, but when the inflammatory process spreads to desmodontium own tissue, the occlusal trauma becomes a co-destruction factor of support structures, protecting the periodontal pockets of bones. A periodontal pockets is pathological deepening of the gingivodental fosse which is formed gradually, resulting the destruction of tooth support tissue and its mobility, finally leading to its expulsion of [19].

Destructive alveolar processes represent another consequence of the occlusal trauma phenomenon. Alveolar bone, despite of its appearance rigidity, is less stable than periodontal tissue, as is continuous-changing structure by obvious resorption phenomenon in the pressure area and by apposition ones manifested within traction territory. In the case of occlusal trauma, the destructive effect on alveolar bone is directly proportional to the overload degree, their frequency and duration being inversely proportional to the resistance of the tissue. On such a field, under the action of repeated occlusion constraints, the negative effects of occlusal trauma occur more easily, periodontal disease having a fast and serious evolution. In conjunction of any occlusal trauma caused by bruxism amid a normal gum, first the bone destruction presents the characteristic of an aseptic process, lytic, of some areas that cannot be radiologically detected yet. In later stages, due to parafunction persistence, destructive phenomena complicate, the blood nutrition being even more deficient, due to prolonged action of pressure forces, amid local irritations (tartar and plaque) will contribute to the failure of the epithelial barrier to invasion of microorganisms and toxins. The existing bone bags, along with the gum ones installed will progress simultaneously, adding also the gingival retraction [20]. Another result of the occlusion dysfunction is represented by the opening of the interproximal contacts. The consequence of periodontal changes caused by occlusal trauma is represented by dental mobility, dental migrations, and gingivorragia. Mobility is due to an occlusal trauma exerted on that tooth, the tooth receiving abnormal forces which pressure it during protrusion and laterotrusion movements.

The more frequently there are affected the monoradiculars that are subjected to occlusal trauma producing bone lysis in the support periodontium level. Because of dental mobility is difficult to detect when occlusal trauma occurs, requiring consideration of occlusion, both in centric relation and maximum intercuspation and also in protrusion and laterotrusion movements. Pathological tooth migration is a phenomenon that occurs due to poor periodontal structure, exacerbating existing traumatic occlusion with more pronounced effect of paraxial transmission of masticatory forces so harmful to the entire dento-maxillary system. Changing the position of one or more teeth causes 'contact rupture' between them, creating spaces (trema, diastema) favoring mechanical injury of epithelial insertion with papilla inflammation often accompanied by bleeding. Implantation of the pluriradiculars is more favorable for the capacity of trauma resistance when the roots are divergent. In fact, all aspects mentioned above influence the capacity of occlusal trauma resistance, making a normal request to appear as supraliminal, emphasizing the traumatogenic character of occlusal forces [3, 21].

Coating or superficial periodontium injuries take various clinical forms depending on the intensity, duration and direction on which occlusal trauma manifests. Occlusal trauma can cause a progressive denudation of teeth roots, characterized by moving the gum to the tooth apex. There are two sets of gum retractions: one which is detected on physical examination, another one hidden, and a part of the root being covered by the inflamed wall of a periodontal pocket. It should be noted that gingival retraction may involve all insertion area from the level of dental package, or only partially. The most common areas are the vestibular and oral of one tooth, of a group of teeth or even of a complete dental arch.

Traumatic dental hygiene habits can worsen the gingival recessions at the level of vestibular teeth face, this being associated with the occurrence and emphasis of cuneiform injuries, which is a pathognomonic sign that the tooth / teeth in question are in occlusal trauma [22].

Occlusal trauma causes and aggravates the gingival retraction, thus accelerating the initial epithelial proliferation by a local irritation, clinical form known as Mc Call's garlands or festoons. It also can reveal injuries as cracks (Stillman's fissures). These identities are pathological bag bottoms in which the ulcerative process developed, they could spontaneously cicatrize or persist in the form of deep fissures with rolled edges [23, 24, 25]. Papilla and gingivitis occurring as a result of opening the cervical interproximal space arise as a consequence of the loss of dental contact points in the presence of partial edentation which are accompanied by migrations, tipping or translations of the limiting dental units to edentulous breaches. The opening of interproximal space allows food particles penetration, thus injuring the gingival papillae.

Local examination reveals the presence of gingival inflammation that may be associated with bleeding. In advanced stages there is a junction of the vestibular and oral gums, accompanied by a slight extrusion of the affected tooth. Interradicular space dissection is characterized by roots denudation, gingival epithelium covering the limbus bone top retreating. Reaching bifurcation or trifurcation root is generally due to deepening of vestibular gingivodental or oral channel [26, 27].

Any indiscriminate therapeutic act in terms of ignorance or underestimation the capacity features and adaptive limit capacity, respectively of teeth defense, periodontium, temporomandibular joint, jaw bones, neuromuscular and vascular complexes, is likely to confuse the morphofunctional balance of dento-maxillary system, thus prejudicing the treated subject through iatrogenesis.

2.2. Malocclusions

The interrelation between the periodontal health status, the presence of dento-maxillary anomalies and the orthodontic treatment remains a controversial issue in the literature [28], reflected in the great diversity of the findings of studies that address this issue. Some researchers promote the idea that the presence of dento-maxillary anomalies is a risk factor in the development of periodontal pathology: [29-34];

The dento-maxillary anomalies may represent a risk factor in producing chronic marginal periodontitis as they maintain the periodontal inflammation, while changing the intensity and direction of occlusal forces. Other periodontal changes as insufficient attached gingiva width and low height of the alveolar bone were also observed and associated with the presence of dento-maxillary anomalies in general, or a single misaligned teeth [35, 36], as well as people with evident dento-maxillary anomalies were discovered to whom periodontal changes were minimal or nonexistent [37].

2.2.1. Dento-alveolar disharmony (DAD) with crowding

They are a risk factor for the presence of septic inflammation, because due to the disparity between mesial-distal sizes of permanent teeth and corresponding alveolar arches' perimeter, various dental malposition occur, localized mainly in incisor-canine region (Figure 1), which causes retention of food debris and plaque, and difficulty in removing them by self-cleaning or artificial cleaning [38]. This correlation is weaker in the maxilla compared to the mandible [39].

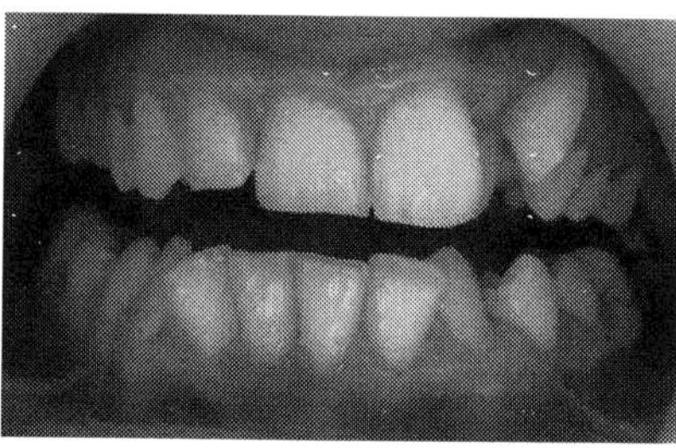

Figure 1. Gingival inflammation with papillae hypertrophy in lower and upper incisors, thin periodontium at 23 (eruption in buccal position) in a patient with dental crowding

The fact that malocclusion with crowding is a risk factor in the development of periodontal pathology is supported by studies that have reported the existence of a strong correlation between the presence of this anomaly and the occurrence of periodontal pockets, [40]; [41]; or the reduction of alveolar bone[42].

Anatomical conditions specific to this anomaly are unfavorable because interdental septa are thin, interdental papillae are laminated, with low volume and with poor blood circulation, unfavorable for a good gingival-periodontal nutrition [43].

2.2.2. Dento-alveolar disharmony (DAD) with spacing

DAD cause periodontal adaptive phenomena such as: hiperkeratinized epithelium, gingival chorion fibrosis, flattening dental papilla (which become a plateau or even concave aspect) (Figure 2). The presence of this anomaly may favor direct trauma on interdental papillae by food fragments.

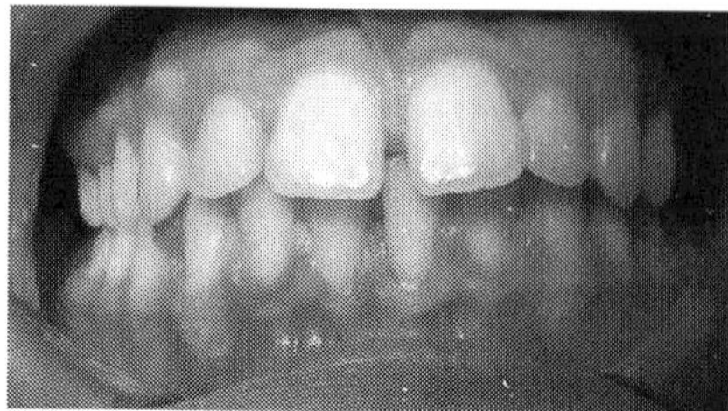

Figure 2. Gingival retractions with a thin periodontium at 31, 41, aplatized papillae between 11 and 21

Many specialized studies could not establish any positive correlation between incongruence with spacing and periodontal parameters in conditions of a rigorous hygiene, so that there are authors who consider that the indication for closure of interdental spaces is aesthetic rather than for periodontal dental health maintaining. [39]

2.2.3. Open bite

In the anterior open bite teeth are not functionaly requested during mastication (missing the food cut), and the self-cleaning phenomenon is absent favoring installation of gingival inflammation and hyperplastic changes. In contrast, lateral teeth are in occlusal contact and they are overworked during masticatory effort, they being almost in a state of permanent occlusal trauma due to the transfer of mandibular movements' previous guide of the lateral teeth [44].

We thus witness the periodontal space widening, gingival retraction emergence and horizontal bone atrophy of these teeth.

According to Macht and Zubery [45], in this syndrome we are witnessing a significant increase in the gingival inflammation, consequence of the enhancing virulence of the dehydrated plaque (due to lack of labial competence), and an increase in the length of the clinical crowns of incisors, which may suggest that open bite predisposes patients to the development of gingival retractions localized in the incisor segment (Figure 3).

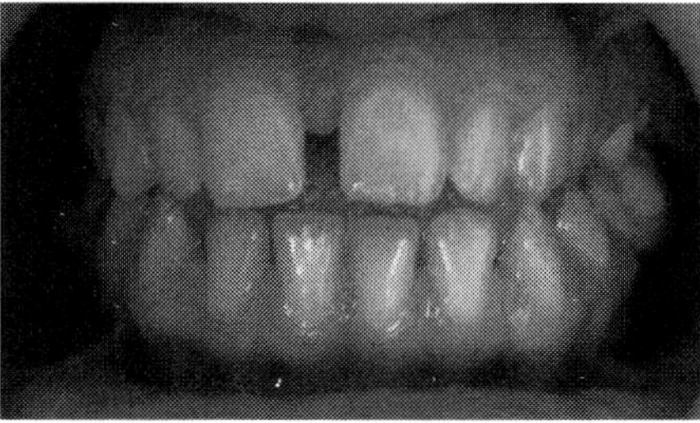

Figure 3. Open bite in a 19 years patient-thin periodontium predisposed at gingival recessions

2.2.4. Deep bite (class II division 2 malocclusion)

In the deep bite syndrome, anterior teeth don't have stable occlusal stops, and their implantation remains normal just as long as inflammation isn't installed due to the presence of plaque. When gingival-periodontal injuries of microbial cause occur, the anterior teeth implantation degrades, it begins a process of accelerated active eruption of the anterior inferior teeth, with the possibility of their direct trauma to the incisive upper periodontium [43], and the progression of periodontal lesions. Deep bite syndrome will lead in these conditions to increased periodontal pocket depth and marginal gingival retractions appearance [39]

2.2.5. Overbite (class II division 1 malocclusions)

Due to inocclusion lips and upper lip hypotrophy, bacterial accumulation occurs in the anterior dental area, the immunological role of saliva is reduced, and on long-term increases the frequency of periodontal lesions [46]. Similar to open bite, in the anterior dental regions, a fragile periodontal can be structured (Figure 4), prone to periodontal lesions because of unstable interdental contacts. The same fragile periodontium can be observed in the side areas, due to unilateral or bilateral crossbite (consequences of a different degree of compression of the two jaws).

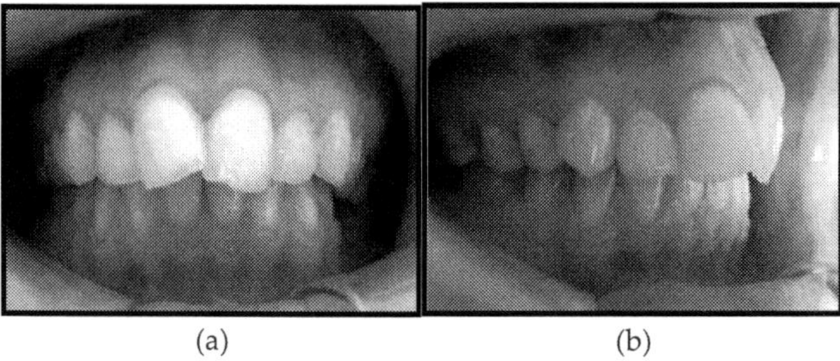

(a)   (b)

Figure 4. Fragile periodontium with gingival recessions in lower incisors (a-frontal b-lateral view) in a patient with maxillary compression

There is no concordance of views regarding correlations between sagittal inocclusion (overjet) and periodontal parameters. Authors such as Davies et al. 1991, [47] or Geiger et al., 1976, [48] support the existence of a significant correlation between plaque index, periodontal diseases and severe anterior overjet (> 6 mm), while Buckley, 1981 [49] considers that there is no significant correlation between the presence of overjet and plaque index, or gingival inflammation index.

According to Torres et al., 2006, [50] an increase in the plaque index occurs only in subjects with sagittal inocclusion > 6, and after Bjornaas et al. 1994 [51], to adulthood, in the presence of a severe sagittal inocclusion (overjet ≥8mm), there is a reduction of alveolar bone level with ≈0,96mm in the upper anterior area, and with ≈0,35 mm in the lower area.

2.2.6. Mandibular prognathism (class III malocclusions)

In mandibular prognathism, the lingual pressure (of the protrude tongue and low positioned) continuously exercised on the lower incisors' lingual face and the occlusal trauma due to anterior crossbite can lead to important vestibulo-version of the mandibular incisors with fine periodontal biotypes inducing and the presence of a very thin vestibular cortical bone, located away from the cemento-enamel junction.

Transferring anterior guide on the lateral teeth, found in this group of anomalies, leads to the lateral dental area overloading concurrent to a less loading of the front area (no food incision)

[44]. Therefore we can expect the emergence of periodontal changes like horizontal bone atrophy and epithelial insertion's descent [52].

Periodontal changes occur early in reverse gear and consist of the occurrence of significant gingival retraction of the lower incisors' vestibular face ("disposal trench"), possibly a tooth mobility, following a permanent occlusal trauma.

These periodontal changes can regress spontaneously if orthodontic treatment is instituted early [53].

There is no uniformity of opinion or about the association between anterior crossbite with different periodontal parameters. Ngom et al. researches 2005, [39] have reported the presence of a significant correlation between anterior crossbite and the percentage of gingival retraction, but not with the plaque index and the gingival pockets depth, while Hashim and Al-Jasser's researches, 1996, [54] have found a significant correlation between crossbite, the plaque index and the periodontal pocket depth. The difference between the two studies may be due to differences in age and dental hygiene of the subjects investigated. Silness and Roynstrand, 1984, [55] opines that the crossbite teeth show more frequently signs of periodontal disease compared to those dealing a normal occlusion.

2.2.7. Congenital malformations of the lip, maxilla and palate(clefts)

Next to specific anatomical defects, the delays in the formation and timing of tooth eruption, the need for long orthodontic treatment [56, 57] and the presence of prosthetic restorations are factors contributing to the reduction of the alveolar bone level in areas adjacent to dehiscence [58].

Multiple dental malposition, segmental alveolar gaps, soft tissue folds made before palatoplasty, the presence of scar tissue or oro-nasal communications persisting after surgical closure of the defect, make oral hygiene maintenance a difficult task, increasing risk and progression of periodontal disease [59, 60, 61].

Comparing the periodontium from patients with cleft lip and cleft palate, to the one from patients with cleft palate only, Gaggl et al., 1999, [62 found that the first have a predisposition to deep periodontal destructions in the teeth adjacent to the splicing area, while in patients that only have cleft palate, clinical peridental appearance may be similar to that of subjects without malformations. However, Dewinter and Quirynen state that the periodontium of the teeth from the splicing zone or near it, in patients with unilateral cleft, can cope relatively well to a long orthodontic treatment or to a combined periodontal-orthodontic treatment [63].

2.3. Orthodontic treatment

The three main reasons justifying the need for orthodontic treatment are: to improve facial and dental aesthetics, oro-dental health and the normal oral functions [36].

In the absence of periodontal diseases and in the presence of a proper oral hygiene, a well led orthodontic treatment should not have, on long-term, significant effects on periodontal supportive structures. According to Graber et al., 2005, [64] it is possible to occur a decrease in the alveolar bone's volume and height, as an adaptive process to the trauma.

The main clinical periodontal effects that can be seen in the oral cavity after insertion of orthodontic appliances are: gingival hyperplasia, marginal gingival retraction, irreversible loss of bone support and excessive fibrous tissue that prevents complete closure of the post extraction spaces [65].

2.3.1. Gingival overgrowth (hypertrophy and hyperplasia)

A periodontal change frequently observed during orthodontic treatment, especially with fixed appliances, is the emergence of gingival overgrowth [66].

Scope, they can be localized or generalized, but seem to be more common in mandibular incisors region (67, 68) (Figure 5).

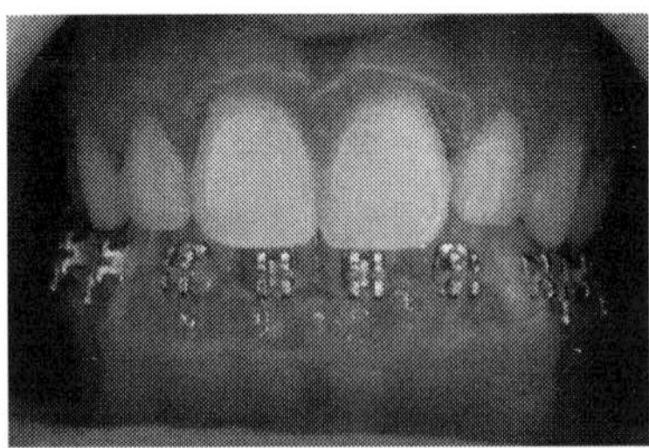

Figure 5. Gingival overgrowth with inflammation and plaque accumulation in the lower incisors

Other authors (69) believe that overgrowths may be marginal, diffuse, papillary, or discrete and have four degrees of severity:

- 0-no gingival overgrowth;

- I – gingival overgrowth extended only to the dental papilla;

- II-gingival overgrowth covering the papilla and marginal gingiva;

- III-gingival overgrowth covers three quarters or more of the dental crown.

Since gingival overgrowth is a factor limiting or preventing orthodontic tooth movement, it often requires its removal by gingivectomy, which removes all fibrous tissues around the tooth and at the same time allows gum's reshaping or remodeling [69]. After gingivectomy, periodontal condition is improving, so the orthodontic mechanic's normal course is possible. If it does not prevent the effectiveness of orthodontic treatment and causes no discomfort to the patient, gum volume enlargement can be removed after the completion of orthodontic treatment, if it does not regress spontaneously.

2.3.2. Marginal gingival retractions and losses of bone support

Sometimes, the incidence of gingival recessions in patients with a fixed orthodontic appliance can be up to 10% [70]. In addition, repeated trauma on marginal gingiva by teeth movements and plaque accumulation, inherent with the application of orthodontic appliances, can lead to the formation of marginal gingival retractions. Moreover, mucogingival problems prior to the initiation of orthodontic treatment could be exacerbated by the application of orthodontic force [70]. It seems that the lower incisors are the teeth most likely to develop marginal gingival retractions, the mechanism of their occurrence being the excessive force applying, which does not allow bone's repairing or remodeling during teeth movement with the existence of a thin or non-existent vestibular cortical and an inadequate or absent keratinized gum [40].

2.3.3. Assesment of periodontal changes using immunological analysis in Gingival Crevicular Fluid (GCF)

During the initial phase of orthodontic treatment, orthodontic forces induce a response to the mechanical stress from periodontium and a net of events it is produced: angiogenesis, aseptic inflammation and periodontal remodeling [71].

Gingival crevicular fluid (GCF) is used to determine the presence and levels of biomarkers expressed during the first phase of orthodontic treatment, this cascade of substances comprising cytokines, metalloproteinases and other mediators of complex transformations in the periodontium [72, 73].

In studies funded by the grant ID573/2008 of the Ministry of Education and Research of Romania, we measured the levels of Pentraxin-3 (PTX3), Thrombospondin1 (TSP1), Lipocalin2/Matrix metalloproteinase 9 (MMP9/NGAL) complex and Matrix metalloproteinase 9 (MMP9) in GCF at different time points of the first 2 weeks of orthodontic treatment, to determine the relationship between these values and theirs implication in inflammation and angiogenesis balance, in the situation of a good control of the bacterial plaque [74, 75].

GCF samples were collected from orthodontic patients requiring upper canine distalization with first premolar extraction. For the orthodontic appliance, there are placed brackets Roth 0.018 inch (GAC Intl, Bohemia, USA) with 0.012 inch NiTi archwire (GAC Intl, Bohemia, USA) and a laceback made from 0.010 inch stainless wire, placed and activated 21 days after the premolar extraction.

Using the statistical analysis, our results show a change in time of PTX3, TSP1, MMP9/NGAL and MMP9 levels in GCF of patients with this method of orthodontic treatment and suggest their stronger involvement in inflammation and angiogenesis processes in PDL during orthodontic periodontal remodeling, in the situation of a healthy periodontium and a good control of the bacterial plaque.

2.3.4. Assessment of periodontal changes using immunohistochemical analysis of gingival tissue

The gingival overgrowth as a reaction of the orthodontic treatment was longtime considered by the clinicians as an inflammatory result of the retention of the bacterial plaque by the orthodontic devices. Clinical observations showed that the gingival overgrowth appear also in patients with good oral hygiene, without any clinical signs of gingival inflammation.

Our studies [76,77] in the grant ID573/2008 funded by the Ministry of Education and Research in Romania showed that the gingival overgrowth during the fixed orthodontic treatment appears at the beginning, without any inflammatory signs, as a result of the mechanical stress and periodontal remodeling during the orthodontic movement, the MMP8 and MMP9 acting as indicators of this situation.The inflammation of gingiva occurs as a consequence of the accumulation of the bacterial plaque favorized by the orthodontic devices.

Gingivectomy was performed in patient with gingival overgrowth in the first eight weeks of the orthodontic treatment and the material obtained was used for histologic and immunohistochemical study.

3. Systemic factors and periodontal changes

3.1. Diabetes and obesity

Diabetes mellitus (DM) and periodontitis are both chronic inflammatory disorders and which enhances their severity, worsen each other prognosis and share a number of pathogenic mechanisms with common inflammatory mediators which have been investigated as possible biomarkers of disease status.These improved diagnostic efforts resulting from utilization of biomarkers should enable optimal treatment planning, also assist in monitoring clinical response to treatment and more focused prevention of common human conditions. The most important inflammatory mediators linked to initiation and progression of periodontal disease is a complex network of pro-inflammatory cytokines, matrix metalloproteinases (MMPs) and prostaglandins [78]. The vast majority of studies of cytokines, adipokines and other mediators in periodontitis and diabetes have been small-scale clinical studies using GCF(gingival crevicular fluid), saliva or gingival tissues samples which have focused on limited number of mediators and many inconclusive because of limitation in study design. Nevertheless there are promising data on certain mediators such IL-1β, IL-6, TNF-α and emerging data on RANKL and OPG; these are likely to have a central role in the pathogenesis of periodontitis in diabetic patients [79, 80]. Complex interactions between individual mediators and emergent pathways, for example, synergy in cytokine signaling, will not be apparent from simple disease association studies of a limited number of molecules [79, 80].

There are studies suggesting that pro-inflammatory cytokines which induce chronic inflammatory diseases including periodontitis, could increase insulin resistance [81, 82]. Both TNF-α and IL-6 are produced in adipose tissue, and a large quantity of circulating IL-6 is derived [83]. There are also studies which correlate periodontitis to obesity [84, 85]. These directions of research suggest that obesity, diabetes and periodontitis may be related to each other.

Effective periodontal treatment in patients with DM significantly reduced GCF [86, 87] and serum levels of several mediators, such as IL6, TNF, adiponectin [88, 89, 90], MMP2, MMP9 [91], thus leading to reduced systemic inflammation.

In the effort to establish a pathway for the periodontitis-DM-obesity co-morbidity, some studies have determined genetic polymorphisms for IL6 and IL1 [92, 93]. These cytokines have been previously measured in blood and GFC from patients with these diseases.

Because fatty tissue serves as a reservoir for inflammatory cytokines, an increase in body fat may determine an increase of the inflammatory response of the host in periodontal disease [94].

In 2014, a study concerning the low fibers rich and fat poor diet for 8 weeks, demonstrated an improvement of the periodontal disease's markers, their levels returning to the initial value after follow-up period [95]. A study proposed the hyperinflammatory state observed in obesity, determined by the increase in cytokine levels, as mechanism to explain this relation [96].

Aknowledgment

Immunological and immunohistochemical studies of MMP9/NGAL, TSP1, PTX3, MMP8 and MMP9 in CCF and gingival tissue of orthodontic patients were funded by the grant ID573/2008 of the Ministry of Education and Research of Romania, IDEAS competition of CNCSIS.

Author details

Petra Surlin[1], Anne Marie Rauten[2], Mihai Raul Popescu[3], Constantin Daguci[4] and Maria Bogdan[5]

1 University of Medicine and Pharmacy of Craiova, Faculty of Dental Medicine, Department of Periodontology, Romania

2 University of Medicine and Pharmacy of Craiova, Faculty of Dental Medicine, Department of Orthodontics, Romania

3 University of Medicine and Pharmacy of Craiova, Faculty of Dental Medicine, Department of Occlusal Sciences, Romania

4 University of Medicine and Pharmacy of Craiova, Faculty of Dental Medicine, Department of Oral Health, Romania

5 University of Medicine and Pharmacy of Craiova, Faculty of Pharmacy, Department of Pharmacology, Romania

References

[1] ASH. Dental Anatomy Phisiology and Occlusion. W. B. Saunders Co.1993; 45-68,89-146.

[2]   Gray HS. Occlusion and restorative dentistry: Part1.NZDent J1993; 89(395):61-5.

[3]   Calandriello M, Carnevale G, Ricci G. Parodontologia, Ed. Martina Bologna 1996; 20-45,156-193,549-587.

[4]   Dawson PE. Position paper regarding diagnosis, management, and treatment of temporomandibular disorders. The American Equilibration Society. J Prosth Dent 1999; 81(2):174-8.

[5]   Lund JP Occlusion: the "science-based" approach. J Can Dent Assoc 2001; 67(2):84.

[6]   Millstein P, Maya A. An evaluation of occlusal contact marking indicators. A descriptive quantitative method. J Am Dent Ass 2001; 132(9):1280-6; quiz 1319.

[7]   Gremillion HA. The relationship beetwen occlusion and TMJ: an evidence-based discussion. J Evid Based Dent Pract 2006; 6:43-47.

[8]   Genco RJ. Current view of risk factors for periodontal diseases. J Periodontol 1996 Oct; 67(10 Suppl):1041-9.

[9]   Armitage GC. Periodontal diagnoses and classification of periodontal diseases. Periodontology 2004; 34:9-21.

[10] Harrel SK, Nunn ME, Hallmon WW. Is there an association betwen occlusion and periodontal destruction? Yes-occlusal forces can contribute to periodontal destruction. J Am Dent Assoc 2006; 137:1380-1384.

[11] Greenstein G, Greenstein B, Cavallaro J. Prerequisite for treatment planning implant dentistry: periodontal prognostication of compromised teeth. Compend Contin Educ Dent 2007; 28:436-437.

[12] MC Neill C. Occlusion: what it is and what it is not. J Calif Dent Assoc 2000; 28(10): 748-58.

[13] Dale R. Occlusion: the standard of care. J Can Dent Assoc 2003; 67(2):83-92.

[14] Telles D, Pegoraro LF, Pereira JC, et al. Incidence of noncarios cervical lesions and their relation to the presence of wear facets. J Esthet Restor Dent 2006; 18: 178-183.

[15] Grippo JO, Simring M, Schreiner S. Attrition, abrasion, corrosion and abfraction revisited: a new perspective on tooth surface lesions. J AM Dent Assoc 2004; 135:1109-1118

[16] Abrahamsen TC, The worn dentition-pathognomonic patterns of abrasion and erosion. Int Dent J 2005; 55:268-276.

[17] Coleman TA, Grippo JO, Kinderknecht KE. Cervical dentin hypersensitivity, Part III: resolution following occlusal equilibration. Quintessence Int 2003; 34:427-434.

[18] Dawson PE. Functional occlusion: from TMJ to Smile Design. St. Louis 2007:27-32.

[19] Ruiz Jl. Achieving Longevity in esthetic dentistry by proper diagnosis and management of occlusal disease. Contemporary Esthetics 2007;11:24-27.

[20] Williams Dm, Hughes FJ, Osell Ew, Farthing PM. Pathology of Periodontal Disease. Oxford University Press, 1992.

[21] Williams RC. Periodontal disease. N Engl J Med 1990; 8:322: 373-82

[22] Papapanou PN. Periodontal Disease: epidemiology. Ann Periodontol 1996; 1(1):1-36.

[23] Okesson J.P. Management of Temporomandibular Disorders and Occlusion, St. Louis, Mosby1993; 111, 125, 569;

[24] Armitage GC. Development of a classification system for periodontal diseases and conditions. Ann Perio 1999; 4:1-6.

[25] Avery JC. Oral development and hystology. Third edition, Ed. Thieme, Stuttgart, 2002.

[26] Wilson TG, Kornman KS. Fundamentals of Periodontics. Quintessence Publishing Co. Chicago, 1996

[27] Zaslansky P, Friesam AA, Weiner S. Structure and mechsnical properties of the soft zone separating bulk dentin and enamel in crown of human teeth. J Struct Biol 2006; 153:188-99.

[28] Johal A, Katsaros C, Kiliaridis S, Leitao P, Rosa M, Sculean A, Weiland F, Zachrisson B. State of the science on controversial topics: orthodontic therapy and gingival recession (a report of the Angle Society of Europe 2013 meeting). In: Johal et al. Progress in Orthodontics 2013;14-16.

[29] Helm S, Petersen PE. Causal relation between malocclusion and periodontal health. Acta Odontol Scand 1989 ;47(4):223-228.

[30] Abu Alhaija ES, Al-Wahadni AM. Relationship between tooth irregularity and periodontal disease in children with regular dental visits. J Clin Pediatr Dent 2006; 30(4): 296-8.

[31] Pugaca Jolanta, Urtane Ilga, Liepa Andra, Laurina Z. The relationship between the severity of malposition of the frontal teeth and periodontal health in age 15-21 and 35-44. Stomat Baltic Dent Maxillofac J 2007;9:86-90.

[32] Mtaya M, Brudvik P, Åstrøm AN. Prevalence of malocclusion and its relationship with socio-demographic factors, dental caries, and oral hygiene in 12-to 14-year-old Tanzanian schoolchildren. European Journal of Orthodontics 2009;31(5):467–476.

[33] Chandrasekhara Reddy V., Ashok Kumar BR., Ankola Anil. Relationship Between Gingivitis and Anterior Teeth Irregularities Among 18 to 26 Years Age Group: A Hospital Based Study in Belgaum, Karnataka. JOHCD 2010;4(3):61-66.

[34] Gusmão S Estela, Coutinho de Queiroz RD, de Souza Coelho Renata, Cimões Renata, Lima dos Santos Rosenês. Association between malpositioned teeth and periodontal disease. Dental Press J Orthod 2011;16(4):87-94

[35] Bimstein, E., Needleman, H.L., Karimbux, N., Van Dyke, T.E. Malocclusion, orthodontic intervention, and gingival and periodontal health-Periodontal and Gingival Health and Diseases – Children, Adolescents, and Yong Adults. Ed Martin Dunity 2001;17-31, 251-273.

[36] Ngom P.I, Benoist, H.M., Thiam, F., Diagne, F., Diallo, P.D. Influence of orthodontic anomalies on periodontal condition. Odontostomatol Tropic 2007;30(118):9-16.

[37] Onyeaso, C.O., Arowojolu, M.O., Taiwo, J.O. Periodontal status of orthodontic patients and the relationship between dental aesthetic index and community periodontal index of treatment need. Am J Orthod Dentofacial Orthop 2003;124(6):714-20

[38] Ashley FP, Usiskin LA, Wilson RF, Wagaiyu E. The relationship between irregularity of the incisor teeth, plaque, and gingivitis: a study in a group of schoolchildren aged 11-14 years. Eur J Orthop 1998;20:65-72.

[39] Ngom PI, Benoist, H.M., Thiam, F., Diagne, F., Diallo, P.D. Intraarch and interarch relationships of the anterior teeth and periodontal conditions. Angle Orthod 2005;76(2):236-242.

[40] EL-Mangoury NH, Gaafar SM, Mostafa YA. Mandibular anterior crowding and periodontal disease. Angle Orthod 1987;1:33-38.

[41] Staufer K, Landmesser H. Effects of crowding in the lower anterior segment—a risk evaluation depending upon the degree of crowding. J Orofac Orthop 2004;65:13-25.

[42] Jensen L, Birgit, Solow B. Alveolar bone loss and crowding in adult periodontal patients. Community Dent Oral Epidemiol 1989;17(1):47–51.

[43] Dumitiu HT. *Parodontologie*. Ed Viaţa Medical Rom 1998;92-94

[44] Dorobăţ Valentina, Stanciu D. Ortodonţie şi ortopedie dento-facială. Ed Med 2009:363-457.

[45] Machtei EE, Zubery Y, Bimstein E, Becker A. Anterior open bite and gingival recession in children and adolescents. Int Dent J, 1990;40(6):369-373.

[46] Bassigny F. Manuel d'orthopedie dento-faciale. Paris: Masson: 1991.

[47] Davies TM, Shaw WC, Worthington HV, Addy M, Dummer P, Kingdon A. The effect of orthodontic treatment on plaque and gingivitis. Am J Orthod Dentofac Orthop 1991;99:155-161.

[48] Geiger AM, Wasserman BH. Relationship of occlusion and periodontal disease: part IX. Incisor inclination and periodontal status. Angle Orthod 1976;46(2):99-110.

[49] Buckley LA. The relationships between irregular teeth, plaque, calculus and gingival disease. A study of 300 subjects. British Dental Journal 1980:148(3):67-69.

[50] Torres H., Corrêa S. Daniela, Zenóbio EG. Avaliação da condição periodontal em pacientes de 10 a 18 anos com diferentes más oclusões. R Dental Press Ortodon Ortop Facial 2006;11(6):73-80.

[51] Bjornaas T, Rygh P, Boe OE. Severe overjet and overbite reduced alveolar bone height in 19-year-old men. Am J Orthod Dentofacial Orthop 1994;106(2):139-45.

[52] Glăvan Florica, Jianu Rodica. Ortodonţie. Ed Miron 1999;229

[53] Boboc G. Anomaliile dento-maxilare. Ed Medicală, Bucureşti, 1971;9-146.

[54] Hashim HA, Al-Jasser NM. Periodontal findings in cases of posterior cross-bite. J Clin Pediatr Dent 1996;20:317-320.

[55] Silness J, Roynstrand T. Effects on dental health of spacing of teeth in anterior segments. J Clin Periodontol 1984;11:387-398.

[56] Lages EM., Marcus B., Pordeus IA. Oral health of individuals with cleft lip, cleft palate, or both. Cleft Palate Craniofac J 2004;41:59-63.

[57] Quirynen M., Dewinter G., Avontoodt P., Heidbuchel K., Verdonck A., Carels C. A split mouth study on periodontal and microbiological parameters in children with complete unilateral cleft lip and palate. J Clin Periodontol 2003;30:49-56.

[58] Stec Magdalena, Szczepańska Joanna, Pypeć J., Hirschfelder Ursula. Periodontal Status and Oral Hygiene in Two Populations of Cleft Patients. The Cleft Palate-Craniofac J 2007;44(1):73-78.

[59] Boloor V., Thomas B. Comparison of periodontal status among patients with cleft lip, cleft palate, and cleft lip along with a cleft in palate and alveolus. J Indian Soc Periodontol 2010;14(3):168-172.

[60] Costa B., Lima JE., Gomide MR., Rosa OP. Clinical and microbiological evaluation of the periodontal status of children with unilateral complete cleft lip and palate. Cleft Palate Craniofac J 2003;40:585–589.

[61] Wong F., King N. The oral health of children with clefts: a review. Cleft Palate-Craniofac J 1998;35:248-254.

[62] Gaggl A, Schultes G, Kärcher H, Mossböck R. Periodontal disease in patients with cleft palate and patients with unilateral and bilateral clefts of lip, palate and alveolus. J Periodontol 1999;70(2):171-8.

[63] Dewinter G, Quirynen M, Heidbüchel K, Verdonck A, Willems G, Carels C. Dental abnormalities, bone graft quality and periodontal conditions in patients with unilateral cleft lip and palate at different phases of orthodontic treatment. Cleft Palate Cranoifacial J 2003;40(4):343-50.

[64] Graber TM., Vanarsdall RL., Vig KW. Orthodontics-Current Principles and Techniques-5th ed. St Louis, Elsevier Mosby, 2012; 807-842.

[65] Krishnan V, Ambili R, Davidovitch Z, Murphy NC. Gingiva and Orthodontic Treatment. Semin Orthod 2007;13:257-271.

[66] Kouraki E., Bissada NF., Palomo JM., Ficara AJ. Gingival enlargement and resolution during and after orthodontic therapy. N Y State Dent J 2005;71(4):34-37.

[67] Zachrisson BU., Alnaes L. Periodontal condition in orthodontically treated and untreated individuals-I. Loss of attachment, gingival pocket depth and clinical crown height. Angle Orthod 1973;43:402-411.

[68] Zachrisson S., Zachrisson BU. Gingival condition associated with orthodontic treatment. Angle Orthod 1972;42:26-34.

[69] Newman MG., Takei HH., Klokkevold PR., Caranzza F. Carranza's Clinical Periodontology-9th edition. W.B. Saunders Co, Philadelphia 2002;279-297.

[70] Geiger AM. Mucogingival problems and the movement of mandibular incisors-a clinical review. Am J Orthod 1980;78:511-527.

[71] V. Krishnan and Z. Davidovitch, "On a path to unfolding the biological mechanism of orthodontic tooth movement", Journal of Dental Research, vol.88, no. 7, pp. 597-609, 2009

[72] J. Jr. Capelli, A. Kantarci, A. Haffajee et al., "Matrix metalloproteinases and chemokines in gingival crevicular fluid during orthodontic tooth movement", European Journal of Orthodontics, vol. 33, no. 6, pp. 705-711, 2011

[73] M.M. Bildt , M. Bloemen , A.M. Kuijpers-Jagtman , J.W. Von den Hoff, "Matrix metalloproteinases and tissue inhibitors of metalloproteinases in gingival crevicular fluid during orthodontic tooth movement", European Journal of Orthodontics, vol. 31, no. 5, pp. 529-537, 2010.

[74] Surlin P, Rauten AM, Silosi I, Foia L. Pentraxin-3 levels in gingival crevicular fluid during orthodontic tooth movement in young and adult patients. Angle Orthod. 2012 Sep; 82(5):833-8. doi: 10.2319/072911-478.1. Epub 2012 Jan 3.

[75] Surlin P, Silosi I, Rauten AM, Cojocaru M, Foia L. Involvement of TSP1 and MMP9/ NGAL in angiogenesis during orthodontic periodontal remodeling. ScientificWorldJournal. 2014; 2014:421029. doi: 10.1155/2014/421029. Epub 2014 May 20.

[76] Surlin P, Rauten AM, Mogoantă L, Siloşi I, Oprea B, Pirici D. Correlations between the gingival crevicular fluid MMP8 levels and gingival overgrowth in patients with fixed orthodontic devices. Rom J Morphol Embryol. 2010; 51(3):515-9.

[77] Şurlin P, Rauten AM, Pirici D, Oprea B, Mogoantă L, Camen A. Collagen IV and MMP-9 expression in hypertrophic gingiva during orthodontic treatment. Rom J Morphol Embryol. 2012; 53(1):161-5.

[78] Hanes PJ, Krishna R Characteristics of inflammation common to both diabetes and periodontitis: are predictive diagnosis and targeted preventive measures possible? EPMA J. 2010 Mar; 1(1):101-16. doi: 10.1007/s13167-010-0016-3

[79] P.M. Preshaw, A.L. Alba, D.Herrera, S. Jepsen, A. Konstantinidis, K. Makrilakis, R. Taylor Periodontitis and diabetes: a two-way relationship. Diabetologia 2012; 55:21-31

[80] Taylor JJ, Preshaw PM, Lalla E. A review of the evidence for pathogenic mechanisms that may link periodontitis and diabetes. J Clin Periodontol 2013; 40 (Suppl. 14)

[81] Hotamisligil GS, Peraldi P, Budavari A, Ellis R, White MF, Spiegelman BM. IRS-1-mediated inhibition of insulin receptor tyrosine kinase activity in TNF-alpha-and obesity-induced insulin resistance. Science 1996; 271: 665-668.

[82] Uysal KT, Wiesbrock SM, Marino MW, Hotamisligil GS. Protection from obesity-induced insulin resistance in mice lacking TNFalpha function. Nature 1997; 389: 610-614.

[83] Mohamed-Ali V, Goodrick S, Rawesh A et al. Subcutaneous adipose tissue releases interleukin-6, but not tumor necrosis factoralpha, in vivo. J Clin Endocrinol Metab 1997; 82: 4196-4200.

[84] Franchini R, Petri A, Migliario M, Rimondini L Poor oral hygiene and gingivitis are associated with obesity and overweight status in paediatric subjects. J Clin Periodontol 2011; 38: 1021–1028

[85] Haffajee AD, Socransky SS. Relation of body mass index, periodontitis and Tannerella forsythia. J Clin Periodontol 2009; 36: 89–99.

[86] Duarte PM, Szeremeske de Miranda T, Lima JA, Dias Gonçalves, Expression of Immune-Inflammatory Markers in Sites of Chronic Periodontitis in Type 2 Diabetic Subjects. J Periodontol 2011; DOI:10.1902/jop.2011.110324

[87] Hardy DC, Ross JH, Schuyler CA, Leite RS, Matrix metalloproteinase-8 expression in periodontal tissues surgically removed from diabetic and non-diabetic patients with periodontal disease. J Clin Periodontol 2011; DOI: 10.1111/j.1600-051X.2011.01788.x

[88] Chen L, Luo G, Xuan D, Wei B, Liu F, Li J, Zhang J, Effects of Non-surgical Periodontal Treatment on Clinical Response, Serum Inflammatory Parameters, and Metabolic Control in Type 2 Diabetic Patients: A Randomized Study J Periodontol 2011; DOI: 10.1902/jop.2011.110327.

[89] Kardeşler L, Buduneli N, Çetinkalp S, Lappin D, Kinane DF, Gingival crevicular fluid IL-6, tPA, PAI-2, albumin levels following initial periodontal treatment in chronic periodontitis patients with or without type 2 diabetes. Inflamm Res 2011; 60(2): 143-51.

[90] Sun WL, Chen LL, Zhang SZ, Wu YM, Ren YZ, Qin GM, Inflammatory cytokines, adiponectin, insulin resistance and metabolic control after periodontal intervention

in patients with type 2 diabetes and chronic periodontitis. Intern Med 2011; 50(15): 1569-74.

[91] Panagiotis A Koromantzos, Konstantinos Makrilakis, Xanthippi Dereka, Steven Offenbacher, Nicholas Katsilambros, Effect of Non-Surgical Periodontal Therapy on CRP, Oxidative Stress, MMP-9 and MMP-2 Levels in Patients With Type 2 Diabetes. A Randomized Controlled Study J Periodontol DOI:10.1902/jop.2011.110148

[92] Xiao LM, Yan YX, Xie CJ, Fan WH, Xuan DY, Association among interleukin-6 gene polymorphism, diabetes and periodontitis in a Chinese population Oral Diseases 2009; 15(8):547–553.

[93] López NJ, Valenzuela CY, Jara L, Interleukin-1 gene cluster polymorphisms associated with periodontal disease in type 2 diabetes. J Periodontol 2009; 80(10):1590-8.

[94] Ritchie CS. Obesity and periodontal disease. Periodontol 2000 2007; 44: 154-63

[95] Kondo K, Ishikado A, Morino K, Nishio Y, Ugi S, Kajiwara S, Kurihara M,Iwakawa H, Nakao K, Uesaki S, Shigeta Y, Imanaka H, YoshizakiT, Sekine O, Makino T, Maegawa H, King GL, Kashiwagi A. A high fiber, low-fat diet improves periodontal disease markers in high-risk subjects: a pilot study. Nutr Res 2014 Jun; 34(6):491-8.

[96] Sophia S, Jaideep M. Multifactorial Relationship of Obesity and Periodontal Disease. J Clin Diagn Res Apr 2014; 8(4): ZE01–ZE03